*The Most Complete, Accessible
Reference of Its Kind…*

THE BANTAM MEDICAL DICTIONARY

Designed for easy use and written especially with the general reader in mind, this invaluable reference brings the latest in medical science to your fingertips. In this fifth edition you'll find:

Easy-to-understand definitions of key terms in anatomy, physiology, biochemistry, and pharmacology, as well as all the major medical and surgical specialties

Updates on recent medical advances, including those in genetics, cancer, organ transplantation, telemedicine, nuclear medicine, emergency medicine, and more

New entries for therapeutic and diagnostic techniques such as brachytherapy, Chart, multislice CT scanning, photodynamic therapy, transrectal ultrasonography, and videokymography

Newly developed drugs for cancer (including angiogenesis inhibitors), AIDS and HIV, diabetes, glaucoma, depression, and more

Information on conditions such as chronic fatigue syndrome, fibromyalgia, SARS, sleep paralysis, and West Nile fever

Expanded and updated information on U.S. health organizations and services such as DAWN (Drug Abuse Warning Network), MEDLARS, MEDLINE, USAN, and USP

And much more.

The Bantam Medical Dictionary provides the key to understanding the wealth of health information now available.

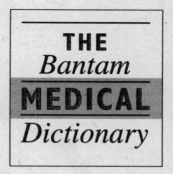

THE *Bantam*
MEDICAL
Dictionary

BANTAM BOOKS

New York
Toronto
London
Sydney
Auckland

THE
Bantam
MEDICAL
Dictionary

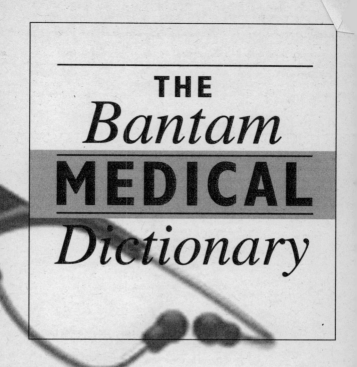

Fifth Edition

**PREPARED BY THE EDITORS OF
MARKET HOUSE BOOKS, LTD.**

THE BANTAM MEDICAL DICTIONARY
A Bantam Book

PUBLISHING HISTORY
John Wiley & Sons edition published January 1981
First Bantam edition / October 1982
Bantam revised edition / March 1990
Bantam second revised edition / March 1996
Bantam third revised edition / April 2000
Bantam fifth edition / November 2004

Published by
Bantam Dell
A Division of Random House, Inc.
New York, New York

ISBN 0-553-58736-6

Manufactured in the United States of America
Published simultaneously in Canada

OPM 10 9 8 7 6 5 4 3 2 1

CONTENTS

This edition is dedicated to Alan Isaacs, founder of Market House Books, Ltd., who died on April 5, 2004. Throughout his long career in publishing, Alan's guiding principles for the compilation of reference books were simplicity of language and clarity of expression. We believe that *The Bantam Medical Dictionary*, with which Alan was closely involved since it was first published in 1981, exemplifies these principles and is a fitting memorial to him.

CONTRIBUTORS AND ADVISORS

Rajesh Aggarwal BM, MRCP, FRCS, FRCOphth

David Ahearne MB, ChB

W. Leslie Alexander FRCS, FRCOphth

J. A. D. Anderson MA, MD, FRCP, FFPHM, FFOM, FRCGP

J. H. Angel MD, FRCP

Dr Andrea Atherton MA, MSc, MRCP(UK)

John R. Bennett MD, FRCP

Stuart Anthony Bentley MB, BS

Dr J. N. Bowles BSc, MRCP, FRCR

Dr Peter Bradbury FRCP

Bruce M. Bryant MB, ChB, MRCP

Philip Chan MA, MChir, FRCS

Robert E. Coleman

Patrick Collins MD, MRCP

J. A. Cullen BSc, MSc

W. J. Dinning FRCS, MRCP

Ivan T. Draper MB, ChB, FRCPEd

J. C. Gingell MB, BCh, FRCSEd, FRCS

John M. Goldman DM, FRCP, FRCPath

Dr Helen K. Gordon FRCOG, MFFP

W. J. Gordon MD, FRCS(G), FRCOG

T. Q. Howes MA, MB, BS, MD, MRCP(I)

Dr J. Craig Jobling MA, MB, BChir, FRCS, FRCR

Michael Klaber MA, MB, FRCP

Marc E. Laniado MD, FRCS(Urol)

Alexander J. Lewis BSc, MB, BS, MRCPsych

D. J. McFerran MA, FRCS

Gordon Macpherson MB, BS

H. Manji MA, MD, FRCP

Charles V. Mann MA, MCh, FRCS

J. E. Nicholl MA, FRCS(Orth)

Heather E. Pitt Ford FDS

T. R. Pitt Ford PhD, BDS, FDS

D. L. Phillips FRCR, FRCOG

Helen Phillips MB, BS, MRCGP, DCH, DRCOG

Amin Rahemtulla PhD, FRCP

Dr John R. Sewell MA, MB, MRCP

Dr Mary Sibellas MD, FFPHM, DTM&H

B. F. Sizer BSc, MB, ChB, FRACR

Dr Tony Smith MA, BM, BCh

Dr Steve Stanaway BSc(Hons), MB, ChB, MRCP

Eric Taylor MA, MB, MRCP, MRCPsych

William F. Whimster MRCP, MRCPath

Paul Watson MA, MB, BChir, DSH, MPH, FFPHM

Robert M. Youngson MB, ChB, DRM&H, DO, FRCOphthal

Editors

Elizabeth A. Martin

Barbara Guidos

INTRODUCTION AND GUIDE
TO THE DICTIONARY

The fifth edition of this dictionary provides full definitions for all the terms that practitioners and students in the health sciences are likely to need to know. *The Bantam Medical Dictionary* was prepared by a distinguished team of specialists and medical writers and is written in clear, concise English without the use of unnecessary jargon. Each entry contains a basic definition, followed, where appropriate, by a more detailed explanation or description.

VOCABULARY

Coverage is provided in the basic sciences of anatomy, physiology, biochemistry, and pharmacology, as well as all the major specialties of clinical medicine and surgery. Treatment of psychology, psychiatry, community medicine, and dentistry is unusually comprehensive, and this edition includes many new entries covering the latest developments in diagnostic radiology and radiotherapy, endocrinology, pediatrics, urology, and emergency and advanced life support systems. Many new drugs have also been added. To make room for this additional material, many of the more obscure and obsolescent terms found in larger medical dictionaries have been omitted. The meanings of many such terms, however, can be readily deduced from definitions of medical prefixes and suffixes, which are included in this work. Derivative words, such as adjectives of nouns that are defined, are listed at the end of the relevant entries in order to avoid cluttering the entry list with unnecessary terms. Synonyms of main entries appear in bold type in parentheses immediately following the main entry.

SUBENTRIES

An extraordinary feature of this work is the inclusion of thousands of terms that are defined within the definitions of other terms. These subentries appear in italic type. For example, the definition for *enterostomy* includes within it definitions of two types of enterostomy (*gastroenterostomy* and *enteroenterostomy*), as well as referring the reader to three other related terms:

an operation in which the small intestine is brought through the abdominal wall and opened (*see* duodenostomy, jejunostomy, ileostomy) or is joined to the stomach (*gastroenterostomy*) or to another loop of small intestine (*enteroenterostomy*).

CROSS-REFERENCES

An asterisk (*) immediately preceding a word in a definition indicates that the term is entered and defined in its own alphabetic place, where additional information may be found.

By providing the reader with copious cross-references, often within definitions (e.g., *duodenostomy, jejunostomy*, and *ileostomy* in the example above), this dictionary can be used as a learning device by which the reader can increase his or her command of medical terminology. *The Bantam Medical Dictionary* attempts to lead the reader, by means of its unique cross-reference system, to many other terms. Although each term is fully defined in its own alphabetic place, longer articles also function as a core of meaning that branches out, like the spokes of a wheel, to related terms. The starred words and *see* cross-references invite the reader to follow these extensions and by-ways of meaning, often employing the same word roots as the entry term, and thus enlarge his or her vocabulary. Perhaps it is not too much to say that this dictionary, though designed primarily as a reference, can also be "read" with profit.

ILLUSTRATIONS

Wherever the editors felt that an illustration would be helpful, a clear and fully labeled line drawing has been provided. Approximately 150 illustrations are included.

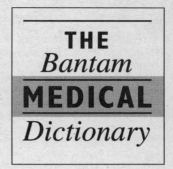

THE *Bantam* **MEDICAL** *Dictionary*

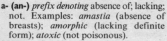

A

a- (an-) *prefix denoting* absence of; lacking; not. Examples: *amastia* (absence of breasts); *amorphic* (lacking definite form); *atoxic* (not poisonous).

AABB *see* American Association of Blood Banks.

AB *see* Aid to the Blind.

ab- *prefix denoting* away from. Example: *abembryonic* (away from or opposite the embryo).

abarticulation *n.* **1.** the dislocation of a joint. **2.** a synovial joint (*see* diarthrosis).

abasia *n.* an inability to walk for which no physical cause can be identified. *See also* astasia.

abbreviated injury scale a quick method for determining the severity of a case of serious trauma. It can be used for purposes of *triage and *medical (clinical) audit.

abciximab *n.* a *monoclonal antibody that inhibits platelet aggregation and is used as an *adjunct to lessen the chance of a heart attack during surgery to open blocked arteries of the heart (*see* coronary angioplasty). It is administered by intravenous infusion; side effects include bleeding, blurred vision, confusion, dizziness, sweating, and unusual tiredness or weakness. Trade name: **ReoPro.**

abdomen *n.* the part of the body cavity below the chest (*see* thorax), from which it is separated by the *diaphragm. The abdomen contains the organs of digestion – stomach, liver, intestines, etc. – and excretion – kidneys, bladder, etc.; in women it also contains the ovaries

and uterus. The regions of the abdomen are shown in the illustration. —**abdominal** *adj.*

abdomin- (abdomino-) *combining form denoting* the abdomen. Examples: *abdominalgia* (pain in the abdomen); *abdominothoracic* (relating to the abdomen and thorax).

abducens nerve the sixth *cranial nerve (VI), which supplies the lateral rectus muscle of each eyeball, responsible for turning the eye outward.

abduct *vb.* to move a limb or any other part away from the midline of the body. —**abduction** *n.*

abductor *n.* any muscle that moves one part of the body away from another or from the midline of the body.

aberrant *adj.* abnormal: usually applied to a blood vessel or nerve that does not follow its normal course.

aberration *n.* (in optics) a defect in the image formed by a lens. In *chromatic aberration* the image formed by a lens has colored fringes as a result of the different extent to which light of different colors is refracted by glass. It is corrected by using an *achromatic lens. In *spherical aberration*, the image is blurred because rays from the object come to a focus in slightly different positions as a result of the curvature of the lens: the rays passing more peripherally through the lens are bent more than those passing through centrally. This occurs even with monochromatic light.

abiotrophy *n.* degeneration or loss of function without apparent cause; for example, *retinal abiotrophy* is progressive degeneration of the retina leading to im-

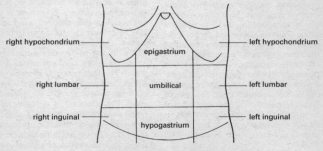

Regions of the abdomen

paired vision, occurring in genetic disorders such as *retinitis pigmentosa.

ablatio *n.* separation; abruptio. *See* detached retina (ablatio retinae).

ablation *n.* the removal of tissue, a part of the body, or an abnormal growth, especially by cutting. *See also* endometrial ablation.

ablepharia *n.* absence of or reduction in the size of the eyelids.

abortifacient *n.* a drug that induces abortion or miscarriage. *See* prostaglandin.

abortion *n.* the expulsion or removal of an embryo or fetus from the uterus at a stage of pregnancy when it is incapable of independent survival (i.e. at any time between conception and the 24th week of pregnancy). In *threatened abortion* there is abdominal pain and bleeding from the uterus but the fetus is still alive; once the fetus is dead abortion becomes *inevitable.* Abortion is *incomplete* so long as the uterus still contains some of the fetus or its membranes. Abortion may be *spontaneous* (a miscarriage) or it may be *induced* for medical or social reasons (termination of pregnancy). *Habitual abortion* is the occurrence of three consecutive pregnancy losses before 20 weeks' gestation with fetuses weighing under 500 grams. The presence of a uterine abnormality, such as *bicornuate uterus or *cervical incompetence, may account for 10–15% of recurrent abortions.

After January 1973, induced abortions during the first three months of pregnancy became legal in the US, requiring only agreement between the woman and her doctor. During the remaining six months, voluntary termination of a pregnancy may be permitted under terms of state laws. Methods in current use include "salting out," in which a saline solution is injected through the cervix into the membranes surrounding the fetus; vacuum *aspiration of the products of conception through a thin cannula; *dilation and curettage; opening the womb through an abdominal incision (hysterotomy); or the use of *prostaglandins or other drugs to induce premature labor. Termination carries little risk early in pregnancy, but complications are more likely after the 13th week.

Nonmedical people make a distinction between abortion and *miscarriage*, the former being a procedure deliberately carried out to end the pregnancy, the latter being an accidental occurrence. The medical profession increasingly recognizes this useful distinction.

abortus *n.* a fetus, weighing less than 500 grams, that is expelled from the mother's body either dead or incapable of surviving.

ABO system *see* blood group.

abrasion *n.* **1.** a graze: a minor wound in which the surface of the skin or a mucous membrane is worn away by rubbing or scraping. **2.** the wearing of the teeth, particularly at the necks by overvigorous brushing. It is frequently enhanced by *erosion. **3.** any rubbing or scraping action that produces surface wear.

abreaction *n.* the release of strong emotion associated with a buried memory. While this can happen spontaneously, it is usually deliberately produced by a therapist using psychotherapy or hypnosis. The technique is used as a treatment for conversion disorder, anxiety state, and other neurotic conditions, especially when they are thought to be caused by *repression of memories or emotions.

abruptio (ablatio) *n.* separation. In *abruptio placentae* (*ablatio placentae*) the placenta separates from the lining of the uterus before the usual time. Bleeding and pain are experienced at the point of separation, and the uterus undergoes constant contraction. Severe cases involve shock, and *hypofibrinogenemia is a further complication. The condition is often associated with high blood pressure or *preeclampsia. If the neck of the uterus is firm and undilated, a live fetus may be delivered by *cesarean section.

abscess *n.* a localized collection of pus anywhere in the body, surrounded and walled off by damaged and inflamed tissues. A *boil is an example of an abscess within the skin. The usual cause is local bacterial infection, often by staphylococci, that the body's defenses have failed to overcome. In a *cold abscess*, sometimes due to tubercle organisms, there is swelling, but little pain or inflammation (as in acute abscesses). Antibiotics, aided by surgical incision to release pus when necessary, are the usual forms of treatment.

The brain and its meninges have a low resistance to infection and a *cerebral abscess* is liable to follow any penetration of these by microorganisms. The condition is fatal unless relieved by aspiration or surgical drainage.

absence *n.* (in neurology) *see* epilepsy.

Absidia *n.* a genus of fungi that sometimes cause disease in humans (*see* phycomycosis).

absorption *n.* (in physiology) the uptake of fluids or other substances by the tissues of the body. Digested food is absorbed into the blood and lymph from the alimentary canal. Most absorption of food occurs in the small intestine – in the jejunum and ileum – although alcohol is readily absorbed from the stomach. The small intestine is lined with minute fingerlike processes (*see* villus), which greatly increase its surface area and therefore the speed at which absorption can take place. *See also* assimilation, digestion.

abulia *n.* absence ·or impairment of willpower. The individual still has desires but they are not put into action; initiative and energy are lacking. Abulia is commonly a symptom of *schizophrenia.

abutment *n.* (in dentistry) a component of a dental *bridge or *implant.

acalculia *n.* an acquired inability to make simple mathematical calculations. It is a symptom of disease in the *parietal lobe of the brain. *See* Gerstmann's syndrome.

acantha *n.* **1.** a spine projecting from a *vertebra. **2.** the *backbone.

Acanthamoeba *n.* a genus of amebas that are commonly found in soil and contaminated water and cause painful corneal infection and ulcers in humans, usually resulting from improper sterilization of contact lenses.

acanthion *n.* the tip of the nasal spine formed where projecting processes of the upper jawbones (maxillae) meet at the front of the face.

acanthoma *n.* a tumor composed of epidermal or squamous cells. *See also* keratoacanthoma.

acanthosis *n.* generalized thickening of the innermost (prickle-cell) layer of the *epidermis, with abnormal increase in the number of cells. In *acanthosis nigricans*

dark warty growths occur, especially in skin folds such as the groin, armpits, and mouth. It is believed to be associated with insulin resistance and may be benign or malignant. *Pseudoacanthosis nigricans* is more common and is associated with obesity.

acapnia (hypocapnia) *n.* a condition in which there is an abnormally low concentration of carbon dioxide in the blood. This may be caused by breathing that is exceptionally deep in relation to the physical activity of the individual.

acarbose *n.* *see* alpha-glucosidase inhibitor.

acardia *n.* congenital absence of the heart. The condition may occur in conjoined twins; the twin with the heart controls the circulation for both.

acariasis *n.* an infestation of mites and ticks and the symptoms, for example allergy and dermatitis, that their presence may provoke.

acaricide *n.* any chemical agent used for destroying mites and ticks.

acarid *n.* a *mite or *tick.

Acarina *n.* the group of arthropods that includes the *mites and *ticks.

Acarus (Tyroglyphus) *n.* a genus of mites. The flour mite, *A. siro* (*T. farinae*), is nonparasitic, but its presence in flour can cause a severe allergic dermatitis in flour-mill workers.

acatalasia *n.* an inborn lack of the enzyme *catalase, leading to recurrent infections of the gums (gingivitis) and mouth. It is most common in the Japanese.

acceptor *n.* (in biochemistry) a substance that helps to bring about oxidation of a reduced *substrate by accepting hydrogen ions.

accessory nerve (spinal accessory nerve) the eleventh *cranial nerve (XI), which arises from two roots, cranial and spinal. Fibers from the cranial root travel with the nerve for only a short distance before branching to join the vagus and then forming the recurrent laryngeal nerve, which supplies the internal laryngeal muscles. Fibers from the spinal root supply the sternomastoid and trapezius muscles, in the neck region (front and back).

accident *n.* an unexpected and traumatic event that results in bodily injury or death. *See also* emergency medicine.

accommodation *n.* adjustment of the shape

of the lens to change the focus of the eye. When the ciliary muscle (*see* ciliary body) is relaxed, suspensory ligaments attached to the ciliary body and holding the lens in position are stretched, which causes the lens to be flattened. The eye is then able to focus on distant objects. To focus the eye on near objects, the ciliary muscles contract and the tension in the ligaments is thus lowered, allowing the lens to become rounder.

accommodation reflex (convergence reflex) the constriction of the pupils and inward turning of the eyes that occurs when an individual focuses on a near object.

accommodative insufficiency a weakness of the *accommodation reflex, resulting in the inability of the eye to focus properly on an object. It can be a result of injury, disease, or the effect of medication and is usually associated with *convergence insufficiency.

accouchement *n.* delivery of a baby. *See also* hydrostatic accouchement.

acebutolol *n.* a *beta blocker drug commonly used to treat high blood pressure, angina pectoris, and irregular heart rhythms. It is administered by mouth. Possible side effects include breathing difficulty, especially in asthmatics, and fatigue. Trade name: **Sectral.**

ACE inhibitor (angiotensin-converting enzyme inhibitor) any one of a group of drugs used in the treatment of high blood pressure and heart failure. ACE inhibitors act by interfering with the action of the enzyme that converts the inactive *angiotensin I to the powerful artery constrictor angiotensin II. The absence of this substance allows arteries to widen and the blood pressure to drop. ACE inhibitors are administered by mouth; they include (among others) *captopril, *enalapril, *lisinopril, *perindopril* (Aceon), and *ramipril* (Altace). Possible side effects include weakness, dizziness, loss of appetite, coughing, and skin rashes.

acentric *n.* (in genetics) a chromosome or fragment of a chromosome that has no *centromere. Since acentrics cannot attach to the *spindle they are usually lost during cell division. They are often found in cells that have been damaged by radiation. —**acentric** *adj.*

acephalus *n.* a fetus without a head.

acervulus cerebri a collection of granules of calcium-containing material that is sometimes found within the *pineal body as its calcification proceeds (normally after the 17th year): "brain sand."

acetabulum (cotyloid cavity) *n.* a cup-shaped socket on the outer surface of the *hip bone, into which the head of the thigh bone (femur) fits at the *hip joint.

acetaminophen (paracetamol) *n.* an *analgesic drug that also reduces fever. It is used to treat mild or moderate pain, such as headache, toothache, and rheumatic pain, and as an antipyretic in colds, influenza, etc. It is administered by mouth and may cause digestive upsets; overdosage causes liver damage. Trade names: **Datril, Panadol, Phenaphen, Tapar, Tempra, Tylenol**.

acetazolamide *n.* a *carbonic anhydrase inhibitor used mainly in the treatment of glaucoma to reduce the pressure inside the eyeball and as a preventive for epileptic seizures and altitude sickness. It is administered by mouth or injection; side effects include drowsiness and numbness and tingling of the hands and feet. Trade name: **Diamox**.

acetoacetic acid an organic acid produced in large amounts by the liver under metabolic conditions associated with a high rate of fatty acid oxidation (for example, in starvation). The acetoacetic acid thus formed is subsequently converted to acetone and excreted. *See also* ketone.

acetohexamide *n.* a sulfonylurea and hypoglycemic drug that is used in the treatment of noninsulin-dependent *diabetes mellitus. It is administered by mouth; side effects include headache, dizziness, and nervousness. *See also* chlorpropamide, glipizide, glyburide, tolazamide, tolbutamide. Trade name: **Dymelor.**

acetone *n.* an organic compound that is an intermediate in many bacterial fermentations and is produced by fatty acid oxidation. In certain abnormal conditions (for example, starvation) acetone and other *ketones may accumulate in the blood (*see* ketosis). Acetone is a volatile liquid that is miscible with both fats and water and therefore of great value as a solvent. It is used in chromatography and in the preparation of tissues for enzyme extraction.

acetone body (ketone body) see ketone.

acetonuria n. see ketonuria.

acetylcholine n. the acetic acid ester of the organic base choline: the *neurotransmitter released at the synapses of parasympathetic nerves and at *neuromuscular junctions. After relaying a nerve impulse, acetylcholine is rapidly broken down by the enzyme *cholinesterase. *Anticholinergic drugs block the action of acetylcholine at receptor sites; *anticholinesterases and *acetylcholinesterase inhibitors prolong the activity of acetylcholine by blocking cholinesterase.

acetylcholinesterase n. see cholinesterase.

acetylcholinesterase inhibitor any one of a class of drugs that block the action of acetylcholinesterase (see cholinesterase), an enzyme that quickly breaks down the neurotransmitter acetylcholine. This neurotransmitter is central to the functional interconnection between nerve cells in the outer layer (cortex) of the brain; the early impairment of cognitive function found in *Alzheimer's disease is associated with a reduction in acetylcholine levels. By inhibiting acetylcholine breakdown, acetylcholinesterase inhibitors have been found helpful in slowing down the rate of cognitive decline in the early stages of the dementia; they do not halt the progress of the disease. The group includes donepezil (Aricept), galantamine (Reminyl), and rivastigmine (Exelon); these drugs are given by mouth.

acetylcysteine n. a drug used to break down thick mucous secretions. It is administered as an aerosol, primarily for the treatment of respiratory diseases, such as bronchitis and cystic fibrosis; it is also used as an oral preparation to prevent liver damage in acetaminophen poisoning. Side effects may include spasm of the bronchial muscles, stomatitis, nausea, vomiting, and fever. Trade name: **Mucomyst**.

acetylsalicylic acid see aspirin.

achalasia (cardiospasm) n. a condition in which the normal muscular activity of the esophagus (gullet) is disturbed, which delays the passage of swallowed material. It may occur at any age: symptoms include difficulty in swallowing liquids and solids, slowly increasing over years; sometimes regurgitation of undigested food; and occasionally severe chest pain caused by spasm of the esophagus. Diagnosis is by a barium X-ray examination and sometimes manometric studies (see manometry). Treatment is by forceful stretching of the tight lower end of the esophagus (cardia), by surgical splitting of the muscular ring in that area (cardiomyotomy or Heller's operation), or by injecting *botulinum toxin into the sphincter.

Achilles tendon the tendon of the muscles of the calf of the leg (the *gastrocnemius and *soleus muscles), situated at the back of the ankle and attached to the calcaneus (heel bone).

achlorhydria n. absence of hydrochloric acid in the stomach. Achlorhydria that persists despite large doses of histamine is associated with atrophy of the lining (mucosa) of the stomach. In this condition there is usually an absence of secretion of *intrinsic factor, which will lead to *pernicious anemia. In some people, however, achlorhydria is not associated with any disease, produces no ill-effects, and needs no treatment.

acholia n. absence or deficiency of bile secretion or failure of the bile to enter the alimentary canal (for example, because of an obstructed bile duct).

acholuria n. the absence of the *bile pigments in the urine, which occurs in some forms of jaundice (acholuric jaundice). —**acholuric** adj.

achondroplasia n. a disorder, inherited as a *dominant characteristic, in which the bones of the arms and legs fail to grow to normal size due to a defect in both cartilage and bone. It results in a type of *dwarfism characterized by short limbs, a normal-sized head and body, and normal intelligence. —**achondroplastic** adj.

achromatic adj. without color.

achromatic lenses lenses specially designed for use in the eyepieces of microscopes and other scientific instruments. They give clear images, unblurred by the colored fringes that are produced with ordinary lenses (caused by splitting of the light into different wavelengths and hence its component colors).

achromatopsia n. the inability to perceive color. Such complete *color blindness is very rare and is usually associated with poor *visual acuity; it is usually determined by hereditary factors. *See also* monochromat.

achylia *n.* absence of secretion. The term is usually applied to a nonsecreting stomach (*achylia gastrica*) whose lining (mucosa) is atrophied (*see* achlorhydria).

acid-base balance the balance between the amount of carbonic acid and bicarbonate in the blood, which must be maintained at a constant ratio of 1:20 in order to keep the hydrogen ion concentration of the plasma at a constant value (pH 7.4). Any alteration in this ratio will disturb the acid-base balance of the blood and tissues and cause either *acidosis or *alkalosis. The lungs and the kidneys play an important role in the regulation of the acid-base balance.

acidemia *n.* abnormally high blood acidity. This condition may result from an increase in the concentration of acidic substances and/or a decrease in the level of alkaline substances in the blood. *See also* acidosis. *Compare* alkalemia.

acid-etch technique a technique for bonding resin-based restorative materials to the enamel of teeth; it is used to retain and seal the margins of *fillings, to retain brackets of fixed *orthodontic appliances, and to retain resin-based *fissure sealants and adhesive bridges. A porous surface is created by applying phosphoric acid for one minute or less.

acid-fast *adj.* 1. describing bacteria that have been stained and continue to hold the stain after treatment with an acidic solution. For example, bacteria that cause tuberculosis are acid-fast when stained with a *carbolfuchsin preparation. 2. describing a stain that is not removed from a specimen by washing with an acidic solution.

acidophil (acidophilic) *adj.* 1. (in histology) describing tissues, cells, or parts of cells that stain with acid dyes (such as eosin). 2. (in bacteriology) describing bacteria that grow well in acid media.

acidosis *n.* a condition in which the acidity of body fluids and tissues is abnormally high. This arises because of a failure of the mechanisms responsible for maintaining a balance between acids and alkalis in the blood (*see* acid-base balance). In *gaseous acidosis* more than the normal amount of carbon dioxide is retained in the body, as in drowning. In

renal acidosis, kidney failure results in excessive loss of bicarbonate or retention of phosphoric and sulfuric acids. Patients with diabetes mellitus have *ketoacidosis, in which sodium, potassium, and *ketone bodies are lost in the urine. *See also* lactic acidosis.

acinus *n.* (*pl.* **acini**) 1. a small sac or cavity surrounded by the secretory cells of a gland. Some authorities regard the term as synonymous with *alveolus, but others distinguish an acinus by the possession of a narrow passage (lumen) leading from the sac. 2. (in the lung) the tissue supplied with air by one terminal *bronchiole. *Emphysema is classified by the part of the acinus involved (i.e. *centriacinar*, *panacinar*, or *periacinar*). —**acinous** *adj.*

aclasis *n. see* diaphysial aclasis.

acne *n.* a common inflammatory disorder of the sebaceous glands. These *sebum-producing glands are under androgen control, but the cause of acne is unknown. It involves the face, back, and chest and is characterized by the presence of blackheads with papules, pustules, and – in more severe cases – cysts and scars. Acne is readily treatable. Mild cases respond to topical therapy with *benzoyl peroxide or *tretinoin, whereas more refractory conditions require treatment with long-term antibiotics or (for treating women only) *antiandrogens: severe or cystic acne can be treated with *isotretinoin.

There are many types of acne, some being caused by contact with chemical substances (such as tar). *See also* rosacea.

aconite *n.* the dried roots of the herbaceous plant *Aconitum napellus* (monkshood or wolfsbane), containing three *analgesic substances: *aconine*, *aconitine*, and *picraconitine*. Aconite was formerly used to prepare liniments for muscular pains and a tincture for toothache, but is regarded as too toxic for use today.

acoria *n.* absence of the pupil.

acoustic *adj.* of or relating to sound or the sense of hearing.

acoustic nerve *see* vestibulocochlear nerve.

acquired *adj.* describing a condition or disorder contracted after birth and not attributable to hereditary causes. *Compare* congenital.

acquired immunodeficiency syndrome *see* AIDS.

acrania *n.* congenital absence of the skull, either partial or complete, due to a developmental defect.

acrivastine *n.* an *antihistamine drug used to treat hay fever and urticaria (nettle rash). It is administered by mouth. Possible side effects include drowsiness, headache, dizziness, dry mouth, and urinary retention. Trade name: **Semprex**.

acro- *prefix denoting* **1.** extremity; tip. Example: *acrohypothermy* (abnormal coldness of the hands and feet). **2.** height; promontory. Example: *acrophobia* (morbid dread of heights). **3.** extreme; intense. Example: *acromania* (an extreme degree of mania).

acrocentric *n.* a chromosome in which the *centromere is situated at or very near one end. —**acrocentric** *adj.*

acrocyanosis *n.* bluish-purple discoloration of the hands and feet due to slow circulation of the blood through the small vessels in the skin.

acrodermatitis *n.* inflammation of the skin of the feet or hands. A diffuse chronic variety produces swelling and reddening of the affected areas, followed by atrophy. It is a manifestation of *Lyme disease.

acrodermatitis enteropathica an inherited inability to absorb sufficient *zinc, which causes poor growth, patchy sparse hair, a generalized skin rash, and chronic diarrhea. Management consists of zinc supplements.

acrodynia *n. see* pink disease.

acromegaly *n.* increase in size of the hands, feet, and the face due to excessive production of *growth hormone (somatotropin) by a tumor of the anterior pituitary gland. The tumor can be treated with X-rays or surgically removed. *See also* gigantism.

acromion *n.* an oblong process at the top of the spine of the *scapula, part of which articulates with the clavicle (collar bone) to form the *acromioclavicular joint*. —**acromial** *adj.*

acroparesthesia *n.* a tingling sensation in the hands or feet. *See also* paresthesia.

acrosclerosis *n.* a skin disease thought to be a type of generalized *scleroderma. It also has features of *Raynaud's disease, with the hands, face, and feet being mainly affected.

acrosome *n.* the caplike structure on the front end of a spermatozoon. It breaks down just before fertilization (the *acrosome reaction*), releasing a number of enzymes that assist penetration between the follicle cells that still surround the ovum. Failure of the acrosome reaction is a cause of male infertility. *See also* andrology.

acrylic resin one of a group of polymeric materials used for making denture teeth, denture bases, and formerly as a dental filling material.

ACTH (adrenocorticotropic hormone, adrenocorticotropin, corticotropin) a hormone synthesized and stored in the anterior pituitary gland, large amounts of which are released in response to any form of stress. Its release is stimulated by *corticotropin-releasing hormone. ACTH controls the secretion of *corticosteroid hormones from the adrenal gland. An analogue of ACTH is administered by injection to test adrenal function.

actin *n.* a protein, found in muscle, that plays an important role in the process of contraction. *See* striated muscle.

Actinobacillus *n.* a genus of gram-negative nonmotile aerobic bacteria that are characteristically spherical or rodlike in shape but may occasionally grow into branching filaments. Actinobacilli cause disease in animals that can be transmitted to humans.

Actinomyces *n.* a genus of gram-positive nonmotile fungus-like bacteria that cause disease in animals and humans. The species *A. israelii* is the causative organism of human *actinomycosis.

actinomycin *n.* any of a large group of antibiotic agents, produced from cultures of various species of *Streptomyces*, that have antibacterial, antifungal, and cytotoxic properties. *Dactinomycin (actinomycin D) is an antineoplastic agent.

actinomycosis *n.* a noncontagious disease caused by the bacterium *Actinomyces israelii*, which most commonly affects the jaw but may also affect the lungs, brain, or intestines. The bacterium is normally present in the mouth but it may become pathogenic following an *apical abscess or extraction of a tooth. It is characterized by multiple sinuses that open onto the skin. Treatment is by drainage of pus and a prolonged course of antibiotics.

actinotherapy *n.* the treatment of disorders with *infrared or *ultraviolet radiation.

action potential the change in voltage that occurs across the membrane of a nerve or muscle cell when a *nerve impulse is triggered. It is due to the passage of charged particles across the membrane (*see* depolarization) and is an observable manifestation of the passage of an impulse.

activated partial thromboplastin time (APTT, aPTT) *see* PTT.

active transport (in biochemistry) an energy-dependent process in which certain substances (including ions, some drugs, and amino acids) are able to cross cell membranes against a concentration gradient. The process is inhibited by substances that interfere with cellular metabolism (e.g. high doses of digitalis).

actomyosin *n.* a protein complex formed in muscle between actin and myosin during the process of contraction. *See* striated muscle.

acuity *n. see* visual acuity.

acupuncture *n.* a complementary therapy, based on a traditional Chinese system of healing, in which fine sterile needles are inserted into the skin at specific points on the body. The needles are stimulated either by rotation or, more recently, by an electric current. The healing system was developed by Eastern physicians, who recognize pathways and flows of energy within the body called *chi*. It is suggested that the needling activates deep sensory nerves, which cause the pituitary and midbrain to release *endorphins – the brain's natural painkillers. Acupuncture is used to treat many conditions, especially chronic pain, and in China it has become an alternative to anesthesia for some major operations.

acute *adj.* **1.** describing a disease of rapid onset, severe symptoms, and brief duration. *Compare* chronic. **2.** describing any intense symptom, such as severe pain.

acute abdomen an emergency surgical condition caused by damage to one or more abdominal organs following injury or disease. The patient is in severe pain and often in shock. Perforation of a peptic ulcer or a severely infected appendix, or rupture of the liver or spleen following a crushing injury, all produce an acute abdomen requiring urgent treatment.

acute retinal necrosis (ARN) severe inflammation and necrosis of the retina associated with inflammation and blockage of retinal blood vessels, hemorrhage and death of retinal tissue, and retinal detachment. It may affect both eyes (*bilateral acute retinal necrosis, BARN*), and visual prognosis is poor. ARN is thought to be due to viral infection.

acute rheumatism *see* rheumatic fever.

acyclovir *n.* an antiviral drug that inhibits DNA synthesis in cells infected by *herpesviruses. Administered by mouth, topically, or intravenously, it is used in patients whose immune systems are compromised and also in the treatment of herpes zoster, genital herpes, herpetic eye disease, and herpes encephalitis. Trade name: **Zovirax**.

ad- *prefix denoting* toward or near. Examples: *adaxial* (toward the main axis); *adoral* (toward or near the mouth).

ADA *see* Americans with Disabilities Act (1990).

ADA deficiency *see* adenosine deaminase deficiency.

Adam's apple (laryngeal prominence) a projection, lying just under the skin, of the thyroid cartilage of the *larynx.

Adams-Stokes syndrome *see* Stokes-Adams syndrome.

adaptation *n.* the phenomenon in which a sense organ shows a gradually diminishing response to continuous or repetitive stimulation. The nose, for example, may become adapted to the stimulus of an odor that is continuously present so that in time it ceases to report its presence. Similarly, the adaptation of touch receptors in the skin means that the presence of clothes can be forgotten a few minutes after they have been put on.

addiction *n.* a state of *dependence produced by the habitual taking of drugs. Strictly speaking, the term implies the state of physical dependence induced by such drugs as morphine, heroin, and alcohol, but it is also used for the state of psychological dependence, produced by drugs such as barbiturates. Treatment is aimed at gradual withdrawal of the drug and eventually total abstention. *See also* alcoholism, tolerance.

Addisonian crisis an acute medical emergency due to a lack of corticosteroid production by the body, caused by disease of the adrenal glands or long-term suppression of production by steroid medication. It manifests as low blood pressure and collapse, biochemical abnormalities, hypoglycemia, and (if untreated) coma and death. Treatment is with steroids, administered initially intravenously in high doses and later orally. In patients with poor adrenal function an Addisonian crisis is usually brought on by an acute illness, such as an infection. [T. Addison (1793–1860), British physician]

Addison's disease a syndrome due to inadequate secretion of corticosteroid hormones by the *adrenal glands, sometimes as a result of tuberculous infection. Symptoms include weakness, loss of energy, low blood pressure, and dark pigmentation of the skin. Formerly fatal, the disease is now treatable by replacement hormone therapy. [T. Addison]

adduct *vb.* to move a limb or any other part toward the midline of the body. —**adduction** *n.*

adductor *n.* any muscle that moves one part of the body toward another or toward the midline of the body.

aden- (adeno-) *prefix denoting* a gland or glands. Examples: *adenalgia* (pain in); *adenogenesis* (development of); *adenopathy* (disease of).

adenine *n.* one of the nitrogen-containing bases (*see* purine) that occurs in the nucleic acids DNA and RNA. *See also* ATP.

adenine arabinoside *see* vidarabine.

adenitis *n.* inflammation of a gland or group of glands. For example, *mesenteric adenitis* affects the lymph nodes in the membranous support of the intestines (the mesentery); *cervical adenitis* affects the lymph nodes in the neck.

adenocarcinoma *n.* a malignant epithelial tumor arising from glandular structures, which are constituent parts of most organs of the body. The term is also applied to tumors that show a glandular growth pattern. These tumors may be subclassified according to the substances that they produce, for example *mucus-secreting* and *serous adenocarcinomas*, or to the microscopic arrangement of their cells into patterns, for example *papillary* and *follicular adenocarcinomas*. They may be solid or cystic (*cystadenocarcinomas*). Each organ may produce tumors showing a variety of histological types; for example, the ovary may produce both mucinous and serous cystadenocarcinomas.

adenohypophysis *n.* the anterior lobe of the *pituitary gland.

adenoidectomy *n.* surgical removal of the *adenoids, commonly combined with tonsillectomy in a child who has recurrent sore throats and difficulty in breathing through the nose.

adenoids (pharyngeal tonsils) *n.* the collection of lymphatic tissue at the rear of the nose. Enlargement of the adenoids from recurrent throat infections may cause obstruction to breathing through the nose and can block the eustachian tubes (*see* adenoidectomy).

adenolymphoma *n. see* Warthin's tumor.

adenoma *n.* a benign tumor of epithelial origin that is derived from glandular tissue or exhibits clearly defined glandular structures. Adenomas may undergo malignant change (*see* adenocarcinoma). Some show recognizable tissue elements, such as fibrous tissue (*fibroadenomas*), while others, such as some bronchial adenomas, may produce active compounds giving rise to clinical syndromes (*see* argentaffinoma). Tumors in certain organs, including the pituitary gland, are often classified by their histological staining affinities, for example *eosinophil*, *basophil*, and *chromophobe adenomas*.

adenomyosis *n. see* endometriosis.

adenosine *n.* a *nucleoside that contains adenine and the sugar ribose: it occurs in all cells in the body and is formed by the enzymatic breakdown of *ATP to *AMP. It is also used as an *antiarrhythmic drug to stop *supraventricular tachycardias and restore a normal heart rhythm. As such, it needs to be injected quickly, which may fleetingly make the patient feel faint and develop chest pain. Trade name: **Adenocard**.

adenosine deaminase deficiency (ADA deficiency) a genetic disorder affecting about one baby in 25,000 and characterized by a defect in *adenosine deami-*

nase (ADA), an enzyme that is involved in purine metabolism. Deficiency of this enzyme results in selective damage to the antibody-producing lymphocytes; this in turn leads to a condition known as *severe combined immune deficiency (SCID)*, in which the affected baby has no resistance to infection and must be entirely isolated from birth. Such children have only about a 50% chance of surviving for six months and are considered to be among the most urgent indications for *gene therapy.

adenosine diphosphate *see* ADP.

adenosine monophosphate *see* AMP.

adenosine triphosphate *see* ATP.

adenosis *n.* (*pl.* **adenoses**) 1. excessive growth or development of glands. 2. any disease of a gland, especially of a lymph node.

adenovirus *n.* one of a group of DNA-containing viruses causing infections of the upper respiratory tract that produce symptoms resembling those of the common cold.

ADEPT *n.* antibody-directed enzyme prodrug therapy: a method under development for the treatment of cancer. It involves the patient being injected first with an antibody-enzyme complex that binds specifically to tumor cells, and later with a *prodrug*, which is inactive until it comes into contact with the antibody-enzyme complex. The enzyme converts the prodrug into a *cytotoxic drug, which is concentrated around the tumor and can therefore destroy the cancer cells without damaging normal tissue.

ADH (antidiuretic hormone) *see* vasopressin.

ADHD *see* attention-deficit/hyperactivity disorder.

adhesion *n.* 1. the union of two normally separate surfaces, such as the moving surfaces of joints, by fibrous connective tissue developing in an inflamed or damaged region. (The fibrous tissue itself is also called an adhesion.) Adhesion between loops of intestine may occur following abdominal surgery, possibly obstructing the alimentary canal. If the pericardial sac is affected by adhesion, the movements of the heart may be restricted. 2. a healing process in which the edges of a wound fit together. In *primary adhesion* there is very little *granulation tissue; in *secondary adhesion* the two edges are joined together by granulation tissue.

adhesion molecules *cell-surface molecules that are important for binding cells to neighboring cells (*intercellular adhesion molecules, ICMA*) and tissues. Absence or weakening of intercellular binding facilitates the local spread of cancer.

adhesive capsulitis *see* frozen shoulder.

adiadochokinesis *n. see* dysdiadochokinesis.

Adie's pupil *see* tonic pupil. [W. J. Adie (1886–1935), British physician]

Adie's syndrome (Holmes-Adie syndrome) an abnormality of the pupils of the eyes, often affecting only one eye. The affected pupil is dilated (*tonic pupil) and reacts slowly to light so that the response on convergence of the eyes is also slow. One or more tendon reflexes may be absent. The condition is almost entirely restricted to women. [W. J. Adie; Sir G. M. Holmes (1876–1965), British neurologist]

adipocere *n.* a waxlike substance, consisting mainly of fatty acids, into which the soft tissues of the body can be converted after death. This usually occurs when the body is buried in damp earth or is submerged in water. Adipocere delays postmortem decomposition and is a spontaneous form of preservation without mummification.

adipocyte *n. see* adipose tissue.

adipose tissue fibrous *connective tissue packed with masses of fat cells (*adipocytes*). It forms a thick layer under the skin and occurs around the kidneys and in the buttocks. It serves both as an insulating layer and an energy store; food in excess of requirements is converted into fats and stored within these cells.

adiposis (liposis) *n.* the presence of abnormally large accumulations of fat in the body. The condition may arise from overeating, hormone irregularities, or a metabolic disorder. In *adiposis dolorosa*, a condition affecting women more commonly than men, painful fatty swellings are associated with defects in the nervous system. *See also* obesity.

aditus *n.* an anatomical opening or passage; for example, the opening of the tympanic cavity (middle ear) to the air spaces of the mastoid process.

adjunct *n.* a drug used in combination with

another drug for treating a particular condition. The adjunct "supports" the other (main) drug by providing additional therapeutic effects, often by a mode of action that is different from that of the main drug. —**adjunctive** *adj.*

adjuvant *n.* any substance that is used in conjunction with another to enhance its activity. Aluminum salts are used as adjuvants in the preparation of vaccines from the toxins of diphtheria and tetanus: by keeping the toxins in precipitated form, the salts increase the efficacy of the toxins as antigens.

adjuvant therapy treatment given to patients, usually after surgical removal of their primary tumor when there is known to be a high risk of future tumor recurrence. Adjuvant therapy is aimed at destroying these secondary tumor cells either locally (e.g. adjuvant breast irradiation after breast-conserving surgery) or systemically (e.g. adjuvant chemotherapy may be recommended for patients with breast cancer, colorectal cancer, and other types of cancer). *Compare* neoadjuvant chemotherapy.

admission rate the number of cases of a specified disease or condition admitted to hospitals, related to the population of a given geographical area.

adnexa *pl. n.* adjoining parts. For example, the *uterine adnexa* are the fallopian tubes and ovaries (which adjoin the uterus).

adolescence *n.* the stage of development between childhood and adulthood. It begins with the start of *puberty, which in girls is usually at the age of about 12 and in boys about 14.

ADP (adenosine diphosphate) a compound containing adenine, ribose, and two phosphate groups. ADP occurs in cells and is involved in processes requiring the transfer of energy (*see also* AMP, ATP).

adrenalectomy *n.* the surgical removal of an *adrenal gland, usually performed because of neoplastic disease.

adrenal glands (suprarenal glands) two triangular *endocrine glands, each of which covers the superior surface of a kidney. Each gland has two parts, the *medulla* and *cortex*. The medulla forms the gray core of the gland; it consists mainly of *chromaffin tissue and is stimulated by the sympathetic nervous system to produce *epinephrine and

*norepinephrine. The cortex is a yellowish tissue surrounding the medulla. It is derived embryologically from mesoderm and is stimulated by pituitary hormones (principally *ACTH) to produce three kinds of *corticosteroid hormones, which affect carbohydrate metabolism (e.g. *cortisol), electrolyte metabolism (e.g. *aldosterone), and the sex glands (estrogens and androgens).

adrenaline *n. see* epinephrine.

adrenarche *n.* the start of secretion of *androgens by the adrenal glands, occurring at around 6–7 years of age in girls and 7–8 in boys. It is usually determined by the measurement of urinary 17-ketosteroids rather than direct assay of the androgens themselves. Adrenal androgens are *dehydroepiandrosterone (DHEA), DHEA sulphate, and androstenedione. The age of adrenarche is unrelated to the age of *gonadarche. Premature adrenarche is usually manifested as the early appearance of pubic hair due to levels of the adrenal androgens equivalent to those found in puberty. It does not proceed to full puberty as the gonads do not become active.

adrenergic *adj.* **1.** describing sympathetic nerve cells or fibers of the autonomic nervous system that either release *norepinephrine as a neurotransmitter or act as *receptors at which norepinephrine acts to pass on messages from sympathetic nerves. *Compare* cholinergic. **2.** describing agents that mimic the actions of sympathetic stimulation.

adrenocorticotropic hormone (adrenocorticotropin) *see* ACTH.

adrenogenital syndrome a hormonal disorder resulting from abnormal *steroid production by the adrenal cortex, due to a genetic defect. It may cause masculinization in girls, precocious puberty in boys, and adrenocortical failure (*see* Addison's disease) in both sexes. Treatment is by lifelong steroid replacement.

adrenoleukodystrophy *n.* a genetically determined condition of neurological degeneration with childhood and adult forms affecting males. It is characterized by progressive *spastic paralysis of the legs and sensory loss, associated with adrenal gland insufficiency and small gonads. The demonstration of abnormal fatty-acid metabolism has implications for future possible drug therapies. *Prenatal diagnosis is possible.

adrenolytic *adj.* inhibiting the activity of *adrenergic nerves. Adrenolytic activity is opposite to that of *norepinephrine.

adult respiratory distress syndrome (ARDS) a condition of acute respiratory failure that occurs after a precipitating event, such as trauma, aspiration, or inhalation of a toxic substance; it is particularly associated with septic shock. Lung injury is characterized by reduced oxygen in the arteries, reduced lung volume, and decreased lung compliance, and bilateral infiltrates are seen on a chest X-ray. Treatment is correction of the original cause, volume replacement, diuretics, oxygen, and mechanical ventilation.

advanced glycation end products damaged proteins that result from the *glycation of a large number of body proteins, which can accumulate and cause permanent damage to tissues. This damage is more prevalent in diabetics due to chronic exposure to blood with high concentrations of glucose. It is believed to be partly responsible for the damage to the kidneys, eyes, and blood vessels that characterizes long-standing diabetes.

advance directive a signed statement by a person that gives treatment preferences in the event of incapacitation or inability to communicate. Kinds of advance directives are *durable power of attorney for health care and *living wills.

advancement *n.* the detachment by surgery of a muscle, musculocutaneous flap, or tendon from its normal attachment site and its reattachment at a more advanced (anterior) point while preserving its previous nerve and blood supply. The technique is used, for example, in the treatment of squint, or in repositioning the uterus, and extensively in plastic surgery to cover large defects (*see also* pedicle).

adventitia (tunica adventitia) *n.* **1.** the outer coat of the wall of a *vein or *artery. It consists of loose connective tissue and networks of small blood vessels, which nourish the walls. **2.** the outer covering of various other organs or parts.

adventitious *adj.* **1.** occurring in a place other than the usual one. **2.** relating to the adventitia.

Aëdes *n.* a genus of widely distributed mosquitoes occurring throughout the tropics and subtropics. Most species are black with distinct white or silvery-yellow markings on the legs and thorax. *Aëdes* species are not only important as vectors of *dengue, *yellow fever, *filariasis, and group B viruses causing encephalitis, but also constitute a serious biting nuisance. *A. aegypti* is the principal vector of dengue and yellow fever.

aer- (aero-) *prefix denoting* air or gas. Examples: *aerogastria* (gas in the stomach); *aerogenesis* (production of gas).

aerobe *n.* any organism, especially a microbe, that requires the presence of free oxygen for life and growth. *See also* anaerobe, microaerophilic.

aerobic *adj.* **1.** of or relating to aerobes: requiring free oxygen for life and growth. **2.** describing a type of cellular *respiration in which foodstuffs (carbohydrates) are completely oxidized by atmospheric oxygen, with the production of maximum chemical energy from the foodstuffs.

aerobic exercises *see* exercise.

aerodontalgia *n.* pain in the teeth due to change in atmospheric pressure during air travel or the ascent of a mountain.

aeroneurosis *n.* a syndrome of anxiety, agitation, and insomnia found in pilots flying unpressurized aircraft and attributed to *anoxia.

aerophagia *n.* the swallowing of air. This may be done voluntarily to stimulate belching, accidentally during rapid eating or drinking, or unconsciously as a habit. Voluntary aerophagia is used to permit esophageal speech after surgical removal of the larynx (usually for cancer).

aerosol *n.* a suspension of extremely small liquid or solid particles (about 0.001 mm diameter) in the air. Drugs in aerosol form may be administered by inhalation.

aerotitis media *see* barotitis.

aetiology *n.* *see* etiology.

AFDC *see* Aid to Families with Dependent Children.

afebrile *adj.* without, or not showing any signs of, a fever.

affect *n.* (in psychiatry) **1.** the predominant emotion in a person's mental state.

2. the emotion associated with a particular idea. —**affective** *adj.*

affective disorder any psychiatric disorder featuring abnormalities of mood or emotion (*affect). The most serious of these are *depression and *mania. Other affective disorders include *SAD (seasonal affective disorder).

afferent *adj.* **1.** designating nerves or neurons that convey impulses from sense organs and other receptors to the brain or spinal cord, i.e. any sensory nerve or neuron. **2.** designating blood vessels that feed a capillary network in an organ or part. **3.** designating lymphatic vessels that enter a lymph node. *Compare* efferent.

afibrinogenemia *n.* complete absence of the coagulation factor *fibrinogen in the blood. *Compare* hypofibrinogenemia.

aflatoxin *n.* a poisonous substance produced in the spores of the fungus *Aspergillus flavus*, which infects peanuts. The toxin is known to produce cancer in certain animals and is suspected of being the cause of liver cancers in human beings living in warm and humid regions of the world, where stored nuts and cereals are contaminated by the fungus.

AFP *see* alpha-fetoprotein.

afterbirth *n.* the placenta, umbilical cord, and ruptured membranes associated with the fetus, which normally become detached from the uterus and are expelled within a few hours after birth.

aftercare *n.* long-term surveillance or rehabilitation as an adjunct or supplement to formal medical treatment of those who are chronically sick or disabled, including those with mental illness or learning disability. Aftercare includes the provision of special aids and the adaptation of homes to improve daily living.

afterimage *n.* an impression of an image that is registered by the brain for a brief moment after an object is removed from in front of the eye, or after the eye is closed.

afterpains *pl. n.* pains caused by uterine contractions after childbirth, especially during breast feeding, due to release of the hormone *oxytocin. The contractions help restore the uterus to its nonpregnant size and are more common in women who have given birth twice or more.

agammaglobulinemia *n.* a total deficiency of the plasma protein *gamma globulin. *Compare* hypogammaglobulinemia.

agar *n.* an extract of certain seaweeds that forms a gel suitable for the solidification of liquid bacteriological *culture media. *Blood agar* is nutrient agar containing 5–10% horse blood, used for the cultivation of certain bacteria or for detecting hemolytic (red blood cell-destroying) activity.

agenesis *n.* absence of an organ, usually due to total failure of its development in the embryo.

Agent Orange the US military code name for a herbicide used as a defoliant in Southeast Asia during the Vietnam War. The chemical mixture was contaminated with *dioxin, a toxic agent associated with *chloracne and *porphyria cutanea tarda that also may be carcinogenic and cause birth defects.

age-related macular degeneration (AMD) *see* macular degeneration.

agglutination (clumping) *n.* the sticking together, by serum antibodies called *agglutinins*, of such microscopic antigenic particles as red blood cells or bacteria so that they form visible clumps. Any substance that stimulates the body to produce an agglutinin is called an *agglutinogen*. Agglutination is a specific reaction; in the laboratory, sera containing different known agglutinins provide an invaluable means of identifying unknown bacteria. When blood of different groups is mixed, agglutination occurs because serum contains natural antibodies (*isoagglutinins*) that attack red cells of a foreign group, whether previously encountered or not. This is not the same process as occurs in *blood coagulation.

agglutinin *n.* an antibody that brings about the *agglutination of bacteria, blood cells, or other antigenic particles.

agglutinogen *n.* any antigen that provokes formation of an agglutinin in the serum and is therefore likely to be involved in *agglutination.

aglossia *n.* congenital absence of the tongue.

agnathia *n.* congenital absence of the lower jaw, either partial or complete.

agnosia *n.* a disorder of the brain whereby the patient cannot interpret sensations correctly although the sense organs and nerves conducting sensation to the brain are functioning normally. It is due to a disorder of the *association areas in the parietal lobes. In *auditory agnosia* the patient can hear but cannot interpret sounds (including speech). A patient with *tactile agnosia* (*astereognosis*) retains normal sensation in the hands but cannot recognize three-dimensional objects by touch alone. In *visual agnosia* the patient can see but cannot interpret symbols, including letters (*see also* alexia).

agonal *adj.* describing or relating to the phenomena, such as cessation of breathing or change in the ECG or EEG, that are associated with the moment of death.

agonist *n.* **1. (prime mover)** a muscle whose active contraction causes movement of a part of the body. Contraction of an agonist is associated with relaxation of its *antagonist. **2.** a drug or other substance that acts at a cell-receptor site to produce an effect that is the same as, or similar to, that of the body's normal chemical messenger. Cholinergic drugs (*see* parasympathomimetic) are examples.

agoraphobia *n.* a morbid fear of public places and/or of open spaces. Treatment is with behavioral therapy, psychotherapy, or medication. *Compare* claustrophobia. *See also* phobia.

agranulocytosis *n.* a disorder in which there is a severe acute deficiency of certain blood cells (*neutrophils) as a result of damage to the bone marrow by toxic drugs or chemicals. It is characterized by fever, with ulceration of the mouth and throat, and may rapidly lead to prostration and death. Treatment is by administration of antibiotics in large quantities. When feasible, transfusion of white blood cells may be lifesaving.

agraphia (dysgraphia) *n.* an acquired inability to write, although the strength and coordination of the hand remain normal. It is related to the disorders of language and it is caused by disease in the *parietal lobe of the brain. *See also* Gerstmann's syndrome.

agromania *n.* a pathologically strong impulse to live alone in open country.

ague *n. see* malaria.

agyria (lissencephaly) *n.* a condition in which the brain develops abnormally – it has no grooves on the outside (so that the brain surface is smooth), large ven-

tricles, and generally is smaller than it should be. The condition causes severe mental retardation and *failure to thrive. *See also* Miller-Deiker syndrome.

Aicardi syndrome a syndrome caused by abnormal development of the brain in which the two halves of the brain do not connect. The *corpus callosum is absent. Affected individuals suffer from mental retardation and seizures. They may also have associated abnormalities of the eyes and spine. [J. D. Aicardi (20th century), French neurologist]

AID *see* artificial insemination.

AIDS (acquired immunodeficiency syndrome) a syndrome first identified in Los Angeles in 1981; a description of the causative virus – the human immunodeficiency virus (*HIV) – was available in 1983. The virus destroys a subgroup of lymphocytes, the *helper T cells (or *CD4 lymphocytes), resulting in suppression of the body's immune response (*see* immunity). AIDS is essentially a sexually transmitted disease, either homosexually or heterosexually. The two other main routes of spread are via infected blood or blood products (current processing of blood for transfusion and for hemophiliacs has virtually eliminated this danger) and by the maternofetal route. The virus may be transmitted from an infected mother to the child in the uterus or it may be acquired from maternal blood during parturition; it may also be transmitted in breast milk. Acute infection following exposure to the virus results in the production of antibodies (seroconversion), their presence indicating that infection has taken place. However, not all those who *seroconvert progress to chronic infection. For those who do enter a chronic stage there may be illness of varying severity, including persistent generalized involvement of the lymph nodes; what is termed *AIDS-related complex* (*ARC*), including intermittent fever, weight loss, diarrhea, fatigue, and night sweats; and AIDS itself, presenting as opportunistic infections (especially pneumonia caused by the protozoan *Pneumocystis carinii*) and/or tumors, such as *Kaposi's sarcoma.

HIV has been isolated from semen, cervical secretions, plasma, cerebrospinal fluid, tears, saliva, urine, and breast milk but the concentration shows wide variations. Moreover HIV is a fragile virus and does not survive well outside the body. It is therefore considered that ordinary social contact with HIV-positive subjects involves no risk of infection. However, high standards of clinical practice are required by all health workers in order to avoid inadvertent infection via blood, blood products, or body fluids from HIV-positive patients. Until recently, AIDS has been considered to be fatal, although the type and length of illness preceding death varies considerably. AIDS is pandemic and as yet there is no known cure, although antiviral drugs, initially used singly but more recently used in dual or triple combinations, may well modify the gloomy outlook. These drugs include the *reverse transcriptase inhibitors and the *protease inhibitors.

Aid to Families with Dependent Children (AFDC) a federally funded program designed to provide medical assistance on behalf of families with dependent children. All needy children under the age of 21 are eligible for medical care under provisions of this section of the US *Social Security Act, with states contributing 20–47% of the costs of the program according to the state's per capita income.

Aid to the Blind (AB) a federal program that provides financial aid to states so that medical assistance can be furnished to persons who are blind. Aid to the Blind is covered by Title X of the US *Social Security Act.

Aid to the Permanently and Totally Disabled (APTD) a federal program of medical care for permanently and totally disabled persons who are considered medically indigent although they are not on welfare. Funding is provided under Title XIV of the US *Social Security Act; prior to 1 January, 1974, APTD was administered as a separate category of medical services to persons receiving public assistance.

AIH see artificial insemination.

ainhum *n.* loss of one or more toes due to slow growth of a fibrous band around the toe that eventually causes a spontaneous amputation. The condition is found in Africans and is associated with going barefoot.

air bed a bed with a mattress whose upper surface is perforated with thousands of holes, through which air is forced under pressure. The patient is thus supported on a cushion of air. This type of bed is invaluable for the treatment of patients with large areas of burns.

air embolism an airlock that obstructs the outflow of blood from the right ventricle of the heart. Air may gain access to the circulation as a result of surgery, injury, or intravenous infusions. The patient experiences breathlessness and chest discomfort and develops acute heart failure. Tipping the patient head down, lying on the left side, may move the airlock.

air sickness see motion sickness.

airway *n.* any natural passageway or respiratory device that enables the flow of air into and out of the trachea, lungs, bronchi, and bronchioles.

akathisia *n.* a pattern of involuntary movements induced by antipsychotic drugs, such as *phenothiazines. An affected person is driven to restless overactivity, which can be confused with the agitation for which the drug was originally prescribed.

akinesia *n.* a loss of normal muscular tonicity or responsiveness. *Akinetic rigid syndrome* is used to describe such conditions as *parkinsonism and *progressive supranuclear palsy. In *akinetic epilepsy* there is a sudden loss of muscular tonicity, making the patient fall with momentary loss of consciousness. *Akinetic mutism* is a state of complete physical unresponsiveness although the patient's eyes remain open and appear to follow movements. It is a consequence of damage to the base of the brain. —**akinetic** *adj.*

ala *n.* (*pl.* alae) (in anatomy) a winglike structure; for example, either of the two lateral flared portions of the external nose or the winglike expansion of the ilium.

alactasia *n.* absence or deficiency of the enzyme lactase, which is essential for the digestion of milk sugar (lactose). All babies have lactase in their intestines, but the enzyme disappears during childhood in about 10% of northern Europeans, 40% of Greeks and Italians, and 80% of Africans and Asians. Alactasia causes symptoms only if the diet regularly includes raw milk, when the undigested lactose causes diarrhea and abdominal pain.

Alagille syndrome (arteriohepatic dysplasia) an inherited condition in which the bile ducts, which drain the liver, become progressively smaller, causing increased *jaundice. It is associated with abnormalities of other organs, such as the heart, kidneys, eyes, and spine. [D. Alagille (1925–), French physician]

alanine n. see amino acid.

alanine transaminase (alanine aminotransferase, ALT) an enzyme involved in the transamination of amino acids. Measurement of ALT in the serum is of use in the diagnosis and study of acute liver disease. It was formerly called *serum glutamic pyruvic transaminase (SGPT)*.

alastrim n. a mild form of smallpox that causes only a sparse rash and low-grade fever. Medical name: **variola minor**.

albendazole n. an *anthelmintic drug used to treat infestations of parasitic worms (see strongyloidiasis, creeping eruption) and *hydatid disease. It is administered by mouth. Possible side effects include headache, dizziness, fever, skin rashes, and loss of hair. Trade names: **Albenza, Stromectol**.

Albers-Schönberg disease see osteopetrosis. [H. E. Albers-Schönberg (1865–1921), German radiologist]

Alberti's regimen see GIK regimen. [K. G. M. M. Alberti (1937–), British physician]

albinism n. the inherited absence of pigmentation in the skin, hair, and eyes, resulting in white hair and pink skin and eyes. The pink color is produced by blood in underlying blood vessels, which are normally masked by pigment. Ocular signs are reduced visual acuity, sensitivity to light (see photophobia), and involuntary side-to-side eye movements.

albino n. an individual lacking the normal body pigment (melanin). *See* albinism.

Albright's syndrome (Albright-McCune-Sternberg syndrome, Albright's hereditary osteodystrophy) the skeletal abnormalities, collectively, of *pseudohypoparathyroidism type 1. These include short stature, abnormally short fingers and toes (particularly involving the fourth and fifth metacarpals and metatarsals), and soft-tissue calcifica-

tion. [F. Albright (1900–69), US physician]

albumin n. a protein that is soluble in water and coagulated by heat. An example is *serum albumin*, which is found in blood plasma and is important for the maintenance of plasma volume. Albumin is synthesized in the liver; the inability to synthesize it is a prominent feature of chronic liver disease (*cirrhosis).

albuminuria (proteinuria) n. the presence of serum albumin, serum globulin, or other serum proteins in the urine. This may be associated with kidney or heart disease. Albuminuria is not always associated with disease: it may occur after strenuous exercise or after a long period of standing (*orthostatic albuminuria*).

albumose n. a substance, intermediate between albumin and peptones, produced during the digestion of proteins by pepsin and other endopeptidases (*see* peptidase).

albuterol n. a drug, similar to *isoproterenol, used as a *bronchodilator to relieve asthma, chronic bronchitis, and emphysema. It is administered by mouth, injection, or inhalation; side effects may include dizziness, tremor, and fast heart rate, particularly after large doses. Trade names: **Proventil, Ventolin, Xopenex**.

alcaptonuria n. see alkaptonuria.

alclometasone n. a *corticosteroid drug administered externally as a cream or ointment to treat inflammatory skin disorders. Possible side effects include skin thinning and allergic reactions. Trade name: **Aclovate**.

alcohol n. any of a class of organic compounds formed when a hydroxyl group (–OH) is substituted for a hydrogen atom in a hydrocarbon. The alcohol in alcoholic drinks is *ethyl alcohol (ethanol)*, which has the formula C_2H_5OH. It is produced by the fermentation of sugar by yeast. "Pure" alcohol contains not less than 94.9% by volume of ethyl alcohol. It is obtained by distillation. A solution of 70% alcohol can be used as a preservative or antiseptic. When taken into the body, ethyl alcohol depresses activity of the central nervous system (*see also* alcoholism). *Methyl alcohol (methanol) is extremely poisonous.

Alcohol, Drug Abuse and Mental Health

Administration *see* Substance Abuse and Mental Health Services Administration.

Alcoholic and Narcotic Addict Rehabilitation Amendment (1968) a US law that added new provisions to the Community Mental Health Centers Act, authorizing funds for construction of facilities and the employment of medical personnel needed for the treatment of alcoholics and narcotics addicts as well as for the financing of special training programs and studies to evaluate the problems and treatments.

Alcoholics Anonymous a voluntary agency of self-help that is organized and operated locally among those with alcoholic dependency and has national and international support. Members are expected to admit to their drinking problems, discuss these openly and frankly at the regular meetings of the group, and also to take part in efficient family support schemes to help those members who have lapses.

alcoholism *n.* the syndrome due to physical *dependence on alcohol, such that sudden deprivation may cause withdrawal symptoms – tremor, anxiety, hallucinations, and delusions (*see* delirium tremens). The risk of alcoholism for an individual and its incidence in a society depend on the amount drunk. Countries such as France, where heavy drinking is socially acceptable, have the highest incidence. Usually several years' heavy drinking is needed for addiction to develop, but the range is from one to 40 years. Alcoholism impairs intellectual function, physical skills, memory, and judgment: social skills, such as conversation, are preserved until a late stage. Heavy consumption of alcohol also causes *cardiomyopathy, peripheral *neuritis, *cirrhosis, and *enteritis. Treatment is usually given in a psychiatric hospital, where the alcoholic is first "dried out" and then helped to understand the psychological pressures that led to his heavy drinking. Drugs such as *disulfiram (Antabuse), which cause vomiting if alcohol is taken, may help in treatment.

aldehyde *n.* an organic compound derived from the oxidation of alcohol, as in the conversion of ethyl alcohol (ethanol) to acetaldehyde (ethanal).

aldesleukin *see* interleukin.

Aldomet *n. see* methyldopa.

aldosterone *n.* a steroid hormone (*see* corticosteroid) that is synthesized and released by the adrenal cortex and acts on the kidney to regulate salt (potassium and sodium) and water balance. It may be given by injection as replacement therapy when the adrenal cortex secretes insufficient amounts of the hormone and also to treat shock.

aldosteronism *n.* overproduction of aldosterone, one of the hormones secreted by the adrenal cortex, leading to abnormalities in the amounts of sodium, potassium, and water in the body. It is one cause of high blood pressure (hypertension). *See also* Conn's syndrome.

alemtuzumab *n.* a *monoclonal antibody used to treat chronic lymphocytic *leukemia in patients whose disease has progressed despite treatment with other chemotherapeutic agents. It is administered by intravenous infusion; side effects include diarrhea, dizziness, fever, headache, rash, nausea and vomiting, shortness of breath, unusual bleeding or bruising, and unusual tiredness or weakness. Trade name: **Campath**.

alendronate *n. see* bisphosphonates.

Aleppo boil *see* oriental sore.

aleukemic *adj.* describing a stage of *leukemia in which there is no increase in the number of white cells in the blood. The stage is usually followed by one in which excessive numbers of white cells are produced, as typical in leukemia.

alexia *n.* an acquired inability to read. It is due to disease in the left hemisphere of the brain in a right-handed person. In *agnosic alexia* (*word blindness*) the patient cannot read because he is unable to identify the letters and words, but he retains the ability to write and his speech is normal. This is a form of *agnosia. A patient with *aphasic alexia* (*visual asymbolia*) can neither read nor write and often has an accompanying disorder of speech. This is a form of *aphasia. *See also* dyslexia.

alexin *n.* a former name for the serum component now called *complement.

alexithymia *n.* a lack of psychological understanding of one's own emotions and moods. It is considered by some psychiatrists to be a way in which people develop *psychosomatic symptoms.

alfentanil hydrochloride a narcotic *analgesic drug used for the induction of anesthesia and in the maintenance of general anesthesia. It is administered by injection. Trade name: **Alfenta**.

alfuzosin *n.* an *alpha blocker commonly used in the treatment of men with *lower urinary tract symptoms thought to be due to benign prostatic hyperplasia. Trade name: **Uroxatral**.

ALG antilymphocyte globulin. *See* antilymphocytic serum.

algesimeter *n.* a piece of equipment for determining the sensitivity of the skin to various touch stimuli, especially those causing pain.

-algia *suffix denoting* pain. Example: *neuralgia* (pain in a nerve).

algid *adj.* cold: usually describing the cold clammy skin associated with certain forms of malaria.

algodystrophy *n.* a specific post-traumatic syndrome after nerve injury, in which a limb remains exquisitely sensitive to any stimulus and later develops disuse *atrophy. Overactivity of sympathetic nerves may contribute to the syndrome.

algorithm *n.* a sequential set of instructions used in calculations or problem solving. A *reconstruction algorithm* is a complex mathematical formula used by a computer to construct images from the data acquired by CT, MRI, or other scanners. A *diagnostic algorithm* or a *therapeutic algorithm* consists of a stepwise series of instructions with branching pathways to be followed to assist a physician in coming to a diagnosis or deciding on a treatment strategy, respectively.

alienation *n.* (in psychiatry) **1.** the state of being estranged from society or the feeling of being an outsider. **2.** the experience that one's thoughts are under the control of somebody else, or that other people participate in one's thinking. It is a symptom of *schizophrenia. **3.** an obsolete term for insanity.

alimentary canal the long passage through which food passes to be digested and ab-

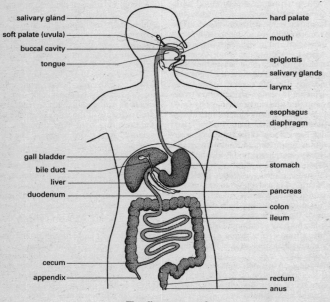

salivary gland — hard palate
soft palate (uvula) — mouth
buccal cavity — epiglottis
tongue — salivary glands
— larynx
— esophagus
— diaphragm
gall bladder — stomach
bile duct — pancreas
liver —
duodenum — colon
— ileum
cecum — rectum
appendix — anus

The alimentary canal

sorbed (see illustration). It extends from the mouth to the anus and each region is specialized for a different stage in the processing of food, from mechanical breakdown in the mouth to chemical *digestion and *absorption in the stomach and small intestine and finally to feces formation and water absorption in the colon and rectum.

alizarin (alizarin carmine) *n.* an orange-red dye derived from coal tar and originally isolated from the plant madder (*Rubia tinctorum*). Alizarin is insoluble in water but dissolves in alkalis, alcohol, and ether. It is used as a pH indicator and as a histochemical reagent for calcium, thallium, titanium, and zirconium.

ALK *see* automated lamellar keratectomy.

alkalemia *n.* abnormally high blood alkalinity. This may be caused by an increase in the concentration of alkaline substances and/or a decrease in that of acidic substances in the blood. *See also* alkalosis. *Compare* acidemia.

alkaloid *n.* one of a diverse group of nitrogen-containing substances that are produced by plants and have potent effects on body function. Many alkaloids are important drugs, including *morphine, *quinine, *atropine, and *codeine.

alkalosis *n.* a condition in which the alkalinity of body fluids and tissues is abnormally high. This arises because of a failure of the mechanisms that usually maintain a balance between alkalis and acids in the arterial blood (*see* acid-base balance). Alkalosis may be associated with loss of acid through vomiting or with excessive sodium bicarbonate intake. Breathing that is abnormally deep in relation to the amount of physical exercise may lead to *respiratory alkalosis*. Alkalosis may produce symptoms of muscular weakness or cramp.

alkaptonuria (alcaptonuria) *n.* congenital absence of an enzyme, homogentisic acid oxidase, that is essential for the normal breakdown of the amino acids tyrosine and phenylalanine. Accumulation of *homogentisic acid causes dark brown discoloration of the skin and eyes (*ochronosis*) and progressive damage to the joints, especially of the spine. The gene responsible for the condition is recessive, so that a child is affected only if both parents are carriers of the defective gene.

alkylating agents a class of drugs used in chemotherapy that includes *cyclophosphamide and *melphalan. These drugs bind to DNA and prevent complete separation of the two DNA chains during cell division.

allantois *n.* the membranous sac that develops as an outgrowth of the embryonic hindgut. Its outer (mesodermal) layer carries blood vessels to the *placenta and so forms part of the *umbilical cord. Its cavity is small and becomes reduced further in size during fetal development (*see* urachus). —**allantoic** *adj.*

allele (allelomorph) *n.* one of two or more alternative forms of a *gene, only one of which can be present in a chromosome. Two alleles of a particular gene occupy the same relative positions on a pair of *homologous chromosomes. If the two alleles are the same, the individual is *homozygous for the gene; if they are different he is *heterozygous. *See also* dominant, recessive. —**allelic** *adj.*

allergen *n.* any *antigen that causes *allergy in a hypersensitive person. Allergens are diverse and affect different tissues and organs. Pollens, fur, feathers, mold, and dust may cause hay fever; house-dust mites (*see* Dermatophagoides) have been implicated in some forms of asthma; drugs, dyes, cosmetics, and a host of other chemicals can cause rashes and dermatitis; some food allergies may cause diarrhea or constipation or simulate acute bacterial food poisoning. When a patient's allergen has been identified (*see* patch test), it may be possible to attempt *desensitization to alleviate or prevent allergic attacks. —**allergenic** *adj.*

allergy *n.* a disorder in which the body becomes hypersensitive to particular antigens (called *allergens), which provoke characteristic symptoms whenever they are subsequently inhaled, ingested, injected, or otherwise contacted. Normally antibodies in the bloodstream and tissues react with and destroy specific antigens without further trouble. In an allergic person, however, the allergens provoke the release of a class of antibodies (IgE) that become bound to *mast cells in the body's tissues. The subsequent reaction of allergen with tissue-bound antibody (see reagin) also leads, as a side effect, to cell damage, release of *histamine and *serotonin, inflammation, and all the symptoms of the particular allergy. Different allergies afflict different tissues and may have either local or general effects, varying from asthma and hay fever to severe dermatitis or gastroenteritis or extremely serious shock (see anaphylaxis). —**allergic** adj.

allied health personnel see paramedical personnel.

Allied Health Professions Personnel Training Act (1966) a US law that established programs for construction of facilities for training personnel in such fields as medical technology and dental hygiene. The act also provided a broad program of student loan funds covering scholarships for nursing students in financial need and cancellation of student loans for physicians, dentists, and optometrists who elected to serve in poor rural areas after graduation.

allodynia n. extreme tenderness of the skin. It results from nerve damage causing hypersensitivity of the pain receptors in that area, such as occurs in shingles (postherpetic neuralgia – see herpes).

allogeneic adj. describing grafted tissue derived from a donor of the same species as the recipient but with different *histocompatibility.

allograft (homograft) n. a living tissue or organ graft between two members of the same species; for example, a heart transplant from one person to another. Such grafts will not survive unless the recipient is treated to suppress his body's *immune response to the foreign tissue or the grafted organ is from an identical twin. See also transplantation. Compare xenograft.

alloisoleucine n. one of the isomers of the amino acid isoleucine.

allopathy n. the system of medicine in which the use of drugs is directed to producing effects in the body that will directly oppose and so alleviate the symptoms of a disease. Compare homeopathy.

allopurinol n. a drug used in the treatment of chronic gout. It acts by reducing the level of uric acid in tissues and blood. It is administered by mouth; side effects include nausea, vomiting, diarrhea, headache, fever, stomach pains, and skin rashes. Occasionally, nerve damage and enlargement of the liver may occur. Trade names: **Aloprim, Lopurin, Zyloprim.**

almotriptan n. see 5HT₁ agonist.

alopecia (baldness) n. absence of hair from areas where it normally grows. Non-scarring alopecias include common baldness in men, which is familial, and androgenetic alopecia in women, in which the hair loss is associated with increasing age. Acute hair fall (telogen effluvium), in which much or all of the hair is shed but starts to regrow at once, may occur after pregnancy or a serious illness. Alopecia areata consists of bald patches that may regrow; it is an example of an organ-specific *autoimmune disease. In scarring (or cicatricial) alopecias the hair does not regrow; examples include *lichen planus and discoid *lupus erythematosus. Alopecia totalis is loss of all the hair, due to an autoimmune condition; in some 70% of cases it regrows within a few years.

ALOS see Average Length of Stay.

alpha agonist see sympathomimetic.

alpha blocker (alpha-adrenergic blocker) a drug that prevents the stimulation of alpha-adrenergic receptors at the nerve endings of the sympathetic nervous system by epinephrine and norepinephrine; it therefore causes widening of arteries (vasodilation) and a drop in blood pressure. Alpha blockers include *alfuzosin, *doxazosin, *phentolamine, *phenoxybenzamine, and *prazosin. Overdosage causes a severe drop in blood pressure, a rapid pulse, nausea and vomiting, diarrhea, a dry mouth, flushed skin, convulsions, drowsiness, and coma.

alpha-fetoprotein (AFP) n. a protein formed by the fetal yolk sac, liver, and gastrointestinal tract and present in the *amniotic fluid and secondarily in maternal blood. It can cross the placental barrier and enter the maternal circulation. The level of AFP can be detected by a maternal blood test performed between the 16th and 18th weeks of pregnancy to aid *prenatal diagnosis of certain fetal conditions. Levels are elevated in open *neural tube defects (e.g. spina bifida), twins and triplets, open abdominal wall defects (e.g. *gastroschisis), and fetal death. Levels of AFP are decreased in *Down's syndrome. However, AFP levels are affected by the length of gestation and the mother's weight, and these factors must be considered when interpreting the results. When levels are unexpectedly high or low, further investigations (for example *ultrasound scanning) are indicated. Alpha-fetoprotein is also produced by certain tumors (see tumor marker).

alpha-glucosidase inhibitor any member of a group of *oral hypoglycemic drugs, including *acarbose* (Precose), used for treating type 2 *diabetes mellitus. They reduce the breakdown and absorption of carbohydrates in the intestine by blocking the action of the enzyme α-glucosidase in this process. Side effects include flatulence and diarrhea.

alphavirus n. any member of a genus of *arboviruses transmitted by mosquitoes. Many alphaviruses can cause disease in humans and animals, including *O'nyong-nyong fever.

Alport's syndrome a hereditary disease that causes *nephritis accompanied by deafness and, less commonly, ocular defects, such as cataracts. Affected males usually develop end-stage renal failure and, unless treated with a kidney transplant, die before the age of 40. Females have a better prognosis. [A. C. Alport (1880–1959), South African physician]

alprazolam n. a *benzodiazepine used to relieve anxiety and as a sedative. It is administered by mouth; side effects include drowsiness and lightheadedness. Trade name: **Xanax**.

alprostadil n. a *prostaglandin drug administered by infusion to improve lung blood flow in newborn babies with congenital heart defects who are awaiting surgery; it acts by preventing the closure of the blood vessel connecting the aorta to the pulmonary artery (see ductus arteriosus). Possible side effects include diminished respiratory efforts. Alprostadil is also administered by injection into the corpora cavernosa of the penis or by application into the urethra to treat erectile *impotence in men; side effects may include dizziness and headache. Trade names: **Caverject, MUSE, Prostin VR**.

ALS 1. see antilymphocytic serum. **2.** amyotrophic lateral sclerosis. *See* motor neuron disease.

ALT 1. see alanine transaminase. **2.** argon laser *trabeculoplasty.

alteplase n. a *tissue-type plasminogen activator made by recombinant DNA technology (genetic engineering). Alteplase is used to dissolve blood clots (see fibrinolytic), especially in the coronary arteries of the heart. It is administered by injection. Possible side effects include local bleeding, cerebral hemorrhage, nausea, and vomiting. Trade name: **Activase**.

alternative medicine see complementary medicine.

altitude sickness (mountain sickness) the condition that results from unaccustomed exposure to a high altitude (15,000 feet or more above sea level). Reduced atmospheric pressure and shortage of oxygen cause deep rapid breathing (*hyperventilation), which lowers the concentration of carbon dioxide in the blood (see alkalosis). Symptoms include nausea, exhaustion, and anxiety. In severe cases there may be acute shortness of breath due to fluid collecting in the lungs (pulmonary *edema), which requires treatment by diuretics and return to a lower altitude.

aluminum chloride hexahydrate a powerful antiperspirant used in the treatment of conditions associated with excessive sweating (see hyperhidrosis). It is applied to the skin in the form of a solution and may cause local irritation.

aluminum hydroxide a safe slow-acting antacid. It is administered by mouth, alone or in combination with other antacids, in the treatment of indigestion, gastric and duodenal ulcers, and reflux *esophagitis. Trade names: **Gaviscon, Maalox, Mylanta, Rolaids, Tums**.

alveolitis n. inflammation of an *alveolus or alveoli. Chronic inflammation of the walls of the lung alveoli is usually caused by inhaled inorganic dusts (see pneumoconiosis) or organic dusts (see birdbreeder's lung, farmer's lung). It is sometimes associated with rheumatoid arthritis or systemic sclerosis. The condition progresses slowly to the state of fibrosis, emphysema, and bronchiectasis known as *honeycomb lung*. Alveolitis can be controlled with corticosteroid therapy.

alveolus n. (pl. **alveoli**) **1.** (in the *lung) a blind-ended air sac of microscopic size. About 30 alveoli open out of each *alveolar duct*, which leads from a respiratory *bronchiole. The *alveolar walls*, which separate alveoli, contain capillaries. The alveoli are lined by a single layer of *pneumocytes, which thus form a very thin layer between air and blood so that exchange of oxygen and carbon dioxide is normally rapid and complete. Children are born with about 20 million alveoli. The adult number of about 300 million is reached around the age of eight years. **2.** the part of the upper or lower jawbone that supports the roots of the teeth (*see also* mandible, maxilla). After tooth extraction it is largely absorbed. **3.** the sac of a *racemose gland (*see also* acinus). **4.** any other small cavity, depression, or sac. —**alveolar** *adj*.

alveus *n*. a cavity, groove, or canal. The *alveus hippocampi* is the bundle of nerve fibers in the brain forming a depression in which the hippocampus lies.

Alzheimer's disease a progressive form of *dementia that occurs in middle age or later, characterized by loss of short-term memory, deterioration in behavior and intellectual performance, confusion, and slowness of thought. The condition may be mimicked by severe depression. The demonstration of damage to the cholinergic pathways in the brain has led to great interest in drug treatments (e.g. *anticholinesterases and vasodilators) but to date few of these have proved successful: the *acetylcholinesterase inhibitors, e.g. donepezil, have some benefit in helping to slow down the disease process for 6 to 12 months. Alzheimer's disease is associated with diffuse degeneration of the brain: pathological studies have revealed excess β–*amyloid protein plaques in the brains of Alzheimer's patients. A genetic locus on chromosome 21 has been found for some inherited forms of Alzheimer's disease. *Compare* Pick's disease. [A. Alzheimer (1864–1915), German physician]

AMA *see* American Medical Association.

amalgam *n*. any of a group of alloys containing mercury. In dentistry amalgam fillings are made by mixing a silver-tin alloy with mercury.

Amanita *n*. a genus of fungi that contains several species of poisonous toadstools, including *A. phalloides* (death cap), *A. pantherina* (panther cap), and *A. muscaria* (fly agaric). They produce toxins that cause abdominal pain, violent vomiting, and continuous diarrhea. In the absence of treatment death occurs in approximately 50% of cases, due to severe liver damage.

amantadine *n*. an antiviral drug that probably acts by preventing the penetration of the virus into the host cell. It is used in the treatment of influenza infections and parkinsonism. Common side effects include nervousness, loss of muscular coordination, and insomnia. Trade name: **Symmetrel**.

amaurosis *n*. partial or complete blindness. For example, *amaurosis fugax* is a condition in which loss of vision is transient. *See also* Leber's congenital amaurosis. —**amaurotic** *adj*.

amaurotic familial idiocy *see* Tay-Sachs disease.

ambivalence *n*. (in psychology) the condition of holding opposite feelings (such as love and hate) for the same person or object. Excessive and prevalent ambivalence was thought by Bleuler to be a feature of schizophrenia.

Amblyomma *n*. a genus of hard *ticks, several species of which are responsible for transmitting tick *typhus. The bite of this tick can also give rise to a serious and sometimes fatal paralysis.

amblyopia *n*. poor sight not due to any detectable disease of the eyeball or visual system, known colloquially as *lazy eye*. In practice this strict definition is not always obeyed. For example, in *toxic amblyopia*, caused by tobacco, alcohol, certain other drugs, and vitamin deficiency, there is a disorder of the *optic nerve. The most common type is *amblyopia ex anopsia*, in which factors such as squint (*see* strabismus), cataract, and other abnormalities of the optics of the eye (*see* refraction) impair its normal use in early childhood by preventing the formation of a clear image on the retina.

amblyoscope (orthoptoscope, synoptophore) *n*. an instrument for measuring the angle of a squint and assessing the degree to which a person uses both eyes together. It consists of two L-shaped tubes, the short arms of which are joined by a hinge so that the long arms point away from each other. The subject looks into the short end and each eye sees, via a system of mirrors and lenses, a different picture, which is placed at the other end of each tube. If a squint is present, the tubes may be adjusted so that the short arms line up with the direction of each eye.

AMD age-related *macular degeneration.

ameba n. (pl. **amebas**) any single-celled microscopic animal of jellylike consistency and irregular and constantly changing shape. Found in water, soil and other damp environments, they move and feed by means of flowing extensions of the body (see pseudopodium). Some amebas (see Acanthamoeba, Entamoeba) cause disease in humans. See also protozoa. —**amebic** adj.

amebiasis n. see dysentery.

amebocyte n. a cell that moves by sending out processes of its protoplasm in the same way as an ameba.

ameboma n. a tumor that occurs in the rectum or cecum of the large intestine and is caused by the parasite *Entamoeba histolytica*, a protozoan that invades and destroys the walls of the gut. Tumors may ulcerate and become infected with pus-forming (pyogenic) bacteria, causing severe inflammation of the bowel wall. The tumors usually harden and may even obstruct the bowel.

amelia n. congenital total absence of the arms or legs due to a developmental defect. It is one of the fetal abnormalities induced by the drug *thalidomide taken early in pregnancy. See also phocomelia.

ameloblast n. a cell that forms the enamel of a tooth and disappears before tooth eruption.

ameloblastoma n. a locally malignant tumor in the jaw. It is considered to develop from ameloblasts although it does not contain enamel.

amelogenesis n. the formation of enamel by *ameloblasts, a process that is completed before tooth eruption. *Amelogenesis imperfecta* is a hereditary condition in which enamel formation is disturbed. The teeth have an unusual surface but may not be more prone to decay.

amenorrhea n. the absence or stopping of the menstrual periods. It is normal for the periods to be absent before puberty, during pregnancy and milk secretion, and after the end of the reproductive period (see menopause). In *primary amenorrhea* the menstrual periods fail to appear at puberty, often due to a con-

genital defect, a genetic disorder (e.g. *Turner's syndrome), or hormonal imbalance. In *secondary amenorrhea* the menstrual periods stop after establishment at puberty, for a great variety of reasons, including disorders of the hypothalamus (a part of the brain), diabetes, deficiency of ovarian, pituitary, or thyroid hormones, mental disturbance, depression, anorexia nervosa, change of surroundings, excessive exercise, and removal of the uterus or ovaries.

amentia n. failure of development of the intellectual faculties. See mental retardation.

American Association of Blood Banks (AABB) an international association of blood banks, including hospital and community blood centers and laboratories, transfusion and transplantation services, and individuals involved in activities related to transfusion and transplantation medicine. The AABB was established in 1947 and is dedicated to encouraging the voluntary donation of blood and other tissues and organs through education, public information, and research. AABB member facilities are responsible for collecting virtually all of the blood supply in the US and transfusing more than 80%. More than 2200 institutions, located in all 50 states and 80 foreign countries, and 8500 individuals, including physicians, scientists, administrators, medical technologists, blood donor recruiters, and public relations personnel, are members of the organization.

American Medical Association (AMA) a professional organization for physicians. Membership is made up of approximately half of the licensed physicians in the US. The Association is governed by elected officers, a Board of Trustees, and a House of Delegates who represent state and local medical associations as well as government agencies. Purposes of the organization include dissemination of scientific information, which is done through 11 medical journals, a weekly newspaper, and its Web site; representation of the profession with Congress and state legislatures regarding proposed health care laws, as well as informing members of any pending health and medical legislation; evaluation of prescription and nonprescription drugs; investigation of cases of alleged quackery; and cooperation with other organizations in setting standards for hospitals, medical schools, residency programs, and continuing medical education courses. The AMA also maintains a directory of all physicians in the US, including nonmembers.

American Red Cross a voluntary organization founded by Clara Barton in 1881. It has operated under congressional charter since 1900, and thus it is able to fulfill US obligations under certain international treaties. It serves members of the armed forces, veterans, and their families, aids disaster victims, and cooperates with the International Red Cross whenever need arises anywhere in the world. It is the largest supplier of blood, plasma, and tissue products in the US, supplying half of the blood used in medicine by working with the donors, hospitals, and blood banks through a national network of 36 blood regions. It maintains a large educational program, training volunteers for service in the 3100 chapters, for work in hospitals and community agencies, and for community services. It offers courses to the public on such subjects as parenthood, pre- and postnatal care, venereal disease, including AIDS, and cardiopulmonary resuscitation. It is administered by a 50-member Board of Directors and all funds are obtained from donations.

Americans with Disabilities Act (1990) (ADA) a US law giving civil rights protection to individuals with disabilities, similar to that provided for individuals on the basis of race, sex, national origin, and religion. It guarantees equal opportunity for individuals with disabilities in employment, public accommodations, transportation, state and local government services, and telecommunications. The Act defines disability as any physical or mental impairment that substantially limits one or more of the person's life activities, such as walking, seeing, hearing, speaking, learning, or working. Employers cannot ask if someone has a disability or subject a person to tests that tend to screen out people with disabilities, but they may ask about an individual's ability to perform job-related functions. Employers may require a medical examination, but only following a job offer. Employers must make facilities accessible to individuals with disabilities, restructure jobs, or modify schedules and equipment as required.

American Type Culture Collection (ATCC) a US nonprofit, nongovernmental organization that functions as a repository for reference cultures of microorganisms and cell lines of animal tissues and as a distribution center of these cultures to academic, medical, and scientific research laboratories.

amethocaine n. see tetracaine.

ametropia n. any abnormality of *refraction of the eye, resulting in blurring of the image formed on the retina. See astigmatism, hyperopia, myopia. Compare emmetropia.

amiloride n. a potassium-conserving *diuretic that causes the increased excretion of sodium and chloride; it is often combined with a thiazide or loop diuretic (e.g. hydrochlorothiazide in Moduretic) to reduce the potassium loss that occurs with these drugs. It may produce dizziness and weakness and its continued use may lead to an excessive concentration of potassium in the blood. Trade name: **Midamor**.

amino acid an organic compound containing an amino group ($-NH_2$) and a carboxyl group ($-COOH$). Amino acids are fundamental constituents of all *proteins. Breakdown of proteins found in the body yields the following amino acids: alanine, arginine, asparagine, aspartic acid, cysteine, cystine, glutamic acid, glutamine, glycine, histidine, isoleucine, leucine, lysine, methionine, phenylalanine, proline, serine, threonine, tryptophan, tyrosine, and valine. Some of these amino acids can be synthesized by the body; others, the *essential amino acids, must be obtained from protein in the diet. Certain amino acids that are present in the body are not found in proteins; these include *citrulline, *ornithine, and the neurotransmitters *taurine and *gamma-aminobutyric acid.

aminoacidopathy n. see maple syrup urine disease.

aminobenzoic acid see para-aminobenzoic acid.

aminoglutethimide n. an *aromatase inhibitor used in the treatment of advanced breast and prostate cancer and Cushing's disease due to a malignant tumor. Because it inhibits synthesis of adrenal steroids (medical adrenalectomy), aminoglutethimide is usually given with corticosteroid replacement therapy. Side effects, which are largely dose-related, include drowsiness, dizziness, and a transient skin rash. Trade name: **Cytadren**.

aminoglycosides *pl. n.* a group of antibiotics used against serious infections caused by gram-negative bacteria. Included in the group are *gentamicin, *kanamycin, *neomycin, and *streptomycin. Because of their toxicity (side effects include ear and kidney damage), they are used only when less toxic antibacterials are ineffective or contraindicated. They are usually administered by injection or infusion.

aminopeptidase *n.* any one of several enzymes in the intestine that cause the breakdown of a *peptide, removing an amino acid.

aminophylline *n.* a drug that relaxes smooth muscle and stimulates respiration. It is widely used to dilate the air passages in the treatment of chronic asthma, emphysema, and bronchitis. Administered by injection, orally, or rectally, it may cause nausea, vomiting, dizziness, and fast heart rate. *See also* theophylline. Trade names: **Phyllocontin, Truphylline**.

aminotransferase *n. see* transaminase.

amiodarone *n.* an *antiarrhythmic drug used to control a variety of abnormal heart rhythms, including atrial *fibrillation and abnormally rapid heartbeat, that are life-threatening. It is administered by mouth or by injection. Side effects can include harmless deposits in the cornea, photosensitivity, and peripheral neuropathy. Trade name: **Cordarone**.

amithiozone *n.* a drug used in the treatment of leprosy and (in combination with *isoniazid) tuberculosis. The drug is administered by mouth. Toxic effects, although infrequent, are severe and include anorexia, hepatitis, and exfoliative dermatitis.

amitosis *n.* division of the nucleus of a cell by a process, not involving *mitosis, in which the nucleus is constricted into two.

amitriptyline *n.* a tricyclic *antidepressant

drug that has a mild tranquilizing action. Common side effects include drowsiness, dizziness, numbness, and tingling of limbs. Trade names: **Elavil, Endep**.

amlodipine *n.* a *calcium antagonist used to treat hypertension and angina pectoris. It is administered by mouth. Possible side effects include headache, dizziness, fatigue, nausea, and fluid retention. Trade name: **Norvasc**.

amnesia *n.* total or partial loss of memory following physical injury, disease, drugs, or psychological trauma (*see* confabulation, fugue, repression). *Anterograde amnesia* is loss of memory for events following some trauma; *retrograde amnesia* is loss of memory for events preceding the trauma. Some patients experience both types.

amnihook *n.* a small plastic hooked instrument for performing *amniotomy. The hook is introduced through the cervix.

amniocentesis *n.* withdrawal of a sample of the fluid (amniotic fluid) surrounding an embryo in the uterus by piercing the amniotic sac through the abdominal wall. Since the amniotic fluid contains cells from the embryo (mostly shed from the skin), cell cultures enable chromosome patterns to be studied so that *prenatal diagnosis of chromosomal abnormalities (such as *Down's syndrome) can be made. Metabolic errors and other diseases, such as *spina bifida, can also be diagnosed prenatally from the biochemistry of the cells or that of the fluid (*see* alpha-fetoprotein). Although the risks of amniocentesis, in skilled hands, are extremely low, there is no point in undertaking it unless the parents agree to a termination of the pregnancy if a serious abnormality is discovered.

amnion *n.* the membrane that forms initially over the dorsal part of the embryo but soon expands to enclose it completely within the *amniotic cavity; it is connected to the embryo at the umbilical cord. It expands outward and fuses with the chorion, obliterating virtually all the intervening cavity. The double membrane (*amniochorion*) normally ruptures at birth. —**amniotic** *adj.*

amnioscopy *n.* examination of the inside of the amniotic sac by means of an instrument (*amnioscope*) that is passed through the abdominal wall. This allows the developing fetus within the cavity to be viewed directly. *Cervical amnioscopy*, performed late in pregnancy, enables the amniotic sac to be inspected through the cervix of the uterus, using a different instrument (a fetoscope). When transilluminated, its fluid volume can be appraised without puncture and any meconium can be observed.

amniotic cavity the fluid-filled cavity between the embryo and the *amnion. It forms initially within the inner cell mass of the *blastocyst and later expands over the back of the embryo, eventually enclosing it completely. *See also* amniotic fluid.

amniotic fluid the fluid contained within the *amniotic cavity. It surrounds the growing fetus, protecting it from external pressure. The fluid is initially secreted from the *amnion and is later supplemented by urine from the fetal kidneys. Some of the fluid is swallowed by the fetus and absorbed through its intestine. *See also* amniocentesis.

amniotomy (artificial rupture of membranes, ARM) *n.* a method of surgically inducing labor by puncturing the *amnion surrounding the baby in the uterus using an *amnihook or similar instrument (*see* induction).

amobarbital (amylobarbitone) *n.* an intermediate-acting *barbiturate administered orally as a *hypnotic in the treatment of severe insomnia in patients already taking barbiturates. Prolonged use may lead to *dependence, and overdosage has serious toxic effects (*see* barbiturism). Trade name: **Amytal**.

amodiaquine hydrochloride an antimalarial drug with effects and uses similar to those of *chloroquine. It has also been used for the treatment of lupus erythematosus, leprosy, and rheumatoid arthritis. Doses used to treat malaria have almost no side effects, but prolonged use may cause blue-gray deposits on the cornea of the eye, fingernails, and hard palate. Trade name: **Camoquin**.

amok (amuck) *n.* a sudden outburst of furious and murderous aggression, directed indiscriminately at everybody in the vicinity. It is encountered particularly in certain cultures.

amorolfine *n.* an antifungal drug used to treat ringworm, candidiasis, and other fungal infections of the skin and nails. It is applied externally as a cream or nail lacquer; possible side effects include itching and a transient burning sensation. Trade name: **Loceryl**.

amorphous *adj.* **1.** lacking a definite shape or form. **2.** (in chemistry) describing a substance that is not crystallized.

amoxapine *n.* a tricyclic antidepressant drug similar to *imipramine. It is administered by mouth. Overdosage may cause acute kidney failure, convulsions, and coma. Trade name: **Asendin**.

amoxicillin *n.* an antibiotic used to treat infections caused by a wide range of bacteria and other microorganisms. It is administered by mouth. Side effects include nausea, vomiting, diarrhea, rashes, and anemia. Sensitivity to penicillin prohibits its use. Trade names: **Amoxil**, **Biomox**, **Polymox**, **Trimox**, **Wymox**.

AMP (adenosine monophosphate) a compound containing adenine, ribose, and one phosphate group. AMP occurs in cells and is involved in processes requiring the transfer of energy (*see also* ADP, ATP).

ampakines *pl. n.* agents believed by some researchers to be capable of improving memory in elderly people. They are thought to act by making the receptors on nerve cells for the neurotransmitter glutamate more responsive. The effect has not been fully proved.

ampere *n.* the basic *SI unit of electric current. It is equal to the current flowing through a conductor of resistance 1 ohm when a potential difference of 1 volt is applied between its ends. The formal definition of the ampere is the current that when passed through two parallel conductors of infinite length and negligible cross-section, placed 1 meter apart in a vacuum, produces a force of 2×10^{-7} newton per meter between them. Symbol: A.

amphetamines *pl. n.* a group of *sympathomimetic drugs that have a marked stimulant action on the central nervous system, alleviating fatigue and producing a feeling of mental alertness and well-being. The drugs are used in the treatment of *narcolepsy and especially *attention-deficit/hyperactivity disorder in children. They are administered by mouth; side effects include insomnia and restlessness. *Tolerance to amphetamines develops rapidly, and prolonged use may lead to *dependence. Amphetamines have many street names, including *black beauties*, *pep pills*, and *speed*. *See also* dextroamphetamine, methamphetamine.

amphiarthrosis *n.* a slightly movable joint in which the bony surfaces are separated by fibrocartilage (*see* symphysis) or hyaline cartilage (*see* synchondrosis).

amphoric breath sounds *see* breath sounds.

amphotericin B an *antifungal drug, derived from the bacterium *Streptomyces nodosus*, used to treat deep-seated fungal infections. It can be administered by mouth, but is usually given by intravenous infusion. Common side effects include headache, fever, muscle pains, and diarrhea. In some cases kidney damage may occur. Trade names: **Amphocin**, **Fungizone**.

ampicillin *n.* an *antibiotic used to treat a variety of infections, including those of the urinary, respiratory, biliary, and intestinal tracts. It is inactivated by *penicillinase and therefore cannot be used against organisms producing this enzyme. It is given by mouth or injection; side effects include nausea, vomiting, and diarrhea, and some allergic reactions may occur. Trade names: **Omnipen**, **Polycillin**, **Principen**, **Totacillin**.

ampule (ampoule) *n.* a sealed glass or plastic capsule containing one dose of a drug in the form of a sterile solution for injection.

ampulla *n.* (*pl.* **ampullae**) an enlarged or dilated ending of a tube or canal. The semicircular canals of the inner ear are expanded into ampullae at the point where they join the vestibule. The *ampulla of Vater* is the dilated part of the common bile duct where it is joined by the pancreatic duct.

amputation *n.* the removal of a limb, part of a limb, or any other portion of the body (such as a breast or the rectum). The term is customarily modified by an adjective showing the particular type of amputation. Once a common operation in surgery, it is now usually performed only in cases of severe injury to limbs or, particularly in elderly people, when circulation to a limb is inadequate and gangrene develops. In planning an am-

putation the surgeon takes account of the patient's work and the type of artificial part (prosthesis) that will be fitted.

amsacrine *n.* a *cytotoxic drug administered by injection to treat acute myeloid leukemia. Side effects include nausea, vomiting, hair loss, and bone marrow suppression. Trade names: **AMSA P-D**, **Amsidyl**.

Amsler's chart (Amsler's grid) a chart usually consisting of a grid of black lines on a white background. It is used to detect and monitor problems of central vision, for example in macular disease. [M. Amsler (1891–1968), Swiss ophthalmologist]

amygdala (amygdaloid nucleus) *n.* one of the *basal ganglia: a roughly almond-shaped mass of gray matter deep inside each cerebral hemisphere. It has extensive connections with the olfactory system and sends fibers to the hypothalamus; its functions are apparently concerned with mood, feeling, instinct, and possibly memory for recent events.

amylase *n.* an enzyme that occurs in saliva and pancreatic juice and aids the digestion of starch, which it breaks down into glucose, maltose, and dextrins. Amylase will also hydrolyze *glycogen to yield glucose, maltose, and dextrins.

amyl nitrite a drug that relaxes smooth muscle, especially that of blood vessels. Given by inhalation, amyl nitrite has been used in the treatment of angina pectoris, although it has largely been replaced by other agents. It is also used in the treatment of cyanide poisoning and is often abused as a sexual stimulant and to produce euphoria. Side effects include flushing, faintness, and headache. High doses may cause restlessness, vomiting, and blue coloration of the skin.

amylobarbitone *see* amobarbital.

amyloid *n.* a *glycoprotein, resembling starch, that is deposited in the internal organs in amyloidosis. β-amyloid protein has been found in the brains of Alzheimer's patients but the significance of this is unclear.

amyloidosis *n.* infiltration of the liver, kidneys, spleen, and other tissues with amyloid, a starchlike substance. In *primary amyloidosis* the disorder arises without any apparent cause; *secondary amyloidosis* occurs as a late complication of such chronic infections as tuberculosis or leprosy and may also occur in *Hodgkin's disease. Amyloidosis is also very common in the genetic disease familial Mediterranean fever (*see* polyserositis).

amylopectin *n. see* starch.

amylose *n. see* starch.

amyotonia *n.* a lack of tone, weakness, and wasting of skeletal muscle, usually the result of motor neuron disease. *Amyotonia congenita (floppy baby syndrome)* is a former diagnosis for various conditions, present at birth, in which the baby's muscles are weak and floppy. The term is becoming obsolete as more specific diagnoses are discovered to explain the cause of floppiness in babies.

amyotrophic lateral sclerosis (ALS) Lou Gehrig's disease. *See* motor neuron disease.

amyotrophy *n.* a progressive loss of muscle bulk associated with weakness of these muscles. It is caused by disease of the nerve that activates the affected muscle. Amyotrophy is a feature of any chronic *neuropathy and it may be found in some diabetic patients (*see* diabetic amyotrophy). A combination of amyotrophy and spasticity may be found in various forms of *motor neuron disease.

an- *prefix. see* a-.

anabolic *adj.* promoting tissue growth by increasing the metabolic processes involved in protein synthesis. Anabolic steroids are synthetic forms of male sex hormones (*see* androgen); they include *nandrolone and *stanozolol. They were formerly used to help weight gain in underweight patients, such as the elderly and those with serious illnesses, but are now used mainly to stimulate production of blood cells by the bone marrow in some forms of aplastic *anemia. Some anabolic steroids cause virilization in women and liver damage.

anabolism *n.* the synthesis of complex molecules, such as proteins and fats, from simpler ones by living things. *See also* anabolic, metabolism.

anacidity *n.* a deficiency or abnormal absence of acid in the body fluids. *See also* achlorhydria.

anacrotism *n.* the condition in which there is an abnormal curve in the ascending line of a pulse tracing. It may be seen in cases of aortic stenosis. —**anacrotic** *adj.*

anadipsia *n.* extreme thirst, resulting from dehydration caused by excessive perspiration, continuous urination, or extreme physical activity.

anaerobe *n.* any organism, especially a microbe, that is able to live and grow in the absence of free oxygen. A *facultative anaerobe* is a microorganism that grows best in the presence of oxygen but is capable of some growth in its absence. An *obligate anaerobe* can grow only in the absence of free oxygen. *Compare* aerobe, microaerophilic.

anaerobic *adj.* **1.** of or relating to anaerobes. **2.** describing a type of cellular respiration in which foodstuffs (usually carbohydrates) are never completely oxidized because molecular oxygen is not used. *Fermentation is an example of anaerobic respiration.

anagen *n.* the growth phase of a hair follicle, lasting two to three years. It is followed by a transitional stage, called *catagen*, and then a resting phase, *telogen*, each of which lasts for about two weeks. On average about 80% of hairs are in anagen and hence growing actively. There are about 100,000 hairs on the human scalp and up to 100 may be shed each day.

anákhré *n. see* goundou.

anal *adj.* of, relating to, or affecting the anus; for example an anal *fissure or an anal *fistula.

anal canal the terminal portion of the large intestine, which is surrounded by the muscles of defecation (*anal sphincters*). The canal ends on the surface at the anal orifice (*see* anus).

analeptic (respiratory stimulant) *n.* a drug that restores consciousness to a patient in a coma; for example, *doxapram. Analeptics act on the central nervous system to stimulate the muscles involved in breathing; they are sometimes used in treating patients with chronic obstructive pulmonary disease.

anal fissure a break in the skin lining the anal canal, usually causing pain during bowel movements and sometimes bleeding. Anal fissures occur as a consequence of constipation or sometimes of diarrhea. Treatment is by soothing ointments, but if the condition is severe the operation of *lateral sphincterotomy* (cutting the muscle of the anal sphincter) is required.

analgesia *n.* reduced sensibility to pain, without loss of consciousness and without the sense of touch necessarily being affected. The condition may arise accidentally, if nerves are diseased or damaged, or be induced deliberately by the use of pain-killing drugs (*see* analgesic). Strictly speaking, local *anesthesia should be called *local analgesia*.

analgesic 1. *n.* a drug that relieves pain. Mild analgesics, such as *aspirin and *acetaminophen, are used for the relief of headache, toothache, and mild rheumatic pain. More potent *narcotic* (or *opioid*) *analgesics*, such as *morphine and *meperidine, are used only to relieve severe pain, since these drugs may produce *dependence and *tolerance (*see also* narcotic, opiate). Some analgesics, including aspirin, *ibuprofen, and *indomethacin, also reduce fever and inflammation and are used in rheumatic conditions (*see also* NSAID). **2.** *adj.* relieving pain.

analogous *adj.* describing organs or parts that have similar functions in different organisms although they do not have the same evolutionary origin or development. *Compare* homologous.

analogue *n.* a drug that differs in minor ways in molecular structure from its parent compound. Examples are *calcipotriene (an analogue of vitamin D), *betahistine (an analogue of histamine), and the *LHRH analogues. Useful analogues of existing drugs are either more potent or cause fewer side effects. *Carboplatin, for example, is a less toxic analogue of *cisplatin.

analogue image a traditional X-ray image on film that is in shades that range smoothly from black to white with no appreciable steps from one shade of gray to the next (*see* gray scale). Analogue images can be converted to digital format (*see* digitization) for manipulation and storage by computers and other electronic devices.

analogue insulins a group of relatively new insulin medications with a very fast onset of action. All members of this group are manufactured forms of human insulin, having had slight alterations made to the original amino-acid sequence in order to allow faster absorption from the injection site. The main advantage of these insulins is that they can be injected immediately before eating.

analysand *n.* a person undergoing *psychoanalysis.

analysis *n.* (in psychology) any means of understanding complex mental processes or experiences. There are several systems of analysis used by different schools of psychology; for example, *psychoanalysis; *transactional analysis*, in which people's relationships are explained in psychoanalytic terms; and *functional analysis*, in which a particular kind of behavior is thoroughly described with reference to its frequency, its antecedents, and its consequences.

anamnesis *n.* memory, particularly the recollection by a patient of the symptoms that he noticed at the time when his disease was first contracted.

anancastic *adj.* describing a collection of longstanding personality traits, including stubbornness, meanness, an overmeticulous concern to be accurate in small details, a disposition to check things unnecessarily, severe feelings of insecurity about personal worth, and an excessive tendency to doubt evident facts. *See* personality disorder, obsession.

anaphase *n.* the third stage of *mitosis and of each division of *meiosis. In mitosis and anaphase II of meiosis the chromatids separate, becoming daughter chromosomes, and move apart along the spindle fibers toward opposite ends of the cell. In anaphase I of meiosis the pairs of homologous chromosomes separate from each other. *See* disjunction.

anaphylaxis *n.* an emergency condition resulting from an abnormal and immediate allergic response to a substance to which the body has become intensely sensitized. It results in flushing, itching, nausea and vomiting, swelling of the mouth and tongue and airway that is often enough to cause obstruction, wheezing, a sudden drop in blood pressure, and even sudden death. In this extreme form it is called *anaphylactic shock*. Common causes are peanuts, latex, and wasp or bee stings. Treatment, which must be given immediately, consists of epinephrine injection, oxygen together with possible advanced support of the airway, intravenous fluids, intravenous corticosteroids, and antihistamines. —**anaphylactic** *adj.*

anaplasia *n.* a loss of normal cell characteristics or differentiation, which may be to such a degree that it is impossible to define the origin of the cells. Anaplasia is typical of rapidly growing malignant tumors, which are described as *anaplastic*.

anasarca *n.* massive swelling of the legs, trunk, and genitalia due to retention of fluid (*edema): found in congestive heart failure and some forms of renal failure.

anastomosis *n.* **1.** (in anatomy) a communication between two blood vessels without any intervening capillary network. *See* arteriovenous anastomosis. **2.** (in surgery) an artificial connection between two tubular organs or parts, especially between two normally separate parts of the intestine or two blood vessels. *See also* shunt.

anastrazole *n. see* aromatase inhibitor.

anatomy *n.* the study of the structure of living organisms. In medicine it refers to the study of the form and gross internal and external structure of the various parts of the human body. The term *morphology* is sometimes used synonymously with anatomy but it is usually used for *comparative anatomy*: the study of differences in form between species. *See also* cytology, histology, physiology. —**anatomical** *adj.* —**anatomist** *n.*

anatoxin *n.* a former name for *toxoid.

anconeus *n.* a muscle behind the elbow that assists in extending the forearm.

Ancylostoma (Ankylostoma) *n.* a genus of small parasitic nematodes (*see* hookworm) that inhabit the small intestine and are widely distributed in Europe, America, Asia, and Africa. The worms suck blood from the gut wall, to which they are attached by means of cutting teeth. Humans are the principal and optimum host for *A. duodenale*.

ancylostomiasis *n.* an infestation of the small intestine by the parasitic hookworm *Ancylostoma duodenale*. *See* hookworm disease.

ANDI an acronym for *a*bnormal *d*evelopment and *i*nvolution, used to tabulate benign disorders of the breast.

andr- (andro-) *prefix denoting* men or the male sex. Example: *androphobia* (morbid fear of).

androblastoma (arrhenoblastoma) *n.* a rare tumor of the testis or ovary, composed of Sertoli cells, Leydig cells, or both. It can produce male or female hormones and may give rise to *feminization or *masculinization; in children it may cause precocious puberty. Up to 30% of these tumors are malignant, but probably as many as 85% of all cases are cured by surgery alone.

androgen *n.* one of a group of steroid hormones, including *testosterone*, *androsterone*, and *dihydrotestosterone*, that stimulate the development of male sex organs and male secondary sexual characteristics (e.g. beard growth, deepening of the voice, and muscle development). The principal source of these hormones is the testis (production being stimulated by *luteinizing hormone) but they are also secreted by the adrenal cortex and ovaries in small amounts. In women excessive production of androgens gives rise to *masculinization. *See also* dehydroepiandrosterone.

Naturally occurring and synthetic androgens are used in replacement therapy (to treat such conditions as delayed puberty in adolescent boys, *hypogonadism, and impotence due to testicular insufficiency); as *anabolic agents; and in the treatment of breast cancer. Side effects include salt and water retention, increased bone growth, and masculinization in women. Androgens should not be used in patients with cancer of the prostate gland or in pregnant women. —**androgenic** *adj.*

androgen insensitivity syndrome a form of *pseudohermaphroditism in which an individual who is genetically male (XY) has female external genitalia and secondary sexual characteristics but lacks female reproductive organs; testes are present internally. The syndrome is an X-linked (*see* sex-linked) recessive condition, in which the body does not react to androgens because androgen receptors do not function.

androgenization *n.* the final effects of the exposure of sensitive tissues to androgens, i.e. the development of secondary male sexual characteristics. Androgenization can also occur abnormally in females, who may develop excessive body hair, male-pattern baldness, and *clitoromegaly.

andrology *n.* **1.** the study of male infertility and impotence. *Semen analysis reveals the presence of gross abnormalities in the shape and motility of spermatozoa, as well as their concentration in the semen, but further procedures are required to diagnose the underlying causes of the sperm dysfunction. These include the diagnosis of abnormalities in the genital tract (e.g. varicocele, obstruction of the vas deferens), which may be corrected surgically, and testing for the presence of antisperm antibodies in the semen and for the ability of the sperm to penetrate the cervical mucus, as well as for the presence of hormonal disorders. More sophisticated techniques include computer-assisted quantitative motility measurements, which monitor the precise speed and the motility patterns of individual sperm; biochemical tests for the production of free oxygen radicals, which cause damage to developing sperm; and *acrosome-reaction assays, which reveal the ability of the sperm to penetrate the barriers surrounding the ovum. The development of all these techniques has enabled the identification of several previously undiagnosed causes of infertility and the selection of treatments most likely to succeed in remedying them. **2.** the study of androgen production and the relationship of plasma androgen to androgen action. This study is necessary to understand *hirsutism and other conditions caused by abnormal androgen production.

androstenedione *n. see* adrenarche, dehydroepiandrosterone.

androsterone *n.* a steroid hormone (*see* androgen) that is synthesized and released by the testes and is responsible for controlling male sexual development.

anemia *n.* a reduction in the quantity of the oxygen-carrying pigment *hemoglobin in the blood. The main symptoms are excessive tiredness and fatigability, breathlessness on exertion, pallor, and poor resistance to infection.

There are many causes of anemia. It may be due to loss of blood (*hemorrhagic anemia*), resulting from an accident, operation, etc., or from chronic bleeding, as from an ulcer or hemorrhoids. *Iron-deficiency anemia* results from lack of iron, which is necessary for the production of hemoglobin (*see* sideropenia). *Hemolytic anemias* result from the in-

creased destruction of red blood cells (which contain the pigment). This can be caused by toxic chemicals; *autoimmunity; the action of parasites, especially in *malaria; or conditions such as *thalassemia and *sickle-cell disease, associated with abnormal forms of hemoglobin, or *spherocytosis, which is associated with abnormal red blood cells. (*See also* hemolytic disease of the newborn.) Anemia can also be caused by the impaired production of red blood cells, as in *leukemia (when red-cell production in the bone marrow is suppressed) or *pernicious anemia. *Aplastic anemia* is characterized by a failure of blood cell production resulting in *pancytopenia and reduced bone marrow cellularity.

Anemias can be classified on the basis of the size of the red cells, which may be abnormally large (*macrocytic anemias*), abnormally small (*microcytic anemias*), or normal sized (*normocytic anemias*). (*See also* macrocytosis, microcytosis.) The treatment of anemia depends on the cause. —**anemic** *adj.*

anencephaly *n.* partial or complete absence of the bones of the rear of the skull, the meninges, and the cerebral hemispheres of the brain. It occurs as a developmental defect and most affected infants are stillborn; if born live they do not survive for more than a few hours. Anencephaly is often associated with other defects of the nervous system, such as *spina bifida. Prenatal screening tests for anencephaly include detection of *alpha-fetoprotein levels and ultrasound scanning.

anergy *n.* **1.** lack of response to a specific antigen or allergen. **2.** lack of energy. —**anergic** *adj.*

anesthesia *n.* loss of feeling or sensation in a part or all of the body. Anesthesia of a part of the body may occur as a result of injury to or disease of a nerve; for example in leprosy. The term is usually applied, however, to the medical technique of reducing or abolishing an individual's sensation of pain to enable surgery to be performed. This is effected by administering drugs (*see* anesthetic) or by the use of other methods, such as *acupuncture or hypnosis.

General anesthesia is total unconsciousness, usually achieved by administering a combination of injections and gases (the latter are inhaled through a mask). *Local anesthesia* abolishes pain in a limited area of the body and is used for minor operations, particularly many dental procedures. It may be achieved by injections of substances such as lidocaine (commonly used in dentistry) close to a local nerve, which deadens the area supplied by that nerve. Local anesthesia may be combined with intravenous sedation. An appropriate injection into the spinal column produces *spinal anesthesia or *epidural anesthesia in the lower limbs or abdomen. *Regional anesthesia*, usually of a limb, is achieved by injecting or by direct application of a local anesthetic (*topical anesthesia*) to block a group of sensory nerves.

anesthesiologist *n.* a physician who administers an anesthetic to induce unconsciousness in a patient before a surgical operation. *Compare* anesthetist.

anesthetic 1. *n.* an agent that reduces or abolishes sensation, affecting either the whole body (*general anesthetic*) or a particular region (*local anesthetic*). General anesthetics, used for surgical procedures, depress activity of the central nervous system, producing loss of consciousness. *Anesthesia is induced by short-acting *barbiturates (such as thiopental) and maintained by inhalation anesthetics (such as *halothane). Local anesthetics inhibit conduction of impulses in sensory nerves in the region where they are injected or applied; they include *bupivacaine, *lidocaine, and tetracaine. **2.** *adj.* reducing or abolishing sensation.

anesthetist *n.* a medically qualified person who administers an anesthetic to induce unconsciousness in a patient before a surgical operation. *Compare* anesthesiologist.

aneuploidy *n.* the condition in which the chromosome number of a cell is not an exact multiple of the normal basic (haploid) number. *See* monosomy, trisomy; *compare* euploidy. —**aneuploid** *adj.*, *n.*

aneurin *n. see* vitamin B₁.

aneurysm *n.* a balloon-like swelling in the wall of an artery. This may be due to degenerative disease or infection, which damages the muscular coats of the vessel, or it may be the result of congenital deficiency in the muscular wall. An *aortic aneurysm* most frequently occurs in the abdominal aorta, below the level of the renal arteries. Beyond a certain size it is prone to rupture, presenting as an acute surgical emergency with abdominal and back pain and hemorrhagic shock. A *dissecting aneurysm* usually affects the first part of the aorta and results from a degenerative condition of its muscular coat. This weakness predisposes to a tear in the lining of the aorta, which allows blood to enter the wall and track along (dissect) the muscular coat. A dissecting aneurysm may rupture or it may compress the blood vessels arising from the aorta and produce infarction (localized necrosis) in the organs they supply. The patient complains of severe chest pain that has a tearing quality and often spreads to the back or abdomen. Surgical repair may help in some cases. A *ventricular aneurysm* may develop in the wall of the left ventricle after myocardial infarction. A segment of myocardium becomes replaced by scar tissue, which expands to form an aneurysmal sac. Heart failure may result or thrombosis within the aneurysm may act as a source of embolism. *See also* arteriovenous aneurysm.

Most aneurysms within the brain are congenital: there is a risk that they may burst, causing a *subarachnoid hemorrhage. *Berry aneurysms* are small saccular aneurysms most commonly occurring in the branches of the *circle of Willis. Usually associated with congenital weakness of the vessels, these aneurysms are a cause of fatal intracranial hemorrhage in young adults. *Charcot-Bouchard aneurysms* are small aneurysms found on tiny arteries within the brain of elderly and hypertensive subjects. These aneurysms may rupture, causing cerebral hemorrhage. Options for treatment of cerebral aneurysms include surgical clipping of the aneurysm and placing metallic coils within the aneurysm to establish a clot within it (*endovascular coiling*). —**aneurysmal** *adj.*

Angelman's syndrome (happy puppet syndrome) a disorder of development characterized by severe learning difficulties, absence of speech, seizures, jerky movements, a characteristic facial expression, and a happy social disposition. It is caused by a genetic abnormality on chromosome 15. [H. Angelman (1915–96), British pediatrician]

angi- (angio-) *prefix denoting* blood or lymph vessels. Examples: *angiectasis* (abnormal dilation of); *angiopathy* (disease of); *angiotomy* (cutting of).

angiitis (vasculitis) *n.* a patchy inflammation of the walls of small blood vessels. It may result from a variety of conditions, including *polyarteritis nodosa, acute nephritis, and serum sickness. Symptoms include skin rashes, arthritis, purpura, and kidney failure. In some cases treatment with cortisone derivatives may be beneficial.

angina *n.* a sense of suffocation or suffocating pain. *See* angina pectoris, Ludwig's angina.

angina pectoris pain in the center of the chest, which is induced by exercise and relieved by rest and may spread to the jaws and arms. Angina pectoris occurs when the demand for blood by the heart exceeds the supply of the coronary arteries and it usually results from coronary artery *atheroma. It may be prevented or relieved by such drugs as *nitroglycerin and *propranolol. If drug treatment proves ineffective, *coronary angioplasty or a *coronary bypass graft may be required, the former being less invasive than the latter.

angiocardiography *n.* X-ray examination of the chambers of the heart after the introduction of a radiographic *contrast medium, which is injected directly into the atria, ventricles, or great vessels of the heart by means of a slim sterile flexible tube (*cardiac catheter*) manipulated from an accessible vein or artery, most commonly in the groin (*see* (cardiac) catheterization). A recording (*angiocardiogram*) is made by a rapid-sequence *digital subtraction technique. Angiocardiography is now usually performed in conjunction with *coronary angiography; similar information can be obtained noninvasively by the technique of *echocardiography.

angiodysplasia *n.* an abnormal collection of small blood vessels in the wall of the bowel, which may bleed. Angiodysplasia is diagnosed by *colonoscopy, enteroscopy (*see* enteroscope), or *angiography and may be treated by *diathermy coagulation or surgical removal.

angioedema (angioneurotic edema) an acute allergic condition producing transient or persistent swelling of areas of skin accompanied by itching, which may be severe. It is caused by *allergy to food substances, drugs, or other allergens or it may be precipitated by heat, cold, or emotional factors. *See also* urticaria.

angiogenesis *n.* the formation of new blood vessels. This process is essential for the development of a tumor and is promoted by *growth factors; it is becoming a target for new anticancer therapy (*see* angiogenesis inhibitor).

angiogenesis inhibitor an agent that interferes with the development of new blood vessels (angiogenesis). Angiogenesis inhibitors are being developed for use as anticancer drugs, since growing cancers have a greater need for blood supply than normal tissue and must develop new blood vessels before progressing beyond a very small size. The first angiogenesis inhibitor to be approved for clinical use was *bevacizumab* (Avastin), a monoclonal antibody that inhibits the action of vascular endothelial *growth factor and has been licensed for treating advanced colorectal cancer.

angiography *n.* imaging of blood vessels (*see also* coronary angiography, lymphangiography). *Fluoroscopic angiography* is performed by injection of contrast medium during X-ray fluoroscopy. Positive (*radiopaque) contrast medium containing iodine or, more recently, negative (*radiolucent) gas (carbon dioxide) may be used. *Digital subtraction increases the visibility of the vessels. *Magnetic resonance angiography* (MRA) can be performed either by injection of a magnetic resonance contrast agent (*see* contrast medium), which gives an increased signal from the blood, or by relying on the movement of blood to give a lack of signal in the plane being examined. These images can be reconstructed in two or three dimensions. *Computerized tomographic angiography* (CTA) uses a radiographic contrast agent, usually injected into a vein, to enhance the density of the blood. This can then be clearly seen on either two- or three-dimensional images, with surrounding tissues hidden by the computer. *Fluorescein angiography* is a common method of investigation in ophthalmology. *Fluorescein sodium is injected into a vein in the arm, from which it circulates throughout the body. Light of an appropriate wavelength is shone into the eye, causing the dye in the retinal blood vessels to fluoresce. This allows the circulation through the retinal blood vessels to be observed and photographed. *Indocyanine green (ICG) angiography*, using a newer dye, gives much better visualization of the choroidal circulation. It is particularly useful for visualization and treatment of choroidal neovascular membranes (*see* neovascularization).

angioid *adj.* resembling a blood vessel.

angioid streaks reddish to dark-brown irregular streaks radiating outward from the optic disk underneath the retinal vessels. They represent irregular linear cracks in *Bruch's membrane and can be the site for the development of new vessels from the choroid that leak. They are seen in such systemic conditions as pseudoxanthoma elasticum, Paget's disease, and sickle-cell disease.

angiokeratoma *n.* a localized collection of thin-walled blood vessels covered by a cap of warty material. It is most often seen as an isolated malformation in the genital skin of the elderly or on the hands and feet of children. Angiokeratomas are not malignant and their cause is unknown. They may be removed surgically. Multiple angiokeratomas affecting the viscera and skin are seen as a rare inherited and fatal disease (*Fabry's disease*).

angiology *n.* the branch of medicine concerned with the structure, function, and diseases of blood and lymph vessels.

angioma *n.* a benign tumor composed of blood vessels or lymph vessels. *Cherry angiomas* (or *De Morgan spots*) are small red spots on the trunk in middle-aged or elderly people. They are completely harmless and consist of a minor vascular malformation. An *arteriovenous angioma* (or *malformation*) is a knot of distended blood vessels overlying and compressing the surface of the brain. It may cause epilepsy or one of the vessels may burst, causing a *subarachnoid hemorrhage or a hemorrhage within the brain (intracerebral hemorrhage). This type of angioma may be suitable for surgical removal or stereotactic radiotherapy. It may be associated with a purple birthmark on the face: this is

called the *Sturge-Weber syndrome*. Arteriovenous malformations may occur in many other parts of the body, where they are often asymptomatic. *See also* hemangioma, lymphangioma.

angioneurotic edema *see* angioedema.

angioplasty *n.* repair or reconstruction of a narrowed or completely obstructed blood vessel. Traditionally, this was performed during open surgery, but in modern practice angioplasty commonly refers to *percutaneous transluminal angioplasty* (*PTA; balloon angioplasty*), in which an inflatable balloon, mounted on the tip of a flexible catheter, is placed within the lumen of the affected vessel at the site of the narrowing/blockage, under X-ray control. On inflation of the balloon the lumen is reopened. In an artery this disrupts the *intima (which reduces the chances of the stenosis recurring). This procedure may be performed before introducing a vascular *stent. Common sites for PTA are coronary, carotid, renal, and leg arteries. *See also* coronary angioplasty.

angiospasm *n. see* Raynaud's disease.

angiotensin *n.* either of two peptides: *angiotensin I* or *angiotensin II*. Angiotensin I is derived, by the action of the enzyme *renin, from a protein (alpha globulin) secreted by the liver into the bloodstream. As blood passes through the lungs, another enzyme acts on angiotensin I to form angiotensin II. This peptide causes constriction of blood vessels and stimulates the release of the hormones *vasopressin and *aldosterone, which increase blood pressure. *See also* ACE inhibitor, angiotensin II antagonist.

angiotensin II antagonist any one of a class of drugs that block the action of the hormone *angiotensin II, which constricts blood vessels; they are therefore useful in treating *hypertension. These drugs include *candesartan* (Atacand), *irbesartan* (Avapro), *losartan* (Cozaar), *telmisartan* (Micardis), and *valsartan* (Diovan). They are taken by mouth and side effects are usually mild.

angle *n.* **1.** (in anatomy) a corner. For example, the *angle of the eye* is the outer or inner corner of the eye; the *angle of the mouth* is the site where the upper and lower lips join on either side. **2.** the degree of divergence of two lines or planes that meet each other; the space between two such lines. The *carrying angle* is the obtuse angle formed between the forearm and the arm when the forearm is fully extended and the hand is supinated.

angstrom *n.* a unit of length equal to one ten millionth of a millimeter (10^{-10} m). It is not a recommended *SI unit but is sometimes used to express wavelengths and interatomic distances: the *nanometer (1 nm = 10 Å) is now the preferred unit. Symbol Å.

anhedonia *n.* the inability to feel pleasure in acts that normally give pleasure.

anhidrosis (anidrosis) *n.* the absence of sweating in the presence of an appropriate stimulus for sweating, such as heat. A reduction in sweating is known as *hypohidrosis*. Anhidrosis and hypohidrosis may accompany disease or occur as a congenital defect.

anhidrotic 1. *n.* any drug that inhibits the secretion of sweat, such as *anticholinergic drugs. **2.** *adj.* inhibiting sweating.

anhydrase *n.* an enzyme that catalyzes the removal of water from a compound.

anhydremia *n.* a decrease in the proportion of water, and therefore plasma, in the blood.

anima *n.* (in Jungian psychology) an *archetype that is the feminine component of a male's personality.

animus *n.* (in Jungian psychology) the *archetype that is the masculine component of a female's personality.

anion *n.* an ion of negative charge, such as a bicarbonate ion (HCO_3^-) or a chloride ion (Cl^-) (*see also* electrolyte). The *anion gap* is the difference between the concentrations of cations (positively charged ions) and anions, calculated from the formula: $(Na^+ + K^+) - (HCO_3^- + Cl^-)$. It is used to estimate the unaccounted-for anions in the blood in cases of metabolic disturbance. The normal anion gap is 10–16 mmol/l.

aniridia *n.* congenital absence of the iris (of the eye). It may be caused by a *deletion on the short arm of chromosome no. 11 and it may be associated with other abnormalities, such as macular dysplasia, sensory nystagmus, and congenital cataract. *See also* WAGR syndrome.

aniseikonia *n.* a condition in which the image of an object differs markedly in size or shape in each eye.

anisocoria *n.* inequality in the size of the pupils of the two eyes, usually a difference of more than 1 mm in diameter.

anisocytosis *n.* an excessive variation in size between individual red blood cells. Anisocytosis is measured by some automatic analyzers; these automated instruments calculate the red cell distribution width (RDW), which reflects anisocytosis. Anisocytosis may be a feature of almost any disease affecting the blood.

anisomelia *n.* a difference in size or shape between the arms or the legs.

anisometropia *n.* the condition in which the power of *refraction in one eye differs from that in the other.

anistreplase *n.* a *fibrinolytic drug consisting of a complex of *streptokinase and *plasminogen. It is administered by injection in the treatment of coronary thrombosis. Possible side effects include local bleeding, slowing of the heart, flushing, low blood pressure, fever, nausea, vomiting, and allergic reactions. Trade name: **Eminase**.

ankle *n.* **1.** the hinge joint between the leg and the foot. It consists of the *talus (ankle bone), which projects into a socket formed by the lower ends of the *tibia and *fibula. **2.** the whole region of the ankle joint, including the *tarsus and the lower parts of the tibia and fibula.

ankyloblepharon *n.* an abnormal fusion (partial or complete) of the upper and lower eyelid margins.

ankylosing spondylitis *see* spondylitis.

ankylosis *n.* pathological fusion of the bones across a joint space, either by bony tissue (*bony ankylosis*) or by shortening of connecting fibrous tissue (*fibrous ankylosis*). Ankylosis is a complication of prolonged joint inflammation, as may occur in chronic infection (e.g. tuberculosis) or rheumatic disease (e.g. ankylosing *spondylitis).

Ankylostoma *n. see* Ancylostoma.

annulus *n.* (in anatomy) a circular opening or ring-shaped structure. —**annular** *adj.*

anodontia *n.* absence of the teeth because they have failed to develop. It is more common for only a few teeth to fail to develop (*see* hypodontia).

anodyne *n.* any treatment or drug that soothes and eases pain.

anomaloscope *n.* an instrument for testing color discrimination. By adjusting the controls the subject has to produce a mixture of red and green light to match a yellow light. The matching is done on a brightly illuminated disk viewed through a telescope.

anomalous pulmonary venous drainage a congenital abnormality in which the pulmonary veins enter the right atrium or vena cava instead of draining into the left atrium. The features are those of an *atrial septal defect.

anomaly *n.* any deviation from the normal, especially a congenital or developmental defect.

anomia *n.* a form of *aphasia in which the patient is unable to give the names of objects, although retaining an understanding of their use and the ability to put words together into speech.

anonychia *n.* congenital absence of one or more nails.

Anopheles *n.* a genus of widely distributed mosquitoes, occurring in tropical and temperate regions, with some 350 species. The malarial parasite (*see* Plasmodium) is transmitted to humans solely through the bite of female *Anopheles* mosquitoes. Some species of *Anopheles* may transmit the parasites of bancroftian *filariasis.

anophthalmos *n.* congenital absence of the eye.

anoplasty *n.* a surgical technique used to repair a weak or injured anal sphincter.

anorchism *n.* congenital absence of one or both testes.

anorexia *n.* loss of appetite.

anorexia nervosa a psychological illness, most common in female adolescents, in which the patients starve themselves or use other techniques, such as vomiting or taking laxatives, to induce weight loss. They are motivated by a false perception of their bodies as being fat and/or a phobia of becoming fat. The result is severe loss of weight, usually *amenorrhea, and sometimes even death from starvation. The cause of the illness is complicated – problems within the family and rejection of adult sexuality are often factors involved. Patients must be persuaded to eat enough to maintain a normal body weight and their emotional disturbance is usually treated by *psychotherapy. *See also* bulimia.

anosmia *n.* loss or impairment of the sense of smell. This can be temporary, as with a cold or other forms of *rhinitis, or it

can be permanent, following certain viral infections, head injuries, and tumors affecting the *olfactory nerve. If loss of the sense of smell is partial rather than total, the condition is called *hyposmia*.

anovular (anovulatory) *adj.* not associated with the development and release of a female germ cell (ovum) in the ovary, as in *anovular menstruation*.

anoxemia *n.* a condition in which there is less than the normal concentration of oxygen in the blood. *See also* anoxia, hypoxemia.

anoxia *n.* a condition in which the tissues of the body receive inadequate amounts of oxygen. This may result from low atmospheric pressure at high altitudes; a shortage of circulating blood, red blood cells, or hemoglobin; or disordered blood flow, such as occurs in heart failure. It can also result from insufficient oxygen reaching the blood in the lungs due to poor breathing movements or because disease, such as pneumonia, is reducing the effective surface area of lung tissue. *See also* hypoxia. —**anoxic** *adj.*

ANS *see* autonomic nervous system.

ansa *n.* (in anatomy) a loop; for example, the *ansa hypoglossi* is the loop formed by the descending branch of the hypoglossal nerve.

ansiform *adj.* (in anatomy) shaped like a loop. The term is applied to certain lobules of the cerebellum.

ant- (anti-) *prefix denoting* opposed to; counteracting; relieving. Examples: *antarthritic* (relieving arthritis); *antibacterial* (destroying or stopping the growth of bacteria).

Antabuse *n.* *see* disulfiram.

antacid *n.* a drug that neutralizes the hydrochloric acid secreted in the digestive juices of the stomach. Antacids, which include *aluminum hydroxide, calcium carbonate, *magnesium hydroxide, and *sodium bicarbonate, are used to relieve pain and discomfort in disorders of the digestive system, including peptic ulcer.

antagonist *n.* **1.** a muscle whose action (contraction) opposes that of another muscle (called the *agonist* or *prime mover*). Antagonists relax to allow the agonists to effect movement. **2.** a drug or other substance with opposite action to that of another drug or natural body chemical, which it inhibits. Examples are the *antimetabolites.* —**antagonism** *n.*

antazoline *n.* a short-acting *antihistamine drug, applied topically in combination with the sympathomimetic drug *naphazoline to treat allergic conjunctivitis.

ante- *prefix denoting* before. Examples: *antenatal* (before birth); *anteprandial* (before meals).

anteflexion *n.* the bending forward of an organ. A mild degree of anteflexion of the uterus is considered to be normal.

antemortem *adj.* before death. *Compare* postmortem.

antenatal diagnosis *see* prenatal diagnosis.

antepartum *adj.* occurring before the onset of labor.

antepartum hemorrhage bleeding from the genital tract after the 24th week of pregnancy until the birth of the baby.

anterior *adj.* **1.** describing or relating to the front (ventral) portion of the body or limbs. **2.** describing the front part of any organ. For example, the *anterior chamber* of the eye is that part of the eye between the cornea and the lens, which is filled with aqueous humor.

anteversion *n.* the normal forward inclination of an organ, especially of the uterus.

anthelix *n. see* antihelix.

anthelmintic **1.** *n.* any drug or chemical agent used to destroy parasitic worms (helminths), e.g. tapeworms, roundworms, and flukes, and/or remove them from the body. Anthelmintics include *albendazole, *mebendazole, *niclosamide, *quinacrine, *praziquantel, and *piperazine. **2.** *adj.* having the power to destroy or eliminate helminths.

anthracosis (coal worker's pneumoconiosis) *n.* a lung disease – a form of *pneumoconiosis – caused by coal dust. It affects mainly coal miners but also other exposed workers, such as bargemen, if the lungs' capacity to accommodate and remove the particles is exceeded.

anthracycline *n.* any of 500 or so antibiotics synthesized or isolated from species of *Streptomyces.* *Doxorubicin is the most important member of this group of compounds, which have wide activity against tumors.

anthralin *n.* a drug applied to the skin as a cream to treat psoriasis, ringworm infections, and other skin conditions. It may irritate the skin on application.

Trade names: **Drithocreme, Dritho-Scalp, Micanol, Psoriatec.**

anthrax *n.* an acute infectious disease of farm animals caused by the bacterium *Bacillus anthracis,* which can be transmitted to humans by contact with animal hair, hides, or excrement. In humans the disease attacks either the lungs, causing pneumonia, or the skin, producing severe ulceration (known as *malignant pustule*). *Woolsorter's disease* is a serious infection of the skin or lungs by *B. anthracis,* affecting those handling wool or pelts (*see* occupational disease). Untreated anthrax can be fatal but administration of large doses of penicillin or tetracycline is usually effective.

anthrop- (anthropo-) *prefix denoting* the human race. Examples: *anthropogenesis* (origin and development of); *anthropoid* (resembling); *anthropology* (science of).

anthropometry *n.* the taking of measurements of the human body or its parts. Comparisons can then be made between individuals of different sexes, ages, and races to determine the difference between normal and abnormal development. —**anthropometric** *adj.*

anthropozoonosis *n.* a disease that is transmissible from an animal to a human, or vice versa, under natural conditions. Diseases that are found primarily in animals and sometimes affect humans include *anthrax, *rabies, and *leptospirosis.

antiandrogen *n.* any one of a group of drugs that block the cellular uptake of testosterone by the prostate gland and are therefore used in the treatment of prostate cancer, which is an androgen-dependent tumor, and various sexual disorders in man. Antiandrogens include *bicalutamide, *cyproterone acetate, *finasteride, and *flutamide.

antiarrhythmic *n.* any of a group of drugs used to correct irregularities in the heartbeat (*see* arrhythmia). They include *adenosine, *amiodarone, *atropine, *verapamil, *quinidine, *disopyramide, *lidocaine, *encainide, and *propafenone.

antibacterial *adj.* describing an antibiotic that is active against bacteria.

antibiotic *n.* a substance, produced by or derived from a microorganism, that destroys or inhibits the growth of other microorganisms. Antibiotics are used to treat infections caused by organisms that are sensitive to them, usually bacteria or fungi. They may alter the normal microbial content of the body (e.g. in the intestine, lungs, bladder) by destroying one or more groups of harmless or beneficial organisms, which may result in infections due to overgrowth of resistant organisms. These side effects are most likely to occur with *broad-spectrum antibiotics* (those active against a wide variety of organisms). Resistance may also develop in the microorganisms being treated (for example, through incorrect dosage or overprescription – *see also* superinfection). Antibiotics should not be used for minor infections, which will clear up unaided. Some antibiotics may cause allergic reactions. *See also* aminoglycosides, antifungal, antiviral drug, cephalosporin, chloramphenicol, penicillin, streptomycin, tetracycline.

antibody *n.* a special kind of blood protein that is synthesized in lymphoid tissue in response to the presence of a particular *antigen and circulates in the plasma to attack the antigen and render it harmless. The production of specific antibodies against antigens as diverse as invading bacteria, inhaled pollen grains, and foreign red blood cells is the basis of both *immunity and *allergy. Antibody formation is also responsible for tissue or organ rejection following transplantation. Chemically, antibodies are proteins of the globulin type; they are classified according to their structure and function (*see* immunoglobulin).

anticholinergic *adj.* inhibiting the action of *acetylcholine, the neurotransmitter that conveys information in the parasympathetic nervous system. Anticholinergic drugs block the effects of certain (muscarinic) receptors; hence they are also called *antimuscarinic* drugs. The actions of these drugs include relaxation of smooth muscle, decreased secretion of saliva, sweat, and digestive juices, and dilation of the pupil of the eye. *Atropine and similar drugs have these effects; they are used in the treatment of gastrointestinal spasms (e.g. *propantheline) and of parkinsonism (e.g. *trihexyphenidyl hydrochloride, *benztropine), as bronchodilators (e.g. *ipratropium, *theophylline), and as *mydriatics. Characteristic side effects

include dry mouth, thirst, blurred vision, dry skin, increased heart rate, and difficulty in urination.

anticholinesterase *n.* any substance that inhibits the action of *cholinesterase, the enzyme responsible for the breakdown of the neurotransmitter acetylcholine, and therefore allows acetylcholine to continue transmitting nerve impulses. Drugs with anticholinesterase activity include *neostigmine, *pyridostigmine, *physostigmine, and *edrophonium; their uses include the diagnosis and treatment of *myasthenia gravis. *See also* parasympathomimetic.

anticoagulant *n.* an agent that prevents the clotting of blood. The natural anticoagulant *heparin directly interferes with blood clotting and is active both within the body and against a sample of blood in a test tube. Synthetic drugs, such as *warfarin, are effective only within the body, since they act by affecting blood *coagulation factors. They take longer to act than heparin. Anticoagulants are used to prevent the formation of blood clots or to break up clots in blood vessels in such conditions as thrombosis and embolism. Incorrect dosage may result in hemorrhage. *See also* fibrinolytic.

anticonvulsant *n.* a drug that prevents or reduces the severity and frequency of seizures in various types of epilepsy; the term *antiepileptic drug* is now preferred since not all seizures involve convulsions. The choice of drug is dictated by the type of seizure and the patient's response. The dosage must be adjusted carefully as individuals vary in their response to these drugs and side effects may be troublesome. Commonly used antiepileptic drugs include *carbamazepine, *ethosuximide, *lamotrigine, *phenytoin, *valproic acid, and *gabapentin; *topiramate, vigabatrin, oxcarbazepine,* and *levetiracetam* are newer drugs. Phenobarbital is no longer commonly prescribed.

antidepressant *n.* a drug that alleviates the symptoms of depression. The most widely prescribed antidepressants are a group of drugs with a basic chemical structure of three benzene rings, called *tricyclic antidepressants,* which include *amitriptyline, *doxepin, and *imipramine. These drugs are useful in treating a variety of different depressive symptoms. Side effects commonly include dry mouth, blurred vision, constipation, drowsiness, and difficulty in urination. Other antidepressants include the *MAO inhibitors, which have more severe side effects, and the serotonin-specific reuptake inhibitors (see SSRI), e.g. *fluoxetine and *fluvoxamine, which generally have less sedative effects than the tricyclic antidepressants.

antidiabetic drugs drugs used to control *diabetes mellitus. Type 1 diabetes is treated with the wide range of formulations of *insulin. Type 2 diabetes is treated mainly with *oral hypoglycaemic drugs but in some cases insulin may be required.

antidiuretic hormone (ADH) see vasopressin.

antidote n. a drug that counteracts the effects of a poison or of overdosage of another drug. For example, *dimercaprol is an antidote to arsenic, mercury, and other heavy metals.

antidromic adj. describing impulses traveling "the wrong way" in a nerve fiber. This is rare but may happen in shingles, when the irritation caused by the virus in the spinal canal initiates impulses that travel outward in normally afferent nerves. The area of skin that the sensory nerves supply (usually a strip on the trunk) becomes painfully blistered. Antidromic impulses cannot pass *synapses, which work in one direction only.

antiemetic n. a drug that prevents vomiting. Various drugs have this effect, including some *antihistamines (e.g. cyclizine, promethazine) and *anticholinergic drugs. They are used for such conditions as motion sickness and vertigo and to counteract nausea and vomiting caused by other drugs. Antiemetics include *buclizine, *domperidone, *metoclopramide, and *ondansetron.

antiepileptic drug see anticonvulsant.

antiestrogen n. one of a group of drugs that oppose the action of *estrogen. The most important of these drugs is currently *tamoxifen, which antagonizes the action of estrogens at the tissue receptors and is used in the treatment of breast cancers dependent on estrogen. Because they stimulate the production of pituitary *gonadotropins, some antiestrogens (e.g. *clomiphene) are used to induce or stimulate ovulation in infertil-

ity treatment. Side effects of antiestrogens include hot flashes, itching of the vulva, nausea, vomiting, fluid retention, and sometimes vaginal bleeding.

antifibrinolytic adj. an agent that inhibits the dissolution of blood clots (see fibrinolysis). Antifibrinolytic drugs include *aprotinin and *tranexamic acid.

antifungal (antimycotic) adj. describing a drug that kills or inactivates fungi and is used to treat fungal (including yeast) infections. Antifungal drugs include *amphotericin B, *griseofulvin, the *imidazoles, *itraconazole, *nystatin, *terbinafine, and *tolnaftate.

antigen n. any substance that the body regards as foreign or potentially dangerous and against which it mounts an *immune response consisting of the production of an *antibody that specifically binds to it. Antigens are usually proteins, but simple substances, even metals, may become antigenic by combining with larger molecules (e.g. proteins). The simple molecules are called *haptens; the larger molecules are called *carriers.
—**antigenic** adj.

antigen-presenting cell see APC.

antihelix (anthelix) n. the curved inner ridge of the *pinna of the ear. See antitragus.

antihemophilic factor see Factor VIII.

antihistamine n. a drug that inhibits the action of *histamine in the body by blocking the receptors for histamine, of which there are two types: H_1 and H_2. When stimulated by histamine, H_1 receptors may produce such allergic reactions as *hay fever, *pruritus (itching), and *urticaria. Antihistamines that block H_1 receptors (H_1-receptor antagonists), such as *acrivastine, *azatadine, and *chlorpheniramine, are used to relieve these conditions. Many H_1-receptor antagonists, e.g. *cyclizine and *promethazine, also have strong *antiemetic activity and are used to prevent motion sickness. The most common side effect of these drugs, especially the older antihistamines (e.g. azatadine, *brompheniramine, *diphenhydramine, promethazine), is drowsiness and because of this they are sometimes used to promote sleep. Newer antihistamines (e.g. acrivastine, cetirizine (Zyrtec), loratidine (Claritin), *terfenadine) are less sedating. Other side effects include dizziness, blurred vision, tremors, digestive upsets, and lack of muscular coordination.

H_2 receptors are mainly found in the stomach, where stimulation by histamine causes secretion of acid gastric juice. H_2-receptor antagonists (e.g. *cimetidine, *famotidine, *nizatidine, *ranitidine) block these receptors and so reduce gastric acid secretion; they are used in the treatment of *peptic ulcers and *gastroesophageal reflux disease.

anti-inflammatory 1. *adj.* describing a drug that reduces *inflammation. The various groups of anti-inflammatory drugs act against one or more of the mediators that initiate or maintain inflammation. Some groups suppress only certain aspects of the inflammatory response. The main groups of anti-inflammatory drugs are the *antihistamines, the glucocorticoids (*see* corticosteroid), and the nonsteroidal anti-inflammatory drugs (*see* NSAID). **2.** *n.* an anti-inflammatory drug.

antiketogenic *n.* an agent that prevents formation of *ketone bodies.

antilymphocytic serum (ALS, antilymphocyte globulin, ALG) an *antiserum, containing antibodies that suppress lymphocytic activity, prepared by injecting an animal with lymphocytes. ALS may be given to a patient to prevent the immune reaction that causes tissue rejection following transplantation of such organs as kidneys or of bone marrow. Administration naturally also impairs other immunity mechanisms, making infection a serious hazard.

antimetabolite *n.* one of a group of drugs that interfere with the normal metabolic processes within cells by combining with the enzymes responsible for them. Some drugs used in the treatment of cancer, e.g. *fluorouracil, *methotrexate, and *mercaptopurine, are antimetabolites that prevent cell growth by interfering with enzyme reactions essential for nucleic acid synthesis. Side effects of antimetabolites can be severe, involving blood cell disorders and digestive disturbances. *See also* chemotherapy, cytotoxic drug.

antimitotic *n.* one of a group of drugs that inhibit cell division and growth, e.g. *doxorubicin, *procarbazine. The drugs used to treat cancer are mainly antimi-

totics. *See also* antimetabolite, cytotoxic drug.

antimutagen *n.* a substance that can either reduce the spontaneous production of mutations or prevent or reverse the action of a *mutagen.

antimycotic *adj. see* antifungal.

antineoplastic 1. *adj.* inhibiting the development or proliferation of malignant cells. **2.** *n.* any substance (especially a chemotherapeutic agent) or procedure with this property. *See also* cytotoxic drug.

antioxidant *n.* a substance capable of neutralizing oxygen free radicals, the highly active and damaging atoms and chemical groups produced by various disease processes and by poisons, radiation, smoking, and other agencies. The body contains its own natural antioxidants but there is growing medical interest in the possibility of controlling cell and tissue damage by means of supplementary antioxidants. Those most commonly used are *vitamin C (ascorbic acid), *vitamin E (tocopherols), and *beta-carotene. Evidence is accumulating that these substances can reduce the incidence of a number of serious diseases.

antiperistalsis *n.* a wave of contraction in the alimentary canal that passes in an oral (i.e. upward or backward) direction (*compare* peristalsis). It was formerly thought that antiperistalsis occurred in vomiting but modern physiological studies indicate that it never takes place in humans.

antiphospholipid-antibody syndrome an autoimmune disease in which the presence of antibody against phospholipid is associated with a tendency to thrombosis and – in women of childbearing age – recurrent (three or more) miscarriages. In pregnant women blood clots form in the placenta, resulting in the fetus being deprived of nourishment. Treatment is by low-dose aspirin or heparin.

antipruritic *n.* an agent that relieves itching (*pruritus). Examples are *calamine and *crotamiton, which are applied in creams or lotions, and some *antihistamine drugs (e.g. *trimeprazine) used if the itching is due to an allergy.

antipsychotic *adj.* describing a group of drugs used to treat severe mental disorders (psychoses), including schizophrenia and mania; some are administered in small doses to relieve anxiety. Formerly known as *major tranquilizers*, antipsychotic drugs include the *phenothiazines (e.g. *chlorpromazine), *butyrophenones (e.g. *haloperidol), and *thioxanthenes (e.g. *thiothixene). The *atypical antipsychotics* are a group of more recently developed drugs that may be helpful in those who do not respond to treatment with other antipsychotics. They include *clozapine, *risperidone, and *olanzapine* (Zyprexa). Side effects of many antipsychotics at high doses include abnormal involuntary movements.

antipyretic *n.* a drug that lowers the body temperature. Several analgesic drugs have antipyretic activity, including *aspirin, *mefenamic acid, and *acetaminophen.

antiretroviral *adj.* inhibiting or slowing the growth or replication of *retroviruses, specifically HIV. Antiretroviral agents used in the treatment of HIV infection and AIDS include *reverse transcriptase inhibitors and *protease inhibitors.

antisecretory drug any drug that reduces the normal rate of secretion of a body fluid, usually one that reduces acid secretion into the stomach. *Anticholinergic drugs, H_2-receptor antagonists (*see* antihistamine), and *proton-pump inhibitors are antisecretory drugs.

antisepsis *n.* the elimination of bacteria, fungi, viruses, and other microorganisms that cause disease by the use of chemical or physical methods.

antiseptic *n.* a chemical that destroys or inhibits the growth of disease-causing bacteria and other microorganisms and is sufficiently nontoxic to be applied to the skin or mucous membranes to cleanse wounds and prevent infections or to be used internally to treat infections of the intestine and bladder. Antiseptics include *cetrimonium, *chlorhexidine, *dequalinium, *gentian violet, and *methenamine.

antiserum *n.* (*pl.* **antisera**) a serum that contains antibodies against antigens of a particular kind; it may be injected to treat, or give temporary protection (passive *immunity) against, specific diseases. Antisera are prepared in large quantities in such animals as horses. In the laboratory, they are used to identify unknown organisms responsible for infection (*see* agglutination).

antisocial personality disorder a *personality disorder characterized by callous unconcern for others, irresponsibility, violence, disregard for social rules, and an incapacity for maintaining enduring relationships. It was formerly known as *dyssocial personality*, *psychopathy*, and *sociopathy*.

antispasmodic *n.* a drug that relieves spasm of smooth muscle, as in the uterus, gastrointestinal system, and urinary tract. *See* spasmolytic. *Compare* antispastic.

antispastic *n.* a drug that relieves spasm of skeletal muscle. *See also* muscle relaxant. *Compare* antispasmodic.

antithrombin *n.* any substance that inhibits or neutralizes the action of thrombin, so that blood does not coagulate.

antitoxin *n.* an antibody produced by the body to counteract a toxin formed by invading bacteria or from any other source.

antitragus *n.* a small projection of cartilage above the lobe of the ear, opposite the *tragus. *See* antihelix, pinna.

antitussive *n.* a drug, such as *dextromethorphan, that suppresses coughing, possibly by reducing the activity of the cough center in the brain and by depressing respiration. Some analgesic drugs also have antitussive activity, e.g. *codeine, diacetylmorphine (*see* heroin), and *methadone.

antivenin (antivenene) *n.* an *antiserum containing antibodies against specific poisons in the venom of such an animal as a snake, spider, or scorpion.

antiviral drug a drug effective against viruses that cause disease. Antiviral drugs include *DNA polymerase inhibitors (e.g. *acyclovir, *foscarnet, *ganciclovir), *idoxuridine and *ribavirin (nucleoside analogues), *amantadine, and *zanamivir; they are used for treating herpes, cytomegalovirus and respiratory syncytial virus infections, and influenza. Antiviral drugs for treating HIV infection and AIDS are *reverse transcriptase inhibitors (e.g. *didanosine, *zidovudine) and *protease inhibitors.

antrectomy *n.* **1.** surgical removal of the bony walls of an *antrum. *See* antrostomy. **2.** a surgical operation in which a part of the stomach (the antrum) is removed. Most secretions of acid, pepsin, and the hormone gastrin occur in the antrum and the operation may be required (usually combined with *vagotomy) in the treatment of peptic ulcers that have recurred after vagotomy and are resistant to H_2-blocking drugs (*see* antihistamine).

antroscopy *n.* inspection of the inside of any cavity, particularly the maxillary sinus (*see* paranasal sinuses), using an *endoscope (called an *antroscope*).

antrostomy *n.* a surgical operation to produce a permanent or semipermanent artificial opening to an *antrum in a bone, so providing drainage for any fluid. The operation is sometimes carried out to treat infection of the *paranasal sinuses.

antrum *n.* **1.** a cavity, especially a cavity in a bone. The *mastoid* (or *tympanic*) *antrum* is the space connecting the air cells of the *mastoid process with the chamber of the inner ear. **2.** the part of the *stomach adjoining the pylorus (*pyloric* or *gastric antrum*).

anuria *n.* failure of the kidneys to produce urine. This can occur in a variety of conditions that produce a sustained drop in blood pressure. Urgent assessment is required to differentiate lack of production of urine from an obstruction to the flow of urine from the kidneys, which can readily be relieved. Anuria is associated with increasing *uremia and may require *hemodialysis.

anus *n.* the opening at the lower end of the alimentary canal, through which the feces are discharged. It opens out from the *anal canal*, below the rectum, and is guarded by two sphincters. The anus is closed except during defecation. —**anal** *adj.*

anvil *n.* (in anatomy) *see* incus.

anxiety *n.* generalized pervasive *fear. *Anxiety state* is a condition in which anxiety dominates the patient's life. Neuroses are now usually called *anxiety disorders* (*see* neurosis, panic disorder, post-traumatic stress disorder) and usually can be treated with psychotherapy, behavior therapy, and tranquilizing drugs. *See also* generalized anxiety disorder.

anxiolytic *adj.* describing a group of drugs used to treat anxiety of various causes. Formerly known as *minor tranquilizers*, they include the *benzodiazepines, *buspirone, and *meprobamate. Common side effects of these drugs are drowsiness and dizziness, and prolonged use may result in *dependence.

aorta *n.* (*pl.* **aortas** or **aortae**) the main artery of the body, from which all others derive. It arises from the left ventricle (*ascending aorta*), arches over the top of the heart (*see* aortic arch) and descends in front of the backbone (*descending aorta*), giving off large and small branches and finally dividing to form the right and left *iliac arteries. The part of the descending aorta from the aortic arch to the diaphragm is called the *thoracic aorta*; the part below the diaphragm is the *abdominal aorta*. —**aortic** *adj.*

aortic aneurysm *see* aneurysm.

aortic arch that part of the aorta that extends from the ascending aorta, upward over the heart and then backward and down as far as the fourth thoracic vertebra. *Stretch receptors in its outer wall monitor blood pressure and form part of the system maintaining this at a constant level.

aortic regurgitation reflux of blood from the aorta into the left ventricle during diastole. Aortic regurgitation most commonly follows scarring of the aortic valve as a result of previous acute rheumatic fever, but it may also result from other conditions, such as syphilis or dissecting aneurysm. Mild cases are symptom-free, but patients more severely affected develop breathlessness, angina pectoris, and enlargement of the heart; all have a diastolic murmur. A badly affected valve may be replaced surgically with a prosthesis.

aortic replacement a surgical technique used to replace a diseased length of aorta, most often the abdominal aorta. It usually involves inserting into the aorta a flexible tube of artificial material, which functions as a substitute for the diseased section.

aortic stenosis narrowing of the opening of the aortic valve due to fusion of the cusps that comprise the valve. It may result from previous rheumatic fever or from calcification and scarring in a valve that has two cusps instead of the normal three, or it may be congenital. Aortic stenosis obstructs the flow of blood from the left ventricle to the aorta during systole. Breathlessness on effort, angina pectoris, and fainting may follow. The patient has a systolic murmur. When symptoms develop, the valve should be replaced surgically with a mechanical prosthesis (such as a *Starr-Edwards ball-cage valve) or with an aortic valve graft.

aortic valve a valve in the heart, lying between the left ventricle and the aorta. It consists of three pockets, shaped like half-moons, that prevent blood returning to the ventricle from the aorta. *See also* semilunar valve.

aortitis *n.* inflammation of the aorta, which was previously common as a late complication of syphilis but is more often now associated with a variety of poorly understood autoimmune conditions (such as *Behçet's syndrome and *Takayasu's disease). Inflammation of the aortic wall may result in the formation of an aneurysm or vascular stenosis, obstructing blood flow to target organs. Chest pain may occur from pressure on surrounding structures or from the reduced blood supply to the heart. *Aortic regurgitation may occur. Surgical repair of the aortic aneurysm or valve may be needed.

aortography *n.* X-ray examination of the aorta, in which a series of images is taken during the injection of a *radiopaque contrast medium (*see* angiocardiography). This technique has been largely replaced as a primary investigation by other *cross-sectional imaging methods.

apathetic hyperthyroidism a condition seen in older patients with *thyrotoxicosis, characterized by weight loss, slow atrial fibrillation, and severe depressive illness, rather than the usual florid symptoms. They have small goiters on examination and the blood tests confirm thyrotoxicosis, which is treated in the standard manner.

APC (antigen-presenting cell) a macrophage that processes antigen for presentation to T lymphocytes (*see* helper T cell).

aperient *n.* a mild *laxative.

apex *n.* the tip or summit of an organ; for example the heart or lung. The apex of a *tooth is the tip of the root, where there is a small hole (the *apical foramen*) through which vessels and nerves pass from the pulp to the periapical tissues. —**apical** *adj.*

apex beat the impact of the heart against the chest wall during *systole. It can be felt or heard to the left of the breastbone, in the space between the fifth and sixth ribs.

Apgar score a method of rapidly assessing the general state of a baby immediately after birth. A maximum of 2 points is given for each of the following signs, usually measured at one and five minutes after delivery: type of breathing, heart rate, color, muscle tone, and response to stimuli. Thus an infant scoring 10 points would be in optimum condition. When the score is low, the test is repeated at intervals as a guide to short-term progress. [V. Apgar (1909–74), US anesthesiologist]

aphakia *n.* absence of the lens of the eye: the state of the eye after a cataract has been removed when no intraocular lens has been inserted. —**aphakic** *adj.*

aphasia (dysphasia) *n.* a disorder of language affecting the generation and content of speech and its comprehension (it is not a disorder of articulation: *see* dysarthria, dyslalia). It is caused by disease in the left half of the brain (the dominant hemisphere) in a right-handed person. It is commonly accompanied by difficulties in reading and writing. —**aphasic** *adj.*

aphonia *n.* absence of or loss of the voice caused by disease of the larynx or mouth: if loss of speech is due to a defect in the brain the disorder is called *aphasia.

aphrenia *n.* failure of development of the intellectual faculties. *See* mental retardation.

aphrodisiac *n.* an agent that stimulates sexual excitement.

aphtha *n.* (*pl.* **aphthae**) a small ulcer, occurring singly or in groups in the mouth as white or red spots. The cause is unknown, and treatment is with topical tetracycline or topical corticosteroids. —**aphthous** *adj.*

apical abscess an abscess in the bone around the apex of a tooth. An acute abscess is extremely painful, causing swelling of the jaw and sometimes also the face. A chronic abscess may cause no pain or swelling. An abscess invariably results from damage to and infection of the pulp of the tooth. Treatment is drainage and *root canal treatment or extraction of the tooth; antibiotics may give temporary relief.

apicectomy *n.* (in dentistry) surgical removal of the apex of the root of a tooth, now often referred to as *root resection*. It is usually accompanied by placement of a filling in a cavity prepared in the root end and is carried out when *root canal treatment cannot be done or has failed.

aplasia *n.* the total or partial failure of development of an organ or tissue. *See also* agenesis. —**aplastic** *adj.*

aplasia cutis congenita the congenital absence of skin on the scalp, usually in one or more small patches. The area is usually covered by a thin, translucent membrane or scar tissue. It may result from an infection in the uterus or from a developmental abnormality.

aplastic anemia *see* anemia.

APMPPE acute posterior multifocal placoid *pigment epitheliopathy.

apnea *n.* temporary cessation of breathing from any cause. The presence of more than five episodes of apnea per hour of sleep, in which nasal airflow is less than 30% of normal for more than 10 seconds per episode, is indicative of obstructive *sleep apnea. The number of apnea episodes per hour of sleep is called the *apnea index*. Attacks of apnea are common in newborn babies and should be taken seriously although they do not necessarily indicate serious illness. Monitors are available that are activated if the baby does not breathe over a specified length of time. *See also* crib death. —**apneic** *adj.*

apneusis *n.* a state in which prolonged inhalation occurs when the appropriate inhibitory influences are prevented from reaching the inspiratory center of the brain.

apocrine *adj.* **1.** describing sweat glands that occur only in hairy parts of the body, especially the armpit and groin. These glands develop in the hair follicles and appear after puberty. The strong odors associated with sweating result from the action of bacteria on the sweat produced by apocrine glands. Inflammation of these glands is called *apocrinitis*. *Compare* eccrine. **2.** describing a type of gland that loses part of its protoplasm when secreting. *See* secretion.

apolipoprotein (Apo) *n.* a protein constituent of *lipoproteins involved in the transport of lipids in plasma. There are four classes: A, B, C, and E. A, B, and C are further classified as A-I, A-II, A-III, A-IV; B-48 and B-100; and C-I, C-II, and C-III. Each forms part of high-density lipoprotein, low-density lipoprotein, or very-low-density lipoprotein, except Apo E, which is part of all of the lipoproteins. Apolipoproteins have a range of molecular weights and perform a variety of functions during the life cycle of the lipoproteins in which they are found. These include acting as ligands for the binding of enzymes (Apo B) and as cofactors for the action of other enzymes (Apo A and C). Apo E may be involved in Alzheimer's disease.

apomorphine *n.* a *dopamine receptor agonist used in the treatment of parkinsonism that is poorly controlled by *levodopa. It is given by subcutaneous injection, infusion, or orally (*see* entacapone); side effects include involuntary movements and instability of posture. Apomorphine is also used as an *emetic, administered subcutaneously, in the treatment of poisoning by noncorrosive substances that have been taken by mouth, and is given orally for the treatment of erectile *impotence.

aponeurosis *n.* a thin but strong fibrous sheet of tissue that replaces a *tendon in muscles that are flat and sheetlike and have a wide area of attachment (e.g. to bones). —**aponeurotic** *adj.*

apophysis *n.* **1.** a protuberance of bone to which a tendon is attached. It ossifies separately from the rest of the bone and fuses with it at maturity. **2.** a projection of any other part, e.g. of the brain (*apophysis cerebri*: the *pineal body).

apophysitis *n.* inflammation of any *apophysis, caused by excessive pull of a tendon to which it is attached. It occurs, for example, in *Osgood-Schlatter disease and *Sever's disease.

apoplexy *n.* *see* stroke.

apoprotein *n.* the protein part only of a conjugated protein or complex protein, e.g. apohemoglobin (the protein of hemoglobin without its heme group). *See also* apolipoprotein.

apoptosis *n.* programmed cell death, which

results in the ordered removal of cells and occurs naturally as part of the normal development, maintenance, and renewal of cells, tissues, and organs. During embryonic development, for example, the fingers are "sculpted" from the embryonic spadelike hand by apoptosis of the cells between them. Failure of apoptosis has been implicated in the uncontrolled cell division that occurs in cancer. Abnormal apoptosis, due to failure of the mechanisms that control it, may be a causative factor in autoimmune disease.

apotreptic *adj.* describing *response prevention therapy for obsessional neurosis.

appendectomy *n.* surgical removal of the vermiform appendix. *See also* appendicitis.

appendicectomy *n.* the usual British term for *appendectomy.

appendicitis *n.* inflammation of the vermiform *appendix. *Acute appendicitis*, which became common in the 20th century, usually affects young people. The chief symptom is abdominal pain, first central and later (with tenderness) in the right lower abdomen, over the appendix. Unusual positions of the appendix may cause pain in different sites, leading to difficulty in diagnosis. Vomiting and diarrhea sometimes occur, but fever is slight. If not treated by surgical removal (appendectomy) the condition usually progresses to cause an abscess or generalized *peritonitis. Conditions that mimic appendicitis include mesenteric *lymphadenitis, acute ileitis (*see* Crohn's disease), *pyelonephritis, and pneumonia.

appendicostomy *n.* an operation in which the vermiform appendix is brought through the abdominal wall and opened in order to drain or decompress the intestine. It is now rarely performed, *ileostomy, *cecostomy, or *colostomy being preferred.

appendicular *adj.* 1. relating to or affecting the vermiform appendix. 2. relating to the limbs: the *appendicular skeleton* comprises the bones of the limbs.

appendix (vermiform appendix) *n.* the short thin blind-ended tube, 7–10 cm long, that is attached to the end of the cecum (a pouch at the start of the large intestine). It has no known function in humans and is liable to become infected and inflamed, especially in young adults (*see* appendicitis).

apperception *n.* (in psychology) the process by which the qualities of an object, situation, etc., perceived by an individual are correlated with his or her preexisting knowledge.

appestat *n.* a region in the brain that controls the amount of food intake. Appetite suppressants probably decrease hunger by changing the chemical characteristics of this center.

applanation *n.* a method of flattening the cornea that is used to determine the intraocular pressure in applanation tonometry (*see* tonometer).

applicator *n.* any device used to apply medication or treatment to a particular part of the body.

apposition *n.* the state of two structures, such as parts of the body, being in close contact or side by side. For example, the fingers are brought into apposition when the fist is clenched, and the eyelids when the eyes are closed.

apraclonidine *n.* an alpha agonist (*see* sympathomimetic) administered in the form of eye drops to reduce or prevent raised intraocular pressure after laser surgery. Trade name: **Iopidine**.

apraxia (dyspraxia) *n.* an inability to make skilled movements with accuracy. This is a disorder of the *cerebral cortex resulting in the patient's inability to organize the movements rather than clumsiness due to weakness, sensory loss, or disease of the *cerebellum. It is most often caused by disease of the *parietal lobes of the brain and sometimes by disease of the frontal lobes.

aproctia *n.* congenital absence of the anus or its opening. *See* imperforate anus.

aprosexia *n.* inability to fix the attention on any subject, due to poor eyesight, defective hearing, or mental weakness.

aprotinin *n.* a drug that prevents the breakdown of blood clots (*see* fibrinolysis) by blocking the action of the enzyme plasmin, i.e. it is an *antifibrinolytic drug. It is administered by injection to control the severe bleeding that may occur in certain cancers, with *fibrinolytic treatments, and during open-heart surgery. Trade name: **Trasylol**.

APTD *see* Aid to the Permanently and Totally Disabled.

APTT (aPTT) activated partial thromboplastin time (*see* PTT).

APUD cells *a*mine *p*recursor *u*ptake and *de*carboxylation cells: a group of loosely related cells in different organs that synthesize and release amines and polypeptides. They are located in several tissues of the body, including the alimentary tract, pancreas, central nervous system, and urinary tract. They secrete polypeptide hormones, such as gastrin, secretin, and somatostatin. The cells contain amines, take up precursors of these amines, and remove the carboxyl group from the precursors to form their respective amines. They are often known as the *diffuse endocrine system*.

apudoma *n* a tumor containing *APUD cells, usually occurring in the alimentary tract, pancreatic islets, adrenal medulla, and pituitary and thyroid glands. The tumor produces excessive amounts of hormones and other peptides. *Argentaffinomas are a good example of this group of tumors, but there are many others (e.g. *gastrinomas, *somatostatinomas, and *VIPomas).

apyrexia *n*. the absence of fever.

aqueduct *n*. (in anatomy) a canal containing fluid. For example, the *aqueduct of the midbrain* (*cerebral aqueduct, aqueduct of Sylvius*) connects the third and fourth *ventricles.

aqueous humor the watery fluid that fills the chamber of the *eye immediately behind the cornea and in front of the lens. It is continually being formed – chiefly by capillaries of the ciliary processes – and it drains away into Schlemm's canal, at the junction of the cornea and sclera.

arachidonic acid *see* essential fatty acid.

arachnidism *n*. poisoning from the bite of a spider. Toxins from the less venomous species of spider cause only local pain, redness, and swelling. Toxins from more venomous species, such as the black widow (*Lactrodectus mactans*), cause muscular pains, convulsions, nausea, and paralysis.

arachnodactyly *n*. abnormally long and slender fingers: usually associated with excessive height and congenital defects of the heart and eyes in *Marfan's syndrome.

arachnoid (arachnoid mater) *n*. the middle of the three membranes covering the brain and spinal cord (*see* meninges), which has a fine, almost cobweblike, texture. Between it and the pia mater within lies the subarachnoid space, containing cerebrospinal fluid and large blood vessels; the membrane itself has no blood supply.

arachnoiditis *n*. an inflammatory process causing thickening and scarring (fibrosis) of the membranous linings (*see* meninges) of the spinal canal. The resulting entrapment of nerve roots may result in weakness, pain, and numbness in the affected area. The condition may result from infection of the meninges, surgery, or as a response to the oil-based dyes previously used in *myelography. The reaction to myelography is prevented by the current use of water-soluble dyes.

arachnoid villus one of the thin-walled projections outward of the arachnoid membrane into the blood-filled sinuses of the dura, acting as a one-way valve for the flow of cerebrospinal fluid from the subarachnoid space into the bloodstream. Large villi, known as *arachnoid granulations* (or *pacchionian bodies*), are found in the region of the superior sagittal sinus. They may be so distended as to cause pitting of the adjacent bone.

arbor *n*. (in anatomy) a treelike structure. *Arbor vitae* is the treelike outline of white matter seen in sections of the cerebellum; it also refers to the treelike appearance of the inner folds of the cervix of the uterus.

arbovirus *n*. one of a group of RNA-containing viruses that are transmitted from animals to humans by insects (i.e. arthropods; hence *a*rthropod-*bo*rne viruses) and cause diseases resulting in encephalitis or serious fever, such as dengue and yellow fever.

ARC AIDS-related complex: *see* AIDS.

arc-eye *n*. a painful condition of the eyes caused by damage to the surface of the cornea by ultraviolet light from arc welding. It usually resolves if the eyes are padded for 24 hours. It is similar to *snow blindness and the condition caused by overexposure of the eye to sun-tanning lamps.

arch- (arche-, archi-, archo-) *prefix denoting* first; beginning; primitive; ancestral. Example: *archinephron* (first-formed embryonic kidney).

archenteron *n*. a cavity that forms in the

arm

very early embryo as the result of gastrulation (*see* gastrula). In humans it forms a tubular cavity, the *archenteric canal*, which connects the amniotic cavity with the yolk sac. —**archenteric** *adj.*

archetype *n.* (in Jungian psychology) an inherited idea or mode of thought supposed to be present in the *unconscious mind and to derive from the experience of the whole human race, not from the life experience of the individual.

arcuate keratotomy a curved incision made in the periphery of the cornea. It is usually performed in the region of greatest curvature of the cornea in order to flatten it and hence reduce *astigmatism.

arcus *n.* (in anatomy) an arch; for example the *arcus aortae* (*aortic arch).

arcus senilis a grayish line in the periphery of the cornea, concentric with the edge but separated from it by a clear zone. It begins above and below but may become a continuous ring. It consists of an infiltration of fatty material and is common in the elderly. When it occurs in younger people it may indicate abnormal fat metabolism, but there is great racial variation in its incidence. It never affects vision.

ARDS *see* adult respiratory distress syndrome.

areola *n.* **1.** the brownish or pink ring of tissue surrounding the nipple of the breast. **2.** the part of the iris that surrounds the pupil of the eye. **3.** a small space in a tissue. —**areolar** *adj.*

areolar tissue loose *connective tissue consisting of a meshwork of collagen, elastic tissue, and reticular fibers that is interspersed with numerous connective tissue cells. It binds the skin to underlying muscles and forms a link between organs while allowing a high degree of relative movement.

Argasidae *n. see* tick.

argentaffin cells cells that stain readily with silver salts. Such cells occur, for example, in the crypts of Lieberkühn in the intestine and other regions of the gastrointestinal tract.

argentaffinoma (carcinoid) *n.* a tumor of the *argentaffin cells in the glands of the intestine (*see* apudoma). Argentaffinomas typically occur in the tip of the appendix and are among the most common tumors of the small intestine. They may also occur in the rectum and other parts of the digestive tract and in the bronchial tree (*bronchial carcinoid adenoma*). Argentaffinomas sometimes produce 5-hydroxytryptamine (*see* serotonin), prostaglandins, and other physiologically active substances, which are inactivated in the liver. If the tumor has spread to the liver, excess amounts of these substances are released into the systemic circulation and the *carcinoid syndrome* results – flushing, headache, diarrhea, asthmalike attacks, and in some cases damage to the right side of the heart.

arginine *n.* an *amino acid that plays an important role in the formation of *urea by the liver.

argon laser a type of *laser that produces a beam of intense light, used especially in eye surgery to treat disease of the retina (e.g. diabetic retinopathy) or glaucoma (as in argon laser *trabeculoplasty). *See also* photocoagulation.

Argyll Robertson pupil a disorder of the eyes, common to several diseases of the central nervous system (such as *syphilis), in which the *pupillary (light) reflex is absent. Although the pupils contract normally for near vision (the accommodation reflex), they fail to contract in bright light. [D. Argyll Robertson (1837–1909), Scottish ophthalmologist]

argyria (argyrosis) *n.* a form of silver poisoning in which the skin becomes dark bluish-gray due to the accumulation of the metal in the tissues, either resulting from industrial exposure or following ingestion or long-term administration of silver salts. The mucous membranes and internal organs are also affected. Argyria is now rare, due to the decline in the use of silver compounds in medicine and industry (except the photographic industry).

ariboflavinosis *n.* the group of symptoms caused by deficiency of riboflavin (vitamin B_2). These symptoms include inflammation of the tongue and lips and sores in the corners of the mouth.

arm *n.* technically, the part of the upper limb between the shoulder joint and the elbow, as distinguished from the forearm; the term is commonly used to denote the entire upper limb from shoulder to hand.

ARM artificial rupture of (fetal) membranes. *See* amniotomy.

ARMD age-related *macular degeneration.

ARN *see* acute retinal necrosis.

Arnold-Chiari malformation a congenital disorder in which there is distortion of the base of the skull with protrusion of the lower brainstem and parts of the cerebellum through the opening for the spinal cord at the base of the skull. It is commonly associated with *neural tube defects and *hydrocephalus and sometimes with *syringomyelia. [J. Arnold (1835–1915) and H. Chiari (1851–1916), German pathologists]

aromatase inhibitor any one of a class of drugs used in the treatment of advanced breast cancer in postmenopausal women. These drugs act by inhibiting the action of aromatase, an enzyme that promotes the conversion of testosterone to estradiol. They therefore reduce estrogen levels, which can be helpful in the control of estrogen-dependent tumors. Aromatase inhibitors include *aminoglutethimide, which requires replacement corticosteroid therapy, and newer drugs, whose side effects may include any of those due to estrogen deficiency but which are better tolerated than aminoglutethimide. These newer drugs include *anastrazole* (Arimidex), *exemestane* (Aromasin), *formestane* (Lentaron), and *letrozole* (Femara).

arousal *n.* **1.** a state of alertness and of high responsiveness to stimuli. It is produced by strong motivation, by anxiety, and by a stimulating environment. **2.** physiological activation of the *cerebral cortex by centers lower in the brain, such as the *reticular activating system, resulting in wakefulness and alertness. It is hypothesized that unduly high or low degrees of arousal lead to neuropsychiatric problems, such as *mania and *narcolepsy.

arrhenoblastoma *n. see* androblastoma.

arrhythmia *n.* any deviation from the normal rhythm (sinus rhythm) of the heart. The natural pacemaker of the heart (the sinoatrial node), which lies in the wall of the right atrium, controls the rate and rhythm of the whole heart under the influence of the autonomic nervous system. It generates electrical impulses that spread to the atria and ventricles, via specialized conducting tissues, and cause them to contract normally. Arrhythmias result from a disturbance of the generation or the conduction of these impulses and may be intermittent or continuous. They include *ectopic beats (extrasystoles), ectopic *tachycardias (*see* supraventricular tachycardia, ventricular tachycardia), *fibrillation, and *heart block (which is often associated with slow heart rates). Symptoms include palpitations, breathlessness, and chest pain. In more serious arrhythmias the *Stokes-Adams syndrome or *cardiac arrest may occur. Arrhythmias may result from most heart diseases but they also occur without apparent cause.

arsenic *n.* a poisonous grayish metallic element producing the symptoms of nausea, vomiting, diarrhea, cramps, convulsions, and coma when ingested in large doses. Drugs used as antidotes to arsenic poisoning include *dimercaprol. Arsenic was formerly readily available in the form of rat poison and in flypapers and was the poisoner's first choice during the 19th century, its presence in a body being then difficult to detect. Today detection is relatively simple. Arsenic was formerly used in medicine, the most important arsenical drugs being *arsphenamine* (*Salvarsan*) and *neoarsphenamine*, used in the treatment of syphilis and dangerous parasitic diseases. Symbol: As.

artefact *n. see* artifact.

arter- (arteri-, arterio-) *prefix denoting* an artery. Examples: *arteriopathy* (disease of); *arteriorrhaphy* (suture of); *arteriovenous* (relating to arteries and veins).

arteriectomy *n.* surgical excision of an artery or part of an artery. This may be performed as a diagnostic procedure (for example, to take an arterial biopsy in the diagnosis of arteritis) or during reconstruction of a blocked artery when the blocked segment is replaced by a synthetic graft.

arteriogram *n.* the image produced during arteriography, which is usually stored on photographic film or electronic media.

arteriography *n.* imaging of arteries (*see* angiography). The major roles of arteriography are to demonstrate the site and extent of atheroma, especially in the coronary arteries (*see* coronary angiography) and leg arteries (*peripheral arte-*

riography), and to demonstrate the anatomy of aneurysms within the skull (*carotid* and *vertebral arteriography*).

arteriole *n.* a small branch of an *artery, leading into many smaller vessels – the *capillaries. By their constriction and dilation, under the regulation of the sympathetic nervous system, arterioles are the principal controllers of blood flow and pressure.

arteriolitis *n.* inflammation of the arterioles (the smallest arteries), which may complicate severe hypertension. This produces *necrotizing arteriolitis*, which may result in kidney failure. A similar condition may affect the lung in pulmonary hypertension.

arterioplasty *n.* surgical reconstruction of an artery; for example, in the treatment of *aneurysms or trauma.

arteriosclerosis *n.* an imprecise term used for any of several conditions affecting the arteries. The term is often used as a synonym for atherosclerosis (*see* atheroma). It may also be used for *Mönckeberg's degeneration*, in which calcium is deposited in the arteries as part of the aging process, and *arterioloscle- rosis*, in which the walls of small arteries become thickened due to aging or hypertension.

arteriotomy *n.* an incision into, or a needle puncture of, the wall of an artery. This is most often performed as a diagnostic procedure in the course of *arteriography or cardiac *catheterization. It may also be required to remove an embolus (*see* embolectomy).

arteriovenous anastomosis a thick-walled blood vessel that connects an arteriole directly with a venule, thus bypassing the capillaries. Arteriovenous anastomoses are commonly found in the skin of the lips, nose, ears, hands, and feet; their muscular walls can constrict to reduce blood flow or dilate to allow blood through to these areas.

arteriovenous aneurysm a direct communication between an artery and vein, without an intervening capillary bed. It can occur as a congenital abnormality or it may be acquired following injury or surgery. It may affect the limbs, lungs, or viscera and may be single or multiple. If the connection is large, the short-circuiting of blood may produce heart failure. Large isolated arteriovenous aneurysms may be closed surgically.

arteriovenous malformation (AVM) *see* angioma.

arteritis *n.* an inflammatory disease affecting the muscular walls of the arteries. It may be part of a *connective tissue disease or it may be due to an infection, such as syphilis. The affected vessels are swollen and tender and may become blocked. *Temporal* (or *giant-cell*) *arteritis* occurs in the elderly and most commonly affects the arteries of the scalp. The patient complains of severe headache, and double vision or scalp tenderness may be present; blindness may result from thrombosis of the arteries to the eyes. Treatment with cortisone derivatives is rapidly effective.

artery *n.* a blood vessel carrying blood away from the heart (see illustrations). All arteries except the *pulmonary artery carry oxygenated blood. The walls of arteries contain smooth muscle fibers, which contract or relax under the control of the sympathetic nervous system. *See also* aorta, arteriole.

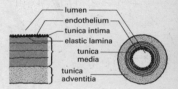

Transverse section through an artery

arthr- (arthro-) *prefix denoting* a joint. Examples: *arthrology* (science of); *arthrosclerosis* (stiffening or hardening of).

arthralgia (arthrodynia) *n.* severe pain in a joint, without swelling or other signs of arthritis. *Compare* arthritis.

arthrectomy *n.* surgical excision of a joint. It is usually performed on a painful joint that has ceased to function, as may result from intractable infection, or after a failed joint replacement. *See also* (excision) arthroplasty.

arthritis *n.* inflammation of one or more joints, characterized by swelling, warmth, redness of the overlying skin, pain, and restriction of motion. Over 200 diseases may cause arthritis, including *rheumatoid arthritis, *osteoarthritis, *gout, *tuberculosis and other infections. Diagnosis is assisted by examination of the pattern of distribution of affected joints, X-rays, blood tests, and examination of synovial fluid obtained by *aspiration of a swollen joint. *Mono- or oligoarthritis* is inflammation of one joint, *pauciarthritis* of a few (four or less), and *polyarthritis* of many joints, either simultaneously or in sequence. Any disease involving the synovial mem-

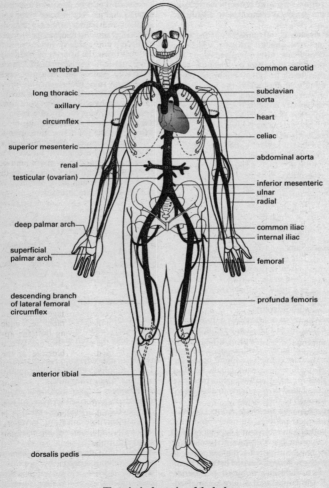

vertebral

long thoracic

axillary

circumflex

superior mesenteric

renal

testicular (ovarian)

deep palmar arch

superficial palmar arch

descending branch of lateral femoral circumflex

anterior tibial

dorsalis pedis

common carotid

subclavian

aorta

heart

celiac

abdominal aorta

inferior mesenteric

ulnar

radial

common iliac

internal iliac

femoral

profunda femoris

The principal arteries of the body

branes or causing degeneration of cartilage may cause arthritis. Treatment of arthritis depends on the cause, but aspirin and similar analgesics are often used to suppress inflammation, and hence reduce pain and swelling. *See also* juvenile rheumatoid arthritis, psoriatic arthritis, septic arthritis, hemarthrosis, pyarthrosis, hydrarthrosis. —**arthritic** *adj.*

arthrocentesis *n.* aspiration of fluid from a joint through a puncture needle.

arthrodesis *n.* artificial ankylosis: the fusion of bones across a joint space by surgical means, a procedure that eliminates movement. This operation is performed when a joint is very painful, highly unstable, grossly deformed, or chronically infected, or when an *arthroplasty would be inadvisable or impossible. *See also* Charnley clamps.

arthrodic joint (gliding joint) a form of *diarthrosis (freely movable joint) in which the bony surfaces slide over each other without angular or rotational movement. Examples are the joints of the carpus and tarsus.

arthrodynia *n. see* arthralgia.

arthrography *n.* an X-ray imaging technique for examining joints. A *contrast medium (either *radiolucent gas or a *radiopaque material) is injected into the joint space, outlining its contents and extent accurately. Arthrography has now largely been replaced by *magnetic resonance imaging (MRI).

arthrogryposis *n.* congenital defects of limbs characterized by *contractures, both flexion and extension, causing fixed deformities of the joints if untreated. *Arthrogryposis multiplex congenita* is a congenital disease with multiple causes in which there are contractures, stiff joints, and absent skin creases, as a result of the muscles being replaced by fibrous tissue. Treatment is by manipulation and splintage of deformed joints; surgical correction is sometimes required.

arthropathy *n.* any disease or disorder involving a joint.

arthroplasty *n.* surgical remodeling of a diseased joint. To prevent the ends of the bones fusing after the operation, a large gap may be created between them (*gap* or *excision arthroplasty*), a barrier of artificial material may be inserted (*interposition arthroplasty*), or one or

both bone ends may be replaced by a *prosthesis of metal or plastic (*replacement arthroplasty*). This operation may replace both joint surfaces (*total arthroplasty*) or only one (*see* hemiarthroplasty). *See also* hip replacement.

arthropod *n.* any member of a large group of animals that possess a hard external skeleton and jointed legs and other appendages. Many arthropods are of medical importance, including the *mites, *ticks, and *insects.

arthroscope *n.* an instrument for insertion into the cavity of a joint through a small incision (arthrotomy) in order to inspect the contents (*see* arthroscopy).

arthroscopy *n.* inspection of a joint cavity with an *arthroscope, enabling percutaneous surgery (such as *meniscectomy) and *biopsy to be performed.

arthrostomy *n.* a procedure to enable a temporary opening to be made into a joint cavity.

arthrotomy *n.* surgical incision of a joint in order to inspect the contents or to drain pus in *septic arthritis.

articulation *n.* (in anatomy) the point or type of contact between two bones. *See* joint.

articulator *n.* (in dentistry) an apparatus for relating the upper and lower models of a patient's dentition in a fixed position, usually with maximum tooth contact. Some articulators can reproduce jaw movements. They are used in the construction of crowns, bridges, and dentures.

artifact (artefact) *n.* **1.** (in radiography) an appearance on an image reflecting a problem with the radiographic technique rather than representing the true appearance of the patient. For example, a movement artifact is blurring of the image due to movement of the patient or organ during the exposure. All imaging techniques are susceptible to a range of artifacts. *See also* partial volume artifact. **2.** (in microscopy) a structure seen in a tissue under a microscope that is not present in the living tissue. Artifacts, which are produced by faulty *fixation or staining of the tissue, may give a false impression that disease or abnormality is present in the tissue when it is not.

artificial heart a titanium pump that is implanted into the body to take over the function of a failing left ventricle in patients with heart disease. This allows the diseased ventricle time to recover its function. The pump is powered by an external battery, strapped to the patient's body, to which it is connected by wires passed through the patient's skin. Originally pumps were implanted into the abdomen, but the most recent devices are small enough to fit into the heart itself.

artificial insemination instrumental introduction of semen into the vagina in order that the woman may conceive. Insemination is timed to coincide with the day on which the woman is expected to ovulate (*see* menstrual cycle). The semen specimen may be provided by the husband (*AIH – artificial insemination husband*) in cases of *impotence or by an anonymous donor (*AID – artificial insemination donor; DI – donor insemination*), usually in cases in which the husband is sterile.

artificial kidney (dialyzer) *see* hemodialysis.

artificial respiration an emergency procedure for maintaining a flow of air into and out of a patient's lungs when the natural breathing reflexes are absent or insufficient. This may occur after drowning, poisoning, etc., or during a surgical operation on the thorax or abdomen when muscle-relaxing drugs are administered. The simplest and most efficient method is the mouth-to-mouth technique (the "kiss of life"). In the hospital the breathing cycle is maintained by means of a *respirator.

artificial rupture of membranes (ARM) *see* amniotomy.

artificial sphincter an apparatus designed to replace or support a *sphincter that is either absent or ineffective. *See also* neosphincter.

arytenoid cartilage either of the two pyramid-shaped cartilages that lie at the back of the *larynx next to the upper edges of the cricoid cartilage.

arytenoidectomy *n*. surgical excision of the arytenoid cartilage of the larynx in the treatment of paralysis of the vocal cords.

asbestosis *n*. a lung disease – a form of *pneumoconiosis – caused by fibers of asbestos inhaled by those who are exposed to large amounts of the mineral. The incidence of lung cancer is high in

such patients, particularly if they smoke cigarettes. *See also* mesothelioma.

A-scan *n*. examination of ocular tissue, including measurement of the length of the eye (axial length), by means of a high-frequency ultrasound machine. *See also* B-scan.

ascariasis *n*. a disease caused by an infestation with the parasitic worm *Ascaris lumbricoides*. Adult worms in the intestine can cause abdominal pain, vomiting, constipation, diarrhea, appendicitis, and peritonitis; in large numbers they may cause obstruction of the intestine. The presence of the migrating larvae in the lungs can provoke pneumonia. Ascariasis occurs principally in areas of poor sanitation; it is treated with *albendazole, *mebendazole, or *piperazine.

Ascaris *n*. a genus of parasitic nematode worms. *A. lumbricoides*, widely distributed throughout the world, is the largest of the human intestinal nematodes – an adult female measures up to 35 cm in length. Eggs, passed out in the stools, may be transmitted to a new host in contaminated food or drink. Larvae hatch out in the intestine and then undergo a complicated migration, via the hepatic portal vein, liver, heart, lungs, trachea, and pharynx, before returning to the intestine where they later develop into adult worms (*see also* ascariasis).

ascites (hydroperitoneum) *n*. the accumulation of fluid in the peritoneal cavity, causing abdominal swelling. Causes include infections (such as tuberculosis), heart failure, *portal hypertension, *cirrhosis, and various cancers (particularly of the ovary and liver). Obstruction to the drainage of lymph from the abdomen results in *chylous ascites* (*see* chyle). *See also* edema.

ascorbic acid *see* vitamin C.

ASD *see* atrial septal defect.

-ase *suffix denoting* an enzyme. Examples: *lactase*; *dehydrogenase*.

asepsis *n*. the complete absence of bacteria, fungi, viruses, or other microorganisms that could cause disease. Asepsis is the ideal state for the performance of surgical operations and is achieved by using *sterilization techniques. —**aseptic** *adj*.

Asherman syndrome a condition in which *amenorrhea and infertility follow a major hemorrhage in pregnancy. It may result from overvigorous curettage of the uterus in an attempt to control the bleeding. This removes the lining, the walls adhere, and the cavity is obliterated to a greater or lesser degree. Some 50% of such patients are infertile, and of those who become pregnant, only a minority achieve an uncomplicated delivery. *Compare* Sheehan's syndrome. [J. G. Asherman (20th century), Czechoslovakian gynecologist]

asparaginase *n.* an enzyme that inhibits the growth of certain tumors. A preparation of this enzyme isolated from *Escherichia coli* is used almost exclusively in the treatment of acute lymphoblastic leukemia. It may cause allergic reactions and *anaphylaxis. Trade name: **Elspar**.

asparagine *n.* *see* amino acid.

aspartate transaminase (aspartate aminotransferase, AST) an enzyme involved in the transamination of amino acids. Measurement of AST in the serum may be used in the diagnosis of acute myocardial infarction and acute liver disease. It was formerly called *serum glutamic oxaloacetic transaminase* (*SGOT*).

aspartic acid (aspartate) *see* amino acid.

Asperger's syndrome a form of abnormal personality characterized by social aloofness, lack of interest in other people, stilted and pedantic styles of speech, and an excessive preoccupation with a very specialized interest (such as timetables). It is often considered to be a mild form of *autism. Intelligence may be normal or enhanced. [H. Asperger (1906–80), Austrian pediatrician]

aspergillosis *n.* a group of conditions caused by fungi of the genus *Aspergillus*, usually *Aspergillus fumigatus*. These conditions nearly always arise in patients with preexisting lung disease and fall into three categories. The allergic form most commonly affects asthmatic patients and may cause collapse of segments or lobes of a lung. The colonizing form leads to the formation of a fungus ball (*aspergilloma*), usually within a preexisting cavity in the lung (such as an emphysematous *bulla or a healed tuberculous cavity). Similar fungus balls may be found in other cavities, such as the eye or the sinuses around the nose. The third form of aspergillosis, in which the fungus spreads throughout the lungs

and may even disseminate throughout the body, is rare but potentially fatal. It is usually associated with deficiency in the patient's immunity. Treatment is with *prednisone, *amphotericin B, *nystatin, or *itraconazole.

Aspergillus *n.* a genus of fungi, including many common molds, some of which cause infections of the respiratory system in humans. The species *A. fumigatus* causes *aspergillosis. *A. niger* is commonly found in the external ear and can become pathogenic.

aspermia *n.* strictly, a lack or failure of formation of semen. More usually, however, the term is used to mean the total absence of sperm from the semen (*see* azoospermia).

asphyxia *n.* suffocation: a life-threatening condition in which oxygen is prevented from reaching the tissues by obstruction of or damage to any part of the respiratory system. Drowning, choking, and breathing poisonous gas all lead to asphyxia. Unless the condition is remedied by removing the obstruction (when present) and by artificial respiration if necessary, there is progressive *cyanosis leading to death. Brain cells cannot live for more than about four minutes without oxygen.

aspiration *n.* the withdrawal of fluid or cells from the body by means of suction using an instrument called an *aspirator*. There are various types of aspirators: some employ hollow needles for removing fluid from cysts, inflamed joint cavities, etc.; another kind is used to suck debris and water from the patient's mouth during dental treatment. *See also* fine-needle aspiration cytology.

aspiration cytology the *aspiration of specimens of cells from tumors or cysts through a hollow needle, using a syringe, and their subsequent examination under the microscope after suitable preparation (by staining, etc.). The technique is now used widely, especially for superficial cysts or tumors, and has become a specialized branch of diagnostic pathology. *See also* fine-needle aspiration cytology.

aspirin (acetylsalicylic acid) *n.* a widely used drug that relieves pain and also reduces inflammation and fever. It is taken by mouth – alone or in combination with other analgesics – for the relief of the less severe types of pain, such as headache, toothache, neuralgias, and the pain of rheumatoid arthritis. It is also taken to reduce fever in influenza and the common cold. Daily doses are used for the prevention of coronary thrombosis and strokes in those at risk, and it has been shown to have a protective effect against a range of other conditions, including cataracts, colorectal cancer, and Behçet's syndrome. Aspirin acts by inhibiting *prostaglandin synthesis; it may irritate the lining of the stomach, causing nausea, vomiting, pain, and bleeding. Tablets should not be held on the gum adjacent to a painful tooth because ulceration may occur. High doses cause dizziness, disturbed hearing, mental confusion, and overbreathing. Aspirin has been implicated as a cause of *Reye's syndrome and should therefore only be given to children below the age of 12 if specifically indicated. *See also* analgesic.

assay *n.* a test or trial to determine the strength of a solution, the proportion of a compound in a mixture, the potency of a drug, or the purity of a preparation. *See also* bioassay.

assimilation *n.* the process by which food substances are taken into the cells of the body after they have been digested and absorbed.

assistive listening device *see* environmental hearing aid.

association area an area of *cerebral cortex that lies away from the main areas that are concerned with the reception of sensory impulses and the start of motor impulses but is linked to them by many neurons known as *association fibers*. The areas of association are thought to be responsible for the elaboration of the information received by the primary sensory areas and its correlation with the information fed in from memory and from other brain areas. They are thus responsible for the maintenance of many higher mental activities. *See also* body image.

association of ideas (in psychology) linkage of one idea to another in a regular way according to their meaning. In *free association* the linkage of ideas arising in dreams or fantasy may be used to discover the underlying motives of the individual. In *word association tests*

stimulus words are produced to which the subject has to respond as quickly as possible.

AST *see* aspartate transaminase.

astasia *n.* an inability to stand for which no physical cause can be found. *Astasia-abasia* is an inability to stand or walk in the absence of any recognizable physical illness. The patient's attempts are bizarre and careful examination reveals contradictory features. It is most commonly an expression of *conversion disorder.

astemizole *n.* an H₁-receptor antagonist formerly used to treat hay fever and allergic skin conditions. It has been withdrawn in many countries because of interactions with other drugs and food, especially grapefruit juice, and potentially serious side effects.

aster *n.* a star-shaped object in a cell that surrounds the *centrosome during *mitosis and *meiosis and is concerned with the formation of the *spindle.

astereognosis *n. see* agnosia.

asteroid hyalosis a degenerative condition, formerly known as *asteroid hyalitis*, in which tiny deposits of calcium are suspended in the vitreous humor. They are more commonly seen in the elderly and usually cause no decrease in vision.

asthenia *n.* weakness or loss of strength.

asthenic *adj.* describing a personality disorder characterized by low energy, susceptibility to physical and emotional stress, and a diminished capacity for pleasure.

asthenopia *n. see* eyestrain.

asthma *n.* a condition characterized by widespread narrowing of the bronchial airways that leads to cough, wheezing, and difficulty in breathing. *Bronchial asthma* may be precipitated by exposure to one or more of a large range of stimuli, including *allergens, drugs (such as aspirin and other *NSAIDs and *beta blockers), exertion, emotions, air pollution, and infections. The first attacks can occur at any age but are normally in early life, when – in allergic people – they may be associated with other manifestations of hypersensitivity, such as eczema and hay fever. The usual treatment is with *bronchodilators, usually in the form of aerosol inhalers; corticosteroids are used to control severe asthmatic attacks, which may be very serious and prolonged (*see* status asthmaticus). Selection of treatment for individual cases is made using stepped guidelines issued by respiratory organizations, e.g. the American and British Thoracic Societies, the National Heart, Lung, and Blood Institute, and the American Association for Respiratory Care. Avoidance of known allergens, as well as *desensitization to them, may help to reduce the frequency of attacks, as will cessation of smoking. *Cardiac asthma* occurs in left ventricular *heart failure and must be distinguished from bronchial asthma, for which the treatment is different. —**asthmatic** *adj.*

astigmatism *n.* a defect of vision in which the image of an object is distorted, usually in either the vertical or the horizontal axis, because not all the light rays come to a focus on the retina. Some parts of the object may be in focus but light from other parts may be focused in front of or behind the retina. This is usually due to abnormal curvature of the cornea and/or lens (*see* refraction), whose surface resembles part of the surface of an egg (rather than a sphere). The defect can be corrected by wearing *cylindrical lenses*, which produce exactly the opposite degree of distortion and thus cancel out the distortion caused by the eye itself. —**astigmatic** *adj.*

astragalus *n. see* talus.

astringent *n.* a drug that causes cells to shrink by precipitating proteins from their surfaces. Astringents are used in lotions to harden and protect the skin and to reduce bleeding from minor abrasions. They are also used in mouth washes, throat lozenges, eye drops, etc., and in antiperspirants.

astrocyte (astroglial cell) *n.* a type of cell with numerous sheet-like processes extending from its cell body, found throughout the central nervous system. It is one of the several different types of cell that make up the *glia. The cells have been ascribed the function of providing nutrients for neurons and possibly of taking part in information storage processes.

astrocytoma *n.* a brain tumor derived from nonnervous cells (*glia), which – unlike the neurons – retain the ability to reproduce themselves by mitosis. All grades of malignancy occur, from slow-growing tumors whose histological structure re-

sembles normal glial cells, to rapidly growing highly invasive tumors whose cell structure is poorly differentiated (*see* glioblastoma). In adults astrocytomas are usually found in the cerebral hemispheres but in children they also occur in the cerebellum.

asymbolia *n. see* alexia.

asymmetric tonic neck reflex *see* tonic neck reflex.

asymptomatic *adj.* not showing any symptoms of disease, whether disease is present or not.

asynclitism *n.* the entry of the head of the baby at birth into the vagina at an oblique angle, which enables it to pass more easily through the maternal pelvis.

asyndesis *n.* a disorder of thought, in which the normal *association of ideas is disrupted so that thought and speech become fragmentary. It is a symptom of schizophrenia, dementia, or confusion.

asynergia *n. see* dyssynergia.

asystole *n.* a condition in which the heart no longer beats, accompanied by the absence of complexes in the electrocardiogram. The clinical features, causes, and treatment are those of *cardiac arrest.

ataraxia *n.* a state of calmness and freedom from anxiety, especially the state produced by tranquilizing drugs.

atavism *n.* the phenomenon in which an individual has a character or disease known to have occurred in a remote ancestor but not in his parents.

ataxia *n.* the shaky movements and unsteady gait that result from the brain's failure to regulate the body's posture and the strength and direction of limb movements. It may be due to disease of the sensory nerves or the *cerebellum. In *cerebellar ataxia* there is clumsiness of willed movements. The patient staggers when walking; he cannot pronounce words properly and may have *nystagmus. *Friedreich's ataxia* is an inherited disorder appearing first in adolescence. It has the features of cerebellar ataxia (*Nonne's syndrome*), together with spasticity of the limbs. The unsteady movements of *sensory ataxia* are exaggerated when the patient closes his eyes (*see* Romberg's sign). *See also* ataxia telangiectasia, tabes dorsalis (locomotor ataxia). —**ataxic** *adj.*

ataxia telangiectasia an inherited (autosomal *recessive) neurological disorder.

*Ataxia is usually noted early in life. Mental retardation, growth retardation, abnormal eye movements, skin lesions, and immune deficiency may be found. Affected individuals may develop malignant disease. A raised level of *alphafetoprotein is found in the blood, and a key feature is the presence of prominent blood vessels visible on the sclerae of the eyes.

ATCC *see* American Type Culture Collection.

atel- (atelo-) *prefix denoting* imperfect or incomplete development. Examples: *atelencephaly* (of the brain); *atelocardia* (of the heart).

atelectasis *n.* failure of part of the lung to expand. This occurs when the cells lining the air sacs (alveoli) are too immature, as in premature babies, or unable to produce the wetting agent (surfactant) with which the surface tension between the alveolar walls is overcome. It also occurs when the larger bronchial tubes are blocked from within by retained secretions, inhaled foreign bodies, or bronchial cancers, or from without by enlarged lymph nodes, such as are found in patients with tuberculosis and lung cancers. The lung can usually be helped to expand by physiotherapy and removal of the internal block (if present) with a *bronchoscope, but prolonged atelectasis becomes irreversible.

ateleiosis *n.* failure of sexual development owing to lack of pituitary hormones. *See* infantilism, dwarfism.

atenolol *n.* a drug (*see* beta blocker) used to treat angina and high blood pressure. It is administered by mouth or intravenous injection and the most common side effects are fatigue, depression, and digestive upsets. Trade names: **Tenoretic, Tenormin**.

atherectomy *n.* a technique for the treatment of atherosclerosis. A rotary blade mechanism is attached to a catheter and both are inserted into an artery occluded with *plaque, but with space enough to pass over the plaque. The rotating blade shaves off the plaque particles, which are then removed through the catheter.

atheroma *n.* degeneration of the walls of the arteries due to the formation in them of fatty plaques and scar tissue. This limits blood circulation and predisposes to thrombosis. It is common in adults in Western countries. A diet rich in animal fats (*see* cholesterol) and refined sugar, cigarette smoking, obesity, and inactivity are the principal causes. It may be symptomless but often causes complications from arterial obstruction in middle and later life (such as angina pectoris, heart attack, stroke, and gangrene). Treatment is by prevention, but some symptoms may be ameliorated by drug therapy (e.g. angina by nitroglycerin) or by surgical bypass of the arterial obstruction. —**atheromatous** *adj.*

atherosclerosis *n.* a disease of the arteries in which fatty plaques develop on their inner walls, with eventual obstruction of blood flow. *See* atheroma.

athetosis *n.* a writhing involuntary movement especially affecting the hands, face, and tongue. It is usually a form of *cerebral palsy. It impairs the child's ability to speak or use his hands; intelligence is often unaffected. Such movements may also be caused by drugs used to treat *parkinsonism or by the withdrawal of phenothiazines. *See also* tardive dyskinesia. —**athetotic** *adj.*

athlete's foot a fungus infection of the skin between the toes: a type of *ringworm. Medical name: **tinea pedis**.

athyreosis *n.* absence of or lack of function of the thyroid gland, causing *cretinism in infancy and *myxedema in adult life.

atlas *n.* the first *cervical vertebra, by means of which the skull is articulated to the backbone.

ATLS advanced trauma life support, which comprises the treatment programs for patients who have been subjected to major trauma (e.g. serious traffic accidents, natural disasters, or terrorist attacks). Doctors, nurses, and paramedical personnel involved in ATLS receive special training for dealing with such emergencies. *See also* EMS.

atony *n.* a state in which muscles are floppy, lacking their normal elasticity. —**atonic** *adj.*

atopen *n.* any substance responsible for *atopy.

atopy *n.* a form of *allergy in which there is a genetic predisposition to develop hypersensitivity reactions (e.g. hay fever, allergic asthma, or atopic *eczema) in response to allergens (*atopens*). Individuals with this predisposition – and the conditions provoked in them by contact with allergens – are described as *atopic*.

atorvastatin *n.* a drug used to reduce abnormally high levels of *cholesterol and other lipids in the blood (*see* statin). It is administered by mouth; side effects include insomnia, abdominal pain, flatulence, diarrhea, and nausea. Trade name: **Lipitor**.

ATP (adenosine triphosphate) a compound that contains adenine, ribose, and three phosphate groups and occurs in cells. The chemical bonds of the phosphate groups store energy needed by the cell, for muscle contraction; this energy is released when ATP is split into ADP or AMP. ATP is formed from ADP and AMP using energy produced by the breakdown of carbohydrates or other food substances. *See also* mitochondrion.

atresia *n.* **1.** congenital absence or abnormal narrowing of a body opening. *See* biliary atresia, duodenal atresia, tricuspid atresia. **2.** the degenerative process that affects the majority of ovarian follicles. Usually only one graafian follicle will ovulate in each menstrual cycle. —**atretic** *adj.*

atri- (atrio-) *prefix denoting* an atrium, especially the atrium of the heart. Example: *atrioventricular* (relating to the atria and ventricles of the heart).

atrial fibrillation *see* fibrillation.

atrial natriuretic peptide a protein hormone (of 28 amino acids) produced by the cells of the atria of the heart in response to a rise in atrial pressure. Its action is to cause a fall in blood pressure by dilating blood vessels and inducing increased water loss from the kidneys.

atrial septal defect (ASD) a congenital defect of the heart in which there is a hole in the partition (septum) separating the two atria (*see* septal defect). There are two kinds of ASD – *ostium primum* and *ostium secundum*. Ostium primum defects are rarer but more serious as the defect lies low down near the valves of the heart. Affected children often have heart failure, although in some a heart murmur detected at routine medical examinations is the only indication of the defect. Ostium secundum defects lie away from the valves and most children have no symptoms; the defect is most commonly indicated by the detection of

a heart murmur, and may not be apparent until adulthood. Small defects may close spontaneously. Moderate and large ostium secundum and all ostium primum defects require surgery.

Intrauterine surgical techniques now enable a fetus in which an ASD has been detected to proceed to full term by using the placental circulation as a substitute for the *extracorporeal circulation that would otherwise be required.

atrioventricular bundle (AV bundle, bundle of His) a bundle of modified heart muscle fibers (*Purkinje fibers*) passing from the *atrioventricular (AV) node forward to the septum between the ventricles, where it divides into right and left bundles, one for each ventricle. The fibers transmit contraction waves from the atria, via the AV node, to the ventricles.

atrioventricular node (AV node) a mass of modified heart muscle situated in the lower middle part of the right atrium. It receives the impulse to contract from the *sinoatrial node, via the atria, and transmits it through the *atrioventricular bundle to the ventricles.

atrium *n.* (*pl.* **atria**) **1.** either of the two upper chambers of the *heart. Their muscular walls are thinner than those of the ventricles; the left atrium receives oxygenated blood from the lungs via the pulmonary vein; the right atrium receives deoxygenated blood from the venae cavae. *See also* auricle. **2.** any of various anatomical chambers into which one or more cavities open. —**atrial** *adj.*

atrophy *n.* the wasting away of a normally developed organ or tissue due to degeneration of cells. This may occur through undernourishment, disuse, or aging. Forms of atrophy peculiar to women include the shrinking of the ovary at the menopause and of the *corpus luteum during the menstrual cycle. *Muscular atrophy* is associated with various diseases, such as poliomyelitis.

atropine *n.* an *anticholinergic drug that occurs in deadly nightshade (*see* belladonna). Atropine relaxes smooth muscle and is used to treat biliary colic and renal colic. It also reduces secretions of the bronchial tubes, salivary glands, stomach, and intestines and is used before general *anesthesia and to relieve peptic ulcers. It is also used to dilate the pupil of the eye (*see* mydriatic). Atropine is administered by mouth, injection, or as eye drops; common side effects include dryness of the throat, thirst, and impaired vision. Trade names: **Isopto Atropine**, **Minims Atropine**.

attachment *n.* (in psychology) the process of developing the first close selective relationship of a child's life, most commonly with the mother. The relationship acts to reduce anxiety in strange settings and forms a base from which children develop further relationships.

attachment disorder a psychiatric disorder in infants and young children that results from *institutionalization, emotional neglect, or *child abuse. Affected children are either withdrawn, aggressive, and fearful or attention-seeking and indiscriminately friendly. Treatment requires the provision of stable caring adults as parents over a long period of time.

attention-deficit/hyperactivity disorder (ADHD, hyperkinetic syndrome, hyperactive child syndrome) a mental disorder, usually of children, characterized by a grossly excessive level of activity and a marked impairment of the ability to attend. Learning is impaired as a result, and behavior is disruptive and may be defiant or aggressive. The disorder is more common in the intellectually subnormal, the epileptic, and the brain-damaged. Treatment usually involves drugs (such as amphetamines and *methylphenidate) and behavior therapy; the family needs advice and practical help.

attenuation *n.* reduction of the disease-producing ability (virulence) of a bacterium or virus by chemical treatment, heating, drying, by growing under adverse conditions, or by passing through another organism. Treated (*attenuated*) bacteria or viruses are used for many *immunizations.

atticotomy *n.* a surgical operation to remove *cholesteatoma from the ear. It is a form of limited *mastoidectomy.

attrition *n.* (in dentistry) the wearing of tooth surfaces by the action of opposing teeth. A small amount of attrition occurs with age but accelerated wear may occur in *bruxism and with certain diets.

atypical antipsychotics *see* antipsychotic.

atypical facial pain a *neuralgia that has no known cause and is typified by pain in the face that does not fit the distribution of nerves. It may be stress-related, and in some cases appears to be associated with defective metabolism of *tyramine. Treatment may involve the use of antidepressants.

atypical mole syndrome (dysplastic nevus syndrome) a condition in which affected patients have numerous moles, some of which are relatively large and irregular in shape or pigmentation. There may be a family history of this syndrome or of malignant *melanoma.

atypical pneumonia any of a group of community-acquired *pneumonias that do not respond to penicillin but do respond to such antibiotics as tetracycline and erythromycin. They include infection with *Mycoplasma pneumoniae*, *Chlamydia psittaci* (*see* psittacosis), and *Coxiella burnetii* (*see* Q fever).

audi- (audio-) *prefix denoting* hearing or sound.

audiogram *n.* the graphic record of a test of hearing carried out on an audiometer.

audiology *n.* the study of disorders of hearing.

audiometer *n.* an apparatus for measuring hearing at different sound frequencies, so helping in the diagnosis of deafness. —**audiometry** *n.*

audit *n. see* medical audit.

auditory *adj.* relating to the ear or to the sense of hearing.

auditory canal (auditory meatus) the canal leading from the pinna to the eardrum.

auditory nerve *see* vestibulocochlear nerve.

auditory verbal therapy (AVT) a technique for teaching deaf children to communicate that focuses on speech and residual hearing rather than sign language.

Auerbach's plexus (myenteric plexus) a collection of nerve fibers – fine branches of the *vagus nerve – within the walls of the intestine. It supplies the muscle layers and controls the movements of *peristalsis. [L. Auerbach (1828–97), German anatomist]

AUR acute urinary retention (*see* retention).

aura *n.* a sensation that forewarns of an attack of a neurological condition. An *epileptic aura* takes many forms, including the feeling of a breeze, coldness passing over the body, or an odd smell or taste. The *migrainous aura* usually affects the patient's eyesight with brilliant flickering lights or blurring of vision, but it may also result in pins and needles or numbness or weakness of the limbs.

aural *adj.* relating to the ear.

auranofin *n.* a *gold preparation administered by mouth to treat rheumatoid arthritis. Side effects include nausea, abdominal pain, diarrhea, rash, and mouth ulcers. Trade name: **Ridaura**.

Aureomycin *n. see* chlortetracycline.

auricle *n.* **1.** a small pouch in the wall of each *atrium of the heart: the term is also used incorrectly as a synonym for *atrium*. **2.** *see* pinna.

auriscope *n. see* otoscope.

auscultation *n.* the process of listening, usually with the aid of a *stethoscope, to sounds produced by movement of gas or liquid within the body. Auscultation is an aid to diagnosis of abnormalities of the heart, lungs, intestines, and other organs according to the characteristic changes in sound pattern caused by different disease processes. —**auscultatory** *adj.*

auscultatory gap a silent period in the knocking sounds heard with a stethoscope over an artery, between the systolic and diastolic blood pressures, when the blood pressure is measured with a *sphygmomanometer.

Australia antigen another name for the *hepatitis B antigen, which was first discovered in the blood of an Australian aborigine. This disease is due to a virus of which the Australia antigen forms part.

aut- (auto-) *prefix denoting* self. Example: *autokinesis* (voluntary movement).

autism *n.* **1. (Kanner's syndrome, infantile autism)** a rare and severe psychiatric disorder of childhood, with an onset before the age of 2½ years. It is marked by severe difficulties in communicating and forming relationships with other people, in developing language, and in using abstract concepts; repetitive and limited patterns of behavior (*see* stereotypy); and obsessive resistance to tiny changes in familiar surroundings. Autistic children find it hard to understand how other people feel, and so tend to remain isolated even into adult life. Many have learning difficulties, but some are very intelligent and may even be gifted in specific areas (*see* idiot savant). The cause is unknown, but genetic factors and brain damage are probably important. The condition often progresses into adulthood, and independent living is uncommon. Treatment is not specific, but lengthy specialized education is usually necessary. Behavior problems and anxiety can be controlled with behavior therapy and drugs (such as *phenothiazines). **2.** the condition of retreating from realistic thinking to self-centered fantasy thinking. This is a symptom of personality disorder and schizophrenia. —**autistic** *adj.*

autoagglutination *n.* the clumping together of the body's own red blood cells by antibodies produced against them, which occurs in acquired hemolytic anemia (an *autoimmune disease).

autoantibody *n.* an antibody formed against one of the body's own components in an *autoimmune disease.

autochthonous *adj.* **1.** remaining at the site of formation. A blood clot that has not been carried in the bloodstream from its point of origin is described as autochthonous. **2.** originating in an organ without external stimulus, like the beating of the heart.

autoclave 1. *n.* a piece of equipment for sterilizing surgical instruments, dressings, etc. It consists of a chamber, similar to a domestic pressure cooker, in which the articles are placed and treated with steam at high pressure. **2.** *vb.* to sterilize in an autoclave.

autocrine *adj.* describing the production by a cell of substances, such as hormones or *growth factors, that can influence the growth of the cell that produces them.

autogenous *adj.* originating within the body of the patient. For example, an autogenous vein graft, to bypass a blocked artery, is made from material derived from the body of the patient receiving the graft.

autogenous vaccine *see* autovaccine.

autograft *n.* a tissue graft taken from one part of the body and transferred to another part of the same individual. The repair of burns is often done by grafting on strips of skin taken from elsewhere on the body, usually the upper arm or thigh. Unlike *allografts, autografts are not rejected by the body's immunity defenses. *See also* skin graft, transplantation.

autoimmune disease one of the growing number of otherwise unrelated disorders now usually accepted as being caused by inflammation and destruction of tissues by the body's own *immune response. These disorders include acquired hemolytic anemia, pernicious anemia, rheumatic fever, rheumatoid arthritis, glomerulonephritis, systemic lupus erythematosus, myasthenia gravis, Sjögren's syndrome, and several forms of thyroid dysfunction, among them Hashimoto's disease. It is not known why the body should lose the ability to distinguish between substances that are "self" and those that are "non-self."

autoimmunity n. a disorder of the body's defense mechanisms in which an immune response is generated against certain components or products of its own tissues, treating them as foreign material and attacking them. See autoimmune disease, immunity.

autoinoculation n. the accidental transfer of inoculated material from one site in the body to another. Following vaccination, for example, satellite lesions may occur around the site of inoculation.

autointoxication n. poisoning by a toxin formed within the body.

autologous adj. denoting a graft that is derived from the recipient of the graft.

autolysis n. the destruction of tissues or cells brought about by the actions of their own enzymes. See lysosome.

automated lamellar keratectomy (ALK) excision of the outer layers of the cornea using an automated *keratome. It is usually used as part of a surgical procedure, to alter the shape of the cornea to correct errors of refraction.

automated perimeter see perimeter.

automatism n. behavior that may be associated with an epileptic seizure, in which the patient performs well-organized movements or tasks without conscious knowledge of doing so. These movements may be simple and repetitive, such as hand clapping or lip smacking, or they may be so complex as to mimic a person's normal conscious activities.

autonomic nervous system (ANS) the part of the *peripheral nervous system responsible for the control of involuntary muscles (e.g. the heart, bladder, bowels) and thus those bodily functions that are not consciously directed, including regular beating of the heart, intestinal movements, sweating, salivation, etc.

The autonomic system is subdivided into *sympathetic* and *parasympathetic nervous systems*. Sympathetic nerves lead from the middle section of the spinal cord and parasympathetic nerves from the brain and lower spinal cord. The heart, smooth muscles, and most glands receive fibers of both kinds: the interplay of sympathetic and parasympathetic reflex activity (the actions are often antagonistic) governs their working. For example, the parasympathetic system is responsible for slowing the heart rate and constricting the pupillary muscles; the sympathetic system increases the heart rate and dilates the pupil. Sympathetic nerve endings liberate *norepinephrine as a neurotransmitter, while parasympathetic nerve endings release *acetylcholine.

autoploidy n. the normal condition in cells or individuals, in which each cell has a chromosome set consisting of *homologous pairs, enabling cells to divide normally. —**autoploid** adj., n.

autopsy (necropsy, postmortem) n. dissection and examination of a body after death in order to determine the cause of death or the presence of disease processes.

autoradiography (radioautography) n. a technique for examining the distribution of a radioactive *tracer in the tissues of an experimental animal. The tracer is injected into the animal, which is killed after a certain period. Thin sections of its organs are placed in close contact with a radiation-sensitive material, such as a photographic emulsion, and observed under a microscope. Blackening of the film indicates a high concentration of radioactive material.

autorefractor n. see optometer.

autoscopy n. the experience of seeing one's whole body as though from a vantage point some distance away. It can be a symptom in *epilepsy. See also out-of-the-body experience.

autosomal dominant see dominant.

autosomal recessive see recessive.

autosome n. any chromosome that is not a *sex chromosome and occurs in pairs in diploid cells. —**autosomal** adj.

autosuggestion n. self-suggestion or self-conditioning that involves repeating ideas to oneself in order to change physiological or psychological states. Autosuggestion is used primarily in *autogenic training*, a technique used to help patients control their anxiety or their habits. *See* suggestion.

autotransfusion *n.* reintroduction into a patient of his or her own blood. This may be blood previously drawn and stored in the blood bank or blood that has been lost from the patient's circulation during surgical operation. The blood is collected by suction during the operation, filtered to remove bubbles and small blood clots, and returned into one of the patient's veins through a drip.

autotrophic (lithotrophic) *adj.* describing organisms (known as *autotrophs*) that synthesize their organic materials from carbon dioxide and nitrates or ammonium compounds, using an external source of energy. *Photoautotrophic* organisms, including green plants and some bacteria, derive their energy from sunlight; *chemoautotrophic (chemosynthetic)* organisms obtain energy from inorganic chemical reactions. All autotrophic bacteria are nonparasitic. *Compare* heterotrophic.

autovaccination *n.* the use of an *autovaccine.

autovaccine (autogenous vaccine) *n.* a *vaccine prepared from cultures of organisms isolated from a patient's own tissues or secretions, which is then reinjected into the patient to stimulate resistance to the infection.

aux- (auxo-) *prefix denoting* increase; growth. Example: *auxocardia* (enlargement of the heart).

auxiliaries persons who volunteer to assist and do complementary tasks at hospitals or clinical settings. Teenage girls who work as auxiliaries are sometimes identified as "candy stripers" because of the colorful striped uniforms they wear.

auxotroph *n.* a strain of a microorganism, derived by mutation, that requires one or more specific factors for growth not needed by the parent organism.

avascular *adj.* lacking blood vessels or having a poor blood supply. The term is usually used with reference to cartilage.

Avastin *n. see* angiogenesis inhibitor.

AV bundle *see* atrioventricular bundle.

Average Length of Stay (ALOS) (in hospital administration) the average number of days of care per patient. It is calculated by dividing the number of days of inpatient care by the number of admissions for a given period.

aversion therapy a form of *behavior therapy that is used to reduce the occurrence of undesirable behavior, such as sexual deviations or drug addiction. *Conditioning is used, with repeated pairing of some unpleasant stimulus with a stimulus related to the undesirable behavior. An example is pairing the taste of beer with electric shock in the treatment of alcoholism. Aversion therapy is little used today. *See also* sensitization.

avitaminosis *n.* the condition caused by lack of a vitamin. *See also* deficiency disease.

AVM arteriovenous malformation (*see* angioma).

AV node *see* atrioventricular node.

avoidant *adj.* describing a personality type characterized by self-consciousness, hypersensitivity to rejection and criticism from others, avoidance of normal situations because of their potential risk, high levels of tension and anxiety, and consequently a restricted life.

AVPU a system for assessing the depth of unconsciousness: A = alert; V = voice responses present; P = pain responses present; U = unresponsive. It is useful for judging the severity of head injury and the need for specialized neurosurgical assistance. *See also* Glasgow Coma Scale.

AVT *see* auditory verbal therapy.

avulsion (evulsion) *n.* **1.** the tearing or forcible separation of part of a structure. For example, a tendon may be torn from the bone to which it attaches or the skin of the scalp may be torn from the underlying tissue and bone. **2.** (in dentistry) the knocking out of a tooth by trauma. The tooth may be reimplanted (*see* replantation).

axilla *n.* (*pl.* **axillae**) the armpit. —**axillary** *adj.*

axis *n.* **1.** a real or imaginary line through the center of the body or one of its parts or a line about which the body or a part rotates. **2.** the second *cervical vertebra, which articulates with the atlas vertebra above and allows rotational movement of the head.

axolemma *n.* the fine cell membrane, visible only under the electron microscope, that encloses the protoplasm of an *axon.

axon *n.* a nerve fiber: a single process extending from the cell body of a *neuron and carrying nerve impulses away from it. An axon may be over a meter in length in certain neurons. In large nerves the axon has a sheath (*neurilemma*) made of *myelin; this is interrupted at intervals by gaps called *nodes of Ranvier*, at which branches of the axon leave. An axon ends by dividing into several branches called *telodendria*, which make contact with other nerves or with muscle or gland membranes.

axonotmesis *n.* rupture of nerve fibers (axons) within an intact nerve sheath. This may result from prolonged pressure or crushing and it is followed by degeneration of the nerve beyond the point of rupture. The prognosis for *nerve regeneration is good. *Compare* neurapraxia, neurotmesis.

axoplasm *n.* the semifluid material of which the *axon of a nerve cell is composed. It flows slowly outward from the cell body.

azatadine *n.* an *antihistamine drug used to treat hay fever, urticaria, itching, and stings. It is administered by mouth. Possible side effects include drowsiness, headache, nausea, and loss of appetite. Trade names: **Optimine, Trinalin**.

azathioprine *n.* an *immunosuppressant drug, used mainly to prevent rejection after organ or tissue transplants. It has also been used in the treatment of inflammatory bowel disease (e.g. ulcerative colitis), rheumatoid arthritis, and myasthenia gravis. Azathioprine may damage bone marrow, causing blood disorders. It may also cause muscle wasting and skin rashes. Trade names: **Azasan, Imuran**.

azelaic acid an antibacterial drug applied externally as a cream in the treatment of acne. Possible side effects include local irritation and light sensitivity. Trade names: **Azelex, Finevin**.

azelastine *n.* an *antihistamine drug administered as a metered-dose nasal spray for the treatment of hay fever and as eye drops to treat allergic conjunctivitis. Possible side effects include nasal irritation and disturbances of taste sensation. Trade names: **Astelin, Optivar**.

azithromycin *n.* an *antibiotic used to treat respiratory, skin, soft-tissue, and other infections, especially those caused by the organism *Chlamydia trachomatis*. It is administered by mouth. Possible side effects include allergic reactions, nausea, and vomiting. Trade name: **Zithromax**.

azlocillin *n.* a penicillin-type antibiotic that is used especially to treat infections caused by *Pseudomonas aeruginosa*. It is administered by intravenous infusion; possible side effects include allergic reactions, nausea, and vomiting. Trade name: **Azlin**.

azo- (azoto-) *prefix denoting* a nitrogenous compound, such as urea. Example: *azothermia* (fever due to nitrogenous substances in the blood).

azoospermia *n.* the complete absence of sperm from the seminal fluid. This is due either to failure of formation of sperm by the seminiferous tubules within the testes or to a blockage in the ducts that conduct sperm from the testes. A biopsy of the testis is necessary to differentiate these two causes of azoospermia; if a blockage is present it may be possible to relieve it surgically (*see* epididymovasostomy). *See also* aspermia.

azotemia *n.* a former name for *uremia.

azoturia *n.* the presence in the urine of an abnormally high concentration of nitrogen-containing compounds, especially urea.

AZT *see* zidovudine.

aztreonam *n.* an antibiotic administered by injection used to treat infections of the lungs, bones, skin, and soft tissues caused by gram-negative organisms (*see* Gram's stain). It is especially useful for treating lung infections in children with cystic fibrosis. Possible side effects include skin rashes, diarrhea, and vomiting. Trade name: **Azactam**.

azygos vein an unpaired vein that arises from the inferior vena cava and drains into the superior vena cava, returning blood from the thorax and abdominal cavities.

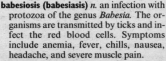

B

babesiosis (babesiasis) *n.* an infection with protozoa of the genus *Babesia*. The organisms are transmitted by ticks and infect the red blood cells. Symptoms include anemia, fever, chills, nausea, headache, and severe muscle pain.

Babinski reflex *see* plantar reflex. [J. F. F. Babinski (1857–1932), French neurologist]

bacille Calmette-Guérin *see* BCG. [A. L. C. Calmette (1863–1933) and C. Guérin (1872–1961), French bacteriologists]

bacillemia *n.* the presence of bacilli in the blood, resulting from infection.

bacilluria *n.* the presence of bacilli in the urine, resulting from a bladder or kidney infection. *See* cystitis.

bacillus *n.* (*pl.* **bacilli**) any rod-shaped bacterium. *See also* Bacillus, Lactobacillus, Streptobacillus.

Bacillus *n.* a large genus of gram-positive spore-bearing rodlike bacteria. They are widely distributed in soil and air (usually as spores). Most feed on dead organic material and are responsible for food spoilage. The species *B. anthracis*, which is nonmotile, causes *anthrax, a disease of farm animals transmissible to humans. *B. polymyxa*, commonly found in soil, is the source of the polymyxin group of antibiotics. *B. subtilis* may cause conjunctivitis in humans; it also produces the antibiotic *bacitracin.

bacitracin *n.* an antibiotic produced by certain strains of bacteria and effective against a number of microorganisms. Combined with other antibiotics, it is applied externally to treat infections of the skin and eyes. Trade names: **Baciguent, Neosporin, Polysporin.**

backbone (spinal column, spine, vertebral column) *n.* a flexible bony column extending from the base of the skull to the end of the trunk. It encloses and protects the spinal cord, articulates with the skull, ribs, and hip girdle, and provides attachment for the muscles of the back. It is made up of individual bones (*see* vertebra) that are connected by disks of fibrocartilage (*see* intervertebral disk) and bound together by ligaments. The backbone of a newborn baby contains 33 vertebrae: seven cervical (neck), 12 thoracic (chest), five lumbar (lower back), five sacral (hip), and four coccygeal. In the adult the sacral and coccygeal vertebrae become fused into two single bones (sacrum and coccyx, respectively); the adult vertebral column therefore contains 26 bones (see illustration). Anatomical name: **rachis.**

baclofen *n.* a skeletal *muscle relaxant drug administered orally or intrathecally to relieve spasm resulting from injury or disease of the brain or spinal cord, including cerebral palsy and multiple scle-

rosis. It may also be used in some cases of trigeminal neuralgia. Most common side effects are drowsiness, weakness, nausea, and vomiting. Trade name: **Lioresal.**

bacteremia *n.* the presence of bacteria in the blood: a sign of infection.

bacteri- (bacterio-) *prefix denoting* bacteria. Example: *bacteriolysis* (dissolution of).

bacteria *pl. n.* (*sing.* **bacterium**) a group of microorganisms all of which lack a distinct nuclear membrane (and hence are considered more primitive than animal and plant cells) and most of which have a cell wall of unique composition (many antibiotics act by destroying the bacterial cell wall). Most bacteria are unicellular; the cells may be spherical (*coccus), rod-shaped (*bacillus), comma-shaped (*Vibrio*), spiral (*Spirillum*), or corkscrew-shaped (*spirochete). Generally, they range in size between 0.5 and 5 μm. Motile species bear one or more fine hairs (flagella) arising from their surfaces. Many possess an outer slimy

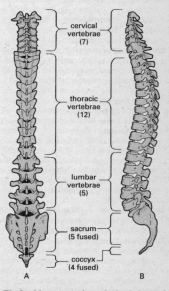

cervical vertebrae (7)

thoracic vertebrae (12)

lumbar vertebrae (5)

sacrum (5 fused)

coccyx (4 fused)

A   B

The backbone, seen from the back (A) and left side (B)

*capsule, and some have the ability to produce an encysted or resting form (*endospore). Bacteria reproduce asexually by simple division of cells; incomplete separation of daughter cells leads to the formation of *colonies of different numbers and arrangements of cells. Some colonies are filamentous in shape, resembling those of fungi. Transfer of DNA from one bacterium to another takes place in the process of *conjugation.

Bacteria are widely distributed. Some live in soil, water, or air, while others are parasites of humans, animals, and plants. Many parasitic bacteria do not harm their hosts; some cause diseases by producing poisons (*see* endotoxin, exotoxin).

bacterial arthritis *see* septic arthritis.

bacterial endocarditis *see* endocarditis.

bactericidal *adj.* being capable of killing bacteria. Substances with this property include antibiotics, antiseptics, and disinfectants; they are known as *bactericides. Compare* bacteriostatic.

bacteriology *n.* the science concerned with the study of bacteria. Bacteriology is a branch of *microbiology. —**bacteriological** *adj.* —**bacteriologist** *n.*

bacteriolysin *n. see* lysin.

bacteriophage (phage) *n.* a virus that attacks bacteria. In general, a phage consists of a head, tail, and tail fibers, all composed of protein molecules, and a core of DNA. The tail and tail fibers are responsible for attachment to the bacterial surface and for injection of the DNA core into the host cell. The phage grows and replicates in the bacterial cell, which is eventually destroyed with the release of new phages. Each phage acts specifically against a particular species of bacterium. This is utilized in *phage typing*, a technique of identifying bacteria by the action of known phages on them. *See also* lysogeny.

bacteriostatic *adj.* capable of inhibiting or retarding the growth and multiplication of bacteria. *Compare* bactericidal.

bacterium *n. see* bacteria.

Bacteroides *n.* a genus of gram-negative, mostly nonmotile, anaerobic rodlike bacteria. They are normally present in the alimentary and urogenital tracts of mammals and are found in the mouth, particularly in dental plaque associated with periodontal disease. Some species have been classified into new genera, *Porphyromonas* and *Prevotella.*

bagassosis *n.* a form of external allergic *alveolitis caused by exposure to the dust of bagasse, the waste product of sugar cane after the sugar has been extracted. It causes *dyspnea, irritant cough, fever, and malaise, especially in the evening after exposure during the day.

Baghdad boil *see* oriental sore.

Baker's cyst a cyst that occurs behind the knee, either originating from a naturally occurring bursa or resulting from a rupture or herniation of the synovial membrane from a knee joint affected by osteoarthritis. [W. M. Baker (1839–96), British surgeon]

BAL 1. *see* bronchoalveolar lavage. **2.** British antilewisite (*see* dimercaprol).

balance *n.* **1.** a state of equilibrium among body constituents, such as *acid-base balance. **2.** the ability to control and maintain the center of the body mass within the support base of the feet. Balance requires visual, vestibular, and somatosensory senses for postural orientation and the appropriate movements to control the motion of the body. Many neurological diseases and disorders of the inner ear result in an imbalance.

balanced salt solution (BSS) a solution made to a physiological pH and having physiological concentrations of salts, including sodium, potassium, calcium, magnesium, and chloride. Such fluids are used during intraocular surgery and to replace intraocular fluids.

balanitis *n.* inflammation of the glans penis, usually associated with tightness of the foreskin (*phimosis). It is more common in childhood than in adult life. An acute attack is associated with redness and swelling of the glans. Treatment is by antibiotics, and further attacks are prevented by *circumcision. In *Zoon's plasma cell balanitis* persistent shiny red patches develop on the glans; the cause is unknown. *Balanitis xerotica obliterans* is an autoimmune condition characterized by ivory-white patches on the glans.

balanoposthitis *n.* inflammation of the foreskin and the surface of the underlying glans penis. It usually occurs as a consequence of *phimosis and represents a more extensive local reaction than simple *balanitis. The affected areas become red and swollen, which further narrows the opening of the foreskin and makes passing urine difficult and painful. Treatment of an acute attack is by administration of antibiotics, and further attacks are prevented by *circumcision.

balantidiasis *n.* an infestation of the large intestine with the parasitic protozoan *Balantidium coli*. Humans usually become infected by ingesting food or drink contaminated with cysts from the feces of a pig. The parasite invades and destroys the intestinal wall, causing ulceration and *necrosis, and the patient may experience diarrhea and dysentery. Balantidiasis is a rare cause of dysentery, mainly affecting farm workers; it can be treated with various antibiotics.

Balantidium *n.* a genus of one of the largest parasitic *protozoans affecting humans (70 μm or more in length). The oval body is covered with threadlike cilia (for locomotion). *B. coli*, normally living in the gut of pigs as a harmless *commensal, occasionally infects humans (*see* balantidiasis).

baldness *n. see* alopecia.

ball-and-cage valve (ball valve, caged-ball valve) any of a variety of prosthetic devices, consisting of a ball within a retaining cage, commonly used for replacing damaged heart valves.

ball-and-socket joint *see* enarthrosis.

ballistocardiograph *n.* an instrument for recording the displacement of the whole body produced by the ejection of blood with each heartbeat. The normal record produced by such an instrument (*ballistocardiogram*) may be altered by disease of the heart or aortic valve (*see* aortic regurgitation, aortic stenosis).

balloon *n.* an inflatable plastic cylinder of variable size that is mounted on a thin tube and used for dilating narrow areas in blood vessels (*see* coronary angioplasty) or in the alimentary tract (*strictures).

ballottement *n.* the technique of examining a fluid-filled part of the body to detect a floating object. During pregnancy, a sharp tap with the fingers, applied to the uterus through the abdominal wall or the vagina, causes the fetus to move away and then return to impart an answering tap to the examiner's hand as it floats back to its original position. This confirms that swelling of the uterus is due to a fetus rather than a tumor or other abnormality.

balneotherapy *n.* the treatment of disease by bathing, usually in the mineral-rich waters of hot springs. The once fashionable "water cures," taken at spas, certainly had a more psychological than physical effect. Today, specialized remedial treatment in baths, under the supervision of physiotherapists, is used to alleviate pain and improve blood circulation and limb mobility in arthritis and in nerve and muscle disorders.

bandage *n.* a piece of material, in the form of a pad or strip, applied to a wound or used to bind around an injured or diseased part of the body.

band keratopathy the deposition of calcium in the superficial layers of the cornea, usually as a horizontal band starting peripherally and moving centrally. It is associated with chronic eye disease, e.g. chronic *uveitis.

Bandl's ring *see* retraction ring. [L. Bandl (1842–92), German obstetrician]

Banti's syndrome a disorder in which enlargement and overactivity of the spleen occurs as a result of increased pressure within the splenic vein. The most common cause is *cirrhosis of the liver. [G. Banti (1852–1925), Italian pathologist]

barbiturate *n.* any of a group of drugs, derived from barbituric acid, that depress activity of the central nervous system and were formerly used as sedatives and hypnotics. They are classified into three groups according to their duration of action – short, medium, and long. Because they produce *tolerance and psychological and physical *dependence, have serious toxic side effects (*see* barbiturism), and can be fatal following large overdosage, barbiturates have been largely replaced in clinical use by safer drugs. The main exception is the short-acting drug *thiopental used to induce anesthesia. *See also* amobarbital, butabarbital, phenobarbital.

barbiturism *n.* addiction to drugs of the barbiturate group. Signs of intoxication include confusion, slurring of speech, yawning, sleepiness, loss of memory, loss of balance, and reduction in muscular reflexes. Withdrawal of the drugs must be undertaken slowly, over 1–3 weeks, to avoid the withdrawal symptoms of tremors and convulsions, which can prove fatal.

bariatrics *n.* the field of medicine concerned with the study of obesity – its causes, prevention, and treatment.

baritosis *n.* a lung disease – a form of *pneumoconiosis – caused by inhaling barium dust. It gives dramatic shadows on chest X-rays but no respiratory disability.

barium enema a technique for examination of the large intestine. A tube is inserted into the rectum through the anus, and barium sulfate is run into the intestine to the cecum. For *double contrast, gas is then pumped through the tube to distend the colon. A series of radiographs is then taken, usually on a tilting table with the patient in a lying and standing position. Barium enema is used mainly to identify tumors, polyps, and diverticular disease and to see the extent of mucosal damage in *inflammatory bowel disease. Its role has been partially taken over by endoscopy.

barium meal a technique for examining the esophagus, stomach, and duodenum. The patient swallows barium sulfate to coat the lining of the organs. Granules that produce gas to distend the stomach may be given to produce a *double-contrast effect. A series of X-rays is taken. A barium meal can be used to diagnose tumors, gastric and duodenal ulcers, hiatus *hernia, and *gastroesophageal reflux disease. Many indications for this examination have been replaced by the use of endoscopy.

barium sulfate a barium salt, insoluble in water, that is opaque to X-rays and is used as a contrast medium in radiography of the gastrointestinal tract (*see* barium enema, barium meal). *See also* enema.

Barlow maneuver (Ortolani's sign) a test for *congenital dislocation of the hip that detects whether or not a hip can be readily dislocated. With the baby lying supine and the pelvis steadied with one hand, the hip being tested is gently *adducted and backward pressure is applied to the head of the femur. If the hip is dislocatable, a clunk will be felt and sometimes heard. If the hip is gently *abducted, it will usually relocate. [T. Barlow (1845–1945), British physician]

BARN bilateral *acute retinal necrosis.

baroreceptor (baroceptor) *n.* a collection of sensory nerve endings specialized to monitor changes in blood pressure. The main receptors lie in the *carotid sinuses and the *aortic arch; others are found in the walls of other large arteries and veins and some within the walls of the heart. Impulses from the receptors reach centers in the medulla; from here autonomic activity is directed so that the heart rate and resistance of the peripheral blood vessels can be adjusted appropriately.

barotitis *n.* discomfort in the ears due to changing air pressure during air travel or while in a rapidly moving elevator. *Barotitis media* (*aerotitis media*) is acute or chronic inflammation of the middle ear caused by changing air pressure.

barotrauma *n.* damage to the middle ear, paranasal sinuses, or *eustachian tube due to changes in ambient pressure associated with air travel or deep-sea diving.

Barr body *see* sex chromatin. [M. L. Barr (1908–95), Canadian anatomist]

Barrett's esophagus a condition in which the normal squamous *epithelium lining the esophagus is replaced by columnar epithelium because of damage caused by *gastroesophageal reflux or (occasionally) corrosive esophagitis. The condition may be associated with an ulcer (*Barrett's ulcer*), and the epithelium has an abnormally high likelihood of undergoing malignant change. [N. R. Barrett (1903–79), British surgeon]

barrier cream a preparation used to protect the skin against water-soluble irritants (e.g. detergents, breakdown products of urine). Usually applied in the form of a cream or ointment and often containing a silicone, barrier creams are useful in the alleviation of various skin disorders, including diaper rash and bedsores.

bartholinitis *n.* inflammation of the mucus-secreting glands alongside the vaginal opening (*Bartholin's glands). In *chronic bartholinitis* cysts may form in the glands. In *acute bartholinitis* the glands are blocked and an abscess develops.

Bartholin's glands (greater vestibular glands) a pair of glands that open at the junction of the vagina and the external genitalia (vulva). Their secretions lubricate the vulva and so assist penetration by the penis during coitus. The *lesser vestibular glands*, around the vaginal opening, perform the same function. [C. Bartholin (1655–1748), Danish anatomist]

Bartonella *n.* a genus of parasitic rod-shaped or rounded microorganisms, usually regarded as *rickettsiae. They occur in the red blood cells and cells of the lymphatic system, spleen, liver, and kidneys. *B. bacilliformis* causes *bartonellosis in humans.

bartonellosis *n.* an infectious disease, confined to high river valleys in Peru, Ecuador, and Colombia, caused by *Bartonella bacilliformis*. The parasite, present in red blood cells and cells of the lymphatic system, is transmitted to humans by sandflies. There are two clinical stages of the disease: *Oroya fever* (*Carrion's disease*), whose symptoms include fever, anemia, and enlargement of the liver, spleen, and lymph nodes; and *verruga peruana*, characterized by wartlike eruptions on the skin that can bleed easily and ulcerate. Oroya fever accounts for nearly all fatalities. Bartonellosis can be treated successfully with penicillin and other antibiotics, and blood transfusions may be given in order to relieve the anemia.

Bartter's syndrome an inherited condition of the kidney, which causes abnormalities in the excretion and reabsorption of salts from the blood. This results in lowered levels of potassium and chloride and an increased level of calcium. The baby fails to grow properly and becomes progressively weaker and dehydrated. Treatment consists of correcting the salt imbalance with appropriate supplements. [F. C. Bartter (1914–83), US physician]

basal cell carcinoma (BCC) the most common form of skin cancer, which grows very slowly. BCC usually occurs on the central area of the face, especially in fair-skinned people; the prevalence increases greatly with exposure to sunlight. The initial sign is a spot or lump that fails to heal, enlarging to a diameter of 1 cm over five years or so. Treatment is with *curettage and cautery, surgical excision, *cryotherapy, or *radiotherapy. Only if

neglected for decades does a BCC eventually become a so-called *rodent ulcer* and destroy the surrounding tissue. However, the term "rodent ulcer" is still sometimes used to mean any basal cell carcinoma.

basal ganglia several large masses of gray matter embedded deep within the white matter of the *cerebrum (see illustration). They include the *caudate* and *lenticular* (or *lentiform*) *nuclei* (together known as the *corpus striatum*) and the *amygdaloid nucleus*. The lenticular nucleus consists of the *putamen* and *globus pallidus*. The basal ganglia have complex neural connections with both the cerebral cortex and thalamus: they are involved with the regulation of voluntary movements at a subconscious level.

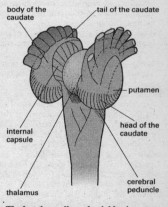

The basal ganglia and neighboring parts (seen from the front)

basal metabolism the minimum amount of energy expended by the body to maintain vital processes, e.g. respiration, circulation, and digestion. It is expressed in terms of heat production per unit of body surface area per day (*basal metabolic rate – BMR*), and for an average man the BMR is 1.7 Calories (7.115 kilojoules) per day. BMR may be determined by the direct method, in which the subject is placed in a respiratory chamber and the amount of heat evolved is measured, or (more normally) by the indirect method, based on the *respiratory quotient. Measurements are best taken during a period of least activity, i.e. during sleep and 12–18 hours after a meal, under controlled temperature conditions. Various factors, such as age, sex, and particularly thyroid activity, influence the value of the BMR.

basement membrane the thin delicate membrane that lies at the base of the *epithelium. It is composed of mucopolysaccharide and fibers of protein.

base pairing the linking of the two strands of a DNA molecule by means of hydrogen bonds between the bases of the nucleotides. Adenine always pairs with thymine and cytosine with guanine. See DNA.

basic life support the provision of treatment designed to maintain adequate circulation and ventilation to a patient in *cardiac arrest, without the use of drugs or specialist equipment.

basilar artery an artery in the base of the brain, formed by the union of the two vertebral arteries. It extends from the lower to the upper border of the pons Varolii and then divides to form the two posterior cerebral arteries.

basilar membrane a membrane in the *cochlea of the ear that separates two of the three channels (scalae) that run the length of the spiral cochlea. The organ of Corti is situated on the basilar membrane, inside the scala media.

basilic vein a large vein in the arm, extending from the hand along the back of the forearm, then passing forward to the inner side of the arm at the elbow.

basion n. the midpoint of the anterior border of the large hole (foramen magnum) at the base of the *skull.

basophil n. a variety of white blood cell distinguished by a lobed nucleus and the presence in its cytoplasm of coarse granules that stain purple-black with *Romanovsky stains. Basophils are capable of ingesting foreign particles and contain *histamine and *heparin.

basophilia n. 1. a property of a microscopic structure whereby it shows an affinity for basic dyes. 2. an increase in the number of certain white blood cells (*basophils) in the blood, which may occur in a variety of blood diseases.

basophilic adj. readily stainable by basic dyes: showing *basophilia.

bathyesthesia n. sensation experienced in the deeper parts of the body, such as the joints and muscles.

Batten's disease one of a group of rare hereditary disorders (known as the *neuronal ceroid lipofuscinoses*) that also includes *Tay-Sachs disease. Fatty substances accumulate in the cells of the nervous system, causing progressive dementia, epilepsy, spasticity, and visual failure. The condition starts in late infancy or childhood. There is no treatment. [F. E. Batten (1865–1918), British neurologist]

battered baby syndrome (battered child syndrome) injuries inflicted on babies or young children by their parents or other care-givers, who are often emotionally disturbed or have themselves suffered from physical abuse in infancy or early childhood. The highest incidence of battering occurs in the first six months of life; it commonly takes the form of bruising (particularly on the face), burns or scalds (especially cigarette burns), bites, head injuries (often with brain damage), and fractured bones. Internal injuries may be fatal. Frequently, signs of older bruises, fractures, etc., indicating long-term abuse, are revealed when the child is brought for treatment. If discharged from the hospital without the intensive support of a social worker and surveillance of family doctor and health-care services, 60% of battered children experience further injury, usually with serious consequences for the child, including *failure to thrive and behavioral problems. A court order is often necessary to safeguard a child from further abuse. Child abuse may be precipitated by many factors, including relationship difficulties, social problems, and ill health.

Bazin's disease a rare disease of young women in which tender nodules develop under the skin in the calves. The nodules may break down and ulcerate, although they may clear up spontaneously. The cause is unknown. Medical name: **erythema induratum**. [A. P. E. Bazin (1807–78), French dermatologist]

BCC see basal cell carcinoma.

B cell see lymphocyte.

BCG (bacille Calmette-Guérin) a strain of tubercle bacillus that has lost the power to cause tuberculosis but retains its antigenic activity; it is therefore used to prepare a vaccine against the disease.

Beau's lines transverse depressions on the nails appearing some weeks after a severe illness, such as pneumonia or a heart attack. [J. H. S. Beau (1806–65), French physician]

Becker muscular dystrophy *see* muscular dystrophy. [P. E. Becker (20th century), German geneticist]

Beck's triad *see* cardiac tamponade. [C. S. Beck (1894–1971), US surgeon]

Beckwith-Wiedemann syndrome an inherited condition characterized by neonatal hypoglycemia, an enlarged body, advanced bone age, large tongue, facial and skull abnormalities, enlargement of internal organs, and diaphragmatic hernia. Treatment is mainly by correcting the hypoglycemia. [J. B. Beckwith (1933–), US pediatric pathologist; H. R. Wiedemann (1915–), German pediatrician]

beclomethasone *n.* a *corticosteroid drug that reduces inflammation and is administered by oral or nasal inhaler or nasal spray to treat asthma, bronchitis, or hay fever. Side effects include hoarseness, dry mouth, and nasal irritation. Trade names: **Beclovent**, **Beconase**, **QVAR**, **Vancenase**, **Vanceril**.

becquerel *n.* the *SI unit of activity of a radioactive source, being the activity of a radionuclide decaying at a rate of one spontaneous nuclear transition per second. It has replaced the curie. Symbol: Bq.

bedbug *n.* a bloodsucking insect of the genus *Cimex*. *C. hemipterus* of the tropics and *C. lectularius* of temperate regions have reddish flattened bodies and vestigial wings. They live and lay their eggs in the crevices of walls and furniture and emerge at night to suck blood; although bedbugs are not known vectors of disease, their bites leave a route for bacterial infection. Premises can be disinfested with appropriate insecticides.

bed occupancy the number of hospital or nursing home beds occupied by patients, expressed as a percentage of the total beds available in the ward, specialty, hospital, facility, area, or region. It may be recorded in relation to a defined point in time or more usefully for a period, when the calculation is based on bed-days. It is used with other indices (such as *admission rate and *discharge rate) to assess the demands for hospital beds in relation to diseases, specialties, or populations and hence to gauge an appropriate balance between health needs and resources.

bedsore (decubitus ulcer, pressure sore) *n.* an ulcerated area of skin caused by continuous pressure on a part of the body: a hazard to be guarded against in all bedridden (especially unconscious) patients. Healing is hindered by the reduced blood supply to the area, and careful nursing is necessary to prevent local gangrene. The patient's position should be changed frequently, and the buttocks, heels, elbows, and other regions at risk kept dry and clean.

bedwetting *n. see* enuresis.

behaviorism *n.* an approach to psychology postulating that only observable behavior need be studied, thus denying any importance to unconscious processes. Behaviorists are concerned with the laws regulating the occurrence of behavior (*see* conditioning). —**behaviorist** *n.*

behavior modification the use of the methods of behaviorist psychology (*see* behaviorism) – especially operant *conditioning – to alter people's behavior. Behavior modification has wider applications than *behavior therapy, since it is also used in situations in which the client is not ill; for example, in education. *See also* chaining, prompting.

behavior therapy treatment based on the belief that psychological problems are the products of faulty learning and not the symptoms of an underlying disease. Treatment is directed at the problem or target behavior and is designed for the particular patient, not for the particular diagnostic label that has been attached to him. *See also* aversion therapy, conditioning, desensitization, exposure, response prevention.

Behçet's syndrome a recurrent multisystem disease characterized by oral and genital ulcerations and inflamed iris with accumulations of pus in the anterior chamber of the eye (*see* uveitis, retrobulbar neuritis). It may also involve the joints and cause inflammation of the large and small veins; skin lesions occur in the majority of patients. The condition, whose cause is unknown, occurs more often in men than women. Treatment is with *azathioprine. [H. Behçet (1889–1948), Turkish dermatologist]

bejel (endemic syphilis) *n.* a long-lasting nonvenereal form of *syphilis that occurs in the Balkans, Turkey, eastern Mediterranean countries, and the dry savannah regions of North Africa; it is particularly prevalent where standards of personal hygiene are low. The disease is spread among children and adults by direct body contact. Early skin lesions are obvious in the moist areas of the body (mouth, armpits, and groin) and later there may be considerable destruction of the tissues of the skin, nasopharynx, and long bones. Wartlike eruptions in the anal and genital regions are common. Bejel, which is rarely fatal, is treated with penicillin.

bel *n. see* decibel.

belladonna *n.* **1.** deadly nightshade (*Atropa belladonna*): the plant from which the drug *atropine is obtained. **2.** the poisonous alkaloid derived from deadly nightshade, from which atropine and hyoscyamine are extracted. Belladonna has *anticholinergic action and is used only in combination with other drugs, especially preparations for treating *diarrhea because of its *antispasmodic effects.

bell and pad a psychological method of treating bed-wetting. When the subject starts to urinate, the urine is detected by a pad (or by sheets of metallic mesh) and this sets off a bell (or loud buzzer). The modern form of the apparatus has a small electronic sensor worn under the underclothes and produces a loud bleep. The purpose of the alarm is to waken the subject, who then empties his bladder fully. A process of conditioning leads to his learning to be dry. It is effective in about 80% of cases.

belle indifference a symptom of *conversion disorder in which an apparently grave physical affliction (which has no physical cause) is accepted in a smiling and calm fashion.

Bell's palsy paralysis of the *facial nerve causing weakness of the muscles of one side of the face and an inability to close the eye. *Bell's phenomenon*, the outward and upward rotation of the eyeball, occurs when the patient tries to close the eyelid. In some patients hearing may be affected so that sounds seem abnormally loud, and a loss of taste sensation may occur. The cause of this condition is usually a viral infection, and recovery normally occurs spontaneously. [Sir C. Bell (1774–1842), Scottish physiologist]

belly *n.* **1.** the *abdomen or abdominal cavity. **2.** the central fleshy portion of a muscle.

Bence-Jones protein a protein of low molecular weight found in the urine of patients with multiple *myeloma, and rarely in patients with *lymphoma, *leukemia, and *Hodgkin's disease. [H. Bence-Jones (1814–73), British physician]

bendroflumethazide (bendrofluazide) *n.* a potent thiazide *diuretic used in the treatment of conditions involving retention of fluid, such as congestive heart failure, hypertension, and *edema. Side effects include dizziness, lethargy, dry mouth, and muscle cramps. Trade name: **Naturetin**.

bends *n. see* compressed air illness.

Benedict's test a test for the presence of sugar in urine or other liquids. A few drops of the test solution are added to *Benedict's solution*, prepared from sodium or potassium citrate, sodium carbonate, and copper sulfate. The mixture is boiled and shaken for about two minutes, then left to cool. The presence of up to 2% glucose is indicated by the formation of a reddish, yellowish, or greenish precipitate, the highest levels corresponding to the red coloration, the lowest (about 0.05%) to the green. [S. R. Benedict (1884–1936), US surgeon]

benign *adj.* **1.** describing a tumor that does not invade and destroy the tissue in which it originates or spread to distant sites in the body, i.e. a tumor that is not cancerous. **2.** describing any disorder or condition that does not produce harmful effects. *Compare* malignant.

benign intracranial hypertension (pseudotumor cerebri) a syndrome of raised pressure within the skull caused by impaired reabsorption of cerebrospinal fluid. The symptoms include headache, vomiting, double vision, and *papilledema. It normally subsides spontaneously but neurosurgical treatment or drug therapy may be required to protect the patient's vision.

benign paroxysmal positional vertigo a common cause of vertigo in which the patient complains of brief episodes of rotary vertigo precipitated by sudden head movements. It is thought to be due to microscopic debris in the posterior semicircular canal. Treatment is with a predetermined set of head movements to move the debris from the posterior semicircular canal.

benign prostatic hyperplasia a condition in which the prostate is enlarged; this results in pressure being exerted on the urethra. The most common symptoms are a frequent need to urinate and the reduced force of the stream, urinary-tract infection, and blood in the urine. If severe and untreated, backup of urine can cause kidney damage. The condition frequently coexists with *prostate cancer. Treatment consists of transurethral *resection of the prostate, using a balloon device to reduce the size of the prostate, or the use of drugs (*finasteride or *alpha blockers).

benserazide n. a drug that prevents the breakdown of *levodopa to dopamine outside the brain by inhibiting the enzyme dopa decarboxylase. Administered by mouth in combination with levodopa (as *Madopar*), it is used to treat Parkinson's disease. Possible side effects include nausea, vomiting, loss of appetite, involuntary movements, and faintness on standing up.

benzalkonium n. a detergent disinfectant with the same uses and effects as *cetrimonium.

benzethonium n. a detergent disinfectant with uses similar to those of *cetrimonium. Trade name: **Phemerol**.

benzhexol n. see trihexyphenidyl hydrochloride.

benzocaine n. a local anesthetic used in the form of an ointment, suppository, or aerosol to relieve painful conditions of the skin and mucous membranes. Virtually nontoxic, it can also be given by mouth in the form of lozenges to treat such conditions as lacerations of the mouth or the tongue and gastric ulcers. Trade names: **Americaine**, **Anbesol**.

benzodiazepines pl. n. a group of pharmacologically active compounds used as *anxiolytics and hypnotics. The group includes *bromazepam, *chlordiazepoxide, *diazepam, *lorazepam, and *oxazepam.

benzoic acid an antiseptic, active against fungi and bacteria, used as a preservative in foods and pharmaceutical preparations, as well as for the treatment of fungal infections of the skin.

benzoyl peroxide a preparation used in the treatment of acne and fungal skin conditions. It acts by removing the surface layers of the epidermis and unblocking skin pores and has an antiseptic effect on skin bacteria. It is administered as a cream, lotion, or gel. Side effects may include skin irritation, excessive peeling, and (occasionally) blistering. Trade names: **Benoxyl**, **Benzac**, **Brevoxyl**, **Fostex**, **Loroxide**, **PanOxyl**.

benzphetamine n. a drug of the *amphetamine group that is given by mouth in the treatment of obesity. Side effects include palpitations, restlessness, and allergic reactions. Trade name: **Didrex**.

benzthiazide n. a thiazide *diuretic used in the treatment of conditions involving fluid retention, such as congestive heart failure, *edema, and hypertension. Trade name: **Exna**.

benztropine n. a drug that is similar to *atropine but also acts as an antihistamine, local anesthetic, and sedative. Given by mouth, it is used mainly in the treatment of *parkinsonism to reduce rigidity and muscle cramps. It is well tolerated, but produces drowsiness and confusion. Trade name: **Cogentin**.

benzyl benzoate an oily aromatic liquid that is applied to the body – in the form of a lotion – for the treatment of scabies. It is also useful in treating pediculosis. Trade name: **Ascabiol**.

bepridil n. a drug used in the treatment of *angina. It increases the oxygen supply to the heart and reduces the oxygen demand. Most common side effects include weakness, dizziness, and nervousness. Because it may rarely cause heart rhythm irregularities and agranulocytosis, it is usually reserved for patients in whom the condition has not been controlled by other drugs. Trade name: **Vascor**.

beractant n. a modified extract derived from bovine lung. This *surfactant is used in the prevention and treatment of respiratory distress syndrome in high-risk premature infants. Trade name: **Survanta**.

Beradinelli-Seip syndrome see lipodystrophy. [W. Beradinelli (1903–56), Argentinian physician; M. Seip (20th century), Scandinavian physician]

Berger's disease (IgA nephropathy) an abnormality of the kidney in which there is a focal area of inflammation (*glomerulonephritis). This causes microscopic amounts of blood in the urine. A quarter of the patients with this condition may develop kidney failure. [J. Berger (20th century), French nephrologist]

beriberi *n.* a nutritional disorder due to deficiency of vitamin B₁ (thiamine). It is widespread in rice-eating communities in which the diet is based on polished rice, from which the thiamine-rich seed coat has been removed. Beriberi takes two forms: *wet beriberi*, in which there is an accumulation of tissue fluid (*edema), and *dry beriberi*, in which there is extreme emaciation. There is nervous degeneration in both forms of the disease and death from heart failure is often the outcome.

berry aneurysm *see* aneurysm.

berylliosis *n.* poisoning by beryllium or its compounds, either by inhalation or by skin contamination. This may be acute and sometimes fatal, but is more often chronic with the development of *fibrosis affecting all parts of the lungs. At low levels of exposure, granulomas may form in the lungs or skin that are similar to those seen in *sarcoidosis.

Best's disease *see* vitelliform degeneration. [F. Best (20th century), German physician]

beta agonist *see* sympathomimetic.

beta blocker (beta-adrenergic blocker) a drug that prevents stimulation of the beta-adrenergic receptors of the nerves of the sympathetic nervous system. There are two kinds of beta receptors: beta 1 receptors are in the heart, and blockade causes a decrease in heart rate and force; beta 2 receptors are in the airways and the arteries, in both of which blockade causes constriction. Beta blockers include *acebutolol, *betaxolol, *nadolol, *oxprenolol, *propranolol, and *sotalol, which are used to control abnormal heart rhythms, to treat angina, and to reduce high blood pressure. Beta blockers that block both beta 1 and beta 2 receptor sites cause constriction of air passages in the lungs, and care has to be taken with the use of these drugs in patients with any bronchial conditions.

Other beta blockers are relatively selective for the heart (cardioselective) and are less likely to constrict the airways. Some beta blockers (e.g. *carteolol, *levobunolol, and *timolol) reduce the production of aqueous humor and therefore the pressure inside the eye; they are administered as eye drops in the treatment of *glaucoma.

beta-carotene *n.* a *vitamin A precursor found in such foods as carrots, dark-green leafy vegetables, sweet potatoes, broccoli, cantaloupe, and winter squash (*see also* carotene). It is an *antioxidant and also used as a dietary supplement, especially for patients with pancreatic and liver conditions and cystic fibrosis. Trade names: **Lemitene, Max-Caro.**

beta cell a type of cell in the *islets of Langerhans of the pancreas that produces *insulin. *See also* diabetes mellitus.

betahistine *n.* a drug that is an *analogue of *histamine and increases blood flow through the inner ear. It is administered by mouth to treat *Ménière's disease. A common side effect is nausea. Trade name: **Serc.**

beta-lactam antibiotic one of a group of drugs that includes the *penicillins and the *cephalosporins. All have a four-membered *beta-lactam* ring that forms part of their molecular structure. Beta-lactam antibiotics function by interfering with the growth of the cell walls of multiplying bacteria. Bacteria become resistant to these antibiotics by producing *beta-lactamases*, enzymes (such as *penicillinase) that disrupt the beta-lactam ring. To counteract this, *beta-lactamase inhibitors* (e.g. *clavulanate potassium) may be added to beta-lactam antibiotics. For example, *co-amoxiclav* (Augmentin) is a mixture of amoxicillin and clavulanate potassium.

betamethasone *n.* a synthetic corticosteroid drug with effects and uses similar to those of *prednisolone. The side effects are those of *cortisone. Trade name: **Celestone.**

betatron *n.* a device used to accelerate a stream of electrons (*beta particles*) into a beam of radiation that can be used in *radiotherapy.

betaxolol *n.* a *beta blocker drug used to treat high blood pressure and chronic simple *glaucoma. It is administered by mouth and as eye drops. Possible side

bilateral

effects include breathing difficulty, fatigue, cold extremities, and sleep disturbances. Trade names: **Betoptic**.

bethanechol *n.* a cholinergic drug (*see* parasympathomimetic) that acts mainly on the bowel and bladder, stimulating these organs to empty. It is administered by mouth. Possible side effects include nausea, vomiting, and abdominal cramps. Trade names: **Duvoid, Myotonachol, Urecholine**.

bevacizumab *n. see* angiogenesis inhibitor.

bezafibrate *n. see* fibrates.

bezoar *n.* a mass of swallowed foreign material within the stomach. The material, which is usually swallowed by psychiatrically disturbed patients, accumulates and ultimately causes gastric obstruction. Its removal often requires a surgical operation. *See also* trichobezoar.

bi- *prefix denoting* two; double. Examples: *biciliate* (having two cilia); *binucleate* (having two nuclei).

bicalutamide *n.* an *antiandrogen commonly used to treat prostate cancer because in men it blocks androgen receptors without reducing levels of testosterone in the blood, preserving libido and general energy levels. It is taken by mouth; side effects include breast enlargement, tenderness, and pain. Trade name: **Casodex**.

biceps *n.* a muscle with two heads. The *biceps brachii* extends from the shoulder joint to the elbow (see illustration). It flexes the arm and forearm and

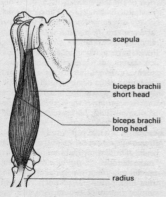

scapula

biceps brachii short head

biceps brachii long head

radius

The biceps muscle of the arm

supinates the forearm and hand. The *biceps femoris* is situated at the back of the thigh and is responsible for flexing the knee, extending the thigh, and rotating the leg outward.

BiCNU *see* carmustine.

biconcave *adj.* having a hollowed surface on both sides. Biconcave lenses are used to correct nearsightedness. *Compare* biconvex.

biconvex *adj.* having a surface on each side that curves outward. Biconvex lenses are used to correct farsightedness. *Compare* biconcave.

bicornuate *adj.* having two hornlike processes or projections. The term is applied to an abnormal uterus that is divided into two separate halves at the upper end.

bicuspid 1. *adj.* having two *cusps, as in the mitral valve of the heart. **2.** *n.* a premolar tooth.

bicuspid valve *see* mitral valve.

b.i.d. abbreviation for the Latin *bis in die*, meaning twice a day.

bifid *adj.* split or cleft into two parts.

bifocal lens a lens with two principal focal lengths: the upper part of the lens gives a sharp image of distant objects and the lower part gives a sharp image of near objects, as when reading. Examples are bifocal glasses, bifocal contact lenses, and bifocal intraocular lenses. *See also* trifocal lenses, multifocal lenses.

bifurcation *n.* (in anatomy) the point at which division into two branches occurs; for example in blood vessels or in the trachea.

bigeminal body one of the two swellings that develop in the roof of the midbrain during its development in the embryo.

bigeminy *n.* the condition in which alternate *ectopic beats of the heart are transmitted to the pulse and felt as a double pulse beat (*pulsus bigeminus*). It is a common manifestation of digitalis poisoning.

biguanide *n.* one of the group of drugs including *metformin, which is used to treat noninsulin-dependent (type 2) diabetes mellitus. Biguanides are *oral hypoglycemic drugs: they act by reducing the release of glucose from the liver and increasing glucose uptake by muscles.

bilateral *adj.* (in anatomy) relating to or affecting both sides of the body or of a tissue or organ or both of a pair of organs (e.g. the eyes, breasts, or ovaries).

bilateral uterine arterial embolization a method of embolizing the uterine artery under radiodiagnostic control, usually performed using Tras/Acryl gelatin microspheres (see embolization). It has been successful in controlling postpartum hemorrhage in 94.9% of cases and can also be used in correcting arterial or venous malformations and in terminating abdominal and cervical pregnancies. The technique has recently been introduced as a treatment for uterine fibroids; although it controlled bleeding in about 82–92% of cases, further studies are required to evaluate issues relating to necrosis of tumors, sepsis, and the long-term effect on size and recurrence rates of fibroids.

bile n. a thick alkaline fluid that is secreted by the *liver and stored in the *gallbladder, from which it is ejected intermittently into the duodenum via the common *bile duct. Bile may be yellow, green, or brown, according to the proportions of the *bile pigments (excretory products) present; other constituents are *lecithin, *cholesterol, and *bile salts. The bile salts help to emulsify fats in the duodenum so that they can be more easily digested by pancreatic *lipase into fatty acids and glycerol. Bile salts also form compounds with fatty acids, which can then be transported into the *lacteals. Bile also helps to stimulate *peristalsis in the duodenum.

bile acids the organic acids in bile; mostly occurring as bile salts (sodium glycocholate and sodium taurocholate). They include cholic (or cholalic) acid, *chenodeoxycholic acid, glycocholic acid, and taurocholic acid.

bile-acid sequestrant a drug that binds to bile acids, forming a complex that is excreted in the feces. Bile acids are formed in the liver from *cholesterol and the effect of loss of bile acids is a reduction in total body cholesterol and a decrease in low-density *lipoprotein serum levels. These drugs, which include *cholestyramine and *colestipol, are used to treat patients with abnormally high blood cholesterol levels who are liable to develop coronary heart disease.

bile duct any of the ducts that convey bile from the liver. Bile is drained from the liver cells by many small ducts that unite to form the main bile duct of the liver, the *hepatic duct*. This joins the *cystic duct*, which leads from the *gallbladder, to form the *common bile duct*, which drains into the duodenum.

bile pigments colored compounds – breakdown products of the blood pigment *hemoglobin – that are excreted in *bile. The two most important bile pigments are *bilirubin*, which is orange or yellow, and its oxidized form *biliverdin*, which is green. Mixed with the intestinal contents, they give the brown color to the feces (see urobilinogen).

bile salts sodium glycocholate and sodium taurocholate – the alkaline salts of *bile – necessary for the emulsification of fats. After they have been absorbed from the intestine, they are transported to the liver for reuse.

Bilharzia n. see Schistosoma.

bilharziasis n. see schistosomiasis.

bili- prefix denoting bile.

biliary adj. relating to or affecting the bile duct or bile. See also fistula.

biliary atresia a congenital or acquired condition in which the bile ducts do not drain. Babies usually present within the first few weeks of life with jaundice that does not improve with time. Some forms of biliary atresia can be corrected surgically, but if diagnosis has been delayed the condition may lead to irreversible liver damage.

biliary colic pain resulting from obstruction of the gallbladder or common bile duct, usually by a stone. The pain, which is very severe, is usually felt in the upper abdomen (in the midline or to the right). It often occurs about an hour after a meal (particularly if fatty), may last several hours, and is usually steady in severity (unlike other forms of *colic). Vomiting often occurs simultaneously.

bilious adj. 1. containing bile; for example *bilious vomiting* is the vomiting of bile-containing fluid. 2. a lay term used to describe attacks of nausea or vomiting.

bilirubin n. see bile pigments.

bilirubinemia n. an excess of the *bile pigment bilirubin in the blood. Normally, there is under 0.8 mg bilirubin per 100 ml blood; when the concentration of bilirubin is above 1–1.5 mg per 100 ml, visible *jaundice occurs. See also van den Bergh's test.

biliuria (choluria) n. the presence of bile in the urine: a feature of certain forms of jaundice.

biliverdin n. see bile pigments.

Billings method a method of family planning involving the daily examination of cervical mucus, which varies in consistency and color throughout the menstrual cycle. [J. and E. Billings (20th century), Australian physicians]

bimanual adj. using two hands to perform an activity, such as a gynecological examination.

binaural adj. relating to or involving the use of both ears.

binder n. a bandage that is wound around a part of the body, usually the abdomen, to apply pressure or to give support or protection.

binge–purge syndrome see bulimia.

binocular adj. relating to or involving the use of both eyes.

binocular vision the ability to focus both eyes on an object at the same time, so that a person sees one image of the object being looked at. It is not inborn, but acquired during the first few months of life. Binocular vision enables judgment of distance and perception of depth. See also stereoscopic vision.

bio- prefix denoting life or living organisms. Example: biosynthesis (formation of a compound within a living organism).

bioassay n. estimation of the activity or potency of a drug or other substance by comparing its effects on living organisms with effects of a preparation of known strength. Bioassay is used to determine the strength of preparations of hormones or other material of biological origin when other physical or chemical methods are not available.

bioavailability n. the proportion of a drug that is delivered to its site of action in the body. This is usually the amount entering the circulation and may be low when drugs are given by mouth.

biochemistry n. the study of the chemical processes and substances occurring in living things. —**biochemical** adj. —**biochemist** n.

bioengineering n. the application of biological and engineering principles to the development and manufacture of equipment and devices for use in biological systems. Examples of such products include orthopedic prostheses and heart pacemakers.

biofeedback n. the giving of immediate information to a subject about his bodily processes (such as heart rate), which are usually unconscious. These processes can then be subject to operant *conditioning. This is an experimental treatment for disturbances of bodily regulation, such as hypertension.

biological response modifier a therapeutic agent, such as *interferon or *interleukin, that influences the body's defense mechanisms to act against a cancer cell. These substances are normally produced in small amounts by the body; relatively large doses are being studied for cancer treatment, especially in melanoma and renal cancer.

biology n. the study of living organisms – plants, animals, and microorganisms – including their structure and function and their relationships with one another and with the inanimate world. —**biological** adj.

biometry n. the measurement of living things and the processes associated with life, including the application of mathematics, particularly statistics, to problems in biology.

bionics n. the science of mechanical or electronic systems that function in the same way as, or have characteristics of, living systems. Compare cybernetics. —**bionic** adj.

bionomics n. see ecology.

biophysical profile a physiological assessment of fetal wellbeing, including ultrasound scans, cardiographs, and fetal movements.

biopsy n. the removal of a small piece of living tissue from an organ or part of the body for microscopic examination. Biopsy is an important means of diagnosing cancer from examination of a fragment of tumor. It is often carried out with a special hollow needle, inserted into the liver, kidney, or other organ, with relatively little discomfort to the patient.

biostatistics n. statistical information and techniques used with special reference to studies of health and social problems. It embraces, overlaps, and to some extent is synonymous with the fields of vital statistics (e.g. *mortality and *fertility rates) and *demography. *Compare* biometry.

biotechnology n. the development of techniques for the application of biological processes to the production of materials of use in medicine and industry. For example, the production of many antibiotics relies on the activity of various fungi and bacteria. Recent techniques of *genetic engineering, in which human genes are cloned in bacterial cells, have enabled the large-scale production of hormones (notably insulin), vaccines, interferon, and other useful products.

biotin n. a vitamin of the B complex that is essential for the metabolism of fat, being involved in fatty acid synthesis and *gluconeogenesis. A biotin deficiency is extremely rare in humans; it can be induced by eating large quantities of raw egg white, which contains a protein – avidin – that combines with biotin, making it unavailable to the body. Rich sources of the vitamin are egg yolk and liver.

biperiden n. an anticholinergic drug used in the treatment of *parkinsonism. It is given by mouth; side effects are those of *atropine. Trade name: **Akineton**.

bipolar adj. 1. (in neurology) describing a neuron (nerve cell) that has two processes extending in different directions from its cell body. 2. (in psychiatry) denoting a disorder characterized by both manic and depressive episodes (*see* manic-depressive psychosis).

bird-breeder's lung a form of extrinsic allergic *alveolitis caused by the inhalation of avian proteins present in the droppings and feathers of certain birds, especially pigeons and caged birds (such as budgerigars). As in *farmer's lung, there is an acute and a chronic form.

birefringence n. the property possessed by some naturally occurring substances (such as cell membranes) of doubly refracting a beam of light, i.e. of bending it in two different directions. —**birefringent** adj.

birth n. (in obstetrics) *see* labor.

birth control the use of *contraception or *sterilization (male or female) to prevent unwanted pregnancies.

birthing chair a chair specially adapted to allow childbirth to take place in a sitting position. Its recent introduction in the Western world followed the increasing demand by women for greater mobility during labor. The chair is electronically powered and can be tilted back quickly and easily should the need arise.

birthmark n. a skin blemish or mark present at birth. The cause is unknown. *See* nevus.

birth rate the number of live births occurring in a year per 1000 total population (the *annual crude birth rate*). *See also* fertility rate.

bisacodyl n. a *laxative that acts on the large intestine to cause reflex movement and bowel evacuation. It is administered by mouth or as a suppository to empty the colon for an examination. The most common side effect is the development of abdominal cramps. Trade names: **Bisco-Lax, Correctol, Fleet Laxative**.

bisexual adj. 1. describing an individual who is sexually attracted to both men and women. 2. describing an individual who possesses the qualities of both sexes.

Bismarck brown a basic aniline dye used for staining and counterstaining histological and bacterial specimens. [O. von Bismarck (1815–98), German statesman]

bisoprolol n. a *beta blocker drug used in the treatment of *hypertension. It is administered by mouth. Possible side effects include breathing difficulty, fatigue, cold extremities, and sleep disturbances. Trade names: **Zebeta, Ziac**.

bisphosphonates (diphosphonates) pl. n. a class of drugs that inhibit the resorption of bone by blocking the action of *osteoclasts. This property makes them useful for treating certain bone disorders, such as *Paget's disease and *osteoporosis, as well as malignant disease – especially in terms of pain relief but also in the treatment of hypercalcemia due to cancer. Bisphosphonates include *etidronate disodium, *pamidronate* (Aredia), *alendronate* (Fosamax), and *clodronate*.

bistoury n. a narrow surgical knife, with a

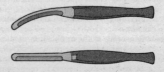

Types of bistoury

straight or curved blade (see illustration).

bite-raiser *n.* an appliance to prevent normal closure of the teeth in orthodontic treatment and in the treatment of the *temporomandibular joint syndrome.

bite-wing *n.* a dental X-ray film that provides a view of the crowns of the teeth in part of both upper and lower jaws. This view is used in the diagnosis of caries and periodontal disease.

Bitot's spots cheesy foamy grayish spots that form on the surface of dry patches of conjunctiva at the sides of the eyes. They consist of fragments of keratinized epithelium. A common cause is vitamin A deficiency. [P. A. Bitot (1822–88), French physician]

bivalent *n.* (in genetics) a structure consisting of homologous chromosomes that are attached to each other by chiasmata during the first division of *meiosis. —**bivalent** *adj.*

blackdamp (chokedamp) *n.* (in mining) the poisonous gas containing carbon dioxide, carbon monoxide, or other suffocating material, sometimes found in pockets in underground workings. *Compare* firedamp.

Black Death *see* plague.

black eye bruising of the eyelids and surrounding area.

black fly a small widely distributed bloodsucking insect of the genus *Simulium*. Black flies are also known as buffalo gnats from their humpbacked appearance. Female black flies can inflict painful bites and constitute a serious pest at certain times of the year. *S. damnosum* in Africa and *S. ochraceum* in Central America and Venezuela transmit the parasites causing *onchocerciasis.

blackhead *n.* a plug formed of fatty material (sebum and keratin) in the outlet of a *sebaceous gland in the skin; the black color is due to *melanin. *See also* acne. Medical name: **comedo**.

Black Lung Benefits Reform Act a law passed by the US Congress in 1977 to provide monthly cash benefits to coal miners totally disabled by pneumoconiosis that resulted from working in coal mines. The Act also provides monthly cash benefits to the widow, child, parents, brother, or sister of a miner who died from pneumoconiosis. The amount of the cash benefits varies according to the number of dependents of the coal miner and other sources of income, such as state workmen's compensation, unemployment insurance, or disability insurance payments.

blackwater fever a rare and serious complication of malignant tertian (falciparum) *malaria in which there is massive destruction of the red blood cells, leading to the presence of the blood pigment hemoglobin in the urine. The condition is probably brought on by inadequate treatment with *quinine; it is marked by fever, bloody urine, jaundice, vomiting, enlarged liver and spleen, anemia, exhaustion, and – in fatal cases – a reduced flow of urine resulting from a blockage of the kidney tubules. Treatment involves rest, administration of alkaline fluids and intravenous glucose, and blood transfusions.

bladder *n.* **1. (urinary bladder)** a sac-shaped organ that has a wall of smooth muscle and stores the urine produced by the kidneys. Urine passes into the bladder through the *ureters; the release of urine from the bladder is controlled by a sphincter at its junction with the *urethra. The *bladder neck* is the outlet of the bladder where it joins the urethra and in males it is in contact with the *prostate gland: it is under the control of the autonomic nerves of the pelvis. The neck of the bladder is the most common site for *retention or urine, usually by an enlarged prostate or a urethral *stricture. **2.** any of several other hollow organs containing fluid, such as the *gallbladder. *See also* cystectomy.

bladder augmentation (bladder enhancement) a surgical method of increasing the capacity of the urinary bladder. This is usually achieved by ileocecocystoplasty (*see* cystoplasty).

bladder neck incision an operation that involves an incision through the bladder neck and prostate to relieve *lower urinary tract symptoms. This is usually performed under a general or spinal anesthetic through a cystoscope and is smaller than a transurethral resection of the prostate.

bladder outflow obstruction blockage caused usually by an enlarged *prostate gland but also by a high bladder neck or uncoordinated contraction of the urinary sphincters and detrusor muscle of the bladder.

bladder pressure study a combined X-ray and manometry examination of the bladder to look for abnormal function. The bladder is filled slowly with contrast medium using a small urinary catheter and the pressure is monitored during filling and voiding (micturition). X-ray images of the bladder and urethra (*see* urethrography) are taken. The test is used to differentiate between obstruction to bladder outflow and abnormal contractions of the muscle in the bladder wall.

bladder replacement *see* cystectomy.

bladderworm *n. see* cysticercus.

Blalock-Taussig operation (or procedure) surgical construction of a *shunt as a temporary measure in infants with congenital heart defects associated with insufficient pulmonary arterial flow, such as *tetralogy of Fallot. Blood from the systemic circulation is directed to the pulmonary circulation by connecting the subclavian artery to the pulmonary artery (*see* anastomosis). [A. Blalock (1899–1964), US surgeon; H. B. Taussig (1898–1986), US pediatrician]

-blast *suffix denoting* a formative cell. Example: *osteoblast* (formative bone cell).

blastema *n.* any zone of embryonic tissue that is still differentiating and growing into a particular organ. The term is usually applied to the tissue that develops into the kidneys and gonads.

blasto- *prefix denoting* a germ cell or embryo. Example: *blastogenesis* (early development of an embryo).

blastocoele *n.* the fluid-filled cavity that develops within the *blastocyst. The cavity increases the surface area of the embryo and thus improves its ability to absorb nutrients and oxygen.

blastocyst *n.* an early stage of embryonic development that consists of a hollow ball of cells with a localized thickening (the *inner cell mass*) that will develop into the actual embryo; the remainder of the blastocyst is composed of *trophoblast (see illustration). At first the blastocyst is unattached, but it soon implants in the wall of the uterus. *See also* implantation.

blastomere *n.* any of the cells produced by *cleavage of the zygote, comprising the earliest stages of embryonic devel-

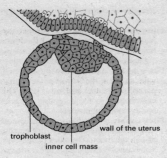

wall of the uterus
trophoblast
inner cell mass

Section through a blastocyst

opment until the formation of the *blastocyst. Blastomeres divide repeatedly without growth and so decrease in size.

blastomycosis *n.* any disease caused by parasitic fungi of the genus *Blastomyces*, which may affect the skin (forming wartlike ulcers and tumors on the face, neck, hands, arms, feet, and legs) or involve various internal tissues, such as the lungs, bones, liver, spleen, and lymphatics. There are two principal forms of the disease: *North American blastomycosis (Gilchrist's disease)*, caused by *B. dermatitidis*; and *South American blastomycosis*, caused by *B. brasiliensis*. Both diseases are treated with antifungal drugs (such as amphotericin B).

blastopore *n.* the opening that forms as a result of invagination of the surface layer of the early embryo (*gastrula). It is very much reduced in humans, in which it gives rise to the archenteric canal (*see* archenteron).

blastula *n.* an early stage of the embryonic development of many animals. The equivalent stage in mammals (including humans) is the *blastocyst.

bleb *n.* a blister or large vesicle (also called *bulla*). A *filtering bleb* is a blisterlike cyst underneath the conjunctiva resulting from *trabeculectomy, a surgical procedure commonly used in the treatment of glaucoma.

bleeding *n. see* hemorrhage.

blenn- (blenno-) *prefix denoting* mucus. Example: *blennemesis* (vomiting of).

blennorrhea (blennorrhagia) *n.* a copious discharge of mucus, particularly from the urethra or vagina. This usually accompanies *urethritis and sometimes occurs with acute *prostatitis. Treatment is directed to clearing the underlying causative organism by antibiotic administration.

bleomycin *n.* an antibiotic with action against cancer cells (*see* cytotoxic drug) that is used in the treatment of Hodgkin's disease and other lymphomas and in squamous-cell carcinoma. It is usually used in combination therapy, administered by injection, and can cause toxic side effects in the skin and lungs; it should not be used in patients with impaired kidney function or lung disease. Trade name: **Blenoxane**.

blephar- (blepharo-) *prefix denoting* the eyelid. Example: *blepharotomy* (incision into).

blepharitis *n.* inflammation of the eyelids. In *squamous blepharitis*, often associated with dandruff of the scalp, white scales accumulate among the eyelashes. *Chronic ulcerative blepharitis* is characterized by yellow crusts overlying ulcers of the lid margins. The lashes become matted together and tend to fall out or become distorted. *Allergic blepharitis* may occur in response to drugs or cosmetics put in the eye or on the eyelids.

blepharochalasis *n.* excessive eyelid skin resulting from recurrent episodes of edema and inflammation of the eyelid. It occurs in young people, causing drooping of the lid. *Compare* dermatochalasis.

blepharoconjunctivitis *n.* inflammation involving the eyelid margins and conjunctiva.

blepharon *n. see* eyelid.

blepharophimosis *n.* narrowing of the aperture between the eyelids.

blepharoplasty (tarsoplasty) *n.* any operation to repair or reconstruct the eyelid. It involves either rearrangement of the tissues of the lid or the use of tissue from other sites (e.g. skin or mucous membrane).

blepharoptosis *n. see* ptosis.

blepharospasm *n.* involuntary tight contraction of the eyelids, either in response to painful conditions of the eye or as a form of *dystonia.

blind loop syndrome (stagnant loop syndrome) a condition of stasis of the small intestine allowing the overgrowth of bacteria, which causes *malabsorption and the passage of fatty stools (*see* steator-rhea). It is usually the result of chronic obstruction (resulting, for example, from *Crohn's disease, a *stricture, or intestinal tuberculosis), or surgical bypass operations producing a stagnant length of bowel, or conditions (e.g. a jejunal *diverticulum) in which a segment of intestine is out of continuity with the rest.

blindness *n.* the inability to see. Lack of all light perception constitutes total blindness but there are degrees of visual impairment far less severe that may be classed as blindness for administrative or statutory purposes. For example, marked reduction in the *visual field is classified as blindness, even if objects are still seen sharply. The most common causes of blindness are *trachoma, *onchocerciasis, and vitamin A deficiency (*see* night blindness) but there is wide geographic variation. Among the most common causes in the US are diabetic *retinopathy, myopic retinal degeneration, age-related *macular degeneration, and *glaucoma.

For purposes of disability benefits provided by US laws, a person must have central visual acuity in the better eye of 20/200 or less when using a correcting lens or a visual field of 20 degrees or less at the widest diameter. However, a blind person who engages in substantial gainful employment despite the handicap is not entitled to disability benefits.

blind spot the small area of the *retina of the eye where the nerve fibers from the light-sensitive cells (*see* cone, rod) lead into the optic nerve. There are no rods or cones in this area and hence it does not register light. Anatomical name: **punctum caecum**.

blind trial *see* intervention study.

blinking *n.* the action of closing and opening the eyelids, which wipes the front of the eyeball and helps to spread the *tears. Reflex blinking may be caused by suddenly bringing an object near to the eye: the eyelids close involuntarily in order to protect the eye.

blister *n.* a swelling containing watery fluid (serum) and sometimes also blood (*blood blister*) or pus, within or just beneath the skin. Blisters commonly develop as a result of unaccustomed friction on the hands or feet or at the site of a burn. Blisters may be treated with antiseptics and dressings. An unduly painful blister may be punctured with a sterile needle so that the fluid is released.

block *n.* any interruption of physiological or mental function, brought about intentionally (as part of a therapeutic procedure) or by disease. *See also* heart block, nerve block.

block grants government funds that are allocated for health care purposes without a stipulation that the money be used for any narrowly defined health function. A block grant may be awarded for general public health services in a community, and the precise application of the funds can be determined by local administrators.

blocking *n.* (in psychiatry) **1.** a sudden halting of the flow of thought or speech. Blocking of thought, accompanied by the sensation of thoughts being removed from the mind, is a symptom of *schizophrenia. Blocking of speech may be a consequence of thought block or a result of a mechanical impediment in speech, such as *stammering. **2.** failure to recall a specific event, or to explore a specific train of thought, because of its unpleasant associations.

blood *n.* a fluid that circulates throughout the body, via the arteries and veins, providing a vehicle by which an immense variety of different substances are transported between the various organs and tissues. It is composed of *blood cells, which are suspended in a liquid medium, the *plasma. An average individual has approximately 70 ml of blood per kilogram body weight (about 5 liters in an average adult male).

blood bank a department within a hospital or blood transfusion center in which blood collected from donors is stored prior to transfusion. Blood must be kept at a temperature of 4°C and may be used up to four weeks after collection.

blood-brain barrier the mechanism that controls the passage of molecules from the blood into the cerebrospinal fluid and the tissue spaces surrounding the cells of the brain. The endothelial cells lining the walls of the brain capillaries are more tightly joined together at their edges than those lining capillaries supplying other parts of the body. This allows the passage of solutions and fat-soluble compounds but excludes particles and large molecules. The importance of the blood-brain barrier is that it protects the brain from the effect of many substances harmful to it. A disadvantage, however, is that many useful drugs pass only in small amounts into the brain, and much larger doses may have to be given than normal. Brain cancer, for example, is relatively insensitive to chemotherapy, although drugs such as *diazepam, alcohol, and fat-soluble general anesthetics pass readily and quickly to the brain cells.

blood cell (blood corpuscle) any of the cells that are present in the blood in health or disease. The cells may be subclassified into three major categories, namely, red cells (*erythrocytes), white cells (*leukocytes), which include granulocytes, lymphocytes, and monocytes, and *platelets (see illustration). Blood cells account for approximately 40% of the total volume of the blood in health; red cells comprise the vast majority.

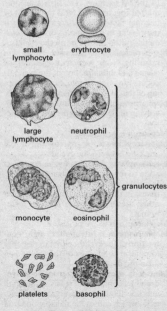

small lymphocyte — erythrocyte

large lymphocyte — neutrophil

monocyte — eosinophil — granulocytes

platelets — basophil

Types of blood cells

blood clot a solid mass formed as the result of *blood coagulation, either within the blood vessels and heart or elsewhere (*compare* thrombus). A blood clot consists of a meshwork of the protein *fibrin in which various blood cells are trapped.

blood coagulation (blood clotting) the process whereby blood is converted from a liquid to a solid state. The process may be initiated by contact of blood with a foreign surface (*intrinsic system*) or with damaged tissue (*extrinsic system*). These systems involve the interaction of a variety of substances (*coagulation factors) and lead to the production of the enzyme thrombin, which converts the soluble blood protein *fibrinogen to the insoluble protein *fibrin. Blood coagulation is an essential mechanism for the arrest of bleeding (*hemostasis).

blood corpuscle see blood cell.

blood count the numbers of different blood cells in a known volume of blood, usually expressed as the number of cells per liter. A sample of blood at known dilution is passed through a narrow opening in an electronic counting device. Blood-count investigations are important in the diagnosis of blood diseases. *See also* differential leukocyte count.

blood donor a person who gives blood for storage in a *blood bank. The blood can then be used for *transfusion into another patient. *See also* blood group.

blood group any one of the many types into which a person's blood may be classified, based on the presence or absence of certain inherited antigens on the surface of the red blood cells. Blood of one group contains antibodies in the serum that react against the cells of other groups.

There are more than 30 blood group systems, one of the most important of which is the *ABO system*. This system is based on the presence or absence of antigens A and B: blood of groups A and B contains antigens A and B, respectively; group AB contains both antigens and group O contains neither. Blood of group A contains antibodies (*isoagglutinins) to antigen B; group B blood contains anti-A antibodies; group AB has neither antibody and group O has both. A person whose blood contains either (or both) of these antibodies cannot receive a transfusion of blood containing the corresponding antigens. The table illustrates which blood groups can be used in transfusion for each of the four groups.

blood plasma see plasma.

blood poisoning the presence of either bacterial toxins or large numbers of bacteria in the bloodstream causing serious illness. *See* pyemia, septicemia, toxemia.

blood pressure (BP) the pressure of blood against the walls of the main arteries. Pressure is highest during *systole, when the ventricles are contracting (*systolic pressure*), and lowest during *diastole, when the ventricles are relaxing and refilling (*diastolic pressure*). Blood pressure is measured – in millimeters of mercury – by means of a *sphygmomanometer at the brachial artery of the arm, where the pressure is most similar to that of blood leaving the heart. The normal range varies with age, but a young adult would be expected to have a systolic pressure of around 120 mm and a diastolic pressure of 80 mm. These are recorded as 120/80.

Individual variations are common. Muscular exertion and emotional factors, such as fear, stress, and excitement, all raise systolic blood pressure (*see* hypertension). Systolic blood pressure is normally at its lowest during sleep. Severe shock may lead to an abnormally low blood pressure and possible circulatory

Donor's blood group	Blood group of people donor can receive blood from	Blood group of people donor can give blood to
A	A, O	A, AB
B	B, O	B, AB
AB	A, B, AB, O	AB
O	O	A, B, AB, O

failure (*see* hypotension). Blood pressure is adjusted to its normal level by the *sympathetic nervous system and hormonal controls. *See* baroreceptor.

blood serum *see* serum.

blood sugar the concentration of glucose in the blood, normally expressed in millimoles per liter. The normal range is 3.5–5.5 mmol/l. Blood-sugar estimation is an important investigation in a variety of diseases, most notably in diabetes mellitus. *See also* hyperglycemia, hypoglycemia.

blood test any test designed to discover abnormalities in a sample of a person's blood, such as the presence of alcohol, drugs, or microorganisms, or to determine the *blood group.

blood transfusion *see* transfusion.

blood vessel a tube carrying blood away from or toward the heart. Blood vessels are the means by which blood circulates throughout the body. *See* artery, arteriole, vein, venule, capillary.

Bloom's syndrome a specific abnormality of chromosome 15 in which the individual suffers from recurrent infections, blistering areas of the hands and lips, and poor growth. Such children have a much higher than normal risk of developing cancer. [D. Bloom (20th century), US dermatologist]

Blount disease (tibia vara) a condition causing *bowlegs as a result of abnormal growth at the *epiphysis at the top of the tibia (shin bone). It is more common in Africans and is most noticeable in childhood. The condition may affect one or both legs, and affected children are often obese. Treatment depends upon the severity and the age of the child but usually involves surgery. [W. P. Blount (1900–92), US orthopedic surgeon]

blue baby a colloquial name, becoming obsolete, for an infant with congenital malformation of the heart, such as *tetralogy of Fallot and *transposition of the great vessels, as a result of which some or all of the blue (deoxygenated) blood is pumped around the body instead of passing through the lungs to be oxygenated. This gives the skin and lips a purple color. Advances in cardiac surgery have enabled remedial operations or even total correction to be performed, usually in the first few days or weeks of life. Those who cannot be corrected or improved may survive for months or years with persistent *cyanosis.

Blue Cross and Blue Shield a nonprofit private insurance corporation that offers protection against costs of hospital treatment and surgery and related medical care for members of a group. Members are assessed prepayment premiums that are adjusted periodically to represent current hospital use by those participating in the plan. Blue Cross originated in 1929 as a hospital insurance plan for teachers in Texas and was endorsed four years later by the American Hospital Association. Blue Shield plans evolved after World War II from a program called Associated Medical Care Plans, sponsored by the *American Medical Association. There are 42 different Blue Cross and Blue Shield organizations in the US with an arrangement through a central Blue Cross and Blue Shield Association that permits members of one plan to utilize services of another affiliated plan in a different geographic area.

Blues *see* Blue Cross and Blue Shield.

B lymphocyte *see* lymphocyte.

BMI *see* body mass index.

Boards of Health local health units found in states, counties, cities, and towns throughout the US. Members of Boards of Health are usually appointed by elected officials, such as governors, county commissioners, or mayors, and membership generally includes at least one physician. The members may have advisory or administrative functions, depending on local laws. In some instances the Board of Health functions somewhat independently of an official state or local Department of Health, which is primarily responsible for public health in the area.

Boari flap an operation in which a tube of bladder tissue is constructed to replace the lower third of the ureter when this has been destroyed or damaged or has to be removed because of the presence of a tumor. *See also* ureteroplasty. [A. Boari (19th century), Italian surgeon]

Boas' sign excessive sensitivity in the region of the wing of the right scapula, associated with *cholecystitis. [I. I. Boas (1858–1938), German gastroenterologist]

body *n.* 1. an entire animal organism. 2.

the trunk of an individual, excluding the limbs. **3.** the main or largest part of an organ (such as the stomach or uterus). **4.** a solid discrete mass of tissue; e.g. the carotid body. *See also* corpus.

body dysmorphic disorder *see* dysmorphophobia.

body image (body schema) the individual's concept of the disposition of his limbs and the identity of the different parts of his body, as well as the overall shape and size. It is a function of the *association areas of the brain. *See also* Gerstmann's syndrome.

body mass index (BMI) a formula for determining whether or not a person is overweight or underweight: the weight of a person (in kilograms) divided by the square of the height of that person (in metres). For example, a person who is 1.7 m (5.6 ft) tall and weighs 65 kg (143 lb) has a BMI of $65/1.7^2 = 22.5$. A BMI of between 18.5 and 25 is considered normal, between 25 and 30 is overweight, and greater than 30 indicates clinical *obesity. A BMI of less than 18.5 is considered underweight.

body temperature the degree of heat of the body, as measured by a thermometer. Body temperature is accurately controlled by a small area at the base of the brain (the *hypothalamus); in normal individuals it is maintained at about 37°C (98.6°F). Heat production by the body arises as the result of vital activities (e.g. respiration, heartbeat, circulation, secretion) and from the muscular effort of exercise and shivering. *See also* fever.

body type (somatotype) the characteristic anatomical appearance of an individual, based on the predominance of the structures derived from the three germ layers (ectoderm, mesoderm, endoderm). The three types are described as *ectomorphic, *mesomorphic, and *endomorphic.

Boeck's disease *see* sarcoidosis. [C. P. M. Boeck (1845–1913), Norwegian dermatologist]

boil *n.* a tender inflamed area of the skin containing pus. The infection is usually caused by the bacterium *Staphylococcus aureus* entering through a hair follicle or a break in the skin, and local injury or lowered constitutional resistance may encourage the development of boils. Boils usually heal when the pus is re-

leased or with antibiotic treatment, although occasionally they may cause more widespread infection. Medical name: **furuncle**.

bolus *n.* a soft mass of chewed food or a pharmaceutical preparation that is ready to be swallowed.

bonding *n.* **1.** (in psychology) the development of a close and selective relationship, such as that of *attachment. *Parental bonding* is the process in which physical contact between parents and child in the child's first hours of life supposedly promotes a strong mutual attachment. **2.** (in dentistry) the attachment of dental restorations, sealants, and orthodontic brackets to teeth. Bonding may be mechanical (*see* acid-etch technique) or chemical, by the use of adhesive *cements or resins. Dentine bonding agents are increasingly used to attach dental fillings to dentine as well as to enamel. In certain artificial *crowns porcelain is bonded to a metal substructure to produce a bonded porcelain crown.

bone *n.* the hard extremely dense connective tissue that forms the skeleton of the body. It is composed of a matrix of collagen fibers impregnated with bone salts (chiefly calcium carbonate and calcium phosphate; *see* hydroxyapatite) in which are embedded bone cells (*see* osteocyte). *Compact* (or *cortical*) *bone* forms the outer shell of bones; it consists of a hard virtually solid mass made up of bony tissue arranged in concentric layers (*Haversian systems*). *Spongy bone*, found beneath compact bone, consists of a meshwork of bony bars (*trabeculae*) with many interconnecting spaces containing marrow. (See illustration.)

Individual bones may be classed as long, short, flat, or irregular. The outer layer of a bone is called the *periosteum. The *medullary cavity* is lined with *endosteum and contains the marrow. Bones not only form the skeleton but also act as stores for mineral salts and play an important part in the formation of blood cells.

bone-anchored hearing aid a specialized form of *hearing aid for patients with certain forms of conductive *deafness. A small titanium screw is surgically fixed into the bone of the skull behind the external ear using a process called *osseointegration. Sound energy is passed from a miniature microphone and amplifier to the screw, through the bone, to the *cochlea.

bone graft *see* graft.

bone growth factor any of a group of *growth factors that act to regulate the stages of bone growth and development. An example is *bone morphogenetic protein*, which has been manufactured by genetic engineering techniques and used in trials to stimulate bone formation and fracture healing.

bone marrow (marrow) the tissue contained within the internal cavities of the bones. At birth, these cavities are filled entirely with blood-forming *myeloid tissue* (*red marrow*) but in later life the marrow in the limb bones is replaced by fat (*yellow marrow*). Samples of bone marrow may be obtained for examination by *aspiration through a stout needle or by *trephine biopsy. *See also* hemopoiesis.

bony labyrinth *see* labyrinth.

BOOP *see* bronchiolitis obliterans organizing pneumonia.

borax *n.* a mild astringent with a weak antiseptic action, applied externally to skin and mucous membranes. Borax and *boric acid* are used in mouth and nasal washes, gargles, eye lotions and contact-lens solutions, and in dusting powder. Side effects from external application are rare; most reported cases of poisoning are in infants.

borborygmus *n.* (*pl.* **borborygmi**) an abdominal gurgle due to movement of fluid and gas in the intestine. Excessive borborygmi occur when intestinal movement is increased, for example, in the *irritable bowel syndrome and in intestinal obstruction.

borderline *adj.* **1.** describing a personality disorder characterized by unstable and intense relationships, exploiting and manipulating other people, rapidly changing moods, recurrent suicidal or self-injuring acts, and a pervasive inner feeling of emptiness and boredom. **2.** *see* schizotypal.

Bordetella *n.* a genus of tiny gram-negative aerobic bacteria. *B. pertussis* causes *whooping cough, and all the other species cause diseases resembling whooping cough.

boric acid *see* borax.

Bornholm disease (devil's grip, epidemic myalgia, epidemic pleurodynia) a disease caused by *coxsackieviruses. It is spread by contact, and epidemics usually occur during warm weather in temperate regions and at any time in the tropics. Symptoms include fever, headache, and attacks of severe pain in the lower chest. The illness lasts about a week and is

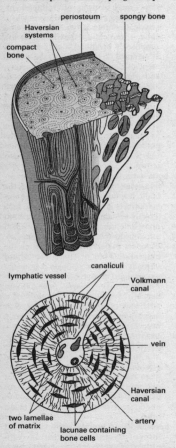

Section of the shaft of a long bone (above) with detail of a single Haversian system (below)

rarely fatal. There is no specific treatment. The disease is named after the island in Denmark where the first documented cases occurred.

Borrelia *n.* a genus of large parasitic *spirochete bacteria. The species *B. duttonii*, *B. persica*, and *B. recurrentis* cause *relapsing fever in Africa, Asia, North America, and Europe. The species *B. burgdorferi* causes *Lyme disease.

bosentan *n. see* endothelin.

bottom shuffling a normal variant of crawling in which babies sit upright and move on their bottoms, usually by pulling forward on their heels. Babies who bottom-shuffle tend to walk slightly later. There is often a family history of bottom shuffling.

botulinum toxin a powerful nerve toxin, produced by the bacterium *Clostridium botulinum*, that has proved effective, in minute dosage, for the treatment of various conditions of muscle overaction, such as strabismus (squint) and various dystonic conditions (*see* dystonia), including spasm of the orbicularis muscle in patients who have *blepharospasm. It is administered by injection. It is also used to treat *achalasia, being injected through an endoscope into the gastroesophageal sphincter. The drug is undergoing clinical trials for its effectiveness in relieving the spastic paralysis associated with cerebral palsy. Possible side effects include prolonged local muscle paralysis. Trade names: **Botox**, **Myobloc**.

botulism *n.* a serious form of *food poisoning from foods containing the toxin *botulin* produced by the bacterium *Clostridium botulinum*. The toxin selectively affects the central nervous system; in fatal cases, death is often caused by heart and lung failure resulting from a malfunction of the cardiac and respiratory centers of the brain. The bacterium thrives in improperly preserved foods, typically canned raw meats. The toxin, being rather unstable to heat, is invariably destroyed in cooking.

Bouchard's node a cartilage-covered bony thickening arising at the proximal interphalangeal joint of a finger in osteoarthritis. It is often found together with *Heberden's nodes. [J. C. Bouchard (1837–1915), French physician]

bougie *n.* a hollow or solid cylindrical instrument, usually flexible, that is inserted into tubular passages, such as the esophagus, rectum, or urethra. Bougies are used in diagnosis and treatment, particularly by enlarging *strictures (for example, in the urethra).

Bourneville's disease *see* tuberous sclerosis. [D.-M. Bourneville (1840–1909), French neurologist]

bovine spongiform encephalopathy (BSE) *see* spongiform encephalopathy.

bowel *n. see* intestine.

Bowen's disease a type of carcinoma of the squamous epidermal cells of the skin that does not spread to the basal layers. [J. T. Bowen (1857–1941), US dermatologist]

bowlegs *pl. n.* abnormal out-curving of the legs, resulting in a gap between the knees on standing. A certain degree of bowing is normal in small children, but persistence into adult life, or later development of this deformity, results from abnormal growth of the *epiphysis or arthritis. The condition can be corrected by *osteotomy or by interposition *arthroplasty. Medical name: **genu varum**.

Bowman's capsule the cup-shaped end of a *nephron, which encloses a knot of blood capillaries (*glomerulus*). It is the site of primary filtration of the blood into the kidney tubule. [Sir W. P. Bowman (1816–92), British physician]

BP *see* blood pressure.

brachi- (brachio-) *prefix denoting* the arm. Example: *brachialgia* (pain in).

brachial *adj.* relating to or affecting the arm.

brachial artery an artery that extends from the axillary artery, at the armpit, down the side and inner surface of the arm to the elbow, where it divides into the radial and ulnar arteries.

brachialis *n.* a muscle that is situated at the front of the arm and contracts to flex the forearm (see illustration). It works against the triceps brachii.

brachial plexus a network of nerves, arising from the spine at the base of the neck, from which arise the nerves supplying the arm, forearm and hand, and parts of the shoulder girdle (see illustration). *See also* radial nerve.

brachiocephalic artery (innominate artery) a short artery originating as the first large branch of the *aortic arch, passing upward to the right, and ending at the

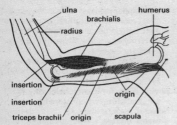

Brachialis and triceps muscles of the forearm

lower neck near the right sternoclavicular joint. Here it divides into the right common carotid and the right subclavian arteries.

brachiocephalic vein (innominate vein) either of two veins, one on each side of the neck, formed by the junction of the external jugular and subclavian veins. The two veins join to form the superior vena cava.

brachium n. (pl. **brachia**) the arm between the shoulder and the elbow.

brachy- prefix denoting shortness. Exam-

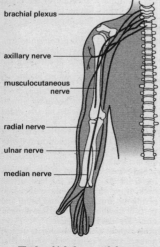

The brachial plexus and the nerves arising from it

ple: *brachydactyly* (shortness of the fingers or toes).

brachycephaly n. shortness of the skull, with a *cephalic index of about 80. —**brachycephalic** adj.

brachytherapy n. radiotherapy administered by implanting radioactive wires or grains into or close to a tumor. This technique is used in the treatment of many accessible tumors, such as breast and cervical cancers, and is increasingly used in the treatment of localized prostate cancer. *Intravascular brachytherapy* has recently been used in the construction of radioactive metallic *stents for arterial procedures, to delay or prevent *restenosis.

bracket n. (in dentistry) the component of a fixed *orthodontic appliance that is bonded to the tooth.

brady- prefix denoting slowness. Example: *bradylalia* (abnormally slow speech).

bradycardia n. slowing of the heart rate to less than 50 beats per minute. *Sinus bradycardia* is often found in healthy individuals, especially athletes, but it is also seen in some patients with reduced thyroid activity, jaundice, hypothermia, or *vasovagal attacks. Bradycardia may also result from *arrhythmias, especially complete *heart block, when the slowing is often extreme and often causes loss of consciousness.

bradykinesia n. a symptom of *parkinsonism comprising a difficulty in initiating movements, slowness in executing movements, and an inability to make adjustments to or to maintain the posture of the body.

bradykinin n. a naturally occurring polypeptide that consists of nine amino acids. Bradykinin is a very powerful vasodilator and causes contraction of smooth muscle; it is formed in the blood under certain conditions and is thought to play an important role as a mediator of inflammation. *See* kinin.

braille n. an alphabet, developed in 1837 by Louis Braille (1809–52) in which each letter is represented by a pattern of raised dots, which are read by feeling with the finger tips. It is the main method of reading used by the blind today.

brain n. the enlarged and highly developed mass of nervous tissue that forms the upper end of the *central nervous system

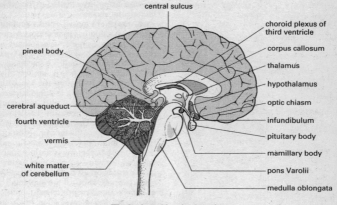

central sulcus

choroid plexus of third ventricle

corpus callosum

thalamus

hypothalamus

optic chiasm

infundibulum

pituitary body

mamillary body

pons Varolii

medulla oblongata

pineal body

cerebral aqueduct

fourth ventricle

vermis

white matter of cerebellum

The brain (midsagittal section)

(see illustration). The average adult human brain weighs about 1400 g (approximately 2% of total body weight) and is continuous below with the spinal cord. It is invested by three connective tissue membranes, the *meninges, and floats in *cerebrospinal fluid within the rigid casing formed by the bones of the skull. The brain is divided into the hindbrain (the rhombencephalon), consisting of the *medulla oblongata, *pons Varolii, and *cerebellum; the *midbrain (the mesencephalon); and the forebrain (the prosencephalon), subdivided into the *cerebrum and the *diencephalon (including the *thalamus and *hypothalamus). Anatomical name: **encephalon**.

brain death *see* death.

brainstem *n.* the enlarged extension upward within the skull of the spinal cord, consisting of the medulla oblongata, the pons, and the midbrain. The pons and medulla are together known as the *bulb*, or *bulbar area*. Attached to the midbrain are the two cerebral hemispheres. *See* brain.

brain tumor *see* cerebral tumor.

branchial arch *see* pharyngeal arch.

branchial cleft *see* pharyngeal cleft.

branchial cyst a cyst that arises at the site of one of the embryonic *pharyngeal pouches due to a developmental anomaly.

branchial pouch *see* pharyngeal pouch.

Brandt Andrews maneuver a technique for expelling the placenta from the uterus. Upward pressure is applied to the uterus through the abdominal wall while holding the umbilical cord taut. When the uterus is elevated in this way, the placenta will be in the cervix or upper vagina and is then expelled by applying pressure below the base of the uterus. [T. Brandt (1819–95), Swedish obstetrician; H. R. Andrews (1872–1942), British gynecologist]

BRCA1 and BRCA2 genes associated with susceptibility to breast and ovarian cancer. Women with mutations in either of these genes have a 56–85% risk of developing breast cancer at a relatively young age.

breakbone fever *see* dengue.

breast *n.* **1.** the mammary gland of a woman: one of two compound glands that produce milk. Each breast consists of glandular lobules – the milk-secreting areas – that are embedded in fatty tissue (see illustration). The milk passes from the lobules into ducts, which connect to form 15–20 *lactiferous ducts*. Near the front of the breast the lactiferous ducts are dilated into *ampullae*, which act as reservoirs for the milk. Each lactiferous duct discharges through a separate orifice in the nipple. The dark area surrounding the nipple is called the

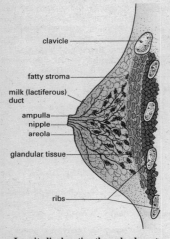

clavicle

fatty stroma

milk (lactiferous) duct

ampulla
nipple
areola

glandular tissue

ribs

Longitudinal section through a breast

areola. See also lactation. Anatomical name: **mamma. 2.** the front part of the chest (thorax).

breastbone *n. see* sternum.

breast cancer a malignant tumor of the breast, usually a *carcinoma (rarely a *sarcoma). It is unusual in men but is the most common form of cancer in women, in some cases involving both breasts. Despite extensive research, the cause is not known but it tends to run in families. The classic sign is a lump in the breast, usually painless; bleeding or discharge from the nipple may occur infrequently. Sometimes the first thing to be noticed is a lump in the armpit, which is due to spread of the cancer to the drainage lymph nodes. The tumor may also spread to the bones, lungs, and liver. Current treatment of a localized tumor is usually by surgery (*see* lumpectomy, mastectomy), with or without radiotherapy; cytotoxic drugs and hormone therapy are used as *adjuvant therapy and for widespread (metastatic) disease. *Tamoxifen is the hormonal treatment of choice for breast cancer in postmenopausal women with metastatic disease; it is also increasingly used as first-line treatment for premenopausal women. COX-2 inhibitors (*see* NSAID)

are also being investigated as possible therapeutic agents.

breast implant a prosthesis to replace breast tissue that has been removed surgically during a simple *mastectomy in the treatment of breast cancer. The type of implant in current use is a silicone sac filled with silicone gel; it has recently been found that coating the sac with polyurethane to give a textured surface reduces the incidence of fibrosis around the implant and consequent hardening of breast tissue. The implant is inserted subcutaneously at the time of operation (the skin and nipple are retained), and follow-up radiotherapy is not normally required. Implants are also used to augment existing breast tissue. Controversy exists over the safety of the implants.

breast-milk jaundice prolonged jaundice lasting several weeks after birth in breast-fed babies for which no other cause can be found. It improves with time and is not an indication to stop breast-feeding.

breath-holding attacks episodes in which a child cries, holds its breath, and goes blue. They are common in toddlers and are usually precipitated by temper tantrums resulting from not getting their own way. The attacks may cause loss of consciousness. Drug treatment is not necessary and the attacks cease spontaneously.

breathing *n.* the alternation of active *inhalation* (or *inspiration*) of air into the lungs through the mouth or nose with the passive *exhalation* (or *expiration*) of the air. During inhalation the *diaphragm and *intercostal muscles contract, which enlarges the chest cavity and draws air into the lungs. Relaxation of these muscles forces air out of the lungs at exhalation. (See illustration.) Breathing is part of *respiration and is sometimes called external respiration. There are many types of breathing in which the rhythm, rate, or character is abnormal. *See also* apnea, bronchospasm, Cheyne-Stokes respiration, dyspnea, stridor.

breathlessness *n. see* dyspnea.

breath sounds the sounds heard through a stethoscope placed over the lungs during breathing. Normal breath sounds are soft and called *vesicular* – they may be increased or decreased in disease states.

The sounds heard over the larger bronchi are louder and harsher. Breath sounds transmitted through consolidated lungs in pneumonia are louder and harsher; they are similar to the sounds heard normally over the larger bronchi and are termed *bronchial breath sounds*. *Crepitations and *rhonchi are sounds added to the breath sounds in abnormal states of the lung. *Amphoric* or *cavernous* sounds have a hollow quality and are heard over cavities in the lung; the amphoric quality may also be heard in voice sounds and on percussion.

breech presentation the position of a baby in the uterus so that it will be delivered buttocks first (instead of the normal head-first position). This type of delivery increases the risk of damage to the baby. *See also* cephalic version.

bregma n. the point on the top of the skull at which the coronal and sagittal *sutures meet. In a young infant this is an opening, the anterior *fontanelle.

Breslow's measurement (or thickness) the distance (in millimeters) between the surface and the deepest extent of a malignant *melanoma. The measurement correlates with prognosis: tumors that are less than 0.76 mm thick have a good prognosis. [A. Breslow (1928–80), US pathologist]

bretylium tosylate an *antiarrhythmic drug used in patients with cardiac arrest to reverse ventricular *fibrillation that has failed to respond to electrical *defibrillation. It is administered by intravenous injection. Side effects include hypotension, nausea, and vomiting. Trade name: **Bretylol.**

bridge n. (in dentistry) a fixed replacement for missing teeth. The artificial tooth is attached to one or more natural teeth, usually by a crown. Bridges may also be fitted on dental *implants. The supporting teeth (or implants) are referred to as *abutments*, and the artificial teeth that fit over them are referred to as *retainers*. The replacements of missing teeth are known as *pontics*. *Adhesive bridges* are attached to one or more adjacent teeth by a metal plate that adheres to the enamel on the tooth surface prepared by the *acid-etch technique; these bridges require minimal tooth preparation compared with conventional types of bridges.

Bright's disease *see* nephritis. [R. Bright (1789–1858), British physician]

brimonidine n. an alpha agonist (*see* sympathomimetic) used in the form of eye drops in the treatment of *glaucoma. The drug reduces the production of aqueous humor and increases its outflow from the eye; it may be used when beta-blocker eye drops are medically undesirable or are ineffective in controlling the glaucoma. Trade name: **Alphagan.**

brinzolamide n. a *carbonic anhydrase in-

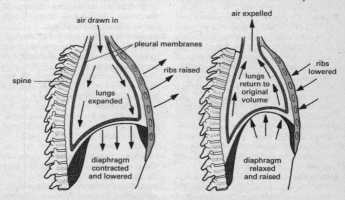

Position of the diaphragm (from the side) during breathing

hibitor used to reduce intraocular pressure in the treatment of *glaucoma: it decreases the production of aqueous humor. Administered as eye drops, it may cause local irritation and taste disturbance. Trade name: **Azopt**.

Briquet's syndrome *see* somatization disorder. [P. Briquet (1796–1881), French psychiatrist]

British thermal unit a unit of heat equal to the quantity of heat required to raise the temperature of 1 pound of water by 1°F. 1 British thermal unit = 1055 joules. Abbreviation: BTU.

brittle diabetes type 1 *diabetes mellitus that constantly causes disruption of lifestyle due to recurrent attacks of hypo- or hyperglycemia from whatever cause. The most common reasons are therapeutic errors, emotional disorders, intercurrent illnesses, and self- or carer-induced episodes.

Broca's area the area of cerebral motor cortex responsible for the initiation of speech. It is situated in the left frontal lobe in most (but not all) right-handed people, in the region of *Brodmann's areas 44 and 45. [P. P. Broca (1824–80), French surgeon]

Brodie's abscess a chronic abscess of bone that develops from acute bacterial *osteomyelitis. The classic appearance on X-ray is a small walled-off cavity in the bone with little or no periosteal reaction. Treatment is by surgical drainage and antibiotics. [Sir B. C. Brodie (1783–1862), British surgeon]

Brodmann's areas the numbered areas (1–47) into which a map of the *cerebral cortex may conveniently be divided for descriptive purposes, based on the arrangement of neurons seen in stained sections under the microscope. On the map, area 4, for example, corresponds to primary motor cortex, whereas the primary visual cortex is in area 17. [K. Brodmann (1868–1918), German neurologist]

bromazepam *n.* a long-acting *benzodiazepine drug used in the short-term treatment of disabling anxiety. It is administered by mouth. Trade name: **Lectopam**.

bromhexine *n.* an *expectorant and mucolytic agent that acts by increasing the volume and reducing the viscosity of bronchial secretions. It is used in the treatment of bronchitis and may cause nausea.

bromides *pl. n.* salts of bromine, including potassium bromide, once widely used as sedatives because of their depressant action on the central nervous system. *See also* bromism.

bromidrosis (bromhidrosis) *n.* bacterial breakdown of sweat, usually in the armpit or on the feet, which causes an unpleasant odor.

bromism *n.* a group of symptoms caused by excessive intake of *bromides, formerly used as sedatives. Overuse for long periods leads to mental dullness, weakness, drowsiness, loss of sensation, slurred speech, and sometimes coma. A form of acne may also develop. Treatment is by immediate withdrawal.

bromocriptine *n.* a *dopamine receptor agonist, derived from ergot, that is used in the treatment of *parkinsonism. It is also used to prevent lactation and to treat disorders associated with excessive secretion of *prolactin (such as *prolactinoma), since it inhibits the secretion of this hormone by the pituitary gland, and to treat *acromegaly, as it suppresses the release of growth hormone. The drug is administered by mouth. Fairly common side effects are dizziness and confusion. Trade name: **Parlodel**.

brompheniramine *n.* an *antihistamine given by mouth to relieve the symptoms of allergic reactions, especially hay fever and rhinitis. Common side effects include drowsiness, dizziness, dryness of the throat, and digestive upsets. Trade names: **Dimetane, Dimetapp**.

Brompton cocktail a mixture of alcohol, morphine, and cocaine sometimes given to control severe pain in terminally ill people, especially those dying of cancer. The mixture was developed at the Brompton Hospital, London, and has given relief to thousands.

bronch- (broncho-) *prefix denoting* the bronchial tree. Examples: *bronchopulmonary* (relating to the bronchi and lungs); *bronchotomy* (incision into).

bronchial carcinoma cancer of the bronchus, one of the most common causes of death in smokers. *See also* lung cancer, oat cell.

bronchial tree a branching system of tubes conducting air from the trachea (windpipe) to the lungs: includes the bronchi (see bronchus) and their subdivisions and the *bronchioles.

bronchiectasis n. widening of the bronchi or their branches. It may be congenital or it may result from infection (especially whooping cough or measles in childhood) or from obstruction, either by an inhaled foreign body or by a growth (including cancer). Pus may form in the widened bronchus so that the patient coughs up purulent sputum, which may contain blood. Diagnosis is based on the clinical symptoms and by X-ray and computed tomography (CT) scan. Treatment consists of antibiotic drugs to control the infection and physiotherapy to drain the sputum. Surgery may be used if only a few segments of the bronchi are affected.

bronchiole n. a subdivision of the bronchial tree that does not contain cartilage or mucous glands in its wall. Bronchioles open from the fifth or sixth generation of bronchi and extend for up to 20 more generations before reaching the *terminal bronchioles*. Each terminal bronchiole divides into a number of *respiratory bronchioles*, from which the *alveoli open. Each terminal bronchiole conducts air to an *acinus in the *lung. —**bronchiolar** adj.

bronchiolitis n. inflammation of the small airways in the lung (see bronchiole) due to viral infection, usually the *respiratory syncytial virus. Bronchiolitis is most common in infants of less than one year old. The bronchioles become swollen, the lining cells die, and the tubes become blocked with debris and mucopus. This prevents air reaching the alveoli and the child becomes short of oxygen (hypoxic), breathless, and possibly cyanosed. In mild cases no treatment is necessary; more severe cases require supportive treatment – administration of oxygen and feeding via a nasogastric tube. Antibiotics are indicated only if there is evidence of a secondary infection. If the child is particularly vulnerable, specific treatment with *ribavirin or artificial ventilation may be beneficial. Recurrent attacks of bronchiolitis may herald the onset of *asthma.

bronchiolitis obliterans organizing pneumonia (BOOP) a disease entity characterized clinically by a flulike illness with cough, fever, shortness of breath, and late inspiratory crackles; there are specific histological features and patchy infiltrates on X-ray. It is sometimes the result of a viral infection, but may follow medication with certain drugs or be associated with connective-tissue disease, such as rheumatoid arthritis. The condition usually responds to oral corticosteroids; however, if a drug is implicated, it must be withdrawn.

bronchitis n. inflammation of the bronchi (see bronchus). *Acute bronchitis* is caused by viruses or bacteria and is characterized by coughing, the production of mucopurulent sputum, and narrowing of the bronchi due to spasmodic contraction (see bronchospasm). In *chronic bronchitis* the patient coughs up excessive mucus secreted by enlarged bronchial mucous glands; the bronchospasm cannot always be relieved by bronchodilator drugs. It is not primarily an inflammatory condition, although it is frequently complicated by acute infections. The disease is particularly prevalent in association with cigarette smoking, air pollution, and *emphysema.

bronchoalveolar lavage (BAL) a method of obtaining cellular material from the lungs that is used particularly in the investigation and monitoring of interstitial lung disease and in the investigation of pulmonary infiltrates in immunosuppressed patients. Examination of the cells in the lavage fluid may help to identify the cause of interstitial lung disease. The combination of cytological and microbiological examination can lead to a very high rate of diagnostic accuracy in such conditions as *Pneumocystis carinii pneumonia.

bronchoconstrictor n. a drug that causes narrowing of the air passages by producing spasm of bronchial smooth muscle.

bronchodilator n. an agent that causes widening of the air passages by relaxing bronchial smooth muscle. *Sympathomimetic drugs that stimulate beta receptors, e.g. *ephedrine, *isoproterenol, *terbutaline, and *albuterol, are potent bronchodilators and are used for relief of bronchial asthma and chronic bronchitis. These drugs are often administered as aerosols, giving rapid relief, but at high doses they may stimulate the heart. Some anticholinergic drugs (e.g. *ipratropium and *theophylline) are also used as bronchodilators.

bronchography n. X-ray examination of the bronchial tree after it has been made visible by the injection of *radiopaque dye or contrast medium. It was used in the diagnosis of *bronchiectasis, but has been superseded by computed tomography (CT) scanning.

bronchophony n. see vocal resonance.

bronchopneumonia n. see pneumonia.

bronchopulmonary dysplasia a condition, seen usually in premature babies as a result of *respiratory distress syndrome, requiring prolonged treatment with oxygen beyond the age of 28 days. The babies have overexpanded lungs, which on X-rays show characteristic changes. Management consists of oxygen support and treating infections. Recovery is slow, sometimes over several years, but most babies do recover.

bronchoscope n. an instrument used to look into the trachea and bronchi. In addition to the rigid tubular metal type, used for many years, there is now a narrower flexible fiberoptic instrument (see fiberoptics) with which previously inaccessible bronchi can be inspected. With either instrument the bronchial tree can be washed out (see bronchoalveolar lavage), and samples of tissue and foreign bodies can be removed with long forceps. —**bronchoscopy** n.

bronchospasm n. narrowing of bronchi by muscular contraction in response to some stimulus, as in *asthma and *bronchitis. The patient can usually inhale air into the lungs, but exhalation may require visible muscular effort and is accompanied by expiratory noises that are clearly audible (see wheeze) or detectable with a stethoscope. The condition in which bronchospasm can usually be relieved by bronchodilator drugs is known as *reversible obstructive airways disease* and includes asthma; that in which bronchodilator drugs usually have no effect is *irreversible obstructive airways disease* and includes chronic bronchitis.

bronchospirometry n. a technique used to assess the efficiency of ventilation of a lung or of a segment of the lung. A catheter with an inflatable cuff is passed into the appropriate airway, through a *bronchoscope, and the volume and rate of gas exchange is determined.

bronchus n. (pl. **bronchi**) any of the air passages beyond the *trachea that has cartilage and mucous glands in its wall (see illustration). The trachea divides into two main bronchi, which divide successively into five *lobar bronchi*, 20 *segmental bronchi*, and two or three more divisions. See also bronchiole. —**bronchial** adj.

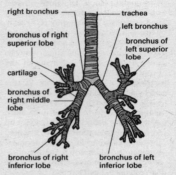

The bronchi and their principal (lobar) branches

bronze diabetes see hemochromatosis.

brown fat a form of fat in adipose tissue that is a rich source of energy and can be converted rapidly to heat. There is speculation that a rapid turnover of brown fat occurs to balance excessive intake of food and unnecessary production of white fat (making up the bulk of adipose tissue). Some forms of obesity may be linked to lack of – or inability to synthesize – brown fat.

Brown-Séquard's syndrome the neurological condition resulting when the spinal cord has been damaged. In those parts of the body supplied by the damaged segment there is a flaccid weakness and loss of feeling in the skin. Below the lesion there is a spastic paralysis on the same side and a loss of pain and temperature sensation on the opposite side. The causes include trauma and multiple sclerosis. [C. E. Brown-Séquard (1818–94), French physiologist]

Brown-Séquard's treatment see organotherapy. [C. E. Brown-Séquard]

Brucella *n.* a genus of gram-negative aerobic spherical or rodlike parasitic bacteria responsible for *brucellosis (undulant fever) in humans and contagious abortion in cattle, pigs, sheep, and goats. The principal species are *B. abortus* and *B. melitensis*.

brucellosis (Malta fever, Mediterranean fever, undulant fever) *n.* a chronic disease of farm animals caused by bacteria of the genus *Brucella*, which can be transmitted to humans either by contact with an infected animal or by drinking nonpasteurized contaminated milk. Symptoms include headache, fever, aches and pains, loss of appetite, and weakness; occasionally a chronic form develops, with recurrent symptoms. Untreated, the disease may last for years but prolonged administration of tetracycline or streptomycin antibiotics is effective. *Brucella ring test* is diagnostic for brucellosis, involving the clumping together of a standard *Brucella* strain by antibodies in an infected person's serum.

Bruch's membrane the transparent innermost layer of the *choroid, which is in contact with the retinal pigment epithelium (*see* retina). [K. W. L. Bruch (1819–84), German anatomist]

Brudzinski's sign a sign present when there is irritation of the meninges (the membranes covering the brain); it is present in meningitis. As the neck is pulled forward, the hips and knees bend involuntarily. [J. von Brudzinski (1874–1917), Polish physician]

Brugia *n.* a genus of threadlike parasitic worms (*see* filaria). *B. malayi* infects humans throughout southeast Asia, causing *filariasis and *elephantiasis (especially of the feet and legs). *B. pahangi*, a parasite of wild cats and domestic animals, produces an allergic condition in humans, with coughing, breathing difficulty, and an increase in the number of *eosinophils in the blood. *Brugia* undergoes part of its development in mosquitoes of the genera *Anopheles* and *Mansonia*, which transmit the parasite from host to host.

bruise (contusion) *n.* an area of skin discoloration caused by the escape of blood from ruptured underlying vessels following injury. Initially red or pink, a bruise gradually becomes bluish, and then greenish yellow, as the hemoglobin

in the tissues breaks down chemically and is absorbed. It may be necessary to draw off blood from very severe bruises through a needle to aid healing.

bruit *n.* a sharp or harsh systolic sound, heard on *auscultation, that is due to turbulent blood flow in a peripheral artery, usually the carotid or iliofemoral artery. Bruits can also be heard over arteriovenous *fistulas or malformations. *See also* murmur.

Brunner's glands compound glands of the small intestine, found in the *duodenum and the upper part of the jejunum. They are embedded in the submucosa and secrete an inhibitor of gastric acid secretion. [J. C. Brunner (1856–1927), Swiss anatomist]

brush border *see* microvillus.

Brushfield spots grayish-brown spots seen in the iris of the eye. They can be found in normal individuals but are usually associated with *Down's syndrome. [T. Brushfield (1858–1937), British physician]

bruxism *n.* a habit in which an individual grinds his teeth, which may lead to excessive wear. This usually occurs during sleep.

B-scan *n.* examination of the tissues of the eye in cross section by means of a high-frequency ultrasound machine. It is useful in the diagnosis of eye disease, especially in the posterior segment of the eye when direct viewing is obscured (e.g. by dense cataracts). *See also* A-scan.

BSE bovine *spongiform encephalopathy. *See also* Creutzfeldt-Jakob disease.

BSS *see* balanced salt solution.

bubo *n.* a swollen inflamed lymph node in the armpit or groin, commonly developing in sexually transmitted diseases (e.g. soft sore), plague, and leishmaniasis.

bubonic plague *see* plague.

buccal *adj.* **1.** relating to the mouth or the hollow part of the cheek. **2.** describing the surface of a tooth adjacent to the cheek.

buccal cavity the cavity of the mouth, which contains the tongue and teeth and leads to the pharynx. Here food is tasted, chewed, and mixed with saliva, which begins the process of digestion.

buccal glands small glands in the mucous membrane lining the mouth. They secrete material that mixes with saliva.

buccinator *n.* a muscle of the cheek that has its origin in the maxilla and mandible (jaw bones). It is responsible for compressing the cheek and is important in mastication.

buclizine *n.* an *antihistamine that has marked sedative properties. Given by mouth, it is used to treat mild anxiety states and tension, motion sickness, and vertigo. Side effects include drowsiness, dizziness, dryness of the throat, and gastrointestinal upsets. Occasionally teratogenic effects may occur. Trade name: **Bucladin**.

Budd-Chiari syndrome a rare condition that follows obstruction of the hepatic vein by a blood clot or tumor. It is characterized by ascites and cirrhosis of the liver. [G. Budd (1808–82), British physician; H. Chiari (1851–1916), German pathologist]

budesonide *n.* an anti-inflammatory *corticosteroid administered as a nasal spray or dry powder inhaler for the management of nasal symptoms of seasonal or perennial allergic *rhinitis and for maintenance treatment in asthma. It is also administered orally for the treatment of mild to moderate active Crohn's disease involving the ileum and/or the ascending colon. Side effects are rare but can include dizziness, nausea, and dry mouth. Trade names: **Entocort** (oral), **Pulmicort, Rhinocort**.

Buerger's disease an inflammatory condition affecting the arteries, especially in the legs, of young men who smoke cigarettes. Intermittent *claudication (pain due to reduced blood supply) and gangrene of the limbs may develop. Coronary thrombosis may occur and venous thrombosis is common. The treatment is similar to that of *atheroma but cessation of smoking is essential to prevent progression of the disease. Medical name: **thromboangiitis obliterans**. [L. Buerger (1879–1943), US physician]

buffer *n.* a solution whose hydrogen ion concentration (pH) remains virtually unchanged by dilution or by the addition of acid or alkali. The chief buffer of the blood and of extracellular body fluids is the bicarbonate (H_2CO_3/HCO_3^-) system. *See also* acid-base balance.

bulb *n.* (in anatomy) any rounded structure or a rounded expansion at the end of an organ or part.

bulbar *adj.* **1.** relating to or affecting the medulla oblongata. **2.** relating to a bulb. **3.** relating to the eyeball.

bulbourethral glands *see* Cowper's glands.

bulimia *n.* insatiable overeating. This symptom may be psychogenic, occurring, for example, as a phase of *anorexia nervosa (*bulimia nervosa* or the *binge–purge syndrome*); or it may be due to neurological causes, such as a lesion of the *hypothalamus. The binge eating usually ends with self-induced vomiting.

bulla *n.* (*pl.* **bullae**) **1.** a large blister, containing serous fluid. *See also* bleb. **2.** (in anatomy) a rounded bony prominence. **3.** a thin-walled air-filled space within the lung, arising congenitally or in *emphysema. It may cause trouble by rupturing into the pleural space (*see* pneumothorax), by adding to the air that does not contribute to gas exchange, and/or by compressing the surrounding lung and making it inefficient. —**bullous** *adj.*

bullous keratopathy a pathological condition of the cornea of the eye due to failure in the functioning of its endothelium. It results in corneal edema, seen as small blisters in the cornea that cause blurring of vision. *See* Fuchs' endothelial dystrophy.

bullous pemphigoid *see* pemphigoid.

bull's-eye maculopathy *see* maculopathy.

bumetanide *n.* a quick-acting loop *diuretic used to relieve the fluid retention (edema) occurring in heart failure, kidney disease, and cirrhosis of the liver. It is administered by mouth or by injection. Side effects include muscle cramps, hypotension, and dizziness. Trade name: **Bumex**.

bundle *n.* a group of muscle or nerve fibers situated close together and running in the same direction; e.g. the *atrioventricular bundle.

bundle branch block a defect in the specialized conducting tissue of the heart (*see* arrhythmia) that is recognized as an electrocardiographic abnormality. Left or right bundle branch blocks, affecting the respective ventricles, may be seen. Occasionally both left and right bundle branch blocks occur simultaneously and the patient develops complete *heart block. The causes are similar to those of complete heart block.

bundle of His *see* atrioventricular bundle. [W. His (1863–1934), Swiss anatomist]

bunion *n.* a swelling of the joint between the great toe and the first metatarsal bone. A *bursa often develops over the site and the great toe becomes displaced toward the others (hallux valgus). Bunions are usually caused by ill-fitting shoes and may require surgical treatment.

bunyavirus *n.* any member of a large, widespread group of *arboviruses, named for the town in Uganda where the species was isolated, that are transmitted by mosquitoes and rodents and in humans cause encephalitis and other diseases characterized by headache, low-grade fever, muscle pain, and rash. *See also* hantavirus.

buphthalmos (hydrophthalmos) *n.* infantile or congenital glaucoma: increased pressure within the eye due to a defect in the development of the tissues through which fluid drains from the eye. Since the outer coat (sclera) of the eyeball of children is distensible, the eye enlarges as the inflow of fluid continues. It usually affects both eyes and may accompany congenital abnormalities in other parts of the body. Treatment is by surgical operation, e.g. *goniotomy, in order to improve drainage of fluid from the eye. Spontaneous arrest of buphthalmos may occur before vision is completely lost.

bupivacaine *n.* a potent local anesthetic, used mainly for regional *nerve block. It is significantly longer acting than many other local anesthetics. It has been used in childbirth, but may cause slowing of the baby's heart, with a risk of death. Trade names: **Marcaine, Sensorcaine**.

buprenorphine *n.* a powerful synthetic *opiate painkilling drug; it acts for 6–8 hours and is administered by injection. Side effects include drowsiness, nausea, dizziness, and sweating. Trade name: **Buprenex**.

bupropion *n.* a drug used to help people stop smoking. It is taken by mouth; side effects include insomnia, headaches, dizziness, depression, and rashes. Bupropion should not be taken by those with a history of epilepsy or eating disorders. Trade name: **Zyban**.

bur (burr) *n.* **1.** a cutting drill that fits in a dentist's handpiece. Burs are mainly used for cutting cavities in teeth, removing old restorations, and preparing teeth to receive artificial crowns. **2.** a surgical drill for cutting through bone.

bur hole (burr hole) a circular hole drilled through the skull to release intracranial tension (due to blood, pus, or cerebrospinal fluid) or to facilitate such procedures as needle aspiration or biopsy.

Burkitt's lymphoma (Burkitt's tumor) a malignant tumor of the lymphatic system, most commonly affecting children and largely confined to tropical Africa in a zone 15° north and south of the equator. It is the most rapidly growing malignancy, with a tumor doubling time of about five days. It can arise at various sites, most commonly the facial structures, such as the jaw, and in the abdomen. The Epstein-Barr virus plays a role in the origin and growth of the tumor. Complications affecting the nervous system occur in up to 50% of cases. Non-African Burkitt's lymphoma is increasingly being recognized. All forms are very sensitive to *cytotoxic drug therapy, but cure is uncommon. [D. P. Burkitt (1911–93), Irish surgeon]

burn *n.* tissue damage caused by such agents as heat, chemicals, electricity, sunlight, or nuclear radiation. A *first-degree burn* affects only the outer layer (epidermis) of the skin. In a *second-degree burn* both the epidermis and the underlying dermis are damaged. A *third-degree burn* involves damage or destruction of the skin to its full depth and damage to the tissues beneath. Burns cause swelling and blistering, due to loss of plasma from damaged blood vessels. In serious burns, affecting 15% or more of the body surface in adults (10% or more in children), this loss of plasma results in severe *shock and requires immediate transfusion of blood or saline solution. Burns may also lead to bacterial infection, which can be prevented by administration of antibiotics. Third-degree burns usually require skin grafting.

burr *n. see* bur.

bursa *n.* (*pl.* **bursae**) a small sac of fibrous tissue that is lined with *synovial membrane and filled with fluid (synovia). Bursae occur where parts move over one another; they help to reduce friction. They are normally formed around joints and in places where ligaments and tendons pass over bones. However, they may be formed in other places in response to unusual pressure or friction.

bursitis (bursal synovitis) *n.* inflammation of a *bursa, resulting from injury, infection, or rheumatoid *synovitis. It produces pain and tenderness and sometimes restricts movement at a nearby joint; for example, at the shoulder. Treatment of bursitis not due to infection is by rest and corticosteroid injection. *See also* housemaid's knee.

Busacca nodule a type of nodule seen on the anterior surface of the iris in granulomatous *uveitis. [A. Busacca (20th century), Italian physician]

buserelin *n.* an *LHRH analogue that is administered as a nasal spray for the treatment of endometriosis and to help in the management of advanced cancer of the prostate gland. Possible side effects include hot flashes, headache, emotional upset, and loss of libido. Trade name: **Suprefact**.

buspirone *n.* a drug used to relieve the symptoms of anxiety. It is administered by mouth; common side effects are headache, nausea, dizziness, and nervousness. Trade name: **BuSpar**.

busulfan *n.* an *alkylating agent that destroys cancer cells by acting on the bone marrow. It is administered by mouth, mainly in the treatment of chronic myeloid leukemia. Busulfan may cause blood disorders producing bleeding. Trade names: **Busulfex**, **Myleran**.

butabarbital *n.* an intermediate-acting *barbiturate, used for the treatment of insomnia and for sedation. It produces sleep within 30 minutes when given by mouth and its sedative effect lasts for about six hours. Prolonged administration may lead to *dependence and its use with alcohol should be avoided; overdosage has serious effects (*see* barbiturism). Trade name: **Butisol**.

butyrophenone *n.* one of a group of chemically related *antipsychotic drugs that includes *haloperidol and *droperidol. Butyrophenones inhibit the effects of *dopamine by occupying dopamine receptor sites in the body.

bypass *n.* a surgical procedure to divert the flow of blood or other fluid from one anatomic structure to another; a *shunt. A bypass can be temporary or permanent and is commonly performed

in the treatment of cardiac and gastrointestinal disorders. *See also* cardiopulmonary bypass, coronary bypass graft.

byssinosis *n.* an industrial disease of the lungs caused by inhalation of dusts of cotton, flax, sisal, or hemp. The patient characteristically has chest tightness and *wheeze after the weekend break, which wears off during the working week. The causal agent has not been identified.

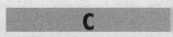

C

cabergoline *n.* a dopamine receptor agonist (*see* dopamine).

CABG coronary artery bypass graft. *See* coronary bypass graft.

cac- (caco-) *prefix denoting* unpleasantness, disease, or deformity. Example: *cacogeusia* (unpleasant taste).

cachet *n.* a flat capsule containing a drug that has an unpleasant taste. The cachet is swallowed intact by the patient.

cachexia *n.* a condition of abnormally low weight, weakness, and general bodily decline associated with chronic disease. It occurs in such conditions as cancer, pulmonary tuberculosis, and malaria.

cacosmia *n.* a disorder of the sense of smell in which scents that are inoffensive to most people are objectionable to the sufferer or in which a bad smell seems to be perpetually present. The disorder is usually due to damage to pathways within the brain rather than in the nose or olfactory nerve.

CAD *see* coronary artery disease.

cadmium *n.* a silvery metallic element that can cause serious lung irritation if the fumes of the molten metal are inhaled. Long-term exposure may also cause kidney damage. Symbol: Cd.

café au lait spots well-defined pale-brown patches on the skin. They are present in up to 20% of the normal population, but the presence of six or more in an individual is strongly suggestive of *neurofibromatosis.

caffeine *n.* an alkaloid drug, obtained from coffee, tea, and chocolate that has a stimulant action, particularly on the central nervous system. It is used to promote wakefulness and increase mental activity; it also possesses diuretic properties and will help relieve certain forms of headache. It is often administered with aspirin and codeine as an analgesic preparation.

Caffey's disease see hyperostosis. [J. Caffey (1895–1966), US pediatrician]

caged-ball valve see ball-and-cage valve.

caisson disease see compressed air illness.

calamine n. a preparation of zinc carbonate used as a mild astringent on the skin in the form of a lotion, cream, or ointment.

calc- (calci-, calco-) prefix denoting calcium or calcium salts.

calcaneus (heel bone) n. the large bone in the *tarsus of the foot that forms the projection of the heel behind the foot. It articulates with the cuboid bone in front and with the talus above.

calcar n. a spurlike projection. The *calcar avis* is the projection in the medial wall of the lateral ventricle of the brain.

calcicosis n. *pneumoconiosis in marble cutters.

calciferol n. see vitamin D.

calcification n. the deposition of calcium salts in tissue. This occurs as part of the normal process of bone formation (see ossification).

calcinosis n. the abnormal deposition of calcium salts in the tissues. This may occur only in the fat layer beneath the skin or it may be more widespread.

calcipotriene n. a vitamin D analogue administered as an ointment for the treatment of psoriasis. It acts by slowing the turnover of cells. Possible side effects include skin irritation and facial dermatitis. Trade name: **Dovonex**.

calcitonin (thyrocalcitonin) n. a hormone, produced by *C cells in the thyroid gland, that lowers the levels of calcium and phosphate in the blood. Calcitonin is given by injection to treat hypercalcemia and Paget's disease of the bone. *Compare* parathyroid hormone.

calcium n. a metallic element essential for the normal development and functioning of the body. Calcium is an important constituent of bones and teeth: the matrix of *bone, consisting principally of calcium phosphate, accounts for about 99% of the body's calcium. It is present in the blood at a concentration of about 10 mg/100 ml, being maintained at this level by hormones (see calcitonin, parathyroid hormone). It is essential for

many metabolic processes, including nerve function, muscle contraction, and blood clotting.

The normal dietary requirement of calcium is about 1 g per day: dairy products (milk and cheese) are the principal sources. Its uptake by the body is facilitated by *vitamin D; a deficiency of this vitamin may therefore result in such conditions as *rickets, *osteoporosis, and *osteomalacia. A deficiency of calcium in the blood may lead to *tetany. Excess calcium may be deposited in the body as *calculi (stones), especially in the gallbladder and kidney. Symbol: Ca.

calcium antagonist (calcium-channel blocker) a drug that inhibits the influx of calcium ions into cardiac and smooth muscle cells; it therefore reduces the strength of heart muscle contraction, reduces conduction of impulses in the heart, and causes vasodilation. Calcium antagonists include *amlodipine, *diltiazem, *nicardipine, *nifedipine, and *verapamil, which are used to treat angina and high blood pressure.

calculosis n. the presence of multiple calculi (stones) in the body. *See* calculus.

calculus n. (*pl.* **calculi**) **1.** a stone: a hard pebblelike mass formed within the body, particularly in the gallbladder (see gallstone) or anywhere in the urinary tract (see cystolithiasis, nephrolithiasis, staghorn calculus). Calculi in the urinary tract are commonly composed of calcium oxalate and are usually visible on X-ray examination. Some of these stones cause pain if they cause obstruction and prevent urine flow in the ureter or kidney, or by direct irritation of the bladder. Stones passing down a duct (such as the ureter) cause severe colicky pain. Most stones pass spontaneously, but some need to be broken into smaller pieces, usually by extracorporeal *lithotripsy, and the remainder by endosurgical techniques (see litholapaxy) or rarely by open surgery. Calculi may also occur in the ducts of the salivary glands. **2.** a calcified deposit that forms on the surface of a tooth as it is covered with dental *plaque. *Supragingival calculus* forms above the *gingivae (gums), principally in relation to the openings of the salivary gland ducts. *Subgingival calculus* forms beneath the crest of the gingivae. Calculus hinders the cleaning of teeth and its presence contributes to *gingivitis and *periodontal disease.

calibrator n. 1. an instrument used for measuring the size of a tube or opening. 2. an instrument used for dilating a tubular part, such as the gullet.

caliectasis (hydrocalycosis) n. dilation or distension of the calyces of the kidney, which is mainly associated with *hydronephrosis or infection and usually demonstrated by *ultrasound or *intravenous urogram.

caliper n. 1. an instrument with two prongs or jaws, used for measuring diameters: used particularly in obstetrics for measuring the diameter of the pelvis. 2. (**caliper splint**) a surgical appliance (see orthosis) that is used to correct or control deformity of a joint in the leg. It consists of a metal bar that is fixed to the shoe and held to the leg by means of straps attached to a padded ring at the top of the leg, taking the weight of the body at the leg. Caliper splints can be used to exert *traction as part of orthopedic treatment.

callosity (callus) n. a hard thick area of skin occurring in parts of the body subject to pressure or friction. The soles of the feet and palms of the hands are common sites, and if much hard dead skin develops a callosity can become painful. A *corn is a type of callosity.

callotasis n. the process of stretching the callus that forms between the ends of a bone that has been divided. It is achieved by means of an external fixator attached to the bone in the procedure for *limb lengthening. The elongated callus consolidates to form new bone.

callus n. 1. the tissue formed between bone ends when a fracture is healing. It initially consists of blood clot and *granulation tissue, which develops into cartilage and then calcifies to form bone. Callus formation is an essential part of the process of healthy union in a fractured bone. 2. see callosity.

calor n. heat: one of the classic signs of inflammation in a tissue, the other three signs being *rubor (redness), *dolor (pain), and *tumor (swelling). An inflamed region has a higher temperature than normal because of the distended blood vessels, which allow an increased flow of blood.

calorie n. a unit of heat equal to the amount of heat required to raise the temperature of 1 gram of water from 14.5°C to 15.5°C (the 15° calorie). One Calorie (also known as the *kilocalorie* or *kilogram calorie*) is equal to 1000 calories; this unit is used to indicate the energy value of foods. Except in this context, the calorie has largely been replaced by the *joule (1 calorie = 4.1855 joules).

calorimeter n. any apparatus used to measure the heat lost or gained during various chemical and physical changes. For example, calorimeters may be used to determine the total energy values of different foods in terms of calories. —**calorimetry** n.

calvaria n. the vault of the *skull.

calyx n. (pl. **calyces**) a cup-shaped part, especially any of the divisions of the pelvis of the *kidney. Each calyx receives urine from the urine-collecting tubes in one sector of the kidney.

camphor n. a crystalline aromatic substance obtained from the tree *Cinnamomum camphora*. It is used in creams, liniments, and sprays as a counterirritant and antipruritic.

campimetry n. a method of assessing the central part of the *visual field. It measures that part of the field of vision within 30° in all directions from the center.

camptodactyly n. congenital and permanent inward bending of a finger, most commonly the little finger; it can occur at one or both interphalangeal joints. It often affects both hands and is first noticed at the age of about ten; no treatment is needed.

Campylobacter n. a genus of curved or spiral rod-shaped gram-negative bacteria. The organisms are found in the intestinal tract of humans and animals and cause diarrhea and enteritis. Treatment is with antibiotics, including streptomycin, erythromycin, and tetracycline.

canal n. a tubular channel or passage; e.g. the *alimentary canal and the auditory canal of the ear.

canaliculitis n. inflammation of a canaliculus, especially a lacrimal canaliculus (see lacrimal apparatus).

canaliculus n. (pl. **canaliculi**) a small channel or canal. Canaliculi occur, for example, in compact bone, linking lacunae containing bone cells. *Bile canaliculi* are minute channels within the liver that transport bile to the bile duct. *Lacrimal* *canaliculi* drain tears into the lacrimal sac (*see* lacrimal apparatus).

cancellous *adj.* latticelike: applied to the bony tissue laid down by *osteoblasts during development of bone and in the *consolidation stage of fracture repair. In a mature bone cancellous bone has a low density and is surrounded by denser cortical bone.

cancer *n.* any *malignant tumor, including *carcinoma and *sarcoma. It arises from the abnormal and uncontrolled division of cells that then invade and destroy the surrounding tissues. Spread of cancer cells (*metastasis) may occur via the bloodstream or the lymphatic channels or across body cavities such as the pleural and peritoneal spaces, thus setting up secondary tumors (metastases) at sites distant from the original tumor. Each individual primary tumor has its own pattern of local behavior and metastasis; for example, bone metastasis is very common in breast cancer and prostate cancer but less common in other tumors.

There are probably many causative factors, some of which are known; for example, cigarette smoking is associated with lung cancer, radiation with some sarcomas and leukemia, and several viruses can cause tumors (*see* oncogenic). A genetic element is implicated in the development of many cancers. In more than half of all cancers a gene called *p53 is deleted or impaired: its normal function is to prevent the uncontrolled division of cells (*see* tumor necrosis factor). Treatment of cancer depends on the type of tumor, the site of the primary tumor, and the extent of spread.

cancrum (canker) *n.* ulceration, mainly of the lips and mouth (*cancrum oris*).

candela (candle) *n.* the *SI unit of luminous intensity, equal to the intensity in a given direction of a surface of 1/60 square centimeter emitting monochromatic radiation at a frequency of 540×10^{12} Hz, of which the radiant intensity is 1/683 watt per steradian. Symbol: cd.

candesartan *n. see* angiotensin II antagonist.

Candida *n.* a genus of *yeasts (formerly called *Monilia*) that inhabit the vagina and alimentary tract and can – under certain conditions – cause *candidiasis.

The species *C. albicans*, a small oval budding fungus, is primarily responsible for candidiasis of the mouth, lungs, intestine, vagina, skin, and nails.

candidiasis (candidosis) *n.* a common *yeast infection caused by fungi of the genus *Candida*, usually the species *C. albicans*. The infection – formerly called *moniliasis* – is usually superficial, occurring in moist areas of the body, such as the skin folds, mouth, respiratory tract, and vagina. Rarely, candidiasis infection may spread throughout the body. Candidiasis of the mouth (popularly known as *thrush*) appears as white patches on the tongue or inside the cheeks. On the skin the lesions are bright red with small satellite pustules, while in the vagina this infection produces itching and sometimes a thick white discharge. Candidiasis sometimes develops in patients receiving broad-spectrum antibiotics and in those who are *immunocompromised. It is treated with topical or oral antifungal drugs – especially *nystatin, *amphotericin B, and *imidazoles.

candle *n. see* candela.

canine *n.* the third tooth from the midline of each jaw. There are thus four canines, two in each jaw, in both the permanent and deciduous (milk) *dentitions. It is known colloquially as the *eye tooth*.

canities *n.* loss of pigment in the hair, which causes graying or whitening. It is usually part of the aging process, when it starts at the temples. White patches may occur as a result of *alopecia areata or *vitiligo.

canker *n. see* cancrum.

cannabis *n.* a drug prepared from the Indian hemp plant (*Cannabis sativa*), also known as *pot*, *marijuana*, *hashish*, and *bhang*. Smoked or swallowed, it produces euphoria and hallucinations and affects perception and awareness, particularly of time. Cannabis has little therapeutic value and its nonmedical use is illegal: there is evidence that prolonged use may cause brain damage and lead the user onto "hard" drugs, such as heroin. *See also* dependence.

cannula *n.* a hollow tube designed for insertion into a body cavity, such as the bladder, or a blood vessel. The tube contains a sharp pointed solid core (*trocar), which facilitates its insertion and is

withdrawn when the cannula is in place.
Fluids may be introduced or withdrawn
via a cannula.

cantharidin *n.* the active principle of *can-
tharides*, or *Spanish fly* (the dried bodies
of a blister beetle, *Lytta vesicatoria*). A
toxic and irritant chemical, cantharidin
causes blistering of the skin and was formerly used in veterinary medicine as a
counterirritant and vesicant. If swallowed it causes nausea, vomiting, and
inflammation of the urinary tract, the
latter giving rise to its reputation as an
aphrodisiac. It is very dangerous and
may cause death.

cantholysis *n.* a surgical procedure to divide the attachment of the *canthus (corner of the eye) from its underlying bone
and tendon. It is performed as part of
some operations on the eyelid.

canthoplasty *n.* a surgical procedure to reconstruct the *canthus (corner of the
eye).

canthus *n.* either corner of the eye; the
angle at which the upper and lower eyelids meet. —**canthal** *adj.*

cap *n.* a covering or a coverlike part. The
duodenal cap is the superior part of the
duodenum as seen on X-ray after a barium meal.

CAPD 1. continuous ambulatory peritoneal
dialysis: a method of treating renal failure on an outpatient basis. *See also*
hemodialysis. **2.** *see* central auditory processing disorder.

capecitabine *n.* a drug that is used in treatment of cancers of the rectum, colon, or
breast that have spread to other sites.
Taken by mouth, it is converted to
*fluorouracil in the body; side effects
may include blood disorders (*see* myelosuppression) and mouth ulcers. Trade
name: **Xeloda.**

Capgras' syndrome (illusion of doubles)
the delusion that a person closely involved with the patient has been replaced by an identical-looking impostor.
It is often, but not necessarily, a form of
paranoid *schizophrenia. [J. M. J. Capgras (1873–1950), French psychiatrist]

capillary *n.* an extremely narrow blood vessel, approximately 5–20 μm in diameter.
Capillaries form networks in most tissues; they are supplied with blood by arterioles and drained by venules. The
vessel wall is only one cell thick, which
enables exchange of oxygen, carbon

dioxide, water, salts, etc., between the
blood and the tissues (see illustrations).

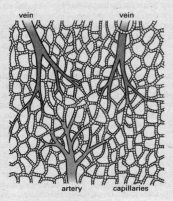

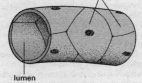

**A network of capillaries (above); a single
capillary (below)**

capitate *adj.* head-shaped; having a
rounded extremity.

capitate bone the largest bone of the wrist
(*see* carpus). It articulates with the
scaphoid and lunate bones behind, with
the second, third, and fourth metacarpal
bones in front, and the trapezoid and
hamate laterally.

capitation fee a system of payment to
physicians for medical care of patients.
The physician receives a fixed sum of
money for each patient assigned to the
doctor's panel of patients, regardless of
the amount of medical care required by
the patient. The patient is charged for
the fixed capitation fee at regular intervals, e.g. monthly or quarterly. A capitation fee system may be used by
*Health Maintenance Organizations.

capitulum *n.* the small rounded end of a

bone that articulates with another bone. For example, the *capitulum humeri* is the round prominence at the elbow end of the humerus that articulates with the radius.

capping *n.* (in dentistry) **1.** colloquial term for crowning: the technique of fitting a tooth with an artificial *crown. **2.** *see* pulp capping.

capreomycin *n.* an antibiotic, derived from the bacterium *Streptomyces capreolus*, that is used in the treatment of tuberculosis. It is given with other antituberculosis drugs to reduce the development of resistance by the infective bacteria. Capreomycin is poorly absorbed from the gastrointestinal tract and therefore must be administered by intramuscular injection. The more serious side effects include ear and kidney damage. Trade name: **Capastat**.

capsaicin a topical analgesic used to relieve the pain associated with neuralgia, osteoarthritis, and rheumatoid arthritis. Capsaicin is the purified extracted alkaloid from red chilli peppers, the substance that makes the peppers hot, and relieves pain by reducing substance P, an amide that is involved in transmitting pain sensations across nerve endings. The most common adverse reaction is a stinging, burning sensation at the site of application, which gradually reduces with continued use. Trade name: **Zostrix**.

capsule *n.* **1.** a membrane, sheath, or other structure that encloses a tissue or organ. For example, the kidney, adrenal gland, and lens of the eye are enclosed within capsules. A *joint capsule* is the fibrous tissue, including the synovial membrane, that surrounds a freely movable joint. **2.** a soluble case, usually made of gelatin, in which certain drugs are administered. **3.** the slimy substance that forms a protective layer around certain bacteria, hindering their ingestion by phagocytes. It is usually composed of *polysaccharide.

capsulitis *n.* inflammation of the capsule surrounding an organ or part, such as a joint. *See also* frozen shoulder.

capsulorrhexis *n.* a surgical procedure in which a continuous circular tear is made in the lens capsule of the eye. In *anterior capsulorrhexis*, performed during cataract surgery, the tear is made in the anterior surface of the capsule. It has the advantage over a *capsulotomy in making the residual capsule much more resilient to being torn during surgery.

capsulotomy *n.* an incision into the capsule of the lens. In modern operations for cataract the lens capsule is not removed and tends, after months or years, to become opaque. Before the advent of laser surgery, a tiny knife (*cystitome*) was inserted into the eye and a hole cut in the center of the capsule, thus providing a clear path for light rays to reach the retina. Currently, this procedure is performed with a *YAG laser as an outpatient procedure.

captopril *n.* a drug used in the treatment of heart failure and hypertension. It acts by inhibiting the action of *angiotensin (*see* ACE inhibitor). Side effects include rash, *neutropenia or *agranulocytosis, hypotension, and loss of taste. Trade names: **Accupril**, **Capoten**.

caput succedaneum a temporary swelling of the soft parts of the head of a newly born infant that occurs during birth, due to compression by the muscles of the cervix (neck) of the uterus.

carbachol *n.* a *parasympathomimetic drug used to relieve pressure within the eye in glaucoma; side effects include headache and local burning and itching. It is also used (now infrequently) after surgical operations to restore the function of inactive bowels or bladder. Side effects may include sweating, nausea, and faintness. Trade names: **Carbastat**, **Carboptic**, **Miostat**.

carbamazepine *n.* an *anticonvulsant drug used in the treatment of epilepsy and to relieve the pain of trigeminal neuralgia. Common side effects include drowsiness, dizziness, and muscular incoordination; abnormalities of liver and bone marrow may occur with long-term treatment. Trade names: **Carbatrol**, **Tegretol**.

carbenicillin *n.* a synthetic penicillin: an antibiotic that is effective against a wide range of bacterial infections, especially of the urinary tract and prostate. It is given orally; side effects include nausea, vomiting, diarrhea, dry mouth, and furry tongue. Trade name: **Geocillin**.

carbenoxolone *n.* a drug that reduces inflammation, used mainly to promote healing in the treatment of gastric ulcers or ulcers of the mouth. It is given by mouth; side effects include the retention of salt and water (see edema), weight gain, and high blood pressure.

carbidopa n. a drug that prevents the breakdown of *levodopa to dopamine outside the brain by inhibiting the enzyme dopa decarboxylase. Administered by mouth in combination with levodopa (as *Sinemet*), it is used to treat Parkinson's disease; side effects are those of *benserazide.

carbimazole n. a drug used to reduce the production of thyroid hormone in cases of overactivity of the gland (thyrotoxicosis). It is administered by mouth; some allergic reactions may occur and high dosage may cause enlargement of the thyroid gland, which may obstruct the windpipe.

carbinoxamine n. a short-acting antihistamine, given by mouth in the treatment of allergic conditions, particularly hay fever and rhinitis, and to prevent motion sickness. Trade name: **Clistin**.

carbohydrate n. any one of a large group of compounds, including the *sugars and *starch, that contain carbon, hydrogen, and oxygen and have the general formula $C_x(H_2O)_y$. Carbohydrates are important as a source of energy: they are manufactured by plants and obtained by animals through the diet, being one of the three main constituents of food (see also fat, protein). All carbohydrates are eventually broken down in the body to the simple sugar *glucose, which can then take part in energy-producing metabolic processes. Excess carbohydrate, not immediately required by the body, is stored in the liver and muscles in the form of *glycogen. In plants carbohydrates are important structural materials (e.g. cellulose) and storage products (commonly in the form of starch). See also disaccharide, monosaccharide, polysaccharide.

carbolfuchsin n. a red stain for bacteria and fungi, consisting of carbolic acid and *fuchsin dissolved in alcohol and water.

carbolic acid see phenol.

carbon dioxide a colorless gas formed in the tissues during metabolism and carried in the blood to the lungs, where it is exhaled (an increase in the concentration of this gas in the blood stimulates respiration). Carbon dioxide occurs in small amounts in the atmosphere; it is used by plants in the process of *photosynthesis. It forms a solid (dry ice) at −75°C (at atmospheric pressure) and in this form is used as a refrigerant. Formula: CO_2.

carbonic anhydrase inhibitor any one of a class of drugs that act by blocking the action of the enzyme carbonic anhydrase. This enzyme greatly speeds up the reaction between carbon dioxide and water to form carbonic acid, a compound needed for the production of many of the body's secretions. Carbonic anhydrase is present in high concentrations in the eye, kidneys, stomach lining, and pancreas. Carbonic anhydrase inhibitors reduce the production of aqueous humor in the eye and are used mainly in treating *glaucoma. They include *acetazolamide, *brinzolamide, and *dorzolamide.

carbon monoxide a colorless almost odorless gas that is very poisonous. When breathed in it combines with hemoglobin in the red blood cells to form *carboxyhemoglobin, which is bright red in color. This compound is chemically stable and thus the hemoglobin can no longer combine with oxygen. Carbon monoxide is present in coal gas and motor exhaust fumes. Formula: CO.

carbon tetrachloride (tetrachloromethane) a pungent volatile fluid used in dry cleaning. When inhaled or swallowed it may severely damage the heart, liver, and kidneys, causing cirrhosis and nephrosis, and it can also affect the optic nerve and other nerves. Treatment is by administration of oxygen. Formula: CCl_4.

carboplatin n. a derivative of platinum that is used in the treatment of certain types of cancer (e.g. ovarian cancer). It is similar to *cisplatin but has fewer side effects; in particular, it causes less nausea and vomiting. Trade name: **Paraplatin**.

carboxyhemoglobin n. a substance formed when carbon monoxide combines with the pigment *hemoglobin in the blood. Carboxyhemoglobin is incapable of transporting oxygen to the tissues and this is the cause of death in carbon monoxide poisoning. Large quantities of carboxyhemoglobin are formed in carbon monoxide poisoning, and low levels are always present in the blood of smokers and city dwellers.

carboxylase n. an enzyme that catalyzes the addition of carbon dioxide to a substance.

carbuncle n. a collection of *boils with multiple drainage channels. The infection is usually caused by *Staphylococcus aureus* and normally results in an extensive slough of skin. Treatment is with antibiotics and sometimes also by surgery.

carcin- (carcino-) *prefix denoting* cancer or carcinoma. Example: *carcinogenesis* (development of).

carcinoembryonic antigen (CEA) a protein produced in the fetus but not in normal adult life. It may be produced by carcinomas, particularly of the colon, and is a rather insensitive marker of malignancy. It is an example of an *oncofetal antigen that is used as a *tumor marker, particularly in the follow-up of colorectal cancer.

carcinogen n. any substance that, when exposed to living tissue, may cause the production of cancer. Known carcinogens include ionizing radiation and many chemicals, e.g. those found in cigarette smoke and those produced in certain industries. They cause damage to the DNA of cells that may persist if the cell divides before the damage is repaired. Damaged cells may subsequently develop into a cancer (*see* carcinogenesis). An inherent susceptibility to cancer may be necessary for a carcinogen to promote the development of cancer. *See also* oncogenic. —**carcinogenic** *adj.*

carcinogenesis n. the evolution of an invasive cancer cell from a normal cell. Intermediate stages, sometimes called *premalignant, preinvasive,* or *noninvasive,* may be recognizable, but the interchangeable use of these terms can be confusing, and they have been replaced by *carcinoma in situ.

carcinoid n. see argentaffinoma.

carcinoma n. any *cancer that arises in epithelium, the tissue that lines the external and internal organs of the body. It may occur in any tissue containing epithelial cells. In many cases the site of origin of the tumor may be identified by the nature of the cells it contains. Organs may exhibit more than one type of carcinoma; for example, an adenocarcinoma and a squamous carcinoma may be found in the cervix (but not usually concurrently). Treatment depends on the nature of the primary tumor, different types responding to different drug combinations. —**carcinomatous** *adj.*

carcinoma in situ (CIS) the earliest stage of cancer spread, in which the tumor is confined to the epithelium and surgical removal of the growth should lead to cure. *See also* cervical cancer, cervical intraepithelial neoplasia, ductal carcinoma in situ.

carcinomatosis n. carcinoma that has spread widely throughout the body. Spread of the cancer cells occurs via the lymphatic channels and bloodstream and across body cavities, for example, the peritoneal cavity.

carcinosarcoma n. a malignant tumor of the cervix, uterus, or vagina containing a mixture of *adenocarcinoma, sarcoma cells, and *stroma. Sarcomatoid differentiation of epithelial cancers often indicates a poor prognosis.

cardi- (cardio-) *prefix denoting* the heart. Examples: *cardiomegaly* (enlargement of); *cardiopathy* (disease of).

cardia n. **1.** the opening at the upper end of the *stomach that connects with the esophagus (gullet). **2.** *Obsolete.* the heart.

cardiac *adj.* **1.** of, relating to, or affecting the heart. **2.** of or relating to the upper part of the stomach (*see* cardia).

cardiac arrest the cessation of effective pumping action of the heart, which most commonly occurs when the muscle fibers of the ventricles start to beat rapidly without pumping any blood (ventricular *fibrillation) or when the heart stops beating completely (*asystole). There is abrupt loss of consciousness, absence of the pulse, and breathing stops. The most common cause is *myocardial infarction. Unless treated promptly, irreversible brain damage and death follow within minutes. Some patients may be resuscitated by massage of the heart, artificial respiration, and *defibrillation.

cardiac catheterization *see* catheterization.

cardiac cycle the sequence of events between one heartbeat and the next, normally occupying less than a second. The atria contract simultaneously and force blood into the relaxed ventricles. The ventricles then contract very strongly and pump blood out through the aorta and pulmonary artery. During ventricular contraction, the atria relax and fill up again with blood. *See* diastole, systole.

cardiac muscle the specialized muscle of the walls of the *heart. It is composed of a network of branching elongated cells (fibers) whose junctions with neighboring cells are marked by irregular transverse bands known as *intercalated disks*.

cardiac output the volume of blood expelled by either ventricle of the heart per unit of time, usually measured as volume per minute. It is equal to the amount of blood ejected at each beat (the stroke output) multiplied by the number of beats per period of time used in the computation. A normal heart in a resting adult ejects from 4.8 to 6.4 liters of blood per minute. A decreased output at rest that does not increase during exercise indicates abnormal cardiac performance.

cardiac reflex reflex control of the heart rate. Sensory fibers in the walls of the heart are stimulated when the heart rate increases above normal. Impulses are sent to the cardiac center in the brain, stimulating the vagus nerve and leading to slowing of the heart rate.

cardiac tamponade a dangerous situation in which there is a build-up of fluid around the heart within the pericardial sac. This causes compression of the heart, which is therefore unable to fill with blood adequately in order to pump effectively. Cardiac tamponade can result in heart failure, a drop in blood pressure, or cardiac arrest. It requires treatment by drainage of the fluid. The classical diagnostic features, known as *Beck's triad*, consist of dilated neck veins, a fall in blood pressure, and muffled heart sounds.

cardinal veins two pairs of veins in the embryo that carry blood from the head (*anterior cardinal veins*) and trunk (*posterior cardinal veins*); they unite to form the *common cardinal vein*, which drains into the sinus venosus of the heart.

cardiology *n.* the science that is concerned with the study of the structure, function, and diseases of the heart. *See also* nuclear cardiology. —**cardiologist** *n.*

cardiomyopathy *n.* any chronic disorder affecting the muscle of the heart. It may be inherited but can also be caused by various conditions, including virus infections, alcoholism, beriberi (vitamin B_1 deficiency), and amyloidosis. The cause is often unknown. It may result in enlargement of the heart, *heart failure, *arrhythmias, and embolism. There is often no specific treatment but patients improve following the control of heart failure and arrhythmias.

cardiomyoplasty *n.* a recent surgical technique to replace or reinforce damaged cardiac muscle with skeletal muscle.

cardiomyotomy *n. see* achalasia, myotomy.

cardioplegia *n.* a technique in which the heart is stopped by injecting it with a solution of salts, by hypothermia, or by an electrical stimulus. This has enabled complex cardiac surgery and transplants to be performed safely.

cardiopulmonary bypass a method by which the circulation to the body is maintained while the heart is deliberately stopped during heart surgery. The function of the heart and lungs is carried out by a pump-oxygenator (*heart-lung machine) until the natural circulation is restored.

cardiopulmonary resuscitation (CPR) an emergency procedure for life support, consisting of artificial respiration and manual external cardiac massage. It is used in cases of cardiac arrest or apparent sudden death resulting from electric shock, drowning, respiratory arrest, or other causes, to establish effective circulation and ventilation in order to prevent irreversible brain damage. External cardiac massage compresses the heart, forcing blood into the systemic and pulmonary circulation; venous blood refills the heart when the compression is released. *Mouth-to-mouth respiration or a mechanical form of ventilation oxygenates the blood being pumped through the circulatory system.

cardiospasm *n. see* achalasia.

cardiotocograph *n.* the instrument used in *cardiotocography to produce a *cardiotocogram*, the graphic printout of the measurements obtained.

cardiotocography *n.* the electronic monitoring of the fetal heart rate and rhythm, either by an external microphone or transducer or by applying an electrode to the fetal scalp, recording the fetal electrocardiogram. The procedure also includes a measurement of the strength and frequency of uterine contractions by means of an external transducer or an intrauterine catheter.

cardiotomy syndrome (postcardiotomy syndrome) a condition that may develop weeks or months after surgery to the heart and the membrane surrounding it (pericardium) and is characterized by fever and *pericarditis. Pneumonia and pleurisy may form part of the syndrome. It is thought to be an *autoimmune disease and may be recurrent. A similar syndrome (*Dressler's syndrome*) may follow myocardial infarction. It may respond to anti-inflammatory drugs.

cardiovascular system (circulatory system, vascular system) the heart together with two networks of blood vessels – the *systemic circulation and the *pulmonary circulation (see illustration). The cardiovascular system effects the circulation of blood around the body, which brings about transport of nutrients and oxygen to the tissues and the removal of waste products.

cardioversion (countershock) *n.* a method of restoring the normal rhythm of the heart in patients with increased heart rate due to arrhythmia. A controlled direct current shock, synchronized with the R wave of the electrocardiograph, is given through electrodes placed on the chest wall of the anesthetized patient. The apparatus is called a *cardiovertor* and is a modified *defibrillator.

caries *n.* decay and crumbling of the substance of a tooth (*see* dental caries) or of a bone. —**carious** *adj.*

carina *n.* a keellike structure, such as the keel-shaped cartilage at the bifurcation of the trachea into the two main bronchi.

cariogenic *adj.* causing caries, particularly

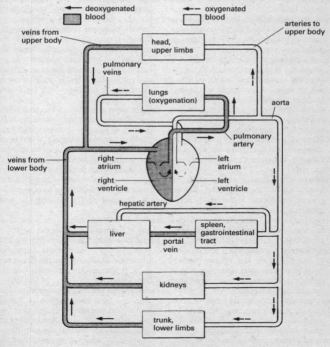

Diagram of the cardiovascular system

dental caries: refers especially to the sugar in food and drinks.

cariology *n.* the branch of dentistry concerned with the study of tooth decay (*see* dental caries).

carisoprodol *n.* a drug with muscle-relaxant, analgesic, and tranquilizing action. It is used in the treatment of spastic conditions, such as parkinsonism, and for back pain, sprains, and other injuries. Carisoprodol is administered by mouth; there are few side effects, but drowsiness or dizziness may occur. Trade names: **Rela, Soma.**

carminative *n.* a drug that relieves flatulence, used to treat gastric discomfort and colic.

carmustine *n.* a drug (an *alkylating agent) used in the treatment of certain cancers, including myeloma, lymphomas, and brain tumors. Administered by injection, it may cause kidney damage. Trade name: **BiCNU.**

carneous mole a fleshy mass in the uterus consisting of blood clots, membranes, pieces of placenta that have not been expelled after abortion.

Caroli's disease an inherited condition in which the bile ducts, which drain the liver, are widened, causing an increased risk of infection or cancer in the gallbladder. *Compare* Caroli's syndrome. [J. Caroli (20th century), French physician]

Caroli's syndrome an inherited condition in which the bile ducts, which drain the liver, are widened and there are fibrous changes in the liver and cysts within the kidneys. *Compare* Caroli's disease. [J. Caroli]

carotene *n.* a yellow or orange plant pigment – one of the carotenoids – that occurs in four forms: alpha (α), beta (β), gamma (γ), and delta (δ). The most important form is *beta-carotene, which is an *antioxidant and can be converted in the body to retinol (vitamin A).

carotenemia (xanthemia) *n.* the presence in the blood of the yellow pigment *carotene, from excessive ingestion of carrots, tomatoes, or other vegetables containing the pigment.

carotenoid *n.* any one of a group of about 100 naturally occurring yellow to red pigments found mostly in plants. The group includes the *carotenes.

carotid artery either of the two main arteries in the neck whose branches supply the head and neck. The *common carotid artery* arises on the left side directly from the aortic arch and on the right from the innominate artery. They ascend the neck on either side as far as the thyroid cartilage (Adam's apple), where they each divide into two branches, the *internal carotid*, supplying the cerebrum, forehead, nose, eye, and middle ear, and the *external carotid*, sending branches to the face, scalp, and neck. *See also* carotid artery stenosis.

carotid artery stenosis (carotid stenosis) narrowing of the carotid artery, which reduces the supply of blood to the brain and is a cause of strokes. Sometimes the condition is due to a tumor of the *carotid body. Many cases can be treated by surgical excision or bypass of the narrowed segment (*see also* endarterectomy).

carotid body a small mass of tissue in the carotid sinus containing *chemoreceptors that monitor levels of oxygen, carbon dioxide, and hydrogen ions in the blood. If the oxygen level falls, the chemoreceptors send impulses to the cardiac and respiratory centers in the brain, which promote increases in heart and respiration rates. It can give rise to carotid body tumors, which are a form of *paraganglioma.

carotid sinus a pocket in the wall of the carotid artery, at its division in the neck, containing receptors that monitor blood pressure (*see* baroreceptor). When blood pressure is raised, impulses travel from the receptors to the vasomotor center in the brain, which initiates a reflex *vasodilation and slowing of heart rate to lower the blood pressure to normal.

carp- (carpo-) *prefix denoting* the wrist (carpus).

carpal 1. *adj.* relating to the wrist. **2.** *n.* any of the bones forming the carpus.

carpal tunnel the space between the carpal bones of the wrist and the connective tissue (retinaculum) over the flexor tendons. It contains the flexor tendons and the median nerve.

carpal tunnel syndrome a condition characterized by a combination of *paresthesia (pins and needles), numbness, and pain affecting all of the hand except the little finger and half of the ring finger. There may also be weakness of the thumb due to wasting of the *thenar eminence. It is caused by pressure on the median nerve as it passes through the wrist (*see* carpal tunnel), which may result from any continuous repetitive movement of the hand, such as typing. The condition is common in rheumatoid arthritis, myxedema, pregnancy, and at the menopause. Treatment is the reduction of any inflammation and immobilization of the wrist by means of a splint. Surgery may become necessary.

carphology (floccillation) *n.* plucking at the bedclothes by a delirious patient. This is often a sign of extreme exhaustion and may be the prelude to death.

carpopedal spasm *see* spasm.

carpus *n.* the eight bones of the wrist (see illustration). The carpus articulates with the metacarpals distally and with the radius and ulna proximally.

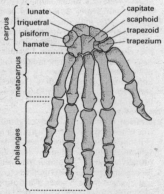

Bones of the left wrist and hand (from the front)

carrier *n.* **1.** a person or animal (usually an insect) that harbors and transmits organisms causing a particular disease without experiencing signs or symptoms of infection. *See also* vector. **2.** (in genetics) a person who bears a gene for an abnormal trait without showing signs of the disorder; the carrier is usually *heterozygous for the gene concerned, which is *recessive. **3.** (in immunology) a molecule to which a *hapten is attached in order to become antigenic and thus produce an *immune response.

carteolol *n.* a *beta blocker used orally to treat high blood pressure; side effects include lightheadedness, dizziness, and weakness. As eye drops it is used in the treatment of *glaucoma; side effects may include local stinging and burning. Trade names: **Cartrol** (oral), **Ocupress** (ophthalmic).

cartilage *n.* a dense connective tissue that is composed of a matrix produced by cells called *chondroblasts*, which become embedded in the matrix as *chondrocytes*. It is a semiopaque gray or white sub-

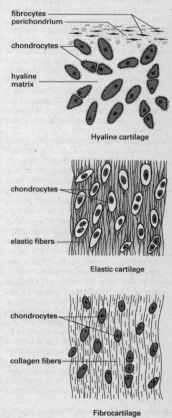

Types of cartilage

stance, consisting chiefly of *chondroitin sulfate, that is capable of withstanding considerable pressure. There are three types: *hyaline cartilage, *elastic cartilage, and *fibrocartilage (see illustration). In the fetus and infant cartilage occurs in many parts of the body, but most of this cartilage disappears during development. In the adult, hyaline cartilage is found in the costal cartilages, larynx, trachea, bronchi, nose, and at the joints of movable bones, where wear and damage result in *osteoarthritis. Elastic cartilage occurs in the external ear, and fibrocartilage in the intervertebral disks and tendons. Cartilage is the precursor of bone following a fracture (*see* callus).

caruncle *n.* a small red fleshy swelling. The *lacrimal caruncle* is the red prominence at the inner angle of the eye. *Hymenal caruncles* occur around the mucous membrane lining the vaginal opening.

caseation *n.* the breakdown of diseased tissue into a dry cheeselike mass: a type of degeneration associated with tubercular lesions.

case control study comparison of a group of people who have a disease with another group free of that disease, in terms of *variables in their backgrounds (e.g. cigarette smoking in those who have died from lung cancer and in those dying from other causes). In the more precise *matched pair study* every individual with the disease is paired with a control matched on the basis of (for example) age, sex, or occupation in order to place greater emphasis on a factor for which the pairs have not been matched. *Compare* cohort study, cross-sectional study.

case fatality ratio the number of fatalities from a specified disease in a given period per 100 episodes of the disease arising in the same period. Unless all such deaths occur rapidly after the onset of the disease (e.g. cholera) they are likely to be the outcome of episodes that started in an earlier period (hence the term "ratio" rather than "rate"). Comparison of the annual number of admissions and fatalities in a given hospital in respect of a specific disease is known as the *hospital fatality ratio*.

casein *n.* a milk protein. Casein is precipitated out of milk in acid conditions or by the action of rennin: it is the principal protein of cheese. Casein is very easily prepared and is useful as a protein supplement, particularly in the treatment of malnutrition.

Casodex *n. see* bicalutamide.

cassette *n.* (in radiography) a thin lightproof box in which a piece of photographic film is placed. It usually contains special screens, which fluoresce on exposure to X-rays, intensifying the image formed on the photographic film when a radiographic exposure is taken. In *computerized radiography the cassette may contain an electrically charged plate.

cast *n.* **1.** a rigid casing for a limb or body part, made of plastic or with openwoven bandage impregnated with plaster of Paris and applied while wet. A plaster cast is designed to protect a broken bone and prevent movement of the aligned bone ends until healing has progressed sufficiently. **2.** a mass of dead cellular, fatty, and other material that forms within a body cavity and takes its shape. It may then be released and appear elsewhere. For example, *granular casts appearing in the urine indicate kidney disease. **3.** (in dentistry) a mold or impression of a part or all of the teeth and surrounding tissue for fitting prostheses or dentures.

castor oil *see* laxative.

castration *n.* removal of the sex glands (the testes or the ovaries). Castration in childhood causes failure of sexual development but when done in adult life (usually as part of hormonal treatment for cancer) it produces less marked physical changes in both sexes. Castration inevitably causes sterility but it need not cause impotence or loss of sexual desire.

CAT computerized axial tomography, now referred to as *computed tomography (CT).

cata- *prefix denoting* downward or against.

catabolism *n.* the chemical decomposition of complex substances by the body in order to form simpler ones, accompanied by the release of energy. The substances broken down include nutrients in food (carbohydrates, proteins, etc.) as well as the body's storage products (such as glycogen). *See also* metabolism. —**catabolic** *adj.*

catagen *n. see* anagen.

catalase *n.* an enzyme, present in many cells (including red blood cells and liver cells), that catalyzes the breakdown of hydrogen peroxide.

catalepsy n. the abnormal maintenance of postures or physical attitudes, occurring in *catatonia. These may have arisen spontaneously or they may be induced by the examiner.

catalyst n. a substance that alters the rate of a chemical reaction but is itself unchanged at the end of the reaction. The catalysts of biochemical reactions are the *enzymes.

cataphoresis n. the introduction into the tissues of positively charged ionized substances (cations) by the use of a direct electric current. *See* iontophoresis.

cataplasia n. degeneration of tissues to an earlier developmental form.

cataplexy n. a sudden onset of muscle weakness that may be precipitated by excitement or emotion. There may be total loss of muscle tone, resulting in collapse, or simply jaw dropping or head nodding. It occurs in most patients with *narcolepsy.

cataract n. any opacity in the lens of the eye, resulting in blurred vision. Cataracts may be congenital or due to metabolic disease (such as *diabetes), direct or indirect injury to the lens, or prolonged exposure of the eye to infrared rays (e.g. *glass-blowers' cataract*) or ionizing radiation, but they are most commonly a result of age (*senile cataract*). A type commonly related to aging is *nuclear sclerotic cataract*, which results from increasing density and yellowing of the center of the lens. A *posterior subcapsular cataract*, which develops at the rear surface of the lens within the lens capsule, is also related to aging but occurs in addition with prolonged use of steroids and chronic ocular inflammation. *Brunescent cataracts* are dark brown and very dense, and a *cortical cataract* is one in which the opacity occurs in the soft outer part (cortex) of the lens. A *Morgagnian cataract* is a longstanding very opaque cataract in which the cortex has started to shrink and liquefy, leaving a central shrunken nucleus. Minor degrees of cataract do not necessarily impair vision seriously.

Cataract is treated by surgical removal of the affected lens (*cataract extraction*; *see also* phacoemulsification); patients may wear a contact lens or appropriate spectacles to compensate for the missing lens but in modern practice a plastic *intraocular lens implant* is routinely placed inside the eye after surgery.

cataract extraction surgical removal of a cataract from the eye. In *extracapsular cataract extraction* the cataract alone is removed, leaving the lens capsule behind to support the remaining lens tissue. *Intracapsular cataract extraction* is the removal of the whole lens, including the capsule that surrounds it.

catarrh n. the excessive secretion of thick phlegm or mucus by the mucous membrane of the nose, nasal sinuses, nasopharynx, or air passages. The term is not used in any precise or scientific sense.

catastrophic illness a health condition that severely affects an individual's physical, social, economic, or mental abilities and usually requires very expensive treatment. In 1978, HEW (now HHS) defined a catastrophic illness as one in which medical expenses exceeded $5000 in a 12-month period. In the US, more than 2,500,000 persons experience a catastrophic illness each year. This segment of slightly more than 1% of the total population accounts for more than 20% of the total national expenditure for health care.

catatonia n. a state in which a person becomes mute or stuporous or adopts bizarre postures. The features include *cerea flexibilitas, in which the limbs may be moved passively by another person into positions that are then retained for hours on end. Catatonia was at one time a noted feature of *schizophrenia but is now hardly ever seen in developed countries. It remains common in developing countries. —**catatonic** adj.

CATCH-22 *see* diGeorge syndrome.

catchment area the geographic area from which a hospital can expect to receive patients. There is no statutory requirement forcing patients to use the hospital(s) of their area.

catecholamines pl. n. a group of physiologically important substances, including *epinephrine, *norepinephrine, and *dopamine, having various different roles (mainly as *neurotransmitters) in the functioning of the sympathetic and central nervous systems. Chemically, all contain a benzene ring with adjacent hydroxyl groups (catechol) and an amine group on a side chain. Catecholamines act at both alpha (α) and beta (β) *adrenergic receptor sites.

catgut *n.* a fibrous material prepared from the tissues of animals, usually from the walls of sheep intestines, twisted into strands of different thicknesses and formerly widely used to sew up wounds (*see* suture) and tie off blood vessels during surgery. The catgut gradually dissolves and is absorbed by the tissues, so that the stitches do not have to be removed later. This also minimizes the possibility of long-term irritation at the site of the operation. Some catgut is treated with chromic acid for different periods during manufacture. This gives catguts that last for different lengths of time before absorption is complete.

catharsis *n.* purging or cleansing out of the bowels by giving the patient a *laxative (cathartic) to stimulate intestinal activity.

cathartic *n. see* laxative.

cathepsin *n.* one of a group of enzymes found in animal tissues, particularly the spleen, that digest proteins.

catheter *n.* a flexible tube for insertion into a narrow opening so that fluids may be introduced or removed. *Urinary catheters* are passed into the bladder through the urethra to allow drainage of urine in certain disorders and to empty the bladder before abdominal operations.

catheterization *n.* the introduction of a *catheter into a hollow organ or vessel. This is most often performed as *urethral catheterization*, when a catheter is introduced into the bladder to relieve obstruction to the outflow of urine (*see also* intermittent self-catheterization). Catheters can also be passed above the pubis through the abdominal wall (*suprapubic catheterization*) directly into an enlarged bladder if urethral catheterization is not possible. *Cardiac catheterization* entails the introduction of special catheters, usually via the femoral blood vessels in the groin, into the chambers of the heart. This allows the measurement of pressures in the chambers and pressure gradients across the heart valves, as well as the injection of contrast medium (*see* angiocardiography). *Vascular catheterization* enables the intro-duction into the arteries or veins of: (1) contrast medium for radiography; (2) drugs to constrict or expand vessels or to dissolve a thrombus (*see* thrombolysis); (3) metal coils or other solid materials to block bleeding vessels or to thrombose *aneurysms (*see* embolization); or (4) devices for monitoring pressures within important vessels (e.g. *Swan-Ganz catheters for monitoring pulmonary artery pressure in critically ill patients).

cation *n.* an ion of positive charge, such as a sodium ion (Na^+). *Compare* anion. *See* electrolyte.

cation-exchange resins complex insoluble chemical compounds that may be administered with the diet to alter the *electrolyte balance of the body in the treatment of heart, kidney, and metabolic disorders. For example, in patients on a strict low-sodium diet such resins combine with sodium in the food so that it cannot be absorbed and passes out in the feces.

CAT scan a scan obtained by computerized axial tomography, now referred to as a CT scan (*see* computed tomography).

cat-scratch fever an infectious disease, probably caused by a gram-negative *bacillus, transmitted to humans following injury to the skin by a cat scratch, splinter, or thorn. Mild fever and swelling of the lymph nodes develop about a week after infection. In some cases, especially in immunocompromised patients, serious abscess formation occurs, but generally recovery is complete.

cauda *n.* a taillike structure. The *cauda equina* is a bundle of nerve roots from the lumbar, sacral, and coccygeal spinal nerves that descend nearly vertically from the spinal cord until they reach their respective openings in the vertebral column.

caudal *adj.* relating to the lower part or tail end of the body.

caul *n.* **1.** (in obstetrics) the *amnion, either as a piece of membrane covering an infant's head at birth or the entire unruptured sac that encloses the fetus during pregnancy. **2.** (in anatomy) *see* omentum.

causal agent a factor associated with the definitive onset of an illness (or other response, including an accident). Examples of causal agents are bacteria, trauma, and noxious agents. The relationship is more direct than in the case of a *risk factor.

causalgia *n.* an intensely unpleasant burning pain felt in a limb where there has been partial damage to the sympathetic and somatic sensory nerves.

caustic *n.* an agent, such as silver nitrate, that causes irritation and burning and destroys tissue. Caustic agents may be used to remove dead skin, warts, etc., but care must be taken not to damage the surrounding area.

caustic soda *see* sodium hydroxide.

cauterize *vb.* to destroy tissues by direct application of a heated instrument, electric current, or caustic agent (known as a *cautery*): used for the removal of small warts or other small growths and to stop bleeding from small vessels. —**cautery** *n.*

Caverject *n.* *see* alprostadil.

cavernitis *n.* inflammation of the corpora cavernosa of the *penis or the corpus cavernosum of the clitoris.

cavernosography *n.* a radiological examination of the erectile tissue of the penis (*see* corpus cavernosum) that entails the infusion of *radiopaque contrast medium into the corpora cavernosa via a small butterfly needle. The contrast medium flow rate needed to maintain erection can be measured, and radiographs taken during the procedure give information regarding the veins draining the penis.

cavernosometry *n.* the measurement of pressure within the corpora cavernosa of the penis during infusion. The flow rate required to produce an erection is recorded and also the flow necessary to maintain the induced erection. The examination is important in the investigation of failure of erection and impotence.

cavernous breathing *see* breath sounds.

cavernous sinus one of the paired cavities within the *sphenoid bone, at the base of the skull behind the eye sockets, into which blood drains from the brain, eye, nose, and upper cheek before leaving the skull through connections with the internal jugular and facial veins. Through the sinus, in its walls, pass the internal carotid artery and the abducens, oculomotor, trochlear, ophthalmic, and maxillary nerves.

cavity *n.* 1. (in anatomy) a hollow enclosed area; for example, the abdominal cavity or the buccal cavity (mouth). 2. (in dentistry) **a.** the hole in a tooth caused by *caries or abrasion. **b.** the hole shaped in a tooth by a dentist to retain a filling.

cavity varnish (in dentistry) a solution of natural or synthetic resin in an organic solvent. It is used as a sealer for amalgam fillings or as a coating over newly inserted cement fillings.

CBW (chemical and biological warfare) the use of poison gases and other chemicals, bacteria, viruses, and toxins during war.

C cells parafollicular cells of the thyroid gland, which are derived from neural crest tissue. They produce *calcitonin. *Medullary carcinoma of the thyroid has its origin in the C cells.

CCU *see* critical care unit.

CD cluster of differentiation: a numerical system for classifying antigens expressed on the surface of lymphocytes. *See also* CD4.

CD4 a surface antigen on *helper T cells that is particularly important for immune resistance to viruses. It is also a receptor for the human immunodeficiency virus (HIV); progressive reduction of CD4-bearing T cells reflects the progression of *AIDS.

CDC *see* Centers for Disease Control and Prevention.

CDH *see* congenital dislocation of the hip.

CEA *see* carcinoembryonic antigen.

cecostomy *n.* an operation in which the cecum is brought through the abdominal wall and opened in order to drain or decompress the intestine, usually when the colon is obstructed or injured.

cecum *n.* a blind-ended pouch at the junction of the small and large intestines, situated below the *ileocecal valve. The upper end is continuous with the colon and the lower end bears the vermiform appendix. *See* alimentary canal.

cefaclor *n.* a *cephalosporin antibiotic used in the treatment of otitis media, upper and lower respiratory tract infections, urinary tract infections, and skin infections. It is administered by mouth; side effects include diarrhea and skin eruptions. Trade name: **Ceclor.**

cefadroxil *n.* a *cephalosporin antibiotic used in the treatment of urinary tract infections, skin infections, pharyngitis, and tonsillitis. It is administered by mouth;

side effects include skin rash and generalized itching. Trade name: **Duricef**.

cefamandole nafate a semisynthetic *cephalosporin antibiotic used in the treatment of certain gram-negative bacterial infections, primarily of the urinary and lower respiratory tracts. It is administered by infusion or injection. Side effects include various hypersensitivity reactions, phlebitis, suprainfection, and pain on intramuscular injection. Trade name: **Mandol**.

cefazolin *n.* a semisynthetic antibiotic, given by intramuscular or intravenous injection in the treatment of a number of serious infections. Side effects are rare. *See* cephalosporin. Trade names: **Ancef**, **Kefzol**, **Zolicef**.

cefixime *n.* a *cephalosporin antibiotic used in the treatment of urinary tract infections, tonsillitis, and otitis media. It is administered by mouth. Side effects include diarrhea, nausea, skin rashes, and headaches. Trade name: **Suprax**.

cefotaxime sodium a *cephalosporin antibiotic used in the treatment of respiratory tract and genitourinary tract infections, bone and skin infections, and central nervous system infections. It is administered by injection or infusion; diarrhea is the most common side effect. Trade name: **Claforan**.

cefotetan a semisynthetic broad-spectrum *cephalosporin antibiotic effective against a wide range of gram-positive, gram-negative, and anaerobic bacteria. It is used in the treatment of urinary tract, lower respiratory tract, gynecologic, intra-abdominal, skin, bone, and joint infections. Adverse effects include hypersensitivity reactions and irritation of the gastrointestinal tract. Trade name: **Cefotan**.

cefoxitin *n.* a *cephalosporin antibiotic used in the treatment of infections of the urinary and lower respiratory tracts, abdomen, skin, bones, and joints, and of septicemia. It is administered by intravenous or intramuscular injection. Side effects include reaction at the site of injection, diarrhea, and rash. Trade name: **Mefoxin**.

cefprozil *n.* a *cephalosporin antibiotic used in the treatment of streptococcal and other infections, rheumatic fever, chronic bronchitis, otitis media, tonsillitis, and lower respiratory infections. It is

administered by mouth. Side effects include nausea, dizziness, diarrhea, and rash. Trade name: **Cefzil**.

ceftazidime *n.* a *cephalosporin antibiotic used in the treatment of urinary and respiratory tract infections, cellulitis, meningitis, and septicemia. It is administered by intravenous or intramuscular injection. Side effects include reaction at the site of injection, diarrhea, and hypersensitivity reactions. Trade names: **Ceptaz**, **Fortaz**, **Tazicef**, **Tazidime**.

ceftriaxone *n.* a *cephalosporin antibiotic used in the treatment of infections of the urinary and lower respiratory tracts and the skin, meningitis, Lyme disease, gonorrhea, and septicemia. It is administered by intravenous or intramuscular injection. Side effects include reaction at the site of injection, diarrhea, and rash. Trade name: **Rocephin**.

cefuroxime *n.* a *cephalosporin antibiotic used in the treatment of infections of the urinary and lower respiratory tracts and the skin, Lyme disease, gonorrhea, tonsillitis, meningitis, and otitis media. It is administered by mouth. Side effects include nausea, diarrhea, and rash. Trade names: **Ceftin**, **Zinacef**.

-cele (-coele) *suffix denoting* swelling, hernia, or tumor. Example: *gastrocele* (hernia of the stomach).

celecoxib *n.* an anti-inflammatory drug (*see* NSAID) that selectively inhibits cyclo-oxygenase 2 (*see* COX-2 inhibitor). It is taken by mouth in the treatment of osteoarthritis and rheumatoid arthritis. Trade name: **Celebrex**.

celi- (celio-) *prefix denoting* the abdomen or belly. Example: *celiectasia* (abnormal distension of).

celiac *adj.* of or relating to the abdominal region. The *celiac trunk* is a branch of the abdominal *aorta supplying the stomach, gallbladder, liver, and spleen.

celiac disease (nontropical sprue) a condition in which the small intestine fails to digest and absorb food. It affects 0.1–0.2% of the population and is due to sensitivity of the intestinal lining to the protein gliadin, which is contained in *gluten in the germ of wheat and rye and causes atrophy of the digestive and absorptive cells of the intestine. Symptoms include stunted growth, distended abdomen, and pale frothy foul-smelling stools; the disease can be diagnosed by

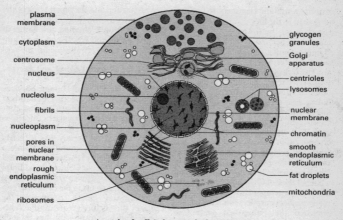

plasma membrane
cytoplasm
centrosome
nucleus
nucleolus
fibrils
nucleoplasm
pores in nuclear membrane
rough endoplasmic reticulum
ribosomes

glycogen granules
Golgi apparatus
centrioles
lysosomes
nuclear membrane
chromatin
smooth endoplasmic reticulum
fat droplets
mitochondria

An animal cell (microscopical structure)

*biopsy of the jejunum and is treated successfully by a strict and lifelong gluten-free diet. Medical name: **gluten enteropathy**.

celioscopy *n.* the technique of introducing an *endoscope through an incision in the abdominal wall to examine the intestines and other organs within the abdominal cavity.

cell *n.* the basic unit of all living organisms, which can reproduce itself exactly (*see* mitosis). Each cell is bounded by a *cell membrane* of lipids and protein, which controls the passage of substances into and out of the cell. Cells contain *cytoplasm, in which are suspended a *nucleus and other structures (*organelles) specialized to carry out particular activities in the cell (see illustration).

Complex organisms are built up of millions of cells that are specially adapted to carry out particular functions. The process of cell differentiation begins early in the development of the embryo and cells of a particular type (e.g. blood cells, liver cells) always give rise to cells of the same type. Each cell has a particular number of *chromosomes in its nucleus (46 in the human). The sex cells (sperm and ova) always contain half the number of chromosomes of all the other cells of the body (*see* meiosis); at fertilization a sperm and ovum combine to form a cell with a complete set of chromosomes that will develop into the embryo.

cell body (perikaryon) the enlarged portion of a *neuron (nerve cell), containing the nucleus. It is concerned more with the nutrition of the cell than with propagation of nerve impulses.

cell division reproduction of cells by division first of the chromosomes (karyokinesis) and then of the cytoplasm (cytokinesis). Cell division to produce more body (somatic) cells is by *mitosis; cell division during the formation of gametes is by *meiosis.

cellophane maculopathy *see* epiretinal membrane.

cell-surface molecules molecules on the surface of cell membranes that are responsible for most cellular functions directly related to their immediate environment. Many have very precise functions of adhesion (*see* adhesion molecules), metabolic exchange, hormone reception, respiration, and immune reactions. Cell-to-cell exchanges involve specialized surface structures (junctions), which form a communicating nexus.

cellulitis *n.* inflammation of the connective tissue between adjacent tissues of the *dermis. This is commonly due to bacterial infection by streptococci (occasionally by staphylococci) and usually requires antibiotic treatment to prevent its spread to the bloodstream. It is most common on the lower legs and there may be associated *lymphangitis and *lymphadenitis. Cellulitis is otherwise similar to *erysipelas, but the margins are less clearly defined because the infection is deeper. Penicillin is the antibiotic of choice for treatment.

cellulose *n.* a carbohydrate consisting of linked glucose units. It is an important constituent of plant cell walls. Cellulose cannot be digested by humans and is a component of *dietary fiber (roughage).

Celsius temperature (centigrade temperature) temperature expressed on a scale in which the melting point of ice is assigned a temperature of 0° and the boiling point of water a temperature of 100°. For many medical purposes this scale has superseded the Fahrenheit scale (*see* Fahrenheit temperature). The formula for converting from Celsius (C) to Fahrenheit (F) is: F = 9/5C + 32. [A. Celsius (1701–44), Swedish astronomer]

cement *n.* **1.** any of a group of materials used in dentistry either as fillings or as *lutes for crowns. Glass ionomer cements are used for filling, and zinc phosphate, zinc polycarboxylate, and glass ionomer cements are used for luting. Zinc oxide–eugenol cements are widely used as temporary fillings or as an impression material. **2.** a fast-setting material used to fix prostheses (e.g. artificial hips) in place. **3.** *see* cementum.

cementocyte *n.* a cell found in cementum.

cementoma *n.* a benign overgrowth of cementum.

cementum (cement) *n.* a thin layer of hard tissue on the surface of the root of a *tooth. It attaches the fibers of the periodontal membrane to the tooth.

censor *n.* (in psychology) the mechanism, postulated by Freud, that suppresses or modifies desires that are inappropriate or feared. The censor is usually regarded as being located in the *superego but was also described by Freud as being in the *ego itself.

center *n.* (in neurology) a collection of neurons (nerve cells) whose activities control a particular function. The *respiratory* and *cardiovascular centers*, for example, are regions in the lower brainstem that control the movements of respiration and the functioning of the circulatory system, respectively.

Center for Drug Evaluation and Research a division of the US *Food and Drug Administration responsible for the regulation of drugs available to patients.

Centers for Disease Control and Prevention (CDC) an agency of the US Department of Health and Human Services located in Atlanta, Georgia, that directs programs for the prevention and control of diseases, particularly infectious diseases, for the US. *Public Health Service. The federal agency was formerly known as the Communicable Disease Center, Center for Disease Control, and Centers for Disease Control. In addition to providing assistance to state and local health departments in the control of epidemiological health problems, the agency directs foreign quarantine functions and has responsibilities in such areas as ecologic investigations, injury control, chronic disease prevention, and occupational health.

-centesis *suffix denoting* puncture or perforation. Example: *amniocentesis* (surgical puncture of the amnion).

centi- *prefix denoting* one hundredth or a hundred.

centigrade temperature *see* Celsius temperature.

centile chart a graph with lines (called *centiles*) showing average measurements of height, weight, and head circumference compared with age and sex, against which a child's physical development can be assessed. The number of a centile predicts the percentage of children who are below a particular measurement at a given age; for example, the 10th centile means 10% of the population will be smaller and 90% larger at that age. A child will normally follow a particular centile line. Children who are above the 97th or below the 3rd centile, or whose growth rapidly changes centiles, should be examined.

central auditory processing disorder (CAPD) hearing difficulty, especially in noisy environments, in an individual with a normal *audiogram. Treatment includes hearing therapy. Children with this condition often have difficulty reading and may exhibit other learning disabilities.

central island an area of significant central

tissue elevation (>1.5 diopters) seen on *corneal topography after laser refractive surgery. It may result in a poor postoperative outcome.

central nervous system (CNS) the *brain and the *spinal cord, as opposed to the cranial and spinal nerves and the *autonomic nervous system, which together form the *peripheral nervous system*. The CNS is responsible for the *integration of all nervous activities.

central venous catheter an intravenous catheter for insertion directly into a large vein, most commonly the subclavian vein, during its passage under the clavicle, or the jugular in the neck. Such catheters can also be inserted into the femoral vein at the groin. They enable intravenous drugs and fluids to be given and intravenous pressures to be measured, which is often useful during operations or in intensive care. Central venous catheters must be inserted under strictly sterile conditions using a local anesthetic.

central venous pressure (CVP) the pressure of blood within the right atrium. Measurement of CVP is obtained by *catheterization of the right side of the heart; the catheter is attached to a manometer. CVP measurements are used to estimate circulatory function and blood volume in cases of shock or severe hemorrhage and to monitor blood replacement. In a recumbent patient, with the zero point of the manometer level with the midaxilla (center of the armpit), CVP should measure between 5 and 8 cm saline under normal conditions.

centrencephalic *adj.* (in electroencephalography) describing discharges that can be recorded synchronously from all parts of the brain. The source of this activity is in the *reticular formation of the midbrain. *Centrencephalic epilepsy* is associated with a congenital predisposition to seizures.

centri- *prefix denoting* center. Example: *centrilobular* (in the center of a lobule (especially of the liver)).

centrifugal *adj.* moving away from a center, as from the brain to the peripheral tissues.

centrifuge *n.* a device for separating components of different densities in a liquid, using centrifugal force. The liquid is placed in special containers that are spun at high speed around a central axis.

centriole *n.* a small particle found in the cytoplasm of cells, near the nucleus. Centrioles are involved in the formation of the *spindle and aster during cell division. During interphase there are usually two centrioles in the *centrosome; when cell division occurs, these separate and move to opposite sides of the nucleus, and the spindle is formed between them.

centripetal *adj.* moving toward a center, as from the peripheral tissues to the brain.

centromere (kinetochore) *n.* the part of a chromosome that joins the two *chromatids to each other and becomes attached to the spindle during *mitosis and *meiosis. When chromosome division takes place the centromeres split longitudinally.

centrosome (centrosphere) *n.* an area of clear cytoplasm, found next to the nucleus in nondividing cells, that contains the *centrioles.

centrosphere *n.* **1.** an area of clear cytoplasm seen in dividing cells around the poles of the spindle. **2.** *see* centrosome.

centrum *n.* (*pl.* **centra**) the solid rod-shaped central portion of a *vertebra.

cephal- (cephalo-) *prefix denoting* the head. Example: *cephalalgia* (pain in).

cephalad *adj.* toward the head.

cephalexin *n.* a *cephalosporin antibiotic used in the treatment of respiratory tract and genitourinary tract infections, bone and skin infections, and otitis media. It is administered by mouth; diarrhea is the most common side effect. Trade names: **Biocef, Keflex, Keftab.**

cephalhematoma *n.* a swelling on the head caused by a collection of bloody fluid between one or more of the skull bones (usually the *parietal bone) and its covering membrane (periosteum). It is most commonly seen in newborn infants delivered with the aid of forceps or subjected to pressures during passage through the birth canal. No treatment is necessary and the swelling disappears in a few months. If it is extensive, blood in the fluid breaks down, releasing bilirubin and resulting in jaundice. A cephalhematoma in an older baby or child is evidence of some recent injury to the head; occasionally an unsuspected fracture is revealed on X-ray.

cephalic *adj.* of or relating to the head.

cephalic index a measure of the shape of a skull, commonly used in *craniometry: the ratio of the greatest breadth, multiplied by 100, to the greatest length of the skull. *See also* brachycephaly, dolichocephaly.

cephalic version a procedure for turning a fetus that is lying in a breech or transverse position so that its head will enter the birth canal first. It may give rise to complications and is therefore only carried out in selected cases.

cephalin *n.* one of a group of *phospholipids that are constituents of cell membranes and are particularly abundant in the brain.

cephalocele *n. see* neural tube defects.

cephalogram *n.* a special standardized X-ray picture that can be used to measure alterations in the growth of skull bones.

cephalometry *n.* the study of facial growth by examination of standardized lateral radiographs of the head. It is used mainly for diagnosis in *orthodontics.

cephalosporin *n.* any one of a group of semisynthetic *beta-lactam antibiotics, derived from the mold *Cephalosporium*, which are effective against a wide range of microorganisms and are therefore used in a variety of infections (*see* cefaclor, cefadroxil, cefazolin, cephalexin, cephalothin sodium). Cross-sensitivity with penicillin may occur and the principal side effects are allergic reactions and irritation of the digestive tract.

cephalothin sodium a semisynthetic antibiotic, given by intramuscular or intravenous injection in the treatment of a number of serious infections. *See* cephalosporin. Trade name: **Keflin**.

cercaria *n.* (*pl.* **cercariae**) the final larval stage of any parasitic trematode (*see* fluke). The cercariae, which have tails but otherwise resemble the adults, are released into water from the snail host in which the parasite undergoes part of its development. Several thousand cercariae may emerge from a single snail in a day.

cerclage *n.* **1.** (in obstetrics) a procedure in which the cervix of the uterus during pregnancy is encircled with nonabsorbable sutures because of weakness of the cervix; spontaneous abortion would otherwise occur. When the pregnancy is at full term, the sutures are released so that labor can begin. **2.** (in orthopedics) the procedure of binding together the ends of a fractured bone with a wire loop or metal ring until healed.

cerea flexibilitas a disorder of posture in which a patient's limbs offer a continuous mild resistance to being moved passively by the examiner and remain for long periods in the position into which the examiner has moved them. It is a feature of *catatonia. *See also* catalepsy.

cerebellar syndrome (Nonne's syndrome) *see* (cerebellar) ataxia.

cerebellum *n.* the largest part of the hindbrain, bulging back behind the pons and the medulla oblongata and overhung by the occipital lobes of the cerebrum. Like the cerebrum, it has an outer gray cortex and a core of white matter. Three broad bands of nerve fibers – the inferior, middle, and superior cerebellar peduncles – connect it to the medulla, the pons, and the midbrain, respectively. It has two hemispheres, one on each side of the central region (the *vermis*), and its surface is thrown into thin folds called *folia* (see illustration). Within lie four pairs of nuclei.

The cerebellum is essential for the maintenance of muscle tone, balance, and the synchronization of activity in groups of muscles under voluntary control, converting muscular contractions into smooth coordinated movement. It does not, however, initiate movement and it plays no part in the perception of conscious sensations or in intelligence. —**cerebellar** *adj.*

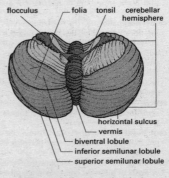

flocculus — folia — tonsil — cerebellar hemisphere

horizontal sulcus
vermis
biventral lobule
inferior semilunar lobule
superior semilunar lobule

The cerebellum (anterior view)

cerebr- (cerebri-, cerebro-) *prefix denoting* the cerebrum or brain.

cerebral abscess *see* abscess.

cerebral aqueduct (aqueduct of Sylvius) the narrow channel, containing cerebrospinal fluid, that connects the third and fourth *ventricles of the brain.

cerebral cortex the intricately folded outer layer of the *cerebrum, making up some 40% of the brain by weight and composed of an estimated 15 thousand million neurons (*see* gray matter). This is the part of the brain most directly responsible for consciousness, with essential roles in perception, memory, thought, mental ability, and intellect, and it is responsible for initiating voluntary activity. It has connections, direct or indirect, with all parts of the body. The folding of the cortex provides a large surface area, the greater part lying in the clefts (*sulci*), which divide the upraised convolutions (*gyri*). On the basis of its microscopic appearance in section, the cortex is mapped into *Brodmann's areas; it is also divided into functional regions; including *motor cortex, *sensory cortex, and *association areas. Within, and continuous with it, lies the *white matter, through which connection is made with the rest of the nervous system.

cerebral hemisphere one of the two paired halves of the *cerebrum.

cerebral hemorrhage bleeding from a cerebral blood vessel into the tissue of the brain. It is commonly caused by degenerative disease of the arteries and high blood pressure, but it may result from bleeding from congenital abnormalities of blood vessels. The extent and severity of the symptoms depend on the type of vessel involved, the site and volume of the hemorrhage, and the cause (traumatic, degenerative); they vary from a transient weakness or numbness to profound coma and death. *See also* atheroma, hypertension, stroke.

cerebral palsy a motor function disorder resulting from permanent, nonprogressive damage to the brain before, during, or immediately after birth. The brain damage has many causes, including an inadequate supply of oxygen to the brain, low levels of glucose in the blood (*hypoglycemia), and infection. It is often associated with other problems, such as learning difficulties, hearing difficulties, poor speech, poor balance, and epilepsy. There are three main types of cerebral palsy: *spastic*, in which the limbs are difficult to control and which may affect the whole body (quadriplegic), one side of the body (hemiplegic), or both legs (diplegic); *ataxic hypotonic*, in which the main problem is poor balance and uncoordinated movements; and *dyskinetic*, in which there is involuntary movement of the limbs. Management requires a multidisciplinary approach, the main components of which are physiotherapy, speech therapy, educational assistance, and appropriate appliances.

cerebral tumor (brain tumor) an abnormal multiplication of brain cells. This forms a swelling that compresses or destroys healthy brain cells surrounding it and – because of the rigid closed nature of the skull – increases the pressure on the brain tissue. Malignant brain tumors, which are much more common in children than in adults, include *medulloblastomas and *gliomas; these grow rapidly, spreading through the otherwise normal brain tissue and causing progressive neurological disability. Benign tumors, such as *meningiomas, grow slowly and compress the brain tissue, and both malignant and benign tumors sometimes cause epileptic seizures. Benign tumors are often cured by total surgical resection. Malignant tumors may be treated by neurosurgery, chemotherapy, and radiotherapy, but the outcome for most patients remains poor.

cerebration *n.* **1.** the functioning of the brain as a whole. **2.** the unconscious activities of the brain.

cerebroside *n.* one of a group of compounds that occur in the *myelin sheaths of nerve fibers. They are *glycolipids, containing *sphingosine, a fatty acid, and a sugar, usually galactose (in galactocerebrosides) or glucose (in glucocerebrosides).

cerebrospinal fever (spotted fever) *see* meningitis.

cerebrospinal fluid (CSF) the clear watery fluid that surrounds the brain and spinal cord. It is contained in the *subarachnoid space and circulates in the *ventricles of the brain and in the central canal of the spinal cord. The brain floats in the fluid (its weight so being reduced from about 1400 g to less than 100 g) and is cushioned by it from contact with the skull when the head is moved vigorously. The CSF is secreted by the *choroid plexuses in the ventricles, circulates through them to reach the subarachnoid space, and is eventually absorbed into the bloodstream through the *arachnoid villi. Its normal contents are glucose, salts, enzymes, and a few white cells, but no red blood cells.

cerebrovascular disease any disorder of the blood vessels of the brain and its covering membranes (meninges). Most cases are due to atheroma and/or hypertension, clinical effects being caused by rupture of diseased blood vessels (*cerebral or *subarachnoid hemorrhage) or inadequacy of the blood supply to the brain (ischemia), due to cerebral thrombosis or embolism. The term *cerebrovascular accident* is given to the clinical syndrome accompanying a sudden and sometimes severe attack, which leads to a *stroke.

cerebrum (telencephalon) *n.* the largest and most highly developed part of the brain, composed of the two *cerebral hemispheres*, separated from each other by the *longitudinal fissure* in the midline (see illustration). Each hemisphere has an outer layer of gray matter, the *cerebral cortex*, below which lies white matter containing the *basal ganglia. Connecting the two hemispheres at the bottom of the longitudinal fissure is the *corpus callosum*, a massive bundle of nerve fibers. Within each hemisphere is a crescent-shaped fluid-filled cavity (lateral *ventricle), connected to the central third ventricle in the *diencephalon. The cerebrum is responsible for the initiation and coordination of all voluntary activity in the body and for governing the functioning of lower parts of the nervous system. The cortex is the seat of all intelligent behavior. —**cerebral** *adj.*

Certificate of Need Law a state law, with specific provisions that may vary in different states of the US, requiring that hospitals and other medical facilities must prove the need for any major expansion or new construction before work is allowed to begin. The law is intended to restrict the duplication of health-care facilities in a geographic area.

ceruloplasmin *n.* a copper-containing protein present in blood plasma. Congenital deficiency of ceruloplasmin leads to abnormalities of the brain and liver (see Wilson's disease).

cerumen (earwax) *n.* the waxy material that is secreted by the sebaceous glands in the external auditory meatus of the outer ear. Its function is to protect the delicate skin that lines the inside of the meatus.

cervic- (cervico-) *prefix denoting* **1.** the neck. Example: *cervicodynia* (pain in). **2.** the cervix, especially of the uterus. Example: *cervicectomy* (surgical removal of).

cervical *adj.* **1.** of or relating to the neck. **2.** of, relating to, or affecting the cervix (neck region) of an organ, especially the cervix of the uterus.

cervical cancer (cervical carcinoma) cancer of the cervix of the uterus. The tumor may develop from the surface epithelium of the cervix (squamous carcinoma) or from the epithelial lining of the cervical canal (adenocarcinoma). In both cases the tumor is invasive, spreading to involve surrounding tissue and subsequently to neighboring lymph nodes and adjacent organs, such as the bladder and rectum. In carcinoma in situ (see cervical intraepithelial neoplasia), there is no invasion of surrounding tissue but, if untreated, it can disseminate. Cancer of the cervix can be detected in an early stage of development (see cervical smear, liquid-based cytology). Features of cervical

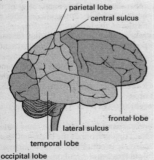

parieto-occipital fissure

parietal lobe

central sulcus

frontal lobe

lateral sulcus

temporal lobe

occipital lobe

Lobes of the cerebrum (from the right side)

cancer include vaginal discharge, often foul-smelling and usually blood-stained. Treatment is by irradiation or surgery, or a combination of both, and cytotoxic drugs may also be used. *See also* human papillomavirus.

cervical fracture a fracture of a vertebra in the neck (*see* cervical vertebrae). Cervical fractures range from minor, requiring no treatment, to those associated with paralysis and instant death. Treatment can be support with a collar, skull traction, an *orthosis attached to the skull, or surgery, depending on the severity of the fracture.

cervical intraepithelial neoplasia (CIN) cellular changes in the cervix of the uterus leading to the preinvasive stage of cervical cancer. The CIN grading system distinguishes three stages: *CIN 1* (mild dysplasia); *CIN 2* (moderate dysplasia); *CIN 3* (severe dysplasia, *carcinoma in situ*). CIN is uncommon after the menopause. Treatment may be by *laser beam, which destroys the tissue, or by large loop excision of the *transformation zone of the cervix, a procedure performed through a colposcope, under local anesthetic, using diathermy.

cervical smear (Papanicolaou [Pap] test) a specimen of cellular material scraped from the cervix of the uterus that is stained and examined under a microscope in order to determine whether cancer or precancerous changes are present. The *transformation zone of the cervix is most likely to produce evidence of *cervical intraepithelial neoplasia if present.

cervical vertebrae the seven bones making up the neck region of the *backbone. The first cervical vertebra – the *atlas* – consists basically of a ring of bone that supports the skull by articulating with the occipital condyles (*see* occipital bone). The second vertebra – the *axis* – has an upward-pointing process (the *odontoid process* or *dens*) that forms a pivot on which the atlas can rotate, enabling the head to be turned. *See also* vertebra.

cervicitis *n.* inflammation of the cervix of the uterus.

cervix *n.* a necklike part, especially the *cervix uteri* (neck of the uterus), which projects into the vagina. The cervical canal passes through it, linking the cavity of the uterus with the vagina. The canal normally contains mucus, the viscosity of which changes throughout the menstrual cycle. The cervix is capable of very wide dilation during childbirth.

cesarean section a surgical operation for delivering a baby through the abdominal wall. The operation most commonly performed is *lower uterine segment cesarean section* (*LUSCS*), carried out through an incision (usually transverse) in the lower segment of the uterus. *Classical cesarean section*, in which the upper segment of the uterus is incised vertically, is now rarely performed. In addition to its use in cases of obstructed labor, *malpresentation (breech, brow, and shoulder) and in severe *antepartum hemorrhage, cesarean section is being performed increasingly when the baby is at risk and is exhibiting signs of distress. Because of improved techniques of postnatal care, the operation may now be performed at 28 weeks or even earlier, with a good chance of survival of the premature child.

cesium-137 *n.* an artificial radioactive isotope of the metallic element cesium. The radiation given off by cesium-137 can be employed in the technique of *radiotherapy, but now is rarely used. Symbol: ^{137}Cs. *See also* teletherapy.

cestode *n. see* tapeworm.

cetirizine *n. see* antihistamine.

cetrimonium *n.* a detergent disinfectant, used for cleansing skin surfaces and wounds, sterilizing surgical instruments and babies' diapers, and in shampoos. There are few adverse reactions from external application; most toxic effects are due to poisoning from ingestion.

cetylpyridinium *n.* a detergent disinfectant, used for the disinfection of skin, wounds, and burns, as a mouthwash, and in the form of throat lozenges. Trade name: **Cepacol**.

CFS *see* chronic fatigue syndrome.

Chagas' disease a disease caused by the protozoan parasite *Trypanosoma cruzi*. It is transmitted to humans when the trypanosomes, present in the feces of nocturnal bloodsucking *reduviid bugs, come into contact with wounds and scratches on the skin or the delicate internal tissues of the nose and mouth. The presence of the parasite in the heart muscles and central nervous system results in serious inflammation and lesions, which can prove fatal. The disease, limited to poor rural areas of South and Central America, is especially prevalent in children and young adults. It may be treated with nifurtimox. *See also* trypanosomiasis. [C. Chagas (1879–1934), Brazilian physician]

chaining *n.* a technique of *behavior modification in which a complex skill is taught by being broken down into its separate components, which are gradually built up into the full sequence. Usually the last component in the sequence is taught first, as it is this component that is followed by *reinforcement: this is termed *backward chaining*.

chalasia *n.* abnormal relaxation of a sphincter, especially the cardiac sphincter in infants, causing reflux of the gastric contents into the esophagus with subsequent regurgitation.

chalazion (meibomian cyst) *n.* a swollen sebaceous gland in the eyelid, caused by chronic inflammation following blockage of the gland's duct. The gland becomes converted into a jellylike mass, producing disfigurement of the lid. It may become secondarily infected, when it will be painful and may discharge. Treatment is by application of antibiotic ointments or surgical incision and curettage of the gland.

chalcosis *n.* the deposition of copper in the tissues of the eye, usually resulting from the presence of a copper foreign body within the eye.

chalicosis *n.* pneumoconiosis that results from the inhalation of calcium dusts and occurs in stone cutters: a variety of *silicosis.

CHAMPUS an acronym for *C*ivilian *H*ealth *A*nd *M*edical *P*rograms of the *U*niformed *S*ervices: a federally funded program that provides health and hospitalization insurance for dependents of US military personnel. The program also helps finance care in private hospitals for retired military personnel.

chancre *n.* a painless ulcer that develops at the site where infection enters the body, e.g. on the lips, penis, urethra, or eyelid. It is the primary symptom of such infections as sleeping sickness and syphilis.

chancroid *n. see* soft sore.

Charcot-Leyden crystals fine colorless sharp-pointed crystals seen in the spu-

tum of asthmatics. [J. M. Charcot (1825–93), French neurologist; E. V. von Leyden (1832–1910), German physician]

Charcot-Marie-Tooth disease (peroneal muscular atrophy) a group of inherited diseases of the peripheral nerves, now more commonly known as *hereditary sensory-motor neuropathy*, causing a gradually progressive weakness and wasting of the muscles of the legs and the lower part of the thighs. The hands and arms are eventually affected. The genetic defect responsible for the most common form, type Ia, is a duplication on chromosome 17. This can be detected by a simple blood test. [J. M. Charcot; P. Marie (1853–1940), French physician; H. H. Tooth (1856–1925), British physician]

Charcot's joint a damaged, swollen, and deformed joint, often the knee, resulting from repeated minor injuries of which the patient is unaware because the nerves that normally register pain are not functioning. The condition may occur in syphilis, diabetes mellitus, and syringomyelia. [J. M. Charcot]

Charcot's triad the combination of fever, rigors, and jaundice that indicates acute *cholangitis. [J. M. Charcot]

charity patients hospital patients whose income is not sufficient to meet daily needs for food, housing, clothing, or medical care. Patients who can afford most daily needs except for medical care are often classified as medically indigent, rather than charity (or indigent) patients.

Charnley clamps parallel metal rods driven through the ends of two bones that are to be joined to form an *arthrodesis. The rods are connected on each side of the joint by bolts bearing wing nuts; tightening of the screw arrangements forces the surfaces of the bones together. When the two bones have joined, by growth and reshaping, the clamps can be removed. [Sir J. Charnley (1911–82), British orthopedic surgeon]

Chart *n. c*ontinuous *h*yperfractionated *ac*celerated *radio*therapy: a recently developed radiotherapy technique aimed at the rapid destruction of tumor cells when they are actively proliferating and therefore most sensitive to radiation. The technique continues to be evaluated at research level: it has been shown to be of benefit in the treatment of lung cancer and may also be useful for locally advanced head and neck cancer.

Chediak-Higashi syndrome a rare fatal hereditary disease in children, inherited as an autosomal *recessive condition, causing enlargement of the liver and spleen, albinism, and abnormalities of the eye. The cause is unknown but thought to be due to a disorder of glycolipid metabolism. [A. Chediak (20th century), Cuban physician; O. Higashi (20th century) Japanese pediatrician]

cheil- (cheilo-) *prefix denoting* the lip(s). Example: *cheiloplasty* (plastic surgery of).

cheilitis *n.* inflammation of the lips. *See also* perlèche.

cheiloplasty *n. see* labioplasty.

cheiloschisis *n. see* cleft lip.

cheilosis *n.* swollen cracked bright-red lips. This is a common symptom of many nutritional disorders, including ariboflavinosis (vitamin B_2 deficiency).

cheir- (cheiro-) *prefix denoting* the hand(s). Examples: *cheiralgia* (pain in); *cheiroplasty* (plastic surgery of).

cheiroarthropathy *n.* the restricted hand movement seen in long-standing diabetes. Due to chronic thickening of the skin limiting joint flexibility, it is part of the *diabetic hand syndrome.

cheiropompholyx *n.* a type of *eczema affecting the palms and fingers. The thickness of the skin in these areas prevents the eczema vesicles from breaking and eventually the skin peels after a period of intense itching. *See* pompholyx.

chelating agent a chemical compound that forms complexes by binding metal ions. Some chelating agents, including *deferoxamine and *penicillamine, are drugs used to treat metal poisoning: the metal is bound to the drug and excreted safely. Chelating agents often form the active centers of enzymes.

cheloid *n. see* keloid.

chem- (chemo-) *prefix denoting* chemical or chemistry.

chemabrasion (chemical peel, chemexfoliation) *n.* a method of removing scars, tattoos, pigmented spots, and other skin blemishes by applying caustic chemical substances that destroy or peel away the upper layers of the epidermis. *Compare* dermabrasion.

chemexfoliation *n. see* chemabrasion.

chemical peel *see* chemabrasion.

chemodectoma *n.* a former name for *paraganglioma.

chemoreceptor *n.* a cell or group of cells that responds to the presence of specific chemical compounds by initiating an impulse in a sensory nerve. Chemoreceptors are found in the taste buds and in the mucous membranes of the nose. *See also* receptor.

chemosis *n.* swelling (edema) of the *conjunctiva. It is usually due to inflammation but may occur if the drainage of blood and lymph from around the eye is obstructed.

chemotaxis *n.* movement of a cell or organism in response to the stimulus of a gradient of chemical concentration.

chemotherapy *n.* the prevention or treatment of disease by the use of chemical substances. The term is increasingly restricted to the treatment of cancer with antimetabolites and similar drugs (in contrast to *radiotherapy), but is also still sometimes used for antibiotic and other treatment of infectious diseases.

chenodeoxycholic acid any of the major bile acids synthesized in the liver. It usually occurs conjugated with glycine or taurine and facilitates fat absorption and the excretion of cholesterol. The pharmaceutical preparation is *chenodiol.

chenodiol *n.* a preparation of *chenodeoxycholic acid. Administered by mouth, it is used in the treatment of cholesterol gallstones, which it gradually dissolves over a period of up to 18 months. A common side effect is diarrhea. Potential hepatotoxicity requires monitoring of liver function. Trade name: **Chenix**.

cherry angioma *see* angioma.

chest *n. see* thorax.

Cheyne-Stokes respiration a striking form of breathing in which there is a cyclical variation in the rate, which becomes slower until breathing stops for several seconds before speeding up to a peak and then slowing down again. It occurs when the sensitivity of the respiratory centers in the brain is impaired, particularly in states of coma. [J. Cheyne (1777–1836), Scottish physician; W. Stokes (1804–78), Irish physician]

chiasma *n.* (*pl.* **chiasmata**) **1.** (in genetics) the point at which homologous chromosomes remain in contact after they have started to separate in the first division of *meiosis. Chiasmata occur from the end of prophase to anaphase and represent the point at which mutual exchange of genetic material takes place (*see* crossing over). **2.** (**chiasm**) (in anatomy) an X-shaped structure. *See* optic chiasm.

chickenpox *n.* a mild highly infectious disease caused by a *herpesvirus (the varicella-zoster virus) that is transmitted by airborne droplets. After an incubation period of 11–18 days a mild fever develops, followed within 24 hours by an itchy rash of dark red pimples. The pimples spread from the trunk to the face, scalp, and limbs; they develop into blisters and then scabs, which drop off after about 12 days. Treatment is aimed at reducing the fever and controlling the itching (e.g. by the application of calamine lotion); scarring is unusual. Complications are rare but include secondary infections and *encephalitis. The patient is infectious from the onset of symptoms until all the spots have gone. Since an attack in childhood generally confers lifelong immunity, chickenpox is rare among adults, although the virus may reactivate to cause shingles (*see* herpes). In adult patients who are particularly vulnerable, e.g. those with AIDS or who are otherwise immunosuppressed, chickenpox can be a serious disease, which may be treated with *acyclovir or *famciclovir. Medical name: **varicella**.

chiclero's ulcer a form of *leishmaniasis of the skin caused by the parasite *Leishmania tropica mexicana*. The disease, occurring in Panama, Honduras, and the Amazon, primarily affects men who visit the forests to collect chicle (gum) and takes the form of an ulcerating lesion on the ear lobe. The sore usually heals spontaneously within six months.

chigger *n. see* Trombicula.

chigoe *n. see* Tunga.

chikungunya fever a disease, occurring in Africa and Asia, caused by an *arbovirus and transmitted to humans by mosquitoes of the genus *Aëdes*. The disease is similar to *dengue and symptoms include fever, headache, generalized body pain, and an irritating rash. The patient is given drugs to relieve the pain and reduce the fever.

chilblain *n.* a dusky red round itchy swelling of the skin, occurring generally on the fingers or toes in cold weather. Chilblains form part of a group of related conditions (*see* perniosis). Treatment is by keeping the limbs warm, although vasodilator drugs may help. Medical name: **pernio**.

child abuse the maltreatment of children. It may take the form of *sexual abuse*, when a child is involved in sexual activity by an adult; *physical abuse*, when physical injury is caused by cruelty or undue punishment (*see* battered baby syndrome); *neglect*, when basic physical provision for needs is lacking; and *emotional abuse*, when lack of affection and/or hostility from caregivers damage a child's emotional development (*see* attachment disorder).

childbirth *n. see* labor.

Child Health Act an amendment to the US *Social Security Act. It provides funds for maternal and infant care as well as for preschool and school-age children. Specific provisions cover such items as dental health of children, services for crippled children, family planning services, research into child health problems, and training of personnel needed to implement authorized child health projects.

chir- (chiro-) *prefix denoting* the hand(s). *See also* cheir-.

chiropody *n. see* podiatry.

chiropractic *n.* a system of treating diseases by manipulation, mainly of the vertebrae of the backbone. It is based on the theory that nearly all disorders can be traced to the incorrect alignment of bones, with consequent malfunctioning of nerves and muscle throughout the body.

Chlamydia *n.* a genus of gram-negative bacteria that are obligate intracellular parasites of humans and other animals, in which they cause disease. Some *Chlamydia* infections of birds can be transmitted to humans (*see* psittacosis). *Chlamydia trachomatis* is the causative agent of the eye disease *trachoma and of sexually transmitted diseases, being responsible for nonspecific *urethritis in men, *pelvic inflammatory disease in women, and *inclusion conjunctivitis in the newborn. *Chlamydia pneumoniae* causes pneumonia. —**chlamydial** *adj.*

chloasma (melasma) *n.* patchy brown coloration of the skin, mainly on the forehead, temples, and cheeks, that occurs sometimes in pregnancy and in some women taking oral contraceptive pills; it rarely occurs in men. It is a photosensitivity reaction that can usually be prevented by sunscreens.

chlor- (chloro-) *prefix denoting* **1.** chlorine or chlorides. **2.** green.

chloracne *n.* an occupational acnelike skin disorder that occurs after regular contact with chlorinated hydrocarbons. These chemicals are derived from oil and tar products; "cutting oils" used in engineering also cause the disease. The skin develops blackheads, papules, and pustules, mainly on hairy parts (such as the forearm). Warts and skin cancer may develop after many years of exposure to these chemicals.

chloral hydrate a sedative and hypnotic drug used, mainly in children and the elderly, to induce sleep or as a daytime sedative. It is rapidly absorbed from the alimentary canal and is usually given by mouth as a syrup, although it can be administered rectally. Toxic effects are usually only seen with overdosage. Prolonged use may lead to *dependence. Trade names: **Aquachloral, Noctec**.

chlorambucil *n.* an *alkylating agent used in chemotherapy. It is given by mouth and used mainly in the treatment of chronic leukemias. Prolonged large doses may cause damage to the bone marrow. Trade name: **Leukeran**.

chloramphenicol *n.* an antibiotic, derived from the bacterium *Streptomyces venezuelae* and also produced synthetically, that is effective against a wide variety of microorganisms. However, due to its serious side effects, especially damage to the bone marrow, it is usually reserved for serious infections (such as typhoid fever) when less toxic drugs are ineffective. It is also used as eye drops or ointment to treat bacterial conjunctivitis. Trade names: **Chloromycetin, Chloroptic**.

chlorcyclizine *n.* an *antihistamine drug that is administered orally as a component of various cold and allergy preparations and topically as an *antipruritic.

chlordiazepoxide *n.* a *benzodiazepine drug with *muscle relaxant properties, used to relieve tension, fear, and anxiety and in the treatment of alcoholism. It is administered by mouth. Common side effects are nausea, skin reactions, and muscular incoordination. Trade name: **Librium**.

chlorhexidine *n.* an antiseptic used as a general disinfectant for skin and mucous membranes or as a preservative (for example, in eye drops). Chlorhexidine is used in solution, creams, gels, and lozenges and in some preparations is combined with *cetrimonium. In very dilute solution it can be used as an effective mouthwash for the prevention and control of infections of the mouth. Skin sensitivity to chlorhexidine occurs rarely. Trade names: **Betasept, Hibiclens, Peridex, PerioGard**.

chlorination *n.* the addition of noninjurious traces of chlorine (often one part per million) to water supplies before human consumption to ensure that disease-causing organisms are destroyed. *See also* fluoridation.

chlorine *n.* an extremely pungent gaseous element with antiseptic and bleaching properties. It is widely used to sterilize drinking water and purify swimming pools. In high concentrations it is toxic; it was used in World War I as a poison gas in the trenches. Symbol: Cl.

chlormadinone *n.* a synthetic sex hormone (*see* progestogen) that was formerly used in oral contraceptives as a sequential and progestogen-only pill. Chlormadinone produces variations in the length of the menstrual cycle and abnormal bleeding; nausea, vomiting, and weight gain may also occur.

chlormethiazole *n.* a *sedative and hypnotic drug used to treat insomnia in the elderly (when associated with confusion, agitation, and restlessness) and drug withdrawal symptoms (especially in alcoholism). It is administered by mouth or injection and the most common side effects are tingling sensations in the nose and sneezing. Trade name: **Distraneurin**.

chlormezanone *n.* a tranquilizing drug used in the treatment of mild anxiety and tension, including premenstrual tension. It is also used to relieve pain and muscle spasm. Chlormezanone is administered by mouth; the most common side effects are drowsiness and dizziness. Trade name: **Trancopal**.

chlorobutanol *n.* an antibacterial and antifungal agent used as a preservative in injection solutions, in eye and nose drops, in powder form for topical use in irritational skin conditions, and occasionally by mouth as a mild sedative in motion sickness. Trade name: **Chloretone**.

chloroform n. a volatile liquid formerly widely used as a general anesthetic. Because its use as such causes liver damage and affects heart rhythm, chloroform is now used only in low concentrations as a flavoring agent and preservative, in the treatment of flatulence, and in liniments as a *rubefacient.

chloroguanide (proguanil) n. a drug that kills malaria parasites and is used in the prevention and treatment of malaria. It is administered by mouth and rarely causes side effects. The malarial parasite has developed resistance to this drug in the US.

chloroma n. a tumor that arises in association with *myeloid leukemia and consists essentially of a mass of leukemic cells. A freshly cut specimen of the tumor appears green, but the color rapidly disappears on exposure to air. It shows red fluorescence with ultraviolet light and responds to specific antileukemic treatment.

chlorophenothane n. see DDT.

chlorophyll n. one of a group of green pigments, found in all green plants and some bacteria, that absorb light to provide energy for the synthesis of carbohydrates from carbon dioxide and water (photosynthesis). The two major chlorophylls, a and b, consist of a porphyrin/magnesium complex.

chloropsia n. green vision: a rare symptom of digitalis poisoning.

chloroquine n. a drug used principally in the treatment and prevention of malaria but also used in rheumatoid arthritis, extraintestinal amebiasis, and lupus erythematosus. Chloroquine is administered by mouth or injection; a side effect of prolonged use in large doses is eye damage. Trade name: **Aralen**.

chlorothiazide n. a *diuretic used to treat fluid retention (edema) and high blood pressure (hypertension). It is administered by mouth and may cause skin sensitivity reactions, stomach pains, nausea, and reduced blood potassium levels. Trade name: **Diuril**.

chlorotrianisene n. a synthetic *estrogen administered by mouth to treat symptoms of the menopause, to suppress lactation in mothers not breast feeding, and to relieve symptoms in inoperable cancer of the prostate gland. Trade name: **TACE**.

chloroxylenol n. an *antiseptic, derived from *phenol but less toxic and more selective in bactericidal activity, used mainly in solution as a skin disinfectant.

chlorphenesin n. a compound with sedative properties used to treat painful musculoskeletal conditions. Side effects include dizziness, fever, allergic reactions, and blood diseases. Trade name: **Maolate**.

chlorpheniramine n. a potent *antihistamine that is used to treat such allergies as hay fever, rhinitis, and urticaria. It is administered by mouth or, in order to relieve severe conditions, by injection. Trade names: **Aller-Chlor, Chlor-Trimeton, Teldrin**.

chlorpromazine n. an *antipsychotic drug used in the treatment of *schizophrenia and *mania, to control severe anxiety and agitation, and to control nausea and vomiting. It also enhances the effects of *analgesics and is used in terminal illness and preparation for anesthesia. Chlorpromazine is administered by mouth or injection or as a rectal suppository; common side effects are drowsiness and dry mouth. It also causes abnormalities of movement, especially *dystonias, *dyskinesia, and *parkinsonism. Trade name: **Thorazine**.

chlorpropamide n. a drug that reduces blood sugar levels and is used to treat diabetes in adults. It is administered by mouth and can cause such side effects as skin sensitivity reactions and digestive upsets. Trade name: **Diabinese**. See also sulfonylurea.

chlorprothixene n. an *antipsychotic drug used to treat agitation, anxiety, insomnia, delusions, and hallucinations. It is administered by mouth; common side effects are dry mouth and drowsiness. Trade names: **Navane, Taractan**.

chlortetracycline n. an *antibiotic active against many bacteria and fungi. It is administered by mouth or injection or as ointment or cream (for skin and eye infections); side effects are those of the other *tetracyclines. Trade name: **Aureomycin**.

chlorthalidone n. a *diuretic used to treat

fluid retention (edema) and high blood pressure (hypertension). It is administered by mouth and may cause skin sensitivity reactions, stomach pains, nausea, and reduced blood potassium levels. Trade names: **Hygroton, Thalitone**.

choana n. (*pl.* **choanae**) a funnel-shaped opening, particularly either of the two openings between the nasal cavity and the pharynx.

chokedamp n. *see* blackdamp.

choking n. the condition in which respiration is prevented by obstruction or compression of the trachea or larynx. There is sudden coughing and the face turns red, then purple. Emergency treatment requires removal of the obstruction (*see* Heimlich maneuver) and resuscitation, if necessary.

chol- (chole-, cholo-) *prefix denoting* bile. Example: *cholemesis* (vomiting of).

cholagogue n. a drug that stimulates the flow of bile from the gallbladder and bile ducts into the duodenum.

cholangiocarcinoma n. a malignant tumor of the bile ducts. It is particularly likely to occur at the junction of the two main bile ducts within the liver, causing obstructive jaundice. Treatment is directed at relieving the jaundice and other symptoms. Then surgery is done to remove the tumor or for liver transplantation.

cholangiography n. X-ray examination of the bile ducts, used to demonstrate the site and nature of any obstruction to the ducts or to show the presence of stones within them. A medium that is opaque to X-rays is introduced into the ducts either by injection into the bloodstream (*intravenous cholangiography*); by direct injection into the liver (*percutaneous transhepatic cholangiography*); by direct injection into the bile ducts at operation (*operative cholangiography*); or by injection into the duodenal opening of the ducts through a *duodenoscope (endoscopic retrograde cholangiopancreatography; see* ERCP). *See also* percutaneous transhepatic cholangiopancreatography.

cholangiolitis n. inflammation of the smallest bile ducts (*cholangioles*). *See* cholangitis.

cholangioma n. a rare tumor originating from the bile duct.

cholangitis n. inflammation of the bile ducts. It usually occurs when the ducts are obstructed, especially by stones, or after operations on the bile ducts. Symptoms of acute cholangitis include intermittent fever, usually with *rigors, and intermittent jaundice (a combination known as *Charcot's triad*). Initial treatment is by antibiotics, but removal of the obstruction is essential for permanent cure. Liver abscess is a possible complication, and recurrent episodes of cholangitis lead to secondary biliary *cirrhosis. *Sclerosing cholangitis* is a characteristic but rare complication of ulcerative colitis in which all the bile ducts develop irregularities and narrowing.

cholecalciferol n. *see* vitamin D.

cholecyst- *prefix denoting* the gallbladder. Example: *cholecystotomy* (incision of).

cholecystectomy n. surgical removal of the gallbladder, usually for *cholecystitis or gallstones. Formerly always performed by *laparotomy, the operation is now often done by *laparoscopy (*percutaneous laparoscopic cholecystectomy*). *See also* minimally invasive surgery.

cholecystenterostomy n. a surgical procedure in which the gallbladder is joined to the small intestine. It is performed in order to allow bile to pass from the liver to the intestine when the common bile duct is obstructed by an irremovable cause.

cholecystitis n. inflammation of the gallbladder. *Acute cholecystitis* is due to bacterial infection, causing fever and acute pain over the gallbladder. It is usually treated by rest and antibiotics. *Chronic cholecystitis* is often associated with *gallstones and causes recurrent episodes of upper abdominal pain. It is also associated with *cholecystitis glandularis proliferans* – thickening of the gallbladder wall and epithelial changes (crypt formation, hypertrophy). Recurrent bacterial infection may be the cause of chronic cholecystitis, but the physical processes leading to gallstone formation may also be important. It may require treatment by *cholecystectomy. *See also* cholesterosis, Murphy's sign.

cholecystoduodenostomy n. a form of *cholecystenterostomy in which the gallbladder is joined to the duodenum.

cholecystogastrostomy n. a form of *cholecystenterostomy in which the gallbladder is joined to the stomach. It is rarely performed.

cholecystography *n.* X-ray examination of the gallbladder. A compound that is opaque to X-rays is taken by mouth, absorbed by the intestine, and excreted by the liver into the bile, which is concentrated in the gallbladder. An X-ray photograph (*cholecystogram*) of the gallbladder indicates whether or not it is functioning, and gallstones may be seen as contrasting (nonopaque) areas within it. A fatty meal is usually also given, to demonstrate the ability of the gallbladder to contract. This technique has largely been replaced by ultrasound scanning.

cholecystokinin (pancreozymin) *n.* a hormone secreted by the cells of the duodenum in response to partly digested food in the duodenum. It causes contraction of the gallbladder and expulsion of bile into the intestine and stimulates the production of digestive enzymes by the pancreas (*see also* pancreatic juice). In the brain cholecystokinin functions as a neurotransmitter, involved in the control of satiety.

cholecystotomy *n.* a surgical operation in which the gallbladder is opened, usually to remove gallstones. It is performed only when *cholecystectomy would be impracticable or dangerous.

choledoch- (choledocho-) *prefix denoting* the common bile duct. Example: *choledochoplasty* (plastic surgery of).

choledocholithiasis *n.* stones within the common bile duct. The stones usually form in the gallbladder and pass into the bile duct, but they may develop within the duct after *cholecystectomy.

choledochotomy *n.* a surgical operation in which the common bile duct is opened, to search for or to remove stones within it. It may be performed at the same time as *cholecystectomy or if stones occur in the bile duct after cholecystectomy.

cholelithiasis *n.* the formation of stones in the gallbladder (*see* gallstone).

cholelithotomy *n.* removal of gallstones by *cholecystotomy.

cholera *n.* an acute infection of the small intestine by the bacterium *Vibrio cholerae*, which causes severe vomiting and diarrhea (known as *ricewater stools*) leading to dehydration. The disease is contracted from food or drinking water contaminated by feces from a patient. Cholera often occurs in epidemics; outbreaks are rare with good sanitary conditions. After an incubation period of 1–5 days symptoms commence suddenly; the resulting dehydration and imbalance in the concentration of body fluids can cause death within 24 hours. Initial treatment involves replacing the fluid loss by *oral rehydration therapy; *tetracycline eradicates vibrios and hastens recovery. The mortality rate in untreated cases is over 50%. Vaccination against cholera is effective for only 6–9 months.

choleresis *n.* the production of bile by the liver.

choleretic *n.* an agent that stimulates the secretion of bile by the liver thereby increasing the flow of bile.

cholestasis *n.* failure of normal amounts of bile to reach the intestine, resulting in obstructive *jaundice. The cause may be a mechanical block in the bile ducts, such as a stone (*extrahepatic biliary obstruction*), or liver disease, such as that caused by the drug *chlorpromazine in some hypersensitive individuals (*intrahepatic cholestasis*); it may also occasionally occur in pregnancy. The symptoms are jaundice with dark urine, pale feces, and usually itching (pruritus).

cholesteatoma *n.* an epithelial-lined sac containing mainly cellular debris in which cholesterol crystals generally may be demonstrated. Cholesteatomas are benign; they occur mainly in the middle ear and mastoid region and, by pressure, cause destruction of surrounding structures. They may also occur in other parts of the skull and nervous system. Left untreated, meningitis or a cerebral abscess may occur. Treatment is with surgery (*see* mastoidectomy).

cholesterol *n.* a fatlike material (a *sterol) present in the blood and most tissues, especially nervous tissue. Cholesterol and its esters are important constituents of cell membranes and are precursors of many steroid hormones and bile salts. Western dietary intake is approximately 500–1000 mg/day. Cholesterol is synthesized in the body from acetate, mainly in the liver, and blood concentration is normally 140–300 mg/100 ml (3.6–7.8 mmol/l). Elevated blood concentration (*hypercholesterolemia*) is frequently associated with *atheroma, of which cholesterol is a major component.

Hypercholesterolemia and the resulting atheroma have been linked with a high dietary intake of saturated fats and cholesterol. However, current thinking suggests that the damage to blood vessels is actually caused by high levels (over 4.4 mmol/l) of low-density *lipoprotein (LDL), one of the forms in which cholesterol is transported in the bloodstream, in its oxidized form. Therefore increasing the dietary intake of *antioxidants would appear to protect against atherosclerosis. People with *primary* (or *familial*) *hypercholesterolemia* have a genetic defect causing a lack of LDL receptors, which remove cholesterol from the bloodstream. Drugs are available that lower serum cholesterol and LDL levels. Cholesterol is also a constituent of *gallstones.

cholesterosis *n.* a form of chronic *cholecystitis in which small crystals of cholesterol are deposited on the internal wall of the gallbladder, like the pips of a strawberry: hence its descriptive term *strawberry gallbladder*. The crystals may enlarge to become *gallstones.

cholestyramine *n.* a drug that binds with bile salts so that they are excreted (*see* bile-acid sequestrant). It is administered by mouth to relieve conditions due to irritant effects of bile salts (such as the itching that occurs in obstructive jaundice), to treat diarrhea, and to lower the blood levels of *cholesterol and other fats in patients with hyperlipidemia. Common side effects include constipation, heartburn, and nausea. Trade names: **Prevalite, Questran, Questran Light**.

cholic acid (cholalic acid) *see* bile acids.

choline *n.* a basic compound important in the synthesis of phosphatidylcholine (lecithin) and other *phospholipids and of *acetylcholine. It is also involved in the transport of fat in the body. Choline is sometimes classed as a vitamin of the B complex; it can be synthesized in the body or obtained in the diet.

cholinergic *adj.* **1.** describing nerve fibers that release *acetylcholine as a neurotransmitter or act as *receptors at which acetylcholine acts to pass on messages from cholinergic nerve fibers. **2.** describing drugs that mimic the actions of acetylcholine (*see* parasympathomimetic). *Compare* adrenergic.

cholinergic urticaria *see* urticaria.

cholinesterase *n.* an enzyme that breaks down a choline ester into its choline and acid components. The term usually refers to *acetylcholinesterase*, which breaks down the neurotransmitter *acetylcholine into choline and acetic acid. It is found in all *cholinergic nerve junctions, where it rapidly destroys the acetylcholine released during the transmission of a nerve impulse so that subsequent impulses may pass. Other cholinesterases are found in the blood and other tissues.

choluria *n.* bile in the urine, which occurs when the level of bile in the blood is raised, especially in obstructive *jaundice. The urine becomes dark brown or orange, and bile pigments and bile salts may be detected in it.

chondr- (chondro-) *prefix denoting* cartilage. Example: *chondrogenesis* (formation of).

chondrin *n.* a material that resembles gelatin, produced when cartilage is boiled.

chondriosome *n. see* mitochondrion.

chondroblast *n.* a cell that produces the matrix of *cartilage.

chondroblastoma *n.* a benign tumor derived from *chondroblasts, having the appearance of a mass of well-differentiated cartilage.

chondrocalcinosis *n.* the presence of calcium pyrophosphate crystals in joint cartilage, which is usually demonstrated radiologically or crystographically and is seen in *pseudogout.

chondroclast *n.* a cell that is concerned with the absorption of cartilage.

chondrocranium *n.* the embryonic skull, which is composed entirely of cartilage and is later replaced by bone. *See also* meninx.

chondrocyte *n.* a *cartilage cell, found embedded in the matrix.

chondrodermatitis nodularis helicis a fairly common painful nodule on the upper part of the ear, which may become ulcerated. It occurs principally in middle-aged or elderly men and characteristically prevents the person from sleeping on the affected side; it is readily treated by surgery.

chondrodysplasia (chondro-osteodystrophy, chondrodystrophy) *n.* any of various conditions in which there is an abnormality in cartilage development. It affects long bones and can cause short-limb dwarfism, overgrowth of the *epiphysis, or other deformities. One particular form is an autosomal *recessive syndrome most commonly found in Old Order Amish populations. *See also* achondroplasia.

chondrodystrophy *n.* see chondrodysplasia.

chondroitin sulfate a mucopolysaccharide that forms an important constituent of cartilage, bone, and other connective tissues. It is composed of glucuronic acid and N-acetyl-D-galactosamine units.

chondroma *n.* a relatively common benign tumor of cartilage-forming cells, which may occur at the growing end of any bone but is found most commonly in the bones of the feet and hands. It may be a chance finding on X-ray.

chondromalacia *n.* softening, inflammation, and degeneration of cartilage at a joint. *Chondromalacia patellae* is the most common kind, affecting the undersurface of the kneecap and commonly seen in athletes; it results in pain in the front of the knee and grating, which is made worse by kneeling, squatting, and climbing stairs. Treatment is physiotherapy and avoidance of aggravating factors.

chondro-osteodystrophy *n.* see chondrodysplasia.

chondrosarcoma *n.* a malignant tumor of cartilage cells, occurring in a bone, usually the pelvis, ribs, sternum, or femur. Such tumors have a typical "snowstorm" appearance on X-ray, are slow-growing but infiltrate adjacent structures, and are often fatal. Treatment is by surgical removal; these tumors are not usually sensitive to radiotherapy or chemotherapy.

chord- (chordo-) *prefix denoting* **1.** a cord. **2.** the notochord.

chorda *n.* (*pl.* **chordae**) a cord, tendon, or nerve fiber. The *chordae tendineae* are stringlike processes in the heart that attach the margins of the mitral and tricuspid valve leaflets to projections of the wall of the ventricle (*papillary muscles*). Rupture of the chordae, through injury, endocarditis, or degenerative changes, results in *mitral incompetence.

chordee *n.* acute angulation of the penis. In *Peyronie's disease, this is due to a lo-

calized fibrous plaque in the penis, which fails to engorge on erection. As a result, the penis angulates at this point making intercourse impossible. In a child, downward chordee is an associated deformity in *hypospadias and the more severe forms are corrected surgically.

chorditis *n.* inflammation of a vocal or spermatic cord. *See* laryngitis.

chordoma *n.* a rare tumor arising from remnants of the embryologic *notochord consisting of a grayish white gelatinous material that displaces surrounding tissue. The classic sites are the base of skull and the region of the sacrum. Treatment is with surgery.

chorea *n.* a jerky involuntary movement particularly affecting the head, face, or limbs. Each movement is sudden but the resulting posture may be prolonged for a few seconds. The symptoms are usually due to disease of the *basal ganglia but may result from drug therapy for *parkinsonism or on withdrawal of phenothiazines. In *Huntington's disease (or chorea) the involuntary movements are accompanied by a progressive *dementia. *Senile chorea* occurs sporadically in elderly people and there is no dementia. *Sydenham's chorea affects children and is associated with rheumatic fever.

chorion *n.* the embryonic membrane that totally surrounds the embryo from the time of implantation. It is formed from *trophoblast lined with mesoderm and becomes closely associated with the *allantois. The blood vessels (supplied by the allantois) are concentrated in the region of the chorion that is attached to the wall of the uterus and forms the *placenta. *See also* villus. —**chorionic** *adj.*

chorionepithelioma (choriocarcinoma, malignant deciduoma) *n.* a rare form of cancer originating in the outermost of the membranes (chorion) surrounding the fetus. Chorionepithelioma, which rapidly invades and causes secondary deposits in the lungs, is highly malignant; it usually follows a *hydatidiform mole, but it may follow abortion or even a normal pregnancy. It is relatively sensitive to *cytotoxic drugs.

chorionic gonadotropin (human chorionic gonadotropin, hCG) a hormone, similar to the pituitary *gonadotropins, produced by the placenta during pregnancy.

Large amounts are excreted in the urine, and this is used as the basis for most *pregnancy tests. hCG maintains the secretion of *progesterone by the corpus luteum of the ovary, the secretion of pituitary gonadotropins being blocked during pregnancy. hCG is given by injection to treat delayed puberty, undescended testes, premenstrual tension, and (with *follicle-stimulating hormone) sterility due to lack of ovulation.

chorionic villus sampling (CVS) a fetal monitoring technique in which a sample of chorionic *villus is taken between the eighth and eleventh weeks of pregnancy. The sample is extracted through the cervix or abdomen under ultrasound visualization. The cells so obtained are subjected to chromosome analysis and biochemical studies to determine if the fetus has any abnormalities. This enables the *prenatal diagnosis of such congenital disorders as Down's syndrome and thalassemia.

chorioretinopathy *n.* any eye disease involving both the choroid and the retina.

choristoma *n.* a tumor or mass of tissue composed of tissue not normally found at the affected site. A *dermoid cyst is an example.

choroid *n.* the layer of the eyeball between the retina and the sclera (*see also* Bruch's membrane). It contains blood vessels and a pigment that absorbs excess light and so prevents blurring of vision. *See* eye. —**choroidal** *adj.*

choroidal detachment the separation of the *choroid from the *sclera of the eye as a result of leakage of fluid from the vessels of the choroid. It occurs when pressure inside the eyeball is very low, usually after trauma or intraocular surgery.

choroideremia *n.* a sex-linked hereditary condition in which the retinal pigment epithelium (*see* retina) and the choroid begin to degenerate in the first few months or years of life. In males this results in blindness, but in females it rarely causes any significant visual loss.

choroiditis *n.* inflammation of the choroid layer of the eye. It may be inflamed together with the iris and ciliary body, but often is involved alone and in patches (*focal* or *multifocal choroiditis*). Vision becomes blurred but the eye is usually painless. *See* uveitis.

choroid plexus a rich network of blood vessels, derived from those of the pia mater, in each of the brain's ventricles. It is responsible for the production of *cerebrospinal fluid.

Christmas disease (hemophilia B) a genetic disorder that is similar in its effects to classic *hemophilia (hemophilia A), but is due to a deficiency of a different blood coagulation factor, the *Christmas factor* (Factor IX). [S. Christmas (20th century), in whom the factor was first identified]

chrom- (chromo-) *prefix denoting* color or pigment.

chromaffin *n.* tissue in the medulla of the *adrenal gland consisting of modified neural cells containing granules that are stained brown by chromates. Epinephrine and norepinephrine are released from the granules when the adrenal gland is stimulated by its sympathetic nerve supply. *See also* neurohormone.

-chromasia *suffix denoting* staining or pigmentation.

chromat- (chromato-) *prefix denoting* color or pigmentation.

chromatid *n.* one of the two threadlike strands formed by longitudinal division of a chromosome during *mitosis and *meiosis. They remain attached at the *centromere. Chromatids can be seen between early prophase and metaphase in mitosis and between diplotene and the second metaphase of meiosis, after which they divide at the centromere to form daughter chromosomes.

chromatin *n.* the material of a cell nucleus that stains with basic dyes and consists of DNA and protein: the substance of which the chromosomes are made. *See* euchromatin, heterochromatin.

chromatography *n.* any of several techniques for separating the components of a mixture by selective absorption. Two such techniques are quite widely used in medicine, for example to separate mixtures of amino acids. In one of these, *paper chromatography*, a sample of the mixture is placed at the edge of a sheet of filter paper. As the solvent soaks along the paper, the components are absorbed to different extents and thus move along the paper at different rates. In *column chromatography* the components separate out along a column of a powdered absorbent, such as silica or aluminum oxide.

chromatolysis *n.* the dispersal or disintegration of the microscopic structures within the nerve cells that normally produce proteins. It is part of the cell's response to injury.

chromatophore *n.* a cell containing pigment. In humans chromatophores containing *melanin are found in the skin, hair, and eyes.

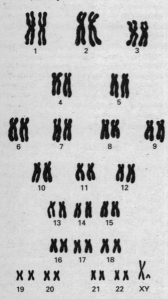

Human male chromosomes, arranged in numbered pairs according to a standard classification. The female set differs only in the sex chromosomes (XX instead of XY).

chromatopsia *n.* abnormal colored vision: a rare symptom of various conditions. Sometimes everything looks reddish to patients after removal of their cataracts; patients with digitalis poisoning may see things in green or yellow. Similar disturbances of color may be experienced by people recovering from inflammation of the optic nerve.

chromoblastomycosis (chromomycosis) *n.* a chronic fungal infection of the skin usually occurring at the site of an injury; for example, a wound from a wood splinter. It produces pigmented wartlike lumps on exposed areas that sometimes ulcerate. In the immunocompromised it may spread rapidly and even prove fatal.

chromosome *n.* one of the threadlike structures in a cell nucleus that carry the genetic information in the form of *genes. It is composed of a long double filament of *DNA coiled into a helix together with associated proteins, with the genes arranged in a linear manner along its length. It stains deeply with basic dyes during cell division (*see* meiosis, mitosis). The nucleus of each human somatic cell contains 46 chromosomes, 23 being of maternal and 23 of paternal origin (see illustration). Each chromosome can duplicate an exact copy of itself between each cell division (*see* interphase) so that each new cell formed receives a full set of chromosomes. *See also* chromatid, centromere, sex chromosome. —**chromosomal** *adj.*

chron- (chrono-) *prefix denoting* time. Example: *chronophobia* (abnormal fear of).

chronic *adj.* describing a disease of long duration, sometimes involving very slow changes. Such disease is often of gradual onset. The term does not imply anything about the severity of a disease. *Compare* acute. —**chronicity** *n.*

chronic fatigue syndrome (CFS) a condition characterized by extreme disabling fatigue that has lasted for at least six months, is made worse by physical or mental exertion, does not resolve with bed rest, and cannot be attributed to other disorders. The fatigue is accompanied by at least some of the following: muscle pain or weakness, poor coordination, joint pain, sore throat, slight fever, painful lymph nodes in the neck and armpits, depression, inability to concentrate, and general malaise. The condition was formerly known as *myalgic encephalomyelitis* (*ME*); it is also called *CFS/ME* and – because it often occurs as a sequel to such viral infections as glandular fever – is sometimes called *postviral fatigue syndrome*. Since the cause is unknown, treatment is limited to relieving the symptoms; graded physiotherapy and cognitive behavioral therapy may be helpful in some cases.

chronic obstructive pulmonary disease (COPD, chronic obstructive airways disease) a disease of adults, especially those over the age of 45 with a history of smoking or inhalation of airborne pollution, characterized by diminished inspiratory and expiratory capacity of the lungs. The disease has features of *emphysema and chronic *bronchitis. It is diagnosed when the *forced expiratory volume in 1 second (FEV$_1$) is less than 60% of the predicted value for the patient's age and height and the patient does not respond to corticosteroids or bronchodilators. Compared to asthma, there is less response to inhaled steroids, which may only be indicated for patients with frequent exacerbations.

chrys- (chryso-) *prefix denoting* gold or gold salts.

chrysiasis *n.* an abnormal condition characterized by the deposition of gold in the eye and other tissues as a result of prolonged or excessive treatment with gold salts.

Chrysops *n.* a genus of bloodsucking flies, commonly called deer flies. Female flies, found in shady wooded areas, bite humans during the day. Certain species in Africa may transmit the tropical disease *loiasis to humans. In the US *C. discalis* is a vector of *tularemia.

chrysotherapy *n.* the treatment of disease by the administration of gold or its compounds. The injection or oral administration of gold salts is extremely effective in the treatment of arthritis in some patients. However, some patients develop potentially severe side effects, including blood disorders, dermatitis, and impairment of kidney function.

Churg-Strauss syndrome (allergic granulomatous angiitis, allergic granulomatosis) a clinical syndrome comprising severe asthma associated with an increased *eosinophil count in the peripheral blood and eosinophilic deposits in the small vessels of the lungs. It usually responds to oral corticosteroids. Untreated, it may result in severe and widespread systemic *angiitis. [J. Churg (1910–) and L. Strauss (1913–), US pathologists]

Chvostek's sign twitching of the facial muscles elicited by stimulation of the facial nerve by tapping. This indicates muscular irritability, usually due to calcium depletion (*see* tetany). [F. Chvosteck (1835–84), Austrian surgeon]

chyle *n.* an alkaline milky liquid found within the *lacteals after a period of absorption. It consists of lymph with a suspension of minute droplets of digested fats, which have been absorbed from the small intestine. It is transported in the lymphatic system to the thoracic duct, which drains into the subclavian vein. *See also* ascites.

chylomicron *n.* a microscopic particle of fat present in the blood after fat has been digested and absorbed from the small intestine.

chyluria *n.* the presence of *chyle in the urine.

chyme *n.* the semiliquid acid mass that is the form in which food passes from the stomach to the small intestine. It is produced by the action of *gastric juice and the churning movements of the stomach.

chymopapain *n.* an enzyme used in the treatment of *prolapsed intervertebral disk. It is a plant protein obtained from the latex of the tropical tree *Carica papaya*. When injected into the intervertebral disk, it breaks up the proteoglycans into smaller glycosamines, thus reducing the disk's ability to retain water. This causes the disintegration of the disk, which in turn reduces the pressure on the nerve root from the disk. Trade name: **Chymodiactin.**

chymotrypsin *n.* a protein-digesting enzyme (*see* peptidase). It is secreted by the pancreas in an inactive form, *chymotrypsinogen*, that is converted into chymotrypsin in the duodenum by the action of *trypsin.

chymotrypsinogen *n. see* chymotrypsin.

cicatrix *n.* a *scar. —**cicatricial** *adj.*

-cide *suffix denoting* killer or killing. Examples: *bactericide* (of bacteria); *infanticide* (of children).

ciliary body the part of the *eye that connects the choroid with the iris. It consists of three zones: the *ciliary ring*, which adjoins the choroid; the *ciliary processes*, a series of about 70 radial ridges behind the iris to which the suspensory ligament of the lens is attached; and the *ciliary muscle*, contraction of which alters the curvature of the lens (*see* accommodation).

cilium *n.* (*pl.* **cilia**) **1.** a hairlike process, large numbers of which are found on certain epithelial cells and on certain (ciliate) protozoa. Cilia are particularly characteristic of the epithelium that lines the upper respiratory tract, where their beating serves to remove particles of dust and other foreign material. **2.** an eyelash or eyelid. —**ciliary** *adj.*

cimetidine *n.* an H₂-receptor antagonist (*see* antihistamine) that reduces secretion of acid in the stomach and is used to treat stomach and duodenal ulcers, gastroesophageal reflux, and other digestive disorders. It is administered by mouth or injection and the most common side effects are dizziness, diarrhea, muscular pains, and rash. Trade name: **Tagamet**.

Cimex *n. see* bedbug.

CIN *see* cervical intraepithelial neoplasia.

cinchona *n.* the dried bark of *Cinchona* trees, formerly used in medicine to treat malaria, to stimulate the appetite, and to prevent hemorrhage and diarrhea. Taken over prolonged periods, it may cause *cinchonism. Cinchona is the source of *quinine.

cinchonism *n.* poisoning caused by an overdose of cinchona or the alkaloids quinine, quinidine, or cinchonine derived from it. The symptoms are commonly ringing noises in the ears, dizziness, blurring of vision (and sometimes complete blindness), rashes, fever, and low blood pressure. Treatment with *diuretics increases the rate of excretion of the toxic compounds from the body.

cine- *prefix denoting* any technique of recording a rapid series of X-ray images on cine film for later analysis. Examples: *cineangiography; cinefluorography.* Cine film is now being replaced by electronic storage media. *See also* video-.

cingulectomy *n.* surgical excision of the cingulum, the part of the brain concerned with anger and depression. The procedure has occasionally been carried out as *psychosurgery for intractable mental illness.

cingulum *n.* (*pl.* **cingula**) **1.** a curved bundle of nerve fibers in each cerebral hemisphere, nearly encircling its connection with the corpus callosum. *See* cerebrum. **2.** a small protuberance on the lingual surface of the crowns of incisor and canine teeth.

ciprofibrate *n. see* fibrates.

ciprofloxacin *n.* a broad-spectrum *quinolone antibiotic that can be given orally and is particularly useful against gram-negative bacteria, such as *Pseudomonas*, that are resistant to all other oral antibiotics. It is used in the treatment of lower respiratory and urinary tract infections and skin, bone, and joint infections. It is administered by mouth; side effects are nausea and vomiting, diarrhea, abdominal pain, and headache. It is also given as eye drops for eye infections. Trade names: **Ciloxan, Cipro**.

circadian *adj.* denoting a biological rhythm or cycle of approximately 24 hours. *Compare* nyctohemeral, ultradian.

circle of Willis a circle on the undersurface of the brain formed by linked branches of the arteries that supply the brain (see illustration). This helps to maintain the blood supply in the event that a vessel supplying blood to the brain becomes blocked. Most cerebral *aneurysms occur on or near the circle of Willis. [T. Willis (1621–75), English anatomist]

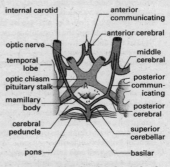

internal carotid — anterior communicating — anterior cerebral — optic nerve — temporal lobe — optic chiasm — pituitary stalk — mamillary body — cerebral peduncle — pons — middle cerebral — posterior communicating — posterior cerebral — superior cerebellar — basilar

Arterial branches forming the circle of Willis (seen from below)

circulatory system *see* cardiovascular system.

circum- *prefix denoting* around; surrounding. Example: *circumanal* (around the anus).

circumcision *n.* surgical removal of the foreskin of the penis. This operation is usually performed for religious and ethnic reasons but is sometimes required for medical conditions, mainly *phimosis and *paraphimosis. *Female circumci-*

sion involves removal of the clitoris, *labia minora, and labia majora. The extent of excision varies from tribe to tribe and from country to country. The simplest and least damaging form is *clitoridectomy* (removal of the clitoris); the next form entails excision of the *prepuce, clitoris, and all or part of the labia minora. The most extensive form, *infibulation*, involves excision of clitoris, labia minora, and labia majora. The vulval lips are sutured together and a piece of wood or reed is inserted to preserve a small passage for urine and menstrual fluid. In the majority of women who are circumcised, *episiotomy, often extensive, is required to allow delivery of a child.

circumduction *n.* a circular movement, such as that made by a limb.

circumflex nerve a mixed sensory and motor nerve of the upper arm. It arises from the fifth and sixth cervical segments of the spinal cord and is distributed to the deltoid muscle of the shoulder and the overlying skin.

circumoral *adj.* situated around the mouth.

circumstantiality *n.* a disorder of thought in which thinking and speech proceed slowly and with many unnecessary trivial details. It is sometimes seen in organic *psychosis, in *schizophrenia, and in people of pedantic and obsessional personality.

cirrhosis *n.* a condition in which the liver responds to injury or death of some of its cells by producing interlacing strands of fibrous tissue between which are nodules of regenerating cells. The liver becomes tawny and characteristically knobbly (due to the nodules). Causes include *alcoholism (*alcoholic cirrhosis*), viral *hepatitis (*postnecrotic cirrhosis*), chronic obstruction of the common bile duct (*secondary biliary cirrhosis*), autoimmune diseases (*chronic aggressive hepatitis, primary biliary cirrhosis*), and chronic heart failure (*cardiac cirrhosis*). In at least half the cases of cirrhosis no cause is found (*cryptogenic cirrhosis*). Complications include *portal hypertension, *ascites, *hepatic encephalopathy, and *hepatoma. Cirrhosis cannot be cured but its progress may be stopped if the cause can be removed. This particularly applies in alcoholism (when all alcohol must be prohibited); in chronic

hepatitis (in which corticosteroid treatment may reduce inflammation); in secondary biliary cirrhosis (in which surgery may relieve obstruction); and in cardiac failure that can be treated. —**cirrhotic** *adj.*

cirs- (cirso-) *prefix denoting* a varicose vein. Example: *cirsectomy* (excision of).

cirsoid *adj.* describing the distended knotted appearance of a varicose vein. The term is used to indicate a type of tumor of the scalp (*cirsoid aneurysm*), which is an arteriovenous aneurysm.

CIS *see* carcinoma in situ.

cisapride *n.* a drug that treats nocturnal *heartburn associated with gastroesophageal reflux by increasing the strength of esophageal contractions and promoting emptying of the stomach. It is administered by mouth. Side effects include headache, diarrhea, and nausea. Trade name: **Propulsid**.

cisplatin *n.* a heavy-metal compound: a *cytotoxic drug that impedes cell division by damaging DNA. Administered intravenously, it is important in the treatment of testicular and ovarian tumors. It is highly toxic; side effects include nausea, vomiting, kidney damage, peripheral neuropathy, and hearing loss. Less toxic analogues of cisplatin are now available. Trade name: **Platinol**.

cisterna *n.* (*pl.* **cisternae**) **1.** one of the enlarged spaces beneath the *arachnoid that act as reservoirs for cerebrospinal fluid. The largest (*cisterna magna*) lies beneath the cerebellum and behind the medulla oblongata. **2.** a dilation at the lower end of the thoracic duct, into which the great lymph ducts of the lower limbs drain.

cistron *n.* the section of a DNA or RNA chain that controls the amino acid sequence of a single polypeptide chain in protein synthesis. A cistron can be regarded as the functional equivalent of a *gene.

citalopram *n.* an antidepressant drug that acts by prolonging the action of the neurotransmitter serotonin (5-hydroxytryptamine) in the brain (*see* SSRI). It is taken by mouth; side effects may include dizziness, agitation, tremor, nausea, diarrhea, and drowsiness. Trade name: **Celexa**.

citric acid an organic acid found naturally in citrus fruits. Citric acid is formed in the first stage of the *Krebs cycle, the important energy-producing cycle in the body.

citric acid cycle *see* Krebs cycle.

Citrobacter *n.* a genus of gram-negative anaerobic rod-shaped bacteria widely distributed in nature. The organisms cause infections of the intestinal and urinary tracts, gallbladder, and the meninges that are usually secondary, occurring in the elderly, newborn, debilitated, and immunocompromised.

citrulline *n.* an *amino acid produced by the liver as a by-product during the conversion of ammonia to *urea.

citrullinemia *n.* an inborn lack of one of the enzymes concerned with the chemical breakdown of proteins to urea: in consequence both the amino acid citrulline and ammonia accumulate in the blood. Affected children fail to thrive and show signs of mental retardation.

CJD *see* Creutzfeldt-Jakob disease.

CK *see* creatine kinase.

cladribine *n.* a drug used in the treatment of hairy cell leukemia. It acts on malignant cells that are resting as well as those that are dividing. Cladribine is administered by intravenous injection for seven days, resulting in complete or partial remission for 8–25 months. Side effects include suppression of bone marrow function, which is reversible and dose-dependent. Trade name: **Leustatin**.

clamp *n.* a surgical instrument designed to compress a structure, such as a blood vessel or a cut end of the intestine (see illustration). A variety of clamps have been designed for specific surgical procedures. Blood vessel clamps are used to stop bleeding from the cut vessels. Intestinal clamps prevent the intestinal

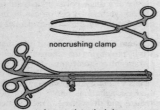

noncrushing clamp

twin gastrointestinal clamp

Intestinal clamps

contents from leaking into the abdominal cavity during operations on the intestines and are designed either not to damage the intestinal wall (noncrushing clamps) or to close the open end (crushing clamps) prior to suturing.

Clark's levels the five vertical levels of skin that are successively penetrated by an invading *melanoma. They are: epidermis, papillary dermis, intervening zone, reticular dermis, and subcutaneous tissue. They usually correlate with *Breslow's measurement. [W. H. Clark (1924–   ), US dermatologist]

clasmatocyte *n. see* macrophage.

clasp *n.* (in dentistry) the part of a *denture that keeps it in place. It is made of flexible metal.

claudication *n.* limping. *Intermittent claudication* is a cramping pain, induced by exercise and relieved by rest, that is caused by an inadequate supply of blood to the affected muscles. It is most often seen in the calf and leg muscles as a result of *atheroma of the leg arteries. The leg pulses are often absent and the feet may be cold. The treatment is that of atheroma.

claustrophobia *n.* a morbid fear of enclosed places. *Compare* agoraphobia. *See also* phobia.

claustrum *n.* a thin vertical layer of gray matter in each cerebral hemisphere, between the surface of the *insula and the lenticular nucleus (*see* basal ganglia).

clavicle *n.* the collar bone: a long slender curved bone, a pair of which form the front part of the shoulder girdle. Each clavicle articulates laterally with the *scapula and medially with the manubrium of the sternum (breastbone). Fracture of the clavicle is a common *sports injury: the majority of cases require no treatment other than supporting the weight of the arm in a sling. —**clavicular** *adj.*

clavulanate potassium a drug that interferes with the *penicillinases that inactivate *beta-lactam antibiotics, such as *amoxicillin or *ticarcillin. Combined with the antibiotic (in *Augmentin* or *Timentin*), clavulanate potassium can overcome drug resistance.

clavus *n.* **1.** *see* corn. **2.** a sharp pain in the head, as if a nail were being driven in.

clawfoot *n.* an excessively arched foot, giving an unnaturally high instep. In most cases the cause is unknown, but the deformity may sometimes be due to an imbalance between the muscles flexing the toes and the shorter muscles that extend them; this type is found in some neuromuscular diseases, such as Friedreich's *ataxia. Surgical treatment is effective in childhood but less so in adult life. Medical name: **pes cavus**.

clawhand *n.* flexion and contraction of the fingers with extension at the joints between the fingers and the hand, giving a clawlike appearance. Any kind of damage to the nerves or muscles may lead to clawhand; causes include injuries, *syringomyelia, and leprosy. *See also* Dupuytren's contracture.

clearance (renal clearance) *n.* a quantitative measure of the rate at which waste products are removed from the blood by the kidneys. It is expressed in terms of the volume of blood that could be completely cleared of a particular substance in one minute.

clearing *n.* (in microscopy) the process of removing the cloudiness from microscopical specimens after *dehydration by means of a *clearing agent*. This increases the transparency of the specimens. Xylene, cedar oil, methyl benzoate plus benzol, and methyl salicylate plus benzol are commonly used as clearing agents.

cleavage *n.* (in embryology) the process of repeated cell division of the fertilized egg to form a ball of cells that becomes the *blastocyst. The cells (*blastomeres*) do not grow between divisions and so they decrease in size.

cleft lip (harelip) the congenital deformity of a cleft in the upper lip, on one or both sides of the midline. It occurs when the three blocks of embryonic tissue that go to form the upper lip fail to fuse and it is often associated with a *cleft palate. Medical name: **cheiloschisis**.

cleft palate a fissure in the midline of the palate due to failure of the two sides to fuse in embryonic development. Only part of the palate may be affected, or the cleft may extend the full length with bilateral clefts at the front of the maxilla; it may be accompanied by a *cleft lip and disturbance of tooth formation. Cleft palates are corrected by surgery.

cleid- (cleido-, clid-, clido-) *prefix denoting*

the clavicle (collar bone). Example: *cleidocranial* (of the clavicle and cranium).

cleidocranial dysostosis a congenital defect of bone formation in which the skull bones ossify imperfectly and the collar bones (clavicles) are absent.

clemastine *n.* an antihistamine used for the treatment of symptoms of hay fever and urticaria. It is administered by mouth; the most common side effects are dizziness, sleepiness, and stomach upset. Trade name: **Tavist**.

client-centered therapy (Rogerian therapy) a method of psychotherapy in which the therapist refrains from directing his client in what he should do and instead concentrates on communicating understanding and acceptance. Frequently, he reflects the client's own words or feelings back to him. The aim is to enable the client to solve his own problems.

climacteric *n.* **1.** *see* menopause. **2.** (**male climacteric**) declining sexual drive and fertility, usually occurring in middle age.

clindamycin *n.* an *antibiotic used to treat serious bacterial infections. It is administered by mouth, injection, or topically; possible side effects are nausea, vomiting, diarrhea, and occasional hypersensitivity reactions. Trade name: **Cleocin**.

clinic *n.* **1.** an establishment or department of a hospital devoted to the treatment of particular diseases or the medical care of outpatients. **2.** a gathering of instructors, students, and patients, usually in a hospital ward, for the examination and treatment of the patients.

clinical audit *see* medical audit.

clinical medicine the branch of medicine dealing with the study of actual patients and the diagnosis and treatment of disease at the bedside, as opposed to the study of disease by pathologic examination or research in basic sciences.

clinodactyly *n.* congenital inward bending of a finger, usually the little finger, or a toe. Clinodactyly may affect both hands or feet and may be found in association with other congenital malformations. No treatment is necessary.

clioquinol *n.* an antibacterial and antifungal agent used as an anti-infective to treat a wide variety of skin infections, such as *eczema, *athlete's foot, *jock itch, and *ringworm. It is administered in ointments, creams, or lotions. Trade name: **Vioform**.

clitoridectomy n. the surgical removal of the clitoris (see [female] circumcision).

clitoris n. the female counterpart of the penis, which contains erectile tissue (see corpus cavernosum) but is not connected with the urethra. Like the penis it becomes erect under conditions of sexual stimulation, to which it is very sensitive.

clitoromegaly n. abnormal development of the clitoris due to excessive exposure to androgens, either from abnormal endogenous production or exogenous administration.

clivus n. (in anatomy) a surface that slopes, such as occurs in part of the sphenoid bone.

CLL chronic lymphocytic leukemia. See leukemia.

cloaca n. the most posterior part of the embryonic *hindgut. It becomes divided into the rectum and the urogenital sinus, which receives the bladder together with the urinary and genital ducts.

clofibrate n. a drug that reduces the levels of blood lipids, including cholesterol, and is used to treat atherosclerosis and angina. It is administered by mouth; side effects can include stomach discomfort, nausea, and diarrhea. Trade names: **Abitrate**, **Atromid-S**.

clomiphene n. a synthetic nonsteroidal compound (see antiestrogen) that induces ovulation and subsequent menstruation in women who fail to ovulate and is used in the treatment of infertility. It is also used to stimulate ovulation (see superovulation) for some procedures of assisted conception (e.g. IVF) and to treat some cases of male infertility. Trade names: **Clomid**, **Milophene**, **Serophene**.

clomipramine n. a drug used to treat various depressive states (see antidepressant). It is administered by mouth or injection; common side effects are dry mouth and blurred vision. Trade name: **Anafranil**.

clonazepam n. a drug with *anticonvulsant properties, used to treat epilepsy and other conditions involving seizures. It is administered by mouth or injection; drowsiness is a common side effect. Trade name: **Klonopin**.

clone 1. n. a group of cells (usually bacteria) descended from a single cell by asexual reproduction and therefore genetically identical to each other and to the parent cell. **2.** n. an organism derived from a single cell of its parent and therefore genetically identical to it. The first cloned animal, born in 1997, was produced by fusing a somatic cell of the parent with a denucleated egg cell of a second animal. The resulting "embryo" was implanted into the uterus of a third animal to complete its development. **3.** n. (**gene clone**) a group of identical genes produced by techniques of *genetic engineering. The parent gene is isolated using *restriction enzymes and inserted, via a *cloning vector* (e.g. a bacteriophage), into a bacterium, in which it is replicated. See also vector. **4.** vb. to form a clone.

clonic adj. of, relating to, or resembling clonus. The term is most commonly used to describe the rhythmical limb movements seen as part of a convulsive epileptic seizure (see epilepsy).

clonidine n. a drug that acts on receptors in the brain and is used to treat high blood pressure (hypertension) and migraine. It is administered by mouth or injection and commonly causes drowsiness and dry mouth. Trade name: **Catapres**.

clonogenic adj. describing a cell capable of producing a colony of cells of a predetermined minimum size. Such a cell is known as a *colony forming unit* (*CFU*).

clonorchiasis n. a condition caused by the presence of the fluke *Clonorchis sinensis* in the bile ducts. The infection, common in the Far East, is acquired through eating undercooked, salted, or pickled freshwater fish harboring the larval stage of the parasite. Symptoms include fever, abdominal pain, diarrhea, liver enlargement, loss of appetite, emaciation, and – in advanced cases – cirrhosis and jaundice. Treatment is unsatisfactory although *praziquantel and *chloroquine phosphate have proved beneficial in some cases.

Clonorchis n. a genus of liver flukes, common parasites of humans and other fish-eating mammals in the Far East. The adults of *C. sinensis* cause *clonorchiasis. Eggs are passed out through the stools and the larvae undergo their development in two other hosts, a snail and a fish.

clonus n. rhythmical contraction of a muscle in response to a suddenly applied and then sustained stretch stimulus. It is most readily obtained at the ankle when the examiner bends the foot sharply upward and then maintains an upward pressure on the sole. It is caused by an exaggeration of the stretch reflexes and is usually a sign of disease in the brain or spinal cord.

clopidogrel n. a drug that reduces platelet aggregation. It is administered by mouth to prevent strokes or heart attacks in those at risk. Side effects may include gastrointestinal bleeding. Trade name: **Plavix**.

clorazepate dipotassium a *benzodiazepine drug used to relieve anxiety, tension, and agitation. It is administered by mouth; side effects can include dizziness, digestive upsets, blurred vision, and, occasionally, drowsiness. Trade name: **Tranxene**.

closed panel practice a type of medical practice in which the physician limits the patients he will care for to those who are members of a prepayment group. A closed panel practice is usually associated with HMOs or similar group practices in which patients agree to pay a fixed monthly or annual fee to the doctors, who in turn provide a wide range of medical care services for the patients included in the panel.

closed staff a hospital medical staff that limits hospital privileges, including admissions and care of patients, to doctors who are accepted as members of staff. Membership, which may be renewed periodically, is granted by a hospital Board of Trustees on the recommendation of a credentials committee. The applicant for closed staff membership usually must agree to contribute a share of his or her time to certain professional medical duties associated with hospital functions, such as supervising interns or residents.

Clostridium n. a genus of mostly gram-positive anaerobic spore-forming rodlike bacteria commonly found in soil and in the intestinal tract of humans and animals. Many species cause disease and produce extremely potent *exotoxins. *C. botulinum* grows freely in badly preserved canned foods, producing a toxin causing serious food poisoning (*botulism); an extremely dilute form of this toxin is now used to treat muscle spasm

(*see* botulinum toxin). *C. histolyticum*, *C. oedematiens*, and *C. septicum* all cause *gas gangrene when they infect wounds. *C. tetani* lives as a harmless *commensal in the intestine but causes *tetanus on contamination of wounds (with manured soil). The species *C. perfringens* – Welch's bacillus – causes blood poisoning, *food poisoning, and gas gangrene. Overgrowth of *C. difficile*, a normal inhabitant of the human large intestine, is a common complication of some antibiotic therapy and produces a specific condition – *pseudomembranous colitis* – which is life-threatening unless treated promptly.

clotrimazole n. an antiseptic used to treat all types of fungal skin infections, including ringworm and infections of the genital organs. It is applied to the infected part as a cream or solution or as vaginal pessaries and may occasionally cause mild burning or irritation. Trade names: **Femcare**, **Gyne-Lotrimin**, **Lotrimin**, **Mycelex**.

clotting factors *see* coagulation factors.

clotting time *see* coagulation time.

cloxacillin sodium an antibiotic, derived from penicillin, that is used to treat many bacterial infections. It is administered by mouth or injection; diarrhea sometimes occurs and hypersensitivity reactions occur in penicillin-sensitive patients. Trade names: **Cloxapen**, **Tegopen**.

clozapine n. an atypical *antipsychotic drug used in the treatment of schizophrenia and other disorders in patients who are unresponsive to conventional antipsychotics. Administered by mouth, it is notable for the absence of tremors and repetitive movements that are associated with other antipsychotic drugs. Side effects include dizziness, headache, and increased salivation, and in a small proportion of cases the drug may depress levels of white blood cells. Trade name: **Clozaril**.

clubbing n. thickening of the tissues at the bases of the finger- and toenails so that the normal angle between the nail and the digit is filled in. The nail becomes convex in all directions and in extreme cases the digit end becomes bulbous like a club or drumstick. Clubbing is seen in pulmonary tuberculosis, bronchiectasis, empyema, infective endocarditis, cyanotic congenital heart disease, and lung cancer and as a harmless congenital abnormality.

clubfoot (talipes) *n.* a congenital deformity of one or both feet in which the patient cannot stand with the sole of the foot flat on the ground. In the most common variety (*talipes equinovarus*) the foot points downward, the heel is inverted, and the forefoot twisted. It is diagnosed at birth and may be associated with other congenital abnormalities. Treatment is initially by physiotherapy and strapping or a plaster cast, but if this fails to correct the deformity surgical correction is performed. Other varieties are *talipes varus*, inward deviation of the hind foot; and *talipes valgus*, an outward deviation of the hind foot, which is much less common.

clumping *n. see* agglutination.

cluster headache a variant of *migraine more common in men than in women (ratio 9:1). The unilateral pain around one eye is very severe and lasts between 15 minutes and three hours. The attacks commonly occur in the early hours of the morning but may occur eight times a day. The pain is associated with drooping of the eyelid (*ptosis), a bloodshot eye, and/or excessive production of tears in the eye. The acute treatment is with antimigraine drugs (5HT₁ agonists) and prophylaxis is with such drugs as verapamil, lithium, or methysergide.

cluttering *n.* an erratic unrhythmical way of speaking in rapid jerky bursts. It can make speech hard to understand, and speech therapy is usually helpful. Unlike *stammering, there are no repetitions or prolonged hesitations of speech.

Clutton's joint a painless joint effusion in a child, usually in the knee, caused by inflammation of the synovial membranes due to congenital syphilis. [H. H. Clutton (1850–1909), British surgeon]

clyster *n.* an old-fashioned term for an *enema.

CMF cyclophosphamide, methotrexate, 5-fluorouracil: the combination of drugs used in standard chemotherapy for cancer, particularly in *adjuvant therapy.

CMV *see* cytomegalovirus.

CNS *see* central nervous system.

coagulant *n.* any substance capable of converting blood from a liquid to a solid state. *See* blood coagulation.

coagulase *n.* an enzyme, formed by the disease-producing varieties of certain bacteria of the genus *Staphylococcus*, that causes blood plasma to coagulate. Staphylococci that are positive when tested for coagulase production are classified as belonging to the species *Staphylococcus aureus*.

coagulation *n.* the process by which a colloidal liquid changes to a jellylike mass. *See* blood coagulation.

coagulation factors (clotting factors) a group of substances present in blood plasma that, under certain circumstances, undergo a series of chemical reactions leading to the conversion of blood from a liquid to a solid state (*see* blood coagulation). Although they have specific names, most coagulation factors are referred to by an agreed set of Roman numerals (e.g. *Factor VIII, *Factor IX). Lack of any of these factors in the blood results in the inability of the blood to clot. *See also* Christmas disease, hemophilia.

coagulation time (clotting time) the time taken for blood or blood plasma to coagulate (*see* blood coagulation). When measured under controlled conditions and using appropriate techniques, coagulation times may be used to test the function of the various stages of the blood coagulation process.

coagulum *n.* a mass of coagulated matter, such as that formed when blood clots.

coalesce *vb.* to grow together or unite. —**coalescence** *n.*

coal worker's pneumoconiosis *see* anthracosis.

coarctation *n.* (of the aorta) a congenital narrowing of a short segment of the aorta. The most common site of coarctation is just beyond the origin of the left subclavian artery from the aorta. This results in high blood pressure (*hypertension) in the upper part of the body and arms and low blood pressure in the legs. The defect is corrected surgically.

Coats' disease a congenital anomaly of the blood vessels of the retina, which are abnormally dilated and leaking. This results in subretinal hemorrhage and massive exudation. [G. Coats (1876–1915), British ophthalmologist]

cobalamin *n. see* vitamin B₁₂.

cobalt *n.* a metallic element. The artificial radioisotope *cobalt-60*, or *radiocobalt*, is a powerful emitter of gamma radiation and is used in the radiation treatment of cancer (*see* radiotherapy, teletherapy). Cobalt itself forms part of the *vitamin B_{12} molecule. Symbol: Co.

cobalt-chromium *n.* a silver-colored nonprecious alloy of cobalt and chromium used for the metal frame of partial *dentures.

cocaine *n.* an alkaloid, derived from the leaves of the coca plant (*Erythroxylon coca*) or prepared synthetically, sometimes used as a local anesthetic in eye, ear, nose, and throat surgery. It constricts the small blood vessels at the site of application and therefore need not be given with *epinephrine. Since it causes feelings of exhilaration and may lead to psychological *dependence, cocaine has largely been replaced by safer anesthetics.

cocainism *n.* **1.** the habitual use of, or addiction to, *cocaine in order to experience its intoxicating effects. **2.** the mental and physical deterioration resulting from addiction to cocaine.

cocarcinogen *n.* a substance that enhances the effect of a *carcinogen.

coccidioidomycosis *n.* an infection caused by inhaling the spores of the fungus *Coccidioides immitis*. In the primary form there is an influenza-like illness that usually resolves within about eight weeks. In a few patients the disease becomes progressive and resembles tuberculosis. Severe or progressive infections are treated with intravenous injections of amphotericin B. The disease is endemic only in the southwestern US, northwestern Mexico, and parts of Central and South America.

coccobacillus *n.* a rod-shaped bacterium (bacillus) that is so small that it resembles a spherical bacterium (coccus). Examples of such bacteria are *Bacteroides* and *Brucella*.

coccus *n.* (*pl.* **cocci**) any spherical bacterium. *See also* gonococcus, meningococcus, Micrococcus, pneumococcus, Staphylococcus, Streptococcus.

cocci- (coccyg-, coccygo-) *prefix denoting* the coccyx. Example: *coccygectomy* (excision of).

coccygodynia *n.* pain in the lowermost segment of the spine (coccyx) and the neighboring area.

coccyx *n.* (*pl.* **coccyges** or **coccyxes**) the lowermost element of the *backbone:

the vestigial human tail. It consists of four rudimentary *coccygeal vertebrae* fused to form a triangular bone that articulates with the sacrum. *See also* vertebra. —**coccygeal** *adj.*

cochlea *n.* the spiral organ of the *labyrinth of the ear, which is concerned with the reception and analysis of sound. As vibrations pass from the middle ear through the cochlea, different frequencies cause particular regions of the basilar membrane to vibrate: high notes cause vibration in the region nearest the middle ear; low notes cause vibration in the region nearest the tip of the spiral. The *organ of Corti*, which lies within a central triangular membrane-bound canal (*scala media* or *cochlear duct*), contains sensory hair cells attached to an overlying *tectorial membrane* (see illustration). When the basilar membrane vibrates the sensory cells become distorted and send nerve impulses to the brain via the *cochlear nerve. —**cochlear** *adj.*

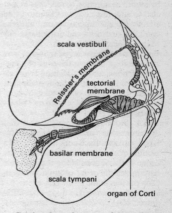

Section through a turn of the cochlea

cochlear duct (scala media) *see* cochlea.

cochlear implant a device to improve the hearing of profoundly deaf people who can derive no benefit from conventional *hearing aids. It consists of an electrode that is permanently implanted into the inner ear (*cochlea). An external device with a microphone and an electronic processing unit passes information to the electrode using radiofrequency waves. The implant is powered by batteries in the external part of the device.

cochlear nerve the nerve connecting the cochlea to the brain and therefore responsible for the nerve impulses relating to hearing. It forms part of the *vestibulocochlear nerve (cranial nerve VIII).

Cockayne's syndrome a hereditary disorder (inherited as an autosomal *recessive condition) associated with *trisomy of chromosome no. 20. Clinical features include *epidermolysis bullosa, dwarfism, mental retardation, and pigmentary degeneration of the retina. [E. A. Cockayne (1880–1956), British physician]

code n. (in hospitals) a discreet signal or announcement that is given over a public address system to call a special team to resuscitate a patient. See also DNR.

codeine n. an *analgesic derived from morphine but less potent as a painkiller and sedative and less toxic. It is administered by mouth or injection to relieve pain and also to suppress coughs. Common side effects include constipation, nausea, vomiting, dizziness, and drowsiness, but *dependence is uncommon.

Codman's triangle a triangular area of new bone seen on X-ray at the edge of a malignant bone tumor resulting from elevation of the *periosteum by malignant tissue. It is most often seen in *osteosarcomas. [E. A. Codman (1869–1940), US surgeon]

codon n. the unit of the *genetic code that determines the synthesis of one particular amino acid. Each codon consists of a section of the DNA molecule, and the order of the codons along the molecule determines the order of amino acids in each protein made in the cell.

-coele suffix denoting **1.** a body cavity. Example: blastocoele (cavity of blastocyst). **2.** see -cele.

coelom n. the cavity in an embryo between the two layers of mesoderm. It develops into the body cavity.

coenzyme n. a nonprotein organic compound that, in the presence of an *enzyme, plays an essential role in the reaction that is catalyzed by the enzyme. Coenzymes, which frequently contain the B vitamins in their molecular structure, include *coenzyme A, *FAD, and *NAD.

coenzyme A (CoA) a *nucleotide containing pantothenic acid, which is an important coenzyme in the Krebs cycle and in the metabolism of fatty acids. See also hydroxymethylglutaryl coenzyme A reductase.

cofactor n. a nonprotein substance that must be present in suitable amounts before certain *enzymes can act. Cofactors include *coenzymes and metal ions (e.g. sodium and potassium ions).

Cogan's syndrome a disorder in which *keratitis and iridocyclitis (see uveitis) are associated with tinnitus, vertigo, and bilateral sensorineural deafness. [D. G. Cogan (1908–93), US ophthalmologist]

cognition n. the mental processes by which knowledge is acquired. These include perception, reasoning, acts of creativity, problem-solving, and possibly intuition. Compare conation.

cognitive psychology the branch of psychology concerned with all human activities relating to knowledge. More specifically, cognitive psychology is concerned with how knowledge is acquired, stored, correlated, and retrieved, by studying the mental processes underlying attention, concept formation, information processing, memory, and speech (psycholinguistics). Cognitive psychology views the brain as an information-processing system operating on, and storing, the data acquired by the senses. It investigates this function by experiments designed to measure and analyze human performance in carrying out a wide range of mental tasks. The data obtained allows possible models of the underlying mental processes to be constructed. These models do not purport to represent the actual physiological activity of the brain. Nevertheless, as they are refined by testing and criticism, it is hoped that they may approach close to reality and gradually lead to a clearer understanding of how the brain operates.

cognitive therapy a form of *psychotherapy based on the belief that psychological problems are the products of faulty ways of thinking about the world. For example, a depressed patient may have come to see him- or herself as powerless to change in any way. The therapist assists the patient to identify these false ways of thinking and to avoid them.

cohort study (longitudinal study) a systematic study of a group of people, which may be conducted prospectively or retrospectively. A *prospective cohort study* involves a systematic follow-up for a defined period of time or until the occurrence of a specified event (e.g. onset of illness, retirement, or death) in order to observe their pattern of disease and/or cause of death. For a *retrospective cohort study*, data on the group's exposure and disease experience are already known.

coinsurance a common form of private medical insurance policy in which the patient or other beneficiary of the policy shares the costs of treatment for injury or disease with the insurance company. A typical coinsurance policy might stipulate that the insurance company would pay 80% of the patient's claim for medical expenses with the patient paying the remaining 20%.

coitus (sexual intercourse, copulation) *n.* sexual contact between a man and a woman during which the erect penis enters the vagina and is moved within it by pelvic thrusts until *ejaculation occurs. *See also* orgasm. —**coital** *adj.*

coitus interruptus a contraceptive method in which the penis is removed from the vagina before ejaculation of semen (orgasm). The method is unreliable (10–20 pregnancies per 100 woman-years) and it may lead to sexual disharmony and anxiety in one or both partners.

col- (coli-, colo-) *prefix denoting* the colon. Example: *coloptosis* (prolapse of).

colchicine *n.* a drug obtained from the meadow saffron (*Colchicum autumnale*), used to relieve pain in attacks of gout. It is administered by mouth or injection; common side effects are nausea, vomiting, diarrhea, and stomach pains.

cold (common cold) *n.* a widespread infectious virus disease causing inflammation of the mucous membranes of the nose, throat, and bronchial tubes. The disease is transmitted by coughing and sneezing. Symptoms commence 1–2 days after infection and include a sore throat, stuffy or runny nose, headache, cough, and general malaise. The disease is mild and lasts only about a week but it can prove serious to young babies and to patients with a preexisting respiratory complaint.

cold sore (herpes simplex) *see* herpes.

colectomy *n.* surgical removal of the colon. *Total colectomy* is the removal of the whole colon, usually for extensive *colitis; *partial colectomy* is the removal of a segment of the colon. *See also* hemicolectomy, proctocolectomy.

colestipol *n.* a *bile-acid sequestrant used, in conjunction with dietary reduction of cholesterol, to lower *cholesterol levels in the blood in patients with hyperlipidemia and primary hypercholesterolemia. It is administered by mouth; side effects include headache, constipation, and abdominal discomfort. Trade name: **Colestid**.

colic *n.* severe abdominal pain, usually of fluctuating severity, with waves of pain seconds or a few minutes apart. *Infantile colic* is common among babies, due to gas in the intestine associated with feeding difficulties. *Intestinal colic* is due to partial or complete obstruction of the intestine or to constipation. Colic arising from the small intestine is felt in the upper abdomen; colic from the colon is felt in the lower abdomen. Medical names: **enteralgia, tormina**. *See also* biliary colic.

coliform bacteria a group of gram-negative rodlike bacteria that are normally found in the gastrointestinal tract and have the ability to ferment the sugar lactose. The group includes the genera *Enterobacter*, *Escherichia*, and *Klebsiella*.

colistin sulfate an *antibiotic used in the treatment of various gastrointestinal, urinary tract, ophthalmic, and otic infections caused by gram-negative bacteria. Colistin sulfate is derived from a strain of the bacterium *Bacillus polymyxa*. It is administered orally, topically, or by injection. Trade name: **Coly-Mycin S Otic**.

colitis *n.* inflammation of the colon. The usual symptoms are diarrhea, sometimes with blood and mucus, and lower abdominal pain. It is diagnosed by demonstrating inflammation of the colon's lining (mucosa) by *sigmoidoscopy or *barium enema X-ray. Colitis may be due to infection by *Entamoeba histolytica* (*amebic colitis*) or by bacteria (*infective colitis*); it may also occur in *Crohn's disease (*Crohn's colitis*). Partial or temporary cessation of blood supply to the colon may cause *ischemic colitis*. *Ulcerative colitis* (*idiopathic proctocolitis*) almost always involves the rectum (*see* proctitis) as well as a varying amount of the colon, which become inflamed and ulcerated. Its cause is unknown. It varies in severity from month to month, relapses being treated by drugs, including corticosteroids and *sulfasalazine, and bed rest. Severe, continuous, or extensive colitis may be treated by surgery (*see* colectomy, proctocolectomy). Diarrhea or pain when inflammation is absent is often due to *irritable bowel syndrome.

collagen *n.* a protein that is the principal constituent of white fibrous connective tissue (as occurs in tendons). Collagen is also found in skin, bone, cartilage, and ligaments. It is relatively inelastic but has a high tensile strength.

collagen disease *see* connective tissue disease.

collapsing pulse *see* Corrigan's pulse.

collar bone *see* clavicle.

collateral 1. *adj.* accessory or secondary. **2.** *n.* a branch (e.g. of a nerve fiber) that is at right angles to the main part.

collateral circulation 1. an alternative route provided for the blood by secondary vessels when a primary vessel becomes blocked. **2.** the channels of communication between the blood vessels supplying the heart. At the apex of the heart, where the coronary arteries form *anastomoses, these are very complex.

Colles' fracture a fracture just above the wrist, across the lower end of the *radius, usually caused by a fall on the outstretched hand. The hand and wrist below the fracture are displaced backward. The bone is restored to its normal position under anesthesia, and a plaster cast is applied. The fracture usually unites within six weeks. Complications are residual deformity resulting from *malunion and stiffness of the wrist. [A. Colles (1773–1843), Irish surgeon]

colliculus *n.* (*pl.* **colliculi**) a small protuberance or swelling. Two pairs of colliculi, the *superior* and *inferior colliculi*, protrude from the roof of the midbrain (*see* tectum).

collimator *n.* a device used in diagnostic radiology or radiotherapy to produce a narrow beam of radiation by means of metallic slits that control the size of the beam from a radiation source. Many new *linear accelerators use a *multi-leaf*

collimator, a specialized form of collimator using individual "leaves" (1 cm or smaller) to shape the radiation *treatment field around the tumor. Collimators are also used on radiation detectors, in particular in *gamma cameras, for which the exact source of radioactivity needs to be known to produce an accurate image.

collodion *n.* a syrupy solution of nitrocellulose in a mixture of alcohol and ether. When applied to the surface of the body, it evaporates to leave a thin clear transparent film, useful for the protection of minor wounds. Flexible collodion also contains camphor and castor oil, which allow the skin to stretch a little more.

colloidian baby the distinctive appearance of a newborn baby that is covered in a shiny membrane, resembling a sausage skin. Although the baby is occasionally normal it is more likely that it will suffer from chronic skin disorders, such as *ichthyosis.

collyrium *n.* a medicated solution used to bathe the eyes.

coloboma *n.* a defect in the development of the eye causing abnormalities ranging in severity from a notch in the lower part of the iris, making it pear-shaped, to defects behind the iris in the *fundus. The enlarged pupil causes dazzle symptoms. A coloboma of the eyelid is a congenital notch in the lid margin.

colon *n.* the main part of the large intestine, which consists of four sections – the *ascending*, *transverse*, *descending*, and *sigmoid colons* (see illustration). The colon has no digestive function but it absorbs large amounts of water and electrolytes from the undigested food passed on from the small intestine. At intervals strong peristaltic movements move the dehydrated contents (feces) toward the rectum. —**colonic** *adj.*

colonic irrigation washing out the contents of the large bowel by means of copious enemas, using either water, with or without soap, or other medication.

colonoscopy *n.* a procedure for examining the interior of the entire colon and rectum using a flexible illuminated *fiberscope (*colonoscope*) introduced through the anus and guided up the colon by a combination of visual and X-ray control. It is possible to obtain specimens for microscopic examination using flex-

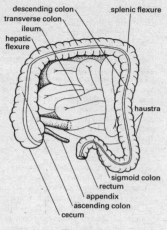

The colon

ible forceps passed through the colonoscope and to remove polyps using a *diathermy snare.

colony *n.* a discrete population or mass of microorganisms, usually bacteria, all of which are considered to have developed from a single parent cell. Bacterial colonies that grow on agar plates differ in shape, size, color, elevation, translucency, and surface texture, depending on the species. This is used as a means of identification. *See also* culture.

colony-stimulating factor (CSF) one of a group of substances produced in the bone marrow that stimulates the production of specific blood cells. Genetically engineered granulocyte-colony stimulating factor (G-CSF) stimulates neutrophil production and also limits bone marrow toxicity from chemotherapy.

color blindness any of various conditions in which certain colors are confused with one another. True lack of color appreciation is extremely rare (*see* monochromat), but some defect of color discrimination is present in about 8% of Caucasian males, and 0.4% of Caucasian females. The most common type of color blindness is *Daltonism* (*protanopia*) – red-blindness – in which the person cannot distinguish between reds and greens.

Occasional cases are due to acquired disease of the retina but in the vast majority it is inherited. The defect is thought to be in the functioning of the light-sensitive cells in the retina responsible for color perception (*see* cone). *See also* deuteranopia, trichromatic.

color flow ultrasound imaging *see* Doppler ultrasonography.

colorimeter *n.* an instrument for determining the concentration of a particular compound in a preparation by comparing the intensity of color in it with that in a standard preparation of known concentration. The instrument is used particularly for measuring the amount of hemoglobin in the blood.

colostomy *n.* a surgical operation in which a part of the colon is brought through the abdominal wall in order to drain or decompress the intestine. The part of the colon chosen depends on the site of obstruction. An *iliac colostomy* opens onto the left lower abdomen; a *transverse colostomy* on the upper abdomen. The colostomy may be temporary, eventually being closed after weeks or months to restore continuity; or permanent, usually when the rectum or lower colon has been removed. An appliance is usually worn over the colostomy opening (*stoma) to prevent soiling the clothes.

colostrum *n.* the first secretion from the breast, occurring shortly after, or sometimes before, birth, before the formation of true milk is established. It is a relatively clear fluid containing serum, white blood cells, and protective antibodies.

colp- (colpo-) *prefix denoting* the vagina. Example: *colpoplasty* (plastic surgery of).

colpoperineorrhaphy (colpoperineoplasty) *n.* an operation for repairing tears in the vagina and the muscles surrounding its opening, particularly posteriorly.

colporrhaphy *n.* an operation to remove lax and redundant vaginal tissue and so reduce the diameter of the vagina in cases of prolapse of the anterior vaginal wall (*anterior colporrhaphy*) or posterior vaginal wall (*posterior colporrhaphy*).

colposcope (vaginoscope) *n.* an instrument that is inserted into the vagina and permits visual examination of the cervix and the upper part of the vagina in which it lies. It is used in the diagnosis of premalignant and early malignant changes in the cervix. —**colposcopy** *n.*

colposuspension *n.* a surgical operation in which the upper part of the vaginal wall is fixed to the anterior abdominal wall by nonabsorbable suture material. Performed through an abdominal incision, it is used in the surgical treatment of prolapse of the vaginal wall, particularly when stress incontinence exists. *See also* Stamey procedure.

colpotomy *n.* an incision made into the wall of the vagina, usually the posterior wall, close to the cervix (*posterior colpotomy*). This was formerly used to confirm the diagnosis of ectopic pregnancy but has now been replaced by *laparoscopy. Colpotomy is sometimes referred to as *culdocentesis.*

columella *n.* (in anatomy) a part resembling a small column. For example, the *columella cochleae* (*modiolus*) is the central pillar of the cochlea, around which the spiral cochlear canal winds. The *columella nasi* is the anterior part of the nasal septum.

column *n.* (in anatomy) any pillar-shaped structure, especially any of the tracts of gray matter found in the spinal cord.

coma *n.* a state of unrousable unconsciousness. Its severity is sometimes graded according to the presence or absence of withdrawal responses to painful stimuli and pupillary and corneal reflexes. *See also* Glasgow Coma Scale.

combined agency a medical facility that may be staffed jointly by representatives of a voluntary health agency and a government agency. A combined agency might provide nursing services contributed by a city health department and a local Visiting Nurses Association.

combined therapy therapy that combines several types of treatment in order to improve results. It is usually a combination of surgery with radiotherapy and/or chemotherapy for the treatment of malignant tumors (*see* adjuvant therapy). *See also* sandwich therapy.

comedo *n.* (*pl.* **comedones**) *see* blackhead.

commando operation a major operation performed to remove a malignant tumor from the head and neck. Extensive dissection, often involving the face, is followed by reconstruction to restore function and cosmetic acceptability.

commensal *n.* an organism that lives in close association with another of a different species without either harming or benefiting it. For example, some microorganisms living in the gut obtain both food and a suitable habitat but neither harm nor benefit humans. *Compare* symbiosis. —**commensalism** *n.*

comminuted fracture a fracture in which the bone is broken into more than two pieces. A crushing force is usually responsible and there is often extensive injury to surrounding soft tissues.

commissure *n.* **1.** a bundle of nerve fibers that crosses the midline of the central nervous system, often connecting similar structures on each side. **2.** any other tissue connecting two similar structures.

commotio *n.* *concussion or violent shock. *Commotio retinae* is swelling of the retina associated with sudden reduction of vision, usually resulting from blunt trauma to the eye. *Commotio cerebri* is concussion of the brain and *commotio spinalis* is concussion of the spinal cord.

communicable disease (contagious disease, infectious disease) any disease that can be transmitted from one person to another. This may occur by direct physical contact, by common handling of an object that has picked up infective microorganisms (*see* fomes), through a disease *carrier, or by spread of infected droplets coughed or exhaled into the air. The most dangerous communicable diseases are on the list of *notifiable diseases. *See also* Centers for Disease Control and Prevention.

communicans *adj.* communicating or connecting. The term is applied particularly to blood vessels or nerve fibers connecting two similar structures.

Community Action Programs programs authorized by the Economic Opportunity Act (1964) to provide federal financial assistance for such health-related activities as Neighborhood Health Centers, family planning, and drug rehabilitation. The programs are supervised by the *Public Health Service.

community medicine the branch of medicine concerned with assessing needs and trends in health and disease of populations as distinct from individuals. Formerly known as *social medicine*, it includes *epidemiology, public health, *preventive medicine, health care planning, and evaluation of services.

Community Mental Health Centers facilities providing services for the diagnosis, treatment, and care of mentally ill persons who reside in or near the community where the facility is located. The original legislation leading to the development of community mental health centers was passed by the US Congress in 1946; since then it has been amended many times to broaden the services provided. Amendments extend coverage to include services for mentally retarded and handicapped children, for those who abuse drugs (including alcoholics), and for people living in poverty areas.

comorbidity *n.* the simultaneous occurrence of two or more unrelated diseases or conditions in a patient or given population. —**comorbid** *adj.*

comparative mortality figure *see* occupational mortality.

compartment *n.* (in anatomy) any one of the spaces in a limb that are bounded by bone and thick sheets of fascia and enclose the muscles and other tissues of the limb.

compartmental syndrome the condition that results from swelling of the muscles in a *compartment of a limb, which raises the pressure within the compartment so that the blood supply to the muscle is cut off, causing *ischemia and further swelling. If it persists, the muscles and nerves within the compartment die, leading to *Volkmann's contracture. Causes are trauma, damage to blood vessels, reperfusion after ischemia, and tight casts or bandages. Treatment is to release any tight dressings and to divide the fascia surrounding the compartment to relieve the pressure.

compatibility *n.* the degree to which the body's defense systems will tolerate the presence of intruding foreign material, such as blood when transfused or a kidney when transplanted. Complete compatibility exists between identical twins: a blood transfusion between identical twins will evoke no *antibody formation in the recipient. In severe *incompatibility*, for example between completely unrelated people, there are likely to be swift immune reactions as antibodies attack and destroy any offending antigenic material. *See also* histocompatibility, immunity. —**compatible** *adj.*

compensation *n.* the act of making up for a functional or structural deficiency. For example, compensation for the loss of a diseased kidney is brought about by an increase in size of the remaining kidney, so restoring the urine-producing capacity.

compensation neurosis a fixed preoccupation with real or imaginary disability or injury, when there is a possibility of financial compensation. The condition tends to deprive the affected person of the motive to overcome the alleged disability and to acknowledge the natural processes of recovery. Uncompensated disability often persists for many years, but the disorder often clears up soon after a satisfactory settlement.

complement *n.* a system of functionally linked proteins that interact with one another to aid the body's defenses when *antibodies combine with *antigens. Complement is involved in the breaking-up (*lysis) and *opsonization of foreign organisms. It is also involved in inflammation and clearing immune (antigen-antibody) complexes. *See also* immunity, phagocytosis.

complementary medicine various forms of therapy that are viewed as complementary to conventional medicine. These include (but are not limited to) *osteopathy, *acupuncture, *homeopathy, *biofeedback, *massage, *reflexology, and *reiki. Previously, such therapies were regarded as an alternative to conventional therapies, and the two types were considered to be mutually exclusive (hence the former names *alternative medicine* and *fringe medicine*). However, many practitioners now have dual training in conventional and complementary therapies.

complement fixation the binding of *complement to the complex that is formed when an antibody reacts with a specific antigen. Because complement is taken up from the serum only when such a reaction has occurred, testing for the presence of complement after mixing a suspension of a known organism with a patient's serum can give confirmation of infection with a suspected organism. The *Wassermann reaction for diagnosis of syphilis is a complement-fixation test.

complex *n.* (in psychoanalysis) an emotionally charged and repressed group of ideas and beliefs that is capable of influencing the behavior of an individual. The term in this sense was originally used by Jung, but it is now widely used in a looser sense to denote an unconscious motive.

complication *n.* a disease or condition arising during the course of or as a consequence of another disease.

composite resin a tooth-colored filling material for teeth. It is composed of two different materials: an inorganic filler chemically held in an organic resin. Composite resins are usually hardened by polymerization initiated by intense light.

compound 1. *n.* (in chemistry and pharmacy) any substance composed of two or more different elements or ingredients. **2.** *adj.* indicating an injury or condition characterized by multiple factors, such as a compound *fracture.

compress *n.* a pad of material soaked in hot or cold water and applied to an injured part of the body to relieve the pain of inflammation.

compressed air illness (caisson disease) a syndrome occurring in people working under high pressure in diving bells or at great depths with breathing apparatus. On return to normal atmospheric pressure nitrogen dissolved in the bloodstream expands to form bubbles, causing pain (the *bends*) and blocking the circulation in small blood vessels in the brain and elsewhere (*decompression sickness*). Pain, paralysis, and other features may be eliminated by returning the patient to a higher atmospheric pressure and reducing this gradually, so causing the bubbles to redissolve. Chronic compressed air illness may cause damage to the bones (*avascular necrosis*), heart, and lungs.

compression syndrome *see* crush syndrome.

compression venography an *ultrasound technique used to look for blockages in leg veins, usually deep vein *thrombosis. Pressing the vein with the ultrasound probe usually causes it to empty and flatten, which does not occur if there is a thrombus in the lumen. *See also* venography.

compulsion *n.* an *obsession that takes the form of a motor act, such as repetitive washing based on a fear of contamination.

computed tomography (CT) a form of X-ray examination in which the X-ray source and detector (*CT scanner*) rotate around the object to be scanned and the information obtained can be used to produce cross-sectional images (*see* cross-sectional imaging) by computer (a *CT scan*). A higher radiation dose is received by the patient than with some conventional X-ray techniques, but the diagnostic information obtained is far greater and should outweigh the risk. CT scanning can be used for all parts of the body, but is particularly useful in the head, chest, and abdomen. The data obtained can be used to construct three-dimensional images of structures of interest. *See also* multislice CT scanning, spiral CT scanning, tomography. *Compare* positron emission tomography (PET).

computerized radiography (CR) a system for replacing photographic film with a charged plate. Exposure to X-rays knocks charge off the plate. The resultant image can be read by a laser beam and stored digitally or printed out as required. This system is widely used in conjunction with *PACS systems.

conation *n.* the group of mental activities (including drives, will, and *instincts) that leads to purposeful action. *Compare* cognition.

conception *n.* **1.** (in gynecology) the start of pregnancy, when a male germ cell (sperm) fertilizes a female germ cell (ovum) in the *fallopian tube. **2.** (in psychology) an idea or mental impression.

conceptus *n.* the products of conception: the developing fetus and its enclosing membrane at all stages in the uterus.

concha *n.* (*pl.* **conchae**) (in anatomy) any part resembling a shell. For example, the *concha auriculae* is a depression on the outer surface of the pinna (auricle), which leads to the external auditory meatus of the outer ear. *See also* nasal concha.

concordance *n.* similarity of any physical characteristic that is found in both of a pair of twins.

concretion *n.* a stony mass formed within such an organ as the kidney, especially the coating of an internal organ (or a foreign body, such as a urinary catheter) with calcium salts. *See also* calculus.

concussion *n.* a condition caused by injury to the head, characterized by headache, confusion, and amnesia. These symptoms may be prolonged and constitute a *post-concussional syndrome*. There may be no recognizable structural damage to the brain, but scans may reveal evidence of *contusion (bruising) within the brain. Repeated concussion eventually causes symptoms suggesting brain damage. Medical name: **commotio cerebri**. *See also* punch-drunk syndrome.

condenser *n.* (in microscopy) an arrangement of lenses beneath the stage of a microscope. It can be adjusted to provide correct focusing of light on the microscope slide.

conditioned reflex a reflex in which the response occurs not to the sensory stimulus that normally causes it but to a separate stimulus, which has been learned to be associated with it. In Pavlov's classic experiments, dogs learned to associate the sound of a bell with feeding time and would salivate at the bell's sound whether food was then presented to them or not.

conditioning *n.* the establishment of new behavior by modifying the stimulus/response associations. In *classic conditioning* a stimulus not normally associated with a particular response is presented together with the stimulus that evokes the response automatically. This is repeated until the first stimulus evokes the response by itself (*see* conditioned reflex). In *operant conditioning* a response is rewarded (or punished) each time it occurs, so that in time it comes to occur more (or less) frequently (*see* reinforcement).

condom *n.* a sheath made of latex rubber, plastic, or silk that is fitted over the penis during sexual intercourse. Use of a condom protects both partners against sexually transmitted diseases (including AIDS) and, when carefully used, it is a reasonably reliable contraceptive (between 2 and 10 pregnancies per 100 woman-years). A more recent development is the *female condom*, which is fitted into the vagina. Manufactured from similar materials as male condoms, they too act as both contraceptives and as barriers to sexually transmitted diseases.

conduct disorder a repetitive and persistent pattern of aggressive or otherwise antisocial behavior. It is usually recognized in childhood or adolescence and can lead to *antisocial personality disorder. Treatment is usually with *behavior therapy or *family therapy.

condylarthrosis (condyloid joint) *n.* a form of *diarthrosis (freely movable joint) in which an ovoid head fits into an elliptical cavity. Examples are the knee joint and the joint between the mandible (lower jaw) and the temporal bone of the skull.

condyle *n.* a rounded protuberance that occurs at the ends of some bones, e.g. the *occipital bone, and forms an articulation with another bone.

condyloma *n.* (*pl.* **condylomata**) a raised wartlike growth. *Condylomata accuminata* (*sing. condyloma acuminatum*) are warts caused by *human papillomavirus and are found on the vulva, under the foreskin, or on the skin of the anal region. They may be treated with podophyllin or trichloroacetic acid; patients should be checked for the presence of other sexually transmitted diseases. *Condylomata lata* (*sing. condyloma latum*) are flat plaques found in the secondary stage of syphilis, occurring in the anogenital region.

cone *n.* one of the two types of light-sensitive cells in the *retina of the eye (*compare* rod). The human retina contains 6–7 million cones; they function best in bright light and are essential for acute vision (receiving a sharp accurate image). The area of the retina called the *fovea contains the greatest concentration of cones. Cones can also distinguish colors. It is thought that there are three types of cones, each sensitive to the wavelength of a different primary color – red, green, or blue. Other colors are seen as combinations of these three primary colors.

cone biopsy surgical removal, via a colposcope, of a cone-shaped segment of tissue from the cervix of the uterus. It may be performed if a cervical smear reveals evidence of *cervical intraepithelial neoplasia (CIN): the affected tissue is removed and examined microscopically for confirmation of the diagnosis.

confabulation *n.* the invention of circumstantial but fictitious detail about events supposed to have occurred in the past. Usually this is to disguise an inability to remember past events. It may be a symptom of any form of loss of memory, but typically occurs in *Korsakoff's syndrome.

confection *n.* (in pharmacy) a sweet substance that is combined with a medicinal preparation to make it suitable for administration.

conflict *n.* (in psychology) the state produced when a stimulus produces two opposing reactions. The basic types of conflict situation are *approach–approach*, in which the individual is drawn toward two attractive, but mutually incompatible, goals; *approach–avoidance*, where the stimulus evokes reactions both to approach and to avoid; and *avoidance–avoidance*, in which the avoidance reaction to one stimulus would bring the individual closer to an equally unpleasant stimulus. Conflict has been used to explain the development of neurotic disorders, and the resolution of conflict is an important part of psychoanalysis. *See also* conversion.

confluence *n.* a point of coalescence. The *confluence of the sinuses* is the meeting point of the superior sagittal, transverse, straight, and occipital venous sinuses in the dura mater in the occipital region of the skull.

congenital *adj.* describing a condition that is recognized at birth or that is believed to have been present since birth. Congenital malformations include all disorders present at birth whether they are inherited or caused by an environmental factor.

congenital adrenal hyperplasia a family of autosomal *recessive genetic disorders causing decreased activity of any of the enzymes involved in the synthesis of *cortisol from *cholesterol. The most commonly affected enzymes are 21-hydroxylase and 11-hydroxylase; each enzyme deficiency can itself be due to a variety of genetic mutations. The clinical manifestations depend on which enzyme is affected and the resultant deficiencies and build-up products produced. The most serious consequence is adrenal crisis and/or severe salt wasting due to lack of cortisol and/or aldosterone, which may prove fatal if undiagnosed. The condition is often easier to spot at birth

in females, who may exhibit ambiguous genitalia due to high levels of *testosterone in utero. This is not seen in males, and suspicions of the condition are thus not raised. Adrenal hyperplasia is the result of excessive stimulation of the glands by *ACTH (adrenocorticotropic hormone) in response to the resultant cortisol deficiency of these conditions.

congenital dislocation of the hip (CDH) one of the most common abnormalities present at birth, in which the head of the femur is displaced or easily displaceable from the acetabulum (socket) of the ilium, which is poorly developed; it frequently affects both hip joints. CDH occurs in about 1.5 per 1000 live births, being more common in first-born girls, in breech deliveries, and if there is a family history of the condition. The leg is shortened and has a reduced range of movement, and the skin creases may be asymmetrical. All babies are routinely screened for CDH at birth and at developmental check-ups by gentle manipulation of the hip causing it to be reduced and dislocated with a clunk (*see* Barlow maneuver). The diagnosis is confirmed by X-ray or ultrasound scan. Treatment is with a special harness holding the hip in the correct position. If this is unsuccessful, the hip is reduced under anesthetic and held with a plaster of Paris cast or the defect is corrected by surgery. Successful treatment of an infant can give a normal hip; if the dislocation is not detected, the hip does not develop normally and osteoarthritis develops at a young age.

congenital macular degeneration *see* vitelliform degeneration.

congestion *n.* an accumulation of blood within an organ, which is the result of back pressure within its veins (for example congestion of the lungs and liver occurs in heart failure). Congestion may be associated with *edema. It is relieved by treatment of the cause.

Congo red a dark-red or reddish-brown pigment that becomes blue in acidic conditions. It is used as a histological *stain. *Amyloidosis is indicated if over 60% of the dye disappears from the blood within one hour of injection.

coniine *n.* an extremely poisonous alkaloid, found in hemlock (*Conium maculatum*), that paralyses the nerves, mainly the motor nerves. Coniine has been included in drug preparations for the treatment of asthma and whooping cough.

conization *n.* surgical removal of a cone of tissue. The technique is commonly used in excising a portion of the cervix of the uterus (*see* cone biopsy) for the treatment of cervicitis or early cancer (carcinoma in situ).

conjoined twins *see* Siamese twins.

conjugate (conjugate diameter, true conjugate) *n.* the distance between the front and rear of the pelvis measured from the most prominent part of the sacrum to the back of the pubic symphysis. Since the true conjugate cannot normally be measured during life, it is estimated by subtracting 1.3–1.9 cm from the *diagonal conjugate*, the distance between the lower edge of the symphysis and the sacrum (usually about 12.7 cm). If the true conjugate is less than about 10.2 cm, delivery of an infant through the natural passages may be difficult or impossible, and *cesarean section may have to be performed.

conjugation *n.* the union of two microorganisms in which genetic material (DNA) passes from one organism to the other. In bacteria minute projections on the donor "male" cell (*pili*) form a bridge with the recipient "female" cell through which the DNA is presumed to be transferred. Conjugation is comparable to sexual reproduction in higher organisms.

conjunctiva *n.* the delicate mucous membrane that covers the front of the eye and lines the inside of the eyelids. The conjunctiva lining the eyelids contains many blood vessels but that over the eyeball contains few and is transparent. —**conjunctival** *adj.*

conjunctivitis (pink eye) *n.* inflammation of the conjunctiva, which becomes red and swollen and produces a watery or pus-containing discharge. It causes discomfort rather than pain and does not usually affect vision. Conjunctivitis may be caused by infection by bacteria or viruses (in which case it usually spreads rapidly to the other eye) or physical or chemical irritation. The patient usually recovers with no after effects in one to three weeks; bacterial infections respond to antibiotic eye drops. *Allergic* (or *vernal*) *conjunctivitis* is acute or chronic inflammation of the cornea usually due to

a specific allergen, such as pollen, animal danders, or dust. It is characterized by itching, irritation, redness, watering of the eyes, and light sensitivity. *See also* inclusion conjunctivitis, ophthalmia neonatorum, trachoma.

connective tissue the tissue that supports, binds, or separates more specialized tissues and organs or functions as a packing tissue of the body. It consists of an amorphous *ground substance* of mucopolysaccharides in which may be embedded white (collagenous), yellow (elastic), and reticular fibers, fat cells, *fibroblasts, *mast cells, and *macrophages (see illustration). Variations in chemical composition of the ground substance and in the proportions and quantities of cells and fibers give rise to tissues of widely differing characteristics, including bone, cartilage, tendons, and ligaments as well as *adipose, *areolar, and *elastic tissues.

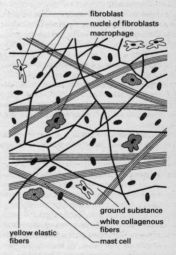

Loose (areolar) connective tissue

connective tissue disease any one of a group of diseases that are characterized by degenerative changes in connective tissue and can affect any part of the body. Formerly known as *collagen diseases* (connective tissue disease is now the preferred term), they include *dermatomyositis, systemic and discoid *lupus erythematosus, *morphea, *polyarteritis nodosa, and *rheumatoid arthritis.

Conn's syndrome the combination of muscular weakness, abnormally intense thirst (polydipsia), the production of large volumes of urine (polyuria), and hypertension, resulting from excessive production of the hormone aldosterone by the adrenal cortex. Some 2% of cases of hypertension are due to it. [W. J. Conn (1907–94), US physician]

consanguinity n. relationship by blood; the sharing of a common ancestor within a few generations.

conservative treatment treatment aimed at preventing a condition from becoming worse, in the expectation that either natural healing will occur or progress of the disease will be so slow that no drastic treatment will be justified. *Compare* radical treatment.

consolidation n. **1.** the state of the lung in which the alveoli (air sacs) are filled with fluid produced by inflamed tissue, as in *pneumonia. It is diagnosed from its dullness to *percussion, bronchial breathing (*see* breath sounds) in the patient, and from the distribution of shadows on the chest X-ray. **2.** the stage of repair of a broken bone following *callus formation, during which the callus is transformed by *osteoblasts into mature bone.

constipation n. a condition in which bowel evacuations occur infrequently, or in which the feces are hard and small, or where passage of feces causes difficulty or pain. The frequency of bowel evacuation varies considerably from person to person and the normal cannot be precisely defined. Constipation developing in a person of previously regular bowel habit may be a symptom of intestinal disease. Recurrent or longstanding constipation is treated by increasing *dietary fiber (roughage), *laxatives, or *enemas. *Fecal impaction*, the end-result of chronic constipation common in senile patients, often requires manual removal of the fecal bolus under an anesthetic.

constrictor n. any muscle that compresses an organ or causes a hollow organ or part to contract.

consultant n. a physician or specialist in a branch of medicine who does not accept total responsibility for a patient but acts in an advisory capacity.

consumption n. any disease causing wasting of tissues, especially (formerly) pulmonary tuberculosis. —**consumptive** adj.

contact n. transmission of an infectious disease by touching or handling an infected person or animal (*direct contact*) or by *indirect contact* with airborne droplets, feces, etc., containing the infective microorganism.

contact lenses lenses worn directly against the eye, separated from it only by a film of tear fluid. *Corneal microlenses* cover only the cornea, while *haptic lenses* cover some of the surrounding sclera as well. Contact lenses are used mainly in place of glasses to correct far- and nearsightedness and other errors of refraction, but they may be used in a protective capacity in some types of corneal disease. Contact lenses may be made of hard or soft materials, which have very different properties. Hard lenses have been partly replaced by newer gas-permeable lenses, which allow oxygen to pass from the atmosphere to the cornea.

contact therapy a form of *radiotherapy in which a radioactive substance is brought into close contact with the part of the body being treated. Needles or capsules of the isotope may be implanted in or around a tumor so that the radiation they emit will destroy it. *Compare* teletherapy.

contagious disease originally, a disease transmitted only by direct physical contact: now usually taken to mean any *communicable disease.

continent diversion *see* urinary diversion.

continuous insulin infusion pump a device used to deliver a continuous infusion of fast-acting insulin to the body instead of using repeated injections throughout the day. It is worn under the clothing and connected to the skin by a tube and a fine needle. These devices have had limited successes in some individuals but require careful usage, particularly when exercise levels unexpectedly differ from usual. They require further evaluation and experience before becoming widely available.

continuous positive airways pressure (CPAP) a method of noninvasive ventilation in which a flow of air is delivered at a constant pressure throughout the respiratory cycle. It is used to optimize oxygen delivery to patients who are being weaned from ventilators, on patients at home with *sleep apnea syndrome, and for *respiratory distress syndrome in infants. It works by improving nasopharyngeal airways, reducing the work of breathing, and preventing basal *atelectasis during sleep.

contra- *prefix denoting* against or opposite. Example: *contraversion* (turning away from).

contraception *n.* the prevention of unwanted pregnancy, which can be achieved by various means. Hormonal contraceptives (estrogen and progestogen or progestogen only) act by preventing ovulation. They are usually taken in regular doses in the form of the Pill (*see* oral contraceptive), but may also be administered through the skin, by means of an adhesive patch impregnated with the hormones, or by three- or two-monthly injections of a long-acting progestogen. Recently developed methods for continuous administration of these hormones are subcutaneous implants of progestogen and vaginal rings containing progestogen. Methods that aim to prevent fertilization of the ovum include *coitus interruptus, the *condom, the *diaphragm, and surgical intervention (tubal occlusion and vasectomy: *see* sterilization). Methods that aim to prevent implantation of a fertilized ovum in the uterus include the intrauterine contraceptive device (*see* IUD); these methods can be used after intercourse but before implantation (*see* postcoital contraception). Couples whose religious beliefs forbid the use of mechanical or hormonal contraceptives may use the *rhythm method, in which intercourse is limited to those days in the menstrual cycle when conception is least likely.

contraction *n.* the shortening of a muscle in response to a motor nerve impulse. This generates tension in the muscle, usually causing movement.

contracture *n.* *fibrosis of muscle or connective tissue producing shrinkage and shortening of the muscle without generating any strength. It is usually a conse-

quence of pain in or disuse of a muscle or limb and may result in deformity of a joint. *See also* Dupuytren's contracture, Volkmann's contracture.

contraindication *n.* any factor in a patient's condition that makes it unwise to pursue a certain line of treatment or to prescribe a particular drug. For example, the presence of pneumonia in a patient would be a strong contraindication against the use of a general anesthetic.

contralateral *adj.* on or affecting the opposite side of the body: applied particularly to paralysis (or other symptoms) occurring on the opposite side of the body from the brain lesion that caused them.

contrast *n.* **1.** short for *contrast medium, e.g. *post-contrast CT scan*. **2.** the difference in the shade of gray between different tissues on a diagnostic image, such as a radiograph or CT scan (*see* gray scale).

contrast medium (contrast agent) a substance that is administered to enhance the visibility of structures (i.e. increase the contrast) during imaging. In *radiography a positive contrast agent (e.g. *barium sulfate or a water-soluble iodine-containing compound) increases the density of a structure. Gas is a negative contrast agent. Positive and negative contrast media can be used together (e.g. barium sulfate and gas in a double-contrast *barium enema). Magnetic resonance (MR) contrast agents contain either a positive contrast atom (usually gadolinium) to increase the signal or a negative contrast atom (such as iron) to decrease it. Ultrasound contrast medium consists of tiny (1–10 μm diameter) bubbles of gas, which reflect back the sound waves strongly. They can also be made to resonate or rupture to increase the signal to the ultrasound probe.

contrecoup *n.* injury of a part resulting from a blow on its opposite side. This may happen, for example, if a blow on the back of the head causes the front of the brain to be pushed against the inner surface of the skull.

Controlled Substances Act legislation passed by the US Congress in 1970 to establish control over narcotics and other drugs of abuse. The law provides classifications for various substances that are known to be addictive and restrictions as to their use. It also authorizes the expenditure of public funds for programs related to addiction treatment and rehabilitation and for public education about the effects of drugs of abuse.

contusion *n.* **1.** *see* bruise. **2.** any of various degrees of bruising of the brain (*cerebral contusion*), resulting from *head injury or surgery. Clinical signs range from *concussion to *coma, reflecting the severity of the trauma.

conus arteriosus the front upper portion of the right ventricle of the heart adjoining the pulmonary arteries.

conus medullaris the conical end of the spinal cord, at the level of the lower end of the first lumbar vertebra.

convergence *n.* **1.** (in neurology) the formation of nerve tracts by fibers coming together into one pathway from different regions of the brain. **2.** (in ophthalmology) the ability of the eyes to turn inward to focus on a near point so that a single image is formed on both retinas. The closer the object, the greater the degree of convergence.

convergence reflex *see* accommodation reflex.

convergence insufficiency an acquired condition in which the eyes fail to turn inward enough to achieve fusion of separate images during near vision.

conversion *n.* (in psychiatry) the expression of *conflict as physical symptoms. Psychoanalysts believe that the repressed instinctual drive is manifested as motor or sensory loss, such as paralysis, rather than as speech or action. This is thought to be one of the ways in which *conversion disorder is produced.

conversion disorder a psychological conflict or need that manifests itself as an organic dysfunction or physical symptom. The person may display symptoms of blindness, deafness, loss of sensation, gait abnormalities, or paralysis of various parts of the body. None of these can be accounted for by organic disease. Conversion disorder was formerly known as *hysteria. It is classified with *dissociative disorders (as dissociative (conversion) disorders) in ICD-10 (*see* International Classification of Diseases). It is also included under the classification of *somatoform disorders.

convolution *n.* a folding or twisting, such as one of the many that cause the fis-

sures, sulci, and gyri of the surface of the *cerebrum.

convulsion *n.* an involuntary contraction of the muscles producing contortion of the body and limbs. Rhythmic convulsions of the limbs are part of major *epilepsy. *Febrile convulsions* are provoked by fever in otherwise healthy infants and young children. Afebrile *infantile convulsions* (*salaam convulsions*) are likely to be due to birth injury or a developmental defect of the brain.

Cooley's anemia *see* thalassemia. [T. B. Cooley (1871–1945), US pediatrician]

Coombs' test a means of detecting rhesus antibodies on the surface of red blood cells that precipitate proteins (globulins) in the blood serum. The test is used in the diagnosis of hemolytic *anemia in babies with rhesus incompatibility in whom there is destruction of red blood cells. [R. R. A. Coombs (1921–   ), British immunologist]

COPD *see* chronic obstructive pulmonary disease.

copr- (copro-) *prefix denoting* feces. Example: *coprophobia* (abnormal fear of).

coprolalia *n.* the repetitive speaking of obscene words. It can be involuntary, as part of the *Gilles de la Tourette syndrome.

coprolith *n.* a mass of hard feces within the colon or rectum, due to chronic constipation. It may become calcified.

coproporphyrin *n.* a *porphyrin compound that is formed during the synthesis of protoporphyrin IX, a precursor of *heme. Coproporphyrin is excreted in the feces in *hereditary coproporphyria*.

copulation *n.* *see* coitus.

cor *n.* the heart.

coracoid process a beaklike process that curves upward and forward from the top of the *scapula, over the shoulder joint.

cord *n.* any long flexible structure, which may be solid or tubular. Examples include the spermatic cord, spinal cord, umbilical cord, and vocal cord.

cordectomy *n.* surgical removal of all or part of a cord, especially the vocal cord.

cordocentesis *n.* the removal of a sample of fetal blood by inserting a hollow needle through the abdominal wall of a pregnant woman, under ultrasound guidance, into the umbilical vein. The blood is subjected to chromosome analysis and biochemical and other tests to determine the presence of abnormalities. *See also* prenatal diagnosis.

cordotomy *n.* a surgical procedure for the relief of severe and persistent pain in the pelvis or lower limbs. The nerve fibers transmitting the sensation of pain to consciousness pass up the spinal cord in special tracts (the *spinothalamic tracts*). In cordotomy the spinothalamic tracts are severed in the cervical (neck) region.

Cordylobia *n. see* tumbu fly.

corectopia *n.* displacement of the pupil toward one side from its normal position in the center of the iris. When present from birth, the displacement is usually inward toward the nose. Scarring of the iris from inflammation may also draw the pupil out of position.

corium *n. see* dermis.

corn *n.* an area of hard thickened skin on or between the toes: a type of *callosity produced by ill-fitting shoes. The horny skin layers form an inverted pyramid that presses down into the deeper skin layers, causing pain. A corn may be treated by soaking in hot water, by using softening agents, or by applying salicylic acid. Medical name: **clavus**.

cornea *n.* the transparent circular part of the front of the eyeball. It refracts the light entering the eye onto the lens, which then focuses it onto the retina. The cornea contains no blood vessels and it is extremely sensitive to pain. The innermost layer (*corneal endothelium*) consists of a single layer of cells that cannot regenerate. —**corneal** *adj.*

corneal graft *see* keratoplasty.

corneal ring a ring designed to be inserted into the peripheral tissue of the cornea in order to alter the curvature of the corneal surface and thus correct errors of refraction. In myopia (nearsightedness), for example, the ring would be required to stretch the corneal tissue peripherally and thus flatten the central corneal curvature in order to correct the myopia.

corneal topography (videokeratography) an imaging technique used to study the shape and refractive power of the cornea in detail. An image projected onto the cornea is analyzed by a computer to produce a representation of the shape and refractive power of the corneal surface. Corneal topography has an important

role in the management of corneal disease and refractive surgery.

cornification *n. see* keratinization.

cornu *n.* (*pl.* **cornua**) (in anatomy) a horn-shaped structure, such as the horn-shaped processes of the hyoid bone and thyroid cartilage. *See also* horn.

corona *n.* a crown or crownlike structure. The *corona capitis* is the crown of the head.

coronal *adj.* relating to the crown of the head or of a tooth. The *coronal plane* divides the body into dorsal and ventral parts (see illustration).

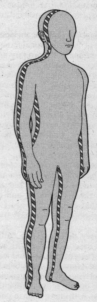

Coronal plane of section through the body

coronal suture *see* suture (def. 1).

corona radiata 1. a series of radiating fibers between the cerebral cortex and the internal capsule of the brain. **2.** a layer of follicle cells that surrounds a freshly ovulated ovum. The cells are elongated radially to the ovum when seen in section.

coronary angiography an X-ray technique for examination of the coronary arteries, often taken to also include examination of the chambers of the heart. A catheter is introduced, usually into a vessel in the groin, and manipulated into the heart. *Contrast medium is then injected to outline the atria, ventricles, and coronary arteries. Video images are recorded during contrast-medium injection, either on film or electronic media, often using *digital subtraction techniques. Coronary angiography is used to diagnose cardiac disease, specifically narrowing or blockage in the coronary arteries, and plan treatment by surgery or radiological interventional techniques (see coronary bypass graft, coronary angioplasty).

coronary angioplasty (balloon angioplasty) a technique of *interventional radiology in which a segment of coronary artery narrowed by *atheroma is stretched by the inflation of a balloon introduced into it by means of cardiac *catheterization under X-ray screening (see angioplasty). The site of the obstruction is identified by prior *coronary angiography. Not all narrowed segments can be improved by angioplasty, but results may be improved by placement of metallic *stents. See also coronary bypass graft.

coronary arteries the arteries supplying blood to the heart. The *right* and *left* *coronary arteries* arise from the aorta, just above the aortic valve, and form branches that encircle the heart. See coronary angioplasty, coronary bypass graft.

coronary artery disease (CAD) *atherosclerosis of the coronary arteries, which may cause *angina pectoris and lead to *myocardial infarction. One of the leading causes of death in Western countries, the disease occurs most frequently in populations with diets high in cholesterol, saturated fats, and refined carbohydrates. Other risk factors include hypertension, diabetes mellitus, obesity, lack of exercise, smoking, excessive alcohol and coffee intake, and high levels of stress. Therapy includes dietary and lifestyle changes, treatment with such medications as *nitroglycerin, *beta blockers, and *calcium antagonists, and interventional measures, such as *coronary bypass surgery or *coronary angioplasty.

coronary bypass graft *coronary revascu-

larization in which a segment of a coronary artery narrowed by *atheroma is bypassed by an autologous section of healthy saphenous vein or internal mammary artery at *thoracotomy. The improved blood flow resulting from one or more such grafts relieves *angina pectoris and reduces the risk of *myocardial infarction. Recently developed techniques of *minimally invasive surgery have enabled the operation to be performed without the need for thoracotomy.

coronary revascularization a surgical method of improving the blood flow through coronary arteries narrowed by *atheroma. See coronary bypass graft.

coronary thrombosis the formation of a blood clot (thrombus) in the coronary artery, which obstructs the flow of blood to the heart. This is usually due to *atheroma and results in the death (infarction) of part of the heart muscle. For symptoms and treatment, see myocardial infarction.

coroner *n.* see medical examiner.

coronoid process 1. a process on the upper end of the *ulna. It forms part of the notch that articulates with the humerus. **2.** the process on the ramus of the *mandible to which the temporalis muscle is attached.

cor pulmonale enlargement of the right ventricle of the heart that results from diseases of the lungs or the pulmonary arteries. Such diseases include those affecting the structure of the lungs (e.g. emphysema) or their function (e.g. obesity) except when these changes result from congenital heart disease or diseases primarily affecting the left side of the heart.

corpus *n.* (*pl.* **corpora**) any mass of tissue that can be distinguished from its surroundings.

corpus albicans the residual body of scar tissue that remains in the ovary at the point where a *corpus luteum has regressed after its secretory activity has ceased.

corpus callosum the broad band of nervous tissue that connects the two cerebral hemispheres, containing an estimated 300 million fibers. See cerebrum.

corpus cavernosum either of a pair of cylindrical blood sinuses that form the erectile tissue of the *penis and clitoris. In the penis a third sinus, the corpus spongiosum, encloses the urethra and extends into the glans. All these sinuses have a spongelike structure that allows them to expand when filled with blood.

corpuscle *n.* any small particle, cell, or mass of tissue.

corpus luteum the glandular tissue in the ovary that forms at the site of a ruptured *graafian follicle after ovulation. It secretes the hormone *progesterone, which prepares the uterus for implantation. If implantation fails the corpus luteum becomes inactive and degenerates. If an embryo becomes implanted the corpus luteum continues to secrete progesterone until the fourth month of pregnancy, by which time the placenta has taken over this function.

corpus spongiosum the blood sinus that surrounds the urethra of the male. Together with the corpora cavernosa, it forms the erectile tissue of the *penis. It is expanded at the base of the penis to form the urethral bulb and at the tip to form the glans penis.

corpus striatum the part of the *basal ganglia in the cerebral hemispheres of the brain consisting of the caudate nucleus and the lentiform nucleus.

correlation *n.* (in statistics) the extent to which one of a pair of characteristics affects the other in a series of individuals. Such pairs of observations can be plotted as a series of points on a graph. If all the points on the resulting *scatter diagram* are in a straight line (which is neither horizontal nor vertical), the *correlation coefficient* may vary within the range of +1, where an increase of one variable is always associated with the corresponding increase in the other, to −1, where an increase of one variable is associated with a constant decrease of the other; a coefficient of 0 indicates no dependence of the one characteristic on the other of a straight line type. The *regression coefficient* is the average extent to which a unit increase of one characteristic influences the increase/decrease of the other. Where several factors appear to correlate with the onset of disease the relative importance of each may be calculated by the statistical technique known as *multivariate analysis*.

Corrigan's pulse (collapsing pulse) a type of pulse that has an exaggerated rise followed by a sudden fall. It is typical of aortic valve incompetence. [Sir D. J. Corrigan (1802–80), Irish physician]

cortex *n.* (*pl.* **cortices**) the outer part of an organ, situated immediately beneath its capsule or outer membrane; for example, the *adrenal cortex* (*see* adrenal glands), *renal cortex* (*see* kidney), or *cerebral cortex*. —**cortical** *adj*.

cortical Lewy body disease a disorder characterized by a combination of parkinsonism and dementia, which typically fluctuates; abnormal proteins called *Lewy bodies* are found within the nerve cells of the cortex and the basal ganglia. It is the second most common cause of dementia (*dementia with Lewy bodies*) after *Alzheimer's disease.

corticosteroid (corticoid) *n.* any steroid hormone synthesized by the adrenal cortex. There are two main groups of corticosteroids. The *glucocorticoids* (e.g. cortisol, *cortisone, and corticosterone) are essential for the utilization of carbohydrate, fat, and protein by the body and for a normal response to stress. Both naturally occurring and synthetic glucocorticoids have very powerful antiinflamatory effects and are used to treat conditions involving inflammation. The *mineralocorticoids* (e.g. *aldosterone) are necessary for the regulation of salt and water balance.

corticosterone *n.* a steroid hormone (*see* corticosteroid) synthesized and released in small amounts by the adrenal cortex.

corticotropin *n.* *see* ACTH.

corticotropin-releasing hormone (CRH) a peptide hypothalamic hormone (of 41 amino acids) stimulating the release of *ACTH (adrenocorticotropic hormone) from the anterior pituitary. Its own release is suppressed by a *negative feedback loop involving cortisol, and its action is increased by antidiuretic hormone (*see* vasopressin) and *angiotensin II. It can be administered intravenously as part of the *CRH test*, during which blood is analyzed at 15-minute intervals for one hour for the ACTH response, which is excessive in cases of primary adrenal failure and suppressed in cases of anterior *hypopituitarism.

cortisol *n.* a steroid hormone: the major glucocorticoid synthesized and released by the human adrenal cortex (*see* corticosteroid). It is important for normal carbohydrate metabolism and for the normal response to any stress. *See also* hydrocortisone.

cortisone *n.* a naturally occurring *corticosteroid that is used mainly to treat deficiency of corticosteroid hormones in *Addison's disease and following surgical removal of the adrenal glands. It is administered by mouth or injection and may cause serious side effects such as stomach ulcers and bleeding, nervous and hormone disturbances, muscle and bone damage, and eye changes.

cor triloculare a rare congenital condition in which there are three instead of four chambers of the heart due to the presence of a single common ventricle. *Cyanosis (blueness) is common. Most patients die in infancy.

Corynebacterium *n.* a genus of gram-positive, mostly aerobic, nonmotile rod-like bacteria that frequently bear club-shaped swellings. Many species cause disease in humans, domestic animals, birds, and plants; some are found in dairy products. The species *C. diphtheriae* (*Klebs-Loeffler bacillus*) is the causative organism of *diphtheria, producing a powerful *exotoxin that is harmful to heart and nerve tissue. It occurs in one of three forms: *gravis*, *intermedius*, and *mitis*.

coryza (cold in the head) *n.* a catarrhal inflammation of the mucous membrane in the nose due to either a *cold or *hay fever. *See also* catarrh.

cost- (costo-) *prefix denoting* the rib(s). Example: *costectomy* (excision of).

costal *adj.* of or relating to the ribs.

costal cartilage a cartilage that connects a *rib to the breastbone (*sternum). The first seven ribs (true ribs) are directly connected to the sternum by individual costal cartilages. The next three ribs are indirectly connected to the sternum by three costal cartilages, each of which is connected to the one immediately above it.

costalgia *n.* pain localized to the ribs. This term is now rarely used.

cost effectiveness a public health strategy employed to estimate the costs of different diagnostic or treatment approaches in controlling a disease. In screening women for cervical cancer, for example,

the cost effectiveness is determined by measuring the expense of the *cervical smear tests against lives saved or years of life extended by detecting the presence of cancer at a stage when the condition can be corrected. More frequent testing might save more lives but the additional cost per additional life saved would rise sharply. The concept is based on the assumption that health-care resources and money should be applied to the medical procedure that would appear to be most productive.

costive *adj.* constipated.

costochondritis *n.* *see* Tietze's syndrome.

co-trimoxazole *n.* an antibacterial drug consisting of *sulfamethoxazole and *trimethoprim. Since both these drugs are well absorbed and rapidly excreted – and each potentiates the action of the other – co-trimoxazole is taken by mouth and is particularly useful for treating urinary tract, respiratory tract, and gastrointestinal infections. Because of the severity of the side effects, which are those of the *sulfonamides, co-trimoxazole is now less frequently prescribed than formerly. Trade names: **Bactrim, Cotrim, Septra, Sulfatrim**.

cotton-wool spots accumulations of *axoplasm in the nerve-fiber layer of the retina, which indicate disease (e.g. hypertension, connective tissue disease, or AIDS).

cotyledon *n.* any of the major convex subdivisions of the mature *placenta. Each cotyledon contains a major branch of the umbilical blood vessels, which branch further into the numerous villi that make up the surface of the cotyledon.

cotyloid cavity *see* acetabulum.

couching *n.* an operation for cataract in which the lens is pushed out of the pupil downward and backward into the jelly-like vitreous humor by a small knife inserted through the edge of the cornea. It was widely used in ancient Hindu civilizations and has been practiced ever since. Its sole advantage is speed of performance, but modern developments in surgery and anesthesia leave little place for it today. The complication rate is very high.

coughing *n.* a form of violent exhalation by which irritant particles in the airways can be expelled. Stimulation of the cough reflexes results in the glottis being kept closed until a high expiratory pressure has built up, which is then suddenly released. Medical name: **tussis**.

coulomb n. the *SI unit of electric charge, equal to the quantity of electricity transferred by 1 ampere in 1 second. Symbol: C.

coumarin n. a substance whose derivatives are used in *anticoagulants for the treatment of such disorders as thrombophlebitis and pulmonary embolism.

counseling n. 1. a method of approaching psychological difficulties in adjustment that aims to help the client work out his own problems. The counselor listens sympathetically, attempting to identify with the client, tries to clarify current problems, and sometimes gives advice. It involves less emphasis on insight and interpretation than does psychotherapy or psychoanalytic therapy. *See also* client-centered therapy. 2. *see* genetic counseling.

counterextension n. an orthopedic procedure consisting of *traction on one part of a limb, while the remainder of the limb is held steady: used particularly in the treatment of a fractured femur (thigh bone).

counterirritant n. an agent, such as methyl salicylate, that causes irritation when applied to the skin and is used in order to relieve more deep-seated pain or discomfort. —**counterirritation** n.

countershock n. *see* cardioversion.

countertraction n. the use of opposing force to balance that being applied during *traction, when a strong continuous pull is applied to a limb so that broken bones can be kept in alignment during healing.

couvade n. 1. a custom in some tribes in which a father takes to his bed during or after the birth of his child. 2. a symptom of abdominal pain experienced by a man in relation to his wife's giving birth. It may be due to *conversion disorder, anxiety, or sympathy.

cover glass an extremely thin square or circle of glass used to protect the upper surface of a preparation on a microscope slide.

cover test a test used to detect a suppressed *strabismus (squint) in children. The child is asked to look fixedly at an object with one eye while the other is kept open but covered by the hand of the observer. The hand is then withdrawn: if the eye that had been covered is seen to move toward the nose to adjust to the focus of the uncovered eye, the child is assumed to have a divergent squint; movement of the eye away from the nose implies a convergent squint.

Cowper's glands (bulbourethral glands) a pair of small glands that open into the urethra at the base of the penis. Their secretion contributes to the seminal fluid, but less than that of the prostate gland or seminal vesicles. [W. Cowper (1660–1709), English surgeon]

cowpox n. a virus infection of cows' udders, transmitted to humans by direct contact, causing very mild symptoms similar to *smallpox. An attack conferred immunity to smallpox before smallpox was eradicated. Medical name: **vaccinia**.

cox- (coxo-) *prefix denoting* the hip. Example: *coxalgia* (pain in).

coxa n. (*pl.* **coxae**) 1. the hip bone. 2. the hip joint.

Coxiella n. a genus of *rickettsiae that cause disease in animals and humans. They are usually transmitted by airborne droplets that are inhaled, and they produce diseases characterized by inflammation of the lungs, without a rash (*compare* typhus). The species *C. burnetii* causes *Q fever.

COX-2 inhibitor any one of a group of anti-inflammatory drugs (*see* NSAID) that block the action of the enzyme cyclo-oxygenase 2 (COX-2), which mediates the production of *prostaglandin at sites of inflammation, especially in joints; they are less likely to inhibit COX-1, which controls the production of prostaglandin in the stomach (where it is involved in the production of protective mucus), and therefore less likely than other NSAIDs to cause peptic ulceration. COX-2 inhibitors are used in the treatment of arthritis and are under investigation for the treatment and prevention of certain cancers, primarily colorectal, breast, and lung cancer. They include *celecoxib and *rofecoxib. Side effects include fluid retention (edema), intestinal upset, dizziness, insomnia, and sore throat.

coxsackievirus n. one of a group of RNA-containing viruses that are able to multiply in the gastrointestinal tract (*see* enterovirus). About 30 different types exist. *Type A coxsackieviruses* generally cause less severe and less well-defined diseases, such as *hand, foot, and mouth disease, although some cause meningitis and severe throat infections (*see* herpangina). *Type B coxsackieviruses* cause inflammation or degeneration of heart tissue, resulting in pericarditis or myocarditis, or brain tissue, producing meningitis or encephalitis. They can also attack the muscles of the chest wall, the bronchi, pancreas, thyroid, or conjunctiva and recent evidence suggests they may be implicated in diabetes in children and in motor neuron disease. *See also* Bornholm disease.

CPAP *see* continuous positive airways pressure.

C peptide *n.* a peptide (so called because of its C shape) formed when insulin is produced from its precursor molecule, proinsulin. It is secreted in equal molar amounts to insulin. However, since it remains detectable in the plasma much longer than insulin, it can be more easily assayed as a marker of the degree of insulin secretion. This can be useful in assessing the ability of the pancreas to secrete insulin, for example when trying to determine whether a patient has type 1 or type 2 diabetes or to distinguish an insulin-secreting tumor (an *insulinoma) from surreptitious insulin usage in unexplained hypoglycemia.

CPR *see* cardiopulmonary resuscitation.

crab louse *see* Phthirus.

cradle *n.* a framework of metal strips or other material that forms a cage over an injured part of the body of a patient lying in bed, to protect it from the pressure of the bedclothes.

cradle cap a common condition in young babies in which crusty white or yellow scales form a "cap" on the scalp. It is treated by applying oil or using a special shampoo and usually resolves in the first year of life, although it may represent the start of seborrhoeic *eczema. Medical name: **crusta lactea**.

cramp *n.* prolonged painful contraction of a muscle. It is sometimes caused by an imbalance of the salts in the body, but is more often a result of fatigue, imperfect posture, or stress. Spasm in the muscles making it impossible to perform a spe-

cific task but allowing the use of these muscles for any other movement is called *occupational cramp*. It most often affects the hand muscles for writing (*writer's cramp*), a form of *dystonia.

crani- (cranio-) *prefix denoting* the skull. Example: *cranioplasty* (plastic surgery of).

cranial nerves the 12 pairs of nerves that arise directly from the brain and leave the skull through separate apertures; they are conventionally given Roman numbers, as follows: I *olfactory; II *optic; III *oculomotor; IV *trochlear; V *trigeminal; VI *abducens; VII *facial; VIII *vestibulocochlear; IX *glossopharyngeal; X *vagus; XI *accessory; XII *hypoglossal. *Compare* spinal nerves.

craniometry *n.* the science of measuring the differences in the size and shape of skulls. *See also* cephalic index.

craniopagus (dicephalus) *n.* *Siamese twins united by their heads.

craniopharyngioma *n.* a brain tumor, situated above the *sella turcica, that is derived from remnants of *Rathke's pouch*, an embryologic structure from which the pituitary gland is partly formed. The patient may show raised intracranial pressure and *diabetes insipidus due to reduced secretion of the hormone *vasopressin. An X-ray of the skull typically shows calcification within the tumor and loss of the normal skull structure around the pituitary gland.

craniostenosis *n.* premature closing of the *sutures and *fontanelles between the cranial bones during development, resulting in deformities of the skull. *Compare* craniosynostosis.

craniosynostosis *n.* premature fusion of some of the cranial bones, usually before birth, so that the skull is unable to expand in certain directions to assume its normal shape under the influence of the growing brain. Depending on which cranial *sutures fuse early, the skull may become elongated from front to back, broad and short, peaked (*oxycephaly* or *turricephaly*), or asymmetrical. *Compare* craniostenosis.

craniotomy *n.* **1.** surgical removal of a portion of the skull (cranium), performed to expose the brain and *meninges for inspection or biopsy or to relieve excessive intracranial pressure (as in a subdural *hematoma). **2.** surgical perforation of the skull of a dead fetus during difficult labor, so that delivery may continue.

For both operations the instrument used is called a *craniotome*.

cranium *n.* the part of the skeleton that encloses the brain. The cranium consists of eight bones connected together by immovable joints (*see* skull). —**cranial** *adj.*

cream *n.* a preparation for use on the skin consisting of an emulsion of oil in water, which may or may not contain medication. It rubs into the skin easily, tends to dry the skin, and also contains preservatives, which may be allergenic. *Compare* ointment.

creatine *n.* a product of protein metabolism found in muscle. Its phosphate, *creatine phosphate* (*phosphocreatine, phosphagen*), acts as a store of high-energy phosphate in muscle and serves to maintain adequate amounts of *ATP (the source of energy for muscular contraction).

creatine kinase (CK) an enzyme involved in the metabolic breakdown of creatine to creatinine. Isomers of creatine kinase originate from brain (BB), skeletal muscle (MM), and myocardium (MB). Any damage to these tissues causes an increase of the isomer in the serum, which can be used in diagnosis, particularly of myocardial injury.

creatinine *n.* a substance derived from creatine and creatine phosphate in muscle. Creatinine is excreted in the urine.

creatinuria *n.* an excess of the nitrogenous compound creatine in the urine.

creatorrhea *n.* the passage of excessive nitrogen in the feces due to failure of digestion or absorption in the small intestine. It is found particularly in pancreatic failure. *See* cystic fibrosis, pancreatitis.

Credé's method 1. a technique for expelling the placenta from the uterus. Downward pressure is applied to the uterus through the abdominal wall in the direction of the birth canal. *See also* Brandt Andrews maneuver. **2.** a method of expressing urine from the bladder through manual pressure on the lower abdominal wall. **3.** the application of 1% silver nitrate solution to the eyes of a newborn baby whose mother has gonorrhea. The treatment aims to prevent the development of *ophthalmia neonatorum in the infant. [K. S. F. Credé (1819–92), German gynecologist]

creeping eruption (larva migrans) a skin disease caused either by larvae of certain nematode worms (e.g. *Ancylostoma braziliense*) normally parasitic in dogs and cats or by the maggots of certain flies (*see* Hypoderma, Gasterophilus). The larvae burrow within the skin tissues, their movements marked by long thin red lines that cause the patient intense irritation. The nematode infections are treated with albendazole or ivermectin; maggots can be surgically removed.

crenation *n.* an abnormal appearance of red blood cells seen under a microscope, in which the normally smooth cell margins appear crinkly or irregular. Crenation may be a feature of certain blood disorders, but most commonly occurs as a result of prolonged storage of a blood specimen prior to preparation of a blood film.

crepitation (rale) *n.* a soft fine crackling sound heard in the lungs through the stethoscope. Crepitations are made either by air passages and alveoli (air sacs) opening up during inspiration or by air bubbling through fluid. They are not normally heard in healthy lungs.

crepitus *n.* **1.** a crackling sound or grating feeling produced by bone rubbing on bone or roughened cartilage, detected on movement of an arthritic joint. Crepitus in the knee joint is a common sign of *chondromalacia patellae in the young and *osteoarthritis in the elderly. **2.** a similar sound heard with a stethoscope over an inflamed lung when the patient breathes in.

cresol *n.* a strong antiseptic effective against many microorganisms and used mostly in soap solutions as a general disinfectant. It is sometimes used in low concentrations as a preservative in injections. Cresol solutions irritate the skin and if taken by mouth are corrosive and cause pain, nausea, and vomiting.

crest *n.* a ridge or linear protuberance, particularly on a bone. Examples include the crest of fibula and the iliac crest (of the ilium).

CREST syndrome a disease characterized by the association of *calcinosis, *Raynaud's phenomenon, *esophageal malfunction, sclerodactyly (tapering fingers), and telangiectasia (*see* telangiectasis). It represents a variant of *systemic sclerosis and may be associated with severe pulmonary hypertension.

cretinism *n.* a syndrome of *dwarfism, mental retardation, and coarseness of the skin and facial features due to lack of thyroid hormone from birth (congenital *hypothyroidism). *Compare* myxedema.

Creutzfeldt-Jakob disease (CJD) a rapidly progressive rare neurological disease, a form of human *spongiform encephalopathy in which dementia progresses to death after a period of 3–12 months. There is no effective treatment. The causative agent is currently believed to be an abnormal *prion protein that accumulates in the brain and causes widespread destruction of tissue. CJD typically affects middle-aged to elderly people. Some 15% of cases are due to a form of the disease that is inherited as an autosomal *dominant trait but most cases are sporadic, susceptibility being genetically determined. A few cases of CJD are acquired: the agent is known to have been transmitted by tissue and organ transplantation and by human growth hormone injections, but the disease may take years to manifest itself. A variant form of acquired CJD (vCJD) affecting younger people has been linked with the consumption of meat products containing tissue from cattle infected with bovine spongiform encephalopathy (BSE). [H. G. Creutzfeldt (1885–1964) and A. M. Jakob (1884–1931), German psychiatrists]

CRH *see* corticotropin-releasing hormone.

crib death (sudden infant death syndrome, SIDS) the sudden unexpected death of an infant less than two years old (peak occurrence between two and six months) from an unidentifiable cause. There appear to be many factors involved, including the position in which the baby is laid to sleep: babies who sleep on their fronts (the prone position) have an increased risk. About half the affected infants will have had a viral upper respiratory tract infection within the 48 hours preceding their death, many of these being due to the *respiratory syncytial virus. *See also* apnea.

cribriform plate *see* ethmoid bone.

cricoid cartilage the cartilage, shaped like a signet ring, that forms part of the anterior and lateral walls and most of the posterior wall of the *larynx.

cricoid pressure a technique in which pressure is applied downward on the *cricoid cartilage of a supine patient to aid endotracheal *intubation.

cricothyroid membrane the fibrous tissue in the anterior aspect of the neck between the lower border of the *thyroid cartilage (the "Adam's apple") and the upper border of the *cricoid cartilage, lying immediately below it. It is the site where certain emergency airway devices can be inserted.

cricothyroidotomy *n.* a technique for obtaining an emergency airway through the *cricothyroid membrane when standard airway techniques have failed. There are two main techniques. In *needle cricothyroidotomy*, a large-bore intravenous cannula is inserted directly through the membrane. Ventilation by this technique can only be through a high-pressure system, must only be performed by trained personnel, and must only continue for a maximum of 45 minutes. Damage to the lungs can ensue. In *surgical cricothyroidotomy*, a surgical hole is made in the membrane and a cuffed tube, similar to a short endotracheal tube (*see* intubation), is inserted directly. This affords much better airway protection.

cri du chat syndrome a congenital condition of severe mental retardation that is associated with multiple physical abnormalities and an abnormal catlike cry in infancy. It results from a chromosomal abnormality in which there is a loss (*deletion) of part of the short arm of chromosome no. 5.

Crigler-Najjar syndrome a genetic disease in which the liver enzyme glucuronyl transferase, responsible for dealing with bilirubin, is absent. Large amounts of bilirubin accumulate in the blood, and the child becomes progressively more jaundiced. The only treatment is a liver transplant, without which life expectancy is usually less than two years. [J. F. Crigler (1919–) and V. A. Najjar (1914–), US pediatricians]

Crile's procedure (or operation) the standard radical operation for en-bloc removal of malignant lymph nodes of the neck. [G. W. Crile (1864–1943), US surgeon]

Crimean Congo hemorrhagic fever a disease caused by bunyaviruses that has occurred in Russia, the Middle East, and Africa. It causes bleeding into the intestines, kidneys, genitals, and mouth with up to 50% mortality. The virus is spread by various types of tick from wild animals and birds to domestic animals (especially goats and cattle) and thus to humans.

crippled children's services funds provided under the US *Child Health Act for the location, diagnosis, and treatment of children who are either crippled or have a condition that leads to crippling. A crippled child is defined as "an individual under the age of 21 who has an organic disease, defect, or condition which may hinder the achievement of normal growth and development."

crisis *n.* **1.** the turning point of a disease, after which the patient either improves or deteriorates. Since the advent of antibiotics, infections seldom reach the point of crisis. **2.** the occurrence of sudden severe pain in certain diseases. *See also* Dietl's crisis.

crista *n.* (*pl.* **cristae**) **1.** the sensory structure within the ampulla of a *semicircular canal within the inner ear (see illustration). The cristae respond to changes in the rate of movement of the head, being activated by pressure from the fluid in the semicircular canals. **2.** one of the infoldings of the inner membrane of a *mitochondrion. **3.** any anatomical structure resembling a crest.

critical care unit (CCU) a specially equipped section of a hospital or treatment center designated for the treatment of patients with life-threatening conditions, predominantly serious cardiac cases who require specialist monitoring equipment and specially trained staff. *See also* intensive care unit.

Crohn's disease a condition in which segments of the alimentary tract become inflamed, thickened, and ulcerated. It usually affects the terminal part of the ileum; its acute form (*acute ileitis*) may mimic *appendicitis. Chronic disease often causes partial obstruction of the intestine, leading to pain, diarrhea, and *malabsorption. *Fistulas around the anus, between adjacent loops of intestine, or from intestine to skin, bladder, etc., are characteristic complications. The cause is unknown but it is thought that an infectious agent might initiate the process (*see* Mycobacterium). Treatment includes rest, corticosteroids, immunosuppressant drugs, antibiotics, dietary modification, or (in some cases) surgical removal of the affected part of the intestine. Alternative names: **regional enteritis, regional ileitis.** [B. B. Crohn (1884–1983), US physician]

cromolyn sodium (sodium cromoglicate) a drug used to prevent asthma attacks and hay fever and to treat other allergic conditions, including allergic conjunctivitis. It is administered by inhalation as a nasal spray, or as eye drops, and may cause local irritation. Trade names: **Gastrocrom, Intal, Nasalcrom, Opticrom.**

crossbite *n.* a condition in which some or all of the lower teeth close outside the upper teeth during normal closure.

cross-dressing *n.* *see* transvestism.

crossing over (in genetics) the exchange of sections of chromatids between pairs of homologous chromosomes, which results in the recombination of genetic material. It occurs during *meiosis at a *chiasma.

crossmatching *n.* **1.** (in blood transfusion) a test to determine compatibility of a donor's blood with that of a recipient before transfusion. Red cells from the blood of the donor are mixed with the serum of the recipient (*major crossmatch*) and red cells from the blood of

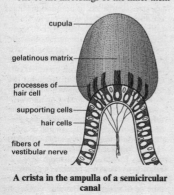

cupula

gelatinous matrix

processes of hair cell

supporting cells

hair cells

fibers of vestibular nerve

A crista in the ampulla of a semicircular canal

the recipient with the serum of the donor (*minor crossmatch*). If agglutination occurs, an antigenic substance is present and the bloods are not compatible, indicating a potentially lethal hemolytic reaction if transfused. **2.** (in transplantation) a test for the presence of cytotoxic antibodies in the serum of a prospectus transplant recipient against donor tissue antigens. Donor lymphocytes are mixed in the serum of the recipient; the presence of cytolysis indicates incompatibility and the likelihood of rejection.

crossover trial *see* intervention study.

cross-sectional imaging any technique that produces an image in the form of a plane through the body with the structures cut across. The main techniques are *ultrasonography, *computed tomography, *magnetic resonance imaging, and some *nuclear medicine techniques (*see* positron emission tomography, SPECT scanning). If a series of thin-section images is stacked they can be "cut" through to show other planes or allow reconstruction of three-dimensional images.

cross-sectional study the collection and analysis of information relating to persons in a population or group at a defined point in time or within a defined period, with particular reference to their individual characteristics and exposure to factors thought likely to predispose to disease. *See also* prevalence rate.

crotamiton *n.* a drug that destroys mites and is used to treat scabies and similar skin infections and also to relieve itching. It is applied to the skin as a lotion or ointment and sometimes causes reddening and hypersensitivity reactions. Trade name: **Eurax.**

croup *n.* acute inflammation and obstruction of the respiratory tract, involving the larynx and the main air passages (trachea and bronchi), in young children (usually aged between six months and three years). The usual cause is a virus infection (*see* laryngotracheobronchitis) but bacterial secondary infection can occur. The symptoms are those of *laryngitis, accompanied by signs of obstruction – harsh difficult breathing (*see* stridor), a characteristic barking cough, a rising pulse rate, restlessness, and *cyanosis. Treatment by humidification

of inspired air and mild sedation usually reverses the alarming symptoms. In severe cases the obstruction may require treatment by steroid nebulizers, *tracheostomy, or nasotracheal *intubation. *See also* epiglottitis.

crown *n.* **1.** the part of a tooth normally visible in the mouth and usually covered by enamel. **2.** a dental *restoration that covers most or all of the natural crown. It may be made of porcelain, gold, a combination of these, or less commonly other materials. Most crowns are like thimbles and are custom made to fit over a trimmed-down tooth. A *post crown* is used to restore a tooth when the natural crown is insufficient. A post is inserted into the root and the missing center of the tooth is built up; over it is fitted a thimblelike crown to restore the natural shape of the tooth. *Root canal treatment is required before such a crown can be made.

crowning *n.* **1.** the stage of labor when the upper part of the infant's head is encircled by, and just passing through, the vaginal opening. **2.** (in dentistry) the fitting of an artificial *crown to a tooth.

cruciate ligaments a pair (anterior and posterior) of ligaments inside each knee joint, which help to prevent excessive anteroposterior glide. Damage to the cruciate ligaments is a common *sports injury, especially in football players.

crude rate the total number of events (e.g. cases of lung cancer) expressed as a percentage (or rate per 1000, etc.) of the whole population. When factors such as age structure or sex of populations may seriously affect their rates (as in *mortality or *morbidity rates) it is more meaningful to compare age/sex-specific rates using one or more age groups of a designated sex (e.g. lung cancer in males aged 55–64 years). More complex calculations, which take into account the age bias of a population as a whole, can produce *standardized rates* or *standardized mortality ratios* (SMR). In these the ratios of subgroups are expressed as percentages of that for a designated or standard population, particularly applied to the age bracket 15–64 years.

crural *adj.* **1.** relating to the thigh or leg. **2.** relating to the crura cerebri (*see* crus).

crus *n.* (*pl.* **crura**) an elongated process or part of a structure. The *crus cerebri* is one of two symmetrical nerve tracts situated between the medulla oblongata and the cerebral hemispheres.

crush syndrome (compression syndrome) kidney failure following massive trauma to, and necrosis of, muscle. It results from acute necrosis of the renal tubules associated with the presence in the blood of *myohemoglobin, released from the damaged muscle.

cry- (cryo-) prefix denoting cold.

cryesthesia n. 1. exceptional sensitivity to low temperature. 2. a sensation of coldness.

cryoglobulin n. an abnormal protein – an *immunoglobulin (see paraprotein) – that may be present in the blood in certain diseases. Cryoglobulins become insoluble at low temperatures, leading to obstruction of small blood vessels in the fingers and toes in cold weather and producing a characteristic rash. The presence of cryoglobulins (cryoglobulinemia) may be a feature of a variety of diseases, including *macroglobulinemia, systemic *lupus erythematosus, and certain infections.

cryoprecipitate n. a precipitate produced by freezing and thawing under controlled conditions. An example is the residue obtained from fresh-frozen blood plasma that has been thawed at 4°C. This residue is extremely rich in a clotting factor, *Factor VIII (antihemophilic factor), and was used in the control of bleeding in *hemophilia prior to the development of recombinant technology to produce Factor VIII.

cryopreservation n. preservation of tissues or organs by freezing. Cryopreservation of embryos may be used as part of *in vitro fertilization procedures, for example, if there are medical reasons for delaying the pregnancy.

cryoprobe n. see cryosurgery.

cryoretinopexy n. the use of extreme cold to freeze areas of weak or torn retina in order to cause scarring and seal breaks. It is used in *cryosurgery for *detached retina.

cryostat n. 1. a chamber in which frozen tissue is sectioned with a *microtome. 2. a device for maintaining a specific low temperature.

cryosurgery n. the use of extreme cold in a localized part of the body to freeze and destroy unwanted tissues. Cryosurgery is usually undertaken with an instrument called a cryoprobe, which has a fine tip cooled by allowing carbon dioxide or nitrous oxide gas to expand within it. Cryosurgery is commonly used for the treatment of detached retina (cryoretinopexy), the destruction of certain bone tumors, and the obliteration of skin blemishes.

cryotherapy n. the use of cold in the treatment of disorders. See cyclocryotherapy, cryosurgery, hypothermia (def. 2). Compare thermotherapy.

crypt n. a small sac, follicle, or cavity; for example, the crypts of Lieberkühn (see Lieberkühn's glands), which are intestinal glands.

crypt- (crypto-) prefix denoting concealed. Example: cryptogenic (of unknown origin).

cryptococcosis (torulosis) n. an infectious disease of worldwide distribution, caused by the fungus Cryptococcus neoformans. The fungus attacks the lungs, causing tumorlike lesions (torulomas), but produces few or no symptoms referable to the lungs. It may also spread to the brain, causing meningitis, and occasionally to the kidneys, bone, and skin. This may occur as an opportunistic infection in those suffering from AIDS. The condition responds well to treatment with *amphotericin B.

Cryptococcus n. a genus of unicellular yeastlike fungi that cause disease in humans. They are found in soil (particularly when enriched with pigeon droppings), and they are common in pigeon roosts and nests. The species C. neoformans causes *cryptococcosis.

cryptomenorrhea n. absence of blood flow when the internal symptoms of menstruation are present. The condition may arise because the hymen at the entrance to the vagina lacks an opening (*imperforate hymen) or because of some other obstruction.

cryptophthalmos n. apparent absence of the eyes due to failure of normal eyelid formation during embryonic development, resulting in absence of the opening between the upper and lower eyelids.

cryptorchidism (cryptorchism) n. the condition in which the testes fail to descend into the scrotum and are retained within the abdomen or inguinal canal. The operation of *orchiopexy is necessary to bring the testes into the scrotum before puberty to allow subsequent normal development; it is thought that the higher temperature in the abdomen interferes with sperm production. —**cryptorchid** *adj.*, *n.*

cryptosporidiosis *n.* an intestinal infection of mammals and birds caused by parasitic protozoa of the genus *Cryptosporidium*, which is usually transmitted to humans via farm animals. Ingestion of water or milk contaminated with infective oocysts results in severe diarrhea and abdominal cramps, caused by release of a toxin. Most patients recover in 7–14 days, but the disease can persist in the immunocompromised (including AIDS patients), the elderly, and young children.

CSF 1. *see* cerebrospinal fluid. **2.** *see* colony-stimulating factor.

CS gas a powerful incapacitating gas used in warfare and riot control. The person exposed experiences a burning sensation in the eyes, difficulty in breathing, tightness of the chest, nausea, vomiting, and tears streaming from the eyes and nose. In confined spaces the gas can prove fatal.

CT *see* computed tomography.

cubital *adj.* relating to the elbow or forearm; for example the *cubital fossa* is the depression at the front of the elbow.

cuboid bone the outer bone of the *tarsus in the ankle, which articulates with the fourth and fifth metatarsal bones in front and with the calcaneus (heel bone) behind.

cuirass respirator *see* respirator.

culdocentesis *n. see* colpotomy.

culdoscope *n.* a tubular instrument with lenses and a light source, used for direct observation of the uterus, ovaries, and fallopian tubes (*culdoscopy*). The instrument is passed through the wall of the vagina behind the neck of the uterus. It has largely been replaced by the *laparoscope. *See also* endoscope.

Culex *n.* a genus of mosquitoes, worldwide in distribution, of which there are some 600 species. Certain species are important as vectors of filariasis (*see also* Wuchereria) and viral encephalitis.

culicide *n.* an agent that destroys mosquitoes or gnats.

Cullen's sign a bluish bruiselike appearance around the umbilicus, which is seen

in acute *pancreatitis. [T. S. Cullen (1868–1953), US gynecologist]

culmen *n.* an area of the upper surface of the *cerebellum of the brain, anterior to the decline and posterior to the central lobule and separated from them by deep fissures.

culture 1. *n.* a population of microorganisms, usually bacteria, grown in a solid or liquid laboratory medium (*culture medium*), which is usually *agar, broth, or *gelatin. A *pure culture* consists of a single bacterial species. A *stab culture* is a bacterial culture growing in a plug of solid medium within a bottle (or tube); the medium is inoculated by "stabbing" it with a bacteria-coated straight wire. A *stock culture* is a permanent bacterial culture, from which subcultures are made. *See also* tissue culture. **2.** *vb.* to grow bacteria or other microorganisms in cultures.

cumulative action the toxic effects of a drug produced by repeated administration of small doses at intervals that are not long enough for it to be either broken down or excreted by the body.

cumulus oophorus a cluster of follicle cells that surround a freshly ovulated ovum. By increasing the effective size of the ovum they may assist its entrance into the end of the fallopian tube. They are dispersed at fertilization by the contents of the *acrosome.

cuneiform bones three bones in the *tarsus of the ankle – the *lateral* (external), *intermediate* (middle), and *medial* (internal) cuneiform bones – that articulate respectively with the first, second, and third metatarsal bones in front. All three bones articulate with the navicular bone behind.

cuneus *n.* a wedge-shaped area of *cerebral cortex that forms the inner surface of the occipital lobe of the brain.

Cuniculus *n.* a genus of large forest-dwelling rodents, the pacas or spotted cavies, found in South and Central America. In Brazil these animals are a natural reservoir of the parasite *Leishmania braziliensis*, which causes espundia (*see* leishmaniasis).

cupola *n.* **1.** the small dome at the end of the cochlea of the inner ear. **2.** any of several dome-shaped anatomical structures.

cupping *n.* the former practice of applying

a heated cup to the skin and allowing it to cool, which causes swelling of the tissues beneath and an increase in the flow of blood in the area. This was thought to draw out harmful excess blood from diseased organs nearby and so promote healing. In *wet cupping* the skin was previously cut, so that blood would actually flow into the cup and could be removed.

cupula *n.* a small dome-shaped structure consisting of sensory hairs embedded in gelatinous material, forming part of a *crista in the ampullae of the semicircular canals of the ear.

curare *n.* an extract from the bark of South American trees (*Strychnos* and *Chondodendron* species) that relaxes and paralyses voluntary muscle. Used for centuries as an arrow poison by South American Indians, curare was formerly employed to control the muscle spasms of tetanus and as a muscle relaxant in surgical operations. It has now been replaced in surgery by *gallamine or other neuromuscular blocking agents.

curet *n.* a spoon-shaped instrument for scraping tissue from a cavity (*see* curettage, dilation and curettage).

curettage (curettement) *n.* the scraping of the skin or the internal surface of an organ or body cavity by means of a spoon-shaped instrument (*curet*), usually to remove diseased tissue or to obtain a specimen for diagnostic purposes (*see also* dilation and curettage). Curettage of the skin is combined with cauterization; it may be used for the removal of *basal cell carcinoma or seborrheic *keratoses, and usually causes little scarring.

curie *n.* a former unit for expressing the activity of a radioactive substance. It has been replaced by the *becquerel. Symbol: Ci.

Curling's ulcer a gastric or duodenal ulcer associated with stress from severe injury or major burns. [T. B. Curling (1811–88), British surgeon]

Curschmann's spirals elongated *casts of the smaller bronchi, which are coughed up in bronchial asthma. They unroll to a length of 2 cm or more and have a central core ensheathed in mucus and cell debris. [H. Curschmann (1846–1910), German physician]

Cushing's syndrome the condition resulting from excess amounts of *corticosteroid hormones in the body. Symptoms include weight gain, reddening of the face and neck, excess growth of body and facial hair, raised blood pressure, loss of mineral from the bones (osteoporosis), raised blood glucose levels, and sometimes mental disturbances. The syndrome may be due to overstimulation of the adrenal glands by excessive amounts of the hormone ACTH, secreted either by a tumor of the pituitary gland (*Cushing's disease*) or by a malignant tumor in the lung or elsewhere. Other causes include a benign or malignant tumor of the adrenal gland(s) resulting in excess activity of the gland and prolonged therapy with high doses of corticosteroid drugs (such as prednisone). [H. W. Cushing (1869–1939), US surgeon]

cusp *n.* **1.** any of the cone-shaped prominences on teeth, especially the molars and premolars. **2.** a pocket or fold of the membrane (endocardium) lining the heart or of the layer of the wall of a vein, several of which form a *valve. When the blood flows backward the cusps fill up and become distended, so closing the valve.

cutaneous *adj.* relating to the skin.

cuticle *n.* **1.** the *epidermis of the skin. **2.** a layer of solid or semisolid material that is secreted by and covers an *epithelium. **3.** a layer of cells, such as the outer layer of cells in a hair.

cutis *n. see* skin.

CVP *see* central venous pressure.

CVS *see* chorionic villus sampling.

cyan- (cyano-) *prefix denoting* blue.

cyanide *n.* any of the notoriously poisonous salts of hydrocyanic acid. Cyanides combine with and render inactive the enzymes of the tissues responsible for cellular respiration, and therefore they kill extremely quickly; unconsciousness is followed by convulsions and death. Hydrogen cyanide vapor is fatal in less than a minute when inhaled. Sodium or potassium cyanide taken by mouth may also kill within minutes. Prompt treatment with amyl nitrite and sodium thiosulfate or dicobalt edetate may save life. Cyanides give off a smell of bitter almonds.

cyanocobalamin *n. see* vitamin B_{12}.

cyanopsia *n.* a condition in which everything looks bluish.

cyanosis *n.* a bluish discoloration of the skin and mucous membranes resulting from an inadequate amount of oxygen in the blood. Cyanosis is associated with heart failure, lung diseases, the breathing of oxygen-deficient atmospheres, and asphyxia. Cyanosis is also seen in *blue babies, because of congenital heart defects. —**cyanotic** *adj.*

cybernetics *n.* the science of communication processes and automatic control systems in both machines and living things: a study linking the working of the brain and nervous system with the functioning of computers and automated feedback devices. *See also* bionics.

cycl- (cyclo-) *prefix denoting* **1.** cycle or cyclic. **2.** the ciliary body. Example: *cyclectomy* (excision of).

cyclamate *n.* either of two compounds, sodium or calcium cyclamate, that are 30 times as sweet as sugar and, unlike saccharin, stable to heat. Cyclamates were used as sweetening agents in the food industry until 1969, when their use was banned because they were suspected of causing cancer.

cyclandelate *n.* a *vasodilator drug used to improve circulation in cerebrovascular disease and other conditions in which blood flow is reduced. It is administered by mouth; side effects are rare but high doses sometimes cause nausea, digestive upsets, and flushing. Trade name: **Cyclospasmol**.

cyclitis *n.* inflammation of the *ciliary body of the eye (*see* uveitis). *See also* Fuchs' heterochromic cyclitis.

cyclizine *n.* a drug with *antihistamine properties, used to prevent and relieve nausea and vomiting in motion sickness, vertigo, disorders of the inner ear, and postoperative sickness. It is administered by mouth; common side effects are drowsiness and dizziness. Trade name: **Marezine**.

cycloablation *n.* the destruction of part of the *ciliary body of the eye to reduce the production of aqueous humor and hence reduce intraocular pressure. This technique is used in the treatment of advanced glaucoma resistant to other forms of treatment.

cyclobarbital *n.* a *barbiturate drug used as a hypnotic and sedative in cases of insomnia and anxiety. It is administered by mouth. Because prolonged use can cause *dependence, it is used only in special situations. Trade name: **Phanodorn**.

cyclobenzaprine *n.* a skeletal muscle relaxant used in the treatment of muscle spasms in conjunction with rest and physical therapy. It is administered by mouth; the most common side effects are drowsiness, dry mouth, and dizziness. Trade name: **Flexeril**.

cyclocryotherapy *n.* the destruction of part of the *ciliary body (*see* cycloablation) by freezing. It is used to reduce intraocular pressure in the control of glaucoma.

cyclodialysis *n.* an operation for *glaucoma in which part of the *ciliary body is separated from its attachment to the sclera, producing a cleft between the two. The aqueous humor comes into contact with the exposed surface of the ciliary body and some of it is absorbed from this surface. The pressure within the eye will be reduced if this absorption adds significantly to the drainage of fluid from the eye. Separation may also result from trauma.

cyclopentolate *n.* a drug, similar to *atropine, that is used in eye drops to paralyze the ciliary muscles and dilate the pupil for eye examinations and to treat some types of eye inflammation. Trade names: **Cyclogyl, Cylate, Pentolair**.

cyclophoria *n.* a type of squint (*see* strabismus) in which the eye tends to rotate slightly clockwise or counterclockwise.

cyclophosphamide *n.* an *alkylating agent used to treat a variety of cancers, often in combination with other *cytotoxic drugs. It also has *immunosuppressant properties and is used to prevent transplant rejection and in other conditions requiring reduced immune response, notably rheumatoid arthritis. Cyclophosphamide is administered by mouth or by injection; common side effects are nausea, vomiting, and – particularly at high doses – hair loss. Trade names: **Cytoxan, Neosar**.

cyclophotocoagulation *n.* the use of light or lasers to destroy the *ciliary body of the eye in order to reduce production of aqueous humor and hence reduce intraocular pressure. It is used in the treatment of glaucoma.

cycloplegia *n.* paralysis of the ciliary muscle of the eye (*see* ciliary body). This causes inability to alter the focus of the eye and is usually accompanied by paralysis of the muscles of the iris, resulting in fixed dilation of the pupil (*mydriasis*). It is induced by the use of atropine or similar drugs in order to inactivate the muscle in cases of inflammation of the iris and ciliary body. It may also occur after injuries to the eye.

cycloserine *n.* an *antibiotic, active against a wide range of bacteria, used as supporting treatment in tuberculosis and in some infections of the urinary tract. Cycloserine is administered by mouth; side effects, which can be severe, include dizziness, drowsiness, convulsions, and mental confusion. Trade name: **Seromycin**.

cyclosporine *n.* an *immunosuppressant drug used to prevent and treat rejection of a transplanted organ or bone marrow. It is also used to treat rheumatoid arthritis, psoriasis, and atopic eczema. Cyclosporine is administered orally or by intravenous infusion; side effects include nausea, gum swelling, tremor, excessive hair growth, hypertension, and kidney impairment. Trade names: **Gengraf, Neoral, Sandimmune, SangCya**.

cyclothymia *n.* the occurrence of marked swings of mood from cheerfulness to misery. These fluctuations are not as great as those of *manic-depressive psychosis. They usually represent a personality disorder, for which *psychotherapy is sometimes helpful.

cyclotron *n.* a machine in which charged particles following a spiral path within a magnetic field are accelerated by an alternating electric field. It produces very high-energy electromagnetic radiation, which has been used in the treatment of certain cancers, particularly of the eye. It is now little used on account of severe adverse effects on the tissues following treatment. Cyclotrons are now being used to manufacture short-lived radioactive isotopes for nuclear medicine scanning (*see* positron emission tomography).

cyesis *n.* see pregnancy.

cyn- (cyno-) *prefix denoting* a dog or dogs. Example: *cynophobia* (morbid fear of).

cyproheptadine *n.* a potent *antihistamine administered by mouth to treat allergies and itching skin conditions and to stimulate the appetite. It also inhibits the effects of *serotonin and is used to prevent migraine attacks. Drowsiness is a common side effect. Trade name: **Periactin**.

cyproterone acetate a steroid drug that inhibits the effects of male sex hormones (*see* antiandrogen) and is used to treat various sexual disorders and advanced prostate cancer in men. It is administered by mouth and common side effects include tiredness, loss of strength, inhibition of sperm formation, infertility, and breast enlargement (gynecomastia).

cyrtometer *n.* a device for measuring the shape of the chest and its movements during breathing.

cyst *n.* **1.** an abnormal sac or closed cavity lined with *epithelium and filled with liquid or semisolid matter. There are many varieties of cysts occurring in different parts of the body. *Retention cysts* arise when the outlet of a glandular duct is blocked, as in *sebaceous cysts. Some cysts are congenital, due to abnormal embryonic development; for example, *dermoid cysts. Others are tumors containing cells that secrete mucus or other substances, and another type of cyst is formed by parasites in the body (*see* hydatid). Cysts may occur in the jaws: a *dental cyst* occurs at the apex of a tooth, a *dentigerous cyst* occurs around the crown of an unerupted tooth, and an *eruption cyst* forms over an erupting tooth. *See also* fimbrial cyst, ovarian cyst. **2.** a dormant stage produced during the life cycle of certain protozoan parasites of the alimentary canal, including *Giardia and *Entamoeba. Cysts, passed out in the feces, have tough outer coats that protect the parasites from unfavorable conditions. The parasites emerge from their cysts when they are eaten by a new host. **3.** a structure formed by and surrounding the larvae of certain parasitic worms.

cyst- (cysto-) *prefix denoting* **1.** a bladder, especially the urinary bladder. Example: *cystoplasty* (plastic surgery of). **2.** a cyst.

cystadenoma *n.* an *adenoma showing a cystic structure.

cystalgia *n.* pain in the urinary bladder. This is common in *cystitis and when there are stones in the bladder and is occasionally present in bladder cancer. Treatment is directed to the underlying cause.

cystectomy *n.* surgical removal of the urinary bladder. This is necessary in the treatment of certain bladder conditions, notably cancer, and necessitates subsequent *urinary diversion. The ureters that drain the urine from the kidneys are reimplanted into the colon (*see* ureterosigmoidostomy) or into an isolated segment of intestine (usually the ileum), which is brought to the skin surface as a spout (*see* ileal conduit). Alternatively, in *bladder replacement*, a segment of ileum or colon is reconstructed to form a pouch, which is anastomosed to the urethra and acts as a reservoir for the urine. Emptying may be achieved by abdominal straining or *intermittent self-catheterization.

cysteine *n.* a sulfur-containing *amino acid that is an important constituent of many enzymes. The disulfide (S–S) links between adjacent cysteine molecules in polypeptide chains contribute to the three-dimensional molecular structure of proteins.

cystic *adj.* **1.** of, relating to, or characterized by cysts. **2.** of or relating to the gallbladder or urinary bladder.

cystic duct *see* bile duct.

cysticercosis *n.* a disease caused by the presence of tapeworm larvae (*see* cysticercus) of the species *Taenia solium* in any of the body tissues. Humans become infected by ingesting tapeworm eggs in contaminated food or drink. The presence of cysticerci in the muscles causes pain and weakness; in the brain the symptoms are more serious and include mental deterioration, paralysis, giddiness, epileptic attacks, and convulsions, which may be fatal. There is no specific treatment for this cosmopolitan disease, although surgical removal of cysticerci may be necessary to relieve pressure on the brain.

cysticercus (bladderworm) *n.* a larval stage of some *tapeworms in which the scolex and neck are invaginated into a large fluid-filled cyst. The cysts develop in the muscles or brain of the host following ingestion of tapeworm eggs. *See* cysticercosis.

cystic fibrosis (fibrocystic disease of the pancreas, mucoviscidosis) a hereditary disease that affects the exocrine glands (including mucus-secreting glands, sweat glands, and others). The faulty gene responsible has been identified as lying on chromosome no. 7 and is recessive, i.e.

both parents of the patient can be *carriers without being affected by the disease. Affected individuals lack a protein, *cystic fibrosis transmembrane regulator* (*CFTR*), that enables the transport of chloride ions across cell membranes; this results in the production of thick mucus, which obstructs the intestinal glands (causing meconium *ileus in newborn babies), pancreas (causing deficiency of pancreatic enzymes resulting in *malabsorption and *failure to thrive), and bronchi (causing *bronchiectasis). Respiratory infections, which may be severe, are a common complication. Common causative agents include *Haemophilus, *Pseudomonas, *Staphylococcus, and *Burkholderia cepacia*. The sweat contains excessive amounts of sodium and chloride, which is an aid to diagnosis. Treatment consists of minimizing the effects of the disease by administration of pancreatic enzymes and by bronchial physiotherapy, and by preventing and combating secondary infection. Sputum viscosity can be reduced by nebulized recombinant human *DNase. *Genetic counseling is essential, as each subsequent child of carrier parents has a one in four chance of being affected (*see also* mouthwash test). Some patients are benefiting from revolutionary new treatments, including transplantation of heart and lungs and treatment aimed at altering the genetic content of the faulty cells (*see* gene therapy).

cystine *n.* *see* amino acid.

cystinosis *n.* an inborn defect in the metabolism of amino acids, leading to abnormal accumulation of the amino acid cystine in the blood, kidneys, and lymphatic system. *See also* Fanconi's syndrome.

cystinuria *n.* an *inborn error of metabolism resulting in excessive excretion of the amino acid cystine in the urine due to a defect of reabsorption by the kidney tubules. It leads to the formation of cystine stones in the kidney.

cystitis *n.* inflammation of the urinary bladder, often caused by infection (most commonly by the bacterium *Escherichia coli*). It is usually accompanied by the desire to pass urine frequently, with a degree of burning. More severe attacks are often associated with the painful passage of blood in the urine, accompanied by a cramplike pain in the lower abdomen persisting after the bladder has been emptied. An acute attack is treated by antibiotic administration and a copious fluid intake. *See also* interstitial cystitis.

cystitome *n.* a small knife with a tiny curved or hooked blade, used to cut the lens capsule in the type of operation for cataract in which the capsule is left behind (*extracapsular cataract extraction*). *See also* capsulotomy.

cystocele *n.* prolapse of the base of the bladder in women. It is usually due to weakness of the pelvic floor after childbirth and causes bulging of the anterior wall of the vagina on straining. When accompanied by stress incontinence of urine, surgical repair (anterior *colporrhaphy) is indicated.

cystography *n.* X-ray examination of the urinary bladder after the injection of a contrast medium. The X-ray images thus obtained are known as *cystograms*. Cystography is most commonly performed to detect reflux of urine from the bladder to the ureters, usually in children (*see* vesicoureteric reflux). If films are taken during voiding, then the urethra can be observed (*see* urethrography). The examination can also be performed in conjunction with manometry (*see* bladder pressure study).

cystoid macular edema swelling of the central area of the retina (macula), usually occurring as a result of trauma or ocular surgery.

cystolithiasis *n.* the presence of stones (calculi) in the urinary bladder. The stones are either formed in the bladder, due to obstruction, urinary retention, or infection (*primary calculi*), or pass to the bladder after being formed in the kidneys (*secondary calculi*). They cause pain, the passage of bloody urine, and interruption of the urinary stream and should be removed surgically. *See* calculus.

cystometer *n.* an apparatus for measuring the pressure within the bladder. Modern investigations also include measurement of urine flow, and the resultant bladder pressure/flow study (*urodynamic investigation*) provides useful information regarding bladder function.

cystopexy (vesicofixation) *n.* a surgical operation to fix the urinary bladder (or a portion of it) in a different position. It may be performed as part of the repair or correction of a prolapsed bladder.

cystoplasty *n.* the operation of enlarging the capacity of the bladder by incorporating a segment of bowel. In a *clam cystoplasty*, the bladder is cut across longitudinally from one side of the neck to the other side through the dome (fundus) of the bladder and a length of ileum or colon is inserted as a patch. In the operation of *ileocecocystoplasty*, the dome is removed by cutting across the bladder transversely or sagittally above the openings of the ureters; it is replaced by an isolated segment of cecum and terminal ileum. In *ileocystoplasty* the bladder is enlarged by an opened-out portion of small intestine. The bladder may be replaced by a reservoir constructed from either small or large intestine (*see* cystectomy).

cystosarcoma phylloides a malignant tumor of the connective tissue of the breast: it accounts for approximately 1% of all breast cancers. Such tumors may show a wide variation in cell structure and are often a large mass without distant spread. The best treatment for a localized tumor is simple *mastectomy.

cystoscopy *n.* examination of the bladder by means of an instrument (*cystoscope*) inserted via the urethra. The cystoscope consists of either a metal sheath surrounding a telescope and light-conducting bundles or a flexible tube with built-in optical fibers for viewing and illumination. Irrigating fluid is conducted through a channel into the bladder. When using the rigid instrument, additional channels are available for the catheters to be inserted into the ureters, diathermy electrodes for removing polyps, or biopsy forceps for taking specimens of tumors or other growths. When using the flexible cystoscope, only small instruments can be passed through the additional channel, such as biopsy forceps, diathermy electrodes, or laser fibers for the destruction of tumors or stones.

cystostomy *n.* the operation of creating an artificial opening between the bladder and the anterior abdominal wall. This provides a temporary or permanent drainage route for urine.

cystotomy *n.* surgical incision into the urinary bladder, usually by cutting through the abdominal wall above the pubic symphysis (*suprapubic cystotomy*). This is necessary for such operations as removing stones or tumors from the bladder and for gaining access to the prostate gland in the operation of transvesical *prostatectomy.

cyt- (cyto-) *prefix denoting* **1.** cell(s). **2.** cytoplasm.

cytarabine *n.* a *cytotoxic drug used to suppress the symptoms of some types of leukemia. It is administered by injection and can damage the normal bone marrow, leading to various blood cell disorders. Other side effects are nausea, vomiting, mouth ulcers, and diarrhea. Trade names: **Cytosar, Tarabine.**

-cyte *suffix denoting* a cell. Examples: *chondrocyte* (cartilage cell); *osteocyte* (bone cell).

cytidine *n.* a compound containing cytosine and the sugar ribose. *See also* nucleoside.

cytochemistry *n.* the study of chemical compounds and their activities in living cells.

cytochrome *n.* a compound consisting of a protein linked to *heme. Cytochromes act as electron transfer agents in biological oxidation-reduction reactions, particularly those associated with the mitochondria in cellular respiration. *See* electron transport chain.

cytogenetics *n.* a science that links the study of inheritance (genetics) with that of cells (cytology); it is concerned mainly with the study of the *chromosomes, especially their origin, structure, and functions.

cytokines *pl. n.* protein molecules, released by cells when activated by antigen, that are involved in cell-to-cell communications, acting as enhancing mediators for immune responses through interaction with specific cell-surface receptors on leukocytes. Kinds of cytokines include *interleukins (produced by leukocytes), *lymphokines (produced by lymphocytes), *interferons, and *tumor necrosis factor.

cytokinesis *n.* division of the cytoplasm of a cell, which occurs at the end of cell division, after division of the nucleus, to form two daughter cells. *Compare* karyokinesis.

cytology *n.* the study of the structure and function of cells. The examination of cells under a microscope is used in the diagnosis of various diseases. These cells are obtained by scraping an organ, as in *cervical cytology* (*see* cervical smear), by aspiration (*see* fine-needle aspiration cytology), or they are collected from cells already shed (*exfoliative cytology*). *See also* biopsy. —**cytological** *adj.*

cytolysis *n.* the breakdown of cells, particularly by destruction of their outer membranes.

cytomegalovirus (CMV) *n.* a member of the herpes group of viruses (*see* herpesvirus). It commonly occurs in humans and normally produces symptoms that are milder than those of the common cold. However, in individuals whose immune systems are compromised (e.g. by cancer or AIDS) it can cause more severe effects, and it has been found to be the cause of congenital defects in infants born to women who have contracted the virus during pregnancy.

cytometer *n.* an instrument for determining the number of cells in a given quantity of fluid, such as blood, cerebrospinal fluid, or urine. *See* hemocytometer.

cytomorphosis *n.* the changes undergone by a cell in the course of its life cycle.

cytopenia *n.* a deficiency of one or more of the various types of blood cells. *See* eosinopenia, erythropenia, lymphopenia, neutropenia, pancytopenia, thrombocytopenia.

cytophotometry *n.* the study of chemical compounds in living cells by means of a *cytophotometer*, an instrument that is used to measure light intensity through stained areas of cytoplasm.

cytoplasm *n.* the jellylike substance that surrounds the nucleus of a cell. *See also* ectoplasm, endoplasm. —**cytoplasmic** *adj.*

cytoplasmic inheritance the inheritance of characteristics controlled by factors present in the cell cytoplasm rather than by genes on the chromosomes in the cell nucleus. An example of cytoplasmic inheritance is that controlled by mitochondrial genes (*see* mitochondrion).

cytosine *n.* one of the nitrogen-containing bases (*see* pyrimidine) that occurs in the nucleic acid DNA.

cytosome *n.* the part of a cell that is outside the nucleus.

cytotoxic drug any drug that damages or

destroys cells: usually refers to those drugs used to treat various types of cancer. There are various classes of cytotoxic drugs, including *alkylating agents (e.g. *chlorambucil, *cyclophosphamide, *melphalan), *antimetabolites (e.g. *fluorouracil, *methotrexate, *mercaptopurine), *anthracycline antibiotics (e.g. *doxorubicin, *daunorubicin, *dactinomycin), *vinca alkaloids, and platinum compounds (e.g. *carboplatin, *cisplatin). (See also taxane, topoisomerase inhibitor.) These drugs offer successful treatment in some conditions and help reduce symptoms and prolong life in others. Cytotoxic drugs destroy cancer cells by interfering with cell division, but they also affect normal cells, causing side effects, particularly in bone marrow, skin, stomach lining, and fetal tissue; dosage must therefore be carefully controlled. See also chemotherapy.

cytotoxic T cell a type of T *lymphocyte that destroys cancerous cells, virus-infected cells, and *allografts. Cytotoxic T cells recognize peptide antigens attached to proteins that are encoded by the *HLA system.

cytotrophoblast n. the part of a *trophoblast that retains its cellular structure and does not invade the maternal tissues. It forms the outer surface of the *chorion.

D

DA see developmental age.

dacarbazine n. a drug used in the treatment of such cancers as *Hodgkin's disease and malignant melanoma. It is administered by intravenous injection. Side effects include severe vomiting. Trade name: **DTIC-Dome**.

dacry- (dacryo-) prefix denoting 1. tears. 2. the lacrimal apparatus.

dacryoadenitis n. inflammation of the tear-producing gland (see lacrimal apparatus). It usually occurs only in people who are in generally poor health.

dacryocystitis n. inflammation of the lacrimal sac (in which tears collect), usually occurring when the duct draining the tears into the nose is blocked (see lacrimal apparatus).

dacryocystorhinostomy n. an operation to relieve blockage of the nasolacrimal duct (which drains tears into the nose), in which a communication is made between the lacrimal sac and the nose by removing the intervening bone. See dacryocystitis, lacrimal apparatus.

dacryops n. Obsolete. a watering eye.

dactinomycin n. a cytotoxic drug, formerly known as actinomycin D, used in the treatment of cancer in children, particularly nephroblastoma. It is administered by intravenous injection. Side effects include nausea, vomiting, blood disorders, and bone marrow damage. Trade name: **Cosmegen**.

dactyl- prefix denoting the digits (fingers or toes). Examples: dactylomegaly (abnormally large); dactylospasm (painful contraction of).

dactylitis n. inflammation of a finger or toe caused by bone infection (as in tuberculous *osteomyelitis) or rheumatic disease, or seen in infants with sickle-cell disease.

dactylology n. the use of finger and hand movements as a means of communication with persons who are deaf and mute.

dalteparin n. a *low molecular weight heparin that is used to prevent deep vein thrombosis and pulmonary embolism in patients undergoing abdominal or hip replacement surgery who are at risk for clotting. It is also used for the prevention of ischemic complications in unstable *coronary artery disease, when concurrently administered with aspirin therapy. The drug is administered intramuscularly; the most common side effect is *hematoma at the injection site. Trade name: **Fragmin**.

Daltonism (protanopia) n. red blindness: a defect in color vision in which a person cannot distinguish between reds and greens. The term has been used to refer to *color blindness in general. [J. Dalton (1766–1844), British chemist]

damp n. (in mining) any gas encountered underground other than air. See blackdamp, firedamp.

danazol n. a synthetic *progestogen that inhibits the secretion by the pituitary gland of gonadotrophins. It is used to treat precocious puberty, breast enlargement in males (gynecomastia), excessively heavy menstrual periods, and *endometriosis. It is administered by mouth. Possible side effects include nausea, swelling of the feet and ankles, weight gain, oiliness of the skin, and, in women, excessive growth of facial and body hair. Trade name: **Danocrine**.

D & C *see* dilation and curettage.

dandruff (scurf) *n.* a common condition in which the scalp is covered with small flakes of dead skin. The flakes, which come away when the hair is brushed or combed, represent an increase in the normal loss of the outermost skin layer. Some types of dandruff, which is associated with the presence of the yeast *Malassezia furfur*, are accompanied by inflammation of the scalp to give a type of seborrheic dermatitis (*see* eczema). If too little sebum is produced, the hair becomes dry and brittle, with the formation of white skin flakes; too much sebum gives greasy hair and yellow flakes. Treatment is by regular washing with a shampoo containing tar, selenium sulfide, zinc pyrithione, or imidazole antifungals. Medical name: **pityriasis capitis**.

Dandy-Walker syndrome a form of *cerebral palsy in which the *cerebellum is usually the part of the brain affected. It leads to unsteadiness of balance and an abnormal gait and may be associated with *hydrocephalus. [W. E. Dandy (1886–1946) and A. E. Walker (1907–95), US surgeons]

dangerous drugs *see* Harrison Antinarcotic Act.

dantrolene *n.* a *muscle relaxant drug used to relieve muscle spasm in such conditions as cerebral palsy, multiple sclerosis, or spinal cord injury. It is administered by mouth or by injection. Possible side effects include weakness, dizziness, drowsiness, and vertigo; liver damage sometimes occurs. Trade name: **Dantrium**.

dapsone *n.* a drug (*see* sulfone) used to treat *leprosy and some types of dermatitis. It is administered by mouth or injection; the most common side effects are allergic skin reactions.

dark adaptation the changes that take place in the retina and pupil of the eye enabling vision in very dim light. Dark adaptation involves activation of the *rods – the cells of the retina that function best in dim light – and the reflex enlargement of the pupil (*see* pupillary reflex). *Compare* light adaptation.

daunorubicin *n.* an *anthracycline antibiotic that interferes with DNA synthesis and is used, in combination with other drugs, in the treatment of acute leukemia. It is administered by intravenous injection. Possible side effects include loss of hair and damage to bone marrow and heart muscle. Trade name: **Cerubidine**.

DAWN (Drug Abuse Warning Network) *n.* a national surveillance system that monitors trends in drug-related emergency department visits and deaths. It is operated by the *Substance Abuse and Mental Health Services Administration (SAMHSA) of the US *Department of Health and Human Services. SAMHSA is required to collect data for DAWN under the Public Health Service Act.

dawn phenomenon (Somogyi phenomenon) the phenomenon of high fasting blood-sugar levels in the morning due to an unrecognized hypoglycemic episode during the night in a person with diabetes. The low blood sugar has resulted in an outpouring of regulatory hormones, such as epinephrine and glucagon, which have raised the blood sugar to supranormal levels by the time of waking. It is important to recognize the cause, since increasing the evening insulin dose, thinking this will bring the morning sugars down, could actually cause a more severe nocturnal hypoglycemic attack, which the body may not be able to counteract: coma might ensue. The condition can be tested for by measuring blood sugars at the time of the assumed low level.

day blindness comparatively good vision in poor light but poor vision in good illumination. The condition is usually congenital and associated with poor visual acuity and defective color vision. Acquired cases occur when the *cones (light-sensitive cells) at the back of the retina are selectively destroyed by disease. Medical name: **hemeralopia**. *Compare* night blindness.

day treatment a system of therapy, usually offered by psychiatric hospitals or psychiatric units of general hospitals, in which the patient spends most of the day in structured activities (such as psychotherapy) or medical treatment but returns home in the evening. Day treatment is intended as a transition service between inpatient and outpatient care. Day-treatment care has increased by nearly tenfold in the US since the 1960s, most of the growth of facilities occurring in urban areas where travel distance between home and treatment center is relatively short.

DCIS *see* ductal carcinoma in situ.

DDST *see* Denver Development Screening Test.

DDT (chlorophenothane, dicophane) *n.* a powerful insecticide that was formerly in wide use for many years against lice, fleas, flies, bedbugs, cockroaches, and other destructive and disease-carrying insects. It is a relatively stable compound that is stored in animal fats, and the quantities now present in the environment – in the form of stores accumulated in animal tissues – have led to its being restricted. Acute poisoning, from swallowing more than 20 g, produces nervous irritability, muscle twitching, convulsions, and coma, but only a few fatalities have been reported.

de- *prefix denoting* **1.** removal or loss. Examples: *demineralization* (of minerals from bones or teeth); *devascularization* (of blood supply). **2.** reversal.

DEA *see* Drug Enforcement Agency.

deactivation *n.* the process by which a substance is made inactive or a reaction is stopped through chemical or physical means. *See also* inactivate. —**deactivate** *vb.*

deafness *n.* partial or total loss of hearing in one or both ears. *Conductive deafness* is due to a defect in the conduction of sound from the external ear to the internal ear, most commonly an infection affecting the small bones (*ossicles*) in the middle ear (*otitis media) but also caused by an abnormal condition of the inner ear (*see* otosclerosis) that affects the conduction of sound. *Sensorineural* (or *perceptive*) *deafness* is due to a lesion of the *cochlea in the inner ear, the auditory nerve, or the auditory centers in the brain. It may be present from birth (for example if the mother was affected with German measles during pregnancy). In adults it may be brought on by injury, disease (e.g. *Ménière's disease), or prolonged exposure to loud noises; progressive sensorineural deaf-

ness (*presbyacusis*) is common with advancing age.

The type of deafness can be diagnosed by a number of hearing tests (*see* Rinne's test, Weber's test, audiogram), and the treatment depends on the cause. *See also* cochlear implant, hearing aid.

deamination *n.* a process, occurring in the liver, that occurs during the metabolism of amino acids. The amino group $(-NH_2)$ is removed from an amino acid and converted to ammonia, which is ultimately converted to *urea and excreted.

death *n.* absence of vital functions. Death is traditionally defined as permanent cessation of the heartbeat. *Brain death* is defined as permanent functional death of the centers in the brainstem that control the breathing, pupillary, and other vital reflexes. Usually two independent medical opinions are required before brain death is agreed, but organs such as kidneys may then legally be removed for transplantation surgery before the heart has stopped.

death certificate a medical certificate stating the cause of a person's death, usually also stating the deceased's marital status, occupation, and age. A doctor's diagnosis of the main cause of death, and any contributory causes of death, and his signature are recorded. Death certificates are required by law in the majority of countries throughout the world.

debridement *n.* the process of cleaning an open wound by removal of foreign material and dead tissue, so that healing may occur without hindrance.

dec- (deca-) *prefix denoting* ten.

decalcification *n.* loss or removal of calcium salts from a bone or tooth.

decapitation *n.* removal of the head, usually the head of a dead fetus to enable delivery to take place. This procedure is very rare nowadays, being undertaken only in dire circumstances when the fetal head is too large to pass through the birth canal, the mother's life is endangered, and cesarean section impossible.

decapsulation *n. see* decortication.

decay *n.* (in bacteriology) the decomposition of organic matter due to microbial action.

decerebrate *adj.* denoting a neurological state in which the functions of the higher centers of the brain are eliminated. This is brought about in experimental animals by cutting across the brain below the cerebrum, but certain injuries to the brain in humans may cause the same severe neurological signs as occur in a decerebrate animal.

deci- *prefix denoting* a tenth.

decibel (db) *n.* one tenth of a bel: a unit for comparing levels of power (especially sound) on a logarithmic scale. A power source of intensity P has a power level of $10 \log_{10} P/P_0$ decibels, where P_0 is the intensity of a reference source. The decibel is much more widely used than the bel. Silence is 0 db; a whisper has an intensity of 30 db, normal speech 60 db, heavy traffic 80–90 db, and a jet aircraft 120 db.

decidua *n.* the modified mucous membrane that lines the wall of the uterus during pregnancy and is shed with the afterbirth at parturition (*see* endometrium). There are three regions: the *decidua capsularis*, a thin layer that covers the embryo; the *decidua basalis*, where the embryo is attached; and the *decidua parietalis*, which is not in contact with the embryo. —**decidual** *adj.*

deciduoma *n.* a mass of tissue within the uterus derived from remnants of *decidua. See also* chorionepithelioma (malignant deciduoma).

deciduous teeth the primary teeth, which develop in infancy and are shed just before eruption of their permanent successors. In the absence of permanent successors they can remain functional for many years. *See* dentition.

declive *n.* an area of the upper surface of the *cerebellum, posterior to the culmen and anterior to the folium of the middle lobe.

decomposition *n.* the gradual disintegration of dead organic matter, usually foodstuffs or tissues, by the chemical action of bacteria or fungi.

decompression *n.* **1.** the reduction of pressure on an organ or part of the body by surgical intervention. Surgical decompression can be effected at many sites: the pressure of tissues on a nerve may be relieved by incision; raised pressure in the fluid of the brain can be lowered by cutting into the *dura mater; and cardiac compression – the abnormal presence of blood or fluid around the heart – can be cured by cutting the sac (pericardium)

enclosing the heart. **2.** the gradual reduction of atmospheric pressure for deep-sea divers, who work at artificially high pressures. *See* compressed air illness.

decompression sickness *see* compressed air illness.

decongestant *n.* an agent that reduces or relieves nasal congestion. Most nasal decongestants are *sympathomimetic drugs, applied either locally, in the form of nasal sprays or drops, or taken by mouth.

decortication *n.* **1.** the removal of the outside layer (cortex) from an organ or structure, such as the kidney. **2.** an operation for removing the blood clot and scar tissue that forms after bleeding into the chest cavity (hemothorax). **3.** (**decapsulation**) the surgical removal of a *capsule from an organ; for example, the stripping of the membrane that envelops the kidney or of the inflammatory capsule that encloses a chronic abscess, as in the treatment of *empyema.

decubitus *n.* the recumbent position.

decubitus ulcer *see* bedsore.

decussation *n.* a point at which two or more structures of the body cross to the opposite side. The term is used particularly for the point at which nerve fibers cross over in the central nervous system.

deep vein thrombosis (DVT) *see* phlebothrombosis.

deer fly *see* Chrysops.

defecation *n.* a bowel movement in which feces are evacuated through the rectum and anus. The amount and composition of the food eaten determine to a large degree the bulk of the feces, and the transit time through the intestinal tract determines the water content. *See* constipation, diarrhea.

defense mechanism the means whereby an undesirable impulse can be avoided or controlled (*see* censor). Many defense mechanisms have been described, including *repression, *projection, *reaction formation, *sublimation, and *splitting. They may be partly responsible for such problems as tics, stammering, and phobias.

deferent *adj.* **1.** carrying away from or down from. **2.** relating to the vas deferens.

deferoxamine *n.* a drug that combines with

iron in body tissues and fluids and is used to treat iron poisoning (including that resulting from prolonged or constant blood transfusion, as for thalassemia), diseases involving iron storage in parts of the body (*see* hemochromatosis), and for the diagnosis of such diseases. It is administered by injection; reactions and pain sometimes occur on injection. Trade name: **Desferal**.

defervescence *n.* the disappearance of a fever, a process that may occur rapidly or take several days, depending upon the cause and treatment given.

defibrillation *n.* administration of a controlled electric shock to restore normal heart rhythm in cases of cardiac arrest due to ventricular *fibrillation. The apparatus used is a *defibrillator.

defibrillation gel pads thin pads of electrically conductive material placed between a patient's skin and the defibrillation paddles to aid the passage of electricity across the patient's chest and to lessen contact burns. There is one pad per paddle and the two pads must not touch during defibrillation or a short circuit will form between the paddles.

defibrillator *n.* the apparatus used for administering a measured electrical current to a patient's heart in *defibrillation. Several types of defibrillator exist, including those that are semi- or fully automated to recognize abnormal rhythms and to deliver the appropriate shock, those that are fully operator-dependent, and those that are implanted into the patient's body in a similar manner to a *pacemaker. Different types can deliver DC or AC currents.

defibrination *n.* the removal of *fibrin, one of the plasma proteins that causes coagulation, from a sample of blood. It is normally done by whisking the blood with a bundle of fine wires, to which the strands of fibrin that form in the blood adhere.

deficiency *n.* (in genetics) *see* deletion.

deficiency disease any disease caused by the lack of an essential nutrient in the diet. Such nutrients include *essential amino acids, *vitamins, and *essential fatty acids.

deflorescence *n.* a disappearance of a rash in those diseases in which a rash is a characteristic part of the illness.

deformity *n. see* malformation.

degeneration *n.* the deterioration and loss of specialized function of the cells of a tissue or organ. The changes may be caused by a defective blood supply or by disease. Degeneration may involve the deposition of calcium salts, fat (*see* fatty degeneration), or fibrous tissue in the affected organ or tissue. *See also* infiltration.

deglutition *n. see* swallowing.

dehiscence *n.* a splitting open, as of a surgical wound.

dehydration *n.* **1.** loss or deficiency of water in body tissues. The condition may result from inadequate water intake or from excessive removal of water from the body; for example, by sweating, vomiting, or diarrhea. Symptoms include great thirst, nausea, and exhaustion. The condition is treated by drinking plenty of water; severe cases require *oral rehydration therapy or intravenous administration of water and salts (which have been lost with the water). **2.** the removal of water from tissue during its preparation for microscopical study, by placing it successively in stronger solutions of ethyl alcohol. Dehydration follows *fixation and precedes *clearing.

dehydroepiandrosterone (DHEA) *n.* a weak androgen that is produced and secreted by the adrenal glands after the stage of adrenal maturation known as *adrenarche. It is produced from 17-hydroxypregnenolone and itself is largely converted to *dehydroepiandrosterone sulfate* and *androstenedione*. All three of these molecules can cause a degree of mild *androgenization but can also be converted in the circulation to the more potent androgens *testosterone and dihydrotestosterone.

dehydrogenase *n. see* oxidoreductase.

déjà vu a vivid psychic experience in which immediately contemporary events seem to be a repetition of previous happenings. It is a symptom of some forms of *epilepsy. *See also* jamais vu.

delavirdine *n.* a *reverse transcriptase inhibitor of the human immunodeficiency virus type 1 (*HIV-1), indicated for the treatment of HIV-1 infection in combination with at least two other active antiretroviral agents when therapy is warranted. This combination of agents blocks the replication of HIV and prevents healthy T cells from becoming infected with the virus. Delavirdine is administered orally; common side effects include rash, muscle and joint aches, oral lesions, headache, excessive tiredness, vomiting and diarrhea. Trade name: **Rescriptor**.

delayed suture (delayed primary closure) a technique used in the closure of contaminated wounds and wounds associated with tissue necrosis, such as are produced by missile injuries. The superficial layers of the wound are left open, to be closed later when the tissues have been cleaned.

deletion (deficiency) *n.* (in genetics) a type of mutation involving the loss of DNA. This may be small, affecting only a portion of a single gene, or large, resulting in loss of a part of a chromosome and affecting many genes.

Delhi boil *see* oriental sore.

delirium *n.* an acute disorder of the mental processes accompanying organic brain disease. It may be manifested by delusions, disorientation, hallucinations, or extreme excitement and occurs in metabolic disorders, intoxication, deficiency diseases, and infections.

delirium tremens a psychosis caused by *alcoholism, usually seen as a withdrawal syndrome in chronic alcoholics. Typically, it is precipitated by a head injury or an acute infection causing abstinence from alcohol. Features include anxiety, tremor, sweating, and vivid and terrifying visual and sensory hallucinations, often of animals and insects. Severe cases may end fatally.

delivery *n.* the birth of a child. *See* labor.

delle *n.* (*pl.* **dellen**) a localized area of reduced corneal thickness, usually at the limbus (the junction of the cornea with the sclera), due to local dehydration. It may occur after surgery to correct a squint, due to elevated conjunctiva at the limbus causing poor wetting of the adjacent cornea.

deltoid *n.* a thick triangular muscle that covers the shoulder joint (see illustration). It is responsible for raising the arm away from the side of the body.

delusion *n.* an irrationally held belief that cannot be altered by rational argument. In mental illness it is often a false belief that the individual is persecuted by others, is very powerful, is controlled by

others, or is a victim of physical disease (*see* paranoia). Delusions may be a symptom of *schizophrenia or other pschotic disorders.

demand-pull theory a theory used to explain increases in the cost of health care. It is based on the premise that rising incomes of patients and the growth of health insurance in the US results in greater purchasing power and, hence, demand for health care, which is in relatively limited supply. *Compare* labor cost-push theory.

demecarium *n.* a *miotic used in the treatment of *glaucoma and convergent *strabismus. It is administered topically as eye drops; common side effects include burning, stinging, redness, and other irritation of the eyes. Trade name: **Humorsol**.

demeclocycline *n.* an antibiotic that is active against a wide range of bacteria and is used to treat various infections. It is also used to treat *syndrome of inappropriate secretion of antidiuretic hormone. Demeclocycline is administered by mouth; common side effects are nausea, diarrhea, and symptoms resulting from the growth of organisms not sensitive to the drug. Trade name: **Declomycin**.

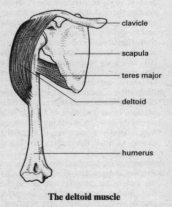

The deltoid muscle

dementia *n.* a chronic or persistent disorder of behavior and higher intellectual function due to organic brain disease. It is marked by memory disorders, changes in personality, deterioration in personal care, impaired reasoning ability, and disorientation. *Presenile dementia* occurs in young or middle-aged people. The most common causes of dementia are *Alzheimer's disease, frontotemporal dementia (e.g. *Pick's disease), and dementia due to diffuse *cortical Lewy body disease. Another common form, *multi-infarct dementia*, results from the destruction of brain tissue by a series of small strokes. It is important to distinguish these organic conditions from psychological disorders that cause the same symptoms (*see* pseudodementia).

demi- *prefix denoting* half.

Demodex *n.* a genus of harmless parasitic mites, the follicle mites, found in the hair follicles and associated sebaceous glands of the face. They resemble tiny worms, about 0.4 mm in length, and their presence may give rise to dermatitis.

demography *n.* the study of populations on a national, regional, or local basis in terms of age, sex, and other *variables, including patterns of migration and survival. It is used in public health medicine to help identify health needs and *risk factors. *See also* biostatistics.

De Morgan spots *see* angioma. [C. G. De Morgan (1811–76), British physician]

demulcent *n.* a soothing agent that protects the mucous membranes and relieves irritation. Demulcents form a protective film and are used in mouth washes, gargles, etc., to soothe irritation or inflammation in the mouth.

demyelination *n.* damage to the *myelin sheaths surrounding nerve fibers in the central or peripheral nervous systems. This in turn affects the function of the nerve fibers, which the myelin normally supports. Demyelination may be the primary disorder, as in *multiple sclerosis, or it may occur after head injury or stroke.

denaturation *n.* the changes in the physical and physiological properties of a protein that are brought about by heat, X-rays, or chemicals. These changes include loss of activity (in the case of enzymes) and loss (or alteration) of antigenicity (in the case of *antigens).

dendrite *n.* one of the shorter branching processes of the cell body of a *neuron, which makes contact with other neurons

at synapses and carries nerve impulses from them into the cell body.

dendritic cell a type of hemopoietic cell with specialized antigen-presenting functions. *See* APC.

dendritic ulcer a branching ulcer of the surface of the cornea caused by *herpes simplex virus. A similar appearance may be produced by a healing corneal abrasion. Dendritic ulcers tend to recur because the virus lies dormant in the tissues; years may elapse between attacks.

denervation *n.* interruption of the nerve supply to the muscles and skin. The muscle is paralyzed and its normal tone (elasticity) is lost. The muscle fibers shrink and are replaced by fat. A denervated area of skin loses all forms of sensation and its subsequent ability to heal and renew its tissues may be impaired.

dengue (breakbone fever) *n.* a disease caused by arboviruses and transmitted to humans principally by the mosquito *Aëdes aegypti*. Symptoms, which last for a few days, include severe pains in the joints and muscles, headache, sore throat, fever, running of the eyes, and an irritating rash. These symptoms recur in a usually milder form after an interval of two or three days. Death rarely occurs, but the patient is left debilitated and requires considerable convalescence. A more severe form, *dengue hemorrhagic fever*, characterized by a breakdown of the blood-clotting mechanism with internal bleeding, often occurs in epidemics and has a high mortality rate, especially in children. Dengue occurs throughout the tropics and subtropics. Patients are given aspirin and codeine to relieve the pain and calamine lotion is helpful in easing the irritating rash.

dens *n.* a tooth or tooth-shaped structure.

dens invaginatus literally, an infolded tooth: a specific type of tooth malformation that mainly affects upper lateral incisors to varying degrees.

dent- (denti-, dento-) *prefix denoting* the teeth. Example: *dentoalveolar* (relating to the teeth and associated jaw).

dental auxiliary any of several assistants to a dentist. A *dental hygienist* performs scaling and instruction in oral hygiene under the supervision of the dentist. A *dental surgery assistant* helps the dentist at the chairside by preparing materials, passing instruments, and aspirating fluids from the patient's mouth. A *dental technician* constructs dentures, crowns, and orthodontic appliances in the laboratory for the dentist.

dental caries decay and crumbling of the substance of a tooth. Dental caries is caused by the metabolism of the bacteria in *plaque attached to the surface of the tooth. Acid formed by bacterial breakdown of sugar in the diet causes demineralization of the enamel of the tooth. If left unrepaired it spreads into the dentine and progressively destroys the tooth completely, first exposing the deeper dentine, causing toothache, and eventually exposing the pulp to allow ingress of infection into the bone and abscess formation (*see* apical abscess). Frequent intake of sugar is a major cause, and the disease is more common in young people and has a predilection for specific sites. It can be most effectively prevented by restricting the frequency of sugar intake and avoiding sweet food and drinks at bedtime or during the night. The resistance of enamel to dental caries can be increased by the application of *fluoride salts to the tooth surface from toothpastes or mouth rinses. *Fluoridation of water also makes teeth resistant to caries during the period of tooth development. Once caries has spread into the dentine, repair consists of removing the decayed part of the tooth using a *drill and replacing it with a *filling.

dental floss fine thread, usually of nylon, used to clean some surfaces of teeth.

dental implant *see* implant.

dental nerve either of two nerves that supply the teeth; they are branches of the trigeminal nerve. The *inferior dental nerve* supplies the lower teeth and for most of its length exists as a single large bundle; thus anesthesia of it has a widespread effect (*see* inferior dental block). The *superior dental nerve*, which supplies the upper teeth, breaks into separate branches at some distance from the teeth and it is possible to anesthetize these individually with less widespread effect for the patient.

dental unit a major piece of dental equipment to which are attached the dental drills, aspirator, compressed air syringe,

and ultrasonic scaler. Frequently, the dental chair is attached to the unit.

dentate *adj.* **1.** having teeth. **2.** serrated; having toothlike projections.

dentifrice *n.* a paste or powder for cleaning the teeth. *See* toothpaste.

dentine (dentin) *n.* a hard tissue that forms the bulk of a tooth. The dentine of the crown is covered by enamel and that of the root by cementum. The dentine is permeated by fine tubules, which close to the center of the tooth contain cellular processes from the pulp. Exposed dentine is sensitive to touch, heat, and cold.

dentinogenesis *n.* the formation of *dentine by *odontoblasts. Although dentine continues to be formed throughout life, very little is formed later than a few years after tooth eruption unless it is stimulated by caries, abrasion, or trauma. *Dentinogenesis imperfecta* is a hereditary condition in which dentine formation is disturbed, resulting in loss of overlying enamel and excessive wear of the dentine.

dentist *n.* a member of the dental profession. To practice dentistry, a license must be obtained from a state board of dental examiners.

dentistry *n.* the study, management, and treatment of diseases and conditions affecting the mouth, jaws, teeth, and their supporting tissues. *See* endodontics, orthodontics, pedodontics, periodontics, preventive dentistry, prosthetic dentistry.

dentition *n.* the arrangement of teeth in the mouth. The *deciduous dentition* comprises the teeth of young children. It consists of 20 teeth, made up of incisors, canines, and molars only. The lower incisor erupts first at about 6 months of age, and all the deciduous teeth have usually erupted by the age of 2½ years. The lower incisors are shed first at about 6 years of age, and from this time until about 12 years old both deciduous and permanent teeth are present; i.e. there is a *mixed dentition*. The *permanent dentition* consists of up to 32 teeth, made up of incisors, canines, premolars, and molars. The first tooth to erupt is the first molar (at the age of 6 years) and most have appeared by the age of 14 years, although the third molars may not erupt

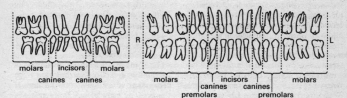

Deciduous dentition	Permanent dentition

until the age of 18–21 years. See illustrations.

denture (prosthesis) *n.* a removable replacement for one or more teeth carried on some type of plate or frame. A *complete denture* replaces all the teeth in one jaw. It is usually made entirely of acrylic resin. A *partial denture* replaces some teeth because others still remain. It is designed to restore function with the least potential damage to the remaining teeth. The framework of the denture base is often made of metal (*cobalt-chromium) because of its strength. *Denture sore mouth* is inflammation of the gum under the denture, caused by a mixed infection of *Candida* and bacteria under a poorly cleaned denture or removable orthodontic appliance. *Denture hyperplasia* is an overgrowth of fibrous tissue covered by mucous membrane, resulting from chronic irritation by a denture.

Denver Development Screening Test (DDST) a test for evaluating the *developmental age of infants and preschool children with regard to levels of motor, social, and language skills in comparison with the average performance of other children. The *Denver II*, released in 1990, is a major revision of the original DDST.

deodorant *n.* an agent that reduces or removes unpleasant body odors by destroying bacteria that live on the skin and break down sweat. Deodorant preparations often contain an antiseptic.

deontology *n.* the study of ethics and correct behavior or duty. In medicine this includes consideration of the proper behavior of a doctor toward his patient, whether a patient should be told if his condition is fatal or not, and similar problems for which there may be no written guidelines. The best-known code of conduct is the *Hippocratic oath.

deoxycholic acid *see* bile acids.

deoxycorticosterone *n.* a hormone, synthesized and released by the adrenal cortex, that regulates salt and water balance. *See also* corticosteroid.

deoxyribonuclease *n.* an enzyme, located in the *lysosomes of cells, that splits DNA at specific places in the molecule.

deoxyribonucleic acid *see* DNA.

Department of Health and Human Services (HHS) the major US Government agency providing health care. The Department was created in 1953 (then called Department of Health, Education and Welfare) to administer the functions of several previously separate agencies, including the Social Security Administration, Public Health Service, Food and Drug Administration, Office of Vocational Rehabilitation, and Office of Education. In 1980, the department was renamed and education was made a separate department. HHS administers more than 300 health or health-related programs, has more than 65,000 federal employees, and provides personal health-care services to more than 15% of the US population, not including *Medicare or *Medicaid beneficiaries. Medicare and Medicaid programs are administered through the Centers for Medicare and Medicaid Services. Other federal agencies with large budgets for health care are the Department of Defense, the Department of Veterans Affairs, the Department of Agriculture, and the Department of Labor.

dependence (drug dependence) *n.* the physical and/or psychological effects produced by the habitual taking of certain drugs, characterized by a compulsion to continue taking the drug. In *physical dependence* withdrawal of the drug causes specific symptoms (*with-*

drawal symptoms), such as sweating, vomiting, or tremors, that are reversed by further doses. Substances that may induce physical dependence include alcohol and the so-called "hard" drugs morphine, heroin, and cocaine. Dependence on these drugs carries a high mortality, partly because overdosage may be fatal and partly because their casual injection intravenously may lead to infections such as *hepatitis and *AIDS. Treatment is difficult and requires specialist skills. Much more common is *psychological dependence*, in which repeated use of a drug induces reliance on it for a state of well-being and contentment, but there are no physical withdrawal symptoms if use of the drug is stopped. Substances that may induce psychological dependence include cannabis and many "soft" drugs, such as barbiturates and amphetamines.

dependent practitioner a paraprofessional or subprofessional health-care worker who is allowed by laws or other regulations to provide a limited amount of treatment to a patient, usually under the supervision or direction of an independent practitioner, such as a physician. An example of a dependent practitioner would be a physician assistant, nurse practitioner, occupational therapist, or dental hygienist.

depersonalization *n.* a state in which a person feels himself becoming unreal or strangely altered, or feels that his mind is becoming separated from his body. Minor degrees of this feeling are common in normal people under stress. Severe feelings of depersonalization occur in anxiety neurosis, in states of *dissociation, in depression and schizophrenia, and in epilepsy (particularly temporal lobe epilepsy). *See also* derealization, out-of-the-body experience.

depilatory *n.* an agent applied to the skin to remove hair.

depolarization *n.* the sudden surge of charged particles across the membrane of a nerve or muscle cell that accompanies a physicochemical change in the membrane and cancels out, or reverses, its resting potential to produce an *action potential. The passage of a *nerve impulse is a rapid wave of depolarization along the membrane of a nerve fiber.

depot injection the administration of a sustained-action drug formulation that allows slow release and gradual absorption, so that the active agent can act for much longer periods than is possible with standard injections. Depot injections are usually given deep into a muscle; some contraceptive hormones are available in a depot formulation.

depressant *n.* an agent that reduces the normal activity of any body system or function. Drugs such as general *anesthetics, *barbiturates, and opiates are depressants of the central nervous system and respiration. *Cytotoxic drugs, such as azathioprine, are depressants of the levels of white blood cells.

depression *n.* a mental state characterized by excessive sadness. Activity can be agitated and restless or slow and retarded. Behavior is governed by pessimistic or despairing beliefs, and sleep, appetite, and concentration are disturbed. There are several causes. *Manic-depressive psychosis causes severe depression, a major *affective disorder, in which there may be delusions of being worthless, ill, wicked, or impoverished and hallucinations of accusing voices. Loss and frustration also cause depression, which may be prolonged and disproportionate in *dysthymic disorder*. Treatment is with *antidepressant drugs, *cognitive therapy, or *psychotherapy. Severe cases may need *electroconvulsive therapy. *See also* puerperal depression.

depressor *n.* **1.** a muscle that causes lowering of part of the body. The *depressor labii inferioris* is a muscle that draws down and everts the lower lip. **2.** a nerve that lowers blood pressure.

deprivation *n. see* sensory deprivation.

dequalinium *n.* an antiseptic, active against some bacteria and fungi, used as lozenges to treat mouth and throat infections.

derealization *n.* a feeling of unreality in which the environment is experienced as unreal and as flat, dull, or strange. The experience is unwelcome and often frightening. It occurs in association with *depersonalization or with the conditions that cause depersonalization.

dereism *n.* undirected fantasy thinking that fails to respect the realities of life. When this becomes markedly dominant it may be a feature of *schizoid personality or of *schizophrenia.

derm- (derma-, dermo-, dermat(o)-) *prefix denoting* the skin.

-derm *suffix denoting* **1.** the skin. **2.** a germ layer.

dermabrasion *n.* a method of removing superficial scars and blemishes from the skin by mechanical means, such as sandpaper or revolving wire brushes. *Compare* chemabrasion.

Dermacentor *n.* a genus of hard *ticks, worldwide in distribution, the adults of which are parasites of humans and other mammals. The wood tick, *D. andersoni*, transmits Rocky Mountain spotted fever to humans in the western US and the dog tick, *D. variabilis*, is the vector of the milder form of this disease in the east.

dermal *adj.* relating to or affecting the skin, especially the *dermis.

Dermanyssus *n.* a genus of widespread parasitic mites. The red poultry mite, *D. gallinae*, is a common parasite of wild birds in temperate regions but can also infest poultry. It occasionally attacks and takes a blood meal from humans, causing itching and mild dermatitis.

dermatitis *n.* inflammation of the skin caused by an outside agent: a condition with many causes (*compare* eczema, which is usually considered an endogenous disease in which such agents do not play a primary role, although in some contexts the terms "dermatitis" and "eczema" are used interchangeably). The skin is red and itchy and small blisters may develop. In most cases (*primary irritant dermatitis*), the condition is associated with certain typical changes in the skin that result from direct irritation by a substance (such as an acid, alkali, solvent, or detergent). It is the most common cause of *occupational dermatitis* in hairdressers, nurses, cooks, etc. (*See also* diaper rash.) In *allergic contact dermatitis* skin changes resembling those of eczema develop as a delayed reaction to contact with a particular allergen, which may be present at low concentrations. The most common example in women is *nickel dermatitis* from jewelery, jeans studs, etc.; in men *chromium dermatitis* is relatively common (cement is the usual source). Treatment of dermatitis depends on removing the cause, which is not always possible.

Dermatitis herpetiformis is an uncommon very itchy rash with symmetrical blistering, especially on the knees, elbows, buttocks, and shoulders. It is associated with *gluten sensitivity and responds well to treatment with dapsone.

Dermatobia *n.* a genus of nonbloodsucking flies inhabiting lowland woods and forests of South and Central America. The parasitic maggots of *D. hominis* can cause a serious disease of the skin in humans (*see* myiasis). The maggots burrow into the skin, after emerging from eggs transported by bloodsucking insects (e.g. mosquitoes), and produce painful boillike swellings. Treatment involves surgical removal of the maggots.

dermatochalasis *n.* redundant eyelid skin, which may cause drooping of the upper lid. It occurs as a result of aging and is therefore seen only in middle-aged and elderly people. *Compare* blepharochalasis.

dermatofibroma *n.* a painless benign skin nodule that is round, firm, and brown to red in color. It is found most commonly on the extremities, especially the legs, of women and requires no treatment. It is sometimes associated with systemic *lupus erythematosus.

dermatofibrosarcoma protuberans a tumor probably derived from *histiocytes that may occur in any part of the body. It is locally invasive but tends not to *metastasize. It often recurs locally despite excision.

dermatoglyphics *n.* the study of the patterns of finger, palm, toe, and sole prints. These patterns are formed by skin ridges, the distribution of which is unique to each individual. As well as being of value in criminology, dermatoglyphics is of interest to anthropologists and to doctors studying genetic disorders since abnormalities in these patterns are characteristic of chromosomal aberrations, such as *Down's syndrome. *See also* fingerprint.

dermatographism *n.* a local allergic reaction caused by pressure on the skin. People with such highly sensitive skin can "write" on it with a finger or blunt instrument, the pressure producing lasting weals.

dermatology *n.* the medical specialty concerned with the diagnosis and treatment

of skin disorders. —**dermatological** *adj.*
—**dermatologist** *n.*

dermatome *n.* **1.** a surgical instrument used for cutting thin slices of skin in some skin grafting operations. **2.** that part of the segmented mesoderm in the early embryo that forms the deeper layers of the skin (dermis) and associated tissues. *See* somite.

dermatomyositis *n.* an inflammatory disorder of the skin and underlying tissues, including the muscles (where breakdown of the muscle fibers occurs); in the absence of a rash it is known as *polymyositis. The condition is one of the *connective tissue diseases. A bluish-red skin eruption occurs on the face, scalp, neck, shoulders, arms, and knuckles and is later accompanied by severe swelling. Dermatomyositis is often associated with internal cancer in adults.

Dermatophagoides *n.* a genus of *mites that have been detected in samples of dust taken from houses in various parts of Europe. The mites may occasionally infest the skin of the scalp and cause dermatitis. Waste products from the mites produce an allergic response that is an important trigger for some forms of *rhinitis and *asthma.

dermatophyte *n.* a fungus that grows on the skin, scalp, and nails and belongs to any one of three genera, *Microsporum*, *Trichophyton*, or *Epidermophyton*. These cause *ringworm (tinea) but do not invade the deeper tissues of the body.

dermatophytosis *n.* any fungus infection of the skin; more specifically, an infection caused by the parasitic fungus *Epidermophyton (see ringworm, athlete's foot).

dermatoplasty *n.* replacement of damaged or destroyed skin by surgery. *See* plastic surgery, skin graft.

dermatosis *n.* any disease of skin, particularly one without inflammation.

dermis (corium) *n.* the true *skin: the thick layer of living tissue that lies beneath the epidermis. It consists mainly of loose connective tissue within which are blood capillaries, lymph vessels, sensory nerve endings, sweat glands and their ducts, hair follicles, sebaceous glands, and smooth muscle fibers. —**dermal** *adj.*

dermoid 1. *adj.* resembling the skin. **2.** *n.* see dermoid cyst.

dermoid cyst (dermoid) a cyst containing hair, hair follicles, and *sebaceous

glands, usually found at sites marking the fusion of developing sections of the body in the embryo. Sometimes a dermoid cyst may develop after an injury. Treatment is by surgical removal (dermoidectomy).

DES *see* diethylstilbestrol.

descemetocele *n.* thinning of the *stroma of the cornea to such an extent that Descemet's membrane is all that is maintaining the integrity of the eyeball. It occurs in severe ulceration of the cornea.

Descemet's membrane the elastic membrane that lines the inner surface of the cornea of the eye, next to the aqueous humor. [J. Descemet (1732–1810), French anatomist]

desensitization *n.* **1.** (*or* **hyposensitization**) a method for reducing the effects of a known allergen by injecting, over a period, gradually increasing doses of the allergen, until resistance is built up. *See* allergy. **2.** a technique used in the *behavior therapy of phobic states. The thing that is feared is very gradually introduced to the patient, first in imagination and then in reality. At the same time, the patient is taught relaxation to inhibit the development of anxiety (*see* relaxation therapy). In this way he is able to cope with progressively closer approximations to the feared object or situation.

deserpidine *n.* a drug that reduces blood pressure and is used to treat essential hypertension (*see* sympatholytic). It is administered by mouth; side effects include stuffiness of the nose, diarrhea, nausea, headache, lethargy, and depression. Trade name: **Harmonyl**.

designer drug a psychoactive drug produced by minor chemical modification of existing illegal substances so as to circumvent prohibitive legislation. These drugs are manufactured in secret laboratories for profit, without regard to any probable medical and social dangers to the consumers.

desipramine *n.* a tricyclic *antidepressant drug administered by mouth; common side effects include dry mouth, blurred vision, insomnia, and unsteadiness in walking. Trade names: **Norpramin**, **Pertofrane**.

desmoid tumor a dense connective tissue tumor with a dangerous propensity for repeated local recurrence after treatment. Intra-abdominal desmoids have an association with familial adenomatous *polyposis (FAP).

desmopressin *n.* a synthetic derivative of *vasopressin that causes a decrease in urine output and is used to treat diabetes insipidus and nocturnal *enuresis. It is also effective in mild hemophilia and von Willebrand's disease. Side effects may include stomach cramps, headache, and flushing of the skin. It is taken orally or intranasally to treat diabetes insipidus and enuresis and intravenously to treat hemophilia and von Willebrand's disease. Trade name: **DDAVP**.

desmosome *n.* an area of contact between two adjacent cells, occurring particularly in epithelia. The cell membranes at a desmosome are thickened and fine fibers (*tonofibrils*) extend from the desmosome into the cytoplasm.

desoximetasone *n.* a corticosteroid applied to the skin as a cream or ointment to reduce inflammation and pruritus. Side effects include burning, itching, and local skin irritation. Trade name: **Topicort**.

desquamation *n.* the process in which the outer layer of the *epidermis of the skin is removed by scaling.

detached retina (retinal detachment) separation in the *retina of the inner nervous layer containing the rods and cones from the pigmented outer layer to which it is attached. It commonly occurs when one or more holes in the retina allow fluid from the vitreous cavity of the eyeball to accumulate under the retina. Vision is lost in the affected part of the retina. The condition can be treated by laser surgery or by application of extreme heat or cold (*see* cryosurgery, photocoagulation), which, combined with *plombage, reattach it. Medical name: **ablatio retinae**.

detergent *n.* a synthetic cleansing agent that removes all impurities from a surface by reacting with grease and suspended particles, including bacteria and other microorganisms. Some detergents, e.g. *cetrimonium, are used solely for cleansing; others may be used as *antiseptics and *disinfectants.

detoxication (detoxification) *n.* **1.** the process whereby toxic substances are removed or toxic effects neutralized. It is

one of the functions of the liver. **2.** the process of bringing about the recovery of a person dependent on alcohol or some other drug.

detrition *n.* the process of wearing away solid bodies (e.g. bones) by friction or use.

detrusor *n.* the muscle of the urinary bladder wall. The functioning of the detrusor and the urethral sphincter is assessed by a urodynamic investigation (*see* urodynamics). This is used to diagnose dysfunction, absent and exaggerated reflexes, and instability in the muscle and lack of coordination between the muscle and the sphincter (bladder sphincter *dyssynergia).

detumescence *n.* **1.** the reverse of erection, whereby the erect penis or clitoris becomes flaccid after orgasm. **2.** subsidence of a swelling.

deut- (deuto-, deuter(o)-) *prefix denoting* two, second, or secondary.

deuteranopia *n.* a defect in color vision in which reds, yellows, and greens are confused. It is thought that the mechanisms for perceiving red light and green light are in some way combined in people with this defect. *Compare* protanopia, tritanopia. *See also* color blindness.

deutoplasm *n. see* yolk.

developmental age (DA) an expression of age based on the degree of physical development, social and psychological functioning, and emotional and mental maturation.

developmental delay considerable delay in the physical or mental development of children when compared with their peers. There are many causes. *Global delay* describes the state of a child whose overall development is slow in all areas.

developmental disorder any one of a group of conditions that arise in infancy or childhood and are characterized by delays in biologically determined psychological functions, such as language. They are more common in males than females and tend to follow a course of handicap with gradual improvement. They are classified into *pervasive* conditions, in which many types of development are involved (e.g. *autism), and *specific* disorders, in which the handicap is an isolated problem (such as *dyslexia).

developmental milestones skills gained by

a developing child, which should be achieved by a given age. Examples of such milestones include smiling by six weeks and sitting unsupported by eight months. Failure to achieve a particular milestone by a given age is indicative of *developmental delay.

deviance n. variation from normal behavior beyond the limits acceptable to the majority of the conforming peer group; particularly (although not exclusively) applied to sexual habits (see also sexual deviation).

deviation n. **1.** (in ophthalmology) any abnormal position of one or both eyes. For example, if the eyes are both looking to one side when the head is facing forward, they are said to be *deviated* to that side. Such deviations of both eyes may occur in brain disease. Deviations of one eye, such as *dissociated vertical deviation, come into the category of squint (see strabismus). **2.** see sexual deviation.

Devic's disease see neuromyelitis optica. [E. Devic (1869–1930), French physician]

devil's grip see Bornholm disease.

devitalization n. (in dentistry) removal of the pulp of a tooth. See root canal treatment.

DEXA (dual-energy X-ray absorptiometry) a method of measuring bone density based on the proportion of a beam of photons that passes through the bone. See osteoporosis.

dexamethasone n. a *corticosteroid drug used principally to treat severe allergies, skin and eye diseases, rheumatic and other inflammatory conditions, and hormone and blood disorders. It is administered by mouth or injection or as eye or ear drops; side effects include sodium and fluid retention, muscle weakness, convulsions, vertigo, headache, and hormonal disturbances (including menstrual irregularities). Failure of injected (0.5 mg) dexamethasone to inhibit ACTH production (the *dexamethasone suppression test*) is a sensitive test for *Cushing's syndrome. Trade names: **Decadron, Dexameth, Dexone, Hexadrol, Maxidex**.

dextr- (dextro-) prefix denoting **1.** the right side. Example: *dextroposition* (displacement to the right). **2.** (in chemistry) dextrorotation.

dextran n. a carbohydrate, consisting of branched chains of glucose units, that is a storage product of bacteria and yeasts. Preparations of dextran solution are used in transfusions, to increase the volume of plasma.

dextrin n. a carbohydrate formed as an intermediate product in the digestion of starch by the enzyme amylase. Dextrin is used in the preparation of pharmaceutical products (as an *excipient) and surgical dressings.

dextroamphetamine n. a drug of the *amphetamine group, used primarily in the treatment of *attention-deficit/hyperactivity disorder. Trade names: **Adderall, Dexedrine, Dexedrine Spansule**.

dextrocardia n. a congenital defect in which the position of the heart is a mirror image of its normal position, with the apex of the ventricles pointing to the right. It may be associated with other congenital defects and is often combined with *situs inversus*, in which the appendix and liver lie on the left side of the abdomen and the stomach lies on the right side. Isolated dextrocardia produces no adverse effects.

dextromethorphan n. a drug used in lozenges, syrups, and linctuses (confections) to suppress coughs (see antitussive). It sometimes causes drowsiness, dizziness, and digestive upsets.

dextrose n. see glucose.

dextrothyroxine n. a *thyroid hormone used to reduce blood cholesterol levels in patients with no known heart disease and normally working thyroid glands and also to treat hypothyroidism. It is administered by mouth and side effects commonly involve chest pains due to angina. Trade name: **Choloxin**.

DHEA see dehydroepiandrosterone.

DI (donor insemination) see artificial insemination.

di- prefix denoting two or double.

dia- prefix denoting **1.** through. **2.** throughout or completely. **3.** apart.

diabetes n. any disorder of metabolism causing excessive thirst and the production of large volumes of urine. Used alone, the term most commonly refers to *diabetes mellitus. See also diabetes insipidus, hemochromatosis (bronze diabetes). —**diabetic** adj., n.

diabetes insipidus a rare metabolic disorder in which the patient produces large quantities of dilute urine and is constantly thirsty. It is due to deficiency of the pituitary hormone *vasopressin (antidiuretic hormone), which regulates reabsorption of water in the kidneys, and is treated by administration of the hormone. *See also* water-deprivation test.

diabetes mellitus a disorder of carbohydrate metabolism in which sugars in the body are not oxidized to produce energy due to lack of the pancreatic hormone *insulin or to resistance to insulin. The accumulation of sugar leads to its appearance in the blood (*hyperglycemia*), then in the urine; symptoms include thirst, loss of weight, and the excessive production of urine. The use of fats as an alternative source of energy leads to disturbances of the *acid-base balance, the accumulation of ketones in the bloodstream (*ketosis), and eventually to convulsions preceding *diabetic coma*. There appears to be an inherited tendency to diabetes; the disorder may be triggered by various factors, including physical stress. Diabetes that starts in childhood or adolescence is usually more severe than that beginning in middle or old age. It is known as *type 1* (or *insulin-dependent, IDD*) *diabetes mellitus* as patients have little or no ability to produce the hormone and are entirely dependent on insulin injections for survival. In *type 2* (or *noninsulin-dependent, NIDD*) *diabetes mellitus*, which usually occurs after the age of 40 but can develop in young people (*see* maturity-onset diabetes of the young), either (1) the pancreas retains some ability to produce insulin but this is inadequate for the body's needs or (2) the body becomes resistant to the effects of insulin. Patients may require treatment with *oral hypoglycemic drugs. *Gestational diabetes mellitus develops during pregnancy. In all types of diabetes the diet must be carefully controlled, with adequate carbohydrate for the body's needs. Lack of balance in the diet or in the amount of insulin taken leads to *hypoglycemia. Long-term complications of diabetes include damage to blood vessels, which can affect the eyes (diabetic *retinopathy), to kidneys (*diabetic nephropathy), and to nerves (*diabetic neuropathy).

diabetic amyotrophy an acute mononeuropathy of the femoral nerve, usually of microvascular origin, associated with chronic poor diabetic control. Symptoms are thigh pain and progressive weakness of knee extension. Examination reveals wasting of the quadriceps muscle group and loss of the knee jerk. It may affect both legs and recovery is usually slow. Treatment is with physiotherapy and improved control of the diabetes; the condition never seems to recur in the same leg. The main *differential diagnosis is of compression of the nerve roots in the spinal canal.

diabetic glomerulosclerosis the characteristic microscopic changes seen in a diabetic kidney after many years of progressive damage.

diabetic hand syndrome the combination of features, often found in the hands of long-standing diabetic subjects, consisting of *Dupuytren's contractures, knuckle pads, *carpal tunnel syndrome, *cheiroarthropathy, and sclerosing *tenosynovitis.

diabetic holiday foot syndrome a condition in which patients with diabetic sensory polyneuropathy (*see* diabetic neuropathy) suffer significant trauma to their insensate feet through holiday activities. These activities may include walking on hot flagstones or sand, wearing ill-fitting shoes or beach shoes, and walking on sharp stones. The condition may be prevented with prior education and advice and by maintaining safe foot-care practices.

diabetic honeymoon period a well-recognized period just after the diagnosis of type 1 *diabetes mellitus when only very low insulin doses are required to control the condition. It will last for a period varying from months to a few years. Inevitably, it will come to an end, and dose requirements will increase quite quickly.

diabetic nephropathy progressive damage to the kidneys seen in some people with long-standing diabetes. It is manifested as an excessive leakage of protein into the urine followed by gradual decline of the kidney function and even kidney failure. *See also* diabetic glomerulosclerosis.

diabetic neuropathy progressive damage to the nerves seen in some people with long-standing diabetes. It most commonly affects the legs, causing pain or numbness working up from the feet. There is no cure but drugs can sometimes be used to control the discomfort experienced, and good diabetic control may prevent worsening. *See also* diabetic holiday foot syndrome.

diabetic retinopathy *see* retinopathy.

diacetylmorphine *n. see* heroin.

diaclasis *n. see* osteoclasis.

diaclast *n.* a surgical instrument used for the destruction of the skull of a fetus. This rare procedure enables a dead fetus to be delivered through the birth canal.

diagnosis *n.* the process of determining the nature of a disorder by considering the patient's *signs and *symptoms, medical history, and – when necessary – results of laboratory tests and X-ray examinations. *See also* differential diagnosis, prenatal diagnosis. *Compare* prognosis. **—diagnostic** *adj.*

diagnostic peritoneal lavage the instillation of saline directly into the abdominal cavity and its subsequent aspiration a few minutes later. If the fluid is blood-stained on recovery an intraabdominal hemorrhage is indicated. This is a useful diagnostic tool in trauma patients.

diagnosis-related group (DRG) a method of payment to hospitals for Medicare and other third-party payment plans that is based on a unit price that is preset according to the principal diagnosis and treatment required. The system was instituted in April 1983 with 470 DRGs under 23 major diagnostic categories, which were derived from the *International Classification of Diseases; the list has now increased to 511 DRGs under 25 categories. Each DRG is based on the principal diagnosis, patient's age and sex, treatment modality, and discharge status. For example, if the length of stay for a condition is 7.1 days and the patient stays 10.5 days, the hospital loses money. The concept of the DRGs was extended to non-Medicare patients in an attempt to reduce hospital costs.

diakinesis *n.* the final stage in the first prophase of *meiosis, in which homologous chromosomes, between which crossing over has occurred, are ready to separate.

dialysis *n.* a method of separating particles of different dimensions in a liquid mixture, using a thin semipermeable membrane whose pores are too small to allow the passage of large particles, such as proteins, but large enough to permit the passage of dissolved crystalline material. A solution of the mixture is separated from distilled water by the membrane; the solutes pass through the membrane into the water while the proteins, etc., are retained. The principle of dialysis is used in the artificial kidney (*see* hemodialysis). In *peritoneal dialysis*, the peritoneum is used as an autogenous semipermeable membrane, which is used when hemodialysis is not appropriate.

dialyzer *n.* a piece of apparatus for separating components of a liquid mixture by *dialysis, especially an artificial kidney (*see* hemodialysis).

diapedesis *n.* migration of cells through the walls of blood capillaries into the tissue spaces. Diapedesis is an important part of the reaction of tissues to injury (*see* inflammation).

diaper rash 1. a painful raw area of skin around the anus and buttocks due to contact with frequent irritant stools. It is common between birth and six months of age. **2.** reddening over the genitals and diaper area due to the formation of ammonia in urine-soaked diapers. A neglected rash will become ulcerated. It is common from six to 16 months. **3.** red raised areas of skin in the diaper region due to candidiasis. It has some resemblance to *psoriasis, hence its alternative name *diaper psoriasis*. Candidal diaper rash is treated with antifungal creams.

diaphoresis *n.* the process of sweating, especially excessive sweating. *See* sweat.

diaphoretic (sudorific) *n.* a drug that causes an increase in sweating, such as *pilocarpine, which stimulates the sweat glands directly. *Antipyretic drugs also have diaphoretic activity, which helps reduce the body temperature in fevers.

diaphragm *n.* **1.** (in anatomy) a thin musculomembranous dome-shaped muscle that separates the thoracic and abdominal cavities. The diaphragm is attached to the lower ribs at each side and to the breastbone and the backbone at the front and back. It bulges upward against the heart and the lungs, arching over the stomach, liver, and spleen. There are openings in the diaphragm through which the esophagus, blood vessels, and nerves pass. The diaphragm plays an important role in *breathing. It contracts with each inspiration, becoming flattened downward and increasing the volume of the thoracic cavity. With each expiration it relaxes and is restored to its dome shape. **2.** a hemispherical rubber cap fitted inside the vagina over the cervix of the uterus as a contraceptive. When combined with the use of a chemical spermicide, the diaphragm provides reliable contraception with a failure rate as low as 2–10 pregnancies per 100 woman-years.

diaphysial aclasis a hereditary abnormality of cartilage and bone growth, resulting in many cartilaginous outgrowths (exostoses) from the long bones. Bone growth may also be retarded, causing stunting and deformity.

diaphysis *n.* the shaft (central part) of a long bone. The diaphysis consists of a thick cylinder of compact bone surrounding a large medullary cavity. *Compare* epiphysis. —**diaphysial** *adj.*

diaphysitis *n.* inflammation of the diaphysis (shaft) of a bone, through infection or rheumatic disease. It may result in impaired growth of the bone and consequent deformity.

diarrhea *n.* frequent bowel evacuation or the passage of abnormally soft or liquid feces. It may be caused by intestinal infections, other forms of intestinal inflammation (such as *colitis or *Crohn's disease), *malabsorption, anxiety, and the *irritable bowel syndrome. Severe or prolonged diarrhea may lead to excess losses of fluid, salts, and nutrients in the feces.

diarthrosis (synovial joint) *n.* a freely movable joint. The ends of the adjoining bones are covered with a thin cartilaginous sheet, and the bones are linked by a ligament (*capsule*) lined with *synovial membrane, which secretes synovial fluid (see illustration). Such joints are classified according to the type of connection between the bones and the type of movement allowed. *See* arthrodic joint, condylarthrosis, enarthrosis, ginglymus, saddle joint, trochoid joint.

diaschisis *n.* a temporary loss of reflex activity in the brainstem or spinal cord following destruction of the cerebral cortex. As time passes this state of suppressed reflex activity is replaced by one of unduly exaggerated reflexes and spasticity of the limbs.

diastase *n.* an enzyme that hydrolyses starch in barley grain to produce maltose during the malting process. It has been used to aid the digestion of starch in some digestive disorders.

diastasis *n.* the separation of two parts that are normally joined, such as the two pubic bones, which are normally joined at the pubic symphysis. In *diastasis recti abdominis*, there is separation of the two rectus muscles that lie along the median line of the abdominal wall, occurring in newborns with incomplete development and in women after repeated pregnancies or multiple births.

diastema *n.* a space between two teeth.

diastole *n.* the period between two contractions of the heart, when the muscle of the heart relaxes and allows the chambers to fill with blood. The term usually refers to *ventricular diastole*, which lasts about 0.5 seconds in a normal heart rate of about 70 beats/minute. During exertion this period shortens, allowing the heart rate to increase. *See also* blood pressure, systole. —**diastolic** *adj.*

diastolic pressure *see* blood pressure.

diathermy *n.* the production of heat in a part of the body by means of a high-frequency electric current passed between two electrodes placed on the patient's skin. The heat generated increases blood flow and can be used in the treatment of deep-seated pain in rheumatic and arthritic conditions. *See also* microwave therapy.

The principle of diathermy is also utilized in various surgical instruments: a *diathermy knife*, for example, is used to coagulate tissues. The knife is itself one electrode, the other being a large moistened pad applied to another part of the patient's body. Because blood is coagu-

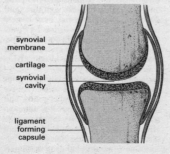

synovial membrane

cartilage

synovial cavity

ligament forming capsule

A synovial joint

lated as the knife is used, and small vessels sealed off, virtually bloodless incisions may be made. *Diathermy snares* and *needles* can be used to destroy unwanted tissue and also to remove small superficial neoplasms. *See also* electrosurgery.

diathesis *n.* a higher than average tendency to acquire certain diseases, such as allergies, rheumatic diseases, or gout. Such diseases may run in families, but they are not inherited.

diatrizoate sodium a water-soluble iodine compound used as a common contrast medium in radiology, especially for studies of the blood vessels and the gastrointestinal and urinary tracts.

diazepam *n.* a *benzodiazepine with *anxiolytic, *anticonvulsant, and *muscle-relaxant properties, used to relieve anxiety and tension and in the treatment of epilepsy and muscular rheumatism. It is also used as a *premedication. It is administered by mouth or injection; common side effects are drowsiness and lethargy, low blood pressure, and rashes. Trade names: **Valium, Valrelease**.

diazoxide *n.* a drug used to lower blood pressure in patients with hypertension and also used to treat conditions in which the levels of blood sugar are low (including *insulinoma). It is intended for short-term use only (10 days or less). It is administered by injection or orally, usually with a diuretic because it causes salt and water retention. Trade names: **Hyperstat, Proglycem**.

dibucaine *n.* a local anesthetic used in dental and other operations and to relieve pain. It is applied directly to the skin or mucous membranes or injected at the site where anesthesia is required or into the spine. Side effects such as yawning, restlessness, excitement, nausea, vomiting, and allergic reactions sometimes occur. Trade name: **Nupercainal**.

DIC *see* disseminated intravascular coagulation.

dicephalus *n.* *see* craniopagus.

dichlorphenamide *n.* a *diuretic used to reduce pressure within the eye in the treatment of glaucoma. It is administered by mouth; side effects include drowsiness, dizziness, digestive upsets, and skin rashes. Trade name: **Daranide**.

dichromatic *adj.* describing the state of color vision of those who can appreciate only two of the three primary colors. People with such vision match any given color by a mixture of the two they can distinguish. *Compare* trichromatic.

DICI (direct intracytoplasmic injection) a former name for *ICSI (intracytoplasmic sperm injection).

Dick test a test for susceptibility to *scarlet fever. If a small quantity of toxin from the bacteria responsible (hemolytic streptococci) is injected under the skin of a person not immune to the disease, a positive reaction results within 24 to 48 hours, causing local reddening of the skin. [G. F. Dick (1881–1967) and G. R. H. Dick (1881–1963), US physicians]

diclofenac *n.* an anti-inflammatory drug (*see* NSAID) taken orally to relieve joint pain in osteoarthritis, rheumatoid arthritis, and ankylosing spondylitis. It is administered in the form of eye drops to treat postoperative inflammation after cataract extraction or corneal refractive surgery. Side effects include headache, abdominal pain, nausea, and diarrhea. Trade names: **Cataflam, Voltaren**.

dicloxacillin *n.* a semisynthetic penicillin used in the treatment of infections caused by staphylococci, especially strains that produce penicillinase. It is administered by mouth; allergic reactions are the most common side effect. Trade names: **Dycill, Dynapen, Pathocil**.

dicophane *n.* *see* DDT.

dicrotism *n.* a condition in which the pulse is felt as a double beat for each contraction of the heart. It may be seen in typhoid fever. —**dicrotic** *adj.*

dicumarol *n.* an *anticoagulant drug used in the treatment of coronary and venous thrombosis. It is administered by mouth and may cause nausea, vomiting, and diarrhea. Dicumarol has now largely been replaced in clinical use by *warfarin and other coumarin derivatives because it is slow acting, has unpredictable effects, and may produce bleeding from overdosage.

dicyclomine *n.* a drug that reduces spasms of smooth muscle and is used to relieve peptic ulcer, infantile colic, colitis, and irritable bowel syndrome. It is administered by mouth and by injection; side effects include dry mouth, thirst, and dizziness. Trade name: **Bentyl**.

didanosine *n.* an antiviral drug that interferes with the action of the enzyme *reverse transcriptase, by means of which HIV, the cause of AIDS, is able to incorporate itself into the human host cell. The drug is administered by mouth. Possible side effects include damage to nerves, severe pancreatitis, nausea, vomiting, and headache. Trade name: **Videx**.

DIDMOAD syndrome *see* Wolfram syndrome.

didym- (didymo-) *prefix denoting* the testis.

dieldrin *n.* an insecticide that attacks the central nervous system of insects and has proved useful in the control of various beetles, flies, and larvae that attack crops. Because of its toxic effects and persistence in the environment, its use is now severely restricted.

diencephalon *n.* an anatomical division of the forebrain, consisting of the epithalamus, thalamus (dorsal thalamus), hypothalamus, and the ventral thalamus (subthalamus). *See* brain.

dienestrol *n.* a synthetic female sex hormone (*see* estrogen) administered topically in the form of a vaginal cream to relieve atrophy, itching, or inflammation of the vagina as part of *hormone replacement therapy. Trade name: **Ortho Dienestrol**.

diet *n.* the mixture of foods that a person eats. A *balanced diet* contains adequate quantities of all the *nutrients, i.e. vitamins, minerals (calcium, phosphorus, potassium, sodium, chlorine, sulfur, magnesium, and the *trace elements), and *dietary fiber, as well as water, carbohydrates and fats (which provide energy), and proteins (required for growth and maintenance).

dietary fiber (roughage) the part of food that cannot be digested and absorbed to produce energy. Dietary fiber falls into four groups: *cellulose, hemicelluloses, lignins,* and *pectins.* Highly refined foods, such as sucrose, contain no dietary fiber. Foods with a high fiber content include wholemeal cereals and flour, root vegetables, nuts, and fruit. Dietary fiber is considered by some to be helpful in the prevention of many of the diseases of Western civilization, such as *diverticulosis, constipation, appendicitis, obesity, and diabetes mellitus. Communities consuming high-fiber diets very rarely have any of these diseases.

dietetics *n.* the application of the principles of *nutrition to the selection of food

and the feeding of individuals and groups.

diethylcarbamazine *n.* an anthelmintic drug that destroys filariae and is therefore used in the treatment of filariasis, loiasis, and onchocerciasis. It is administered as tablets. Side effects may include headache, malaise, joint pains, nausea, and vomiting. Trade name: **Hetrazan**.

diethylpropion *n.* a drug, similar to the *amphetamines, that suppresses the appetite and is used in the treatment of obesity. It is administered by mouth and may cause dry mouth, insomnia, depression, headache, constipation, and allergic rashes. Dependence of the amphetamine type can occur. Trade names: **Tenuate**, **Tepanil**.

diethylstilbestrol (DES) *n.* a synthetic female sex hormone (*see* estrogen) used to treat symptoms of the menopause, menstrual disorders, inflammation of the female genital organs, and cancer of the breast and prostate. It was formerly prescribed for prevention of habitual abortion and premature labor, but it has since been found to be an epigenetic carcinogen and is not recommended for use in pregnant women. It is administered by mouth or injection; side effects include loss of appetite, abdominal pain, and diarrhea. Trade name: **Stilphostrol**.

Dietl's crisis acute obstruction of a kidney causing severe pain in the loins. The obstruction usually occurs at the junction of the renal pelvis and the ureter, causing the kidney to become distended with accumulated urine (*see* hydronephrosis). Sometimes the pelvis drains spontaneously, with relief of pain, but acute decompression of the kidney may be required with surgical relief of the obstruction (*see* pyeloplasty). [J. Dietl (1804–78), Polish physician]

Dieulafoy's lesion an abnormality of small blood vessels in the mucosal lining of the upper region of the stomach that may cause severe spontaneous hemorrhage. The abnormality is difficult to see at gastroscopy or at surgical exploration and therefore may be overlooked. [G. Dieulafoy (1839–1911), French physician]

differential diagnosis *diagnosis of a condition whose signs and/or symptoms are shared by various other conditions. For example, abdominal pain may be due to any of a large number of different disorders, which must be ruled out in arriving at a correct diagnosis.

differential leukocyte count (differential blood count) a determination of the proportions of the different kinds of white cells (leukocytes) present in a sample of blood. Usually 100 white cells are counted and classified under the microscope or by electronic apparatus, so that the results can readily be expressed as percentages of the total number of leukocytes and the absolute numbers per liter of blood. The information often aids diagnosis of disease.

differentiation *n.* **1.** (in embryology) the process in embryonic development during which unspecialized cells or tissues become specialized for particular functions. **2.** (in oncology) the degree of similarity of tumor cells to the structure of the organ from which the tumor arose. Tumors are classified as well, moderately, or poorly differentiated: well-differentiated tumors appear similar to the cells of the organ in which they arose; poorly differentiated tumors do not. Such classification is often of prognostic significance.

diffusion *n.* **1.** the process in which molecules or other particles in a fluid spontaneously move from an area of higher concentration to an area of lower concentration, resulting in an even distribution of the particles throughout the solution. **2.** *see* dialysis.

diflunisal *n.* a nonsteroidal anti-inflammatory, antipyretic, and analgesic drug used in the treatment of mild to moderate pain, osteoarthritis, and rheumatoid arthritis (*see* NSAID). It is administered by mouth; most common side effects are headache, skin rash, nausea, and diarrhea. Trade name: **Dolobid.**

DiGeorge syndrome a hereditary condition resulting in an inability to fight infections (immunodeficiency) associated with absence of the parathyroid and thymus glands, abnormalities of the heart, and low calcium levels. Affected children are prone to *Candida* infections and often present with *failure to thrive. The condition has also been named *CATCH-22*: *C*ardiac abnormalities, *A*bnormal facies, *T*-cell deficiency (from absent thymus), *C*left palate, *H*ypocalcemia,

chromosome *22* (in which the defect lies). [A. M. DiGeorge (1921–), US pediatrician]

digestion *n.* the process in which ingested food is broken down in the alimentary canal into a form that can be absorbed and assimilated by the tissues of the body. Digestion includes mechanical processes, such as chewing, churning, and grinding food, as well as the chemical action of digestive enzymes and other substances (bile, acid, etc.). Chemical digestion begins in the mouth with the action of *saliva on food, but most of it takes place in the stomach and small intestine, where the food is subjected to *gastric juice, *pancreatic juice, and *succus entericus.

digit *n.* any one of the terminal divisions of a limb: a finger or toe.

digital *adj.* **1.** (in anatomy) relating to a digit. **2.** (in radiology) relating to or utilizing *digitization.

digital image an image made up of *pixels. Each pixel has numbers (digits) to describe its position and shade on the *gray scale. The more shades available, described by the number of computer bits required to store the shade of gray, the more accurately the image represents the original tissue contrast. An 8-bit computer image shows 2^8 (256) possible shades of gray, close to the maximum the human eye can differentiate. 12-bit (4096 levels of gray) images are of much higher quality and take up more memory. These images can be manipulated more easily by computer using image enhancement techniques. *Compare* analogue image.

digitalis *n.* an extract from the dried leaves of foxgloves (*Digitalis* species), which contains various substances, including *digitoxin and *digoxin, that stimulate heart muscle and are used to treat heart failure. *See also* digitalization.

digitalization *n.* the administration of a derivative of *digitalis to a patient with heart failure until the optimum level has been reached in the heart tissues. At this stage the control of heart failure should be adequate and there should be few side effects. The process of digitalization may take several days.

digital radiography (DR) an alternative to film radiography, in which X-ray images are acquired from a large number of individual X-ray detectors on a matrix in a digital format directly. This contrasts with *computerized radiography, in which an *analogue image is taken and then put into a reader to be converted into a *digital image. The technique allows the storage of images on hard disk or digital tape and their subsequent retrieval, manipulation, and interpretation using TV monitors rather than photographic film (*see* PACS). Digital detectors are currently expensive but are likely to become the preferred technology.

digital spot imaging (DSI) the production of static images using an *image intensifier and a digital camera, usually during a fluoroscopic examination. The images produced can be stored digitally (*see* digitization) and then either transferred to photographic film or viewed on a TV monitor.

digital subtraction a sophisticated radiological technique in which *digitization allows X-ray examination, most commonly of blood vessels (*see* angiography), to be performed using smaller volumes of contrast material. A digitized image is taken before the contrast medium is added, and this is subtracted by computer from the images taken after contrast injection. Only the outline of the blood vessel or other structure containing contrast medium remains on the image. The technique enables blood vessel anatomy and blood supply to an organ to be demonstrated more clearly. It is very dependent on the patient remaining still, since movement causes severe loss of image (movement *artifact). The technique can also be used in nuclear medicine using two different tracers to look for parathyroid gland tumors.

digitization *n.* (in radiology) the conversion of an *analogue image to a *digital image. The image is broken down to pixels and numerical values assigned to each pixel for its position and to describe its shade on the *gray scale. This allows storage, electronic manipulation, and transfer via computer links of any images, including radiographs or CT, MRI, or ultrasound scans.

digitoxin *n.* a drug that increases heart muscle contraction and is used in heart failure. It is slow-acting but the effects are prolonged. Digitoxin is administered

by mouth; side effects include nausea, vomiting, loss of appetite, diarrhea, abdominal pain, and abnormal heart activity. *See also* digitalization. Trade name: **Crystodigin**.

digoxin *n.* a drug that increases heart muscle contraction and is used in heart failure. It is rapidly effective and the effects are short-lived. Digoxin is administered by mouth or injection; side effects are those of *digitoxin. Trade names: **Digitek, Lanoxicaps, Lanoxin**.

diheterozygote *n.* an individual who is *heterozygous with respect to two gene pairs. —**diheterozygous** *adj.*

dihydrocodeine *n.* a drug used to relieve pain and suppress coughs (*see* analgesic, antitussive). It is administered as a combination drug by mouth or injection and sometimes causes nausea, dizziness, and constipation. Dependence of the *morphine type can also occur, but this is rare. Trade name: **Synalgos-DC**.

dihydroergotamine *n.* a derivative of *ergotamine used to prevent and relieve migraine and headaches. It is administered by injection or as a nasal spray; side effects are rare but nausea sometimes occurs. Trade names: **DHE-45, Migranal**.

dihydrofolate reductase an enzyme that catalyzes the conversion of dihydrofolate into folate. The enzyme is necessary in rapidly growing tissue, such as cancers, so inhibiting its action is one form of cancer therapy. Inhibitors include *pyrimethamine, *triamterene, *trimethoprim, and *methotrexate. When such drugs are necessary, folate deficiency is treated with *folinic acid rather than folic acid.

dihydrotestosterone *n.* a hormone formed from testosterone in tissue, particularly in the secondary sex organs. It is the biologically active form of testosterone except in muscle and bone and it is necessary for male external genital development, such as the formation of the penis, scrotum, and prostate. A synthetic form, called *stanolone, is used in the treatment of disease.

diiodotyrosine *n.* an iodine-containing substance produced in the thyroid gland from which the *thyroid hormones are derived.

dilaceration *n.* a condition affecting some teeth after traumatic injury, in which the incomplete root continues to form at an abnormal angle to the part already formed. In severe cases it may be necessary to remove the tooth.

dilation *n.* the enlargement or expansion of a hollow organ (such as a blood vessel) or cavity.

dilation and curettage (D & C) an operation in which the cervix of the uterus is expanded, using an instrument called a *dilator, and the lining (endometrium) of the uterus is lightly scraped with a curet (*see* curettage). It is performed for a variety of reasons, including the removal of any remaining material left after abortion, removal of small tumors, and obtaining a sample of endometrium for histologic examination in the diagnosis of gynecologic disorders. Special types of curet to which suction is applied are used to obtain tissue samples or remove the products of conception in abortion.

dilator *n.* **1.** an instrument used to enlarge a body opening or cavity. For example, the male urethra may become narrowed by disease and it can sometimes be restored to its original size by inserting a dilator. Dilators are also used to enlarge the canal in the cervix of the uterus in the procedure of *dilation and curettage. **2.** a drug, applied either locally or systemically, that causes expansion of a structure, such as the pupil of the eye or a blood vessel. *See also* vasodilator. **3.** a muscle that, by its action, opens an aperture or orifice in the body.

diltiazem *n.* a *calcium antagonist used in the treatment of effort-associated angina, angina pectoris due to coronary artery spasm, and high blood pressure (hypertension). It acts as a vasodilator and is administered by mouth; side effects include edema, headache, nausea, dizziness, and skin rash. Trade names: **Cardizem, Dilacor XR, Tiazac**.

dimenhydrinate *n.* an *antihistamine used to prevent and treat motion sickness, nausea and vomiting due to other causes, vertigo, and inner ear disturbances. It is administered by mouth or injection and commonly causes drowsiness, dizziness, digestive upsets, dry mouth, and headache. Trade name: **Dramamine**.

dimercaprol (BAL, British antilewisite) *n.* a drug that combines with metals in the body and is used to treat poisoning by antimony, arsenic, bismuth, gold, mercury, and thallium and in Wilson's disease. It is administered by injection and commonly causes nausea, vomiting, and watering of the eyes.

dimethicone *n.* a silicone preparation used externally to prevent undue drying of the skin and to protect it against irritating external agents. It is commonly used to prevent diaper rash in babies. Trade name: **Gerber Diaper Rash Lotion**.

dimethyl sulfoxide (DMSO) a chemical used in an ointment to treat skin inflammations or in combination with other topically applied drugs to improve their absorption. A solution is also available for the symptomatic relief of patients with interstitial cystitis. It may cause skin irritation and a garlic-like taste in the mouth. Trade name: **Rimso-50**.

dinoprostone *n.* a *prostaglandin drug used mainly to induce labor. It is also used to terminate pregnancy or to expel a fetus that has died. It is administered as a vaginal suppository or gel. Trade names: **Cervidil, Prepidil, Prostin E2**.

diode laser a portable laser used for treating diseases of the retina of the eye by producing small burns in the retina. It is used in *photocoagulation of the retina.

diopter *n.* the unit of measurement of the power of *refraction of a lens. One diopter is the power of a lens that brings parallel light rays to a focus at a point one meter from the lens, after passing through it. A stronger lens brings light rays to a focus at a point closer to it than a weaker lens and has a higher diopter power.

dioxin *n.* any of a group of chemical compounds, especially the most toxic member, 2,3,7,8-tetrachlorobenzene-*p*-dioxin (TCDD), that occur as environmental pollutants throughout the world. Released into the environment as byproducts in the manufacture of certain herbicides and bleaching agents and produced during combustion processes, dioxins accumulate in the food chain, being stored in animal fat; the most common adverse effect of exposure to large amounts of dioxins is *chloracne. TCDD was present as a contaminant in the jungle defoliant *Agent Orange, used by the US military during the Vietnam War. Because of their toxicity, strict controls are now in place in the US to limit industrial emissions of dioxins.

dipeptidase *n.* an enzyme, found in digestive juices, that splits certain products of protein digestion (dipeptides) into their constituent amino acids. The latter are then absorbed by the body.

dipeptide *n.* a compound consisting of two amino acids joined together by a peptide bond (e.g. glycylalanine, a combination of the amino acids glycine and alanine). *See* dipeptidase.

diphenhydramine *n.* an *antihistamine used to treat allergic conditions, such as hay fever and rhinitis, in cough mixtures, for motion sickness, and to induce sleep. It is administered by mouth or topically to relieve minor skin irritation. Side effects include drowsiness, dry mouth, dizziness, and nausea. Trade names: **Benadryl, Benylin, Caladryl.**

diphenoxylate *n.* a drug used, often in combination with *atropine, to treat diarrhea. It is also used after *colostomy or *ileostomy to reduce the frequency and fluidity of the stools. It is administered by mouth; side effects can include nausea, drowsiness, dizziness, skin reactions, and restlessness. Trade name: **Lomotil.**

diphosphonates *pl. n. see* bisphosphonates.

diphtheria *n.* an acute highly contagious infection, caused by the bacterium *Corynebacterium diphtheriae*, generally affecting the throat but occasionally other mucous membranes and the skin. The disease is spread by direct contact with a patient or carrier or by contaminated milk. After an incubation period of 2–6 days a sore throat, weakness, and mild fever develop. Later, a soft gray membrane forms across the throat, constricting the air passages and causing difficulty in breathing and swallowing; a *tracheostomy may be necessary. Bacteria multiply at the site of infection and release a toxin into the bloodstream, which damages heart and nerves. Death from heart failure or general collapse can follow within four days but prompt administration of antitoxin and penicillin arrests the disease; complete recovery requires prolonged bed rest. An effective immunization program has now made diphtheria rare in most Western countries (*see also* Schick test).

diphtheroid *adj.* resembling diphtheria (especially the membrane formed in diphtheria) or the bacteria that cause it.

diphyllobothriasis *n.* an infestation of the intestine with the broad tapeworm, *Diphyllobothrium latum*, which sometimes causes nausea, malnutrition, diarrhea, and anemia resulting from impaired absorption of vitamin B_{12} through the gut. The infestation, common in Baltic countries, is contracted following ingestion of uncooked fish infected with the larval stage of the tapeworm. The tapeworm can be expelled from the gut with the anthelmintic *quinacrine.

Diphyllobothrium *n.* a genus of large tapeworms that can grow to a length of 3–10 m. The adult of *D. latum*, the broad (or fish) tapeworm, infects fish-eating mammals, including humans, in whom it may cause serious anemia (*see* diphyllobothriasis). The parasite has two intermediate hosts: a freshwater crustacean and a fish (*see also* plerocercoid).

dipivefrin *n.* a *sympathomimetic drug indicated as initial therapy for the control of intraocular pressure in chronic openangle *glaucoma. It is administered as eye drops; common adverse reactions include eye irritation and blurred vision. Trade name: **Propine.**

dipl- (diplo-) *prefix denoting* double.

diplacusis *n.* perception of a single sound as double owing to a defect of the *cochlea in the inner ear.

diplegia *n.* paralysis involving both sides of the body and affecting the legs more severely than the arms. *Cerebral diplegia* is a form of *cerebral palsy in which there is widespread damage, in both cerebral hemispheres, of the brain cells that control the movements of the limbs. —**diplegic** *adj.*

diplococcus *n.* any of a group of nonmotile parasitic spherical bacteria that occur in pairs. The group includes the *pneumococcus.

diploë *n.* the latticelike tissue that lies between the inner and outer layers of the *skull.

diploid *adj.* describing cells, nuclei, or organisms in which each chromosome except the Y sex chromosome is represented twice. *Compare* haploid, triploid. —**diploid** *n.*

diplopia *n.* double vision: the simultaneous awareness of two images of one object. It is usually due to limitation of movement of one eye so that the two eyes cannot simultaneously look at the same object. This may be caused by a defect of the nerves or muscles controlling eye movement or a mechanical restriction of eyeball movement in the orbit. A flexible plastic prism, called a *Fresnel prism*, can be stuck to spectacle lenses to correct double vision. Double vision that does not disappear on covering one eye can be caused by early cataract (*see also* polyopia).

diplotene *n.* the fourth stage in the first prophase of *meiosis, in which *crossing over occurs between the paired chromatids of homologous chromosomes, which then begin to separate.

diprosopus *n.* a fetal monster with a single trunk and normal limbs but with some degree of duplication of the face.

-dipsia (-dipsy) *suffix denoting* a condition relative to thirst. Examples: *polydipsia* (abnormal intense thirst), *oligodipsia* (diminished or absent thirst).

dipsomania *n.* morbid and insatiable craving for alcohol, occurring in paroxysms. Only a small proportion of alcoholics show this symptom. *See* alcoholism.

Diptera *n.* a large group of insects, including *mosquitoes, gnats, midges, house flies, and *tsetse flies, that possess a single pair of wings. The mouthparts of many species, e.g. mosquitoes and tsetse flies, are specialized for sucking blood; these forms are important in the transmission of disease (*see* vector). *See also* fly.

Dipylidium *n.* a genus of tapeworms. *D. caninum*, a common parasite of the small intestine of dogs and cats, occasionally infects humans but usually produces no obvious symptoms. Fleas are the intermediate hosts, and children in close contact with pets become infected on ingesting fleas harboring the parasite.

dipyridamole *n.* a drug that dilates the blood vessels of the heart and reduces platelet aggregation. It is used to treat postoperative thromboembolic complications after cardiac valve replacement It is given by mouth and may cause headache, stomach upsets, rash, and dizziness. Trade name: **Persantine**.

direct intracytoplasmic injection (DICI) a former name for intracytoplasmic sperm injection (*see* ICSI).

direct observed therapy (DOT) *see* tuberculosis.

director *n.* an instrument used to guide the extent and direction of a surgical incision.

dis- *prefix denoting* separation.

disability *n.* **1.** a loss or restriction of functional ability or activity as a result of impairment of the body or mind. *See also* handicap. **2.** (as defined by the US Department of Health and Human Services) the inability to engage in any substantial gainful activity by reason of any medically determined physical or mental impairment that can be expected to last at least 12 months or result in death. Age, education, and work experience are taken into consideration in determining whether the person might be gainfully employed in a job comparable to the work performed at the time of the disability. Persons who qualify according to the definition are entitled to Disabled Workers' Benefits. *See* Americans with Disabilities Act (1990), handicap.

disaccharide *n.* a carbohydrate consisting of two linked *monosaccharide units. The most common disaccharides are *maltose, *lactose, and *sucrose.

disarticulation *n.* separation of two bones at a joint. This may be the result of an injury or it may be done by the surgeon at operation in the course of amputation; for example of a limb, finger, or toe.

discharge rate the number of cases of a specified disease or condition discharged from hospitals related to the population of the *catchment area: usually expressed regionally per 10,000.

discission *n.* an obsolete operation for cataract in which the front of the lens capsule is cut extensively by a fine knife or needle inserted through the edge of the cornea. Subsequently, the lens is absorbed naturally into the surrounding fluid of the eye. It is usually necessary to perform *capsulotomy later.

discoid lupus erythematosus (DLE) *see* lupus erythematosus.

disease *n.* a disorder with a specific cause and recognizable signs and symptoms; any bodily abnormality or failure to function properly, except that resulting directly from physical injury (the latter, however, may open the way for disease).

disimpaction *n.* the process of separating the broken ends of a bone when they have been forcibly driven together during a fracture. *Traction may be required to keep the bone ends separate but in good alignment.

disinfectant n. an agent that destroys or removes bacteria and other microorganisms and is used to cleanse surgical instruments and other objects. Examples are *cresol, *hexachlorophene, and *phenol. Dilute solutions of some disinfectants may be used as *antiseptics or as preservatives in solutions of eye drops or injections.

disinfection n. the process of eliminating infective microorganisms from contaminated instruments, clothing, or surroundings by using physical means or chemicals (*disinfectants).

disinfestation n. the destruction of insect pests and other animal parasites. This generally involves the use of insecticides applied either topically, as in delousing, or as a spray for eliminating an infestation of fleas or bedbugs in the home.

disintegrative psychosis 1. a pervasive *developmental disorder, often with features of *autism, occurring as a result of a brain disease, such as encephalitis, in childhood. **2.** see Heller's syndrome.

disjunction n. the separation of pairs of homologous chromosomes during meiosis or of the chromatids of a chromosome during *anaphase of mitosis or meiosis. *Compare* nondisjunction.

disk (disc) n. (in anatomy) a rounded flattened structure, such as an *intervertebral disk or the *optic disk.

disk cupping an abnormal enlargement of the central depression of the *optic disk due to loss of nerve fibers, as occurs in glaucoma as a result of raised intraocular pressure.

dislocation (luxation) n. displacement from their normal position of bones meeting at a joint so that there is complete loss of contact of the joint surfaces. It usually results from trauma (dislocation of the shoulder is common in sports injuries) but may be congenital, in which case it usually affects the hip (see congenital dislocation of the hip). In a traumatic dislocation the bones are restored to their normal positions by manipulation under local or general anesthesia (see reduction). *Compare* subluxation.

dismemberment n. the separating of body parts or the amputation of a leg, arm, or part of a limb.

disoma n. a double-bodied fetal monster with a single head.

disopyramide n. an *antiarrhythmic drug administered by mouth; side effects such as dry mouth, blurred vision, difficulty in urination, and digestive upsets may occur. Trade name: **Norpace**.

disorder n. an abnormality of function or structure or both, resulting from a genetic condition, developmental defect, or from an external factor, such as trauma. *See also* disease.

disorientation n. the state produced by loss of awareness of space, time, or personality. It can be the result of drugs, anxiety, or organic disease (such as dementia or *Korsakoff's syndrome).

dispensary n. a place where medicines are made up by a pharmacist according to the doctor's prescription and dispensed to patients. A dispensary is often part of an out-patient department in a hospital.

displacement n. (in psychology) the substitution of one type of behavior for another, usually the substitution of a relatively harmless activity for a harmful one; for example, yelling at the cat instead of one's boss.

dissection n. the cutting apart and separation of the body tissues along the natural divisions of the organs and different tissues in the course of an operation. Dissection of corpses is carried out for the study of anatomy.

disseminated adj. widely distributed in an organ (or organs) or in the whole body. The term may refer to disease organisms or to pathologic changes.

disseminated intravascular coagulation (DIC) a disorder resulting from overstimulation of the blood-clotting mechanisms in response to disease or injury, such as severe infection, malignancy, acute leukemia, severe trauma, burns, abruptio placentae, or intrauterine fetal death. The overstimulation results in generalized blood coagulation and excessive consumption of *coagulation factors and *platelets. The resulting deficiency of these may lead to spontaneous bleeding. Transfusions of plasma are given to replace the depleted clotting factors, and treatment of the underlying cause is essential.

disseminated sclerosis *see* multiple sclerosis.

dissociated vertical deviation (DVD) a condition in which one eye looks upward when the amount of light entering it is reduced, e.g. when it is covered. The eye returns to its original position when the cover is removed. DVD is an acquired condition chiefly associated with infantile esotropia (convergent *strabismus).

dissociation *n.* (in psychiatry) the process whereby thoughts and ideas can be split off from consciousness and may function independently, thus (for example) allowing conflicting opinions to be held at the same time about the same object. Dissociation may be the main factor in cases of dissociative *fugue and multiple personalities.

dissociative disorder any one of a group of extreme *defense mechanisms that include loss of memory for important personal details (*see* amnesia); wandering away from home and the assumption of a new identity (*see* fugue); splitting of the personality into two or more distinct personalities (*see* multiple personality disorder); and trancelike states with severely reduced response to external stimuli. *Conversion disorder is classified with dissociative disorders as dissociative (conversion) disorders in ICD-10 (*see* International Classification of Diseases).

distal *adj.* **1.** (in anatomy) situated away from the origin or point of attachment or from the median line of the body. For example, the term is applied to a part of a limb that is furthest from the body; to a blood vessel that is far from the heart; and to a nerve fiber that is far from the central nervous system. *Compare* proximal. **2.** (in dentistry) describing the surface of a tooth away from the midline of the jaw.

distichiasis *n.* a very rare condition in which there is an extra row of eyelashes behind the normal row. They may rub against and irritate the cornea.

distraction *n.* (in orthopedics) increasing the distance between two points. In *limb lengthening procedures callus can be stretched longitudinally by increasing the distance between pins attached to the bone (*see* callotasis).

distraction test a hearing test used for screening infants between the ages of six and ten months. The infant is placed on its caregiver's knee, one examiner sits in front of the infant and gains its attention, and a second examiner is situated just behind the infant. At a given moment the first examiner becomes very still and the second examiner makes a sound at the level of the infant's ear to one side or the other. If the infant can hear it turns in the direction of the sound. The sounds made should be of different pitches and a given loudness.

disulfiram *n.* a drug used in the treatment of chronic alcoholism. It acts as a deterrent by producing unpleasant effects when taken with alcohol, including flushing, breathing difficulties, headache, palpitations, nausea, and vomiting. It is used in conjunction with supportive and psychotherapeutic treatment. It is administered by mouth; common side effects are fatigue, nausea, and constipation. Trade name: **Antabuse**.

diuresis *n.* increased secretion of urine by the kidneys. This normally follows the drinking of more fluid than the body requires, but it can be stimulated by the administration of a *diuretic.

diuretic *n.* a drug that increases the volume of urine produced by promoting the excretion of salts and water from the kidney. The main classes of diuretics act by inhibiting the reabsorption of salts and water from the kidney tubules into the bloodstream. *Thiazide diuretics* (e.g. *bendroflumethazide, *chlorthalidone) act at the distal convoluted tubules (*see* nephron), preventing the reabsorption of sodium and potassium. *Potassium-sparing diuretics* (such as *amiloride, *spironolactone, *triamterene) prevent excessive loss of potassium at the distal convoluted tubules, and *loop diuretics* (e.g. *furosemide) prevent reabsorption of sodium and potassium in *Henle's loop. Diuretics are used to reduce edema that has been caused by salt and water retention in disorders of the heart, kidneys, liver, or lungs. Thiazides and potassium-sparing diuretics are also used – usually in conjunction with other drugs – in the treatment of high blood pressure. Treatment with thiazide and loop diuretics often results in potassium deficiency; this is corrected by simultaneous administration of potassium salts or a potassium-sparing diuretic.

diurnal *adj.* relating to the daylight hours; daily. *See* circadian.

divagation *n.* rambling discursive thought and speech. It is not specific to any one psychiatric condition.

divarication *n.* the separation or stretching of bodily structures. *Rectus divarication* is stretching of the *rectus abdominis muscle, a common condition associated with pregnancy or obesity.

divaricator *n.* **1.** a scissorlike surgical instrument used to divide portions of tissue into two separate parts during an operation. **2.** a form of retractor used to open out the sides of an abdominal incision and facilitate access.

divergence *n.* (in ophthalmology) abduction of the eyes. *Divergence excess* is a type of squint (divergent *strabismus) in which the eyes are deviated outward more when looking in the distance than for near vision. *Divergence insufficiency* is a type of squint (convergent *strabismus) in which the eyes are deviated slightly inward only when looking in the distance.

diverticular disease a condition in which there are diverticula (*see* diverticulum) in the colon associated with lower abdominal pain and disturbed bowel habit. The pain is due to spasm of the muscles of the intestine and not to inflammation of the diverticula (*compare* diverticulitis).

diverticulitis *n.* inflammation of a *diverticulum, most commonly of one or more colonic diverticula. This type of diverticulitis is caused by infection and causes lower abdominal pain with diarrhea or constipation; it may lead to abscess formation, which often requires surgical drainage. A Meckel's diverticulum sometimes becomes inflamed due to infection, causing symptoms similar to *appendicitis. Diverticula elsewhere in the alimentary tract are not subject to diverticulitis. *Compare* diverticular disease.

diverticulosis *n.* a condition in which diverticula exist in a segment of the intestine without evidence of inflammation (*compare* diverticulitis).

diverticulum *n.* (*pl.* **diverticula**) a sac or pouch formed at weak points in the walls of the alimentary tract. They may be caused by increased pressure from within (*pulsion diverticula*) or by pulling from without (*traction diverticula*). A *pharyngeal diverticulum* occurs in the pharynx and may cause difficulty in swallowing. *Esophageal diverticula* occur in the middle or lower esophagus (gullet); they may be associated with muscular disorders of the esophagus but rarely cause symptoms. *Gastric diverticula* affect the stomach (usually the upper part) and cause no symptoms. *Duodenal diverticula* occur on the concave surface of the duodenal loop; they may be associated with *dyspepsia but usually cause few symptoms. *Jejunal diverticula* affect the small intestine, are often multiple, and may give rise to abdominal discomfort and *malabsorption due to growth of bacteria within them. *Meckel's diverticulum* occurs in the ileum, about 35 cm from its termination, as a congenital abnormality. It may become inflamed, mimicking *appendicitis; if it contains embryonic remnants of stomach mucosa, it may form a *peptic ulcer, causing pain, bleeding, or perforation. *Colonic diverticula*, affecting the colon (particularly the lowest portion), become more common with increasing age and often cause no symptoms. However, they are sometimes associated with abdominal pain or altered bowel habits (*see* diverticular disease) or they may become inflamed (*see* diverticulitis).

division *n.* **1.** the separation of an organ or tissue into parts by surgery. **2.** *see* cell division.

divulsor *n.* a surgical instrument that is used to dilate forcibly any canal or cavity, usually the urethra.

dizygotic twins *see* twins.

DMD Duchenne's muscular dystrophy: *see* muscular dystrophy.

DMSA dimercaptosuccinic acid, which when labeled with *technetium-99m is used as a tracer to obtain *scintigrams of the kidney, by means of a *gamma camera, particularly to show scarring resulting from infection and to assess the relative quantity of functioning tissue in each kidney.

DNA (deoxyribonucleic acid) the genetic material of nearly all living organisms, which controls heredity and is located in the cell nucleus (*see* chromosome, gene). DNA is a *nucleic acid composed of two strands made up of units called *nucleotides (see illustration). The two strands are wound around each other into a double helix and linked together by hydrogen bonds between the bases of the nucleotides (*see* base pairing). The genetic information of the DNA is contained in the sequence of bases along the molecule (*see* genetic code); changes in the DNA cause *mutations. The DNA molecule can make exact copies of itself by the process of *replication, thereby passing on the genetic information to the daughter cells when the cell divides.

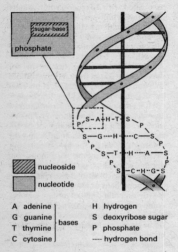

A adenine		H hydrogen
G guanine	bases	S deoxyribose sugar
T thymine		P phosphate
C cytosine		---- hydrogen bond

Structure of part of a DNA molecule

DNA markers segments of chromosomal DNA that are known to be linked with inherited traits or diseases, which are passed on through the genes located on these sites.

DNA polymerase inhibitor any one of a class of antiviral drugs that inhibit the action of DNA polymerase enzymes, which are used by viruses to form their own DNA. These drugs prevent, to a varying degree, the reproduction of viruses. They include *acyclovir, *foscarnet, *ganciclovir, and *valacyclovir.

DNA repair a variety of mechanisms that help to ensure that the genetic sequence, as expressed in the DNA, is maintained and that errors that occur during DNA replication, by mutation, are not allowed

to accumulate. An error in the genetic sequence could cause cell death by interfering with the replication process. DNA repair involves the action of enzymes, which detect damage to DNA and effect the repair. Some genetic diseases, including *ataxia telangiectasia and *xeroderma pigmentosum, are due to deficiencies in these enzymes.

DNase *n.* an enzyme that catalyzes the cleavage of DNA. A genetically engineered form, recombinant human DNase (*dornase alfa*), is used in the treatment of *cystic fibrosis to reduce the viscosity of the sticky secretions in the lungs. Administered by inhalation via a jet nebulizer, it appears to hydrolyze extracellular DNA that accumulates with other neutrophil debris in the airways. Trade name: **Pulmozyme**.

DNR do not resuscitate. This instruction, signed by the patient (or designated representative) and the attending physician, directs that no resuscitation is to be given to the patient in the event of cardiac or respiratory failure. A DNR instruction is usually given only when a person is so gravely ill that death is imminent and inevitable. Also called: **nocode**.

dobutamine *n.* a *sympathomimetic drug used to assist in the management of heart failure. It increases the force of contraction of the ventricles and improves the heart output and it may be given by continuous intravenous drip. Trade name: **Dobutrex**.

docetaxel *n. see* taxane.

Doctor *n.* the title given to the recipient of a *Medicinae Doctor* (MD) degree, which in the US is awarded on qualification. In the US qualified professors, dentists, pharmacists, and others may also use the title Doctor, since they have received a doctorate in dentistry, science, philosophy, education, or other discipline.

docusate sodium a softening agent that is given by mouth or in suppositories, often together with a laxative, to relieve constipation. It is also used in solution to soften ear wax. Trade names: **Colace**, **Dulcolax**, **Senokot-S**.

dolich- (dolicho-) *prefix denoting* long. Example: *dolichocolon* (abnormally long colon).

dolichocephaly *n.* the condition of having

a relatively long skull, with a *cephalic index of 75 or less. —**dolichocephalic** adj.

dolor n. pain: one of the classic signs of inflammation in a tissue, the other three being *calor (heat), *rubor (redness), and *tumor (swelling). The pain in inflammation is thought to be due to the release of chemicals from damaged cells.

dolorimetry n. the measurement of pain. See algesimeter.

dominant adj. (in genetics) describing a gene (or its corresponding characteristic) whose effect is shown in the individual whether its *allele is the same or different. If the allele is different, its effect is masked and it is the *recessive gene of that pair. In genetic diseases showing autosomal dominant inheritance, the defective gene is dominant and will therefore be inherited by 50% of the offspring (of either sex) of a person with the disease. It will always be expressed in these offspring (since the normal allele inherited from the unaffected parent is recessive). —**dominant** n.

domperidone n. an antiemetic drug used especially to reduce the nausea and vomiting caused by other drugs (e.g. anticancer drugs). It inhibits the effects of *dopamine, acting to close the sphincter muscle at the upper opening of the stomach (the cardia) and to relax the sphincter at the lower opening (the pylorus). It is administered by mouth or suppository; possible side effects include breast enlargement and milk secretion. Trade name: **Motilium**.

Donald-Fothergill operation (Manchester operation) a surgical operation consisting of anterior *colporrhaphy, amputation of the cervix, and *colpoperineorrhaphy. It is performed for genital prolapse. [A. Donald (1860–1933) and W. E. Fothergill (1865–1926), British gynecologists]

donepezil n. see acetylcholinesterase inhibitor.

donor n. a person who makes his own tissues or organs available for use by someone else. For example, a donor may provide blood for transfusion (see blood donor), a kidney for transplantation, or sex cells for *artificial insemination or *oocyte donation.

donor insemination (DI) see artificial insemination.

dopa n. dihydroxyphenylalanine: a physio-

logically important compound that forms an intermediate stage in the synthesis of catecholamines (dopamine, epinephrine, and norepinephrine) from the essential amino acid tyrosine. It also plays a role itself in the functioning of certain parts of the brain. The form L-dopa (see levodopa) is administered for the treatment of *parkinsonism, a disease in which there is a deficiency of *dopamine in the brain.

dopamine n. a *catecholamine derived from dopa that functions as a *neurotransmitter, acting on specific dopamine receptors and also on adrenergic receptors throughout the body, especially in the *limbic system and *extrapyramidal system of the brain and in the arteries and the heart. It also stimulates the release of norepinephrine from nerve endings. The effects vary with the concentration. Dopamine is used as a drug to increase the strength of contraction of the heart in heart failure, shock, severe trauma, and septicemia. It is administered by injection in carefully controlled dosage. Possible side effects include unduly rapid or irregular heartbeat, nausea, vomiting, breathlessness, angina pectoris, and kidney damage. Trade name: **Intropin**.

Certain drugs (dopamine receptor agonists) have an effect on the body similar to that of dopamine. They include *apomorphine, *bromocriptine, *pergolide, *ropinirole, and cabergoline (Dostinex) and are used to treat *parkinsonism, *acromegaly (they suppress the release of growth hormone), and to suppress or prevent milk secretion (through their action in blocking the release of prolactin). Drugs that compete with dopamine to occupy and block the dopamine receptor sites in the body are known as dopamine receptor antagonists. They include some *antipsychotic drugs (e.g. the phenothiazines and butyrophenones) and certain drugs (e.g. *domperidone and *metoclopramide) used to treat nausea and vomiting.

dopamine hypothesis the theory that schizophrenia is caused in part by abnormalities in the metabolism of *dopamine and can be treated by drugs (such as *chlorpromazine) that antagonize its action as a neurotransmitter.

Doppler ultrasonography a diagnostic

technique that utilizes the fact that the frequency of *ultrasound waves changes when they are reflected from a moving surface. It is used to study the flow in blood vessels and the movement of blood in the heart. The frequency detector may be part of an ultrasound imaging probe, which displays an image of the anatomy on a TV screen. Simultaneously the Doppler signal from a particular point on the ultrasound image can be displayed next to the anatomical position using a split screen (*duplex imaging*). Using electronic techniques, direction and velocity of blood flow can each be allocated different colors and displayed on a color monitor over the anatomical image (*color flow ultrasound imaging*). *Power Doppler*, a modification of this technique, is more sensitive at detecting flow but does not give information on direction of flow. [C. J. Doppler (1803–53), Austrian physicist]

dornase alfa *n. see* DNase.

dors- (dorsi-, dorso-) *prefix denoting* **1.** the back. Example: *dorsalgia* (pain in). **2.** dorsal.

dorsal *adj.* relating to or situated at or close to the back of the body or to the posterior part of an organ.

dorsiflexion *n.* backward flexion of the foot or hand or their digits; i.e. bending toward the upper surface.

dorsoventral *adj.* (in anatomy) extending from the back (dorsal) surface to the front (ventral) surface.

dorsum *n.* **1.** the back. **2.** the upper or posterior surface of a part of the body; for example, of the hand. *See also* dorsal.

dorzolamide *n.* a *carbonic anhydrase inhibitor used to reduce intraocular pressure in the treatment of *glaucoma: it decreases the production of aqueous humor. Administered as eye drops (sometimes in combination with timolol) it may cause local burning or stinging, blurred vision, increased production of tears, dizziness, and pins and needles. Trade names: **Cosopt, Trusopt**.

dose *n.* a carefully measured quantity of a drug that is prescribed by a doctor to be given to a patient at any one time. The *median effective dose* (*ED$_{50}$*) is the dose of a drug that produces desired effects in 50% of individuals tested. *See also* LD$_{50}$.

dosimeter *n.* **1.** a device used to measure the intensity of a radiation source. **2.** a

device to record the amount of radiation received by workers exposed to X-rays or other radiation. Typically, it consists of a small piece of photographic film in a holder attached to the clothing, but this film badge has now been replaced by *thermoluminescent dosimeters.

dosimetry *n.* **1.** the calculation of appropriate radiation doses for treating given conditions, usually cancer in different parts of the body. *See* radiotherapy. **2.** the measurement of the dose received by a patient having a diagnostic technique involving ionizing radiation or by a radiation worker.

DOT direct observed therapy: *see* tuberculosis.

double-bind *n.* a disordered pattern of family relationships in which one family member gives contradictory instructions to another (as when a mother asks her child verbally for affection but simultaneously, by her gestures, indicates that the child should remain distant). The result is that any action the child makes will be wrong, and furthermore he cannot escape from the situation. This has been supposed, but not proved, to be a factor in causing schizophrenia.

double-blind trial *see* intervention study.

double contrast a technique used in X-ray examinations of the intestine. *Barium sulfate *contrast medium is used to coat the intestinal wall and the intestine is then distended with gas. The X-ray images obtained give exquisite detail of the lining of the intestinal tract. *See also* barium enema, barium meal.

double J stents *see* stent.

double uterus *see* uterus didelphys.

double vision *see* diplopia.

douche *n.* a forceful jet of water used for cleaning any part of the body, most commonly the vagina. A vaginal douche is extremely unreliable as a method of contraception.

Down's syndrome a condition resulting from a genetic abnormality in which an extra chromosome is present (there are three no. 21 chromosomes instead of the usual two), giving a total of 47 chromosomes rather than the normal 46. The chances of having a Down's child are higher with increasing maternal age. Affected individuals share certain clinical features, including a characteristic flat facial appearance with slanting eyes (as in Mongolian races, which gave the former name, *mongolism*, to the condition), broad hands with short fingers and a single crease across the palm, malformed ears, eyes with a speckled iris (*Brushfield spots*), short stature, and *hypotonia. Many individuals also have a degree of mental handicap, although the range of ability is wide and some individuals are of normal intelligence. Associated abnormalities, including heart defects (which affect about 40% of Down's children), intestinal malformation, deafness, and squints, may also be present. *Prenatal diagnosis of Down's syndrome can be obtained by *amniocentesis and *chorionic villus sampling; the condition can be confirmed by chromosomal analysis. Down's syndrome can also occur as a result of chromosomal rearrangement (*translocation) and as part of a *mosaicism. [J. L. H. Down (1828–96), British physician]

doxapram *n.* a drug that stimulates breathing following an operation or after a drug overdosage. It is administered intravenously; side effects include fever, cough, and heart rate changes. Trade name: **Dopram**.

doxazosin *n.* an *alpha blocker drug used to treat high blood pressure. It is administered by mouth. Possible side effects include faintness on standing up, weakness, dizziness, and headache. Trade name: **Cardura**.

doxepin *n.* a drug used to relieve depression, especially when associated with anxiety (*see* antidepressant). Doxepin is administered by mouth; possible side effects include drowsiness, dry mouth, blurred vision, and digestive upsets. It is also applied topically to relieve itching associated with eczema. Trade names: **Adapin**, **Sinequan**, **Zonalon**.

doxorubicin *n.* an *anthracycline antibiotic isolated from the bacterium *Streptomyces peucetius caesius* and used mainly in the treatment of leukemia and various other forms of cancer. Doxorubicin acts by interfering with the production of DNA and RNA (*see also* antimetabolite). It is administered by injection or infusion and can be given as a lipid formulation (*Doxil, see* liposome); side effects include bone marrow depression,

baldness, gastrointestinal disturbances, and heart damage. Trade names: **Adriamycin**, **Rubex**.

doxycycline *n.* an *antibiotic used to treat infections caused by a wide range of bacteria and other microorganisms. It is administered by mouth and side effects are those of the other *tetracyclines. Trade name: **Vibramycin**.

DPT vaccine a combined *vaccine against *d*iphtheria, whooping cough (pertussis), and *t*etanus organisms, prepared from their *toxoids and other antigens. It is given as a course of three doses in the first year of life, at two, three, and four months of age (currently recommended ages). The diphtheria and tetanus components require further boosters.

DR *see* digital radiography.

dracontiasis *n.* a tropical disease caused by the parasitic nematode *Dracunculus medinensis* (*see* guinea worm) in the tissues beneath the skin. The disease is transmitted to humans via contaminated drinking water. The initial symptoms, which appear a year after infection, result from the migration of the worm to the skin surface and include itching, giddiness, difficulty in breathing, vomiting, and diarrhea. Later a large blister forms on the skin, usually on the legs or arms, which eventually bursts and may ulcerate and become infected. Dracontiasis is common in India and West Africa but also occurs in Arabia, Iran, East Africa, and Afghanistan. Treatment involves slowly extracting the adult worm or administration of an *anthelmintic, such as *thiabendazole.

Dracunculus *n. see* guinea worm.

dragee *n.* a *pill that has been coated with sugar.

drain 1. *n.* a device, usually a tube or wick, used to draw fluid from an internal body cavity to the surface. A drain is sometimes inserted during an operation to ensure that any fluid formed immediately passes to the surface, so preventing an accumulation that may become infected or cause pressure in the operation site. **2.** *vb. see* drainage.

drainage *n.* the drawing off of fluid from a cavity in the body, usually fluid that has accumulated abnormally. For example, serous fluid may be drained from a swollen joint, pus removed from an internal abscess, or urine from an overdistended bladder. *See also* drain.

dram (drachm) *n.* **1.** a unit of weight used in pharmacy. 1 dram = 3.883 g (60 grains). **2.** a unit of volume used in pharmacy. 1 fluid dram = 3.696 ml (1/8 fluid ounce).

drastic *n.* any agent causing a major change in a body system or function, e.g. strong laxatives.

draw sheet a sheet placed beneath a patient in bed that, when one portion has been soiled or becomes uncomfortably wrinkled, may be pulled under the patient so that another portion may be used. The bed does not have to be remade, and the patient does not have to leave the bed.

drepanocyte (sickle cell) *n. see* sickle-cell disease.

drepanocytosis *n. see* sickle-cell disease.

dressing *n.* material applied to a wound or diseased part of the body, with or without medication, to give protection and assist healing.

DRG *see* diagnosis-related group.

drill *n.* (in dentistry) a rotary instrument used to remove tooth substance, particularly in the treatment of caries. It consists of a handpiece that takes variously shaped *burs. Most drilling is done with an air-driven turbine handpiece, but some is performed with a much slower mechanically driven handpiece. Drills usually have a water spray coolant and may have a fiberoptic light.

drip (intravenous drip) *n.* apparatus for the continuous injection (*transfusion) of blood, plasma, saline, glucose solution, drugs, or other fluid into a vein. The fluid flows under gravity from a suspended bottle through a tube ending in a hollow needle inserted into the patient's vein. The rate of flow can be adjusted according to the rate of drips seen in a transparent section of the tube, but many *infusions are now controlled by electronically regulated infusion pumps.

drom- (dromo-) *prefix denoting* movement or speed.

dromomania *n.* a pathologically strong impulse to travel, which is said to be present in some vagabonds.

dronabinol *n.* one of the active substances of marijuana. It is used in the treatment of nausea and vomiting associated with cancer chemotherapy in patients who do not respond to conventional antiemetic treatment. It is given by mouth; side effects include drowsiness, dizziness, and impaired coordination, sensations, and perceptions. It can also lead to dependence. Trade name: **Marinol**.

droperidol *n.* a neuroleptic antipsychotic drug that produces a state of emotional quietness and mental detachment. It is used as a premedication before surgery and to maintain general and regional anesthesia. Trade name: **Inapsine**.

dropsy *n. see* edema.

Drosophila *n.* a genus of very small flies, commonly called fruit flies, that breed in decaying fruit and vegetables. *D. melanogaster* has been extensively used in genetic research because it has only four pairs of chromosomes and those in its salivary glands are easily recognizable. Adult *D. repleta* sometimes feeds on fecal matter and may transmit disease organisms.

drug *n.* any substance that affects the structure or functioning of a living organism. Drugs are widely used for the prevention, diagnosis, and treatment of disease and for the relief of symptoms. The term *medicine* is sometimes preferred for therapeutic drugs in order to distinguish them from narcotics and other addictive drugs that are used illegally.

drug dependence *see* dependence.

Drug Enforcement Agency (DEA) a government agency created in 1973 that regulates and enforces the US laws involving the import, export, and traffic across state lines of narcotic drugs and other controlled substances.

drusen *pl. n.* **1.** (macular drusen) white or yellow deposits of *hyalin in *Bruch's membrane of the choroid. They are often associated with *macular degeneration. **2.** (disk drusen) glistening nodules seen on an irregularly raised *optic disk. Consisting of excess *glia (produced congenitally) that has undergone degeneration and calcification, they can be confused with *papilledema.

dry mouth a condition that occurs as a result of reduced salivary flow from a variety of causes, including *Sjögren's syndrome, connective tissue diseases, diabetes, excision or absence of a major salivary gland, or radiotherapy to the head that destroys the salivary glands. It causes swallowing and speech difficulties, inflamed gums and teeth, an increased incidence of dental caries, and loss of denture stability in people who have lost their teeth. Patients with their own teeth should be given sugar-free nonacidic saliva substitutes, strict dietary advice, and chlorhexidine mouthwashes; they require special monitoring by their dentist. Medical name: **xerostomia**.

dry socket a painful condition in which the normal healing of a tooth socket has been disturbed. Instead of being filled with a blood clot the socket is empty. Treatment is palliative and the condition resolves in 10–14 days.

DSI *see* digital spot imaging.

DSM Diagnostic and Statistical Manual: an influential publication of the American Psychiatric Association in which psychiatric disorders are classified and defined. *DSM-IV-TR* is the current (2000) version.

DTPA *see* pentetic acid.

Duane's syndrome a hereditary congenital abnormality of the eye muscles leading most commonly to restricted abduction (outward movement of the eye away from the midline) of one eye. On attempted adduction (inward movement of the eye toward the midline) of that same eye there is retraction of the eye into the orbit and narrowing of the opening between the eyelids. [A. Duane (1858–1926), US ophthalmologist]

Duchenne's muscular dystrophy *see* muscular dystrophy. [G. B. A. Duchenne (1806–75), French neurologist]

duct *n.* a tubelike structure or channel, especially one for carrying glandular secretions.

ductal carcinoma in situ (DCIS) the earliest stage of breast cancer, detectable by mammography, which is confined to the lactiferous (milk) ducts of the breast. *See* carcinoma in situ.

ductions *pl. n.* movements of one eye, i.e. adduction (rotation toward the nose), abduction (rotation toward the temple), elevation, depression, intorsion, and extorsion.

ductless gland *see* endocrine gland.

ductule *n.* a small duct or channel.

ductus *n.* a duct. The *ductus deferens* is the *vas deferens.

ductus arteriosus a blood vessel in the fetus connecting the pulmonary artery directly to the ascending aorta, so bypassing the pulmonary circulation. It normally closes after birth. Failure of the ductus to close (*patent ductus arteriosus*) produces a continuous *murmur, and the consequences are similar to those of a *septal defect. It may close spontaneously in childhood but often requires surgical closure.

Dukes' classification a histological staging system that classifies colorectal tumors according to the degree of tissue invasion and metastasis, which is useful for prognosis. It formed the basis for many later systems of cancer staging and is still used. [Sir C. Dukes (1890–1977), British pathologist]

dumbness *n. see* mutism.

Dumdum fever *see* kala-azar.

dumping syndrome (postgastrectomy syndrome) a group of symptoms that sometimes occur after stomach operations, particularly *gastrectomy. After a meal, especially one rich in carbohydrate, the patient feels faint, weak, and nauseous, and may sweat and become pale. The attack lasts 30 minutes to two hours and is caused by rapid stomach emptying, leading to decrease in blood sugar and the drawing of fluid from the blood into the intestine. Avoidance of carbohydrate meals may relieve the syndrome but further surgery is sometimes required.

Duncan's disease *see* X-linked lymphoproliferative syndrome. [Duncan family, in whom the disease was first studied]

duo- *prefix denoting* two.

duoden- (duodeno-) *prefix denoting* the duodenum. Example: *duodenectomy* (excision of).

duodenal atresia a condition in which the duodenum is narrowed, causing complete obstruction. It presents at birth with vomiting, which is usually bile-stained, and is associated with other congenital abnormalities, particularly *Down's syndrome. Treatment is correction of any fluid imbalance and surgical repair.

duodenal ulcer an ulcer in the duodenum, caused by the action of acid and pepsin on the duodenal lining (mucosa) of a susceptible individual. It is usually associated with an increased output of stomach acid. Infection of the *antrum of the stomach with *Helicobacter py-

lori is almost always present. Symptoms include pain in the upper abdomen, especially when the stomach is empty, which often disappears completely for weeks or months; vomiting may occur. Complications include bleeding, *perforation, and obstruction due to scarring (*see* pyloric stenosis). Symptoms are relieved by antacid medicines; most ulcers heal if treated by an *antisecretory drug, or if *H. pylori* is eradicated by a combination of a *proton-pump inhibitor (or an H₂-receptor antagonist) and antibiotics. Surgery (*see* gastrectomy, vagotomy) is now rarely required.

duodenoscope *n.* a *fiberscope for examining the interior of the duodenum. An end-viewing instrument is used for most examinations, but a side-viewing instrument is used for *ERCP. The end-viewing instrument is also used for examination of the stomach (it is also known as a *gastroduodenoscope*) and it is usual to combine the two examinations (*gastroduodenoscopy*).

duodenostomy *n.* an operation in which the duodenum is brought through the abdominal wall and opened, usually in order to introduce food. *See also* gastroduodenostomy.

duodenum *n.* the first of the three parts of the small *intestine. It extends from the pylorus of the stomach to the jejunum. The duodenum receives bile from the gallbladder (via the common bile duct) and pancreatic juice from the pancreas. Its wall contains various glands (including *Brunner's glands*) that secrete an alkaline juice (*succus entericus), rich in mucus, that protects the duodenum from the effects of the acidic *chyme passing from the stomach. —**duodenal** *adj.*

duplex imaging *see* Doppler ultrasonography.

Dupuytren's contracture forward curvature of one or more fingers (usually the third or fourth) due to fixation of the flexor tendon of the affected finger to the skin of the palm. The condition is treated by surgical *division of the fibrous bands joining tendon and skin. [Baron G. Dupuytren (1777–1835), French surgeon]

dura (dura mater, pachymeninx) *n.* the thickest and outermost of the three *meninges surrounding the brain and spinal cord. It consists of two closely adherent layers, the outer of which is identical with the periosteum of the skull. The inner dura extends downward between the cerebral hemispheres to form the *falx cerebri* and forward between the cerebrum and cerebellum to form the *tentorium*. A thin film of fluid (which is not cerebrospinal fluid) separates the inner dura from the arachnoid. —**dural** *adj.*

durable power of attorney for health care the designation of a surrogate person to make health care decisions for another person who may be incapacitated or incapable of making decisions regarding treatment. *See* advance directive.

DVD *see* dissociated vertical deviation.

DVT (deep vein thrombosis) *see* phlebothrombosis.

dwarfism *n.* abnormally short stature from any cause. The most common type of dwarf is the *achondroplastic dwarf* (*see* achondroplasia). *Pituitary dwarfs* have a deficiency of *growth hormone due to a defect in the pituitary gland; they are well proportioned and show no mental retardation, but may be sexually underdeveloped. *Primordial dwarfs* have a genetic defect in their response to growth hormone. Dwarfism is also associated with thyroid deficiency (*see* cretinism), in which both physical and mental development is retarded; chronic diseases such as rickets; renal failure; and intestinal malabsorption.

dydrogesterone *n.* a synthetic female sex hormone (*see* progestogen) used to treat menstrual abnormalities (such as dysmenorrhea) and infertility and to prevent miscarriage. It is administered by mouth and may cause mild nausea and breakthrough bleeding.

dynamic orthosis a technique that retains the essentials of splinting but allows some controlled movement of the restrained body part.

dynamometer *n.* a device for recording the force of a muscular contraction. A small hand-held dynamometer may be used to record the strength of a patient's grip. A special optical dynamometer measures the action of the muscles controlling the shape of the lens of the eye.

dyne *n.* a unit of force equal to the force required to impart to a mass of 1 gram an acceleration of 1 centimetre per second per second. 1 dyne = 10^{-5} newton.

-dynia *suffix denoting* pain. Example: *proctodynia* (in the rectum).

dyphylline *n.* a drug that relaxes bronchial muscle. It is used to relieve symptoms in asthma and bronchitis and for treating reversible bronchospasm. It is administered by mouth or injection and may cause nausea and vomiting, headache, palpitations, and dizziness, especially following injection. *See also* bronchodilator. Trade names: **Dilor, Lufyllin**.

dys- *prefix denoting* difficult, abnormal, or impaired. Examples: *dysbasia* (difficulty in walking); *dysgeusia* (impairment of taste).

dysarthria *n.* a speech disorder in which the pronunciation is unclear although the language content and meaning are normal.

dysbarism *n.* any clinical syndrome due to a difference between the atmospheric pressure outside the body and the pressure of air or gas within a body cavity (such as the paranasal sinuses or the middle ear). *See* compressed air illness.

dysbulia *n.* any disturbance of the will or of the mental processes that lead to purposeful action.

dyschezia *n.* a form of constipation resulting from a long period of voluntary suppression of the urge to defecate. The rectum becomes distended with feces and bowel movements are difficult or painful.

dyschondroplasia (Ollier's disease) *n.* a condition due to faulty ossification of cartilage, resulting in development of many benign cartilaginous tumors (*see* chondroma). The bones involved may become stunted and deformed. There is an increased risk of developing malignant tumors (*see* chondrosarcoma).

dyschromatopsia *n.* any defect of color vision.

dyscoria *n.* any abnormality in the shape of the pupil.

dyscrasia *n.* an abnormal state of the body or part of the body, especially one due to abnormal development or metabolism. In classical medicine the term was used for the imbalance of the four humors (blood, phlegm, yellow bile, black bile), which was believed to be the basic cause of all diseases.

dysdiadochokinesis (adiadochokinesis) *n.* clumsiness in performing rapidly alternating movements. It is often recognized by asking the patient to tap with his fingers on the back of his other hand. It is a sign of disease of the cerebellum or its intracerebral connections.

dysentery *n.* an infection of the intestinal tract causing severe diarrhea with blood and mucus. *Amebic dysentery (amebiasis)* is caused by the protozoan *Entamoeba histolytica* and results in ulceration of the intestines and occasionally in the formation of abscesses in the liver (*amebic* or *tropical abscesses*), lungs, testes, or brain. The parasite is spread by food or water contaminated by infected feces. Symptoms appear days or even years after infection and include diarrhea, indigestion, loss of weight, and anemia. Prolonged treatment with drugs, including metronidazole, is usually effective in treating the condition. Amebic dysentery is mainly confined to tropical and subtropical countries.

Bacillary dysentery is caused by bacteria of the genus *Shigella* and is spread by contact with a patient or carrier or through food or water contaminated by their feces. Epidemics are common in overcrowded unsanitary conditions. Symptoms, which develop 1–6 days after infection, include diarrhea, nausea, cramping, and fever and they persist for about a week. An attack may vary from mild diarrhea to an acute infection causing serious dehydration and bleeding from the intestine. In most cases, provided fluid losses are replaced, recovery occurs within 7–10 days; antibiotics may be given to eliminate the bacteria. *Compare* cholera.

dysesthesia *n.* the abnormal and sometimes unpleasant sensations felt by a patient with partial damage to a peripheral nerve when his skin is touched. *Compare* paresthesia.

dysfunctional uterine bleeding *see* menorrhagia.

dysgenesis *n.* faulty development; *gonadal dysgenesis* is failure of the ovaries or testes to develop (*see* Turner's syndrome).

dysgerminoma (germinoma, gonocytoma) *n.* a malignant tumor of the ovary, thought to arise from primitive germ cells; it is homologous to the *seminoma of the testis. About 15% of such tumors affect both ovaries; outside the ovary they have been recorded in the anterior mediastinum and in the pineal gland. Dysgerminomas may occur from infancy to old age, but the average age of patients is about 20 years. They are very sensitive to both *radiotherapy and *chemotherapy.

dysgraphia n. see agraphia.

dyshidrosis (dysidrosis) n. any abnormality of sweating or the sweat glands other than excessive sweating (*hyperhidrosis*), diminished sweating (*hypohidrosis*), or absence of sweating (*anidrosis*); for example, changes in the color or smell of sweat.

dyshormonogenesis n. a collection of inherited disorders of thyroid hormone synthesis resulting in low levels of *thyroxine and *triiodothyronine and high levels of *thyroid-stimulating hormone, with consequent *goiter formation. The result may be *cretinism with a goiter or milder forms of *hypothyroidism with a goiter. Several different stages of the production pathway for thyroid hormones can be affected.

dyskariosis n. the abnormal condition of a cell that has a nucleus showing the features characteristic of the earliest stage of malignancy, while retaining relatively normal cytoplasm. It may be seen, for example, in the squamous and columnar epithelial cells of a *cervical smear.

dyskinesia n. a group of involuntary movements that appear to be a fragmentation of the normal smoothly controlled limb and facial movements. They include *chorea, *dystonia, and those involuntary movements occurring as side effects to the use of levodopa and the phenothiazines (*see* tardive dyskinesia).

dyslalia n. a speech disorder in which the patient uses a vocabulary or range of sounds that is peculiar to him. It is a feature of the defective speech acquired by children who have been aphasic from birth (*see* aphasia).

dyslexia n. a developmental disorder selectively affecting a child's ability to learn to read and write. The condition, affecting boys more often than girls, is usually apparent by the age of seven years. It is sometimes called *specific (developmental) dyslexia, developmental (congenital) word blindness,* or *developmental reading disorder* to distinguish it from acquired difficulties with reading and writing. *Compare* alexia. —**dyslexic** *adj.*

dyslogia n. disturbed and incoherent speech. This may be due to *dementia, *aphasia, *mental retardation, or mental illness.

dysmenorrhea n. painful menstruation. *Primary dysmenorrhea* begins with the first period and is often associated with nausea, vomiting, and faintness. The cause is thought to be related to excessive *prostaglandin production. In *secondary dysmenorrhea,* usually affecting older patients, a congested ache and abdominal cramps precede menstruation. Causes include pelvic inflammatory disease, endometriosis, fibroids, and the presence of an IUD.

dysmnesic syndrome a disorder of memory in which new information is not learned but old material is well remembered. *See* Korsakoff's syndrome.

dysmorphophobia (body dysmorphic disorder) n. a fixed distressing belief that one's body is deformed and repulsive, or an excessive fear that it might become so.

dysostosis n. the abnormal formation of bone or the formation of bone in abnormal places, such as a replacement of cartilage by bone.

dyspareunia n. painful or difficult sexual intercourse experienced by a woman. Psychological or physical factors may be responsible (*see* vaginismus).

dyspepsia (indigestion) n. disordered digestion: usually applied to pain or discomfort in the lower chest or abdomen occurring after eating and sometimes accompanied by nausea or vomiting. —**dyspeptic** *adj.*

dysphagia n. a condition in which the action of swallowing is either difficult to perform, painful (*see* odynophagia), or in which swallowed material seems to be held up in its passage to the stomach. It is caused by painful conditions of the mouth and throat, obstruction of the pharynx or esophagus by diseases of the wall or pressure from outside, or by abnormalities in the neurological coordination of the muscular activity of the pharynx or esophagus, as a result of such disorders as motor neuron disease or multiple sclerosis.

dysphasia *n. see* aphasia.

dysphemia *n. see* stammering.

dysphonia *n.* difficulty in speaking. This may be due to a disorder of the larynx, vocal cords, tongue, or mouth, or it may be *psychogenic. Compare* aphasia, dysarthria.

dysplasia (alloplasia, heteroplasia) *n.* abnormal development of skin, bone, or other tissues. *See* bronchopulmonary dysplasia, fibrous dysplasia. **—dysplastic** *adj.*

dysplastic nevus syndrome *see* atypical mole syndrome.

dyspnea *n.* labored or difficult breathing. (The term is often used for a sign of labored breathing apparent to the doctor, *breathlessness* being used for the subjective feeling of labored breathing.) Dyspnea can be due to obstruction to the flow of air into and out of the lungs (as in bronchitis and asthma), various diseases affecting the tissue of the lung (including pneumoconiosis, emphysema, tuberculosis, and cancer), and heart disease.

dyspraxia *n. see* apraxia.

dyssynergia (asynergia) *n.* lack of coordination, especially clumsy uncoordinated movements found in patients with disease of the cerebellum. They include *dysmetria* (the application of inappropriate force for a movement), intention *tremor, *dysdiadochokinesis, and a staggering wide-based gait. *Bladder sphincter dyssynergia* is the incoordination of micturition that occurs due to spinal cord damage in multiple sclerosis.

dysthymic disorder *see* depression, neurosis.

dystocia *n.* difficult birth, caused by abnormalities in the fetus or the mother. The most common causes of *fetal dystocia* are excessive size or *malpresentation. *Maternal dystocia* may result if the pelvis is abnormally small, or the uterus muscles fail to contract, or the cervix of the uterus fails to expand. If the cause of dystocia cannot be eliminated, it may be necessary to deliver the baby by cesarean section or to operate in such a way that it can be removed with the minimum possible risk to the mother.

dystonia *n.* any dysfunction of muscle tone, usually characterized by spasms or abnormal muscle contractions. One form is a postural disorder often associated with disease of the *basal ganglia in the brain. There may be spasm in the muscles of the face, shoulders, neck, trunk, and limbs. The arm is often held in a rotated position and the head is drawn back and to one side. Dystonic conditions, such as *torticollis, *blepharospasm, and writer's *cramp, may be helped by the injection of *botulinum toxin. **—dystonic** *adj.*

dystrophia myotonica (myotonic dystrophy) a type of *muscular dystrophy in which the muscle weakness and wasting is accompanied by an unnatural prolongation of the muscular contraction after any voluntary effort (*see* myotonia). The muscles of the face, temples, and neck are especially wasted. Baldness, endocrine malfunction, and cataracts occur. The disease can affect both sexes (it is inherited as an autosomal dominant character).

dystrophy (dystrophia) *n.* a disorder of an organ or tissue, usually muscle, due to impaired nourishment of the affected part. The term is applied to several unrelated conditions; for example, *muscular dystrophy, *Fuchs' endothelial dystrophy, and *dystrophia adiposogenitalis* (*see* Fröhlich's syndrome).

dysuria *n.* difficult or painful urination. This is usually associated with urgency and frequency of urination if due to *urethritis or *cystitis. The pain is burning in nature and is relieved by curing the underlying cause. A high fluid intake usually helps.

E

Eagle-Barrett syndrome *see* prune belly syndrome. [J. F. Eagle (20th century), US physician; N. R. Barrett (20th century), British physician]

Eales' disease inflammation of the blood vessels of the retina occurring in young adults. It is characterized by leakage from abnormal growths of new vessels as well as recurrent hemorrhages into the vitreous humor. [H. Eales (1852–1913), British physician]

ear *n.* the sense organ for hearing and balance (see illustration). Sound waves, transmitted from the outside into the external auditory meatus, cause the eardrum (tympanic membrane) to vi-

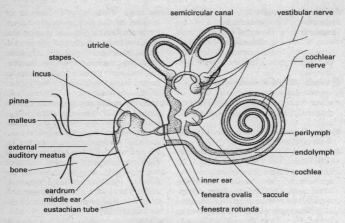

semicircular canal

vestibular nerve

utricle

stapes

incus

pinna

malleus

external auditory meatus

bone

cochlear nerve

perilymph

endolymph

cochlea

eardrum

middle ear

eustachian tube

inner ear

fenestra ovalis

saccule

fenestra rotunda

Structure of the ear

brate. The small bones (ossicles) of the middle ear – the malleus, incus, and stapes – transmit the sound vibrations to the fenestra ovalis, which leads to the inner ear (*see* labyrinth). Inside the *cochlea the sound vibrations are converted into nerve impulses. Vibrations emerging from the cochlea could cause pressure to build up inside the ear, but this is released through the *eustachian tube. The *semicircular canals, *saccule, and *utricle – also in the inner ear – are all concerned with balance.

earache *n. see* otitis, otalgia.

eardrum *n. see* tympanic membrane.

Early and Periodic Screening, Diagnosis and Treatment (EPSDT) programs administered under provisions of the 1972 US Social Security Act amendments relating to Medicaid and Maternal and Child Health. The legislation provides for child-health screening and corrective treatment as needed for children in families receiving aid to dependent children. The law also permits the federal government to reduce the Medicaid matching funds allocated to states that fail to provide such child-health screening programs.

earwax *n. see* cerumen.

eating disorder any of a group of disorders in which abnormal feeding habits are associated with emotional and psycholog-

ical conflicts. *See* anorexia nervosa, bulimia, pica.

Ebola virus a virus responsible for an acute infection in humans with features similar to those of *Marburg disease. Transmission is by contact with infected blood and other body fluids and the incubation period is 2–21 days (7 days on average). The mortality rate is 53–88%, but intensive treatment (including rehydration) in the early stages of the disease can halt its rapid and usually irreversible progression to hemorrhaging of internal organs. Sporadic but short-lived outbreaks have occurred in Africa since 1976, when the virus was first identified during an outbreak in the region of the Ebola River, in Zaïre (now Democratic Republic of Congo). An unknown species of animal is assumed to act as a reservoir for the virus between outbreaks of the disease in humans.

Ebstein's anomaly a form of congenital heart disease affecting the right side of the heart: the muscle is unusually thin and the heart valves are abnormal. It causes breathlessness, *failure to thrive, cyanosis, and abnormalities of heart rhythm, although if mild, it may be asymptomatic and life expectancy is normal. If severe, corrective surgery may be necessary. [W. Ebstein (1836–1912), German physician]

eburnation n. the wearing down of the cartilage at the articulating surface of a bone, exposing the underlying bone and leading to bone sclerosis, in which the bone's surface becomes dense and smooth like ivory. This is an end result of *osteoarthritis.

EB virus (EBV) see Epstein-Barr virus.

ec- prefix denoting out of or outside.

ecbolic n. an agent, such as *oxytocin, that induces childbirth by stimulating contractions of the uterus.

ecchondroma n. a benign cartilaginous tumor (see chondroma) that protrudes beyond the margins of a bone. Compare enchondroma.

ecchymosis n. a bruise: an initially bluish-black mark on the skin, resulting from the release of blood into the tissues either through injury or through the spontaneous leaking of blood from the vessels (as in some blood diseases).

eccrine adj. 1. describing sweat glands that are distributed all over the body. Their ducts open directly onto the surface of the skin and they are most dense on the soles of the feet and the palms of the hands. Compare apocrine. 2. see merocrine.

ecdemic adj. not occurring normally in the population of a country: applied sometimes to unusual diseases brought in from abroad by immigrants or travelers. Compare endemic.

ecdysis n. the act of shedding skin; *desquamation.

ECF see Extended Care Facility.

ECFMG see Educational Council for Foreign Medical Graduates.

ECG n. see electrocardiogram.

echinococciasis (echinococcosis) n. see hydatid disease.

Echinococcus n. a genus of small parasitic tapeworms that reach a maximum length of only 8 mm. Adults are found in the intestines of dogs, wolves, or jackals. If the eggs are swallowed by a human, who can act as a secondary host, the resulting larvae penetrate the intestine and settle in the lungs, liver, or brain to form large cysts, usually 5–10 cm in diameter (see hydatid disease). Two species causing this condition are E. granulosus and E. multilocularis.

echoacousia n. a false sensation of echoing after a normally heard sound due to a defect of the cochlea of the inner ear.

echocardiography n. the use of *ultrasound waves to investigate and display the action of the heart as it beats. Used in the diagnosis and assessment of congenital and acquired heart diseases, echocardiography is safe, painless, and reliable and reduces the need for cardiac *catheterization. M-mode echocardiography uses a single beam of ultrasound. The image produced is not anatomic but permits precise measurement of cardiac dimensions and the diagnosis of valvular, myocardial, and pericardial disease. Real-time echocardiography uses a pulsed array of ultrasound beams to build up a moving image on a TV monitor of the chambers and valves of the heart. In Doppler echocardiography, ultrasound reflected from moving red blood cells is subject to the Doppler effect (change of pitch with velocity relative to the observer), which can be used to calculate blood flow and pressure within the heart and great vessels. It is useful in the diagnosis and assessment of valve disease and intracardial shunts. In transesophageal echocardiography the ultrasound probe is mounted on an esophageal endoscope. The examination from within the esophagus allows the probe to be placed directly against the back of the heart, enabling improved visualization of posterior structures.

echoencephalography n. investigation of structures within the skull by detecting the echoes of ultrasonic pulses. The chief value of the method was in detecting those disorders causing a displacement of the midline structures of the brain. The technique has largely been superseded by *computed tomography (CT) and *magnetic resonance imaging (MRI).

echokinesis n. see echopraxia.

echolalia n. pathologic repetition of the words spoken by another person. It may be a symptom of language disorders, *autism, *catatonia, or *Gilles de la Tourette syndrome.

echo planar imaging (EPI) an imaging technique, based on *nuclear magnetic resonance (NMR), that provides a real-time snapshot with, apparently, the same image quality as NMR. This method, which is still in the early stages of development, may provide new insights into fetal pathology.

echopraxia (echokinesis) n. pathologic imitation of the actions of another person. It may be a symptom of *catatonia or of *latah.

echothiophate iodide a *miotic used in the treatment of *glaucoma and convergent *strabismus. It is administered topically as eye drops; common side effects include burning, stinging, redness, and other irritation of the eyes. Trade name: **Phospholine Iodide**.

echovirus n. one of a group of more than 30 RNA-containing viruses (enteroviruses), originally isolated from the human intestinal tract, that were found to produce pathologic changes in cells grown in culture. These viruses – which were accordingly termed *enteric cytopathic human orphan viruses* – are now thought to be the cause of nonspecific meningitis, many gastrointestinal and respiratory tract infections, and of motor paralysis. They are now more commonly known as *coxsackieviruses. *Compare* reovirus.

eclabium n. the turning outward of a lip.

eclampsia n. the occurrence, during pregnancy or shortly after childbirth, of one or more convulsions not caused by other conditions, such as epilepsy or cerebral hemorrhage, in a woman with *preeclampsia. The onset of convulsions may be preceded by a sudden rise in blood pressure and/or a sudden increase in *edema and development of *oliguria. The convulsions are usually followed by coma. Eclampsia is a threat to both mother and baby and must be treated immediately.

ECMO *see* extracorporeal membrane oxygenation.

ECoG *see* electrocochleography.

ecology (bionomics) n. the study of the relationships between humans, plants and animals, and the environment, including the way in which human activities may affect other animal populations and alter natural surroundings. —**ecological** *adj.* —**ecologist** n.

econazole n. an antifungal drug used to treat ringworm and candidiasis. Econazole is administered as a cream. Possible side effects include local irritation and burning. Trade name: **Spectazole**.

ecraseur n. a surgical device, resembling a *snare, that is used to sever the base of a tumor during its surgical removal.

ecstasy n. a sense of extreme well-being and bliss. The word applies particularly to *trance states dominated by religious thinking. While not necessarily pathologic, it can be caused by epilepsy (especially of the temporal lobe) or by schizophrenia.

Ecstasy n. the street name for methylenedioxymethamphetamine (MDMA), a mildly hallucinogenic drug that generates feelings of euphoria in those who take it. Its most common side effect is hyperthermia; drinking large quantities of water to combat the intense thirst produced by taking the drug may result in fatal damage to the body's fluid balance. Its manufacture, sale, use, and possession are illegal.

ECT *see* electroconvulsive therapy.

ect- (ecto-) *prefix denoting* outer or external.

ectasia (ectasis) n. the dilation of a tube, duct, or hollow organ.

ecthyma n. an infection of the skin, caused by both *Streptococcus pyogenes* and *Staphylococcus aureus*, in which the full thickness of the epidermis is involved (*compare* impetigo, which is a superficial infection). Ecthyma heals more slowly than impetigo and causes scarring. It may be associated with poor hygiene or depressed immunity.

ectoderm n. the outer of the three *germ layers of the early embryo. It gives rise to the nervous system and sense organs, the teeth and lining of the mouth, and the *epidermis and its associated structures (hair, nails, etc.). —**ectodermal** *adj.*

ectomorphic *adj.* describing a *body type that is relatively thin, with a large skin surface in comparison to weight. *Compare* endomorphic, mesomorphic. —**ectomorph** n. —**ectomorphy** n.

-ectomy *suffix denoting* surgical removal of a segment or all of an organ or part. Examples: *appendectomy* (of the appendix); *prostatectomy* (of the prostate gland).

ectoparasite n. a parasite that lives on the outer surface of its host. Some ectoparasites, such as bedbugs, maintain only periodic contact with their hosts, whereas others, such as the crab louse, have a permanent association. *Compare* endoparasite.

ectopia n. **1.** the misplacement, due either to a congenital defect or injury, of a bodily part. **2.** the occurrence of something in an unnatural location (*see* ectopic beat, ectopic pregnancy). —**ectopic** *adj.*

ectopic beat (extrasystole) a heartbeat due to an impulse generated somewhere in the heart outside the sinoatrial node. Ectopic beats are generally premature in timing; they are classified as *supraventricular* if they originate in the atria and *ventricular* if they arise from a focus in the ventricles. They may be produced by any heart disease, by nicotine from smoking, or by caffeine from excessive tea or coffee consumption; they are common in normal individuals. The patient may be unaware of their presence or may feel that his heart has "missed a beat." Ectopic beats may be suppressed by drugs such as quinidine, propranolol, and lidocaine; avoidance of smoking and reduction in excessive tea or coffee intake may help. *See* arrhythmia.

ectopic hormone a hormone produced by cells that do not usually produce it. Some tumor cells secrete hormones; for example, small-cell lung cancer cells secrete vasopressin and cause *hyponatremia.

ectopic pregnancy (extrauterine pregnancy) the development of a fetus at a site other than in the uterus. This may happen if the fertilized egg cell remains in the ovary or in the tube leading from near the ovary to the uterus (the fallopian tube) or if it lodges in the free abdominal cavity. The most common type of ectopic pregnancy is a *tubal* (or *oviducal*) *pregnancy*, which occurs in fallopian tubes that become blocked or inflamed. The growth of the fetus may cause the tube to burst and bleed. In most cases the fetus dies within three months of conception and the products are absorbed into the maternal circulation. Rarely, the pregnancy may continue until a live baby can be delivered by cesarean section. The condition may be diagnosed by ultrasound and the products of conception may be removed by laparoscopy before damage is done to the fallopian tube. Medical name: **ecyesis.**

ectoplasm *n.* the outer layer of cytoplasm in cells, which is denser than the inner cytoplasm (*endoplasm) and concerned with activities such as cell movement. —**ectoplasmic** *adj.*

ectro- *prefix denoting* congenital absence.

ectrodactyly *n.* congenital absence of all or part of one or more fingers.

ectromelia *n.* congenital absence or gross shortening (aplasia) of the long bones of one or more limbs. *See also* amelia, hemimelia, phocomelia.

ectropion *n.* turning out of the eyelid, away from the eyeball. The most common type is *senile ectropion*, in which the lower eyelid droops because of loss of the elasticity of its tissues in old age. If the muscle that closes the eye (orbicularis oculi) is paralyzed, the lower lid also droops. Ectropion may also occur if the lining membrane (conjunctiva) of the lid is very thickened or if scarring causes contraction of the surrounding facial skin.

eczema *n.* a superficial inflammation of the skin, mainly affecting the *epidermis. Eczema causes itching, with a red rash often accompanied by small blisters that weep and become crusted. Subsequent scaling, thickening, or discoloration of the skin may occur. It is usually considered endogenous, or constitutional, i.e., outside agents do not play a primary role (*compare* dermatitis), but in some contexts the terms "dermatitis" and "eczema" are used interchangeably. The condition is therefore often classified into two major divisions: *eczematous dermatitis*, which results from external factors (*see* dermatitis); and *endogenous* (or *constitutional*) *eczema*, occurring without any obvious external cause. Classification of endogenous eczema is based on its appearance and site. The five main types are: (1) *atopic eczema*, which affects up to 20% of the population and is associated with asthma and hay fever; (2) *seborrheic eczema* (or *dermatitis*), which involves the scalp, eyelids, nose, and lips, is associated with the presence of *Malassezia* yeasts, and is common in patients with AIDS; (3) *discoid* (or *nummular*) *eczema*, which is characterized by coin-shaped lesions and occurs only in adults; (4) *pompholyx, affecting the hands and feet; (5) *gravitational* (or *stasis*) *eczema*, associated with poor venous circulation and incorrectly known as *varicose eczema*.

Treatment of eczema is with topical or systemic corticosteroids but emollients are very important, especially in treating mild cases. Newer treatments include *PUVA or cyclosporin A. —**eczematous** adj.

edema n. excessive accumulation of fluid in the body tissues: popularly known as *dropsy*. The resultant swelling may be local, as with an injury or inflammation, or more general, as in heart or kidney failure. In generalized edema there may be collections of fluid within the chest cavity (*pleural effusions*), abdomen (*see* ascites), or within the air spaces of the lung (*pulmonary edema*). It may result from heart or kidney failure, cirrhosis of the liver, acute nephritis, the nephrotic syndrome, starvation, allergy, or drugs (e.g. phenylbutazone or cortisone derivatives). In such cases the kidneys can usually be stimulated to get rid of the excess fluid by the administration of *diuretic drugs. *Subcutaneous edema* commonly occurs in the legs and ankles due to the influence of gravity and (in women) before menstruation; the swelling subsides with rest and elevation of the legs. —**edematous** adj.

edentulous adj. lacking teeth: usually applied to people who have lost some or all of their teeth.

edetate n. a salt of *ethylenediamine tetraacetic acid* (*EDTA*), which is used as a *chelating agent in the treatment of poisoning. *Edetate calcium disodium* (*Calcium Disodium Versenate, Versene Ca*) is administered by intravenous injection to treat poisoning by heavy metals, such as lead and strontium; side effects are mild. *Edetate disodium* (*Disotate, Endrate, Versene Na*) is used as treatment for increased calcium serum levels and for the control of heart rhythm associated with *digitalis toxicity. It is administered by intravenous injection; side effects include nausea, vomiting, and diarrhea.

edrophonium n. an *anticholinesterase drug that is administered by injection in a test for diagnosis of *myasthenia gravis and to reverse the neuromuscular block produced by curare. Side effects can include nausea and vomiting, increased saliva flow, diarrhea, and stomach pains. Trade names: **Enlon, Reversol, Tensilon**.

EDTA (ethylenediamine tetraacetic acid) *see* edetate.

Educational Council for Foreign Medical Graduates (ECFMG) a council that directs examination procedures for graduates of medical schools outside the US and Canada who wish to enter internship, residency, or practice in the US. The ECFMG represents the American Medical Association, the American Hospital Association, the Association of American Medical Colleges, and the Federation of State Medical Boards.

Edwards' syndrome a condition resulting from a genetic abnormality in which an extra chromosome is present – there are three no. 18 chromosomes instead of the usual two. Affected babies, who rarely survive, have a characteristic abnormally shaped head, low birth weight, prominent heels ("rocker-bottom feet"), heart abnormalities, and severe mental retardation. Prenatal diagnosis can be made by *amniocentesis or *chorionic villus sampling. [J. H. Edwards (1928–), British geneticist]

EEG (electroencephalogram) *see* electroencephalography.

efavirenz n. a *reverse transcriptase inhibitor of the human immunodeficiency virus type 1 (*HIV-1), indicated for the treatment of HIV-1 infection in combination with at least one or two other active antiretroviral agents when therapy is warranted. This combination of agents blocks the replication of HIV and prevents healthy T cells from becoming infected with the virus. Efavirenz is administered orally; common side effects include rash, muscle and joint aches, oral lesions, headache, excessive tiredness, vomiting and diarrhea. Trade name: **Sustiva**.

effacement n. the shortening and obliteration of the vaginal portion of the cervix by the movement of the fetus during labor and birth.

effector n. any structure or agent that brings about activity in a muscle or gland, such as a motor nerve that causes muscular contraction or glandular secretion. The term is also used for the muscle or gland itself.

efferent adj. **1.** designating nerves or neurons that convey impulses from the brain or from the spinal cord to muscles, glands, and other effectors; i.e. any motor nerve or neuron. **2.** designating vessels or ducts that drain fluid (such as lymph) from an organ or part. *Compare* afferent.

effleurage *n.* a form of *massage in which the hands are passed continuously and rhythmically over a patient's skin in one direction only, with the aim of increasing blood flow in that direction and aiding the dispersal of any swelling due to *edema.

effluvium *n.* (*pl.* **effluvia**) **1.** an outflowing or shedding, especially of the hair. **2.** an obsolete term for an exhalation, especially one of bad or noxious odor formerly believed to cause disease.

effort syndrome a condition of marked anxiety about the condition of one's heart and circulatory system. This is accompanied by a heightened consciousness of heartbeat and respiration, which in turn is worsened by the anxiety it induces. Treatment is commonly with reassurance and *anxiolytic drugs; psychotherapy is only occasionally necessary.

effusion *n.* **1.** the escape of pus, serum, blood, lymph, or other fluid into a body cavity as a result of inflammation or the presence of excess blood or tissue fluid in an organ or tissue. **2.** fluid that has escaped into a body cavity.

eflornithine *n.* a drug used against protozoa for the treatment of *sleeping sickness. It is administered by intravenous injection. Possible side effects include diarrhea, hair loss, convulsions, and damage to bone marrow. Trade name: **Ornidyl.**

EGD *see* esophagogastroduodenoscopy.

egg cell *see* ovum.

ego *n.* (in psychoanalysis) the part of the mind that develops from a person's experience of the outside world and is most in touch with external realities. In Freudian terms the ego is said to reconcile the demands of the *id (the instinctive unconscious mind), the *superego (moral conscience), and reality.

Ehlers-Danlos syndrome any one of a rare group of inherited (autosomal *dominant or autosomal *recessive) disorders of the connective tissue involving abnormal or deficient *collagen, the protein that gives the body tissues strength. There are several types of differing severity. The skin of affected individuals is very elastic but also very fragile: it bruises easily and scars poorly, the scars

often being paper-thin. The joints of those affected tend to be very mobile (double-jointed) and dislocate easily. In some types the uterus or intestine can rupture or the valves in the heart can be weaker than normal. [E. L. Ehlers (1863–1937), Danish dermatologist; H. A. Danlos (1844–1912), French dermatologist]

egophony *n. see* vocal resonance.

eidetic *adj. see* imagery.

eikonometer *n.* an instrument for measuring the size of images on the retina of the eye.

Eisenmenger reaction a condition in which *pulmonary hypertension is associated with a *septal defect, so that blood flows from the right to the left side of the heart or from the pulmonary artery to the aorta. This allows blue blood, poor in oxygen, to bypass the lungs and enter the general circulation. This reduces the oxygen content of the arterial blood in the aorta and its branches, resulting in a patient with a dusky blue appearance (*cyanosis) and an increased number of red blood cells (*polycythemia). There is no curative treatment at this stage, but the patient may be helped by the control of heart failure and polycythemia. The condition may be prevented by appropriate surgical treatment of the septal defect before irreversible pulmonary hypertension develops. [V. Eisenmenger (1864–1932), German physician]

ejaculation *n.* the discharge of semen from the erect penis at the moment of sexual climax (orgasm) in the male. The constituents of semen are not released simultaneously, but in the following sequence: the secretion of *Cowper's glands followed by that of the *prostate gland and the spermatozoa and finally the secretion of the *seminal vesicles. *See also* premature ejaculation.

Ekbom syndrome *see* restless legs syndrome. [K. A. Ekbom (1907–77), Swedish neurologist]

elastic cartilage a type of *cartilage in which elastic fibers are distributed in the matrix. It is yellowish in color and is found in the external ear.

elastic tissue strong extensible flexible *connective tissue rich in yellow *elastic fibers*. These are long, thin, and branching and are composed primarily of an albumin-like protein, *elastin*. Elastic tissue is found in the dermis of the skin, in arterial walls, and in the walls of the alveoli of the lungs.

elastin *n.* protein forming the major constituent of *elastic tissue fibers.

elastography *n.* an ultrasonic imaging technique that displays the elasticity of soft tissues. It has been found useful in demonstrating abnormalities of both muscle and breast tissue.

elastosis *n.* degeneration of the yellow fibers in connective tissues and skin (*see* elastic tissue).

elation (exaltation) *n.* a state of cheerful excitement and enthusiasm. Marked elation of mood is a characteristic of *mania or *hypomania.

elbow *n.* the hinge joint (*see* ginglymus) between the bones of the upper arm (humerus) and the forearm (radius and ulna). It is a common site of fractures and dislocation.

electrocardiogram (ECG) *n.* a recording of the electrical activity of the heart on a moving paper strip (see illustration). The ECG tracing is recorded by means of an apparatus called an *electrocardiograph* (*see* electrocardiography). It aids in the diagnosis of heart disease, which may produce characteristic changes in the ECG.

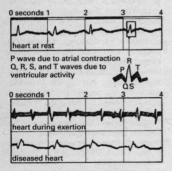

P wave due to atrial contraction
Q, R, S, and T waves due to ventricular activity

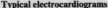

Typical electrocardiograms

electrocardiography *n.* a technique for recording the electrical activity of the heart. Electrodes connected to the recording apparatus (*electrocardiograph*) are placed on the skin of the four limbs and chest wall; the record itself is called an *electrocardiogram (ECG). In con-

ventional *scalar electrocardiography* 12 leads (*see* lead[2]) are recorded, but more may be used in special circumstances (for example, an esophageal lead, from an electrode within the trachea, may be used in the analysis of arrhythmias). *Vectorcardiography* is less common, but this may be used to obtain a three-dimensional impression of electrical activity of the heart.

electrocardiophonography *n.* a technique for recording heart sounds and murmurs simultaneously with the ECG, which is used as a reference tracing. The sound is picked up by a microphone placed over the heart. The tracing is a *phonocardiogram*. It provides a permanent record of heart sounds and murmurs and is useful in their analysis.

electrocautery (galvanocautery) *n.* the destruction of diseased or unwanted tissue by means of a needle or snare that is electrically heated (*see* diathermy). Warts, polyps, and other growths can be burned away by this method.

electrocoagulation *n.* the coagulation of body tissues by means of a high-frequency electric current concentrated at one point as it passes through them. Electrocoagulation, using a *diathermy knife, permits bloodless incisions to be made during an operation.

electrocochleography (ECoG) *n.* a test to measure electrical activity produced within the *cochlea in response to a sound stimulus. It is used in the diagnosis of Ménière's disease and other forms of sensorineural *deafness.

electroconvulsive therapy (ECT, electroshock) a treatment for severe depression and occasionally for schizophrenia and mania. A convulsion is produced by passing an electric current through the brain. The convulsion is modified by giving a *muscle relaxant drug and an *anesthetic, so that in fact only a few muscle twitches are produced. The means by which ECT acts is not yet known. The procedure can also produce confusion, loss of memory, and headache, which almost always pass off within a few hours. These side effects are reduced by unilateral treatment, in which the current is passed only through the nondominant hemisphere of the brain.

electrodesiccation *n. see* fulguration.

electroencephalogram (EEG) n. see electroencephalography.

electroencephalography n. the technique for recording electrical activity from different parts of the brain and converting it into a tracing called an *electroencephalogram* (*EEG*). The machine that records this activity is known as an *encephalograph*. The pattern of the EEG reflects the state of the patient's brain and his level of consciousness in a characteristic manner. Electroencephalography is mostly used in the diagnosis and management of epilepsy and sleep disorders.

electroglottography n. a method of assessing laryngeal function using external recording electrodes.

electrokymography n. the technique of recording the movements of an organ, especially the heart, by means of a fluoroscope and a photoelectric recording system.

electrolarynx n. a battery-powered electrical vibrator that helps people to speak after *laryngectomy.

electrolyte n. a substance that dissociates into ions in a solution (an ion is an atom or group of atoms that conduct electricity); for example, sodium chloride solution consists of free sodium and free chloride ions. The term *serum electrolyte level* means the concentration of separate ions (sodium, potassium, chloride, bicarbonate, etc.) in the circulating blood. Concentrations of various electrolyte levels can be altered by many diseases, in which electrolytes are lost from the body (as in vomiting or diarrhea) or are not excreted and therefore accumulate (as in renal failure). When electrolyte concentrations are severely diminished, they can be corrected by administering the appropriate substance by mouth or by intravenous drip. When excess of an electrolyte exists it may be removed by *dialysis or by special resins in the intestine, taken by mouth or by enema. See also anion.

electromyography n. continuous recording of the electrical activity of a muscle by means of electrodes inserted into the muscle fibers. The tracing is displayed on an oscilloscope. The technique is used for diagnosing various nerve and muscle disorders and assessing progress in recovery from some forms of paralysis.

electronarcosis n. the induction of sleep by passing weak electrical currents through the brain. It is seldom used in Western psychiatry.

electron microscope a microscope that uses a beam of electrons as a radiation source for viewing the specimen. The resolving power (ability to register fine detail) is a thousand times greater than that of an ordinary light microscope. The specimen must be examined in a vacuum, which necessitates special techniques for preparing it, and the electrons are usually focused onto a fluorescent screen (for direct viewing) or onto a photographic plate (for a photograph, or *electron micrograph*). A *transmission electron microscope* is used to examine thin sections at high magnification. A *scanning electron microscope* reveals the surfaces of objects at various magnifications; its great depth of focus is advantageous.

electron transport chain a series of enzymes and proteins in living cells through which electrons are transferred, via a series of oxidation-reduction reactions. This ultimately leads to the conversion of chemical energy into a readily usable and storable form. The most important electron transport chain is the *respiratory chain*, present in mitochondria and functioning in cellular respiration.

electron volt a unit of energy equal to the increase in the energy of an electron when it passes through a rise in potential of one volt. Symbol: eV.

electrooculography n. an electrical method of recording eye movements. Tiny electrodes are attached to the skin at the inner and outer corners of the eye, and as the eye moves an alteration in the potential between these electrodes is recorded. The size of this potential at rest also gives an indication of the health of the retina. The recording itself is called an *electrooculogram* (*EOG*).

electrophoresis n. the technique of separating electrically charged particles, particularly proteins, in a solution by passing an electric current through the solution. The rate of movement of the different components depends upon their charge, so that they gradually separate into bands. Electrophoresis is widely used in the investigation of body chemicals, such as the analysis of the different proteins in blood serum.

electroretinography *n.* a method of recording changes in the electrical potential of the retina when it is stimulated by light. The recording itself is called an *electroretinogram* (*ERG*). One electrode is placed on the eye in a contact lens and the other is usually attached to the back of the head. In retinal disease the pattern of electrical change is altered. The technique is useful in diagnosing retinal diseases when opacities, such as cataract, make it difficult to view the retina or when the disease produces little visible change in the retina.

electroshock *n. see* electroconvulsive therapy.

electrosurgery *n.* surgery using a high-frequency electric current from a fine wire electrode (a *diathermy knife) to cut tissue. The ground electrode is a large metal plate. When used correctly, little heat spreads to the surrounding tissues, in contrast to *electrocautery.

electrotherapy *n.* the passage of electric currents through the body's tissues to stimulate the functioning of nerves and the muscles that they supply. The technique is applied to the muscles of patients with various forms of paralysis due to nerve disease or muscle disorder. *See also* faradism, galvanism.

electuary *n.* a pharmaceutical preparation in which the drug is made up into a paste with syrup or honey.

element *n.* **1.** any of the primary or constituent parts of matter. **2.** (in chemistry) any one of the more than 100 primary substances that are composed of atoms of identical atomic number and that cannot be broken down by chemical means into any other substance. The chemical properties of an element can only be changed by union with some other element or by nuclear reaction. *See* nuclear medicine.

elephantiasis *n.* gross enlargement of the skin and underlying connective tissues caused by obstruction of the lymph vessels, which prevents drainage of lymph from the surrounding tissues. Inflammation and thickening of the walls of the vessels and their eventual blocking is commonly caused by the parasitic filarial worms *Wuchereria bancrofti* and *Brugia malayi*. The parts most commonly affected are the legs but the scrotum, breasts, and vulva may also be involved. Elastic bandaging is applied to the affected parts and the limbs are elevated and rested. Larval forms in the blood are killed with diethylcarbamazine. *See also* filariasis.

elevator *n.* **1.** an instrument that is used to raise a depressed broken bone, for example, in the skull or cheek. A specialized *periosteal elevator* is used in orthopedics to strip the fibrous tissue (periosteum) covering bone. **2.** a lever-like instrument used to ease a tooth or root out of its socket during extraction.

elimination *n.* (in physiology) the entire process of excretion of metabolic waste products from the blood by the kidneys and urinary tract.

ELISA *see* enzyme-linked immunosorbent assay.

elixir *n.* a preparation containing alcohol (ethanol), glycerine, or flavoring substances, which is intended for oral use as the vehicle for bitter or nauseous drugs.

elliptocytosis *n.* the presence of significant numbers of abnormal elliptical red cells (*elliptocytes*) in the blood. Elliptocytosis may occur as a hereditary disorder or be associated with certain blood diseases, such as *myelofibrosis or iron-deficiency *anemia.

Elschnig pearls round or oval transparent cystic structures seen through the pupil of the eye, due to proliferation of lens epithelial cells following extracapsular *cataract extraction. They can grow to occlude the pupil and hence cause reduction in vision. [A. Elschnig (1863–1939), German ophthalmologist]

elutriation *n.* the separation of a fine powder from a coarser powder by mixing them with water and decanting the upper layer while it still contains the finer particles. The heavier coarse particles sink to the bottom more rapidly.

em- *prefix. see* en-.

emaciation *n.* wasting of the body, caused by such conditions as malnutrition, tuberculosis, cancer, or parasitic worms.

emasculation *n.* strictly, surgical removal of the penis, the testes, or both. The term is often used to mean loss of male physical and emotional characteristics, either as a result of removal of the testes (castration) or of emotional stress.

embalming *n.* the preservation of a dead

Emergency Medical Service

body by the introduction of chemical compounds that delay putrefaction. The ancient Egyptians raised the process to a fine art in the production of their mummies. Today embalming is used mainly so that a body can be transported long distances and funeral rites can be conducted without undue haste. In the US embalming is a routine hygienic measure.

embedding n. (in microscopy) the fixing of a specimen within a mass of firm material in order to facilitate the cutting of thin sections for microscopical study. The embedding medium, e.g. paraffin for light microscopy or Araldite for electron microscopy, helps to keep the specimen intact.

embolectomy n. surgical removal of an *embolus in order to relieve arterial obstruction. The embolus may be removed by cutting directly into the affected artery (arteriotomy). In some instances it is removed by a balloon *catheter, which is manipulated beyond the embolus from a small arteriotomy in an accessible artery. The catheter is then withdrawn carrying the embolus with it. In some cases of pulmonary embolism, embolectomy may be life saving. It may also prevent gangrene, with loss of a limb, in cases of a limb artery embolus.

embolism n. the condition in which an embolus becomes lodged in an artery and obstructs its blood flow. The most common form of embolism is *pulmonary embolism, in which a blood clot is carried in the circulation to lodge in the pulmonary artery. An embolus in any other artery constitutes a systemic embolism. In this case a common source of the embolus is a blood clot within the heart in mitral valve disease or following *myocardial infarction. The clinical features depend upon the site at which an embolus lodges (for example, a stroke may result from a cerebral embolism and gangrene from a limb embolism). Treatment is by *anticoagulant therapy with heparin and warfarin. Major embolism is treated by *embolectomy or *streptokinase, *urokinase, or *tissue-type plasminogen activator to remove or dissolve the embolus. See also air embolism.

embolization (therapeutic embolization) n. the introduction of embolic material to reduce or completely obstruct blood flow in such conditions as congenital arteriovenous malformations (see angioma), angiodysplasia, malignant tumors, or arterial rupture. Under X-ray screening control, a cannula is inserted into the artery supplying the affected area and occluding material, such as microspheres, metallic coils, or PVA (polyvinyl alcohol) foam, is injected. The procedure may treat the underlying problem or simplify subsequent surgery. See also bilateral uterine arterial embolization.

embolus n. (pl. emboli) material, such as a blood clot, fat, air, amniotic fluid, or a foreign body, that is carried by the blood from one point in the circulation to lodge at another point (see embolism).

embrasure n. the space formed between adjacent teeth.

embrocation n. a lotion that is rubbed onto the body for the treatment of sprains and strains.

embryo n. an animal at an early stage of development, before birth. In humans the term refers to the products of conception within the uterus up to the eighth week of development, during which time all the main organs are formed (see illustration). Compare fetus. —**embryonic** adj.

embryology n. the study of the growth and development of the embryo and fetus from fertilization of the ovum until birth. —**embryological** adj.

embryonic disk the early embryo before the formation of *somites. It is a flat disk of tissue bounded dorsally by the amniotic cavity and ventrally by the yolk sac. The formation of the *primitive streak and *archenteron in the embryonic disk determines the orientation of the embryo, which then becomes progressively elongated.

embryoscopy n. examination of an embryo or fetus during the first 12 weeks of pregnancy by means of a fiberoptic *endoscope inserted through the cervix; it can be performed as early as five weeks' gestation. Access to the fetal circulation may be obtained through the instrument and direct visualization of the embryo permits the diagnosis of malformations.

embryo transfer the transfer of an embryo from an in vitro culture into the uterus. See also in vitro fertilization.

Emergency Medical Service see EMS.

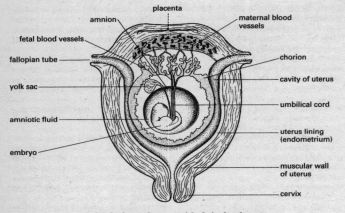

amnion

placenta

fetal blood vessels

maternal blood vessels

fallopian tube

chorion

yolk sac

cavity of uterus

umbilical cord

amniotic fluid

uterus lining (endometrium)

embryo

muscular wall of uterus

cervix

A developing embryo nourished via the placenta

emergency medicine the specialty that deals with acutely injured or ill patients who require immediate medical treatment.

emesis *n. see* vomiting.

emetic *n.* an agent that causes vomiting. Strong emetics, such as *apomorphine, are used to induce vomiting following drug overdose. Substances such as common salt, which irritate the stomach nerves if taken in sufficient quantities, also cause vomiting. Some emetics, e.g. *ipecac, are *expectorants at low doses.

emetine *n.* a drug used to treat infections of the liver, bowel, and intestine caused by amebas, including amebic dysentery. It is administered by injection, which may be painful, and irritates the stomach lining and other mucous membranes.

-emia *suffix denoting* a specified condition of the blood. Example: *hyperglycemia* (excess sugar in the blood).

eminence *n.* a projection, often rounded, on an organ or tissue, particularly on a bone. An example is the *iliopubic eminence* on the hip bone.

emissary veins a group of veins within the skull that drain blood from the venous sinuses of the dura mater to veins outside the skull.

emission *n.* the flow of semen from the erect penis, usually occurring while the subject is asleep (*nocturnal emission*).

EMLA cream a cream containing a *eutectic* mixture of *local anesthetics (hence the name). Applied to the skin as a thick coating and left on for 90 minutes, it gives a helpful degree of local anesthesia, allowing blood samples to be taken and facilitating biopsy procedures in young children.

emmenagogue *n.* an agent that stimulates menstruation.

emmetropia *n.* the state of refraction of the normal eye, in which parallel light rays are brought to a focus on the retina with the accommodation relaxed. Distant objects are seen clearly without any effort to focus. *Compare* ametropia, hyperopia, myopia.

emollient *n.* an agent that soothes and softens the skin. Emollients are fats and oils, such as lanolin and liquid paraffin; they are used alone as moisturizers to lessen the need for active drug therapy (such as corticosteroids for eczema) and in skin preparations as a base for more active drugs, such as antibiotics.

emotion *n.* a state of arousal that can be experienced as pleasant or unpleasant. Emotions can have three components: *subjective, physiological,* and *behavioral.* For example, fear can involve an unpleasant subjective experience, an increase in physiological measures such as heart rate, sweating, etc., and a tendency to flee from the fear-provoking situation.

empathy *n.* the ability to understand the thoughts and emotions of another person. In a psychotherapist empathy is often considered to be one of the necessary qualities enabling successful treatment. *See* alexithymia.

emphysema *n.* air in the tissues. In *pulmonary emphysema* the air sacs (*alveoli) of the lungs are enlarged and damaged, which reduces the surface area for the exchange of oxygen and carbon dioxide. Severe emphysema causes breathlessness, which is made worse by infections. There is no specific treatment, and the patient may become dependent on oxygen. The mechanism by which emphysema develops is not understood, although it is known to be particularly common in men and is associated with chronic bronchitis, smoking, and advancing age.
In *surgical emphysema* air may escape into the tissues of the chest and neck from leaks in the lungs or esophagus; occasionally air escapes into other tissues during surgery, and bacteria may form gas in soft tissues. The presence of gas or air gives the affected tissues a characteristic crackling feeling to the touch, and it may be visible on X-rays. It is easily absorbed once the leak or production is stopped.

empirical *adj.* describing a system of treatment based on experience or observation, rather than of logic or reason.

empty sella syndrome a congenital malformation of the bony structure (the *sella turcica) that houses the pituitary gland so that the space is largely filled with cerebrospinal fluid, which squashes the usually spherical gland into a flattened shape against the floor of the sella. It is usually associated with enlargement of the sella, which can be seen on lateral X-ray. Only 10% of cases of this condition have defective pituitary function.

empyema (pyothorax) *n.* pus in the *pleural cavity, usually secondary to infection in the lung or in the space below the diaphragm. It is a life-threatening condition, which can be relieved by aspiration or drainage of the pus or by decapsulation (*see* decortication).

EMS (Emergency Medical Service) a coordinated national US network of services linked by a vast communications system that provides aid and medical assistance by personnel specially trained in rescue, stabilization, transport, and treatment of medical and traumatic emergencies, from initial response to inpatient critical care treatment.

emulsion *n.* a preparation in which fine droplets of one liquid (such as oil) are dispersed in another liquid (such as water). In the pharmacy, medicines are prepared in the form of emulsions to disguise the taste of an oil, which is dispersed in a flavored liquid.

en- (em-) *prefix denoting* in; inside.

enalapril *n.* a drug used in the treatment of high blood pressure (hypertension) and symptomatic congestive heart failure. It inhibits the action of *angiotensin, which results in decreased vasopressor (blood-vessel constricting) activity and decreased aldosterone secretion. Enalapril is administered by mouth; side effects include headache, dizziness, fatigue, and hypotension. Trade names: **Lexxel, Vaseretic, Vasotec.**

enamel *n.* the extremely hard outer covering of the crown of a *tooth. It is formed before tooth eruption by *ameloblasts and consists of crystalline *hydroxyapatite.

enanthema *n.* an eruption occurring on a mucus-secreting surface, such as the inside of the mouth or vagina.

enarthrosis *n.* a ball-and-socket joint: a type of *diarthrosis (freely movable joint), e.g. the shoulder joint and the hip joint. Such a joint always involves a long bone, which is thus allowed to move in all planes.

encainide *n.* an *antiarrhythmic drug that is used in the treatment of life-threatening ventricular *arrhythmias. It is administered orally; side effects include chest pain, shortness of breath, and swelling in the legs and feet. Trade name: **Enkaid.**

encapsulated *adj.* (of an organ, tumor, bacterium, etc.) enclosed in a capsule.

encephal- (encephalo-) *prefix denoting* the brain.

encephalin *n.* *see* enkephalin.

encephalitis *n.* inflammation of the brain. It may be caused by a viral or bacterial infection or it may be part of an allergic response to a systemic viral illness or vaccination (*see* encephalomyelitis). *Viral encephalitis* is endemic in some parts of the world; it may also occur epidemically or sporadically. One form – *encephalitis lethargica* – reached epidemic proportions shortly after World War I and was marked by headache and drowsiness, progressing to coma (hence its popular name – *sleeping sickness*). Occasional cases may still occur as a complication of mumps. It can cause postencephalitic *parkinsonism. Another type of encephalitis that occurs sporadically is due to herpes simplex.

encephalocele *n. see* neural tube defects.

encephalography *n.* any of various techniques for recording the structure of the brain or the activity of the brain cells. Examples are *echoencephalography, *electroencephalography, and *pneumoencephalography.

encephaloid *adj.* 1. having the appearance of brain tissue. 2. *see* medullary carcinoma.

encephalomyelitis *n.* an acute inflammatory disease affecting the brain and spinal cord. It is sometimes part of an overwhelming virus infection but *acute disseminated encephalomyelitis* is a form of delayed tissue hypersensitivity provoked by a mild infection or vaccination 7–10 days earlier. Survival through the acute phase of the illness is often followed by a remarkably complete recovery.

encephalomyelopathy *n.* any condition in which there is widespread disease of the brain and spinal cord. *Necrotizing encephalomyelopathy of childhood* is a progressive illness with extensive destruction of nerve cells throughout the central nervous system. It is thought to be caused by a disorder of metabolism.

encephalon *n. see* brain.

encephalopathy *n.* any of various diseases that affect the functioning of the brain. *See* hepatic encephalopathy, spongiform encephalopathy, Wernicke's encephalopathy.

enchondroma *n.* a benign cartilaginous tumor (*see* chondroma) that occurs in the growing zone (metaphysis) of a bone and does not protrude beyond its margins. Such tumors are often solitary; when multiple the condition is known as *enchondromatosis*. *Compare* ecchondroma.

encopresis *n.* incontinence of feces not due to organic illness or defect. The term is used for fecal soiling associated with psy-

chiatric disturbance, especially in a child who has gained bowel control but passes formed stools in unacceptable places. The underlying problem is behavioral and treatment is often difficult. Encopresis must be distinguished from chronic constipation with overflow.

encounter group a form of group psychotherapy. The emphasis is on encouraging close relationships between group members and on the expression of feelings. To this end, physical contact and confrontations between group members are arranged by the group leader. The stress of the experience can be damaging to maladjusted people.

encysted *adj.* enclosed in a cyst.

end- (endo-) *prefix denoting* within or inner. Example: *endonasal* (within the nose).

endarterectomy *n.* a surgical technique to open an artery that has become obstructed by *atheroma with or without a blood clot (thrombus); the former operation is known as *thromboendarterectomy*. The inner part of the wall is removed together with any clot that is present. This restores patency and arterial blood flow to the tissues beyond the obstruction. The technique is most often applied to obstruction of the carotid arteries or of the arteries that supply the legs.

endarteritis *n.* chronic inflammation of the inner (intimal) portion of the wall of an artery, which most often results from late syphilis. Thickening of the wall produces progressive arterial obstruction and symptoms from inadequate blood supply to the affected part (*ischemia). The arteries to the brain are often involved, giving rise to meningovascular syphilis. Endarteritis of the aorta may obstruct the openings to the coronary arteries, supplying the heart. Endarteritis of the arteries to the wall of the aorta (the vasa vasorum) contributes to *aneurysm formation. The syphilitic infection may be eradicated with penicillin.

end artery the terminal branch of an artery, which does not communicate with other branches. The tissue it supplies is therefore probably completely dependent on it for its blood supply.

endemic *adj.* occurring frequently in a particular region or population: applied to diseases that are generally or constantly found among people in a particular area. *Compare* ecdemic, epidemic, pandemic.

endemic syphilis *see* bejel.

endocarditis *n.* inflammation of the lining of the heart cavity (endocardium) and valves. It is most often due to rheumatic fever or results from bacterial infection (*bacterial endocarditis*). Temporary or permanent damage to the heart valves may result. The main features are fever, changing heart murmurs, heart failure, and embolism. Treatment consists of rest and antibiotics; surgery may be required to repair damaged heart valves.

endocardium *n.* a delicate membrane, formed of flat endothelial cells, that lines the heart and is continuous with the lining of arteries and veins. At the openings of the heart cavities it is folded back on itself to form the cusps of the valves. The endocardium presents a smooth slippery surface, which does not impede blood flow. —**endocardial** *adj.*

endocervicitis *n.* inflammation of the membrane lining the cervix (neck) of the uterus, usually resulting from infection. Surface cells (epithelium) may die, resulting in a new growth of healthy epithelium over the affected area. The condition is accompanied by a thick mucoid discharge.

endocervix *n.* the mucous membrane (*endometrium) lining the cervix (neck) of the uterus.

endochondral *adj.* within the material of a cartilage.

endocrine gland (ductless gland) a gland that manufactures one or more *hormones and secretes them directly into the bloodstream (and not through a duct to the exterior). Endocrine glands include the pituitary, thyroid, parathyroid, and adrenal glands, the ovary and testis, the placenta, and part of the pancreas.

endocrinology *n.* the study of the *endocrine glands and the substances they secrete (*hormones). —**endocrinologist** *n.*

endoderm *n.* the inner of the three *germ layers of the early embryo, which gives rise to the lining of most of the alimentary canal and its associated glands, the liver, gallbladder, and pancreas. It also forms the lining of the bronchi and alveoli of the lung and most of the urinary tract.

endodermal sinus tumor a rare tumor of fetal remnants of the ovaries or testes.

endodontics *n.* the study, treatment, and prevention of diseases of the pulp of teeth and their sequelae. A major part of treatment is *root canal treatment.

endogenous *adj.* arising within or derived from the body. *Compare* exogenous.

endolymph *n.* the fluid that fills the membranous *labyrinth of the ear.

endolymphatic duct a blind-ended duct that leads from the sacculus and joins a duct from the utriculus of the membranous *labyrinth of the ear.

endolymphatic sac a dilation at the end of the *endolymphatic duct that removes waste products from the inner ear.

endometrial ablation the removal of the entire endometrium by using an ablative technique; the procedure is performed under local anesthesia using a *hysteroscope. It is an alternative to the more traditional hysterectomies that were undertaken for the relief of *menorrhagia. Methods for hysteroscopic endometrial ablation that were introduced in the 1980s included Nd:YAG (neoymium:yttrium–aluminum–garnet) laser ablation, *transcervical resection of the endometrium (TCRE), and rollerball *electrocoagulation (RBE). These first-generation procedures remain the gold standard for the hysteroscopic treatment of menorrhagia. In the 1990s, the second generation of hysteroscopic ablation techniques were developed, including balloon heating methods (Thermachoice), in which a balloon filled with a hot liquid is inserted into the uterus and causes the endometrium to slough off; microwave endometrial ablation (MEA); a radio-frequency method; and a *cryotherapy method. They all seem to be equally effective in achieving their aim.

endometrial hyperplasia an increase in the thickness of the cells of the *endometrium, usually due to prolonged exposure to unopposed estrogen, which can be endogenous, as in *anovular menstrual cycles; or exogenous, deriving, for example, from *hormone replacement therapy or an estrogen-secreting tumor. Atypical cells may or may not be present. The presence of atypical cells may lead to endometrial carcinoma. Treatment can include progestogen therapy or surgery (*see* endometrial ablation).

endometriosis *n.* the presence of tissue similar to the lining of the uterus (*see* endometrium) at other sites in the pelvis or, rarely, throughout the body (e.g. in the lung, rectum, or umbilicus). It is thought to be caused by retrograde *menstruation. When the tissue has infiltrated the wall of the uterus (myometrium) the condition is known as *adenomyosis*. The tissue may also be found in the ovary, fallopian tubes, pelvic ligaments, on the pelvic peritoneum, and even in the cervix and the vagina. This tissue undergoes the periodic changes similar to those of the endometrium and causes pelvic pain and severe *dysmenorrhea. The pain is usually worse immediately before, and at the beginning of, menstruation but usually ceases after menstruation. The symptoms resolve in pregnancy and after the menopause. Treatment is normally to down-regulate ovarian function with analogues of *gonadotropin-releasing hormone (*see* LHRH analogue) or danazol. Surgical treatment may also be necessary, usually by laser or ablative therapy via laparoscope. More radical surgical treatment in the form of a total abdominal hysterectomy and bilateral salpingo-oophorectomy is sometimes required.

endometritis *n.* inflammation of the *endometrium due to acute or chronic infection. It may be caused by foreign bodies, bacteria, viruses, or parasites. In the acute phase it may occur in the period immediately after childbirth (puerperium) but the chronic phase may not be associated with pregnancy (as in tuberculous endometritis). Chronic endometritis in women with IUDs may be responsible for the contraceptive action.

endometrium *n.* the mucous membrane lining the uterus, which becomes progressively thicker and more glandular and has an increased blood supply in the latter part of the menstrual cycle. This prepares the endometrium for implantation of the embryo, but if this does not occur much of the endometrium breaks down and is lost in menstruation. If pregnancy is established, the endometrium becomes the *decidua, which is shed after birth. —**endometrial** *adj.*

endomorphic *adj.* describing a *body type

that is relatively fat, having highly developed viscera and weak muscular and skeletal development. *Compare* ectomorphic, mesomorphic. —**endomorph** *n.* —**endomorphy** *n.*

endomyocarditis *n.* an acute or chronic inflammatory disorder of the muscle and lining membrane of the heart. When the membrane surrounding the heart (pericardium) is also involved the condition is termed *pancarditis*. The principal causes are rheumatic fever and virus infections. There is enlargement of the heart, murmurs, embolism, and frequently arrhythmias. The treatment is that of the cause and complications. *See also* endocarditis.

A chronic condition, *endomyocardial fibrosis*, is seen in black Africans; the cause is unknown.

endomysium *n.* the fine connective tissue sheath that surrounds a single *muscle fiber.

endoneurium *n.* the layer of fibrous tissue that separates individual fibers within a *nerve.

endoparasite *n.* a parasite that lives inside its host, for example in the liver, lungs, intestine, or other tissues of the body. *Compare* ectoparasite.

endopeptidase *n.* a digestive enzyme (e.g. *pepsin) that splits a whole protein into small peptide fractions by splitting the linkages between peptides in the interior of the molecule. *Compare* exopeptidase. *See also* peptidase.

endophthalmitis *n.* inflammation, usually due to infection, confined to the posterior chamber of the eye, i.e. the part behind the lens. *Compare* panophthalmitis.

endoplasm *n.* the inner cytoplasm of cells, which is less dense than the *ectoplasm and contains most of the cell's structures. —**endoplasmic** *adj.*

endoplasmic reticulum (ER) a system of membranes present in the cytoplasm of cells. ER is described as *rough* when it has *ribosomes attached to its surface and *smooth* when ribosomes are absent. It is the site of manufacture of proteins and lipids and is concerned with the transport of these products within the cell (*see also* Golgi apparatus).

end organ a specialized structure at the end of a peripheral nerve, acting as a receptor for a particular sensation. Taste buds, in the tongue, are end organs subserving the sense of taste.

endorphin *n.* one of a group of chemical compounds, similar to the *enkephalins, that occur naturally in the brain and have pain-relieving properties similar to those of the opiates. They are also responsible for sensations of pleasure. The endorphins are derived from a substance found in the pituitary gland called *betalipotropin*; they are thought to be concerned with controlling the activity of the endocrine glands.

endoscope *n.* any instrument used to obtain a view of the interior of the body. Examples of endoscopes include the *auriscope, used for examining the ear canal and eardrum, and the *gastroscope, for examining the inside of the stomach. Essentially, most endoscopes consist of a tube with a light at the end and an optical system, or a miniature video camera, for transmitting an image to the examiner's eye. *See also* fiberscope. —**endoscopic** *adj.* —**endoscopy** *n.*

endoscopic retrograde cholangiopancreatography *see* ERCP.

endospore *n.* the resting stage of certain bacteria, particularly species of the genera *Bacillus* and *Clostridium*. In adverse conditions the nucleus and cytoplasm within the normal vegetative stage of the bacterium can become enclosed within a tough protective coat, allowing the cell to survive. On return of favorable conditions the spore changes back to the vegetative form.

endostapler *n.* a stapling instrument (*see* staple) used endoscopically for purposes of fixing tissues or joining them together.

endosteum *n.* the membrane that lines the marrow cavity of a bone.

endothelin *n.* any one of a class of peptide hormones, consisting of chains of 21 amino acids, that are synthesized by endothelial cells, often of large blood vessels. They are the most powerful known stimulants of smooth muscle (such as that in the walls of arteries) and may possibly be important causes of hypertension. The drug *bosentan*, which blocks receptors for endothelin-1, has been used in treating patients with pulmonary hypertension with encouraging results.

endothelioma *n.* any tumor arising from or resembling endothelium. It may arise from the linings of blood vessels or lymph vessels (*hemangioendothelioma* and *lymphangioendothelioma*, respectively); from the linings of the pleural or peritoneal cavities (*see* mesothelioma); or from the meninges (*see* meningioma).

endothelium *n.* the single layer of cells that lines the heart, blood vessels, and lymphatic vessels. It is derived from embryonic mesoderm. The *corneal endothelium* is the innermost layer of the *cornea. *Compare* epithelium.

endothermic *adj.* describing a chemical reaction associated with the absorption of heat. *Compare* exothermic.

endotoxin *n.* a poison generally harmful to all body tissues, contained within certain gram-negative bacteria and released only when the bacterial cell is broken down or dies and disintegrates. *Compare* exotoxin.

endotracheal *adj.* within or through the trachea (windpipe). *See* intubation.

end-plate *n.* the area of muscle cell membrane immediately beneath the motor nerve ending at a *neuromuscular junction. Special receptors in this area trigger muscular contraction when the nerve ending releases its *neurotransmitter.

end-stage disease a terminal condition due to irreversible damage to vital organs or tissues, such as *end-stage renal failure*, the most advanced stage of kidney failure.

enema *n.* (*pl.* **enemata** or **enemas**) a quantity of fluid infused into the rectum through a tube passed into the anus. An *evacuant enema* (soap or olive oil) is used to remove feces. A *therapeutic enema* is used to insert drugs into the rectum, usually corticosteroids in the treatment of *proctocolitis. *See also* barium enema, small bowel enema.

enervation *n.* **1.** weakness; loss of strength. **2.** the surgical removal of a nerve.

enflurane *n.* a volatile drug used to induce and maintain general anesthesia. It is administered by inhalation. Possible side effects include seizures, hepatitis, and kidney damage. Trade name: **Ethrane**.

engagement *n.* (in obstetrics) the stage of pregnancy that occurs when the presenting part of the fetus has descended into the mother's pelvis. Engagement of the fetal head occurs when the widest part has passed through the pelvic inlet.

engram n. the supposed physical basis of an individual memory.

enkephalin (encephalin) n. a peptide occurring naturally in the brain and having effects resembling those of morphine or other opiates. See also endorphin.

enophthalmos n. a condition in which the eye is abnormally sunken into the socket. It may follow fractures of the floor of the orbit that allow the eye to sink downward and backward.

enoxacin n. see quinolone.

enoxaparin n. see low molecular weight heparin.

enoximone n. an *inotropic drug used in heart failure to increase the force and output of the heart. It is administered by injection. Trade name: **Perfan**.

ensiform cartilage see xiphoid process.

ENT see otorhinolaryngology.

entacapone n. a drug used as an *adjunct to *levodopa and *carbidopa to treat patients with Parkinson's disease who experience the signs and symptoms of end-of-dose "wearing-off." By improving muscle control, this medicine allows more normal movements of the body. It is administered orally; side effects include abdominal pain, nausea, diarrhea, hyperactivity, twitching, dizziness, and fatigue. Trade names: **Comtan, Stalevo**.

Entamoeba n. a genus of widely distributed amebas, of which some species are parasites of the digestive tract of humans. E. histolytica invades and destroys the tissues of the intestinal wall, causing amebic *dysentery and ulceration of the gut wall (see ameboma), and the parasite may spread to the liver, where it produces an abscess (amebic hepatitis). E. coli is a harmless intestinal parasite; E. gingivalis, found within the spaces between the teeth, is associated with periodontal disease and gingivitis.

enter- (entero-) prefix denoting the intestine. Example: enterolith (calculus in).

enteral adj. of or relating to the intestinal tract.

enteral feeding see nutrition.

enteralgia n. see colic.

enterectomy n. surgical removal of part of the intestine.

enteric adj. relating to or affecting the intestine.

enteric-coated adj. describing tablets that are coated with a substance that enables them to pass through the stomach to the intestine unchanged. Enteric-coated tablets contain drugs that are destroyed by the acid contents of the stomach.

enteric fever typhoid or paratyphoid fever.

enteritis n. inflammation of the small intestine, usually causing diarrhea. Infective enteritis is caused by viruses or bacteria; radiation enteritis is caused by X-rays or radioactive isotopes. See also Crohn's disease (regional enteritis), gastroenteritis.

enterobiasis (oxyuriasis) n. a disease, common in children throughout the world, caused by the parasitic nematode Enterobius vermicularis (see pinworm) in the large intestine. The worms do not cause any serious lesions of the gut wall although, rarely, they may provoke appendicitis. The emergence of the female from the anus at night irritates and inflames the surrounding skin, causing the patient to scratch and thereby contaminate fingers and nails with infective eggs. The eggs may reinfect the same child or be spread to other children. Worms may occasionally enter the vulva and cause a discharge from the vagina. Enterobiasis responds well to treatment with *piperazine compounds.

Enterobius (Oxyuris) n. see pinworm.

enterocele n. a hernia of the *pouch of Douglas (between the rectum and uterus) into the upper part of the posterior vaginal wall. It may contain loops of small intestine.

enterocentesis n. a former name for a surgical procedure in which a hollow needle is pushed through the wall of the stomach or intestines to release an abnormal accumulation of gas or fluid or to introduce a catheter for feeding (see enterostomy, gastrostomy).

enteroclysis n. see small bowel enema.

enterocolitis n. inflammation of the colon and small intestine. See also colitis, enteritis, necrotizing enterocolitis.

enterogastrone n. a putative hormone from the small intestine (duodenum) that inhibits the secretion of gastric juice by the stomach. It is said to be released when the stomach contents pass into the small intestine.

enterogenous adj. originating in the intestine.

enterokinase n. the former name for *enteropeptidase.

enterolith n. a stone within the intestine. I

usually builds up around a gallstone or a swallowed fruit stone.

enteromegaly n. Rare. enlargement (usually increased diameter) of the intestine.

enteropathy n. disease of the small intestine. See also celiac disease (gluten enteropathy).

enteropeptidase n. an enzyme secreted by the glands of the small intestine that acts on trypsinogen to produce *trypsin.

enteropexy n. a surgical operation in which part of the intestine is fixed to the abdominal wall. This was formerly performed for visceroptosis (a condition in which the abdominal organs were thought to have descended to a lower than normal position), but it is no longer carried out.

enteroptosis n. a condition in which loops of intestine (especially transverse *colon) are in a low anatomic position. At one time this was thought to cause various abdominal symptoms, and operations were devised to correct it. It is now known that no symptoms result from simple anatomic variations of this sort.

enterorrhaphy n. the surgical procedure of stitching an intestine that has either perforated or been divided during an operation.

enteroscope n. an illuminated optical instrument used to inspect the interior of the small intestine. The image is transmitted through a fiberoptic bundle or by a tiny video camera. The push type, about 280 cm long and of variable stiffness, is introduced by guidance under direct vision. The sonde type, about 280 cm long, has an inflatable balloon that pulls the instrument through the length of the intestine by peristalsis. The enteroscope is useful in diagnosing the cause of hemorrhage of the small intestine or of *strictures. —**enteroscopy** n.

enterospasm n. powerful contraction of the intestine, usually accompanied by pain.

enterostomy n. an operation in which the small intestine is brought through the abdominal wall and opened (see duodenostomy, jejunostomy, ileostomy) or is joined to the stomach (gastroenterostomy) or to another loop of small intestine (enteroenterostomy).

enterotomy n. surgical incision into the intestine.

enterotoxin n. a poisonous substance (toxin) that has a particularly marked effect upon the gastrointestinal tract, causing vomiting, diarrhea, and abdominal pain.

enterovirus n. any virus that enters the body through the gastrointestinal tract, multiplies there, and then (generally) invades the central nervous system. Enteroviruses include *coxsackieviruses, *echoviruses, and *polioviruses.

enterozoon n. any animal species inhabiting or infecting the gut of another. See also endoparasite.

enthesis n. **1.** the site of insertion of tendons or ligaments into bones. **2.** the insertion of synthetic inorganic material to replace lost tissue.

enthesopathy n. any rheumatic disease resulting in inflammation of *entheses. Ankylosing *spondylitis, *Reiter's syndrome, and *psoriatic arthritis are examples.

entoptic phenomena visual sensations caused by changes within the eye itself, rather than by the normal light stimulation process. The most common are tiny floating spots (floaters) that most people can see occasionally, especially when gazing at a brightly illuminated background (such as a blue sky).

entrapment neuropathy pain, muscle wasting, and paralysis resulting from pressure on a nerve in conditions in which it is subjected to compression by surrounding structures. See carpal tunnel syndrome, Morton's neuralgia.

entropion n. inturning of the eyelid toward the eyeball. The lashes may rub against the eye and cause irritation (see trichiasis). The most common type is spastic entropion of the lower eyelid, due to spasm of the muscle that closes the eye (orbicularis oculi). Entropion may also be caused by scarring of the lining membrane (conjunctiva) of the lid.

enucleation n. a surgical operation in which an organ, tumor, or cyst is completely removed. In ophthalmology it is an operation in which the eyeball is removed but the other structures in the socket (e.g. eye muscles) are left in place. Commonly a plastic ball is buried in the socket to provide a better cosmetic result prior to fitting an artificial eye.

enuresis n. the involuntary passing of urine, especially bedwetting by children at night (nocturnal enuresis). This can be caused by underlying disorders of the urinary tract, particularly infection, but is usually behavioral in nature; there is often a family history. The condition is cured spontaneously as the child grows older, although it may persist into teenage – and rarely adult – life. The condition can be treated successfully by behavioral techniques, such as the use of a nocturnal alarm (*see* bell and pad), by *reinforcement of periods of continence with a reward system, or by drug treatment. Enuresis that starts in adulthood is usually associated with a disorder of the bladder or a neurological disease, such as multiple sclerosis. *See also* incontinence. —**enuretic** *adj*.

environment *n*. any or all aspects of the surroundings of an organism, both internal and external, which influence its growth, development, and behavior.

Environmental Protection Agency (EPA) an agency established by the US in 1970 to coordinate various government activities associated with environmental quality control. It is responsible for implementation of the Federal Water Pollution Control Act, the Clean Air Act, and similar laws.

environmental hearing aid (assistive listening device) a device for helping people who have hearing difficulties. Environmental aids include amplified telephones, infrared links to televisions, door bells with visible as well as audible alarms, and vibrating alarm clocks.

enzyme *n*. a protein that, in small amounts, speeds up the rate of a biologic reaction without itself being used up in the reaction (i.e. it acts as a catalyst). An enzyme acts by binding with the substance involved in the reaction (the *substrate*) and converting it into another substance (the *product* of the reaction). An enzyme is relatively specific in the type of reaction it catalyzes; hence there are many different enzymes for the various biochemical reactions. Each enzyme requires certain conditions for optimum activity, particularly correct temperature and pH, the presence of *coenzymes, and the absence of specific inhibitors. Enzymes are unstable and are easily inactivated by heat or certain chemicals. They are produced within living cells and may act either within the cell (as in cellular respiration) or outside

it (as in digestion). The names of enzymes usually end in -*ase*; enzymes are named according to the substrate upon which they act (as in *lactase*), or the type of reaction they catalyze (as in *hydrolase*).

Enzymes are essential for the normal functioning and development of the body. Failure in the production or activity of a single enzyme may result in metabolic disorders; such disorders are often inherited and some have serious effects. —**enzymatic** *adj*.

enzyme-linked immunosorbent assay (ELISA) a sensitive technique for measuring the amount of a substance. An antibody that will bind to the substance is produced; the amount of an easily measured enzyme that then binds to the antibody complex enables accurate measurement.

eonism *n*. the adoption of female manners and dress by a man. *See* transsexualism, transvestism.

eosin *n*. a red acidic dye, produced by the reaction of bromine and fluorescein, used to stain biologic specimens for microscopical examination. Eosin may be used in conjunction with a contrasting blue alkaline dye taken up by different parts of the same specimen.

eosinopenia *n*. a decrease in the number of eosinophils in the blood.

eosinophil *n*. a variety of white blood cell distinguished by a lobed nucleus and the presence in its cytoplasm of coarse granules that stain orange-red with *Romanovsky stains. Eosinophils are capable of ingesting foreign particles, are present in large numbers in lining or covering surfaces within the body, are involved in allergic responses, and may be involved in host defense against parasites. There are normally $40–400 \times 10^6$ eosinophils per liter of blood.

eosinophilia *n*. an increase in the number of eosinophils in the blood. Eosinophilia occurs in response to certain drugs and in a variety of diseases, including allergies, parasitic infestations, and certain forms of leukemia.

EPA *see* Environmental Protection Agency.

eparterial *adj*. situated on or above an artery.

ependyma *n*. the extremely thin membrane, composed of cells of the *glia (*ependymal cells*), that lines the ventricles of the brain and the choroid plexuses. It is responsible for helping to form cerebrospinal fluid. —**ependymal** adj.

ependymoma n. a cerebral tumor derived from the glial (non-nervous) cells lining the cavities of the ventricles of the brain (see ependyma). It may obstruct the flow of cerebrospinal fluid, causing a *hydrocephalus.

ephebiatrics (hebiatrics) n. the branch of medicine concerned with the common disorders of children and adolescents. Compare pediatrics.

ephedrine n. a drug that causes constriction of blood vessels and widening of the bronchial passages (see sympathomimetic). It is used mainly in the treatment of asthma and other allergic conditions and chronic bronchitis. It is administered by mouth or by inhalation and may cause nausea and vomiting, insomnia, headache, and nervousness.

EPI see echo planar imaging.

epi- prefix denoting above or upon.

epiblepharon n. an abnormal fold of skin, present from birth, stretching across the eye just above the lashes of the upper eyelid or in front of them in the lower lid. It may cause the lower lashes to turn upward or inward against the eye. It usually disappears within the first year of life.

epicanthus (epicanthic fold) n. a vertical fold of skin from the upper eyelid that covers the inner corner of the eye. It is normal in Mongolian races and occurs abnormally in certain congenital conditions, e.g. *Down's syndrome. —**epicanthal**, **epicanthic** adj.

epicardia n. the part of the *esophagus, about 2 cm long, that extends from the level of the diaphragm to the stomach.

epicardium n. the outermost layer of the heart wall, enveloping the myocardium. It is a serous membrane that forms the inner layer of the serous *pericardium. —**epicardial** adj.

epicondyle n. the protuberance above a *condyle at the end of an articulating bone.

epicranium n. the structures that cover the cranium, i.e. all layers of the scalp.

epicranius n. the muscle of the scalp. The frontal portion, at the forehead, is responsible for raising the eyebrows and wrinkling the forehead; the occipital portion, at the base of the skull, draws the scalp backward.

epicritic adj. describing or relating to sensory nerve fibers responsible for the fine degrees of sensation, as of temperature and touch. Compare protopathic.

epidemic n. a sudden outbreak of infectious disease that spreads rapidly through the population, affecting a large proportion of people. The most common epidemics today are of influenza. Compare endemic, pandemic. —**epidemic** adj.

epidemiology n. the study of the occurrence, distribution, and control of infectious and noninfectious diseases in populations, which is a basic part of community medicine. Originally restricted to the study of epidemic infectious diseases, such as smallpox and cholera, it now covers all forms of disease that relate to the environment and ways of life. It thus includes the study of the links between smoking and cancer, and diet and coronary disease, as well as *communicable diseases. See also Centers for Disease Control and Prevention.

epidermis n. the outer layer of the *skin, which is divided into four layers (see illustration). The innermost malpighian or germinative layer (stratum germinativum) consists of continuously dividing cells. The other three layers are continually renewed as cells from the germinative layer are gradually pushed outward and become progressively impregnated with keratin (see keratinization). The outermost layer (stratum corneum) consists of dead cells whose cytoplasm has been entirely replaced by keratin. It is thickest on the soles of the feet and palms of the hands. —**epidermal** adj.

epidermoid adj. having the appearance of epidermis (the outer layer of the skin): used to describe certain tumors of tissues other than the skin.

epidermoid cyst see sebaceous cyst.

epidermolysis n. loosening of the outer layer of the skin (epidermis), with the development of large blisters, occurring either spontaneously or after injury. Epidermolysis bullosa is any one of a group of genetically determined disorders characterized by blistering of skin and mucous membranes. In the simple forms the blistering is induced by injury. In the more serious (dystrophic) forms the blis-

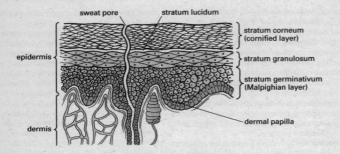

A section of epidermis

tering may occur spontaneously; some of the dystrophic forms of the disease are fatal.

Epidermophyton *n.* a genus of fungi that grow on the skin and produce the skin infections *athlete's foot and *ringworm of the nails. *See also* dermatophyte.

epidiascope *n.* an apparatus for projecting a greatly magnified image of an object, such as a specimen on a microscope slide, on to a screen.

epididymectomy *n.* the surgical removal or excision of the epididymis.

epididymis *n.* (*pl.* **epididymides**) a highly convoluted tube, about seven meters long, that connects the *testis to the vas deferens. The spermatozoa are moved passively along the tube over a period of several days, during which time they mature and become capable of fertilization. They are concentrated and stored in the lower part of the epididymis until ejaculation. —**epididymal** *adj.*

epididymitis *n.* inflammation of the epididymis. The usual cause is infection spreading down the vas deferens from the bladder or urethra, resulting in pain, swelling, and redness of the affected half of the scrotum. The inflammation may spread to the testicle (*epididymo-orchitis*). Treatment is by administration of antibiotics and analgesics.

epididymovasostomy *n.* the operation of making a new connection between the vas deferens and the epididymis in order to bypass obstruction of the latter. It is performed in an attempt to cure *azoospermia caused by this blockage.

epidural (extradural) *adj.* on or over the dura mater (the outermost of the three membranes covering the brain and spinal cord). The *epidural space* is the space between the dura mater of the spinal cord and the vertebral canal. The spinal epidural space is used for anesthetizing spinal nerve roots. *See* epidural anesthesia, spinal anesthesia.

epidural anesthesia suppression of sensation in the lower part of the body by the injection of a local anesthetic into the *epidural space. The injection site is often the sacral or caudal region of the vertebral column, and a special blunt needle with a side hole is used to reduce the chance of penetrating the dura. A fine catheter is passed through the needle to enable repeated or continuous injections of anesthetic solution. Epidural anesthesia is particularly useful for providing pain relief during childbirth or to reduce the need for deep general anesthesia.

epigastrium *n.* the upper central region of the *abdomen. —**epigastric** *adj.*

epigastrocele *n.* a *hernia through the upper central abdominal wall.

epiglottis *n.* a thin leaf-shaped flap of cartilage, covered with mucous membrane, situated immediately behind the root of the tongue. It covers the entrance to the *larynx during swallowing.

epiglottitis *n.* an infection of the epiglottis, which swells and causes obstruction of the upper airways. Epiglottitis usually occurs in children between one and seven years old, who complain of drooling and breathing difficulties and are acutely ill. The main bacterium that causes epiglottitis is *Haemophilus influenzae*, and the infection has become much less common since the *Hib vaccine was introduced. Treatment consists of antibiotics and, if necessary, intubation. Children should be nursed in intensive care until the infection is under control. *See also* croup.

epikeratophakia *n.* eye surgery to correct errors of *refraction in which the curvature of the cornea is altered using donor corneal tissue, which has been frozen and shaped using a lathe to produce a tissue lens that is then sutured onto the cornea.

epilation *n.* the removal of a hair by its roots. This can be done mechanically (by plucking or using wax) or by electrolysis; lasers for epilation are now available.

epilepsy *n.* any one of a group of disorders of brain function characterized by recurrent seizures that have a sudden onset. The term *idiopathic* is used to describe epilepsy that is not associated with structural damage to the brain. Seizures may be generalized or partial. *Generalized epilepsy* may take the form of *major*, or *tonic-clonic*, seizures (formerly called *grand mal*), in which, at the onset, the patient falls to the ground unconscious with the muscles in a state of spasm. The lack of any respiratory movement results in a bluish discoloration of the skin and lips (cyanosis). This – the tonic phase – is replaced by convulsive movements, when the tongue may be bitten and urinary incontinence may occur (the clonic phase). Movements gradually cease and the patient may rouse in a state of confusion, complaining of headache, or may fall asleep.

Partial epilepsy may be idiopathic or a symptom of structural damage to the brain. In one type of partial idiopathic epilepsy, often affecting children, the seizures take the form of *absences* (formerly called *petit mal* in children): brief spells of unconsciousness, lasting for a few seconds, during which posture and balance are maintained. The eyes stare blankly and there may be fluttering movements of the lids and momentary twitching of the fingers and mouth. The electroencephalogram characteristically shows bisynchronous wave and spike discharges (3 per second) during the seizures and at other times. Attacks are sometimes provoked by overbreathing or intermittent photic stimulation. As the stream of thought is completely interrupted, children with frequent seizures may have learning difficulties. This form of epilepsy seldom appears before the age of three or after adolescence. It often subsides spontaneously in adult life, but it may be followed by the onset of major or partial epilepsy.

In partial epilepsy due to brain damage, called *focal epilepsy*, the nature of the seizure depends upon the location of the disease in the brain. In *jacksonian epilepsy* the epileptic discharge spreads over the cerebral cortex, with the resulting manifestations spreading throughout the body. In a jacksonian motor seizure the convulsive movements might spread from the thumb to the hand, forearm, arm, and face (this spread of symptoms is called the *march*). *Temporal lobe* (or *psychomotor*) *epilepsy* is caused by disease in the cortex of the temporal lobe or the adjacent parietal lobe of the brain. Its symptoms include *hallucinations of smell, taste, sight, and hearing, paroxysmal disorders of memory, and *automatism. Throughout an attack the patient is in a state of clouded awareness and afterward may have no recollection of the event (*see also* déjà vu, jamais vu). A number of these symptoms are due to scarring and atrophy (mesial temporal sclerosis) affecting the temporal lobe.

The different forms of epilepsy can be controlled by the use of *anticonvulsant drugs. Surgical resection of focal epileptogenic lesions in the brain is appropriate in a strictly limited number of cases. —**epileptic** *adj.*, *n.*

epileptogenic *adj.* having the capacity to provoke epileptic seizures.

epiloia *n. see* tuberous sclerosis.

epimenorrhagia *n. see* menorrhagia.

epimenorrhea *n.* menstruation at shorter intervals than is normal.

epimysium *n.* the fibrous elastic tissue that surrounds a *muscle.

epinephrine (adrenaline) *n.* an important hormone secreted by the medulla of the adrenal gland. It has the function of preparing the body for "fright, flight, or fight" and has widespread effects on circulation, the muscles, and sugar metabolism. The action of the heart is increased, the rate and depth of breathing are increased, and the metabolic rate is raised; the force of muscular contraction improves and the onset of muscular fatigue is delayed. At the same time the blood supply to the bladder and intestines is reduced, their muscular walls relax, and the sphincters contract. Sympathetic nerves were originally thought to act by releasing epinephrine at their endings, and were called *adrenergic* nerves. In fact the main substance released is the related substance *norepinephrine*, which also forms a portion of the adrenal secretion.

Epinephrine given by injection is used in the emergency treatment of anaphylaxis and cardiac arrest and is valuable for the relief of bronchial asthma, because it relaxes constricted airways. It is also used during surgery to reduce blood loss by constricting vessels in the skin and mucous membranes. It is added to some anesthetic solutions to prolong the anesthesia and is used as eye drops for treating glaucoma.

epineural *adj.* derived from or situated on the neural arch of a vertebra.

epineurium *n.* the outer sheath of connective tissue that encloses the bundles (fascicles) of fibers that make up a *nerve.

epiphenomenon *n.* an unusual symptom or event that may occur simultaneously with a disease but is not necessarily directly related to it. *Compare* complication.

epiphora *n.* watering of the eye, in which tears flow onto the cheek. It is due to some abnormality of the tear drainage system (*see* lacrimal apparatus).

epiphysis *n.* 1. the end of a long bone, which is initially separated by cartilage from the shaft (diaphysis) of the bone and develops separately. It eventually fuses with the diaphysis to form a complete bone. *See also* Salter and Harris classification. 2. *see* pineal body.

epiphysitis *n.* inflammation of the end (epiphysis) of a long bone. It may result in retardation of growth and deformity of the affected bone.

epiplo- *prefix denoting* the omentum. Example: *epiplocele* (hernia containing omentum).

epiploon *n. see* omentum.

epiretinal membrane (cellophane maculopathy) a transparent membrane that forms on the retina, over the *macula.

Contraction of this causes wrinkling of the retina (*macular pucker*) and hence distorted vision.

epirubicin *n.* an *anthracycline cytotoxic drug indicated as a component of *adjuvant therapy in patients with evidence of axillary node tumor involvement following surgical treatment of primary breast cancer. It is administered by intravenous infusion. Side effects include nausea and vomiting, diarrhea, hair loss, and hot flashes. Trade name: **Ellence**.

episclera *n.* the outermost covering of the *sclera of the eye, which provides nutritional support to the sclera.

episcleritis *n.* inflammation of the *episclera, resulting in a red painful eye that is sensitive to light. It is usually a benign condition, which will settle without treatment.

episio- *prefix denoting* the vulva. Example: *episioplasty* (plastic surgery of).

episiotomy *n.* an incision into the tissues surrounding the opening of the vagina (perineum) during a difficult birth, at the stage when the infant's head has partly emerged through the opening of the birth passage. The aim is to enlarge the opening in a controlled manner so as to make delivery easier and to avoid extensive tearing of adjacent tissues.

epispadias *n.* a congenital abnormality in which the opening of the *urethra is on the dorsal (upper) surface of the penis. Surgical correction is carried out in infancy.

epistasis *n.* 1. the stoppage of a flow or discharge, such as blood. 2. a type of gene action in which one gene suppresses the action of another (nonallelic) gene. The term is sometimes used for any interaction between nonallelic genes. —**epistatic** *adj.*

epistaxis *n. see* nosebleed.

epithalamus *n.* part of the forebrain, consisting of a narrow band of nerve tissue in the roof of the third ventricle (including the region where the choroid plexus is attached) and the *pineal body. *See also* brain.

epithalaxia *n.* loss of layers of epithelial cells from the skin or the lining of the intestine.

epithelial ingrowth abnormal healing of a corneal wound or incision in which the conjunctival/corneal epithelium invades the internal surface of the healing wound. The consequences of this can be devastating to the eye and difficult to treat.

epithelioma *n.* a tumor of *epithelium, the covering of internal and external surfaces of the body: a former term for *carcinoma, but now also used to describe benign tumors.

epithelium *n.* the tissue that covers the external surface of the body and lines hollow structures (except blood and lymphatic vessels). It is derived from embryonic ectoderm and endoderm. Epithelial cells may be flat and scalelike (*squamous*), *cuboidal*, or *columnar*. The latter may bear cilia or brush borders or secrete mucus or other substances (*see* goblet cell). The cells rest on a common *basement membrane*, which separates epithelium from underlying *connective tissue. Epithelium may be either *simple*, consisting of a single layer of cells; *stratified*, consisting of several layers; or *pseudostratified*, in which the cells appear to be arranged in layers but in fact share a common basement membrane (see illustration). *See also* endothelium, mesothelium. —**epithelial** *adj.*

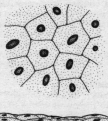

Stratified squamous epithelium, surface view above and sectional view below

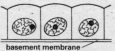

basement membrane

Simple cuboidal epithelium

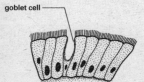

goblet cell

Ciliated columnar epithelium

basement membrane

Pseudostratified ciliated epithelium

Types of epithelium

epitrichium (periderm) *n.* the most superficial layer of the skin, one cell in thickness, that is only present early in embryonic development. It protects the underlying *epidermis until it is fully formed.

epituberculosis *n.* enlargement of lymph nodes in the thorax due to tuberculosis infection, causing the nodes to press upon and occlude a bronchiole, which may result in the collapse of a lung segment (*see* atelectasis).

eponychium *n. see* nail.

eponym *n.* a disease, structure, or species named after a particular person, usually the person who first discovered or described it. Eponyms are widespread in medicine, but they are being replaced as more descriptive terms become necessary. For example the eponyms islets of Langerhans, aqueduct of Sylvius, and Hashimoto's disease are more likely to be designated in textbooks as pancreatic islands, cerebral aqueduct, and autoimmune thyroiditis, respectively. —**eponymous** *adj.*

epoophoron *n. see* paroophoron.

epoprostenol *n.* a *prostaglandin drug used immediately before and during renal dialysis to prevent clotting of blood in the shunt. It is administered by intravenous injection.

EPSDT *see* Early and Periodic Screening, Diagnosis and Treatment.

Epstein-Barr virus (EB virus, EBV) the virus, belonging to the *herpesvirus group, that is the causative agent of *glandular fever. It attacks B *lymphocytes; an imbalance in the immune response to this gives rise to the clinical features of the disease. EB virus is also implicated in hepatitis and in certain cancers (e.g. *Burkitt's lymphoma and *Hodgkin's disease). [Sir M. A. Epstein (1921–) and Y. M. Barr (1932–), British pathologists]

epulis n. a swelling on the gum. Most such swellings are due to fibrous hyperplasia, but an epulis may be the opening of a *sinus tract.

equi- prefix denoting equality.

equinia n. see glanders.

ER see endoplasmic reticulum.

Erb's palsy weakness or paralysis of the shoulder and arm caused by injury to a baby's *brachial plexus during birth. This may happen if – during a difficult delivery – excess traction applied to the head damages the fifth cervical root of the spinal cord. The muscles of the shoulder and the flexors of the elbow are paralyzed and the arm hangs at the side internally rotated at the shoulder. Recovery may be spontaneous, but in some cases nerve grafts or muscle transfers are required. [W. H. Erb (1840–1921), German neurologist]

ERCP (endoscopic retrograde cholangiopancreatography) a technique in which a catheter is passed through a *duodenoscope into the *ampulla of Vater of the common bile duct and injected with a radiopaque medium to outline the pancreatic duct and bile ducts radiologically. It is widely used in the diagnosis of obstructive jaundice and pancreatic disease. See also papillotomy.

erectile adj. capable of causing erection or becoming erect. The penis is composed largely of erectile tissue.

erection n. the sexually active state of the penis, which becomes enlarged and rigid (due to the erectile tissue being swollen with blood) and capable of penetrating the vagina. The term is also applied to the clitoris in a state of sexual arousal.

erepsin n. a mixture of protein-digesting enzymes (see peptidase) secreted by the intestinal glands. It is part of the *succus entericus.

erethism n. 1. a state of abnormal mental excitement or irritation. 2. rapid response to a stimulus.

erg n. a unit of work or energy equal to the work done when the point of application of a force of 1 dyne is displaced through a distance of 1 centimeter in the direction of the force. 1 erg = 10^{-7} joule.

erg- (ergo-) prefix denoting work or activity.

ergocalciferol n. see vitamin D.

ergograph n. an apparatus for recording the work performed by the muscles of the body when undergoing activity. Ergographs are useful for assessment of the capabilities of athletes undergoing training.

ergoloid mesylate an *adrenergic agent with *psychotropic actions used to treat some mood, behavioral, or dementia symptoms that may be due to changes in the brain from Alzheimer's disease or multiple small strokes. It is administered orally; side effects include dizziness, nausea, and gastric distress. Trade names: **Gerimal, Hydergine**.

ergonomics n. the study of people in relation to their work and working surroundings. This broad science involves the application of psychologic as well as physiologic principles to the design of buildings, machinery, vehicles, packaging, implements, and anything else with which people come into contact.

ergonovine n. a drug that stimulates contractions of the uterus. It is administered by injection to assist labor and (combined with oxytocin) to control bleeding following delivery. Trade name: **Ergotrate**.

ergosterol n. a plant sterol that, when irradiated with ultraviolet light, is converted to ergocalciferol (vitamin D_2). See vitamin D.

ergot n. a fungus (Claviceps purpurea) that grows on rye. It produces several important alkaloids, chemically related to LSD, including *ergotamine and *ergonovine, which are used in medicine in the treatment of migraine and in childbirth. Eating bread made with rye infected with the fungus has led to sporadic outbreaks of *ergotism over the centuries.

ergotamine n. a drug that causes constriction of blood vessels and is used to relieve migraine. It is administered by mouth, injection, inhalation, or in suppositories. Common side effects are nausea and vomiting, and ergotism may develop as a result of high doses; because of this it has largely been superseded by *5HT$_1$ agonists. Trade names: **Cafergot, D.H.E. 45, Ergostat, Gynergen**.

ergotism n. poisoning caused by eating rye infected with the fungus *ergot. The chief symptom is gangrene of the fingers and toes, with diarrhea and vomiting, nausea, and headache. In the Middle Ages the disease was known as *St. Anthony's fire*, because of the inflamed appearance of the tissues afflicted with gangrene and the belief that a pilgrimage to St. Anthony's tomb would result in a cure.

erogenous adj. describing certain parts of the body, the physical stimulation of which leads to sexual arousal.

erosion n. **1.** an eating away of surface tissue by physical or chemical processes, including those associated with inflammation. A *cervical erosion* is an abnormal area of epithelium that may develop at the neck of the uterus due to tissue damage caused at childbirth or by attempts at abortion. In the skin an erosion represents a superficial type of ulceration and therefore heals quite readily. **2.** (in dentistry) loss of surface tooth substance, usually caused by repeated application of acid, which softens the enamel surface. It may result from excessive intake of citrus drinks, citrus fruits, or carbonated drinks or by regurgitation of acid from the stomach, as in bulimia nervosa, hiatus hernia, alcoholism, or stress. The teeth become very sensitive. The cause should be corrected; severe cases may require extensive dental restoration.

erot- (eroto-) prefix denoting sexual desire or love. Example: *erotophobia* (morbid dread of).

eroticism n. **1.** those elements in thought, imagination, pictorial imagery, literature, or the arts that tend to arouse sexual excitement or desire. **2.** actual sexual arousal. **3.** a greater than average disposition for sex and all its manifestations. **4.** sexual interest or excitement that is prompted by contemplation or stimulation of areas of the body not normally associated with sexuality. The terms *anal eroticism* and *oral eroticism* are used both in a theoretical Freudian sense and in reference to adult physical sexual activity.

erotomania n. a delusion that the individ-

ual is loved by some person, often a person of importance. Sometimes, but not always, this progresses to schizophrenia.

eructation n. belching: the sudden raising of gas from the stomach.

eruption n. **1.** any lesion or rash that appears at the surface of the skin and is characterized by its prominence and redness. A *bullous eruption* is an outbreak of blisters. **2.** (in dentistry) the emergence of a growing tooth from the gum into the mouth.

erysipelas n. a streptococcal infection of the skin, especially the face (although the arms and legs are often affected), characterized by redness and swelling; it usually has a sharply defined margin, which can differentiate erysipelas from the otherwise similar *cellulitis. The patient is ill, with a high temperature. *Penicillin V is the treatment of choice.

erysipeloid n. an infection of the skin and underlying tissues with *Erysipelothrix rhusiopathiae*, developing usually in people handling fish, poultry, or meat. Infection enters through scratches or cuts on the hands, and is normally confined to a finger or hand, which becomes reddened; sometimes systemic illness develops. Treatment is with antibiotics, particularly penicillin.

Erysipelothrix n. a genus of gram-positive nonmotile rod-shaped bacteria with a tendency to form filaments. They are parasites of mammals, birds, and fish. *E. rhusiopathiae* (also called *E. insidiosa*) is a widely distributed species causing the disease *erysipeloid.

erythema n. abnormal flushing of the skin caused by dilation of the blood capillaries. Erythema may be produced by various conditions – it is often a sign of inflammation and infection. For example, *erythema nodosum* is a disease of sudden onset, often associated with streptococcal infection, characterized by fever, joint pains, and an eruption of painful bruiselike swellings on the legs. In *erythema multiforme* the eruption consists of circular or irregular red patches, commonly occurring on the backs of the arms and hands and sometimes accompanied by systemic disease. Although no cause is found in the majority of cases, often viral infections, particularly herpes simplex, may be implicated. *Erythema infectiosum* is a benign infectious disease of children, caused by a *parvovirus, in which there is an abrupt onset of rash, first on the cheeks and later on the trunk and limbs, which disappears spontaneously after several days. *Erythema ab igne* is a reticular pigmented rash on the lower legs or elsewhere caused by persistent exposure to radiant heat.

erythr- (erythro-) *prefix denoting* 1. redness. Example: *erythuria* (excretion of red urine). 2. erythrocytes.

erythrasma *n.* a chronic skin infection due to the bacterium *Corynebacterium minutissimum*, occurring in such areas as the armpits, groin, and toes, where skin surfaces are in contact. It fluoresces coral-pink under *Wood's light and can be treated with antifungal creams or with antibiotics.

erythredema *n. see* pink disease.

erythremia *n. see* polycythemia vera.

erythroblast *n.* any of a series of nucleated cells (*see* normoblast, proerythroblast) that pass through a succession of stages of maturation to form red blood cells (*erythrocytes). Erythroblasts are normally present in the blood-forming tissue of the bone marrow, but they may appear in the circulation in a variety of diseases (*see* erythroblastosis). *See also* erythropoiesis.

erythroblastosis *n.* the presence in the blood of the nucleated precursors of the red blood cells (*erythroblasts). This may occur when there is an increase in the rate of red cell production, as in hemorrhagic or hemolytic *anemia, or in infiltrations of the bone marrow by tumors, etc.

erythroblastosis fetalis a severe but rare hemolytic *anemia affecting newborn infants due to destruction of the infant's red blood cells by factors present in the mother's serum. It is usually caused by incompatibility of the rhesus blood groups between mother and infant (*see* rhesus factor).

erythrocyanosis *n.* mottled purplish discoloration on the legs and thighs, usually of adolescent girls or fat boys before puberty. The disorder sometimes occurs in older women. The condition is worse in cold weather and there is no satisfactory treatment apart from weight loss, which reduces the insulating effect of a thick layer of fat.

erythrocyte (red blood cell) *n.* a *blood cell containing the red pigment *hemoglobin, the principal function of which is the transport of oxygen. A mature erythrocyte has no nucleus and its shape is that of a biconcave disk, approximately 7 μm in diameter. There are normally about 5×10^{12} erythrocytes per liter of blood. *See also* erythropoiesis.

erythrocyte sedimentation rate *see* ESR.

erythrocytic *adj.* describing those stages in the life cycle of the malarial parasite (*see* Plasmodium) that develop inside the red blood cells (*see* trophozoite). *Compare* exoerythrocytic.

erythroderma (exfoliative dermatitis) *n.* abnormal reddening, flaking, and thickening of the skin, typically affecting a wide area of the body. It is more common after the age of 50 years and affects men three times as often as women; it frequently develops from a preexisting skin disease, such as psoriasis or eczema, or is caused by drugs or lymphoma.

erythrogenesis *n. see* erythropoiesis.

erythromelalgia *n.* painful paroxysmal dilation of the blood vessels of the skin, usually affecting the extremities, especially the feet; the skin feels hot. Some patients may respond to aspirin.

erythromycin *n.* an *antibiotic used to treat infections caused by a wide range of bacteria and other microorganisms. It is administered by mouth or injection or topically. Side effects are rare and mild, although nausea, vomiting, and diarrhea occur occasionally. Trade names: **Emgel, E-Mycin, ERYC, Erycette, EryDerm, Erygel, Erymax, Ery-Tab, Erythrocin, Ilotycin**.

erythron *n.* the circulating red blood cells in the bloodstream and all the elements of the body that are involved in their production. The erythron is not a single organ but is dispersed throughout the blood-forming tissue of the *bone marrow. *See also* erythropoiesis.

erythropenia *n.* a reduction in the number of red blood cells (*erythrocytes) in the blood. Erythropenia usually, but not invariably, occurs in *anemia.

erythroplasia *n.* an abnormal red patch of skin that occurs primarily in the mouth or on the genitalia and is precancerous. *Compare* leukoplakia.

erythropoiesis (erythrogenesis) *n.* the process of red blood cell (*erythrocyte) production, which normally occurs in the blood-forming tissue of the *bone marrow. The ultimate precursor of the red cell is the *hemopoietic stem cell, but the earliest precursor that can be identified microscopically is the *proerythroblast. This divides and passes through a series of stages of maturation termed, respectively, early, intermediate, and late *normoblasts, the latter finally losing its nucleus to become a mature red cell. *See also* hemopoiesis.

erythropoietin *n.* a hormone secreted by certain cells in the kidney in response to a reduction in the amount of oxygen reaching the tissues. Erythropoietin increases the rate of red cell production (*erythropoiesis) and is the mechanism by which the rate of erythropoiesis is controlled.

erythropsia *n.* red vision: a rare symptom in which objects appear to be tinged red, sometimes experienced after removal of a cataract and also in snow blindness.

eschar *n.* a scab or slough, as produced by the action of heat or a corrosive substance on living tissue.

escharotic *n.* a *caustic agent that produces a dry scab, or slough, when applied to the skin.

Escherichia *n.* a genus of gram-negative, generally motile, rodlike bacteria that have the ability to ferment carbohydrates, usually with production of gas, and are found in the intestines of humans and many animals. *E. coli* – a lactose-fermenting species – is usually not harmful but some strains can cause gastrointestinal infections. Ingestion of the pathogenic serotype *E. coli* O157, derived from infected meat, causes colitis with bloody diarrhea, which may give rise to the complications of *hemolytic uremic syndrome or thrombocytopenic *purpura (*see also* food poisoning). *E. coli* is also widely used in laboratory experiments for bacteriologic and genetic studies.

eserine *n. see* physostigmine.

esomeprazole *n.* a *proton-pump inhibitor that is used to treat heartburn, acid indigestion, sour stomach, *gastroesophageal reflux disease, and (in combination with antibiotics) gastric and duodenal ulcers. It is administered orally; common side effects include

headache, diarrhea, flatulence, and dry mouth. Trade name: **Nexium.**

esophag- (esophago-) *prefix denoting* the esophagus. Example: *esophagectomy* (surgical removal of).

esophageal ulcer *see* peptic ulcer, esophagitis.

esophageal varices dilated veins in the lower esophagus due to *portal hypertension. These may rupture and bleed, resulting in *hematemesis; serious bleeding may endanger life. Bleeding may be arrested by a compression balloon, by *sclerotherapy, by applying elastic bands via an endoscope, or by injections of *vasopressin or *somatostatin.

esophagitis *n.* inflammation of the esophagus (gullet). Frequent regurgitation of acid and peptic juices from the stomach causes *reflux esophagitis*, the most common form, which may be associated with a hiatus *hernia. The main symptoms are heartburn, regurgitation of bitter fluid, and sometimes difficulty in swallowing; complications include bleeding, narrowing (*stricture) of the esophageal canal, ulceration, and *Barrett's esophagus. It is treated by antacid medicines, drugs to reduce acid secretion, weight reduction, and avoidance of bending; in severe cases surgery may be required. *Corrosive esophagitis* is caused by the ingestion of caustic acid or alkali. It is often severe and may lead to perforation of the esophagus or to extensive stricture formation. Treatment includes avoidance of food and administration of antibiotics and corticosteroids; later dilation of the stricture may be needed. *Infective esophagitis* is most commonly due to a fungus (*Candida*) infection in debilitated patients, especially those being treated with antibiotics, corticosteroids, and immunosuppressant drugs, but is occasionally due to viruses (such as cytomegalovirus or herpes virus). All of these infections are common in patients with AIDS.

esophagocele *n.* protrusion of the lining (mucosa) of the esophagus (gullet) through a tear in its muscular wall.

esophagogastroduodenoscopy (EGD) *n.* endoscopic examination of the upper alimentary tract using a fiberoptic or video instrument. *See also* gastroscope.

esophagoscope *n.* an illuminated optical instrument used to inspect the interior of the esophagus (gullet), dilate its canal (in cases of stricture), obtain material for biopsy, or remove a foreign body. It may be a rigid metal tube or a flexible fiberoptic or videocamera instrument (see gastroscope). —**esophagoscopy** n.

esophagostomy n. a surgical operation in which the esophagus (gullet) is opened onto the neck. It is usually performed after operations on the throat as a temporary measure to allow feeding.

esophagotomy n. surgical opening of the esophagus (gullet) in order to inspect its interior or to remove or insert something.

esophagus n. the gullet: a muscular tube, about 23 cm long, that extends from the pharynx to the stomach. It is lined with mucous membrane, whose secretions lubricate food as it passes from the mouth to the stomach. Waves of *peristalsis assist the passage of food.

Diseases of the esophagus include *achalasia, carcinoma, hiatus hernia, *esophageal varices, *esophagitis, and *peptic ulcer. —**esophageal** adj.

esophoria n. a tendency to squint in which the eye, when covered, tends to turn inward toward the nose. See also heterophoria.

esotropia n. convergent *strabismus: a type of squint.

ESP see extrasensory perception.

espundia (mucocutaneous leishmaniasis) n. a disease of the skin and mucous membranes caused by the parasitic protozoan Leishmania braziliensis (see leishmaniasis). Occurring in South and Central America, espundia takes the form of ulcerating lesions on the arms and legs; the infection may also spread to the mucous membranes of the nose and mouth, causing serious destruction of the tissues.

ESR (erythrocyte sedimentation rate) the rate at which red blood cells (erythrocytes) settle out of suspension in blood plasma, measured under standardized conditions. The ESR increases if the level of certain proteins in the plasma rises, as in rheumatic diseases, chronic infections, and malignant disease, and thus provides a simple but valuable screening test for these conditions.

essence n. a solution consisting of an essential oil dissolved in alcohol.

essential adj. describing a disorder that is not apparently attributable to an outside cause; for example, essential *hypertension.

essential amino acid an *amino acid that is essential for normal growth and development but cannot be synthesized by the body. Essential amino acids are normally obtained from protein-rich foods in the diet, such as liver, eggs, and dairy products. There are nine essential amino acids: tryptophan, lysine, phenylalanine, histidine, threonine, valine, methionine, leucine, and isoleucine.

essential fatty acid one of a group of unsaturated fatty acids that are essential for growth but cannot be synthesized by the body. The essential fatty acids are linoleic, linolenic, and arachidonic acids; of these, only linoleic acid needs to be included in the diet because the other two can be synthesized from it in the body. Large amounts of linoleic acid occur in corn oil and soybean oil; smaller amounts in pork fat.

essential oil a volatile oil derived from an aromatic plant. Essential oils are used in various pharmaceutical preparations.

esterase n. an enzyme that catalyzes the hydrolysis of esters into their constituent acids and alcohols. For example, fatty-acid esters are broken down to form fatty acids plus alcohol.

estradiol n. the major female sex hormone produced by the ovary. See estrogen.

estriol n. one of the female sex hormones produced by the ovary. See estrogen.

estrogen n. one of a group of steroid hormones (including estriol, estrone, and estradiol) that control female sexual development, promoting the growth and function of the female sex organs (see menstrual cycle) and female secondary sexual characteristics (such as breast development). Estrogens are synthesized mainly by the ovary; small amounts are also produced by the adrenal cortex, testes, and placenta. In men excessive production of estrogen gives rise to *feminization.

Naturally occurring and synthetic estrogens, given by mouth or injection, are used to treat *amenorrhea, menopausal symptoms (see hormone replacement therapy), androgen-dependent cancers (e.g. cancer of the prostate), and to inhibit lactation. Synthetic estrogens are a major constituent of *oral contraceptives. Side effects of estrogen therapy may include nausea and vomiting, headache and dizziness, irregular vaginal bleeding, fluid and salt retention, and feminization in men. Estrogens should not be used in patients with a history of cancer of the breast, uterus, or genital tract. —**estrogenic** adj.

estrogen receptor a specific site on the surface of a cell that binds to *estrogen; the binding triggers responses of the cell to the hormone. *Antiestrogens, used for treating breast cancer, act by preventing the binding of estrogen to these *receptors.

estrone n. one of the female sex hormones produced by the ovary. See estrogen.

ESWL extracorporeal shock-wave lithotripsy. See lithotripsy.

ethacrynic acid a loop *diuretic used to treat fluid retention (edema), such as that associated with heart failure and kidney and liver disorders. It is administered by mouth or injection. Common side effects are loss of appetite, difficulty in swallowing, nausea, vomiting, and diarrhea. Trade name: **Edecrin**.

ethambutol n. a drug used in the treatment of tuberculosis, in conjunction with other drugs. It is administered by mouth and occasionally causes visual disturbances, which cease when the drug is withdrawn. Allergic rashes and digestive upsets may also occur. Trade name: **Myambutol**.

ethanol (ethyl alcohol) n. see alcohol.

ethchlorvynol n. a drug used in the short-term treatment of insomnia (see hypnotic). It is administered by mouth; side effects include temporary giddiness, muscle incoordination, nausea, and vomiting. Trade name: **Placidyl**.

ether n. a volatile liquid formerly used as an anesthetic administered by inhalation, although now largely replaced by safer and more efficient drugs. It also has laxative action when administered by mouth. Ether irritates the respiratory tract and affects the circulation.

ethical committee a group of senior doctors and other experts set up (especially in a hospital) to monitor any problems of ethics, including withholding treatment, use of fetal tissue, and investigations, concerned with teaching or research, that involve the use of human subjects. It is responsible for ensuring

that patients are adequately informed of the procedures involved in a research project (including the use of dummy or placebo treatments as controls), that the tests and/or therapies are safe, and that no one is pressured into participating.

ethinyl estradiol a synthetic female sex hormone (see estrogen) used mainly in combination with a progestogen, in *oral contraceptives. Trade names: **Estinyl**, **Feminone**.

ethionamide n. a drug used to treat tuberculosis, usually after other drugs have failed, and in conjunction with other drugs. It is administered by mouth. Loss of appetite, nausea, and vomiting are common side effects. Trade name: **Trecator-SC**.

ethmoid bone a bone in the floor of the cranium that contributes to the nasal cavity and orbits. The part of the ethmoid forming the roof of the nasal cavity – the cribriform plate – is pierced with many small holes through which the olfactory nerves pass. See also nasal concha, skull.

ethnology n. the study of the different races of mankind and their variations: a branch of anthropology that deals mainly with cultural and social differences between groups and the problems, medical and otherwise, that arise from their particular ways of life. —**ethnic** adj.

ethopropazine n. a drug that has effects similar to those of *atropine and is used to treat parkinsonism. It is administered by mouth and may cause lethargy and drowsiness in the early stages of treatment. Trade name: **Parsidol**.

ethosuximide n. an *anticonvulsant drug used to control epileptic seizures. It is administered by mouth; side effects such as drowsiness, depression, and digestive disturbances may occur but are usually temporary. Trade name: **Zarontin**.

ethotoin n. an *anticonvulsant drug used, usually in conjunction with other anticonvulsants, to treat tonic-clonic and partial epileptic seizures. It is administered by mouth; possible side effects include digestive and visual disturbances and drowsiness. Trade name: **Peganone**.

ethyl alcohol (ethanol) see alcohol.

ethylene n. an inflammable gas sometimes used as an anesthetic administered by inhalation. There are usually no toxic effects, but nausea and vomiting commonly occur after its use.

ethynodiol n. a synthetic female sex hormone (see progestogen) that is used to treat menstrual disorders and in *oral contraceptives. It is administered by mouth, usually in combination with an *estrogen. Side effects can include nausea, vomiting, headache, breast swelling, weight gain, fluid retention, and breakthrough bleeding. Trade names: **Demulen**, **Zovia**.

etidronate disodium a *bisphosphonate drug used to treat *Paget's disease and to improve mineralization of bone in women with postmenopausal osteoporosis, especially those who have already had fractures. It is administered by mouth or injection. Possible side effects include nausea, diarrhea, and a metallic taste in the mouth. Trade name: **Didronel**.

etiology (aetiology) n. **1.** the study or science of the causes of disease. **2.** the cause of a specific disease.

etoposide n. a *cytotoxic drug derived from an extract of the mandrake plant; it inhibits topoisomerase, an enzyme involved in DNA replication. It is administered intravenously or by mouth, primarily in the treatment of bronchial carcinoma, lymphomas, and testicular tumors. Side effects include alopecia, nausea, and marrow suppression. Trade names: **Etopophos**, **Toposar**, **VePesid**.

eu- prefix denoting **1.** good, well, or easy. **2.** normal.

eubacteria pl. n. a very large group of bacteria with rigid cell walls and – typically – flagella for movement. The group comprises the so-called "true" bacteria, excluding those, such as spirochetes and mycoplasmas, with flexible cell walls.

eucalyptol n. a volatile oil that has a mild irritant effect on the mucous membranes of the mouth and digestive system. It is taken as pastilles or inhaled as vapor to relieve catarrh. Large doses may cause nausea, vomiting, and diarrhea.

eucaryote n. see eukaryote.

euchromatin n. chromosome material (see chromatin) that stains most deeply during mitosis and represents the major genes. Compare heterochromatin.

eugenics n. the science that is concerned with the improvement of the human race by means of the principles of genetics. It is mainly concerned with the detection and, where possible, the elimination of genetic disease in humans.

eukaryote (eucaryote) n. an organism whose cells have a true nucleus, i.e. a nucleus that is bounded by a nuclear membrane within which are contained the chromosomes of DNA, RNA, and proteins, with cell division occurring by *mitosis. Compare prokaryote.

eumenorrhea n. regular menstruation. This does not necessarily indicate regular ovulation.

eupepsia n. the state of normal or good digestion: freedom from digestive symptoms.

euphoria n. a state of optimism, cheerfulness, and well-being. A morbid degree of euphoria is characteristic of *mania and *hypomania. See also ecstasy, elation.

euplastic adj. describing a tissue that heals quickly after injury.

euploidy n. the condition of cells, tissues, or organisms in which there is one complete set of chromosomes or a whole multiple of this set in each cell. Compare aneuploidy. —**euploid** adj., n.

eustachian tube the tube that connects the middle *ear to the pharynx. It allows the pressure on the inner side of the eardrum to remain equal to the external pressure. [B. Eustachio (1520–74), Italian anatomist]

euthanasia n. the act of taking life to relieve suffering. In voluntary euthanasia the sufferer asks for measures to be taken to end his life. This may be accomplished by active steps, usually the administration of a drug, or by passive euthanasia – the deliberate withholding of treatment. In compulsory euthanasia society or a person acting on authority gives instructions to terminate the life of a person, such as an infant, who cannot express his wishes. In no country is either voluntary or compulsory euthanasia legal, although many organizations exist to promote the cause of voluntary euthanasia.

euthyroid adj. having a thyroid gland that functions normally. Compare hyperthyroidism, hypothyroidism. —**euthyroidism** n.

euthyroid sick syndrome (sick euthyroid syndrome) a syndrome characterized by alteration in the thyroid function tests in which the level of triiodothyronine is markedly reduced, thyroxine is slightly reduced, and thyroid-stimulating hormone is reduced or normal. This syndrome is commonly seen in nonthyroidal illness, due to altered metabolism and transport of the thyroid hormones, but is sometimes mistaken for primary hypothyroidism.

evacuator n. a device for sucking fluid out of a cavity. In its simplest form it consists of a hollow rubber bulb that is attached, via a valve system, to a tube inserted into the cavity. Another valve leads to a discharge tube. Evacuators may be used to empty the bladder of unwanted material during such operations as the removal of a calculus or transurethral *prostatectomy.

evagination n. the protrusion of a part or organ from a sheathlike covering or by eversion of its inner surface.

eventration n. 1. protrusion of the intestines through the abdominal wall. 2. (of the diaphragm) abnormal elevation of part of the diaphragm due to a congenital weakness (but without true herniation), as observed by X-ray.

event sampling (in psychology) a way of recording behavior in which the presence of a particular kind of behavior is noted whenever it occurs. It is used for precise descriptions of behavior and for following the course of *behavior modification. *See also* time sampling.

eversion n. a turning outward; in *eversion of the cervix* the edges of the cervix (neck) of the uterus turn outward after having been torn during childbirth.

evisceration n. 1. protrusion of an organ through a surgical incision. 2. removal of part of the viscera; disembowelment. 3. (in ophthalmology) an operation in which the contents of the eyeball are removed, the empty outer envelope (sclera) being left behind. *Compare* enucleation.

evocation n. *see* induction.

evulsion n. *see* avulsion.

Ewing's sarcoma a highly malignant tumor of bone occurring in children and young adults. Distinguished from *osteosarcoma by J. Ewing in 1921, it commonly arises in the femur but is liable to spread to other bones and to the lung. It usually presents with pain, often associated with fever and *leukocytosis. The tumor is sensitive to radiotherapy, and systemic

therapy with *cytotoxic drugs has greatly improved its prognosis. [J. Ewing (1866–1943), US pathologist]

ex- (exo-) *prefix denoting* outside or outer.

exacerbation n. an increase in the seriousness of a disease or any of its symptoms.

exaltation n. *see* elation.

exanthem n. 1. a skin rash accompanying any eruptive disease or fever. 2. any disease characterized by a skin rash, such as measles. *Exanthem subitum* is another name for *roseola (infantum). —**exanthematous** *adj.*

excavator n. 1. a spoon-shaped surgical instrument that is used to scrape out diseased tissue, usually for laboratory examination. 2. a type of hand instrument with spoon ends used for removing decayed dentine from teeth. It may also be used as a *curet.

exchange transfusion a technique for treating *hemolytic disease in newborn infants. Using a syringe with a three-way tap, blood is withdrawn from the baby (via the umbilical vein), ejected, and replaced by an equal amount of donor blood compatible with the mother's blood, without detaching the syringe. By many repetitions of this exchange, red blood cells liable to be destroyed and bilirubin released from those already destroyed are removed, while keeping the baby's blood volume and number of red cells constant. Exchange transfusion can also be used in *sickle-cell disease, as a temporary treatment during a crisis, or in neonatal jaundice.

excimer laser a laser that can remove very thin sheets of tissue from the surface of the cornea of the eye. This can be done to alter the curvature of the corneal surface, for example to treat near- or farsightedness (*see* LASEK, LASIK), or to remove diseased (e.g. calcified) tissue from the corneal surface. *See* keratectomy.

excipient n. a substance that is combined with a drug in order to render it suitable for administration; for example in the form of pills. Excipients have no pharmacologic action themselves.

excise vb. to cut out tissue, an organ, or a tumor from the body. —**excision** n.

excitation n. (in neurophysiology) the triggering of a conducted impulse in the membrane of a muscle cell or nerve fiber. During excitation a polarized membrane becomes momentarily depolarized and an *action potential is set up.

excoriation *n.* the destruction and removal of the surface of the skin or the covering of an organ by scraping, the application of a chemical, or other means.

excrescence *n.* an abnormal outgrowth on the surface of the body, such as a wart.

excreta *n.* any waste material discharged from the body, especially feces.

excretion *n.* the removal of the waste products of metabolism from the body, mainly through the action of the *kidneys. Excretion also includes the loss of water, salts, and some urea through the sweat glands and carbon dioxide and water vapor from the lungs, and the term is also used to include the egestion of feces.

exemestane *n. see* aromatase inhibitor.

exenteration *n.* (in ophthalmology) an operation in which all the contents of the eye socket (orbit) are removed, leaving only the bony walls intact. The bone is covered by a skin graft. This operation is sometimes necessary when there is a malignant tumor in the orbit.

exercise *n.* any activity resulting in physical exertion that is intended to maintain physical fitness, to condition the body, or to correct a physical deformity. Exercises may be done actively by the person or passively by a therapist. *Aerobic exercises* are intended to increase oxygen consumption (as in running) and to benefit the lungs and cardiovascular system, in contrast to *isometric exercises. In *isotonic exercises*, the muscles contract and there is movement, but the force remains the same; this improves joint mobility and muscle strength.

exflagellation *n.* the formation and release of mature flagellated male sex cells (*see* microgamete) by the *microgametocytes of the malarial parasite (*see* Plasmodium). The process, which is completed in 10–15 minutes, occurs after the microgametocytes have been transferred from a human to the stomach of a mosquito.

exfoliation *n.* **1.** flaking off of the upper layers of the skin. **2.** separation of a surface epithelium from the underlying tissue. **3.** the natural shedding of deciduous teeth. —**exfoliative** *adj.*

exfoliative dermatitis *see* erythroderma.

exhalation (expiration) *n.* the act of breathing air from the lungs out through the mouth and nose. *See* breathing.

exhibitionism *n.* exposure of the genitals to another person, as a sexually deviant act. The word is often broadened to mean public flaunting of any quality of the individual.

exo- *prefix. see* ex-.

exocoelom *n. see* extraembryonic coelom.

exocrine gland a gland that discharges its secretion by means of a duct, which opens onto an epithelial surface. An exocrine gland may be *simple*, with a single unbranched duct, or *compound*, with branched ducts and multiple secretory sacs. The illustration shows some different types of these glands. Examples of exocrine glands are the sebaceous and sweat glands. *See also* secretion.

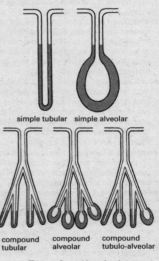

simple tubular   simple alveolar

compound   compound   compound
tubular   alveolar   tubulo-alveolar

Types of exocrine glands

exoenzyme *n.* an *enzyme that acts outside the cell that produced it. Examples of exoenzymes are the digestive enzymes.

exoerythrocytic *adj.* describing those stages in the life cycle of the malarial parasite (*see* Plasmodium) that develop in the cells of the liver. Each parasite (*sporozoite) divides repeatedly to produce a schizont containing many merozoites.

exogenous *adj.* originating outside the body or part of the body: applied particularly to substances in the body that are derived from the diet rather than built up by the body's own processes of metabolism. *Compare* endogenous.

exomphalos *n.* an umbilical *hernia.

exopeptidase *n.* an enzyme (e.g. *trypsin) that takes part in the digestion of proteins by splitting off the terminal amino acids of a polypeptide chain. *Compare* endopeptidase. *See also* peptidase.

exophoria *n.* a tendency to squint in which the eye, when covered, tends to turn outward. *See also* heterophoria.

exophthalmic goiter (Graves' disease) *see* thyrotoxicosis.

exophthalmometer (proptometer) *n.* an instrument for measuring the degree of protrusion of the eyeball, primarily in Graves' disease (*see* thyrotoxicosis). The distance measured is that from the rim of bone at the outer edge of the eye forward to the surface of the front of the cornea.

exophthalmos *n.* protrusion of the eyeballs in their sockets. This can result from injury or disease of the eyeball or socket but is most commonly associated with overactivity of the thyroid gland (*see* thyrotoxicosis).

exosmosis *n.* outward osmotic flow. *See also* osmosis.

exostosis *n.* a benign outgrowth of bone with a cap of cartilage, arising from the surface of a bone. *See* osteoma.

exothermic *adj.* describing a chemical reaction in which energy is released in the form of heat. *Compare* endothermic.

exotic *adj.* describing a disease occurring in a region of the world far from where it might be expected. Thus, malaria and leishmaniasis are regarded as exotic when they are diagnosed in patients in the US.

exotoxin *n.* a highly potent poison, often harmful to only a limited range of tissues, that is produced by a bacterial cell and secreted into its surrounding medium. It is generally unstable, being rendered inactive by heat, light, and chemicals. Exotoxins are produced by such bacteria as those causing *botulism, *diphtheria, and *tetanus. *Compare* endotoxin.

exotropia *n.* divergent *strabismus: a type of squint.

expectorant *n.* a drug that enhances the secretion of sputum by the air passages so that it is easier to cough up. Expectorants are used in cough mixtures; they act by increasing the bronchial secretion or make it less viscous (*see* mucolytic). Drugs such as *ipecac are *stimulant expectorants* in small quantities: they irritate the lining of the stomach, which provides a stimulus for the reflex production of sputum by the glands in the bronchial mucous membrane. At higher doses they produce vomiting.

expectoration *n.* the act of spitting out material brought into the mouth by coughing.

expiration *n.* **1.** the act of breathing out air from the lungs: exhalation. **2.** death.

explant 1. *n.* live tissue transferred from the body (or any organism) to a suitable artificial medium for culture. The tissue grows in the artificial medium and can be studied for diagnostic or experimental purposes. Tumor growths are sometimes examined in this way. **2.** silicone rubber material sutured to the outside of the eyeball over a retinal tear or hole (*see* detached retina, plombage). The resulting indent allows the retina to reattach. **3.** *vb.* to transfer live tissue for culture outside the body. —**explantation** *n.*

exploration *n.* (in surgery) an investigative operation to determine the cause of symptoms. —**exploratory** *adj.*

exposure *n.* **1.** (in radiology) the condition of being subjected to X-ray or gamma radiation. **2.** (in behavior therapy) a method of treating fears and phobias that involves confronting the individual with the situation he has been avoiding, so allowing the fears to wane by *habituation. It can be achieved either gradually by *desensitization or *graded self-exposure or suddenly by *flooding.

expressed emotion a measure of the degree of warmth or hostility in a relationship between two people, assessed when one person is talking about the other. High levels of criticism and hostility from family members can worsen the prognosis of mentally ill patients.

expulsive hemorrhage sudden bleeding from the choroid and retina of the eye, usually during a surgical procedure or trauma. This may force the ocular tissue out of the wound and is potentially one of the most devastating intraoperative complications of ocular surgery.

exsanguination *n.* **1.** depriving the body of blood; for example, as a result of an accident causing severe bleeding or – very rarely – through uncontrollable bleeding during a surgical operation. **2.** a technique for providing a bloodless field to facilitate delicate or hemorrhagic operative procedures. **3.** the removal of blood from a part (usually a limb) prior to stopping the inflow of blood (by tourniquet). —**exsanguinate** *vb.*

exsiccation *n.* drying up, as may occur in tissues deprived of an adequate supply of water during dehydration or starvation.

exstrophy *n.* a severe congenital abnormality in which the bladder fails to close during development: the baby is born with an absent lower abdominal wall and the internal surface of the posterior bladder wall is exposed. It is associated with *epispadias, total urinary incontinence, and undescended testes.

exsufflation *n.* the forcible removal of secretions from the air passages by some form of suction apparatus.

Extended Care Facility (ECF) an institution or part of an institution that provides long-term care for patients undergoing rehabilitation and for chronically ill patients who may not require the usual services of hospital inpatients. ECF support is provided under terms of the Medicare amendments to the US Social Security Act if the facility offers 24-hour nursing service, supervision of care by a physician, and meets other conditions relating to the health and safety of the patients. An ECF also may be identified as a Skilled Nursing Facility.

extension *n.* **1.** the act of extending or stretching, especially the muscular movement by which a limb is straightened. **2.** the application of *traction to a fractured or dislocated limb in order to restore it to its normal position.

extensor *n.* any muscle that causes the straightening of a limb or other part.

exteriorization *n.* a surgical procedure in which an organ is brought from its normal site to the surface of the body. This may be done as a temporary or permanent measure; for example, the intestine may be brought to the surface of the abdomen (*see* colostomy). The process is also sometimes used in physiologic experiments on animals.

external fixator an apparatus consisting of a rigid frame that connects pins passed through the skin into the bone above and below a fracture. This immobilizes the fracture, and is used particularly to treat some compound fractures. An external fixator is also used for *limb lengthening.

exteroceptor *n.* a sensory nerve, ending in the skin or a mucous membrane, that is responsive to stimuli from outside the body. *See also* chemoreceptor, receptor.

extinction *n.* (in psychology) the weakening of a conditioned reflex that takes place if it is not maintained by *reinforcement. This is used as a method of treatment when undesirable behavior (e.g. destructiveness) is reduced simply by withdrawing whatever rewards it (e.g. the fuss made by other people).

extirpation *n.* the complete surgical removal of tissue, an organ, or a growth.

extra- *prefix denoting* outside or beyond.

extracellular *adj.* situated or occurring outside cells; for example, *extracellular fluid* is the fluid surrounding cells.

extracorporeal *adj.* situated or occurring outside the body. *Extracorporeal circulation* is the circulation of the blood outside the body, as through a *heart-lung machine or an artificial kidney (*see* hemodialysis).

extracorporeal membrane oxygenation (ECMO) a technique for otherwise fatal respiratory failure in newborn babies or infants due to prematurity or overwhelming septicemia (e.g. meningococcal septicemia). It involves modified prolonged *cardiopulmonary bypass to support gas exchange, which allows the lungs to rest and recover.

extracorporeal shock wave lithotripsy (ESWL) *see* lithotripsy.

extract *n.* a preparation containing the pharmacologically active principles of a drug, made by evaporating a solution of the drug in water, alcohol, or ether.

extraction *n.* **1.** the surgical removal of a part of the body. Extraction of teeth is usually achieved by applying extraction *forceps to the crown or root of the tooth to dislocate it from its socket. When this is not possible, for example because the tooth or root is deeply buried within the bone, extraction is performed surgically by removing bone and dividing the tooth. **2.** the act of pulling out a baby from the body of its mother during childbirth.

extractor *n.* an instrument used to pull out a natural part of the body, to remove a foreign object, or to assist the delivery of a baby (*see* vacuum extractor).

extradural *adj. see* epidural.

extraembryonic coelom (exocoelom) the cavity, lined with mesoderm, that surrounds the embryo from the earliest stages of development. It communicates temporarily with the coelomic cavity within the embryo (peritoneal cavity). Late in pregnancy, it becomes almost entirely obliterated by the growth of the *amnion, which fuses with the *chorion.

extraembryonic membranes the membranous structures that surround the embryo and contribute to the placenta and umbilical cord. They include the *amnion, *chorion, *allantois, and *yolk sac. In humans the allantois is always very small and by the end of pregnancy the amnion and chorion have fused into a single membrane and the yolk sac has disappeared.

extrapleural *adj.* relating to the tissues of the chest wall outside the parietal *pleura.

extrapyramidal system the system of nerve tracts and pathways connecting the cerebral cortex, basal ganglia, thalamus, cerebellum, reticular formation, and spinal neurons in complex circuits not included in the *pyramidal system. The extrapyramidal system is mainly concerned with the regulation of stereotyped reflex muscular movements.

extrasensory perception (ESP) a supposed way of perceiving that involves none of the known senses. *Clairvoyance* is the extrasensory perception of current events; *precognition* is extrasensory perception of future events; *telepathy* is extrasensory perception of the thoughts of others.

extrasystole *n. see* ectopic beat.

extrauterine *adj.* outside the uterus.

extravasation *n.* the leakage and spread of blood or fluid from vessels into the surrounding tissues, which follows injury, burns, inflammation, and allergy.

extraversion *n. see* extroversion.

extrinsic muscle a muscle, such as any of those controlling movements of the eye-

ball, that has its origin some distance from the part it acts on.

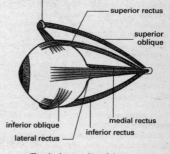

Extrinsic muscles of the eye

extroversion *n.* **1. (extraversion)** an enduring personality trait characterized by interest in the outside world rather than the self. People high in extroversion (*extroverts*), as measured by questionnaires and tests, are gregarious and outgoing, prefer to change activities frequently, and are not susceptible to permanent *conditioning. Extroversion was first described by Carl Jung as a tendency to action rather than thought, to scientific rather than philosophical interests, and to emotional rather than intellectual reactions. *Compare* introversion. **2.** a turning inside out of a hollow organ, such as the uterus (which sometimes occurs after childbirth).

extrovert *n. see* extroversion.

extrusion *n.* (in dentistry) **1.** the forced eruption of a tooth by means of an orthodontic appliance; for example, to realign a tooth that has been accidentally forced into the jaw. **2.** the partial lifting of a tooth from its socket as a result of traumatic injury.

exudation *n.* the slow escape of liquid (called the *exudate*) containing proteins and white cells through the walls of intact blood vessels, usually as a result of inflammation. Exudation is a normal part of the body's defense mechanisms.

eye *n.* the organ of sight: a three-layered roughly spherical structure specialized for receiving and responding to light. The outer fibrous coat consists of the sclera and the transparent cornea; the

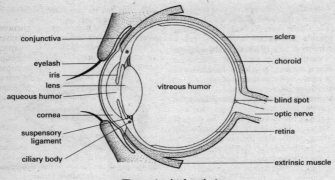

conjunctiva
eyelash
iris
lens
aqueous humor
cornea
suspensory ligament
ciliary body

vitreous humor

sclera
choroid
blind spot
optic nerve
retina
extrinsic muscle

The eye (sagittal section)

middle vascular layer comprises the choroid, ciliary body, and iris; and the inner sensory layer is the retina (see illustration).

Light enters the eye through the cornea, which refracts the light through the aqueous humor onto the lens. By adjustment of the shape of the lens (*see* accommodation) light is focused through the vitreous humor onto the retina. In the retina light-sensitive cells (*see* cone, rod) send nerve impulses to the brain via the optic nerve. The arrangement of the two eyes at the front of the head provides *binocular vision. Each eye is contained in an *orbit, and movement of the eye within the orbit is controlled by *extrinsic muscles.

eyeball *n.* the body of the *eye, which is roughly spherical, is bounded by the *sclera, and lies in the *orbit. It is closely associated with accessory structures – the eyelids, conjunctiva, and lacrimal (tear-producing) apparatus – and its movements are controlled by three pairs of extrinsic eye muscles (see illustration).

eyebrow *n.* the small fringe of hair on the bony ridge just above the eye. It helps to prevent moisture from running into the eye. Anatomic name: **supercilium**.

eyeground *n.* the inside of the eye as seen through an ophthalmoscope; the ocular fundus.

eyelash *n.* one of the long stiff hairs that form a row projecting outward from the front edge of the upper and lower eyelids. The eyelashes help keep dust away from the eye. Anatomic name: **cilium**.

eyelid *n.* the protective covering of the eye. Each eye has two eyelids consisting of skin, muscle, connective tissue (*tarsus*), and sebaceous glands (*meibomian* or *tarsal glands*). Each eyelid is lined with membrane (*conjunctiva) and fringed with eyelashes. Stimulation of the pain receptors in the cornea causes the eyelids to close in a reflex action. Inflammation of a meibomian gland can result in a *chalazion. Anatomic names: **blepharon**, **palpebra**.

eyepiece *n.* the lens or system of lenses of an optical instrument, such as a microscope, that is nearest to the eye of the examiner. It usually produces a magnified image of the previous image formed by the instrument. *Compare* objective.

eyestrain *n.* a sense of fatigue brought on by use of the eyes for prolonged close work or in persons who have an uncorrected error of *refraction or an imbalance of the muscles that move the eyes. Symptoms are usually aching or burning of the eyes, accompanied by headache and even general fatigue if the eyes are not rested. Medical name: **asthenopia**.

F

Fabry's disease *see* angiokeratoma. [J. Fabry (1860–1930), German dermatologist]

face *n.* the front portion of the head, from the forehead to the chin, including the skin, muscles, and structures of the eyes, nose, mouth, cheeks, and jaw, and excluding the ears.

face-bow *n.* (in dentistry) an instrument for transferring the jaw relationship of a patient to an *articulator to allow reproduction of the lateral and protrusive movements of the lower jaw.

face-lift *n.* plastic surgery designed to correct sagging facial tissues. Eyelid drooping can be corrected at the same procedure. Medical names: **rhytidectomy, rhytidoplasty**.

face peel a technique of removing unwanted blemishes from the face. Phenol is applied to the face, which causes cellular destruction in the epidermis and upper dermis. Epithelial regeneration begins by the second day and is usually complete in 10 to 14 days.

facet *n.* a small flat surface on a bone or tooth, especially a surface of articulation.

facial nerve the seventh *cranial nerve (VII): a mixed sensory and motor nerve that supplies the muscles of facial expression, the taste buds of the front part of the tongue, the sublingual salivary glands, and the lacrimal glands. A small branch to the middle ear regulates the tension on the ear ossicles.

facial paralysis paralysis of the facial nerve, causing weakness and loss of function of the muscles it serves. It occurs in *Bell's palsy.

-facient *suffix denoting* causing or making. Example: *abortifacient* (causing abortion).

facies *n.* **1.** facial expression, often a guide to a patient's state of health as well as his emotions. The typical facies seen in a person, especially a child, with enlarged adenoids is the vacant look, with the mouth drooping open. A *Hippocratic facies* is the sallow face, sagging and with listless staring eyes, that is an indication of approaching death. **2.** (in anatomy) a specific surface of a body structure or part.

facilitation *n.* (in neurology) the phenomenon that occurs when a neuron receives, through a number of different synapses, impulses that are not powerful enough individually to start an *action potential but whose combined activity brings about some *depolarization of the membrane. In this facilitated state a small additional depolarization will suffice to trigger an impulse in the cell.

facio- *prefix denoting* the face. Examples: *faciobrachial* (relating to the face and arm); *faciolingual* (relating to the face and tongue); *facioplegia* (paralysis of).

facioscapulohumeral muscular dystrophy *see* muscular dystrophy.

factitious *adj.* produced artificially, either deliberately or by accident, and therefore not to be taken into account when the results of an experiment are considered or a diagnosis is being made.

factor *n.* (in biochemistry) a substance that is essential to a physiologic process, often a substance the nature of which is unknown. *See also* coagulation factors, growth factor.

Factor V Leiden an inherited mutation in the gene coding for coagulation Factor V, which results in an increased susceptibility to develop venous *thrombosis.

Factor VIII (antihemophilic factor) a *coagulation factor normally present in blood. Deficiency of the factor, which is inherited by males from their mothers, results in *hemophilia A (classic hemophilia). Genetically engineered replacement factor is available. *See also* von Willebrand's disease.

Factor IX (Christmas factor) a *coagulation factor normally present in blood. Deficiency of the factor results in *hemophilia B. A concentrate of Factor IX is available for replacement therapy.

Factor XI a *coagulation factor normally present in blood. Deficiency of the factor is inherited, but rarely causes spontaneous bleeding. However, bleeding does occur after surgery or trauma to the blood vessels.

facultative *adj.* describing an organism that is not restricted to one way of life. A *facultative parasite* can live either as a parasite or, in different conditions, as a nonparasite able to survive without a host. *Compare* obligate.

FAD (flavin adenine dinucleotide) a *coenzyme, derived from riboflavin, that takes part in many important oxidation-reduction reactions. It consists of two phosphate groups, adenine, and ribose.

fading n. (in behavior modification) see prompting.

Fahrenheit temperature temperature expressed on a scale in which the melting point of ice is assigned a temperature of 32° and the boiling point of water a temperature of 212°. For most medical purposes the Celsius (centigrade) scale has replaced the Fahrenheit scale. The formula for converting from Fahrenheit (F) to Celsius (C) is: $C = 5/9(F − 32)$. See also Celsius temperature. [G. D. Fahrenheit (1686–1736), German physicist]

failure to thrive (FTT) failure of an infant to grow satisfactorily compared with the average. It is detected by regular measurements and plotting on *centile charts. It can be the first indication of a serious underlying condition, such as kidney or heart disease or malabsorption, or it may result from problems at home, particularly nonaccidental injury (see battered baby syndrome).

fainting n. see syncope.

falciform ligament a fold of peritoneum separating the right and left lobes of the liver and attaching it to the diaphragm and the anterior abdominal wall as far as the umbilicus.

fallopian tube (oviduct, uterine tube) either of a pair of tubes that conduct ova (egg cells) from the ovary to the uterus (see reproductive system). The ovarian end opens into the abdominal cavity via a funnel-shaped structure with finger-like projections (fimbriae) surrounding the opening. Movements of the fimbriae at ovulation assist in directing the ovum to the fallopian tube. The ovum is fertilized near the ovarian end of the tube. [G. Fallopius (1523–63), Italian anatomist]

Fallot's tetralogy see tetralogy of Fallot.

false negative an incorrect result of a diagnostic test or procedure that wrongly indicates the absence of a disease or condition. False negative results are more common than false positive results since failure to observe a finding is more likely to occur than the imagined observation of something that does not exist. Compare false positive.

false positive a diagnostic or procedural test result that wrongly indicates the presence of a disease or other condition, due to inexact methods of testing. Compare false negative.

false pregnancy see pseudocyesis.

false rib see rib.

falx (falx cerebri) n. (pl. **falces**) a sickle-shaped fold of the *dura mater that dips inward from the skull in the midline, between the cerebral hemispheres.

famciclovir n. an antiviral drug, similar to *acyclovir, used to treat *herpes zoster, genital herpes, and recurrent mucocutaneous herpes simplex infections in HIV-infected patients. It is administered orally; side effects include headache, stomach upset, vomiting, and diarrhea. Trade name: **Famvir**.

familial adj. describing a condition or character that is found in some families but not in others. The condition or character is often inherited.

familial adenomatous polyposis (FAP) see polyposis.

family planning 1. the use of *contraception to limit or space out the number of children born to a couple. **2.** provision of contraceptive methods within a community or nation. See also genetic counseling.

family practitioner a doctor who is the main provider of primary medical care of the entire family, from infants to the aged. This includes following each member of the family on a continuing basis, supplying ancillary medical services when needed, and providing techniques that will keep the family in good health. See also general practitioner.

family therapy a form of *psychotherapy based on the belief that psychological problems are the products of abnormalities in communication between family members. All family members are therefore seen together, when possible, in order to clarify and modify the ways they relate together (see genogram, paradox, sculpting).

famotidine n. an H_2-receptor antagonist (see antihistamine) used for the treatment of duodenal ulcers and conditions of excessive gastric acid secretion, such as the Zollinger-Ellison syndrome. Famotidine is administered by mouth and intravenously; side effects are headache, diarrhea, and dizziness. Trade names: **Pepcid, Pepcidine**.

Fanconi's anemia an autosomal *recessive disorder characterized by severe aplastic *anemia (failure of the bone marrow to produce blood cells, either red or white) and an increased predisposition to malignancy. The condition also causes mental retardation, poor growth, skeletal abnormalities, and kidneys of an unusual shape or in an unusual position. The condition is due to a defect in one of a group of genes known as Fanconi's anemia (*FA*) genes. Children are usually diagnosed between five and ten years of age. The only treatment available is *hemopoietic stem cell transplantation; without this, most affected individuals die by the age of 30 from bone marrow failure or leukemia. [G. Fanconi (1892–1979), Swiss pediatrician]

Fanconi's syndrome a disorder of the proximal kidney tubules, which may be inherited or acquired and is most common in children. It is characterized by the urinary excretion of large amounts of amino acids, glucose, and phosphates (although blood levels of these substances are normal). Symptoms may include osteomalacia, rickets, muscle weakness, and *cystinosis. Treatment is directed to the cause. [G. Fanconi]

fantasy *n.* a complex sequence of imagination in which several imaginary elements are woven together into a story. An excessive preoccupation with one's own imaginings may be symptomatic of a difficulty in coping with reality. In psychoanalytic psychology, *unconscious fantasies* are supposed to control behavior, so that psychological symptoms can be symbols of or defenses against such fantasies (*see* symbolism).

farad *n.* the *SI unit of capacitance, equal to the capacitance of a capacitor between the plates of which a potential difference of 1 volt appears when it is charged with 1 coulomb of electricity. Symbol: F.

faradism *n.* the use of induced rapidly alternating electric currents to stimulate nerve and muscle activity. *See also* electrotherapy.

farcy *n. see* glanders.

farmer's lung an occupational lung disease caused by allergy to fungal spores that grow in inadequately dried stored hay, straw, or grain, which then becomes moldy. It is an allergic *alveolitis, such as also results from sensitivity to many other allergens. An acute reversible form can develop a few hours after exposure; a chronic form, with the gradual development of irreversible breathlessness, occurs with or without preceding acute attacks. Avoidance of the allergen is the main principle of treatment.

farsightedness *n. see* hyperopia.

fascia *n.* (*pl.* **fasciae**) connective tissue forming fibrous layers of variable thickness in all regions of the body. Fascia surrounds organs and tissues and is divided into *superficial fascia* (found immediately beneath the skin) and *deep fascia* (which forms sheaths for muscles and muscle groups that separate them into layers).

fasciculation *n.* brief spontaneous contraction of a few muscle fibers, which is seen as a flicker of movement under the skin. It is most often associated with disease of the motor neurons in the spinal cord or of the nerve fibers (*see* motor neuron disease). It may also be seen in the calf muscles of normal persons.

fasciculus (fascicle) *n.* a bundle, e.g. of nerve or muscle fibers.

fasciitis *n.* inflammation of *fascia. It may result from bacterial infection or from a rheumatic disease, such as *Reiter's syndrome or ankylosing spondylitis. *See also* necrotizing fasciitis, plantar fasciitis.

Fasciola *n.* a genus of *flukes. *F. hepatica*, the liver fluke, normally lives as a parasite of sheep and other herbivorous animals but sometimes infects humans (*see* fascioliasis).

fascioliasis *n.* an infestation of the bile ducts and liver with the liver fluke *Fasciola hepatica*. Humans acquire the infection through eating wild watercress on which the larval stages of the parasite are present. Symptoms include fever, dyspepsia, vomiting, loss of appetite, abdominal pain, and coughing; the liver may also be extensively damaged (causing *liver rot*). *Anthelmintics are used in the treatment of fascioliasis.

fasciolopsiasis *n.* a disease, common in the Far East, caused by the fluke *Fasciolopsis buski* in the small intestine. At the site of attachment of the adult flukes in the intestine there may be inflammation

.with some ulceration and bleeding. Symptoms include diarrhea, and in heavy infections the patient may experience loss of appetite, vomiting, and (later) swelling of the face, abdomen, and legs. Death may follow in cases of severe ill health and malnutrition. The flukes can be removed with an anthelmintic, such as praziquantel.

Fasciolopsis *n.* a genus of large parasitic flukes widely distributed throughout eastern Asia and especially common in China. The adults of *F. buski*, the giant intestinal fluke, live in the human small intestine. Infection with the fluke occurs after eating uncooked water chestnuts contaminated with fluke larvae and the resulting symptoms can be serious (*see* fasciolopsiasis).

fastigium *n.* the highest point, as of a fever.

fat *n.* a substance that contains one or more *fatty acids (in the form of *triglycerides) and is the principal form in which energy is stored by the body (in *adipose tissue). It also serves as an insulating material beneath the skin (in the subcutaneous tissue) and around certain organs (including the kidneys). Fat is one of the three main constituents of food (*see also* carbohydrate, protein); it is necessary in the diet to provide an adequate supply of *essential fatty acids and for the efficient absorption of fatsoluble vitamins from the intestine. Excessive deposition of fat in the body leads to *obesity. *See also* brown fat, lipid.

fatal familial insomnia an autosomal *dominant disorder due to a mutation in the gene for the *prion protein (PrP): it is an example of a *spongiform encephalopathy. Patients present with intractable progressive insomnia, disturbances of the autonomic nervous system, and eventually dementia. Death usually occurs within six months to three years of onset.

fatigue *n.* **1.** mental or physical tiredness, following prolonged or intense activity. Muscle fatigue may be due to the waste products of metabolism accumulating in the muscles faster than they can be removed by the venous blood. Incorrect or inadequate food intake or disease may predispose a person to fatigue. **2.** the inability of an organism, an organ, or a tissue to give a normal response to a stimulus until a certain recovery period has elapsed.

fatty acid an organic acid with a long straight hydrocarbon chain and an even number of carbon atoms. Fatty acids are the fundamental constituents of many important lipids, including *triglycerides. Some fatty acids can be synthesized by the body; others, the *essential fatty acids, must be obtained from the diet. Examples of fatty acids are *palmitic acid*, *oleic acid*, and *stearic acid*. *See also* fat, saturated fatty acid, unsaturated fatty acid.

fatty degeneration deterioration in the health of a tissue due to the deposition of abnormally large amounts of fat in its cells. The accumulation of fat in the liver and heart may seriously impair their functioning. The deposition of fat may be linked with incorrect diet, excessive alcohol consumption, or a shortage of oxygen in the tissues caused by poor circulation or a deficiency of hemoglobin.

fauces *n.* the opening leading from the mouth into the pharynx; the throat. It is surrounded by the *glossopalatine arch* (which forms the anterior pillars of the fauces) and the *pharyngopalatine arch* (the posterior pillars).

favism *n.* an inherited defect in the enzyme glucose-6-phosphate dehydrogenase causing the red blood cells to become sensitive to a chemical in broad beans. It results in destruction of red blood cells, which sometimes leads to severe anemia, requiring blood transfusion. Favism occurs in parts of the Mediterranean and Iran. *See also* glucose-6-phosphate dehydrogenase deficiency.

favus *n.* a type of *ringworm of the scalp, caused by the fungus *Trichophyton schoenleinii*. Favus, which is rare in Europe and the United States, is typified by yellow crusts made up of the threads of fungus and skin debris, which form honeycomb-like masses.

FDA *see* Food and Drug Administration.

fear *n.* an emotional state evoked by threat of danger and usually characterized by unpleasant subjective experiences and physiological and behavioral changes. Fear is often distinguished from *anxiety in having a specific object. Physiological changes can include increases in heart rate, blood pressure, sweating, etc. Behavioral changes can include an avoidance of fear-producing objects or situations and may be extremely disabling; for example, fear of open spaces. These specific disabling fears are known as *phobias. Treatment of short-term fears, such as the fear of hearing the results of an examination, can be relieved by *beta blockers or by anxiolytics, such as diazepam. With anxiolytics, however, there is danger of developing dependence, and *behavior therapy or *cognitive therapy are preferred for disabling and persistent fears.

febricula n. a fever of low intensity or short duration.

febrifuge n. a treatment or drug that reduces or prevents fever. See antipyretic.

febrile adj. relating to or affected with fever.

febrile convulsion (febrile seizure) an epileptic-type seizure associated with a fever. Such seizures affect up to 4% of children, usually aged between six months and six years, and generally last less than 10 minutes. Seizures do not lead to mental retardation or cerebral palsy, but the risk of developing *epilepsy is around 2%, especially when other risk factors, such as family history, are present. Seizures may be recurrent, but the risk of this can be minimized by attempts to reduce the fever. The underlying infection is usually viral, but more serious conditions, such as meningitis, should be excluded.

fecal impaction see constipation, impacted.

fecalith n. a small hard mass of feces, found particularly in the vermiform appendix: a cause of inflammation.

feces n. the waste material that is eliminated through the anus. It is formed in the *colon and consists of a solid or semisolid mass of undigested food remains (chiefly cellulose) mixed with *bile pigments (which are responsible for the color), bacteria, various secretions (e.g. mucus), and some water. —**fecal** adj.

feeblemindedness n. a former name for *mental retardation.

feedback n. the coupling of the output of a process to the input. Feedback mechanisms are important in regulating many physiological processes; for example, hormone output and enzyme-mediated reactions. In *negative feedback*, a rise in the output of a substance (e.g. a hormone) will inhibit a further increase in its production, either directly or indirectly (see negative feedback loops). In *positive feedback*, a rise in the output of a substance is associated with an increase in the output of another substance, either directly or indirectly.

fee for service a standard system of charges for personal medical care in which a patient is asked to pay for each procedure performed by the attending physician. The fees charged may differ according to the length and difficulty of the treatment provided for the patient. Compare capitation fee.

Fehling's test a test for detecting the presence of sugar in urine; it has now been replaced by better and easier methods. It uses Fehling's solution, of which there are two components: Fehling's I (a copper sulfate solution) and Fehling's II (a solution of potassium sodium tartrate and sodium hydroxide). Boiling Fehling's solution is added to an equal volume of boiling urine; a yellowish or brownish coloration indicates the presence of sugar. [H. von Fehling (1812–85), German chemist]

Feingold diet a diet that purports to treat many illnesses by the elimination of artificial food colorings, preservatives, and salicylates from the diet. It has been particularly recommended for the treatment of *attention-deficit/hyperactivity disorder, but is of unproved value.

felbamate n. a drug used in the treatment of epilepsy and for partial and generalized seizures associated with the *Lennox-Gastaut syndrome. It is administered by mouth; side effects include nausea, insomnia, and loss of appetite. Because the use of the drug has been associated with marked increases in the incidence of aplastic anemia and acute hepatic failure, it should only be used when the seizure disorder cannot be managed by alternative therapy. Trade name: **Felbatol**.

felodipine n. a *calcium antagonist used in the treatment of hypertension. It is administered by mouth; side effects include edema, headache, and flushing. Trade name: **Plendil**.

felon (whitlow) n. an abscess affecting the pulp of the fingertip. See also paronychia.

feminization n. the development of female secondary sexual characteristics (enlargement of the breasts, loss of facial hair, and fat beneath the skin) in the male, either as a result of an endocrine disorder or of hormone therapy.

femoral *adj.* of or relating to the thigh or to the femur.

femoral artery an artery arising from the external iliac artery at the inguinal ligament. It is situated superficially, running down the front medial aspect of the thigh. Two-thirds of the way down it passes into the back of the thigh, continuing downward behind the knee as the *popliteal artery*.

femoral nerve the nerve that supplies the quadriceps muscle at the front of the thigh and receives sensation from the front and inner sides of the thigh. It arises from the second, third, and fourth lumbar nerves.

femoral triangle (Scarpa's triangle) a triangular depression on the inner side of the thigh bounded by the sartorius and adductor longus muscles and the inguinal ligament. The pulse can be felt here because the femoral artery lies over the depression.

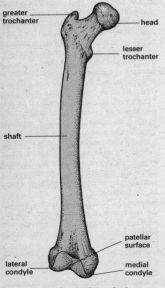

greater trochanter — head

lesser trochanter

shaft

patellar surface

lateral condyle — medial condyle

The femur (front view)

femur (thigh bone) *n.* a long bone between the hip and the knee (see illustration). The head of the femur articulates with the acetabulum of the *hip bone. The *greater* and *lesser trochanters* are protuberances on which the gluteus and psoas major muscles, respectively, are inserted. The *lateral* and *medial condyles* articulate with the *tibia and the concave grooved *patellar surface* accommodates the kneecap (patella). Partial dislocation of the *femoral epiphysis*, the growth area of the upper end of the bone, leads to deformity of the head of the femur and premature degeneration of the hip joint. The narrowed end of the femur (*femoral neck*) is the most common site of fracture of the leg in elderly women.

fenbufen *n.* an anti-inflammatory drug (*see* NSAID) used to relieve inflammation and the resulting pain and stiffness. It is administered by mouth. Possible side effects include nausea, vomiting, and skin rashes.

fenestra *n.* (in anatomy) an opening resembling a window. The *fenestra ovalis* (*fenestra vestibuli*) – the oval window – is the opening between the middle *ear and the vestibule of the inner ear. It is closed by a membrane to which the stapes is attached. The *fenestra rotunda* (*fenestra cochleae*) – the round window – is the opening between the scala tympani of the cochlea and the middle ear. Sound vibrations leave the cochlea through the fenestra rotunda, which, like the fenestra ovalis, is closed by a membrane.

fenestration *n.* a surgical operation in which a new opening is formed in the bony *labyrinth of the inner ear as part of the treatment of deafness due to *otosclerosis. It is rarely performed, having been superseded by *stapedectomy.

fenofibrate *n. see* fibrates.

fenoprofen *n.* an *analgesic drug that also reduces inflammation (*see* NSAID) and is used to treat arthritic conditions. It is administered by mouth and may cause digestive upsets, drowsiness, dizziness, sweating, and headache. Trade name: **Nalfon.**

fermentation *n.* the biochemical process by which organic substances, particularly carbohydrates, are decomposed by the action of enzymes to provide chemical energy. An example is *alcoholic fermentation*, in which enzymes in yeast decompose sugar to form ethyl alcohol and carbon dioxide.

ferning n. a test to determine if the amniotic membrane surrounding the fetus has ruptured in late pregnancy. A typical pattern of amniotic fluid crystallization occurs when the amniotic fluid dries.

ferri- (ferro-) prefix denoting iron.

ferritin n. an iron-protein complex that is one of the forms in which iron is stored in the tissues.

ferrous sulfate an *iron salt that is administered by mouth to treat or prevent iron-deficiency anemia. There are few serious side effects; stomach upsets and diarrhea may be prevented by taking the drug with meals. Similar preparations used to treat anemia include ferrous fumarate and ferrous succinate.

fertility rate the number of live births occurring in a year per 1000 women of child-bearing age (usually 15 to 44 years of age). A less reliable measure of fertility can be obtained from the live birth rate (the number of live births per 1000 of the population) or the natural increase (the excess of live births over deaths). More rarely quoted are the gross reproduction rate (i.e. the rate at which the child-bearing female population is reproducing itself) and the net reproduction rate, which takes into account female mortality before the age of reproduction. Other measures of fertility include the legitimate birth rate (the number of live births per 1000 women married once and aged 16 to 44) and the illegitimate birth rate (the number of illegitimate births per 1000 unmarried women and widows aged 15 to 44).

fertilization n. the fusion of a spermatozoon and an ovum. Rapid changes in the membrane of the ovum prevent other spermatozoa from penetrating. Penetration stimulates the completion of meiosis and the formation of the second polar body. Once the male and female pronuclei have fused, the zygote starts to divide by cleavage.

FESS see functional endoscopic sinus surgery.

festination n. the short tottering steps that characterize the gait of a patient with *parkinsonism.

fetal alcohol syndrome a condition of newborn babies that results from the toxic effects on the fetus of maternal alcohol abuse. Babies have a low birth weight and growth is retarded; there may be head and facial abnormalities and possibly mental retardation. The greater the alcohol abuse, the more severe the fetal manifestations.

fetal blood sampling a technique, usually carried out during labor, in which a sample of blood is withdrawn from a vein in the scalp of the fetus. From this is determined the degree of fetal *acidosis. The normal pH of fetal blood is 7.35 (range 7.45–7.25). The lower the level, the more likely is the fetus to be suffering from *hypoxia, indicating an urgent need to terminate the labor; if the pH is allowed to fall below a level of 7.10, the life of the fetus is endangered.

fetal hydantoin syndrome a complex of birth defects, including craniofacial and skeletal abnormalities, poor growth and development, and mental retardation, caused by prenatal maternal exposure to anticonvulsant *hydantoin derivatives.

fetal implant (fetal graft) the introduction of an ovum, fertilized in vitro and developed to the *blastocyst stage, into the uterus of a postmenopausal woman in order that she may become pregnant. Before this procedure, the woman's uterus must be prepared, by hormone therapy, to receive and nurture the blastocyst. Hormone treatment is continued throughout the pregnancy.

fetal transplant specific cells taken from a healthy newly aborted fetus and transplanted into a person suffering from a specific disease. These fetal cells take over the function of the specific diseased or damaged cells of the host. Examples are fetal brain cells transplanted into the affected part of the brain in a patient suffering from Parkinson's disease, and fetal pancreatic cells transplanted into the pancreas of a juvenile diabetic. Other diseases are being investigated experimentally with a view to using fetal transplants. Potentially, such procedures involve ethical considerations.

feticide n. the destruction of a fetus in the uterus; for example by injection of a lethal substance into the fetal heart to achieve a late-stage termination of pregnancy.

fetishism n. sexual attraction to an inappropriate object (known as a fetish). This may be a part of the body (e.g. the foot or the hair), clothing (e.g. underwear or shoes), or other objects (e.g. leather handbags or rubber sheets). In all these cases the fetish has replaced the normal object of sexual love, in some cases to the point at which sexual relationships with another person are impossible or are possible only if the fetish is either present or fantasized. Treatment can involve *psychotherapy or behavior therapy using *aversion therapy and masturbatory conditioning of desirable sexual behavior. *See also* sexual deviation.

feto- *prefix denoting* a fetus.

fetor *n.* an unpleasant smell. *Fetor oris* is bad breath (*halitosis).

fetoscopy *n.* inspection of the fetus before birth by passing a special fiberoptic instrument known as a *fetoscope* through the abdomen of a pregnant woman into her uterus. Fetoscopy, usually performed in the 18th–20th week of gestation, allows the inspection of the fetus for visible abnormalities and blood sampling by inserting a hollow needle under direct vision into a placental blood vessel. The blood can then be examined for abnormalities and hence the *prenatal diagnosis of blood disorders (such as *thalassemia, hemophilia, and *sickle-cell disease) and Duchenne *muscular dystrophy.

fetus *n.* a mammalian *embryo during the later stages of development within the uterus. In human reproduction it refers to an unborn child from its eighth week of development. —**fetal** *adj.*

fetus papyraceous a twin fetus that has died in the uterus and become flattened and mummified.

Feulgen reaction a method of demonstrating the presence of DNA in cell nuclei. The tissue section under investigation, after hydrolysis with dilute hydrochloric acid, is treated with *Schiff's reagent. A purple coloration develops in the presence of DNA. [R. Feulgen (1884–1955), German chemist]

FEV *see* forced expiratory volume.

fever (pyrexia) *n.* a rise in body temperature above the normal, i.e. above an oral temperature of 98.6°F (37°C) or a rectal temperature of 99°F (37.2°C). Fever may be accompanied by shivering, headache, nausea, constipation, or diarrhea. A rise in temperature above 105°F (40.5°C) may cause delirium and, in young children, *convulsions. Fevers are usually caused by bacterial or viral infections and can accompany any infectious illness, from the common cold to *malaria. An *intermittent fever* is a periodic rise and fall in body temperature, often returning to normal during the day and reaching its peak at night, as in malaria. A *remittent fever* is one in which body temperature fluctuates but does not return to normal. *See also* relapsing fever.

fexofenadine *n.* an *antihistamine used to relieve the symptoms of hay fever and to treat the skin manifestations of chronic *urticaria. It is administered orally; side effects include dizziness, drowsiness, fever, headache, and nausea. Trade name: **Allegra**.

fiber *n.* **1.** (in anatomy) a threadlike structure, such as a muscle cell, a nerve fiber, or a collagen fiber. **2.** (in dietetics) *see* dietary fiber. —**fibrous** *adj.*

fiberoptics *n.* the use of fibers for the transmission of light images. Synthetic fibers with special optical properties can be used in instruments to relay pictures of the inside of the body for direct observation or photography. *See* fiberscope. —**fiberoptic** *adj.*

fiberscope *n.* an *endoscope that uses *fiberoptics for the transmission of images from the interior of the body. Fiberscopes have a great advantage over the older endoscopes because they are flexible and can be introduced into relatively inaccessible cavities of the body.

fibr- (fibro-) *prefix denoting* fibers or fibrous tissue.

fibrates *pl. n.* a class of drugs, chemically related to fibric acid, that are capable of reducing concentrations of *triglycerides and low-density *lipoproteins in the blood; they also tend to raise the levels of the beneficial high-density lipoproteins. Fibrates are used for treating hyperlipidemia; they include *bezafibrate* (Bezalip), *ciprofibrate* (Modalim), *fenofibrate* (Lofibra, Tricor), and *gemfibrozil.

fibril *n.* a very small fiber or a constituent thread of a fiber (for example, a *myofibril of a muscle fiber). —**fibrillar, fibrillary** *adj.*

fibrillation *n.* a rapid and chaotic beating of the many individual muscle fibers of the heart, which is consequently unable to maintain effective synchronous contraction. The affected part of the heart then ceases to pump blood.

Fibrillation may affect the atria or ventricles independently. *Atrial fibrillation*, a common type of *arrhythmia, results in rapid and irregular heart and pulse rates. The main causes are atherosclerosis, chronic rheumatic heart disease, and hypertensive heart disease. It may also complicate various other conditions, including chest infections and thyroid overactivity. The heart rate is controlled by the administration of *digoxin; in some cases the heart rhythm can be restored to normal by *cardioversion. Anticoagulant therapy with *warfarin reduces the risk of blood-clot formation, which could cause a stroke.

When *ventricular fibrillation* occurs, the heart stops beating (*see* cardiac arrest). It is most commonly the result of *myocardial infarction.

fibrin *n.* the final product of the process of *blood coagulation, produced by the action of the enzyme thrombin on a soluble precursor fibrinogen. The product thus formed (*fibrin monomer*) links up (polymerizes) with similar molecules to give a fibrous meshwork that forms the basis of a blood clot, which seals off the damaged blood vessel.

fibrinogen *n.* a substance (*coagulation factor), present in blood plasma, that is acted upon by the enzyme thrombin to produce the insoluble protein fibrin in the final stage of *blood coagulation. The normal level of fibrinogen in plasma is 2–4 g/l (4–6 g/l during pregnancy).

fibrinogenopenia *n. see* hypofibrinogenemia.

fibrinoid *adj.* resembling the protein fibrin.

fibrinokinase *n.* a former name for a group of enzymes now known as *plasminogen activators.

fibrinolysin *n. see* plasmin.

fibrinolysis *n.* the process by which blood clots are removed from the circulation, involving digestion of the insoluble protein *fibrin by the enzyme *plasmin. The latter exists in the plasma as an inactive precursor (plasminogen), which is activated in parallel with the *blood coagulation process. Normally, a balance is maintained between the processes of coagulation and fibrinolysis in the body;

an abnormal increase in fibrinolysis leads to excessive bleeding.

fibrinolytic *adj.* describing a group of drugs that are capable of breaking down the protein fibrin, which is the main constituent of blood clots, and are therefore used to disperse blood clots (thrombi) that have formed within the circulation, particularly after a myocardial infarction. Fibrinolytic drugs include *streptokinase, *alteplase, *anistreplase, *reteplase* (Retavase), and *urokinase. Possible side effects include bleeding at needle puncture sites, headache, backache, blood spots in the skin, and allergic reactions.

fibroadenoma *n. see* adenoma.

fibroblast *n.* a widely distributed cell in *connective tissue that is responsible for the production of both the ground substance and of the precursors of collagen, elastic fibers, and reticular fibers.

fibrocartilage *n.* a tough kind of *cartilage in which there are dense bundles of fibers in the matrix. It is found in the intervertebral disks and pubic symphysis.

fibrocyst *n.* a benign tumor of fibrous connective tissue that contains cystic spaces. —**fibrocystic** *adj.*

fibrocystic disease of the pancreas *see* cystic fibrosis.

fibrocyte *n.* an inactive cell present in fully differentiated *connective tissue. It is derived from a *fibroblast.

fibrodysplasia *n.* abnormal development affecting connective tissue.

fibroelastosis *n.* overgrowth or disturbed growth of the yellow (elastic) fibers in *connective tissue, especially *endocardial fibroelastosis*, overgrowth and thickening of the wall of the heart's left ventricle.

fibroepithelial polyp a fibrous overgrowth covered by epithelium, often occurring in the mouth in response to chronic irritation. It is sometimes called an *epulis.

fibroid 1. *n.* (**fibromyoma, uterine fibroid**) a benign tumor of fibrous and muscular tissue, one or more of which may develop in the muscular wall of the uterus. Fibroids often cause pain and excessive menstrual bleeding and they may become extremely large. They do not threaten life, but render pregnancy unlikely. It is usually women over 30 years of age who are affected. Fibroids can be removed surgically; in some cases removal of the uterus (hysterectomy) may be necessary. If, as frequently happens, discomfort and other symptoms are absent, surgery is not required. **2.** *adj.* resembling or containing fibers.

fibroma *n.* a nonmalignant tumor of connective tissue.

fibromyalgia *n.* a disorder characterized by pain in the fibrous tissue components of muscles without any inflammation (*compare* fibromyositis). Widespread aching and stiffness are accompanied by extreme fatigue and often associated with headache, numbness and tingling, and various other symptoms. Fibromyalgia is frequently triggered by anxiety, stress, sleep deprivation, and straining or overuse of muscles; it appears to be closely related to *chronic fatigue syndrome.

fibromyoma *n.* a tumor of muscular and fibrous material, usually occurring in the uterus (*see* fibroid).

fibromyositis *n.* general inflammation of fibromuscular tissue.

fibronectin *n.* a large glycoprotein that acts as a host defense mechanism. In the plasma it induces phagocytosis and on the cell surface it induces protein linkage, which is important in the formation of new epithelium in wound healing. It is also involved in platelet aggregation. It is concentrated in connective tissue and the endothelium of the capillaries and is a component of the extracellular matrix.

fibroplasia *n.* the production of fibrous tissue, occurring normally during the healing of wounds. *Retrolental fibroplasia* is the abnormal proliferation of fibrous tissue immediately behind the lens of the eye, leading to blindness. It was formerly seen in newborn premature infants due to overadministration of oxygen.

fibrosarcoma *n.* a malignant tumor of connective tissue, derived from *fibroblasts. Fibrosarcomas may arise in soft tissue or bone; they can affect any organ but are most common in the limbs, particularly the leg. They occur in people of all ages and may be congenital. The cells of these tumors show varying degrees of differentiation; the less well-differentiated tumors containing elements of histiocytes have been reclassified as *malignant fibrous histiocytomas.*

fibrosis *n.* thickening and scarring of connective tissue, most often a consequence of inflammation or injury. *Pulmonary interstitial fibrosis* is thickening and stiffening of the lining of the air sacs (alveoli) of the lungs, causing progressive breathlessness. *See also* cystic fibrosis, retroperitoneal fibrosis.

fibrositis *n.* inflammation of fibrous connective tissue, especially an acute inflammation of back muscles and their sheaths, causing pain and stiffness. *See also* muscular rheumatism.

fibrous dysplasia a developmental abnormality in which bony tissue is replaced by fibrous tissue, resulting in aching and a tendency to pathological fracture. In *monostotic fibrous dysplasia* one bone is affected; *polyostotic fibrous dysplasia* involves many bones. There is a small risk (5–10%) of malignant transformation (*fibrosarcoma).

fibula *n.* the long thin outer bone of the lower leg. The head of the fibula articulates with the *tibia just below the knee; the lower end projects laterally as the *lateral malleolus*, which articulates with one side of the *talus.

field of vision *see* visual field.

FIGLU test a test for folic acid or vitamin B_{12} deficiency. A dose of the amino acid histidine, which requires the presence of folic acid or vitamin B_{12} for its complete breakdown, is given by mouth. In the absence of these vitamins, *formiminoglu*tamic acid (FIGLU) – an intermediate product in histidine metabolism – accumulates and can be detected in the urine.

FIGO staging a classification drawn up by the International Federation of Gynecology and Obstetrics to define the extent of spread of cancers of the ovary, uterus, and cervix.

filament *n.* a very fine threadlike structure, such as a chain of bacterial cells. —**filamentous** *adj.*

filaria *n.* (*pl.* **filariae**) any of the long threadlike nematode worms that, as adults, are parasites of human connective and lymphatic tissues capable of causing disease. They include the genera *Brugia, *Loa, *Onchocerca, and *Wuchereria. Filariae differ from the intestinal nematodes (*see* hookworm) in that they undergo part of their development in the body of a bloodsucking insect, e.g. a mosquito, on which they subsequently depend for their transmission to another human host. *See also* microfilaria. —**filarial** *adj.*

filariasis *n.* a disease, common in the tropics and subtropics, caused by the presence in the lymph vessels of the parasitic nematode worms *Wuchereria bancrofti* and *Brugia malayi* (*see* filaria). The worms, transmitted to humans by various mosquitoes (including *Aëdes*, *Culex*, *Anopheles*, and *Mansonia*), bring about inflammation and eventual blocking of lymph vessels, which causes the surrounding tissues to swell (*see* elephantiasis). The rupture of urinary lymphatics may lead to the presence of *chyle in the urine. Filariasis is treated with the drug *diethylcarbamazine.

filiform *adj.* shaped like a thread; for example, the threadlike *filiform papillae* of the *tongue.

filling *n.* (in dentistry) the operation of inserting a specially prepared substance into a cavity drilled in a carious tooth. The filling may be *temporary* or *permanent*, and various materials may be used (*see* amalgam, cement, composite resin, gold).

Filtragometer *n.* a device to measure platelet aggregation in flowing venous blood. The instrument measures the pressure difference across a filter through which heparinized blood from a forearm vein is drawn at a constant rate. Platelets aggregate, obstructing the filter, and cause a pressure difference over the filter that is proportional to the degree of platelet aggregation.

filum *n.* a threadlike structure. The *filum terminale* is the slender tapering terminal section of the spinal cord.

fimbria *n.* (*pl.* **fimbriae**) a fringe or fringelike process, such as any of the fingerlike projections that surround the opening of the ovarian end of the *fallopian tube. —**fimbrial** *adj.*

fimbrial cyst a simple cyst of the *fimbria of the fallopian tube.

finasteride *n.* a drug for the treatment of *benign prostatic hyperplasia. It causes shrinkage of the prostate gland and is administered by mouth for relieving the symptoms caused by an enlarged gland obstructing the outflow of urine from the bladder. The drug acts by reducing androgenic stimulation of the prostate, inhibiting the enzyme responsible for converting testosterone to its more active metabolite, 5-dihydrotestosterone (5-DHT), within the gland. It is sometimes prescribed in men who have recurrent bleeding from the prostate. Finasteride is also used by some balding men to stimulate hair growth. Trade names: **Proscar**, **Propecia**.

fine-needle aspiration cytology a technique using samples obtained by fine-needle aspiration to provide information on the cells of tumors or cysts. It is useful for detecting the presence of malignant cells, particularly in lumps of the breast and thyroid. *See also* aspiration cytology.

fingerprint *n.* the distinctive pattern of minute ridges in the outer horny layer of the skin. Every individual has a unique pattern of loops (70%), whorls (25%), or arches (5%) (see illustration). Fingerprint patterns can show the presence of inherited disorders. *See also* dermatoglyphics.

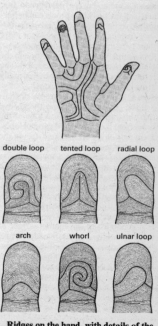

Ridges on the hand, with details of the most common fingerprints

firedamp *n.* (in mining) an explosive mixture of gases, usually containing a high proportion of methane, occasionally encountered in pockets underground. It is distinguished from *blackdamp (chokedamp), which does not ignite.

first aid procedures used in an emergency to help a wounded or ill patient before the arrival of a doctor or admission to the hospital.

first intention *see* intention.

first-pass clearance the metabolism of a drug before it reaches the systemic circulation and the tissues. This usually occurs in the liver.

FISH (fluorescence in situ hybridization) a technique that allows the nuclear DNA of *interphase cells or the DNA of *metaphase chromosomes, which are fixed to a glass microscope slide, to anneal with a fluorescent gene *probe. It is used for detecting and locating gene mutations and chromosome abnormalities.

fission *n.* a method of asexual reproduction in which the body of a protozoan or bacterium splits into two equal parts (*binary fission*), as in the *amebas, or more than two equal parts (*multiple fission*), for example sporozoite formation in the malarial parasite (*see* Plasmodium). The resulting products of fission eventually grow into complete organisms.

fissure *n.* **1.** (in anatomy) a groove or cleft; e.g. the *fissure of Sylvius* is the groove that separates the temporal lobe of the brain from the frontal and parietal lobes. **2.** (in pathology) a cleftlike defect in the skin or mucous membrane caused by some disease process; e.g. an *anal fissure* is a break in the skin lining the anal canal. **3.** (in dentistry) a naturally occurring groove in the enamel on the surface of a tooth, especially a molar. It is a common site of dental caries.

fissure sealant (in dentistry) a material that is bonded to the enamel surface of teeth to seal the fissures, in order to prevent dental caries. Composite resins, unfilled resins, and glass ionomer cements have been used as fissure sealants.

fistula *n.* an abnormal communication between two hollow organs or between a hollow organ and the exterior. Many fistulas are due to infection or injury. For example, an *anal fistula* may develop after an abscess in the rectum has burst (*see* ischiorectal abscess), creating an opening between the anal canal and the surface of the skin. *Crohn's disease has a particular tendency to cause fistulae to form between adjacent loops of bowel or from bowel to bladder, vagina, or skin. Some fistulas result from malignant growths or ulceration: a carcinoma of the colon may invade and ulcerate the adjacent wall of the stomach, causing a *gastrocolic fistula*. Other fistulas develop as complications of surgery: after gallbladder surgery, for example, bile may continually escape to the surface through the wound, producing a *biliary fistula*. Fistulas may also be a form of congenital abnormality; examples include a *tracheoesophageal fistula* (between the windpipe and gullet) and a *rectovaginal fistula* (between the rectum and vagina). *See also* vesicovaginal fistula.

An *arteriovenous fistula* is a surgical connection between an artery and a vein, usually in a limb, to create arterial and venous access for *hemodialysis. It can be a direct *anastomosis between the artery and vein or a loop connecting the two, which may be autogenous or prosthetic.

fit *n.* a sudden attack. The term was previously reserved for the seizures of *epilepsy but it is now used more generally, e.g. a fit of coughing.

fixation *n.* **1.** (in psychoanalysis) a failure of psychological development, in which traumatic events prevent a child from progressing to the next developmental stage. This is said to be a cause of mental illness and of personality disorder. *See also* psychosexual development. **2.** a procedure for the hardening and preservation of tissues or microorganisms to be examined under a microscope. Fixation kills the tissues and ensures that their original shape and structure are retained as closely as possible. It also prepares them for sectioning and staining. The specimens can be immersed in a chemical *fixative or subjected to *freeze-drying.

fixative (fixing agent) *n.* a chemical agent, e.g. alcohol or osmium tetroxide, used for the preservation and hardening of tissues for microscopical study. *See* fixation (def. 2).

FK 506 *see* tacrolimus.

flaccid *adj.* **1.** flabby and lacking in firmness. **2.** characterized by decreased muscle tone (e.g. flaccid *paralysis). —**flaccidity** n.

flagellate n. a type of *protozoan with one or more fine whiplike threads (see flagellum) projecting from its body surface, by means of which it is able to swim. Some flagellates are parasites of humans and are therefore of medical importance. See Trypanosoma, Leishmania, Giardia, Trichomonas.

flagellation n. the act of whipping oneself or others as a means of obtaining sexual pleasure (see masochism, sadism). A person displaying this sexual deviation is called a flagellant or flagellomane.

flagellum n. (pl. **flagella**) a fine long whiplike thread attached to certain types of cell (e.g. spermatozoa and some unicellular organisms). Flagella are responsible for the movement of the organisms to which they are attached.

flail chest a condition of the chest associated with an unstable ribcage following multiple fractures of the ribs and sternum, often associated with underlying lung trauma or pneumothorax. It leads to asphyxia unless corrected promptly.

flap n. **1.** (in surgery) a strip of tissue dissected away from the underlying structures but left attached at one end so that it retains its blood and nerve supply in a *pedicle. The flap is then used to repair a defect in another part of the body. The free end of the flap is sewn into the area to be repaired and after about three weeks, when the flap has "healed into" its new site, the other end is detached and the remainder of the flap is sewn in. Flaps are commonly used by plastic surgeons in treating patients who have severe skin and tissue loss after surgery (e.g. *mastectomy) or after burns or injuries not amenable to repair by split-skin grafting (see skin graft). Skin flaps are also used to cover the end of a bone in an amputated limb. In neurosurgery combined skin and bone (osteoplastic) flaps are commonly raised to provide access to the cranium. **2.** (in dentistry) a piece of mucous membrane and periosteum attached by a broad base. It is lifted back to expose the underlying bone and enable a procedure such as surgical *extraction to be performed. It is subsequently replaced.

flare n. **1.** reddening of the skin that spreads outward from a focus of infection or irritation in the skin. **2.** the red outside part of an urticarial wheal – the skin's response in an allergic or hypersensitivity reaction (see urticaria). **3.** sudden intensification of a disease.

flashback n. vivid involuntary reliving of the perceptual abnormalities experienced during a previous episode of drug intoxication, including *hallucinations and *derealization.

flatfoot n. absence of the arching of the foot, so that the sole lies flat on the ground. It may be present in infancy or be acquired in adult life, usually either from prolonged standing or from excessive weight. Flatfeet need treatment (exercises) only if they cause pain. Medical name: **pes planus.**

flatulence n. **1.** the presence of gas or air in the stomach or intestine. **2.** a sensation of abdominal distension. —**flatulent** adj.

flatus n. intestinal gas, composed partly of swallowed air and partly of gas produced by bacterial fermentation of intestinal contents. It consists of hydrogen, carbon dioxide, and methane in varying proportions. Indigestible nonabsorbable carbohydrates in some foods (e.g. beans) cause increased volumes of flatus.

flatworm (platyhelminth) n. any of the flat-bodied worms, including the *flukes and *tapeworms. Both these groups contain many parasites of medical importance.

flav- (flavo-) prefix denoting yellow.

flavin adenine dinucleotide see FAD.

flavin mononucleotide see FMN.

flavivirus n. any member of a genus (and family) of *arboviruses that cause a wide range of diseases in vertebrates (including humans). Transmitted by ticks or mosquitoes, these include *yellow fever, *dengue, *Kyasanur Forest disease, *Russian spring-summer encephalitis, and *West Nile fever.

flavoprotein n. a compound consisting of a protein bound to either *FAD or *FMN (called flavins). Flavoproteins are constituents of several enzyme systems involved in intermediary metabolism.

flavoxate n. a smooth muscle relaxant used as an antispasmodic for conditions involving the urinary tract, such as *dysuria, *nocturia, and incontinence. It is administered orally; common side effects include nausea, vomiting, dry mouth, dizziness, and drowsiness. Trade name: **Urispas**.

flea n. a small wingless bloodsucking insect with a laterally compressed body and long legs adapted for jumping. Adult fleas are temporary parasites on birds and mammals and those species that attack humans (*Pulex*, *Xenopsylla*, and *Nosopsyllus*) may be important in the transmission of various diseases. Their bites are not only a nuisance but may become a focus of infection. Pyrethrum powder is used to destroy fleas in the home.

flecainide n. a drug used to control irregular heart rhythms. It is administered by mouth. Possible side effects include nausea, vomiting, dizziness, vertigo, jaundice, visual disturbances, and some nerve damage. Trade name: **Tambocor**.

flexibilitas cerea see cerea flexibilitas.

flexion n. the bending of a joint so that the bones forming it are brought toward each other. *Plantar flexion* is the bending of the toes (or fingers) downward, toward the sole (or palm). *See also* dorsiflexion.

flexor n. any muscle that causes bending of a limb or other part.

flexure n. a bend in an organ or part, such as the *hepatic* and *splenic flexures* of the *colon.

floaters pl. n. opacities in the vitreous humor of the eye, which cast a shadow on the retina and are therefore seen as dark shapes against a bright background in good illumination. They are a form of *entoptic phenomenon.

floccillation n. see carphology.

flocculation n. a reaction in which normally invisible material leaves a solution to form a coarse suspension or precipitate as a result of a change in physical or chemical conditions. *See also* agglutination.

flocculus n. a small ovoid lobe of the *cerebellum, overhung by the posterior lobe and connected centrally with the nodulus in the midline.

flooding n. **1.** excessive bleeding from the uterus, as in *menorrhagia or miscarriage. **2.** (**implosion**) (in psychology) a method of treating *phobias in which the patient is exposed intensively and at length to the feared object, either in reality or fantasy. Although it is distressing and needs good motivation if treatment is to be completed, it is an effective and rapid therapy.

floppy baby syndrome see amyotonia (congenita).

flora pl. n. the aggregate of microorganisms that normally occur in or on the bodies of humans and other animals, such as the *intestinal flora, which includes certain strains of *Streptococcus* organisms.

flow cytometry a technique in which cells are tagged with a fluorescent dye and then directed single file through a laser beam. The intensity of *fluorescence induced by the laser beam is proportional to the amount of DNA in the cells.

flowmeter n. an instrument for measuring the flow of a liquid or gas. Anesthetic equipment is fitted with flowmeters so that the administration of anesthetic gases in different proportions can be controlled. Flowmeters are used by asthmatic subjects to measure their ability to expire air.

floxuridine n. an antineoplastic drug, similar in its action and side effects to *fluorouracil, used primarily to treat cancers of the digestive system. It is administered by intra-arterial injection. Trade name: **FUDR**.

fluconazole n. an antifungal drug used to treat candidiasis in any part of the body, externally or internally. It is administered by mouth and injection. Possible side effects include nausea and vomiting. Trade name: **Diflucan**.

fluctuation n. the characteristic feeling of a wave motion produced in a fluid-filled part of the body by an examiner's fingers. If fluctuation is present when a swelling is examined, this is an indication that there is fluid within and that the swelling is not due to a solid growth.

flucytosine n. an antifungal drug that is effective against systemic infections, including cryptococcosis and candidiasis. It can be administered by mouth; side effects may include nausea and vomiting, diarrhea, rashes, and blood disorders. Trade name: **Ancobon**.

fludarabine n. an *antimetabolite that is used in the treatment of B-cell chronic lymphocytic *leukemia. It is administered intravenously; side effects include *myelosuppression, nausea and vomiting, fatigue, fever, and chills. Trade name: **Fludara**.

fludrocortisone *n.* a synthetic mineralocorticoid (*see* corticosteroid) used to treat disorders of the adrenal glands. It is administered by mouth and side effects include muscle weakness, bone disorders, digestive and skin disorders, and fluid retention. Trade name: **Florinef**.

fluke *n.* any of the parasitic flatworms belonging to the group Trematoda. Adult flukes, which have suckers for attachment to their host, are parasites of humans, occurring in the liver (*liver flukes*; *see* Fasciola), lungs (*see* Paragonimus), gut (*see* Heterophyes), and blood vessels (*blood flukes*; *see* Schistosoma) and often cause serious disease. Eggs, passed out with the stools, hatch into larvae called *miracidia, which penetrate an intermediate snail host. Miracidia give rise asexually to *redia larvae and finally *cercariae in the snail's tissues. The released cercariae may enter a second intermediate host (such as a fish or crustacean), form a cyst (*metacercaria) on vegetation, or directly penetrate the human skin.

flumazenil *n.* a *benzodiazepine antagonist drug, used in anesthesia to reverse the effects of benzodiazepines on the nervous system. It is administered by injection. Trade name: **Romazicon**.

flunisolide *n.* an anti-inflammatory corticosteroid drug used in the long-term treatment of asthma and rhinitis. It is administered as an inhalation or a spray; common side effects are nausea and vomiting, headache, and local irritation. Trade names: **Aerobid**, **Bronalide**, **Nasarel**.

fluocinonide *n.* a synthetic corticosteroid used topically to reduce inflammation. It is applied to the skin as a cream, gel, ointment, or solution. Side effects include burning, itching, and local eruptions. Trade names: **Fluonex**, **Leonide**, **Lidex**.

fluorescein sodium a water-soluble dye that glows with a brilliant green color when blue light is shone on it. A dilute solution is used to detect defects in the surface of the cornea, since it stains areas where the *epithelium is not intact. In retinal *angiography it is injected into a vein and its circulation through the blood vessels of the retina is viewed and photographed by a special camera.

fluorescence *n.* the emission of light by a material as it absorbs radiation from outside. The radiation absorbed may be visible or invisible (e.g. ultraviolet rays or X-rays). *See* fluoroscope. —**fluorescent** *adj.*

fluorescence in situ hybridization *see* FISH.

fluoridation *n.* the addition of *fluoride to drinking water in order to reduce *dental caries. Drinking water with a fluoride ion content of one part per million is effective in reducing caries throughout life when given during the years of tooth development. *See also* fluorosis.

fluoride *n.* a compound of fluorine. The incorporation of fluoride ions in the enamel of teeth makes them more resistant to *dental caries. The ions enter enamel during its formation, by surface absorption. The addition of fluoride to public water supplies is called *fluoridation. Fluoride may also be applied topically in toothpaste or by a dentist. If the water supply contains too little fluoride, fluoride salts may be given to children in the form of drops or tablets.

fluoroscope *n.* historically, an instrument by which X-rays were projected through a patient onto a fluorescent screen enabling the resultant image to be viewed directly by the radiologist. However, this resulted in high radiation doses for the radiologist. For diagnostic purposes the screen has been replaced by *image intensifiers and TV monitors (*see* X-ray screening).

fluoroscopy *n.* the use of a *fluoroscope to visualize X-ray images. *Videofluoroscopy is synonymous with *X-ray screening. It is valuable for observing moving structures (e.g. swallowed *barium sulfate) or for guiding *interventional radiology procedures.

fluorosis *n.* a disorder characterized by bony overgrowth, neurologic complications, and arthritis caused by long-term *fluoride intake, such as occurs in industrial workers. *Dental fluorosis* is characterized by mottled enamel, which is opaque and may be stained. Its incidence increases when the level of fluoride in the water supply is above 2 parts per million. The mottled enamel is resistant to dental caries. When the level is over 8 parts per million, systemic fluorosis may occur, with calcification of ligaments.

fluorouracil *n.* a drug that prevents cell

growth (*see* antimetabolite) and is used in the treatment of cancers of the digestive system and breast (*see also* folinic acid). It is usually administered by injection. Side effects, which may be severe, include digestive and skin disorders, mouth ulcers, hair loss, nail changes, and blood disorders. Fluorouracil is also applied as a cream to treat certain skin conditions, including skin cancer. Trade names: **Adrucil, Efudex, Fluoroplex**.

fluoxetine *n.* an *antidepressant drug that acts by prolonging the action of the neurotransmitter serotonin (5-hydroxytryptamine) in the brain (*see* SSRI). It is administered by mouth. Possible side effects include nausea, vomiting, diarrhea, insomnia, anxiety, fever, skin rash, and convulsions. Trade name: **Prozac**.

fluoxymesterone *n.* a synthetic androgenic anabolic steroid hormone used in the treatment of male hypogonadism. It is also used in certain females for the palliative therapy of inoperable breast cancer. The drug is administered orally; common side effects include acne, *gynecomastia, and edema. Trade name: **Halotestin**.

fluphenazine *n.* a phenothiazine *antipsychotic drug used for the treatment of schizophrenia and other psychotic disorders. It is administered by mouth or injection. High doses may cause drowsiness, restlessness, and abnormal muscular movements. Trade names: **Permitil, Prolixin**.

flurazepam *n.* a sedative drug used to treat insomnia and sleep disturbances (*see* hypnotic). It is administered by mouth and sometimes causes morning drowsiness, dizziness, and muscle incoordination. Trade name: **Dalmane**.

flurbiprofen *n.* an analgesic that relieves inflammation (*see* NSAID) used in the treatment of rheumatoid arthritis and osteoarthritis and to prevent contraction of the pupil during eye surgery. Side effects include gastrointestinal upset, diarrhea, and nausea. Trade names: **Ansaid, Ocufen**.

flush *n.* reddening of the face and/or neck. *Hectic flush* occurs in such wasting diseases as pulmonary tuberculosis. *See also* hot flash.

flutamide *n.* an *antiandrogen commonly used in the treatment of prostate cancer, sometimes alone or in combination with *LHRH analogues. It is taken by mouth; side effects include diarrhea. Trade name: **Eulexin**.

flutter *n.* a disturbance of normal heart rhythm that – like *fibrillation – may affect the atria or ventricles. However, the arrhythmia is less rapid and less chaotic. The causes and treatment are similar to those of fibrillation. *See also* cardiac arrest, defibrillation.

fluvastatin *n.* a drug that is used for the treatment of hypercholesterolemia. A *hydroxymethylglutaryl coenzyme A reductase inhibitor (*see* statin), it is administered by mouth; side effects include fatigue, headache, nausea, and vomiting. Trade name: **Lescol**.

fluvoxamine *n.* an *antidepressant drug that acts by prolonging the action of the neurotransmitter serotonin (5-hydroxytryptamine) in the brain (*see* SSRI). It is taken by mouth; side effects may include sleepiness, agitation, tremor, vomiting, and diarrhea. Trade name: **Luvox**.

flux *n.* an abnormally copious flow from an organ or cavity. *Alvine flux* is *diarrhea.

fly *n.* a two-winged insect belonging to a large group called the Diptera. The mouthparts of flies are adapted for sucking and sometimes also for piercing and biting. Fly larvae (maggots) may infest human tissues and cause disease (*see* myiasis).

FMN (flavin monucleotide) a derivative of riboflavin (vitamin B_2) that is the immediate precursor of *FAD and functions as a *coenzyme in various oxidation-reduction reactions.

focal distance (of the eye) the distance between the lens and the point behind the lens at which light from a distant object is focused. In a normal-sighted person this point of focus is on the retina, but distortion of the shape of the eyeball may result in *myopia (nearsightedness) or *hyperopia (farsightedness).

focus 1. *n.* the point at which rays of light converge after passing through a lens. **2.** *n.* the principal site of an infection or other disease. **3.** *vb.* (in ophthalmology) to accommodate (*see* accommodation).

fold *n.* (in anatomy and embryology) the infolding of two surfaces or membranes.

folic acid (pteroylglutamic acid) a B vitamin that is important in the synthesis of nucleic acids. The metabolic role of folic acid is interdependent with that of *vitamin B_{12} (both are required by rapidly dividing cells) and a deficiency of one may lead to deficiency of the other. A deficiency of folic acid results in the condition of megaloblastic anemia. Good sources of folic acid are liver, yeast extract, and green leafy vegetables. The actual daily requirement of folate is not known but the suggested daily intake is 200 µg/day for an adult, which should be doubled shortly before conception and during the first three months of pregnancy to prevent neural tube defects (e.g. spina bifida) and other congenital malformations (e.g. cleft lip and cleft palate) in the fetus.

folie à deux (communicated insanity) a condition in which two people who are closely involved with each other share a system of *delusions. Sometimes one member of the pair has developed a *psychosis and has imposed it on the other by a process of suggestion; sometimes both members are schizophrenic and elaborate their delusions or hallucinations together. More than two people may be involved (*folie à trois, folie à quatre*, etc.). Treatment usually involves separation of the affected people and management according to their individual requirements.

folinic acid (leucovorin) a derivative of folic acid involved in purine synthesis. Administered by mouth or by injection in the form of its calcium salts, it is used to reverse the biological effects of *methotrexate and other *dihydrofolate reductase inhibitors and so to prevent excessive toxicity. This action is termed *folinic acid rescue*. Folinic acid has a potentiating effect with *fluorouracil, with which it is often used. Trade name: **Wellcovorin**.

folium n. (pl. **folia**) a thin leaflike structure, such as any of the folds on the surface of the cerebellum.

follicle n. a small secretory cavity, sac, or gland, such as any of the cavities in the *ovary in which the ova are formed. *See also* graafian follicle, hair follicle. —**follicular** adj.

follicle-stimulating hormone (FSH) a hormone (*see* gonadotropin) synthesized and released by the anterior pituitary gland. FSH stimulates ripening of the

follicles in the ovary and formation of sperm in the testes. It is administered by injection to treat sterility due to lack of ovulation, amenorrhea, and decreased sperm production. Stimulation of ovulation by FSH may, in some cases, lead to multiple pregnancy.

follicular occlusion tetrad the combination of major acne, *pilonidal sinus, chronic scalp *folliculitis, and *hidradenitis suppurativa.

folliculitis n. inflammation of hair follicles in the skin, commonly caused by infection (*see also* sycosis). Folliculitis caused by *Malassezia* yeasts may be a marker for the diagnosis of AIDS.

fomentation n. see poultice.

fomes n. (pl. **fomites**) any object that is used or handled by a person with a *communicable disease and may therefore become contaminated with the infective organisms and transmit the disease to a subsequent user. Common fomites are towels, bedclothes, cups, and money.

fontanelle n. an opening in the skull of a fetus or young infant due to incomplete *ossification of the cranial bones and the resulting incomplete closure of the *sutures. The *anterior fontanelle* occurs where the coronal, frontal, and sagittal sutures meet; the *posterior fontanelle* occurs where the sagittal and lambdoidal sutures meet (see illustration).

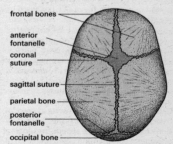

frontal bones
anterior fontanelle
coronal suture
sagittal suture
parietal bone
posterior fontanelle
occipital bone

Fontanelles in the skull of a newborn infant (from above)

Food and Drug Administration (FDA) an agency within the US *Public Health Service division of the *Department of Health and Human Services that is responsible for protecting the public against the health hazards of impure or dangerous substances by controlling and enforcing federal regulations concerned with the manufacture, distribution, and sale of food, cosmetics, biological products, medical devices, radiation-emitting products, such as microwave ovens, and the feed and drugs for farm animals and pets. The FDA is made up of six component organizations: the Center for Biologics Evaluation and Research, the Center for Devices and Radiological Health, the Center for Drug Evaluation and Safety, the Center for Food Safety and Applied Nutrition, the Center for Veterinary Medicine, and the National Center for Toxicology Research.

food handler a person engaged in the preparation, storage, cooking, and serving of food. Such people should be free from infectious conditions, either in the form of overt disease or as carriers. They may be subject to inspection to prove freedom from infection, particularly those who handle food that is either to be eaten raw or has previously been subjected to cooking (e.g. meat pies, paté).

food poisoning an illness affecting the digestive system that results from eating food contaminated either by bacteria or bacterial toxins or, less commonly, by residues of insecticides (on fruit and vegetables) or poisonous chemicals such as lead or mercury. It can also be caused by eating poisonous fungi, berries, etc. Symptoms commence 1–24 hours after ingestion and include vomiting, diarrhea, abdominal pain, and nausea. Food-borne infections are caused by bacteria of the genus *Salmonella*, *Campylobacter*, and *Listeria* in foods of animal origin. The disease is transmitted by human carriers who handle the food, by shellfish growing in sewage-polluted waters, or by vegetables fertilized by manure. Toxin-producing bacteria causing food poisoning include those of the genus *Staphylococcus*, which rapidly multiply in warm foods, pathogenic *Escherichia coli*; and the species *Clostridium perfringens*, which multiplies in reheated cooked meals. A rare form of food poisoning – *botulism* – is caused by toxins produced by the bacterium *Clostridium botulinum*, which may con-

taminate badly preserved canned foods. *See also* gastroenteritis.

foot *n*. the terminal organ of the lower limb. From a surgical point of view, the human foot comprises the seven bones of the *tarsus, the five metatarsal bones, and the phalangeal bones plus the surrounding tissues; anatomically, the ankle bones and tissues are excluded.

foramen *n*. (*pl*. **foramina**) an opening or hole, particularly in a bone. The *apical foramen* is the small opening at the apex of a tooth. The *foramen magnum* is a large hole in the occipital bone through which the spinal cord passes. The *foramen ovale* is the opening between the two atria of the fetal heart, which allows blood to flow from the right to the left side of the heart by displacing a membranous valve.

forced expiratory volume (FEV) the volume of air exhaled in a given period (usually limited to 1 second in tests of vital capacity). FEV is reduced in patients with obstructive airways disease and diminished lung volume.

forceps *n*. a pincerlike instrument designed to grasp an object so that it can be held firm or pulled. Specially designed forceps – of which there are many varieties – are used by surgeons and dentists in operations (see illustration). The forceps used in childbirth are so designed to fit firmly round the baby's head without damaging it. Dental *extraction forceps* are designed to fit the various shapes of teeth. By having long handles and short beaks they provide considerable leverage.

forebrain (prosencephalon) *n*. the furthest forward division of the *brain, consisting of the *diencephalon and the two cerebral hemispheres.

foregut *n*. the front part of the embryonic gut, which gives rise to the esophagus (gullet), stomach, and part of the small intestine (from which the liver and pancreas develop).

forensic medicine the branch of medicine concerned with the scientific investigation of the causes of injury and death in unexplained circumstances, particularly when criminal activity is suspected. Such investigations are carried out chiefly by pathologists at the request of a *medical examiner, in conjunction with other experts and police investigators.

forequarter amputation an operation involving removal of an entire arm, including the scapula and clavicle. It is usually performed for soft tissue or bone sarcomas arising from the upper arm or shoulder. *Compare* hindquarter amputation.

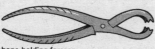

bone-holding forceps

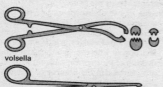

volsella

sinus forceps

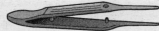

dissecting forceps

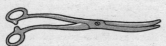

dressing forceps

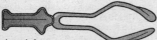

obstetric forceps

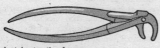

dental extraction forceps

Types of forceps

foreskin *n. see* prepuce.

forewaters *n.* the *amniotic fluid that escapes from the uterus through the vagina when that part of the amnion lying in front of the presenting part of the fetus ruptures, either spontaneously or by *amniotomy. Spontaneous rupture is usual in labor but rupture may occur before labor starts (premature rupture of membranes).

formaldehyde *n.* the aldehyde derivative of formic acid, once used as a vapor to sterilize and disinfect rooms and such items as mattresses and blankets. The toxic vapor is produced by boiling *formalin in an open container or using it in a sealed autoclave.

formalin *n.* a solution containing 37% formaldehyde in water, used as a sterilizing agent and, in pathology, as a fixative. It is lethal to bacteria, viruses, fungi, and spores. It is used to treat wools and hides to kill anthrax spores. Heating the solution produces the irritating vapor of *formaldehyde, which can also be used for disinfection.

forme fruste an atypical form of a disease in which the usual symptoms fail to appear and its progress is stopped at an earlier stage than would ordinarily be expected.

formestan *n. see* aromatase inhibitor.

formication *n.* a prickling sensation said to resemble the feeling of ants crawling over the skin. It is sometimes a symptom of drug intoxication and has also been reported by patients with Parkinson's disease and multiple sclerosis.

formoterol *n.* a *sympathomimetic drug used as a long-acting *bronchodilator to treat asthma. Formoterol is formulated in powder form for administration by inhaler. Side effects include tremor, palpitations, and headache. Trade name: **Foradil**.

formulary *n.* a compendium of formulas used in the preparation of medicinal drugs.

fornix *n.* (*pl.* **fornices**) an arched or vault-like structure, especially the *fornix cerebri*, a triangular structure of white matter in the brain, situated between the hippocampus and hypothalamus. The *fornix of the vagina* is any of three vaulted spaces at the top of the vagina, around the cervix of the uterus.

foscarnet *n.* an antiviral drug used in the treatment of infections caused by herpesviruses, including *cytomegaloviruses, that are resistant to *acyclovir, especially in patients with AIDS. It is administered by intravenous injection.

Possible side effects include thirst and increased urine output, nausea and vomiting, fatigue, headache, and kidney damage. Trade name: **Foscavir**.

fossa n. (pl. **fossae**) a depression or hollow. The *cubital fossa* is the triangular hollow at the front of the elbow joint; the *iliac fossa* is the depression in the inner surface of the ilium; the *pituitary fossa* is the hollow in the sphenoid bone in which the pituitary gland is situated; a *tooth fossa* is a pit in the enamel on the surface of a tooth.

fovea n. (in anatomy) a small depression, especially the shallow pit in the retina at the back of the eye. It contains a large number of *cones and is therefore the area of greatest acuity of vision: when the eye sees an object, the part of the image that is focused on the fovea is the part that is most accurately registered by the brain. *See also* macula (lutea).

foveola n. (in anatomy) a small depression.

fractals pl. n. patterns of chaotic nonlinear systems found in nature in which a part is similar to the whole, such as a fold of the brain.

fracture n. breakage of a bone, either complete or incomplete. A *simple fracture* involves a clean break with little damage to surrounding tissues and no break in the overlying skin. If a bone end pierces the overlying skin and there is a wound extending to the fracture site, the fracture is *compound* or *open*, and there is a risk of infection (*see* osteomyelitis).Fracture of an already diseased bone is termed a *pathological fracture* and may occur after minor injuries. Treatment of a simple fracture includes realignment of the bone ends where there is displacement, immobilization by external splints or internal fixation, followed by *rehabilitation. *See also* Colles' fracture, comminuted fracture, greenstick fracture, scaphoid fracture, Smith's fracture.

fragile-X syndrome a major genetic disorder caused by a constriction near the end of the long arm of an *X chromosome. The fragile-X syndrome is second only to *Down's syndrome as a cause of mental retardation. Affected males have unusually high foreheads, unbalanced faces, large jaws, long protruding ears, and large testicles. They have an IQ below 50 and are prone to violent outbursts. Folic acid helps to control their

behavior. About one-third of the females with this mutation on one of their two X chromosomes are also mentally retarded. Screening for the characteristic chromosome can be done by *amniocentesis or *chorionic villus sampling and tests for the detection of carriers of the disorder have been developed.

fragilitas n. abnormal brittleness or fragility, for example of the hair (*fragilitas crinium*) or the bones (*fragilitas ossium*; *see* osteogenesis imperfecta).

frambesia n. see yaws.

fraternal twins see twins.

freckle n. a small brown spot on the skin commonly found on the exposed areas of red-haired or blond people with a fair complexion. Freckles, which are harmless, appear where there is excessive production of the pigment melanin without any increase in the number of melanocytes after exposure to sunlight. *Compare* lentigo.

free association (in *psychoanalysis) a technique in which the patient is encouraged to pursue a particular train of ideas as they enter consciousness. *See also* association of ideas.

free-floating anxiety an all-pervasive unfocused fear that is not produced by any appropriate cause or attached to any particular idea. Such anxiety is a feature of the *generalized anxiety disorder.

freeze-drying n. a method for the *fixation of histological specimens, involving a minimum of chemical and physical change. Specimens are immersed in isopentane cooled to $-190°C$ in liquid air. This fixes the tissue instantly, without the formation of large ice crystals (which would cause structural changes). The tissue is then dehydrated in a vacuum for about 72 hours at $-32.5°C$.

freeze-etching n. a technique for preparing specimens for electron microscopy. The unfixed tissue is frozen and then split with a knife and a layer of ice is sublimed from the exposed surface. The resultant image is thus not distorted by chemical fixatives.

Frei test a rarely used diagnostic test for the sexually transmitted disease *lymphogranuloma venereum. A small quantity of the virus, inactivated by heat, is injected into the patient's skin. If the disease is present, a small red swelling appears at the site of injection within 48 hours. [W. S. Frei (1885–1943), German dermatologist]

fremitus n. vibrations or tremors in a part of the body, detected by feeling with the fingers or hand (*palpation) or by listening (*auscultation). The term is most commonly applied to vibrations perceived through the chest when a patient breathes, speaks (*vocal fremitus*), or coughs. The nature of the fremitus gives an indication as to whether the chest is affected by disease. For example, loss of vocal fremitus suggests the presence of fluid in the pleural cavity; its increase suggests consolidation of the underlying lung.

frenectomy n. an operation to remove the frenum, including the underlying fibrous tissue.

frenum (frenulum) n. **1.** any of the folds of the mucous membrane under the tongue or between the gums and the upper or lower lips. **2.** any of several other structures of similar appearance.

frequency n. (of urine) the passage of urine more than seven times a day: a *lower urinary tract symptom that usually indicates genitourinary disorders and diseases but also accompanies *polyuria.

frequency distribution (in statistics) presentation of the characteristics (*variables) of a series of individuals (e.g. their heights, weights, or blood pressures) in tabular form or as a histogram (bar chart) so as to indicate the proportion of the series that have different measurements. In a *normal* or *Gaussian distribution* the number of readings and their range on either side of the *mean value is symmetrical; in a *skewed distribution* (e.g. *Poisson*) the measurements are bunched on one side of the mean and spread out over a wider range on the other.

Freudian adj. relating to or describing the work and ideas of Sigmund Freud (1856–1939): applied particularly to the school of psychiatry based on his teachings (*see* psychoanalysis).

friction murmur (friction rub) a scratching sound, heard over the heart with the aid of the stethoscope, in patients who have *pericarditis. It results from the two inflamed layers of the pericardium rubbing together during activity of the heart.

Friedman's test a rarely used pregnancy test based on the ability of the urine of a pregnant woman (containing chorionic gonadotropin) to induce the development of corpora lutea in a female rabbit. [M. Friedman (20th century), US physiologist]

Friedreich's ataxia *see* ataxia. [N. Friedreich (1825–82), German neurologist]

frigidity n. lack of sexual desire or inability to reach the climax of sexual excitement. Frigidity may affect either sex, but the term is almost always applied to women only. In some cases the woman feels revulsion toward sexual activity.

fringe medicine *see* complementary medicine.

Fröhlich's syndrome a disorder of the *hypothalamus (part of the brain) affecting males: the boy is overweight with lack of sexual development and disturbances of sleep and appetite. Medical name: **dystrophia adiposogenitalis**. [A. Fröhlich (1871–1953), Austrian neurologist]

Froin's syndrome a condition in which the cerebrospinal fluid (CSF) displays a combination of yellow color and high protein content. It is characteristic of a block to the spinal circulation of CSF caused by a tumor. [G. Froin (1874–1932), French physician]

frontal adj. **1.** of or relating to the forehead (*see* frontal bone). **2.** denoting the *anterior part of a body or organ.

frontal bone the bone forming the forehead and the upper parts of the orbits; it contains several air spaces (*frontal sinuses: see* paranasal sinuses). At birth, it consists of right and left halves, joined by a suture that usually closes during infancy. *See* skull.

frontal lobe the anterior part of each cerebral hemisphere (*see* cerebrum), extending as far back as the deep central sulcus (cleft) of its upper and outer surface. Immediately anterior to the central sulcus lies the motor cortex, responsible for the control of voluntary movement; the area further forward – the *prefrontal lobe – is concerned with behavior, learning, judgment, and personality.

frontal sinus *see* paranasal sinuses.

frostbite n. damage to the tissues caused by freezing. The affected parts, usually the nose, fingers, or toes, become pale and numb. Ice forms in the tissues, which may thus be destroyed, and amputation may become necessary. Frostbitten parts should not be rubbed, since there is no blood circulation in the tissues, but they may be gently warmed in tepid water. Precautions must be taken against bacterial infection, to which frostbitten skin is highly susceptible.

frottage n. rubbing up against somebody (usually in a crowd) as a means of obtaining sexual pleasure. A person (almost exclusively male) displaying this sexual deviation is called a *frotteur*.

frozen shoulder chronic painful stiffness of the shoulder joint. This may follow injury, a stroke, or *myocardial infarction or may gradually develop for no apparent reason. Treatment is by gentle stretching and exercises, sometimes combined with *corticosteroid injection into the joint. Medical name: **adhesive capsulitis**.

frozen watchfulness the state of a child who is unresponsive to its surroundings but is clearly aware of them. The child is usually expressionless and difficult to engage but of normal intelligence. Frozen watchfulness is usually a marker of *child abuse.

fructose n. a simple sugar found in honey and in such fruit as figs. Fructose is one of the two sugars in *sucrose. Fructose from the diet can be used to produce energy by the process known as *glycolysis, which takes place in the liver. Fructose is important in the diet of diabetics, since, unlike glucose, fructose metabolism is not dependent on insulin.

fructosuria (levulosuria) n. the presence of fructose (levulose) in the urine.

FSH *see* follicle-stimulating hormone.

FTT *see* failure to thrive.

Fuchs' endothelial dystrophy a hereditary condition in which the endothelium of the cornea fails to function with age; small whitish deposits of hyalin are seen on the inner surface of the cornea (*cornea guttata*). It results in thickening and swelling of the cornea (*bullous keratopathy) and hence reduced vision. Treatment is corneal transplantation (*see* keratoplasty), which both improves vision and reduces pain. [E. Fuchs (1851–1913), German ophthalmologist]

Fuchs' heterochromic cyclitis a condition characterized by chronic low-grade inflammation of the ciliary body and iris (anterior *uveitis) affecting one eye and depigmentation of the affected iris (*heterochromia). Glaucoma and cataract can develop in the affected eye. [E. Fuchs]

fuchsin (magenta) n. any one of a group of reddish to purplish dyes used in staining bacteria for microscopic observation and capable of killing various disease-causing microorganisms. *Acid fuchsin* (*acid magenta*) is a mixture of sulfonated fuchsins; *basic fuchsin* (*basic magenta*) and *new* (*trimethyl*) *fuchsin* are basic histological dyes (basic fuchsin is also an antifungal agent).

Fuchs' spots pigmented lesions in the macular area of the retina that are seen in severely myopic (nearsighted) individuals. They are breaks in *Bruch's membrane allowing choroidal *neovascularization and can result in reduced vision. [E. Fuchs]

-fuge *suffix denoting* an agent that drives away, repels, or eliminates. Example: *febrifuge* (a drug that reduces fever).

fugue n. a period of memory loss during which the patient leaves his usual surroundings and wanders aimlessly or starts a new life elsewhere. It is often preceded by psych pnological conflict and depression, and may be associated with organic mental disease. *See also* dissociation, dissociative disorder.

fulguration (electrodesiccation) n. the destruction with a *diathermy instrument of warts, growths, or unwanted areas of tissue, particularly inside the bladder. This latter operation is performed via the urethra and viewed through a cystoscope.

fulminating (fulminant, fulgurant) adj. describing a condition or symptom that is of very sudden onset, severe, and of short duration.

fumigation n. the use of gases or vapors to bring about *disinfestation of clothing, buildings, etc. Sulfur dioxide, formaldehyde, and chlorine are common fumigating agents.

functional disorder a condition in which a patient complains of symptoms for which no physical cause can be found. Such a condition is frequently an indication of a psychiatric disorder. *Compare* organic disorder.

functional endoscopic sinus surgery (FESS) surgery of the *paranasal sinuses using *endoscopes. Routes of sinus drainage and aeration that are blocked by disease are cleared and enlarged, allowing the rest of the sinuses to return to normal.

Functional Independence Measure a table recommended by the World Health Organization for assessing the degree of whole-person disability, being particularly useful for judging the extent of recovery from serious injury. It has five grades, ranging from 0 (fully independent) to 4 (completely dependent).

Functional Limitations Index a system used by the US Social Security Administration to measure the degree of disability of an injured or sick worker. The index is based on such factors as the number of days of restricted activity of a worker during the preceding six months, the type of occupation, and the cause of the worker's disability.

Functional Recovery Index an international index, published by the World Health Organization, that grades the degree of recovery after serious injury.

fundoplication n. a surgical operation for *gastroesophageal reflux disease in which the upper part of the stomach is wrapped around the lower esophagus. The most common technique is named after Rudolf Nissen, a Swiss surgeon.

fundoscopy (ophthalmoscopy) n. examination of the interior of the eye by means of an *ophthalmoscope.

fundus n. 1. the base of a hollow organ: the part farthest from the opening; e.g. the fundus of the stomach, bladder, or uterus. 2. the interior concavity forming the back of the eyeball, opposite the pupil. *Fundus flavimaculatus* is a hereditary disease of the retina in which white material is deposited in the fundus at the level of the retinal pigment epithelium (*see* retina). It usually causes loss of central vision, but good vision may persist into adulthood. *Fundus albipunctatus* is a hereditary disease in which the fundus shows widespread distribution of uniform-sized white dots, resulting in poor *dark adaptation.

fungicide n. an agent that kills fungi. *See also* antimycotic.

fungoid n. 1. *adj.* resembling a fungus. 2. n. a funguslike growth.

fungus n. (*pl.* **fungi**) a simple organism (formerly regarded as a plant) that lacks the green pigment chlorophyll. Fungi include the *yeasts, rusts, molds, and mushrooms. They live either as *sapro-phytes or as *parasites of plants and animals; some species infect and cause disease in humans (*see* blastomycosis). The single-celled microscopic yeasts are a good source of vitamin B and many antibiotics are obtained from the molds (*see* penicillin). —**fungal** *adj.*

funiculitis n. inflammation of the spermatic cord. This usually arises in association with *epididymitis and causes pain and swelling of the involved cord. Treatment is by administration of antibiotics and analgesics.

funiculus n. 1. any of the three main columns of white matter found in each lateral half of the spinal cord. 2. a bundle of nerve fibers enclosed in a sheath; a fasciculus. 3. (formerly) the spermatic cord or umbilical cord.

funis n. (in anatomy) any cordlike structure, especially the umbilical cord.

funnel chest depression of the breastbone and inward curving of the costal cartilages articulating with it, resulting in deformity of the chest. It may displace the heart to the left and can cause slight breathlessness. Medical name: **pectus ex-cavatum.**

furcation n. the place where the roots fork on a multirooted tooth.

furfuraceous *adj.* describing scaling of skin in which the scales resemble bran or dandruff.

furor n. indiscriminate violence and destructiveness, occurring especially during a period of mental confusion due to *epilepsy.

furosemide n. a loop *diuretic used to treat fluid retention (edema) associated with heart, liver, or kidney disease and also high blood pressure. It is administered by mouth or injection; common side effects are nausea and vomiting. Trade name: **Lasix.**

furuncle n. *see* boil.

furunculosis n. the occurrence of several *boils (furuncles) at the same time, usually caused by *Staphylococcus aureus* infection. Treatment includes thorough daily disinfection of the skin and incision (lancing), which may be more effective than antibiotic therapy. The urine should be checked for sugar.

fusiform *adj.* spindle-shaped; tapering at both ends.

fusion n. the joining together of two structures. For example, the surgical fusion of two or more vertebrae is performed to stabilize an unstable spine. Fusion of the *epiphyses during growth is the cause of arrested growth of stature.

Fusobacterium *n.* a genus of gram-negative rodlike bacteria with tapering ends. Most species are normal inhabitants of the mouth of animals and humans and produce no harmful effects, but anaerobic *Fusobacterium* species are associated with *ulcerative gingivitis.

G

GA *see* Gamblers Anonymous.

GABA *see* gamma-aminobutyric acid.

gabapentin *n.* an *anticonvulsant drug used in the management of partial seizures in epilepsy. It is useful in combination therapy because it does not cause adverse reactions with other anticonvulsant drugs. Gabapentin is also used in the management of postherpetic neuralgia (*see* herpes). It is administered by mouth; side effects include dizziness, sedation, and fatigue. Trade name: **Neurotin**.

GAD *see* generalized anxiety disorder, glutamic acid decarboxylase.

gadopentate dimeglumine an injectable contrast medium for *magnetic resonance imaging. It is indicated for enhancing the contrast of brain lesions with abnormal vascularity, an abnormal blood-brain barrier, and in the spine and its associated tissues. Side effects include headache, pain and coldness at the site of injection, and nausea. Trade name: **Magnevist**.

Gaffkya *n.* a genus of bacteria now classified as *Micrococcus*.

gag 1. *n.* an instrument that is placed between a patient's teeth to keep the mouth open. **2.** *vb.* to retch or heave; to strive to vomit.

gag reflex (pharyngeal reflex) a normal reflex action caused by contraction of pharynx muscles when the soft palate or posterior pharynx is touched. The reflex is used to test the integrity of the *vagus and *glossopharyngeal nerves.

gait *n.* the manner in which a person walks. In neurological disease, the gait is often unsteady or uncoordinated. A staggering gait indicates alcohol or bar-

biturate intoxication or cerebellar disease.

galact- (galacto-) *prefix denoting* **1.** milk. Example: *galactosis* (formation of). **2.** galactose.

galactagogue *n.* an agent that stimulates the secretion of milk or increases milk flow.

galactocele *n.* **1.** a breast cyst containing milk, caused by closure of a milk duct. **2.** an accumulation of milky liquid in the sac surrounding the testis (*see* hydrocele).

galactorrhea *n.* **1.** abnormally copious milk secretion. **2.** secretion of milk after breast feeding has been stopped.

galactose *n.* a simple sugar and a constituent of the milk sugar *lactose. Galactose is converted to glucose in the liver. The enzyme necessary for this conversion is missing in infants with a rare inherited metabolic disease called *galactosemia.

galactosemia *n.* an inborn inability to utilize the sugar galactose, which in consequence accumulates in the blood. Untreated, affected infants fail to thrive and become mentally retarded, but if galactose is eliminated from the diet, growth and development may be normal.

galantamine *n. see* acetylcholinesterase inhibitor.

galea *n.* **1.** a helmet-shaped part, especially the *galea aponeurotica*, a flat sheet of fibrous tissue (*see* aponeurosis) that caps the skull and links the two parts of the *epicranius muscle. **2.** a type of head bandage.

galenical *n.* a pharmaceutical preparation of a drug of animal or plant origin.

gallamine *n.* a drug administered by injection to produce muscle relaxation during anesthesia (*see* muscle relaxant). Trade name: **Flaxedil**.

gallbladder a pear-shaped sac (7–10 cm long), lying underneath the right lobe of the liver, in which *bile is stored (see illustration). Bile passes (via the hepatic duct) to the gallbladder from the liver, where it is formed, and is released into the duodenum (through the common bile duct) under the influence of the hormone *cholecystokinin, which is secreted when food is present in the duodenum. The gallbladder is a common site of stone formation (*see* gallstone).

gallium n. a silvery metallic element. A radioisotope of gallium can be used for the detection of lymphomas and areas of infection (such as an abscess) following intravenous injection. This technique is being replaced by other methods of imaging with lower radiation doses and better anatomical resolution.

gallop n. (in cardiology) an abnormal third or fourth heart sound occurring during *diastole in the cardiac cycle. The rhythm resembles the pattern produced when a horse's hooves strike the ground in a gallop, giving the sound its name. The sounds, especially in older adults, are usually indicative of serious heart disease.

gallstone n. a hard mass composed of bile pigments, cholesterol, and calcium salts, in varying proportions, that can form inside the gallbladder. The formation of gallstones (*cholelithiasis*) occurs when the physical characteristics of bile alter so that cholesterol is less soluble, although chronic inflammation of the gallbladder (*see* cholecystitis) or diminished contractility may also be a contributory factor. Gallstones may exist for many years without causing symptoms. However, they may cause severe pain (*see* biliary colic) or they may pass into the common bile duct and cause obstructive *jaundice or *cholangitis. Gallstones are usually diagnosed by ultrasonography, but those containing calcium may be seen on a plain X-ray (opaque stones).

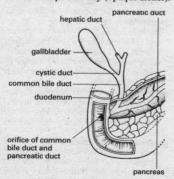

hepatic duct
pancreatic duct
gallbladder
cystic duct
common bile duct
duodenum
orifice of common bile duct and pancreatic duct
pancreas

The gallbladder and pancreas and their associated ducts

Cholelithiasis is treated by surgical removal of the gallbladder (*see* cholecystectomy) or by removing the stones themselves, which can be either dissolved using bile salts given by mouth or shattered by ultrasound waves. There is no need for treatment if the stones are causing no symptoms.

galvanism n. (formerly) any form of medical treatment that uses electricity. *Interrupted galvanism* is a form of *electrotherapy in which direct current, in impulses lasting for 30 to 100 milliseconds, is used to stimulate the activity of nerves or the muscles they supply. *See also* faradism.

galvanocautery n. *see* electrocautery.

Gamblers Anonymous (GA) an international organization, founded in the US in 1957, that seeks to assist compulsive gamblers. The despair, humiliation, and loneliness of compulsive gamblers is neither widely known nor understood. Invariably their addiction leads to bankruptcy, loss of jobs, rejection by family and friends, and ultimately to criminal means of obtaining money with which to gamble. GA offers a form of group therapy similar to that provided by *Alcoholics Anonymous. Senior members help the new members to face their creditors and to work out repayment budgets that will eventually free them from their obligations. The sister organization, *Gam-Anon*, provides advice and encouragement for the families of compulsive gamblers.

gamete n. a mature sex cell: the *ovum of the female or the *spermatozoon of the male. Gametes are haploid, containing half the normal number of chromosomes.

gamete intrafallopian transfer (GIFT) a procedure for assisting conception, suitable only for women with healthy fallopian tubes. In over 50% of women in whom infertility is diagnosed, the tubes are normal but some other factor, such as endometriosis, prevents conception. Using needle *aspiration, under laparoscopic or ultrasonic guidance, ova are removed from the ovary. After being mixed with the partner's spermatozoa, they are introduced into a fallopian tube, where fertilization takes place. The fertilized ovum can subsequently become implanted in the uterus.

gametocide n. a drug that kills *gametocytes. Drugs such as *primaquine destroy gametocytes of the malaria parasite (see Plasmodium), thus interrupting the life cycle and preventing infection of the mosquito.

gametocyte n. any of the cells that are in the process of developing into gametes by undergoing *gametogenesis. See also oocyte, spermatocyte.

gametogenesis n. the process by which spermatozoa and ova are formed. In both sexes the precursor cells undergo *meiosis, which halves the number of chromosomes. However, the timing of events and the size and number of gametes produced are very different in the male and female. See oogenesis, spermatogenesis.

gamma-aminobutyric acid (GABA) an amino acid found in the central nervous system, predominantly in the brain, where it acts as an inhibitory *neurotransmitter.

gamma benzene hexachloride see lindane.

gamma camera a piece of apparatus that detects radioactivity in the form of gamma rays emitted by radioactive isotopes that have been introduced into the body as *tracers. It contains an activated sodium iodide crystal (see scintillator) and a large array of photomultiplier tubes. Using lead *collimators, the position of the source of the radioactivity can be plotted and displayed on a TV monitor or photographic film (see scintigram).

gamma globulin any of a class of proteins, present in the blood *plasma, identified by their characteristic rate of movement in an electric field (see electrophoresis). Almost all gamma globulins are *immunoglobulins. Injection of gamma globulin provides temporary protection against *hepatitis A and has recently been shown to reduce the incidence of coronary artery involvement in *Kawasaki disease. Infusions of gamma globulin are used to treat immunodeficiencies or immune-mediated disorders, such as autoimmune hemolytic *anemia or *idiopathic thrombocytopenic purpura. See also globulin.

gamma rays electromagnetic radiation of wavelengths shorter than X-rays, given off by certain radioactive substances. Gamma rays used in *nuclear medicine tend to have higher energy than diagnostic X-rays, with greater penetration; they are harmful to living tissues and can be used to sterilize certain materials and to kill bacteria as a means of food preservation. Higher doses are used in *radiotherapy to kill tumor cells.

gamo- prefix denoting marriage.

ganciclovir n. an antiviral drug used to treat severe *cytomegalovirus infections, mainly in patients with AIDS. It is administered orally, by injection, or as eye drops. Possible side effects include nausea, vomiting, diarrhea, infertility, confusion, seizures, and disturbance of bone marrow blood-cell production. It is an *orphan drug. Trade names: **Cytovene**, **Vitrasert**.

gangli- (ganglio-) prefix denoting a ganglion.

ganglion n. (pl. **ganglia**) 1. (in neurology) any structure containing a collection of nerve cell bodies and often also numbers of synapses. In the *sympathetic nervous system chains of ganglia are found on each side of the spinal cord, while in the *parasympathetic nervous system ganglia are situated in or nearer to the organs innervated. Swellings in the posterior sensory *roots of the spinal nerves are termed ganglia; these contain cell bodies but no synapses. In the central nervous system, certain well-defined masses of nerve cells are called ganglia (or nuclei); for example, the *basal ganglia. 2. an abnormal but harmless swelling (cyst) that sometimes forms in tendon sheaths, especially at the wrist.

ganglioside n. one of a group of *glycolipids found in the brain, liver, spleen, and red blood cells (they are particularly abundant in nerve cell membranes). Gangliosides are chemically similar to *cerebrosides but contain additional carbohydrate groups.

gangosa n. a lesion that occasionally appears in the final stage of *yaws, involving considerable destruction of the tissues of both the hard palate and the nose.

gangrene n. death and decay of part of the body due to deficiency or cessation of blood supply. The causes include disease, injury, or *atheroma in major blood vessels, frostbite or severe burns, and diseases such as *diabetes mellitus and *Raynaud's disease. Dry gangrene is death and withering of tissues caused simply by a cessation of local blood circulation. *Moist gangrene* is death and putrefactive decay of tissue caused by bacterial infection. *See also* gas gangrene.

Ganser state (pseudodementia) a syndrome characterized by *approximate answers*, i.e. the patient gives grossly and absurdly false replies to questions, but the reply shows that the question has been understood. For example, the question "What color is snow?" may elicit the reply "Green." This can be accompanied by odd behavior or episodes of *stupor. The condition is due to *conversion disorder or to conscious malingering. [S. J. M. Ganser (1853–1931), German psychiatrist]

Gardnerella *n.* a genus of anaerobic bacteria. *G. vaginalis* is a cause of vaginitis and, in pregnant women, of late miscarriage.

Gardner's syndrome a variant form of familial adenomatous *polyposis in which polyps in the colon are associated with fibromas and *osteomas (benign tumors), especially of the skull and jaw, and multiple *sebaceous cysts. [E. J. Gardner (1909–   ), US physician]

gargoylism *n. see* Hunter's syndrome, Hurler's syndrome.

gas gangrene death and decay of wound tissue infected by the soil bacterium *Clostridium perfringens*. Toxins produced by the bacterium cause putrefactive decay of connective tissue with the generation of gas. Treatment is usually by surgery.

Gasterophilus *n.* a genus of widely distributed nonbloodsucking beelike flies. The parasitic maggots normally live in the alimentary canal of horses but, rarely, can also infect humans and cause an inflamed itching eruption of the skin (*see* creeping eruption).

gastr- (gastro-) *prefix denoting* the stomach. Examples: *gastralgia* (pain in); *gastrocolic* (relating to the stomach and colon).

gastrectasia *n.* dilation of the stomach. This may be caused by *pyloric stenosis or it may occur as a complication of some abdominal operations or trauma.

gastrectomy *n.* a surgical operation in which the whole or a part of the stomach is removed. *Total gastrectomy*, in which

the esophagus is joined to the duodenum, is usually performed for stomach cancer but occasionally for the *Zollinger-Ellison syndrome. In *partial* (or *subtotal*) *gastrectomy* the upper third or half of the stomach is joined to the duodenum or small intestine (*gastroenterostomy*): an operation previously carried out in severe cases of *peptic ulcers before the advent of effective drug treatment. After gastrectomy capacity for food is reduced, sometimes leading to weight loss. Other complications of gastrectomy include *dumping syndrome, anemia, and *malabsorption.

gastric *adj.* relating to or affecting the stomach.

gastric glands tubular glands that lie in the mucous membrane of the stomach wall. There are three varieties: the *cardiac*, *fundic*, and *pyloric glands*, and they secrete *gastric juice. *See also* oxyntic cells.

gastric juice the liquid secreted by the *gastric glands of the stomach. Its main digestive constituents are hydrochloric acid, mucin, *rennin, and pepsinogen. The acid acts on pepsinogen to produce *pepsin, which functions best in an acid medium. The acidity of the stomach contents also kills unwanted bacteria and other organisms that have been ingested with the food. Gastric juice also contains *intrinsic factor, which is necessary for the absorption of vitamin B_{12}.

gastric ulcer an ulcer in the stomach, caused by the action of acid, pepsin, and bile on the stomach lining (mucosa). The output of stomach acid is not usually increased. Taking *NSAIDs (nonsteroidal anti-inflammatory drugs) or *corticosteroids is a predisposing factor, and *Helicobacter pylori* is often present. Symptoms include vomiting and pain in the upper abdomen soon after eating, and such complications as bleeding (*see also* hematemesis), *perforation, and obstruction due to scarring may occur. Symptoms are relieved by antacid medicines, and most ulcers heal if treated by an *antisecretory drug and antibiotics. Surgery may be required if the ulcer fails to heal. Since stomach cancer may mimic a gastric ulcer, all gastric ulcers should be examined with a *gastroscope to aid in their differentiation.

gastrin *n.* a hormone produced in the mucous membrane of the pyloric region of the *stomach (*see* G cell). Its secretion is stimulated by the presence of food. It is circulated in the blood to the rest of the stomach, where it stimulates the production of *gastric juice.

gastrinoma *n.* a rare tumor that secretes excess amounts of the hormone *gastrin, causing the *Zollinger-Ellison syndrome. Such tumors most frequently occur in the pancreas; about half of them are malignant.

gastritis *n.* inflammation of the lining (mucosa) of the stomach. *Acute gastritis* is caused by ingesting excess alcohol or other irritating or corrosive substances, resulting in vomiting. *Chronic gastritis* is associated with smoking and chronic alcoholism and may be caused by bile entering the stomach from the duodenum, but most cases are caused by the bacterium *Helicobacter pylori*. It has no definite symptoms, but the patient is liable to develop gastric ulcers or gastric cancer. *Atrophic gastritis*, in which the stomach lining is atrophied, may succeed chronic gastritis but may occur spontaneously as an *autoimmune disease.

gastrocele *n.* a *hernia of the stomach.

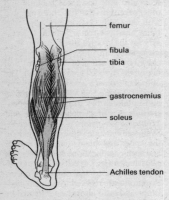

femur
fibula
tibia
gastrocnemius
soleus
Achilles tendon

Gastrocnemius and soleus muscles

gastrocnemius *n.* a muscle that forms the greater part of the calf of the leg (see illustration). It flexes the knee and foot (so that the toes point downward).

gastrocolic reflex a wave of peristalsis produced in the intestine and colon by introducing food into a fasting stomach.

gastroduodenoscope *n. see* duodenoscope, gastroscope.

gastroduodenoscopy *n.* the technique of viewing the inside of the stomach and duodenum with an endoscope. *See also* duodenoscope.

gastroduodenostomy *n.* a surgical operation in which the *duodenum (usually the third or fourth part) is joined to an opening made in the stomach in order to bypass an obstruction (such as *pyloric stenosis) or to facilitate the exit of food from the stomach after vagotomy. *See also* duodenostomy.

gastroenteritis *n.* inflammation of the stomach and intestine. Gastroenteritis is usually due to acute infection by viruses or bacteria or to food-poisoning toxins, which causes vomiting and diarrhea. The illness usually lasts 3–5 days. Fluid loss is sometimes severe, especially in infants, and intravenous fluid replacement may be necessary.

gastroenterology *n.* the study of the gastrointestinal organs and their diseases, which include diseases of any part of the digestive tract and also of the liver, biliary tract, and pancreas.

gastroenterostomy *n.* a surgical operation in which the small intestine is joined to an opening made in the stomach. The usual technique is *gastroduodenostomy.

gastroesophageal reflux a condition in which the stomach contents reflux into the esophagus because of permanent or intermittent impairment of the usual mechanisms preventing this. It may give rise to *esophagitis.

gastroesophageal reflux disease (GERD) the syndrome that is caused by abnormal gastroesophageal reflux, which includes symptoms of *heartburn, regurgitation, and *odynophagia, in which *esophagitis may be present.

gastroesophagostomy *n.* a surgical operation in which the *esophagus (gullet) is joined to the stomach, bypassing the natural junction when this is obstructed by *achalasia, *stricture (narrowing) of the esophagus, or cancer. This operation is rarely performed, because gastric juices entering the esophagus through the artificial junction cause inflammation and stricture.

Gastrografin n. trade name for meglumine diatrizoate, a water-soluble contrast medium used in diagnostic radiology, usually in the gastrointestinal tract. It is used in some conditions as a laxative.

gastroileac reflex the relaxation of the *ileocecal valve caused by the presence of food in the stomach.

gastrojejunostomy n. a surgical operation in which the *jejunum is joined to an opening made in the stomach. This is done in preference to *gastroduodenostomy if the latter operation is technically difficult or in special operations to avoid a backflow of bile into the stomach.

gastrolith n. a stone in the stomach, which usually builds up around a *bezoar.

gastropexy n. surgical attachment of the stomach to the abdominal wall.

gastroplasty n. surgical alteration of the shape of the stomach without removal of any part. The term was originally used for correction of an acquired deformity, e.g. narrowing due to a peptic ulcer, but has more recently been applied to techniques for reducing the size of the stomach in the treatment of morbid obesity, e.g. *vertical banded gastroplasty*.

gastroptosis n. a condition in which the stomach hangs low in the abdomen. Although the diagnosis was once used to explain various abdominal complaints, it is now known that the stomach may assume various anatomical positions without causing any symptoms.

gastroschisis n. a congenital defect in the abdominal wall, which fails to close to the right of a normal umbilical cord. It is diagnosed by ultrasound. Intestine prolapses through the defect and has no covering; treatment is surgical.

gastroscope n. an illuminated optical instrument used to inspect the interior of the stomach. For many years these were rigid or semirigid instruments affording only limited views, but modern fully flexible instruments, which transmit the image through a fiberoptic bundle or by a small video camera, allow all areas of the stomach to be seen and photographed and specimens to be taken for microscopic examination. Therapeutic procedures (e.g. to arrest hemorrhage, remove a polyp, or produce a *gastrostomy) may be performed. Since the same instruments can usually be introduced into the duodenum they are also known

as *gastroduodenoscopes* or *esophagogastroduodenoscopes*. —**gastroscopy** n.

gastrostaxis n. an obsolete term for *hematemesis (bleeding from the stomach).

gastrostomy n. a surgical procedure in which an opening is made into the stomach from the outside. It is usually performed to allow food and fluid to be poured directly into the stomach when swallowing is impossible because of disease or obstruction of the esophagus. Sometimes it is used temporarily after operations on the esophagus, until healing has occurred. Formerly a gastrostomy was always performed surgically, but it can now be done using an *endoscope (*percutaneous endoscopic gastrostomy*) or by direct puncture under radiological guidance.

gastrotomy n. a procedure during abdominal surgery in which the stomach is opened, usually to allow inspection of the interior (e.g. to find a point of bleeding), to remove a foreign body, or to allow the esophagus to be approached from below (e.g. to pull down a tube through a constricting growth).

gastrula n. an early stage in the development of many animal embryos. It consists of a double-layered ball of cells formed by invagination and movement of cells in the preceding single-layered stage (blastula) in the process of *gastrulation*. It contains a central cavity, the *archenteron, which opens through the *blastopore* to the outside. True gastrulation only occurs in the embryos of amphibians and certain fish, but a similar process occurs in the embryonic disk in other vertebrates, including humans.

Gaucher's disease a genetically determined (autosomal *recessive) disease resulting from the deposition of glucocerebrosides (*see* cerebroside) in the brain, liver, spleen, and bone. It causes mental retardation, abnormal limb posture and spasticity, and difficulty with swallowing. Carrier detection and *prenatal diagnosis are possible; enzyme replacement therapy may be used in treatment. [P. C. E. Gaucher (1854–1918), French physician]

gauss n. a unit of magnetic flux density equal to 1 maxwell per square centimeter. 1 gauss = 10^{-4} tesla.

Gaussian distribution *see* frequency distribution, significance. [K. F. Gauss (1777–1855), German mathematician]

gauze *n.* thin open-woven material used in several layers for the preparation of dressings and swabs.

gavage *n.* forced feeding: any means used to get an unwilling or incapacitated patient to take in food by mouth, especially via a stomach tube.

G cell *n.* any of the cells of the mucous membrane of the stomach that are responsible for producing *gastrin. They occur mainly in the gastric *antrum. Increased production of G cells is associated with duodenal ulcer and the *Zollinger-Ellison syndrome: gastrin acts to increase the production of acid by the oxyntic (parietal) cells of the gastric glands.

GCS *see* Glasgow Coma Scale.

gel *n.* a colloidal suspension that has set to form a jelly. Some insoluble drugs are administered in the form of gels.

gelatin *n.* a jellylike substance formed when tendons, ligaments, etc. containing *collagen (a protein) are boiled in water. Gelatin has been used in medicine as a source of protein in the treatment of malnutrition, in pharmacy for the manufacture of capsules and suppositories, and in bacteriology for preparing culture media.

gemfibrozil *n.* a drug used to lower very low density *lipoproteins in patients with high *triglyceride serum levels who have not responded to diet, weight reduction, or exercise (*see* fibrates). It is administered by mouth; side effects include diarrhea, abdominal pain, and nausea and vomiting. Trade name: **Lopid.**

gemmule *n.* one of the minute spines or surface extensions of a *dendrite, through which contact is made with another neuron at a *synapse.

gemtuzumab ozogamicin a *monoclonal antibody used in the treatment of acute *myeloid leukemia in patients who are in first relapse, older than 60 years of age, and who are not considered candidates for other cytotoxic chemotherapy. It is administered intravenously; side effects include *myelosuppression, nausea and vomiting, fever, and fatigue. Trade name: **Mylotarg.**

gene *n.* the basic unit of genetic material, which is carried at a particular place on a *chromosome. Originally, it was regarded as the unit of inheritance and mutation but is now usually defined as a sequence of *DNA or *RNA that acts as the unit controlling the formation of a single polypeptide chain (*see* cistron). In diploid organisms, including humans, genes occur as pairs of *alleles. Various kinds of genes have been discovered: *structural genes* determine the biochemical makeup of the proteins; *regulator genes* control the rate of protein production (*see* operon). *Architectural genes* are responsible for the integration of the protein into the structure of the cell, and *temporal genes* control the time and place of action of the other genes and largely control the *differentiation of the cells and tissues of the body.

gene clone *see* clone.

generalized anxiety disorder (GAD) a state of inappropriate and sometimes severe anxiety, without adequate cause, that lasts for at least six months. It affects women twice as often as men and often develops in early adult life; there is a hereditary tendency to develop the disorder. The condition is thought to be caused by a disturbance of the functions of neurotransmitters, such as epinephrine or GABA, in the frontal lobes or the *limbic system of the brain. Symptoms include shakiness, *bruxism, breathlessness, restlessness, fatigability, palpitations, sweating, clammy hands, dry mouth, lightheadedness, diarrhea, flushing, and *globus pharyngeus. Treatment is with beta blockers, antihistamines, and antidepressants.

general paralysis of the insane (paresis) a late consequence of syphilitic infection. The symptoms are those of a *dementia and spastic weakness of the limbs. Deafness, epilepsy, and *dysarthria (defective pronunciation) may occur. The infecting organism can be detected in the brain cells and the tests for syphilis are usually positive in blood and cerebrospinal fluid. When the symptoms are combined with those of *tabes dorsalis, the condition is called *taboparesis*. Vigorous treatment with procaine penicillin is required, but recovery is likely to be limited.

general practitioner (GP) a doctor who is the main provider of *primary medical care*, through whom patients make first contact with health services for an episode of illness or new developments of chronic diseases. Advice and treatment are provided for those who do not require the services of specialists or hospitals (*secondary medical care*). Two or more practitioners may form a partnership sharing fees and work loads, including cross-cover for each other's patients. When they share premises, secretarial help, and other resources this constitutes a *group practice. *See also* family practitioner.

generic *adj*. **1.** of or relating to a *genus. **2.** denoting a drug name that is not protected by a trademark.

-genesis *suffix denoting* origin or development. Example: *spermatogenesis* (development of spermatozoa).

gene therapy treatment directed to curing genetic disease by introducing normal genes into patients to overcome the effects of defective genes, using techniques of *genetic engineering. The most radical approach would be to do this at a very early stage in the embryo, so that the new gene would be incorporated into the germ cells (ova and sperm) and would therefore be inheritable. However, this approach is not considered to be either safe or ethical, because the consequences would affect all descendants of the patient, and it is not being pursued. In *somatic cell gene therapy* the healthy gene is inserted into *somatic cells (such as the *hemopoietic stem cells of the bone marrow) that give rise to other cells. All the surviving descendants of these modified cells will then be normal and, if present in sufficient numbers, the condition will be cured (the defective gene will, however, still be present in the germ cells).

At present, gene therapy is most feasible for treating disorders caused by a defect in a single recessive gene, so that the deficiency can be overcome by the introduction of a normal allele (therapy for disorders caused by dominant genes, e.g. Huntington's disease, would require the modification or replacement of the defective allele because its effect is expressed in the presence of a normal allele). Examples of such recessive disorders include *adenosine deaminase (ADA) deficiency and *cystic fibrosis. Gene therapy trials have begun for these

and other disorders, such as *severe combined immune deficiency, *sickle-cell disease, and *thalassemia.

Gene therapy for certain types of cancer is also undergoing clinical trials. Here the approach is aimed at introducing into the cancer cells tumor-suppressing genes, such as *p53 (which prevents uncontrolled cell division), or genes that direct the production of substances (such as *interleukin-2) that stimulate the immune system to destroy the tumor cells.

genetic code the information carried by *DNA and *messenger RNA that determines the sequence of amino acids in every protein and thereby controls the nature of all proteins made by the cell. The genetic code is expressed by the sequence of *nucleotide bases in the nucleic acid molecule, a unit of three consecutive bases (a *codon*) coding for each amino acid. The code is translated into protein at the ribosomes (*see* transcription, translation). Changes in the genetic code result in the insertion of incorrect amino acids in a protein chain, giving a *mutation.

genetic counseling the procedure by which patients and their families are given advice about the nature and consequences of inherited disorders, the possibility of becoming affected or having affected children, and the various options that are available to them for the prevention, diagnosis, and management of such conditions. Genetic counseling should be available at prenatal and postnatal clinics, and also through family planning clinics.

genetic drift the tendency for variations to occur in the genetic composition of small isolated inbreeding populations by chance. Such populations become genetically different from the original population from which they were derived.

genetic engineering (recombinant DNA technology) the techniques involved in altering the characteristics of an organism by inserting genes from another organism into its DNA. This altered DNA (known as *recombinant DNA*) is usually produced by isolating foreign genes, often by the use of *restriction enzymes, and inserting them into bacterial DNA, often using viruses as *vectors. Once inserted, the foreign gene may use the cell machinery of its host to synthesize the protein that it originally coded for in the organism it was derived from. For example, the human genes for *insulin, *interferon, and *growth hormone production have been incorporated into bacterial DNA and such genetically engineered bacteria are used in the commercial production of these hormones. Other applications of genetic engineering include DNA analysis, the production of *monoclonal antibodies, and, more recently, *gene therapy.

genetics *n.* the science of inheritance. It attempts to explain the differences and similarities between related organisms and the ways in which characteristics are passed from parents to their offspring. *Human* and *medical genetics* are concerned with the study of inherited diseases. *See also* cytogenetics, Mendel's laws.

genetic screening a *screening test to discover individuals whose *genotypes are associated with specific diseases (*see* mouthwash test). Such individuals may later develop the disease itself or pass it on to their children (*see* carrier). The recent use of genetic screening to diagnose the sex of the fetus so that the parents may "choose" the sex of their children has caused considerable controversy.

geni- (genio-) *prefix denoting* the chin.

-genic *suffix denoting* **1.** producing. **2.** produced by.

genicular *adj.* relating to the knee joint: applied to arteries that supply the knee.

geniculum *n.* a sharp bend in an anatomical structure, such as the bend in the facial nerve in the medial wall of the middle ear.

genion *n.* (in craniometry) the tip of the protuberance of the chin.

genioplasty *n.* an operation performed in plastic surgery to alter the size and shape of the chin. This can be built up with grafted bone, cartilage, or artificial material.

genital *adj.* relating to the reproductive organs or to reproduction.

genital herpes *see* herpes.

genitalia *pl. n.* the reproductive organs of either the male or the female. However, the term is usually used in reference to the external parts of the reproductive system. *See also* vulva.

genito- *prefix denoting* the reproductive organs. Examples: *genitoplasty* (plastic surgery of); *genitourinary* (relating to the reproductive and excretory systems).

genodermatosis *n.* any genetically determined skin disorder, such as *ichthyosis, *neurofibromatosis, or *xeroderma pigmentosum.

genogram *n.* a technique of family *psychotherapy, in which a family tree and family history of a particular psychological disorder are constructed in view of the whole family to help them understand each other better.

genome *n.* the total genetic material of an organism, comprising the genes contained in its chromosomes; sometimes the term is used for the basic *haploid set of chromosomes of an organism. The human genome comprises 23 pairs of chromosomes (*see* Human Genome Project).

genotype *n.* **1.** the genetic constitution of an individual or group, as determined by the particular set of genes it possesses. **2.** the genetic information carried by a pair of alleles, which determines a particular characteristic. **3.** a gene or pattern of genes the precise details of which are defined. *Compare* phenotype.

gentamicin *n.* an *aminoglycoside antibiotic that is used to treat infections caused by a wide range of bacteria. It can be administered by injection or applied in a cream to the skin or in drops to the ears and eyes. Kidney and ear damage may occur at high doses. Trade names: **Garamycin, Genoptic Liquifilm, Genoptic S.O.P., Gentacidin, Gentamar.**

gentian violet a dye used to stain tissues and microorganisms for microscopical study. *See* methyl violet.

genu *n.* **1.** the knee. **2.** any bent anatomical structure resembling the knee. —**genual** *adj.*

genus *n.* (*pl.* **genera**) a category used in the classification of animals and plants. A genus consists of several closely related and similar species; for example the genus *Canis* includes the dog, wolf, and jackal.

genu valgum *see* knock knee.

genu varum *see* bowlegs.

geo- *prefix denoting* the earth or soil.

geophagia *n.* the eating of dirt. *See* pica.

ger- (gero-, geront(o)-) *prefix denoting* old age.

GERD *see* gastroesophageal reflux disease.

geriatrics *n.* the branch of medicine concerned with the diagnosis and treatment of disorders that occur in old age and with the care of the aged. *See also* gerontology.

germ *n.* any microorganism, especially one that causes disease. *See also* infection.

German measles a mild highly contagious virus infection, mainly of childhood, causing enlargement of lymph nodes in the neck and a widespread pink rash. The disease is spread by close contact with a patient. After an incubation period of 2–3 weeks, a headache, sore throat, and slight fever develop, followed by swelling and soreness of the neck and the eruption of a rash of minute pink spots, spreading from the face and neck to the rest of the body. The spots disappear within seven days but the patient remains infectious for a further 3–4 days. An infection usually confers immunity. Because German measles can cause fetal malformations during early pregnancy, girls should be immunized against the disease before puberty. Most children now receive immunization via the *MMR vaccine in their second year. Medical name: **rubella**. *Compare* scarlet fever.

germ cell (gonocyte) any of the embryonic cells that have the potential to develop into spermatozoa or ova. The term is also applied to any of the cells undergoing gametogenesis and to the gametes themselves.

germicide *n.* an agent that destroys microorganisms, particularly those causing disease. *See* antibiotic, antimycotic, antiseptic, disinfectant.

germinal *adj.* **1.** relating to the early developmental stages of an embryo or tissue. **2.** relating to a germ.

germinal epithelium the epithelial covering of the ovary, which was formerly thought to be the site of formation of *oogonia. It is now thought that oogonia persist in a dormant state from the prenatal period until required in reproductive life.

germinal vesicle the nucleus of a mature *oocyte, prior to fertilization. It is considerably larger than the nucleus of other cells.

germ layer any of the three distinct types of tissue found in the very early stages of embryonic development (*see* ectoderm, endoderm, mesoderm). The germ layers

can be traced throughout embryonic development as they differentiate to form the entire range of body tissues.

germ plasm the substance postulated by 19th-century biologists (notably Weismann) to be transmitted via the gametes from one generation to the next and to give rise to the body cells.

gerontology *n.* the study of the changes in the mind and body that accompany aging and the problems associated with them.

Gerstmann's syndrome a group of symptoms that represent a partial disintegration of the patient's recognition of his *body image. It consists of an inability to name the individual fingers, misidentification of the right and left sides of the body, and inability to write or make mathematical calculations (*see* acalculia, agraphia). It is caused by disease in the association area of the left parietal lobe of the brain. [J. G. Gerstmann (1887–1969), Austrian neurologist]

Gerstmann-Sträussler-Scheinker syndrome an autosomal *dominant condition that resembles *Creutzfeldt-Jakob disease (CJD). Patients present with cerebellar dysfunction (*ataxia and *dysarthria) and later develop dementia. They continue to deteriorate over several years, in contrast with patients with CJD, who deteriorate rapidly over periods of less than 12 months. *See also* prion. [J. G. Gerstmann]

gestaltism *n.* a school of psychology that regards mental processes as wholes (*gestalts*) that cannot be broken down into constituent parts. From this was developed *gestalt therapy*, which aims at achieving a suitable gestalt within the patient that includes all facets of functioning.

gestation *n.* the period during which a fertilized egg cell develops into a baby that is ready to be delivered. Gestation averages 266 days in humans (or 280 days from the first day of the last menstrual period). *See also* pregnancy.

gestational diabetes mellitus (type 3 diabetes) diabetes that develops during pregnancy. Only by observing what happens at the end of the pregnancy can it be decided whether or not the condition is persistent. Gestational diabetes is routinely screened for at antenatal appointments; it is important to diagnose the condition, as uncontrolled blood sugars have an adverse effect on the fetus as well as the mother. It often recurs in subsequent pregnancies and affected women in whom it later disappears have a higher risk than others of developing type 2 diabetes during their lifetime. It is treated like standard diabetes, with around 30% of affected women needing insulin.

GFR see glomerular filtration rate.

Ghon's focus the lesion produced in the lung of a previously uninfected person by tubercle bacilli. It is a small focus of granulomatous inflammation, which may become visible on a chest X-ray if it grows large enough or if it calcifies. A Ghon focus usually heals without further trouble, but in some patients tuberculosis spreads from it via the lymphatics, the air spaces, or the bloodstream. [A. Ghon (1866–1936), Czech pathologist]

giant cell any large cell, such as a *megakaryocyte. Giant cells may have one or many nuclei.

giant cell arteritis see arteritis.

Giardia n. a genus of parasitic pear-shaped protozoa inhabiting the small intestine of humans. They have four pairs of *flagella, two nuclei, and two sucking disks used for attachment to the intestinal wall. Giardia is usually harmless but may occasionally cause diarrhea (see giardiasis).

giardiasis (lambliasis) n. a disease that is caused by the parasitic protozoan Giardia lamblia in the small intestine. Humans become infected by eating food contaminated with cysts containing the parasite. Symptoms include diarrhea, nausea, abdominal pain, flatulence, and the passage of pale fatty stools (steatorrhea). Large numbers of the parasite may interfere with the absorption of food through the gut wall. The disease occurs throughout the world and is particularly common in children; it responds well to oral doses of quinacrine and *metronidazole.

gibbus (gibbosity) n. a sharply angled curvature of the backbone, resulting from collapse of a vertebra. Infection with tuberculosis was a common cause.

Giemsa's stain a mixture of *methylene blue and *eosin, used for distinguishing different types of white blood cells and for detecting parasitic microorganisms

in blood smears. It is one of the *Romanovsky stains. [G. Giemsa (1867–1948), German chemist]

GIFT see gamete intrafallopian transfer.

gigantism n. abnormal growth causing excessive height, most commonly due to oversecretion during childhood of *growth hormone (somatotropin) by the pituitary gland. In eunuchoid gigantism the tall stature is due to delayed puberty, which results in continued growth of the long bones before their growing ends (epiphyses) fuse. See also acromegaly.

GIK regimen (Alberti's regimen) a method for controlling blood-sugar levels in diabetic patients who are being fasted for whatever reason. It involves infusing a solution of glucose (G), insulin (I), and potassium (K) chloride intravenously over a standard time period. Blood sugar and potassium are measured frequently so that appropriate adjustments can be made to the mixture to hold things stable.

Gilbert's syndrome familial unconjugated hyperbilirubinemia: a condition due to an inherited congenital deficiency of the enzyme UDP glucuronyl transferase in the liver cells. Patients become mildly jaundiced, especially if they fast or have some minor infection. Occasionally, they have mild abdominal discomfort. The jaundice can be diminished by small doses of phenobarbital, which stimulates enzyme activity. The condition is benign. [N. A. Gilbert (1858–1927), French physician]

Gilles de la Tourette syndrome (Tourette's syndrome, TS) a condition of severe and multiple *tics, including vocal tics, grunts, and involuntary obscene speech (*coprolalia). The patient may also involuntarily repeat the words or imitate the actions of others (see palilalia). The condition usually starts in childhood and becomes chronic; the causes are unknown. Drug treatment (for example, with *pimozide) is sometimes successful. [G. Gilles de la Tourette (1857–1904), French neurologist]

Gimbernat's ligament a portion of the medial end of the *inguinal ligament that is reflected along the upper part of the pubic bone. It is used to hold stitches during repairs of a femoral *hernia. [A. de Gimbernat (1734–1816), Spanish surgeon and anatomist]

gingiv- (gingivo-) *prefix denoting* the gums. Example: *gingivoplasty* (plastic surgery of).

gingiva *n.* (*pl.* **gingivae**) the gum: the layer of dense connective tissue and overlying mucous membrane that covers the alveolar bone and necks of the teeth. —**gingival** *adj.*

gingivectomy *n.* the surgical removal of excess gum tissue. It is a specific procedure of periodontal surgery.

gingivitis *n.* inflammation of the gums (*see* gingiva) caused by *plaque on the surfaces of the teeth at their necks. The gums are swollen and bleed easily. *Chronic gingivitis* is an early stage of *periodontal disease but is reversible with good oral hygiene. *Ulcerative gingivitis is painful and destructive. Gingival overgrowth may be caused by drug therapy, e.g. phenytoin.

ginglymus (hinge joint) *n.* a form of *diarthrosis (freely movable joint) that allows angular movement in one plane only, increasing or decreasing the angle between the bones. Examples are the knee joint and the elbow joint.

girdle *n.* (in anatomy) an encircling or arching arrangement of bones. *See also* pelvic girdle, shoulder girdle.

glabella *n.* the smooth rounded surface of the *frontal bone in the middle of the forehead, between the two eyebrows.

gladiolus *n.* the middle and largest segment of the *sternum.

gland *n.* an organ or group of cells that is specialized for synthesizing and secreting certain fluids, either for use in the body or for excretion. There are two main groups of glands: the *exocrine glands, which discharge their secretions by means of ducts, and the *endocrine glands, which secrete their products – hormones – directly into the bloodstream. *See also* secretion.

glanders (equinia) *n.* an infectious disease of horses, donkeys, and mules that is caused by the bacterium *Pseudomonas mallei* and can be transmitted to humans. Symptoms include fever and inflammation (with possible ulceration) of the lymph nodes (a form of the disease known as *farcy*), skin, and nasal mucous membranes. In the untreated acute form death may follow in 2–20 days. In the more common chronic form, many patients survive without treatment. Administration of antibiotics is usually effective.

glandular fever an infectious disease, caused by the Epstein-Barr virus, that affects the lymph nodes in the neck, armpits, and groin; it mainly affects adolescents and young adults. After an incubation period of 5–7 days, symptoms commence with swelling and tenderness of the lymph nodes, fever, headache, a sore throat, lethargy, and loss of appetite. In some cases the liver is affected, causing *hepatitis, or the spleen is enlarged. Glandular fever is diagnosed by the presence of large numbers of *monocytes in the blood. Complications are rare but symptoms may persist for weeks before recovery. Medical name: **infectious mononucleosis**.

glans (glans penis) *n.* the acorn-shaped end part of the *penis, formed by the expanded end of the corpus spongiosum (erectile tissue). It is normally covered by the prepuce (foreskin), unless this has been removed by circumcision. The term glans is also applied to the end of the *clitoris.

glare *n.* the undesirable effects of scattered stray light on the retina, causing reduced contrast and visual performance as well as annoyance and discomfort.

Glasgow Coma Scale (GCS) a numerical system used to estimate a patient's level of consciousness after head injury. Each of the following are numerically graded: eye opening (1–4), motor response (1–6), and verbal response (1–5). The higher the score, the greater the level of consciousness: a score of 7 indicates a coma.

glatiramer *n.* a drug that modifies the body's immune response and is used to reduce the frequency of relapses in people with relapsing/remitting multiple sclerosis. It is administered by subcutaneous injection; side effects include flushing and palpitations. Trade name: **Copaxone**.

glaucoma *n.* a condition in which loss of vision occurs because of an abnormally high pressure in the eye. In most cases there is no other ocular disease. This is known as *primary glaucoma* and there are two pathologically distinct types: *acute* (or *angle-closure*) *glaucoma*, in which a sudden rise in pressure, due to sudden closure of the angle between the cornea and iris where aqueous humor usually drains from the eye, is accompanied by pain and marked blurring of vision; and the more common *chronic simple* (or *open-angle*) *glaucoma*, in which the pressure increases gradually, usually without producing pain, and the visual loss is insidious. The same type of visual loss may occur in eyes with a normal pressure: this is called *low-tension glaucoma*. Primary glaucoma occurs increasingly with age and is an important cause of blindness. *Secondary glaucoma* may occur when other ocular disease impairs the normal circulation of the aqueous humor and causes the intraocular pressure to rise.

In all types of glaucoma the eventual problem is to reduce the intraocular pressure. Drops are put into the eye at regular intervals to improve the outflow of aqueous humor from the eye and/or to reduce the production of aqueous humor. Drugs used for this purpose include beta blockers (e.g. timolol, levobunolol, carteolol), carbonic anhydrase inhibitors (e.g. acetazolamide, dichlorphenamide), alpha-receptor stimulants (e.g. apraclonidine, brimonidine), and latanoprost. If this treatment is ineffective, conventional or laser surgery may be performed to make an accessory channel through which the aqueous humor may drain from the eye in sufficient quantities to allow the pressure to return to normal. Such operations are known as *drainage* or *filtering operations*.

glaukomflecken *pl. n.* small anterior subcapsular lens opacities seen in acute (angle-closure) glaucoma.

Gleason grade the grade (from one to five) that is given to an area of prostate cancer, reflecting the level of differentiation of the tumor. Higher grades indicate poorer differentiation. [D. F. Gleason (1920–), US pathologist]

Gleason score a numerical score from two to ten, which is the sum of the two *Gleason grades given to the most common and second most common pattern of prostate cancer seen in the tumor. [D. F. Gleason]

gleet *n.* a discharge of purulent mucus from the penis or vagina resulting from chronic *gonorrhea.

Gleevec *n. see* imatinib.

glenohumeral *adj.* relating to the glenoid

cavity and the humerus: the region of the shoulder joint.

glenoid cavity (glenoid fossa) the socket of the shoulder joint: the pear-shaped cavity at the top of the *scapula into which the head of the humerus fits.

gli- (glio-) *prefix denoting* **1.** glia. **2.** a glutinous substance.

glia (neuroglia) *n.* the special connective tissue of the central nervous system, composed of different cells, including the *oligodendrocytes, *astrocytes, ependymal cells (*see* ependyma), and *microglia, with various supportive and nutritive functions (see illustration). Glial cells outnumber the neurons by between five and ten to one, and make up some 40% of the total volume of the brain and spinal cord. —**glial** *adj.*

Ependymal cells

Protoplasmic astrocyte

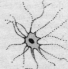

Fibrous astrocyte

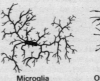

Microglia

Oligodendroglia

Types of glia

gliadin *n.* a protein, soluble in alcohol, that is obtained from wheat. It is one of the constituents of *gluten.

gliding joint *see* arthrodic joint.

glioblastoma (spongioblastoma) *n.* the

most aggressive type of brain tumor derived from non-nervous (glial) tissue (*see* astrocytoma). Its rapid enlargement destroys normal brain cells, with a progressive loss of function, and raises the intracranial pressure, causing headache, vomiting, and drowsiness. Treatment is rarely successful and prognosis is poor.

glioma *n.* any tumor of non-nervous cells (*glia) in the nervous system. The term is sometimes also used for all tumors that arise in the central nervous system, including *astrocytomas and *glioblastomas. Tumors of low-grade malignancy produce symptoms by pressure on surrounding structures; those of high-grade malignancy may be invasive.

gliosome *n.* a *lysosome in an *astrocyte.

glipizide *n.* a drug used to control high blood glucose levels (*hyperglycemia) in patients with noninsulin-dependent diabetes after diet control has failed. It stimulates release of insulin by the pancreas and thus is only effective if the beta cells of the islets of Langerhans are functional. It is administered by mouth; side effects are hypoglycemia, nausea and vomiting, and skin rash. Trade name: **Glucotrol.**

globin *n.* a protein, found in the body, that can combine with iron-containing groups to form *hemoglobin (found in red blood cells) and *myohemoglobin (found in muscle).

globulin *n.* one of a group of simple proteins that are soluble in dilute salt solutions and can be coagulated by heat. A range of different globulins is present in the blood (the *serum globulins*, including alpha (α), beta (β), and *gamma (γ) globulins). Some globulins have important functions as antibodies (*see* immunoglobulin); others are responsible for transport of lipids, iron, or copper in the blood. *See also* hormone-binding globulins.

globulinuria *n.* the presence of globulins in the urine.

globus *n.* a spherical or globe-shaped structure; for example the *globus pallidus*, part of the lenticular nucleus in the brain (*see* basal ganglia).

globus pharyngeus the sense of having a "lump in the throat," in the midline just above the sternum, that can neither be swallowed nor brought up. The condition, which was formerly called *globus*

hystericus, is sometimes related to *gastroesophageal reflux and tends to be worse during periods of stress. It is due to a constriction of the circularly placed muscles around the lower part of the pharynx.

glomangioma (glomus tumor) *n. see* glomus.

glomerular filtration rate (GFR) the rate at which substances are filtered from the blood of the glomeruli into the Bowman's capsules of the *nephrons. It is calculated by measuring the *clearance of specific substances (e.g. creatinine) and is an index of renal function.

glomerulitis *n.* any one of a variety of lesions of the glomeruli (*see* glomerulus) associated with acute or chronic kidney disease. Such lesions are recognized by electron microscopic examination, using immunofluorescent staining techniques, of kidney biopsy specimens taken during the course of the disease.

glomerulonephritis (glomerular nephritis) *n.* any of a group of kidney diseases involving the glomeruli (*see* glomerulus), usually thought to be the result of antibody–antigen reactions that localize in the kidneys because of their filtering function. *Acute nephritis* is marked by blood in the urine and fluid and urea retention. It may be related to a recent streptococcal throat infection and usually resolves completely, with rapid return of normal kidney function. Other forms of nephritis present with chronic *hematuria or with the *nephrotic syndrome; children often eventually recover completely, but adults are more likely to progress to *chronic nephritis* and eventual kidney failure.

glomerulus *n.* (*pl.* **glomeruli**) 1. the network of blood capillaries contained within the cuplike end (*Bowman's capsule*) of a *nephron. It is the site of primary filtration of waste products from the blood into the kidney tubule. 2. any other small rounded mass.

glomus *n.* (*pl.* **glomera**) a small communication between a tiny artery and vein in the skin of the limbs. It is concerned with the regulation of temperature.

glomus jugulare a collection of *paraganglion cells in close relation to the internal jugular vein at its origin at the base of the skull. It is a site of origin for *glomus tumors (*see also* paraganglioma).

glomus tumor 1. a benign tumor arising from *paraganglion cells of the vagus nerve in the neck (*see* paraganglioma). In the middle ear they are called *glomus tympanicum tumors*; around the jugular vein they are called *glomus jugulare tumors*. **2.** (**glomangioma**) a harmless but often painful tumor produced by the malformation and overgrowth of a *glomus, usually occurring in the skin at the ends of the fingers or toes. It may be cauterized or removed surgically.

gloss- (glosso-) *prefix denoting* the tongue. Examples: *glossopharyngeal* (relating to the tongue and pharynx); *glossoplasty* (plastic surgery of).

glossa *n. see* tongue.

glossectomy *n.* surgical removal of the tongue, an operation usually carried out for cancer in this structure.

Glossina *n. see* tsetse.

glossitis *n.* inflammation of the tongue. This can be caused by anemia, candidiasis, or vitamin deficiency. "Geographical tongue" is a benign glossitis characterized by areas of *erythema that change from day to day.

glossolalia *n.* nonsense speech that mimics normal speech in that it is appropriately formed into an imitation of syllables, words, and sentences. It can be uttered in *trance states and during sleep.

glossopharyngeal nerve the ninth *cranial nerve (IX), which supplies motor fibers to part of the pharynx and to the parotid salivary glands and sensory fibers to the posterior third of the tongue and the soft palate.

glossoplegia *n.* paralysis of the tongue.

glottis *n.* the space between the two *vocal cords. The term is often applied to the vocal cords themselves or to that part of the larynx associated with the production of sound.

gluc- (gluco-) *prefix denoting* glucose. Example: *glucosuria* (urinary excretion of).

glucagon *n.* a hormone, produced by the pancreas, that causes an increase in the blood sugar level and thus has an effect opposite to that of *insulin. Glucagon is administered by injection to counteract diabetic *hypoglycemia.

glucagonoma *n.* a pancreatic tumor that secretes glucagon and produces attacks of *hypoglycemia.

glucocorticoid *n. see* corticosteroid.

glucokinase *n.* an enzyme (a *hexokinase), found in the liver, that catalyzes the conversion of glucose to glucose-6-phosphate. This is the first stage of *glycolysis.

gluconeogenesis *n.* the biochemical process in which glucose, an important source of energy, is synthesized from noncarbohydrate sources, such as amino acids. Gluconeogenesis occurs mainly in the liver and kidney and meets the needs of the body for glucose when carbohydrate is not available in sufficient amounts in the diet.

glucosamine *n.* the amino sugar of glucose, i.e. glucose in which the hydroxyl group is replaced by an amino group. Glucosamine is a component of *mucopolysaccharides and *glycoproteins: for example, *hyaluronic acid, a mucopolysaccharide found in synovial fluid, and *heparin.

glucose (dextrose) *n.* a simple sugar containing six carbon atoms (a hexose). Glucose is an important source of energy in the body and the sole source of energy for the brain. Free glucose is not found in many foods (grapes are an exception); however, glucose is one of the constituents of both sucrose and starch, both of which yield glucose after digestion. Glucose is stored in the body in the form of *glycogen. The concentration of glucose in the blood is maintained at around 5 mmol/l by a variety of hormones, principally *insulin and *glucagon. If the blood glucose concentration falls below this level, neurological and other symptoms may result (*see* hypoglycemia). Conversely, if the blood glucose level is raised above its normal level, to 10 mmol/l, the condition of *hyperglycemia develops. This is a symptom of *diabetes mellitus.

glucose-6-phosphate dehydrogenase deficiency a hereditary (X-linked) condition in which the absence of the enzyme glucose-6-phosphate dehydrogenase (G6PD), which functions in carbohydrate metabolism, results in the breakdown of the red blood cells (*hemolysis), usually after exposure to *oxidants, such as drugs, or infections. The breakdown causes acute attacks that are characterized by pallor, loin pain, and rigors. There are several varieties of G6PD deficiency: African (which is sensitive to some antimalarial drugs), European (including *favism), and oriental. Treatment involves identifying and avoiding agents that trigger the hemolysis and treating acute attacks symptomatically.

glucose tolerance test a test used in the diagnosis of *diabetes mellitus and the related condition *impaired glucose tolerance* (IGT). After an overnight fast the blood-sugar level is measured (the fasting level). The patient is then given a drink containing 75 g glucose, and a further blood-sugar measurement is taken after two hours. Diabetes is diagnosed if the fasting level is above 7.0 mmol/l and/or the two-hour level is above 11.1 mmol/l. IGT is diagnosed when the fasting level is below 7.0 mmol/l and the two-hour level is between 7.0 mmol/l and 11.1 mmol/l. Many people with IGT progress to develop diabetes, but this can be prevented with adoption of a diabetic-type diet and weight loss (if overweight).

glucoside n. see glycoside.

glucosuria n. see glycosuria.

glucuronic acid a sugar acid derived from glucose. Glucuronic acid is an important constituent of *chondroitin sulfate (found in cartilage) and *hyaluronic acid (found in synovial fluid).

glue ear (secretory otitis media) see otitis.

glue sniffing inhalation of the fumes from plastic cements, which contain toluene, benzene, and other chemicals that stimulate the central nervous system, causing intoxication and dizziness. Prolonged accidental or occupational exposure or repeated recreational use may result in damage to various organ systems.

glutamate dehydrogenase (glutamic acid dehydrogenase) an important enzyme involved in the *deamination of amino acids.

glutamic acid (glutamate) see amino acid, neurotransmitter.

glutamic acid decarboxylase (GAD) a common enzyme that, because of similarities to certain bacterial proteins, can provoke an autoimmune reaction against the beta cells of the pancreas progressing to type 1 *diabetes mellitus.

glutamic oxaloacetic transaminase (GOT) see aspartate transaminase.

glutamic pyruvic transaminase (GPT) see alanine transaminase.

glutaminase n. an enzyme, found in the kidney, that catalyses the breakdown of

the amino acid glutamine to ammonia and glutamic acid: a stage in the production of urea.

glutamine n. see amino acid.

glutathione n. a peptide containing the amino acids glutamic acid, cysteine, and glycine. It functions as a *coenzyme in several oxidation-reduction reactions. Glutathione serves as an *antioxidant: it reacts with potentially harmful oxidizing agents and is itself oxidized (see also selenium). This is important in ensuring the proper functioning of proteins, hemoglobin, membrane lipids, etc. High levels of glutathione in the blood are associated with longevity.

glutelin n. one of a group of simple proteins found in plants and soluble only in dilute acids and bases. An example is *glutenin*, found in wheat (see gluten).

gluten n. a mixture of the two proteins *gliadin* and *glutenin*. Gluten is present in wheat and rye and is important for its baking properties: when mixed with water it becomes sticky and enables air to be trapped and dough to be formed. Sensitivity to gluten leads to *celiac disease in children.

glutethimide n. a drug used for the short-term treatment of insomnia and other sleep disturbances (see hypnotic). It is administered by mouth. Side effects can include nausea, mental excitement, and skin rashes. It has generally been replaced by safer and more effective treatment of insomnia.

gluteus n. one of three paired muscles of the buttocks (*gluteus maximus*, *gluteus medius*, and *gluteus minimus*). They are responsible for movements of the thigh. —**gluteal** adj.

glyburide n. a drug that lowers blood glucose in patients with noninsulin-dependent diabetes when the condition cannot be controlled by diet alone. Glyburide lowers blood sugar by stimulating the pancreas to secrete insulin and helping the body use insulin more efficiently. Side effects include nausea, heartburn, and skin reactions. Trade names: **Diabeta, Glynase, Micronase**.

glyc- (glyco-) prefix denoting sugar.

glycated hemoglobin see glycosylated hemoglobin.

glycation n. the chemical linkage of glucose to a protein, to form a glycoprotein. Glycation of body proteins has been postulated as a cause of complications of diabetes mellitus. *See* advanced glycation end products, glycosylated hemoglobin.

glyceride *n.* a *lipid consisting of glycerol (an alcohol) combined with one or more fatty acids. *See also* triglyceride.

glycerin (glycerol) *n.* a clear viscous liquid obtained by hydrolysis of fats and mixed oils and produced as a by-product in the manufacture of soap. It is used as an *emollient in many skin preparations, as a laxative (particularly in the form of *suppositories), and as a sweetening agent by the pharmaceutical industry.

glyceryl trinitrate *see* nitroglycerin.

glycine *n.* *see* amino acid.

glycobiology *n.* the study of the chemistry, biochemistry, and other aspects of carbohydrates and carbohydrate complexes, especially *glycoproteins. Elucidation of the structure and role of the sugar molecules of glycoproteins has important medical implications and has led to the development of new drugs, such as *tissue-type plasminogen activators, drugs that affect the immune system, antiviral drugs, and drugs used to treat *rheumatoid arthritis.

glycocholic acid *see* bile acids.

glycogen *n.* a carbohydrate consisting of branched chains of glucose units. Glycogen is the principal form in which carbohydrate is stored in the body: it is the counterpart of starch in plants. Glycogen is stored in the liver and muscles and may be readily broken down to glucose.

glycogenesis *n.* the biochemical process, occurring chiefly in the liver and in muscle, by which glucose is converted into glycogen.

glycogenolysis *n.* a biochemical process, occurring chiefly in the liver and in muscle, by which glycogen is broken down into glucose.

glycolipid *n.* a *lipid containing a sugar molecule (usually galactose or glucose). The *cerebrosides are examples of glycolipids.

glycolysis *n.* the conversion of glucose, by a series of ten enzyme-catalyzed reactions, to lactic acid. Glycolysis takes place in the cytoplasm of cells and the first nine reactions (converting glucose to pyruvate) form the first stage of cellular *respiration. The process involves the production of a small amount of energy (in the form of ATP), which is used for biochemical work. The final reaction of glycolysis (converting pyruvate to lactic acid) provides energy for short periods of time when oxygen consumption exceeds demand; for example, during bursts of intense muscular activity. *See also* lactic acid.

glycoprotein *n.* one of a group of compounds consisting of a protein combined with a carbohydrate (such as galactose or mannose). Examples of glycoproteins are certain enzymes, hormones, and antigens.

glycoside *n.* a compound formed by replacing the hydroxyl (–OH) group of a sugar by another group. (If the sugar is glucose the compound is known as a *glucoside*.) Glycosides found in plants include some pharmacologically important products (such as *digitalis). Other plant glycosides are natural food toxins, present in cassava, almonds, and other plant products, and may yield hydrogen cyanide if the plant is not prepared properly before eating.

glycosuria (glucosuria) *n.* the presence of glucose in the urine in abnormally large amounts. Only very minute quantities of this sugar may be found normally in the urine. Higher levels may be associated with diabetes mellitus, kidney disease, and some other conditions.

glycosylated hemoglobin (glycated hemoglobin) the standard marker of overall diabetes control over the preceding 2–3 months, based on the fact that glucose molecules will attach themselves permanently to hemoglobin molecules and the percentage of all the hemoglobin so affected can be measured in the blood. The higher the levels of blood sugar, the more hemoglobin molecules will have attached glucose molecules. As hemoglobin molecules have a lifespan of 2–3 months in the circulation, the percentage glycosylated gives an indication of the blood-sugar levels over this time period.

gnath- (gnatho-) *prefix denoting* the jaw. Example: *gnathoplasty* (plastic surgery of).

gnathion *n.* the lowest point of the midline of the lower jaw (mandible).

Gnathostoma *n.* a genus of parasitic nematodes. Adult worms are commonly found in the intestines of tigers, leopards, and dogs. The presence of the larval stage of *G. spinigerum* in humans, who are not the normal hosts, causes a skin condition called *creeping eruption.

gnotobiotic *adj.* describing germ-free conditions or a germ-free animal that has been inoculated with known microorganisms.

GnRH *see* gonadotropin-releasing hormone.

GnRH analogues *see* gonadotropin-releasing hormone, LHRH analogue.

goblet cell a column-shaped secretory cell found in the *epithelium of the respiratory and intestinal tracts. Goblet cells secrete the principal constituents of mucus.

goiter *n.* enlargement of the thyroid gland, which causes swelling of the neck. This may be due to lack of dietary iodine, which is necessary for the production of thyroid hormone: the gland enlarges in an attempt to increase the output of hormone. This was the cause of *endemic goiter,* formerly common in regions where the diet lacked iodine. *Sporadic goiter* may be due to simple overgrowth (hyperplasia) of the gland or to a tumor. In *exophthalmic goiter* (*Graves' disease*) the swelling is associated with overactivity of the gland and is accompanied by other symptoms (*see* thyrotoxicosis). Autoimmune thyroiditis can be associated with goiter (*see* Hashimoto's disease).

gold *n.* **1.** a bright yellow metal that is very malleable. In dentistry pure gold is occasionally used as a filling. Alloys are used for *crowns, *inlays, and *bridges, either alone or veneered with a tooth-colored material. Gold alloys are now only rarely used as the metal framework for partial dentures, *cobalt-chromium alloys being used instead. **2.** (in pharmacology) any of several compounds of the metal gold, used in the treatment of rheumatoid arthritis. It is administered by intramuscular injection (as *Myochrysine*) or orally (*see* auranofin). Common side effects (often occurring after treatment has stopped) include mouth ulcers, itching, blood disorders, skin reactions, and inflammation of the colon and kidneys.

Goldmann applanation tonometer *see* tonometer. [H. Goldmann (1899–1991), Swiss ophthalmologist]

golfer's elbow inflammation of the origin of the muscle on the inside of the elbow caused by overuse. Treatment is by rest, anti-inflammatory medication, or steroid injection. *Compare* tennis elbow.

Golgi apparatus a collection of vesicles and folded membranes in a cell, usually connected to the *endoplasmic reticulum. It stores and later transports the proteins manufactured in the endoplasmic reticulum. The Golgi apparatus is well developed in cells that produce secretions, e.g. pancreatic cells producing digestive enzymes. [C. Golgi (1844–1926), Italian histologist]

Golgi cells types of *neurons (nerve cells) within the central nervous system. *Golgi type I neurons* have very long axons that connect different parts of the system; *Golgi type II neurons,* also known as *microneurons,* have only short axons or sometimes none.

Golgi tendon organ *see* tendon organ.

Gomori's method a method of staining for the demonstration of enzymes, especially phosphatases and lipases, in histological specimens. [G. Gomori (1904–57), Hungarian histochemist]

gomphosis *n.* a form of *synarthrosis (immovable joint) in which a conical process fits into a socket. An example is the joint between the root of a tooth and the socket in the jawbone.

gonad *n.* a male or female reproductive organ that produces the gametes. *See* ovary, testis.

gonadarche *n.* the period during which the gonads begin to secrete sex hormones, so triggering puberty. The timing for this event is controlled by the pituitary gland; gonadarche occurs usually between the ages of 10 and 11 in girls and 11 and 12 in boys.

gonadorelin *n.* a synthetic analogue of gonadotropin-releasing hormone (*see* LHRH analogue), administered by intravenous injection to stimulate the production of pituitary gonadotropins. It is used in the treatment of *amenorrhea and certain types of infertility.

gonadotropin (gonadotropic hormone) *n.* any of several hormones synthesized and released by the pituitary gland that act on the testes or ovaries (gonads) to promote production of sex hormones and either sperm or ova. Their production is controlled by *gonadotropin-releasing hormone. The main gonadotropins are *follicle-stimulating hormone and *luteinizing hormone. They may be given by injection to treat infertility. *See also* chorionic gonadotropin.

gonadotropin-releasing hormone (GnRH) a peptide hormone produced in the hypothalamus and transported via the bloodstream to the pituitary gland, where it controls the synthesis and release of pituitary *gonadotropins. *GnRH analogues*, which are also known as *LHRH analogues, are used to treat endometriosis, fibroids, some types of infertility, and prostate cancer.

gonagra *n.* gout in the knee.

goni- (gonio-) *prefix denoting* an anatomical angle or corner.

goniometer *n.* an instrument for measuring angles, such as those made in joint movements.

gonion *n.* the point of the angle of the lower jawbone (mandible).

goniopuncture *n.* a rarely performed operation for congenital glaucoma (*see* buphthalmos) to enable fluid to be drawn from the eye.

gonioscope *n.* a special lens used for viewing the structures around the edge of the anterior chamber of the eye (in front of the iris). These structures are hidden behind the sclera at the edge of the cornea and are not accessible to direct viewing.

goniotomy (trabeculotomy) *n.* an operation for congenital glaucoma (*see* buphthalmos) in which a fine knife is used to make an incision into Schlemm's canal from within the eye. It is the first stage of *goniopuncture.

gonococcus *n.* (*pl.* **gonococci**) the causative agent of gonorrhea: the bacterium *Neisseria gonorrhoeae.* —**gonococcal** *adj.*

gonocyte *n. see* germ cell.

gonorrhea *n.* a sexually transmitted disease, caused by the bacterium *Neisseria gonorrhoeae*, that affects the genital mucous membranes of either sex. Symptoms develop about a week after infection and include pain on passing urine and discharge of pus (known as *gleet*) from the penis (in men) or vagina (in women); some infected women, however, experience no symptoms. If a pregnant woman has gonorrhea, her baby's eyes may become infected during passage through the birth canal (*see* ophthalmia neonatorum). In untreated cases, the infection may spread throughout the reproductive system, causing sterility; severe inflammation of the urethra in men can prevent passage of urine (a condition known as *stricture). Later complications include arthritis, inflammation of the heart valves (*endocarditis), and infection of the eyes, causing conjunctivitis. Treatment with ceftriaxone, doxycycline, or ciprofloxacin is usually effective.

gooseflesh the reaction of the skin to cold or fear. The blood vessels contract and the small muscle attached to the base of each hair follicle also contracts, causing the hairs to stand up: this gives the skin an appearance of plucked goose skin. Medical name: **cutis anserina**.

gorget *n.* an instrument formerly used in the operation for removal of stones from the bladder. It is a *director or guide with a wide groove.

goserelin *n.* an *LHRH analogue used in the treatment of advanced carcinoma of the prostate. The drug is implanted subcutaneously, with release over 28 days. Side effects include sexual dysfunction, decreased erections, and hot flushes. Trade name: **Zoladex**.

gouge *n.* a curved chisel used in orthopedic operations to cut and remove bone (see illustration).

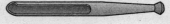

A gouge

goundou (anákhré) *n.* a condition following an infection with *yaws in which the nasal processes of the upper jaw bone thicken (*see* hyperostosis) to form two large bony swellings, about 7 cm in diameter, on either side of the nose. The swellings not only obstruct the nostrils but also interfere with the field of vision. Initial symptoms include persistent headache and a bloody purulent discharge from the nose. Early cases can be treated with injections of penicillin; otherwise surgical removal of the growths is necessary. Goundou occurs in central Africa and South America.

gout *n.* a disease in which a defect in purine metabolism causes an excess of uric acid and its salts (urates) to accumulate in the bloodstream and the joints. It results in attacks of acute gouty arthritis and chronic destruction of the joints and deposits of urates (*tophi*) in the skin and cartilage, especially of the ears. The excess of urates also damages the kidneys, in which stones may form. Treatment with drugs that increase the excretion of urates (*uricosuric drugs) or with *allopurinol, which slows their formation, can control the disease. Acute attacks of gout are treated with anti-inflammatory analgesics. *See also* podagra.

graafian follicle a mature follicle in the ovary prior to ovulation, containing a large fluid-filled cavity that distends the surface of the ovary. The *oocyte develops inside the follicle, attached to one side. [R. de Graaf (1641–73), Dutch physician and anatomist]

graded self-exposure a technique used in the *behavior therapy of phobias. A hierarchy of fears (increasingly fearful stimuli) is set up and the patients expose themselves to each level of the hierarchy in turn. Exposure continues until *habituation occurs before proceeding to the next highest level of the hierarchy. The patient is then ultimately able to cope with the feared object or situation.

graft 1. *n.* any organ, tissue, or object used for *transplantation to replace a faulty part of the body. A *skin graft is a piece of skin cut from a healthy part of the body and used to heal a damaged area of skin. A *bone graft* is healthy bone collected from the patient or from another person and used to fill a defect in a bone or as a stimulus to fracture healing. A healthy kidney removed from one person and transplanted to another individual is described as a *kidney* (or *renal*) *graft*. Corneal grafts are taken from a recently dead individual to repair corneal opacity (*see* keratoplasty). Diseased coronary arteries may be replaced by a *coronary bypass graft. Artificial grafts are used to replace diseased peripheral arteries and heart valves. **2.** *vb.* to transplant an organ or tissue. *See also* allograft, xenograft.

graft-versus-host disease (GVHD) a condition that occurs following bone marrow transplantation and sometimes blood transfusion, in which lymphocytes from the graft attack specific tissues in the host. The skin, gut, and liver are the most severely affected. Drugs that suppress the immune reaction, such as steroids and *cyclosporine, and antibodies directed against lymphocytes reduce the severity of the tissue damage.

grain *n.* a unit of mass equal to 1/7000 of a pound (avoirdupois). 1 grain = 0.0648 gram.

gram *n.* a unit of mass equal to one thousandth of a kilogram. Symbol: g.

-gram *suffix denoting* a record; tracing. Example: *electrocardiogram* (record of an electrocardiograph).

gramicidin *n.* an *antibiotic that acts against a wide range of bacteria. It is used in combination with other antibiotics or steroids in topical preparations for the treatment of skin, ear, and eye infections.

Gram's stain a method of staining bacterial cells, used as a primary means of identification. A film of bacteria spread onto a glass slide is dried and heat-fixed, stained with a violet dye, treated with decolorizer (e.g. alcohol), and then counterstained with red dye. *Gram-negative* bacteria lose the initial stain but take up the counterstain, so that they appear red microscopically. *Gram-positive* bacteria retain the initial stain, appearing violet microscopically. These staining differences are based on variations in the structure of the cell wall in the two groups. [H. C. J. Gram (1853–1938), Danish physician]

grand mal (major epilepsy) *see* epilepsy.

grand multiparity the condition of a woman who has had six or more previous pregnancies. Such women are more prone to the accidents of labor and to some of the diseases of pregnancy.

grants-in-aid funds that are distributed to state and local health agencies in the US by the federal government. The grants are authorized for stated purposes, such as training health personnel, building hospitals, or medical research. The federal funds often are allotted to states according to a formula that is based on the area's population, per capita income, and incidence of disease.

granular cast a cellular *cast derived from a kidney tubule. In certain kidney diseases, notably acute *glomerulonephritis, abnormal collections of renal tubular cells are shed from the kidney, often as a cast of the tubule. The casts can be observed on microscopic examination of the centrifuged deposit of a specimen of urine. Their presence in the urine indicates continued activity of the disease.

granulation *n.* the formation of a multicellular mass of tissue (*granulation tissue*) in response to an injury: this is an essential part of the healing process. Granulation tissue contains many new blood vessels and, in its later stages, large numbers of fibroblasts. The response is most frequently seen in healing open wounds and in the bases of ulcers.

granulocyte *n.* any of a group of white blood cells that, when stained with *Romanovsky stains, are seen to contain granules in their cytoplasm. They can be subclassified on the basis of the color of the stained granules into *neutrophils, *eosinophils, and *basophils.

granulocytopenia *n.* a reduction in the number of *granulocytes (a type of white cell) in the blood. *See* neutropenia.

granuloma *n.* (*pl.* **granulomas** or **granulomata**) a localized collection of cells produced in response to chronic infection, inflammation, a foreign body (e.g. starch, talc), or to unknown causes. It is characterized by the presence of epithelioid *histiocytes, giant cells, monocytes, or other lymphocytes; the types of cells comprising a granuloma (of which there may be many or few) and their arrangement can assist in diagnosing the cause of the response. Conditions giving rise to granulomas include syphilis, tuberculosis, *granuloma inguinale, leprosy, some fungal diseases (e.g. coccidioidomycosis), sarcoidosis, and Crohn's disease. A granuloma may also occur around the apex of a tooth root as a result of inflammation or infection of its pulp. —**granulomatous** *adj.*

granuloma annulare a chronic skin condition of unknown cause. In the common localized type there is a ring or rings of closely set papules, 1–5 cm in diameter, found principally on the hands and arms. If generalized, it may be associated with diabetes mellitus.

granuloma inguinale an infectious disease caused by the bacterium *Calymmatobacterium granulomatis*, transmitted during sexual intercourse. A pimply rash on and around the genital organs develops into a granulomatous ulcer. The disease responds to treatment with tetracyclines and streptomycin.

granulomatosis *n.* any condition marked by multiple widespread *granulomas. *See also* Wegener's granulomatosis.

granulopoiesis *n.* the process of production of *granulocytes, which normally occurs in the blood-forming tissue of the *bone marrow. Granulocytes are ultimately derived from a *hemopoietic stem cell, but the earliest precursor that can be identified microscopically is the *myeloblast. This divides and passes through a series of stages of maturation termed *promyelocyte, *myelocyte, and *metamyelocyte, before becoming a mature granulocyte. *See also* hemopoiesis.

graph- (grapho-) *prefix denoting* handwriting.

-graph *suffix denoting* an instrument that records. Example: *electrocardiograph* (instrument recording heart activity).

graphology *n.* the study of the characteristics of handwriting to obtain indications about a person's psychological makeup or state of health. It is possible to detect certain signs of physical disease, such as fine nervous tremors or irregularity of the pulse.

grattage *n.* the process of brushing or scraping the surface of a slowly healing ulcer or wound to stimulate healing. Grattage removes *granulation tissue, which – although a stage in the healing process – sometimes overgrows or becomes infected and therefore delays healing. Grattage is used in the treatment of *trachoma.

gravel *n.* small stones formed in the urinary tract. The stones usually consist of calcareous debris or aggregations of other crystalline material. The passage of gravel from the kidneys is usually associated with severe pain (*ureteric colic*) and may cause blood in the urine. *See also* calculus.

Graves' disease (exophthalmic goiter) *see* thyrotoxicosis. [R. J. Graves (1797–1853), Irish physician]

gravid *adj.* pregnant.

Grawitz tumor *see* hypernephroma. [P. A. Grawitz (1850–1932), German pathologist]

gray *n.* the *SI unit of absorbed dose of ionizing radiation, being the absorbed dose when the energy per unit mass imparted to matter by ionizing radiation is 1 joule per kilogram. It has replaced the rad. Symbol: Gy.

gray matter the darker colored tissues of

the central nervous system, composed mainly of the cell bodies of neurons, branching dendrites, and glial cells (*compare* white matter). In the brain gray matter forms the *cerebral cortex and the outer layer of the cerebellum; in the spinal cord the gray matter lies centrally and is surrounded by white matter.

gray scale (in radiology) a scale representing the possible gradient of densities from black to white for each *pixel in an image. In an *analogue image this gradient is smooth. A *digital image has many discrete steps. The more steps allowed, the closer to representing the true analogue image it comes, although more steps require more computer memory. Images can be manipulated by *windowing. This concept is particularly valuable in *computed tomography. *See* Hounsfield unit, digitization.

green monkey disease *see* Marburg disease.

greenstick fracture an incomplete break in a long bone in which part of the outer shell (cortex) remains intact. It occurs in children, who have more flexible bones. *See also* fracture.

Grey Turner's sign a bluish bruiselike appearance around the flanks, which is seen in acute *pancreatitis. [G. Grey Turner (1877–1951), British surgeon]

gripe *n.* severe abdominal pain (*see* colic).

grippe *n. see* influenza.

griseofulvin *n.* an *antibiotic administered by mouth to treat fungal infections of the hair, skin, and nails, such as ringworm. Mild and temporary side effects such as headache, skin rashes, and digestive upsets may occur. Trade names: **Fulvicin, Grifulvin V, Grisactin, Gris-PEG**.

groin *n.* the external depression on the front of the body that marks the junction of the abdomen with either of the thighs. *See also* inguinal.

ground substance the matrix of *connective tissue, in which various cells and fibers are embedded.

group practice a voluntary association of two or more doctors who agree to share common diagnostic and treatment facilities and to divide the income from the group practice in a designated manner. Members of a group practice may represent a single type of medical specialty or two or more different specialties. A dental group practice may consist of several dentists who use common facilities and share the income of the practice. The Mayo Clinic, established in the late 19th century, was the first multispecialty group practice in the US.

group therapy 1. (**group psychotherapy**) *psychotherapy involving at least two patients and a therapist. The patients are encouraged to understand and analyze their own and one another's problems. *See also* encounter group, psychodrama. **2.** therapy in which people with the same problem, such as *alcoholism, meet and discuss together their difficulties and possible ways of overcoming them.

growth factor any of various chemicals, particularly polypeptides, that have a variety of important roles in the stimulation of new cell growth and cell maintenance. They bind to the cell surface on receptors. Specific growth factors can cause new cell proliferation (*epidermal growth factor*, *hemopoietic growth factor*) and the migration of cells (*fibroblast growth factor*) and play a role in wound healing (*platelet-derived growth factor*; *PDGF*). Some growth factors act in the embryonic stage of development; for example, *nerve growth factor. It is thought that some growth factors that induce cell proliferation are involved in the abnormal regulation of growth seen in cancer when produced in excessive amounts (e.g. *insulin-like growth factor*, *IGF-I*). Growth factors produced locally around a carcinoma (e.g. *vascular endothelial growth factor*) are important in the encouragement of invasion by the tumor; other factors (e.g. autocrine motility factor, migration-stimulating factor) are also significant. *See also* bone growth factor.

growth hormone (GH, somatotropin) a hormone, synthesized and stored in the anterior pituitary gland, that promotes growth of the long bones in the limbs and increases protein synthesis (via *somatomedin). Its release is controlled by the opposing actions of *growth-hormone releasing factor* and *somatostatin. Excessive production of growth hormone results in *gigantism before puberty and *acromegaly in adults. Lack of growth hormone in children causes *dwarfism.

grumous *adj.* coarse; lumpy; clotted; often

used to describe the appearance of the center of wounds or diseased cells or the surface of a bacterial culture.

guaifenesin *n.* an *expectorant given by mouth to increase respiratory fluid secretions. It is also used in cough mixtures and tablets. There are no serious side effects. Trade names: **Anti-Tuss**, **Robitussin**.

guanethidine *n.* a drug that is used to reduce high blood pressure (*see* sympatholytic). It is administered by mouth; common side effects are diarrhea, faintness, and dizziness. Trade name: **Ismelin**.

guanfacine *n.* a drug used for the treatment of high blood pressure (hypertension). It is administered by mouth; common side effects include headache, dizziness, dry mouth, and constipation. Trade name: **Tenex**.

guanine *n.* one of the nitrogen-containing bases (*see* purine) that occurs in the nucleic acids DNA and RNA.

guanosine *n.* a compound containing guanine and the sugar ribose. *See also* nucleotide.

gubernaculum *n.* (*pl.* **gubernacula**) either of a pair of fibrous strands of tissue that connect the gonads to the inguinal region in the fetus. In the male they guide and possibly move the testes into the scrotum before birth. In the female the ovaries descend only slightly within the abdominal cavity and the gubernacula persist as the round ligaments, connecting the ovaries and uterus to the abdominal wall.

Guillain-Barré syndrome a disease of the peripheral nerves in which there is numbness and weakness in the limbs. It usually develops 10–20 days after a respiratory or gastrointestinal infection (commonly with *Campylobacter*) that provokes an allergic response in the peripheral nerves. A rapidly progressive form of the disease is called *Landry's paralysis* or *acute idiopathic polyneuritis*: paralysis starts in the hands and feet and ascends to the neck; involvement of the respiratory muscles may require mechanical ventilation. Recovery is usually excellent although often prolonged. Treatment with immunoglobulins or with plasma exchange may speed recovery and reduce long-term disability. *See* polyradiculitis. [G. Guillain (1876–1961)

and A. Barré (1880–1967), French neurologists]

guillotine *n.* **1.** a surgical instrument used for removing the tonsils. It is loop-shaped and contains a sliding knife blade (see illustration). **2.** an encircling suture to control the escape of fluid or blood from an orifice or to close a gap.

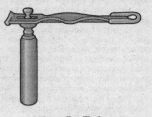

A tonsil guillotine

guinea worm a nematode worm, *Dracunculus medinensis*, that is a parasite of humans. The white threadlike adult female, 60–120 cm long, lives in the connective tissues beneath the skin. It releases its larvae into a large blister on the legs or arms; when the limbs are immersed in water the larvae escape and are subsequently eaten by tiny water fleas (*Cyclops*), in which their development continues. The disease *dracontiasis results from drinking water contaminated with *Cyclops*.

Gulf War syndrome a variety of symptoms, mainly neurological (including chronic fatigue, dizziness, amnesia, digestive upsets, and muscle wasting), that have been attributed to exposure of armed forces personnel to chemicals (e.g. insecticides) used during the Gulf War (1991) or possibly to the effects of vaccines and tablets given to protect personnel against the anticipated threat of chemical and biological warfare during the conflict. Medical research into the syndrome is continuing.

gullet *n.* *see* esophagus.

gum *n.* (in anatomy) *see* gingiva.

gumboil *n.* the opening on the surface of the gum of a *sinus tract from a chronic abscess associated with the roots of a tooth. It may be accompanied by varying degrees of swelling, pain, and discharge and is more often related to deciduous than to permanent teeth.

gumma n. a small soft tumor, characteristic of the tertiary stage of *syphilis, that occurs in connective tissue, the liver, brain, testes, heart, or bone.

gumshield n. a soft flexible cover that fits over the teeth for protection in contact sports. The best type is specially made to fit the individual.

gustation n. the sense of taste or the act of tasting.

gustatory adj. relating to the sense of taste or to the organs of taste.

gut n. **1.** see intestine. **2.** see catgut.

Guthrie test a blood test performed on all newborn infants at the end of the first week of life. The blood is obtained by pricking the heel of the baby. The test can detect several *inborn errors of metabolism (including *phenylketonuria) and *hypothyroidism; it can also be used for detecting *cystic fibrosis, although this is not routinely offered. [R. Guthrie (1916–), US pediatrician]

gutta n. (pl. **guttae**) (in pharmacy) a drop. Drops are the form in which medicines are applied to the eyes and ears.

gutta-percha the juice of an evergreen Malaysian tree, which is hard at room temperature but becomes soft and elastic when heated in boiling water. On cooling, gutta-percha will retain any deformity imparted to it when hot; thus it was used in dentistry as an impression material and as a temporary filling material. It has been superseded for these purposes by better materials but is still used as the principal core of *root fillings.

guttate adj. describing lesions in the skin that are shaped like drops.

GVHD see graft-versus-host disease.

gyn- (gyno-, gynec(o)-) prefix denoting women or the female reproductive organs.

gynecology n. the study of diseases of the genital tract in women and girls. Compare obstetrics. —**gynecological** adj. —**gynecologist** n.

gynecomastia n. enlargement of the breasts in the male, due either to hormone imbalance or to hormone therapy. Treatment is by removal of excess glandular material or with such drugs as *dihydrotestosterone, *danazol, or *clomiphene. Spontaneous regression often occurs.

gypsum n. see plaster of Paris.

gyr- (gyro-) prefix denoting **1.** a gyrus. **2.** a ring or circle.

gyrate atrophy a hereditary condition causing night blindness and constricted visual fields, usually developing in the third decade of life. Clinically it is characterized by a progressive atrophy of the choroid and retina.

gyrus n. (pl. **gyri**) a raised convolution of the *cerebral cortex, between two sulci (clefts).

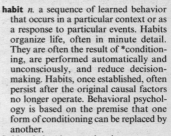

habit n. a sequence of learned behavior that occurs in a particular context or as a response to particular events. Habits organize life, often in minute detail. They are often the result of *conditioning, are performed automatically and unconsciously, and reduce decision-making. Habits, once established, often persist after the original causal factors no longer operate. Behavioral psychology is based on the premise that one form of conditioning can be replaced by another.

habitual abortion see abortion.

habituation n. **1.** (in psychology) a simple type of learning consisting of a gradual waning response by the subject to a continuous or repeated stimulus that is not associated with *reinforcement. **2.** (in pharmacology) the condition of being psychologically dependent on a drug, following repeated consumption, characterized by reduced sensitivity to its effects and a craving for the drug if it is withdrawn. See also dependence.

habitus n. an individual's general physical appearance, especially when this is associated with a constitutional tendency to a particular disease.

Haemaphysalis n. a genus of hard *ticks. Certain species transmit tick *typhus in the Old World; H. spinigera transmits the virus causing *Kyasanur Forest disease in India.

Haemophilus n. a genus of gram-negative aerobic nonmotile parasitic rodlike bacteria frequently found in the respiratory tract. They can grow only in the presence of certain factors in the blood and/or certain coenzymes: they are cultured on fresh blood *agar. Most species are pathogenic: *H. aegyptius* causes conjunctivitis, and *H. ducreyi*, soft sore (chancroid). *H. influenzae* is associated with acute and chronic respiratory infections and is a common secondary cause of *influenza infections; *H. influenzae* type B is an important cause of bacterial *meningitis in young children (*see* Hib vaccine).

hair *n.* a threadlike keratinized outgrowth of the epidermis of the *skin. It develops inside a tubular *hair follicle*. The part above the skin consists of three layers: an outer *cuticle*; a *cortex*, forming the bulk of the hair and containing the pigment that gives the hair its color; and a central core (*medulla*), which may be hollow. The *root* of the hair, beneath the surface of the skin, is expanded at its base to form the *bulb*, which contains a matrix of dividing cells. As new cells are formed the older ones are pushed upward and become keratinized to form the root and shaft. A hair may be raised by a small erector muscle in the dermis, attached to the hair follicle.

hairball *n. see* trichobezoar.

hair follicle a sheath of epidermal cells and connective tissue that surrounds the root of a *hair.

hair papilla a projection of the dermis that is surrounded by the base of the hair bulb. It contains the capillaries that supply blood to the growing *hair.

hairy cell an abnormal white blood cell that has the appearance of an immature lymphocyte with fine hairlike cytoplasmic projections around the perimeter of the cell. It is found in a rare form of leukemia (*hairy cell leukemia*) most commonly occurring in young men.

half-life *n.* **1.** the period of time required for the radioactivity or the number of atoms of a radioactive substance to decrease by half. The term is generally applied to any substance whose quantity decreases exponentially with time. **2.** (**biological half-life**) (in pharmacy) the time required for the body to eliminate one-half of an administered dose of any substance by means of regular physiological processes. **3.** (**effective half-life**) (in radiotherapy) the time required for a radioactive substance in the body to be reduced by one-half as a result of the combined action of radioactive decay and biological elimination.

halfway house a residential home for a group of people where some professional supervision is available. It is used as a stage in the rehabilitation of the mentally ill, usually when they have just been discharged from the hospital and are able to work but are not yet ready for independent life.

halitosis *n.* bad breath. Causes of temporary halitosis include recently eaten strongly flavored food, such as garlic or onions, and drugs such as paraldehyde. Other causes include mouth breathing, *periodontal disease, and infective conditions of the nose, throat, and lungs (especially *bronchiectasis). Constipation, indigestion, and some liver diseases may also cause the condition.

hallucination *n.* a false perception of something that is not really there. Hallucinations may be visual, auditory, tactile, gustatory (of taste), or olfactory (of smell). They may be provoked by psychological illness (such as *schizophrenia) or physical disorders in the brain (such as temporal lobe *epilepsy or stroke) or they may be caused by drugs or sensory deprivation. Hallucinations should be distinguished from dreams and from *illusions (since they occur at the same time as real perceptions and are not based on real stimuli).

hallucinogen *n.* a drug that produces hallucinations, e.g. *cannabis and *lysergic acid diethylamide. Hallucinogens were formerly used in the treatment of certain types of mental illness. —**hallucinogenic** *adj.*

hallux *n.* (*pl.* **halluces**) the big toe.

hallux rigidus painful stiffness of the metatarsophalangeal joint, between the big toe and the first metatarsal bone, usually resulting from osteoarthritis. Conservative treatment is often successful, but in some cases *arthrodesis or *arthroplasty is required.

hallux valgus displacement of the big toe toward the others. It is often associated with a *bunion.

hallux varus displacement of the big toe away from the others.

halo *n.* a colored ring seen around a light by people with acute congestive glaucoma and sometimes by people with cataract.

haloperidol *n.* a *butyrophenone antipsychotic drug used to relieve anxiety and tension in the treatment of schizophrenia and other psychiatric disorders. It is administered by mouth or injection; muscular incoordination and restlessness are common side effects. Trade name: **Haldol**.

halophilic *adj.* requiring solutions of high salt concentration for healthy growth. Certain bacteria are halophilic. —**halophile** *n.*

haloprogin *n.* a synthetic topical antifungal agent used in the treatment of various forms of *ringworm, primarily athlete's foot (tinea pedis). Among the most serious side effects are local irritation, a burning sensation, and vesicle formation. Trade name: **Halotex**.

halothane *n.* a potent general *anesthetic administered by inhalation, used for inducing and maintaining anesthesia in all types of surgical operations. Reduced blood pressure and irregular heartbeat may occur during halothane anesthesia, and it may cause liver damage and is therefore less widely used now than formerly. Trade name: **Fluothane**.

hamartoma *n.* an overgrowth of mature tissue in which the elements show disordered arrangement and proportion in comparison to normal. The overgrowth is benign but malignancy may occur in any of the constituent tissue elements.

hamate bone (unciform bone) a hook-shaped bone of the wrist (*see* carpus). It articulates with the capitate and triquetral bones at the sides, with the lunate bone behind, and with the fourth and fifth metacarpal bones in front.

hammer *n.* (in anatomy) *see* malleus.

hammer toe a deformity of a toe, most often the second, caused by fixed flexion of the first joint. A corn often forms over the deformity, which may be painful. If severe pain does not respond to strapping or corrective footwear, it may be necessary to perform *arthrodesis at the affected joint.

hamstring *n.* any of the tendons at the back of the knee. They attach the *hamstring muscles* (the biceps femoris, semitendinosus, and semimembranosus) to their insertions on the tibia and fibula.

hamulus *n.* (*pl.* **hamuli**) any hooklike _process, such as occurs on the hamate, lacrimal, and sphenoid bones and on the cochlea.

hand *n.* the terminal organ of the upper limb. The human hand comprises the eight bones of the *carpus (wrist), the five metacarpal bones, and the phalangeal bones plus the surrounding tissues; anatomically, the bones and tissues of the wrist are excluded. The hand is a common site of infections and injuries.

handedness *n.* the preferential use of one hand, rather than the other, in voluntary actions. Ambidexterity – the ability to use either hand with equal skill – is rare. About 90% of people are right-handed and this correlates with the half of the brain that is dominant for speech: some 97% of right-handed people have left-hemisphere dominance for speech, whereas only 60% of left-handed people are right-hemisphere dominant for speech.

hand, foot, and mouth disease a self-limiting disease, mainly affecting young children, caused by *coxsackievirus A16. A feeling of mild illness is accompanied by mouth ulcers and blisters on the hands and feet.

handicap *n.* **1.** partial or total inability to perform a social, occupational, or other activity. It reflects the extent to which an individual is disadvantaged by some partial or total *disability* when compared with those in a peer group who have no such disability. A handicap is usually related to an identifiable structural *impairment*, often based on a range of two standard deviations from the *mean observation obtained from studying a large number of apparently healthy subjects. It may also reflect functional impairment, which may be unsuspected by the individual and discovered by clinical observation or testing. The alternative terms *abnormality*, *defect*, or *malformation* (for impairment) and *malfunction* (for disability) are used by many authorities but this may sometimes cause confusion. *See also* Americans with Disabilities Act (1990), International Classification of Diseases. **2.** *see* mental handicap.

Hand-Schüller-Christian disease *see* Langerhans cell histiocytosis. [A. Hand (1868–1949), US pediatrician; A. Schüller (1874–1958), Austrian neurologist; H. A. Christian (1876–1951), US physician]

Hansen's bacillus *see* Mycobacterium. [G.

H. A. Hansen (1841–1912), Norwegian physician]

Hansen's disease *see* leprosy. [G. H. A. Hansen]

hantavirus *n.* one of a genus of viruses that infect rats, mice, and voles and cause disease in humans when the secretions or excreta of these rodents are inhaled or ingested. The disease was first reported from the area of the Hantaan river, which separates North from South Korea, but hantavirus infections also occur in Japan, China, Russia, Europe, and the USA. The symptoms vary according to the strain of the infecting virus. Many patients have a mild influenza-like illness, but severe cases are characterized by high fever, headache, shock, nausea and vomiting, and *petechiae in the skin; there may be kidney pain and rapidly progressive kidney damage leading to kidney failure. A particularly virulent strain in the USA attacks the lungs, leading to rapid respiratory failure. The mortality rate in these severe cases is high.

haploid (monoploid) *adj.* describing cells, nuclei, or organisms with a single set of unpaired chromosomes. In humans the gametes are haploid following *meiosis. *Compare* diploid, triploid. —**haploid** *n.*

haplotype *n.* a complete set of HLA antigens (*see* HLA system) inherited from either parent.

happy puppet syndrome *see* Angelman's syndrome.

hapt- (hapto-) *prefix denoting* touch.

hapten *n.* a nonprotein substance that when bonded to a *carrier protein can induce the formation of antibodies. *See also* antigen.

haptoglobin *n.* a protein present in blood plasma that binds with free hemoglobin to form a complex that is rapidly removed from the circulation by the liver. Depletion of plasma haptoglobin is a feature of anemias in which red blood cells are destroyed inside the circulation with the release of hemoglobin into the plasma and loss in the urine.

harara *n.* a severe and itchy inflammation of the skin occurring in people continuously subjected to the bites of the *sandfly *Phlebotomus papatasii.* The incidence of this allergic skin reaction, prevalent in the Middle East, may be checked by controlling the numbers of sandflies.

harelip *n. see* cleft lip.

Harrison Antinarcotic Act a US federal law restricting the use of dangerous drugs. These controlled drugs include the natural *opiates and their synthetic substitutes, many stimulants (including amphetamine, cocaine, and pemoline) hallucinogens such as LSD and cannabis, and the sedative methaqualone. The law specifies certain requirements for writing prescriptions for these drugs.

Harrison's sulcus a depression on both sides of the chest wall of a child between the pectoral muscles and the lower margin of the ribcage. It is caused by exaggerated suction of the diaphragm when breathing in and develops in conditions in which the airways are partially obstructed (e.g. poorly treated asthma) or when the lungs are abnormally congested due to some congenital abnormality of the heart. [E. Harrison (1789–1838), British physician]

Hartmann's operation (Hartmann's procedure) a method of reconstruction after surgical removal of distal colon and proximal rectum, in which the rectal stump is closed off and the divided end of the colon is brought out as a *colostomy. The technique allows for second-stage joining up of the bowel ends with no colostomy. [H. Hartmann (1860–1952), French surgeon]

Hartmann's pouch a saclike dilation of the gallbladder wall near its outlet; it is a common site for finding *gallstones. [H. Hartmann]

Hartmann's solution (lactated Ringer's solution) a *physiological solution used for infusion into the circulation. In addition to essential ions, it also contains glucose. [A. F. Hartmann (1898–1964) US pediatrician]

Hartnup disease a rare hereditary defect in the absorption of the amino acid tryptophan, leading to mental retardation, thickening and roughening of the skin on exposure to light, and lack of muscular coordination. The condition is similar to *pellagra, and treatment with nicotinamide is usually effective. [Hartnup, the family in whom it was first reported]

harvest mite *see* Trombicula.

Hashimoto's disease chronic inflammation of the thyroid gland (*thyroiditis*) due t the formation of antibodies against normal thyroid tissue (autoantibodies; *see* thyroid antibodies). Its features include a firm swelling of the thyroid and partial or total failure of secretion of thyroid hormones; often there are autoantibodies to other organs, such as the stomach. Women are more often affected than men, and the condition often occurs in families. [H. Hashimoto (1881–1934), Japanese surgeon]

hashish *n. see* cannabis.

haustrum *n.* one of the pouches on the external surface of the *colon.

Haversian canal one of the small canals (diameter about 50 μm) that ramify throughout compact *bone. *See also* Haversian system. [C. Havers (1650–1702), English anatomist]

Haversian system one of the cylindrical units of which compact *bone is made. A *Haversian canal* forms a central tube, around which are alternate layers of bone matrix (*lamellae*) and *lacunae* containing bone cells. The lacunae are linked by minute channels (*canaliculi*). [C. Havers]

hay fever a form of *allergy due to the pollen of grasses, trees, and other plants, characterized by inflammation of the membrane lining the nose and sometimes of the conjunctiva (*vernal conjunctivitis*). The symptoms of sneezing, running or blocked nose, and watering eyes are due to histamine release and often respond to treatment with *antihistamines. If the allergen is identified, it may be possible to undertake *desensitization or remove it from the environment. Medical name: **allergic rhinitis**.

hCG *see* chorionic gonadotropin.

head *n.* **1.** the part of the body that contains the brain and the organs of sight, hearing, smell, and taste. **2.** the rounded portion of a bone, which fits into a groove of another to form a joint; for example, the head of the humerus or femur.

headache *n.* pain felt deep within the skull or in the forehead, temple area, or base of the skull. Most headaches are caused by emotional stress or fatigue but some are symptoms of serious intracranial disease. *See also* cluster headache, migraine.

headgear *n.* (in dentistry) a strap that is fixed round the back of the head and/or the neck and attached to an *orthodontic appliance to aid tooth movement. It is normally worn at night and for part of the day.

head injury an injury usually resulting from a blow to the head and often associated with brain injury. It may result in *contusion or – if the blood vessels in the head are torn – a *hematoma. The level of consciousness of a patient following a head injury can be assessed using the *Glasgow coma scale. Head injuries are an important cause of death due to accidents: legislation to impose protective headgear at industrial sites and on construction workers, motorcyclists, and bicyclists has reduced their incidence.

head-tilt, chin-lift technique a maneuver for opening the airway of an unconscious patient. With the patient lying on his or her back, the neck is extended and the chin simultaneously pulled gently upward to pull the tongue away from the back of the pharynx. This method is often used when mouth-to-mouth respiration is to be given and is an alternative to the *jaw thrust maneuver.

Heaf test a skin test to determine whether or not an individual is immune to tuberculosis. A spring-loaded gun mounted with very short needles produces a circle of six punctures in the forearm through which *tuberculin is introduced. If the test is positive a reaction causes the skin to become red and raised, indicating that the individual is immune. If the test is negative a vaccine (*BCG) should be given. [F. R. G. Heaf (20th century), British physician]

health education persuasive methods used to encourage people (either individually or collectively) to adopt life styles that the educators believe will improve health and to reject habits regarded as harmful to health or likely to shorten life expectancy. The term is also used in a broader sense to include instruction about bodily function, etc., so that the public is better informed about health issues.

Health Interview Survey a system used by the US Public Health Service for collecting health-related data on a regular periodic basis. Interviewers visit homes throughout the nation to question household members about illnesses, disabilities, and utilization of available health services.

Health Maintenance Organization (HMO) a type of prepaid group medical practice with a defined and restricted patient population. Each enrolled patient pays a fixed fee regardless of the amount of physician services used. The HMO physicians assume responsibility for the health care of the enrolled members and provide a wide range of inpatient and outpatient medical services. Part of an HMO agreement with enrolled patients may be a provision that the HMO will absorb the cost of hospitalization when required for further treatment, with the result that HMO physicians tend to recommend hospitalization for patients only when actually necessary.

Health Systems Agency (HSA) a local group of consumers and government leaders empowered by the US federal government to oversee the quality and quantity of health-care services provided in a local area with funds supplied by the federal government under *Medicare and *Medicaid. Attention of HSA members generally is directed toward effectiveness of federally subsidized health care offered to the aged and the poor. The *Social Security Act amendment authorizing the formation of HSAs requires that the consumer-dominated HSAs coordinate their activities with the physician-controlled *Professional Standards Review Organizations.

hearing aid a device to improve the hearing. An *analogue hearing aid* consists of a miniature microphone, an amplifier, and a tiny loudspeaker. The aid is powered by a battery and the whole unit is small enough to fit behind or within the ear inconspicuously. If necessary, aids can be built into the frames of glasses. In a few cases of conductive hearing loss the loudspeaker is replaced by a vibrator that presses on the bone behind the ear and transmits the sound energy through the bones of the skull to the inner ear. *Digital hearing aids* are in some respects similar to analogue aids but in addition to the microphone, amplifier, and loudspeaker, they have digital-to-analogue converters and a tiny computer built into the casing of the aid. This enables the aid to be programmed to the patient's particular requirements and generally offers improved sound quality. *See also* bone-anchored hearing aid, cochlear implant, environmental hearing aid, implantable hearing aid.

heart *n.* a hollow muscular cone-shaped organ, lying between the lungs, with the pointed end (*apex*) directed downward, forward, and to the left. The heart is about the size of a closed fist. Its wall consists largely of *cardiac muscle (myocardium), lined and surrounded by membranes (*see* endocardium, pericardium). It is divided by a *septum* into separate right and left halves, each of which is divided into an upper *atrium

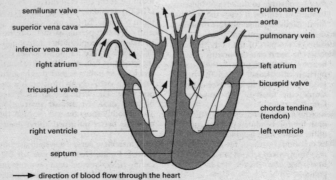

semilunar valve — pulmonary artery
superior vena cava — aorta
inferior vena cava — pulmonary vein
right atrium — left atrium
tricuspid valve — bicuspid valve
chorda tendina (tendon)
right ventricle — left ventricle
septum

➤ direction of blood flow through the heart

Vertical section through the heart

and a lower *ventricle (see illustration). Deoxygenated blood from the *venae cavae passes through the right atrium to the right ventricle. This contracts and pumps blood to the lungs via the *pulmonary artery. The newly oxygenated blood returns to the left atrium via the pulmonary veins and passes through to the left ventricle. This forcefully contracts, pumping blood out to the body via the *aorta. The direction of blood flow within the heart is controlled by *valves.

heart attack *see* myocardial infarction.

heart block a condition in which conduction of the electrical impulses generated by the natural pacemaker of the heart (the *sinoatrial node) is impaired, so that the pumping action of the heart is slowed down. In *partial* or *incomplete heart block* conduction between atria and ventricles is delayed (*first degree heart block*) or not all the impulses are conducted from the atria to the ventricles (*second degree heart block*). In *third degree* or *complete heart block* no impulses are conducted and the ventricles beat at their own slow intrinsic rate (20–40 per minute).

Heart block may be congenital or it may be due to heart disease, including myocardial infarction, myocarditis, cardiomyopathy, and disease of the valves. It is most frequently seen in the elderly as the result of chronic degenerative scarring around the conducting tissue. There may be no symptoms, but when very slow heart and pulse rates occur the patient may develop heart failure or *Stokes-Adams syndrome. Symptoms may be abolished by the use of an artificial *pacemaker.

heartburn (pyrosis) *n.* discomfort or pain, usually burning in character, that is felt behind the breastbone and often appears to rise from the abdomen toward or into the throat. It may be accompanied by the appearance of acid or bitter fluid in the mouth and is usually caused by regurgitation of stomach contents into the gullet or by *esophagitis.

heart failure a condition in which the pumping action of the ventricle of the heart is inadequate. This results in back pressure of blood, with congestion of the lungs and liver. The veins in the neck becomed engorged and fluid accumu-

lates in the tissues (*see* edema). There is a reduced flow of arterial blood from the heart, which in extreme cases results in peripheral circulatory failure (cardiogenic shock). Heart failure may result from any condition that overloads, damages, or reduces the efficiency of the heart muscle. Common causes are coronary thrombosis, hypertension, chronic disease of the valves, and arrhythmias. The patient experiences breathlessness, even when lying flat, and edema of the legs.

Treatment consists of rest, a low salt diet, diuretic drugs (e.g. furosemide), and digitalis derivatives (e.g. digoxin). Structural abnormalities, such as defective valves, may be corrected surgically.

heart-lung machine an apparatus for taking over temporarily the functions of both the heart and the lungs during heart surgery. It incorporates a pump, to maintain the circulation, and equipment to oxygenate the blood. Blood is taken from the body by tubes inserted into the superior and inferior venae cavae, and the oxygenated blood is returned under pressure into a large artery, such as the femoral artery. The surgeon is therefore able to undertake the repair or replacement of heart valves or perform other surgical operations involving the heart and great blood vessels.

heat exhaustion fatigue and collapse due to the low blood pressure and blood volume that result from loss of body fluids and salts after prolonged or unaccustomed exposure to heat. It is most common in new arrivals in a hot climate and is treated by giving drinks or intravenous injections of salted water.

heatstroke (sunstroke) *n.* raised body temperature (pyrexia), absence of sweating, and eventual loss of consciousness due to failure or exhaustion of the temperature-regulating mechanism of the body. It is potentially fatal unless treated immediately: the body should be cooled by applying damp cloths and body fluids restored by giving drinks or intravenous injections of salted water.

hebephrenia *n.* a form of *schizophrenia. It is typically a chronic condition, and the most prominent features are disordered thinking; inappropriate emotions with thoughtless cheerfulness, apathy, or querulousness; and silly behavior. It typically starts in adolescence or young adulthood. Social and occupational rehabilitation are the most important therapies for most patients; drugs such as the *phenothiazines or *butyrophenones can also help. —**hebephrenic** *adj.*

Heberden's node a bony thickening arising at the terminal joint of a finger in *osteoarthritis. It is often inherited. [W. Heberden (1710–1801), British physician]

hebetude *n.* apathy and emotional dullness. This is not a symptom specific to any one condition; extreme degrees are found in *schizophrenia and *dementia.

hebiatrics *n. see* ephebiatrics.

hectic *adj.* occurring regularly. A *hectic fever* typically develops in the afternoons, in cases of pulmonary tuberculosis.

hecto- *prefix denoting* a hundred.

heel *n.* the part of the foot that extends behind the ankle joint, formed by the *heel bone* (*see* calcaneus).

Hegar's sign an indication of pregnancy detectable between the 6th and 12th weeks: used before modern urine tests for pregnancy were available. If the fingers of one hand are inserted into the vagina and those of the other are placed over the pelvic cavity, the lower part of the uterus feels very soft compared with the body of the uterus above and the cervix below. [A. Hegar (1830–1914), German gynecologist]

Heimlich maneuver a method of forcing out food or some other substance that has entered the trachea instead of the esophagus. While standing behind and placing his arms around the choking subject, a person makes a fist with one hand and covers it with the other hand. He then abruptly and forcibly thrusts the fist with an upward movement into the subject's abdomen above the navel. This forces air out of the lungs and pushes the object out. The maneuver may have to be repeated. Although lifesaving, it carries the risk of causing damage to the aorta. [H. J. Heimlich (1920–   ), US surgeon]

helc- (helco-) *prefix denoting* an ulcer.

helical CT scanning *see* spiral CT scanning.

Helicobacter *n.* a genus of spiral flagellated gram-negative bacteria. The species *H. pylori* (formerly classified as *Campylobacter pylori*) is found in the stomach within the mucous layer. It occurs in the majority of middle-aged people and causes progressive gastritis. It is almost invariably present in duodenal ulceration and usually in gastric ulceration. Eradication of the organism (using various combinations of antibiotics and antisecretory drugs) leads to healing of the ulcer. *H. pylori* has also been implicated in some forms of stomach cancer and in heart disease.

helicotrema *n.* the narrow opening between the scala vestibuli and the scala tympani at the tip of the *cochlea in the ear.

helio- *prefix denoting* the sun.

heliotherapy *n.* the use of sunlight to promote healing; sunbathing.

helix *n.* the outer curved fleshy ridge of the *pinna of the outer ear.

Heller's operation *see* achalasia. [E. Heller (1877–1964), Austrian pathologist]

Heller's syndrome (disintegrative psychosis) a rare mental illness of childhood. Abnormalities of behavior may be the only sign at first but the condition progresses to psychotic manifestations, such as *stereotypies and hallucinations, and ultimately to dementia. Nearly always a physical cause can be found. The illness progresses to severe incapacity or death. [T. Heller (20th century)]

Heller's test a test for the presence of protein (albumin) in the urine. A quantity of urine is carefully poured onto the same quantity of pure nitric acid in a test tube. A white ring forms at the junction of the liquids if albumin is present. However, a similar result may be obtained if the urine contains certain drugs or is very concentrated. A dark brown ring indicates the presence of an abnormally high level of potassium indoxyl sulfate in the urine (*see* indicanuria). [J. F. Heller (1813–71), Austrian pathologist]

HELLP syndrome a form of severe *preeclampsia affecting many body systems and characterized by *h*emolysis, elevated *l*iver enzymes, and a *low platelet* count (hence the name). It constitutes an emergency requiring prompt termination of the pregnancy.

Helly's fluid a mixture of potassium dichromate, sodium sulfate, mercuric chloride, formaldehyde, and distilled water, used in the preservation of bone marrow. [K. Helly (20th century), Swiss pathologist]

helminth *n.* any of the various parasitic worms, including the *flukes, *tapeworms, and *nematodes.

helminthiasis *n.* the diseased condition resulting from an infestation with parasitic worms (helminths).

helminthology *n.* the study of parasitic worms.

heloma *n.* a *callosity or *corn on the foot or hand.

helper T cell a type of T *lymphocyte that plays a key role in cell-mediated immunity by recognizing foreign antigen on the surface of antigen-presenting cells (*see* APC) when this is associated with the individual's *MHC antigens, having been processed by antigen-presenting cells. Helper T cells stimulate the production of *cytotoxic T cells, which destroy the target cells.

hem- (hema-, hemo-, hemat(o)-) *prefix denoting* blood. Examples: *hematogenesis* (formation of); *hemophobia* (fear of).

hemagglutination *n.* the clumping of red blood cells (*see* agglutination). It is caused by an antibody–antigen reaction or some viruses and other substances.

hemangioblastoma (Lindau's tumor) *n.* a tumor of the brain or spinal cord arising in the blood vessels of the meninges or brain. It is often associated with pheochromocytoma and syringomyelia. *See also* von Hippel-Lindau disease.

hemangioma *n.* a benign tumor of blood vessels. It often appears on the skin as a type of birthmark (*see* nevus). For example, a *strawberry hemangioma* is seen in newborn babies and infants, usually on the face; it is red and may attain a very large size, but usually disappears spontaneously within the first year of life. For those that do not regress, treatment is with corticosteroids, cryotherapy, and surgery. *Senile hemangiomas* occur in the elderly. *See also* angioma.

hemarthrosis *n.* joint pain and swelling caused by bleeding into a joint. This may follow injury or may occur spontaneously in a disease of the blood, such as *hemophilia. Treatment is by immobilization, cold compresses, and correction of the blood disorder (if present). Removal of blood from the joint may relieve the pain.

hematemesis *n.* the act of vomiting blood.

The blood may have been swallowed (e.g. following nosebleed or tonsillectomy) but more often arises from bleeding in the esophagus, stomach, or duodenum. Common causes are gastric and duodenal ulcers and varicose veins in the esophagus. If much blood is lost, it is usually replaced by blood transfusion. If bleeding does not stop spontaneously it may be arrested by coagulation of the bleeding point using either a *laser or by the injection of epinephrine or a sclerosing material: all these techniques are applied through an *endoscope. *See also* melena.

hematidrosis (hemathidrosis) *n. see* hematohidrosis.

hematin *n.* a chemical derivative of *hemoglobin formed by removal of the protein part of the molecule and oxidation of the iron atom from the ferrous to the ferric form.

hematinic *n.* a drug that increases the amount of *hemoglobin in the blood, e.g. ferrous sulfate and other iron compounds. Hematinics are used, often in combination with vitamins and *folic acid, to prevent and treat anemia due to iron deficiency. They are used particularly to prevent anemia during pregnancy. Digestive disturbances sometimes occur with hematinics.

hematocele *n.* a swelling caused by leakage of blood into a cavity, especially that of the membrane overlying the front and sides of the testis. A *parametric (pelvic) hematocele* is a swelling near the uterus formed by the escape of blood, usually from a fallopian tube in ectopic pregnancy.

hematocolpos *n.* the accumulation of menstrual blood in the vagina because the hymen at the entrance to the vagina lacks an opening. *See* cryptomenorrhea.

hematocrit *n. see* packed cell volume.

hematocyst *n.* a cyst containing blood.

hematogenous (hematogenic) *adj.* **1.** relating to the production of blood or its constituents; hematopoietic. **2.** produced by, originating in, or carried by the blood.

hematohidrosis (hemathidrosis, hematidrosis) *n.* the secretion of sweat containing blood.

hematology *n.* the study of blood and blood-forming tissues and the disorders associated with them. —**hematological** *adj*. —**hematologist** *n*.

hematoma *n*. an accumulation of blood within the tissues that clots to form a solid swelling. Injury, disease of the blood vessels, or a clotting disorder of the blood are usually the causative factors. An *intracranial hematoma* causes symptoms by compressing the brain and by raising the pressure within the skull. A blunt injury to the head, especially the temple, may tear the middle meningeal artery, giving rise to a rapidly accumulating *extradural hematoma* requiring urgent surgical treatment. In elderly people a relatively slight head injury may tear the veins where they cross the space beneath the dura, giving rise to a *subdural hematoma*. Excellent results are obtained by surgical treatment. An *intracerebral hematoma* may be a consequence of severe head injury but is more often due to atheromatous disease of the cerebral arteries and high blood pressure resulting in bleeding into the brain. *See also* perianal hematoma.

hematometra *n*. **1.** accumulation of menstrual blood in the uterus. **2.** abnormally copious bleeding in the uterus.

hematomyelia *n*. bleeding into the tissue of the spinal cord. This may result in acutely developing symptoms that mimic *syringomyelia.

hematopoiesis *n*. *see* hemopoiesis.

hematoporphyrin *n*. a type of *porphyrin produced during the metabolism of hemoglobin.

hematosalpinx (hemosalpinx) *n*. the accumulation of menstrual blood in the *fallopian tubes.

hematoxylin *n*. a colorless crystalline compound extracted from logwood (*Haematoxylon campechianum*) and used in various histological stains. When oxidized hematoxylin is converted to *hematein*, which imparts a blue color to certain parts of cells, especially cell nuclei. *Heidenhain's iron hematoxylin* is used to stain sections that are to be photographed, since it gives great clarity at high magnification.

hematuria *n*. the presence of blood in the urine, which may be seen by the naked eye or detected by urinalysis sticks or urine microscopy. The blood may come from the kidneys, one or both ureters, the bladder, or the urethra, as a result of injury or disease. Hematuria is a very important symptom because it is associated with *transitional cell carcinoma, most commonly in the bladder, and kidney cancer. It may also be due to urinary-tract infections, stone disease, or some forms of *glomerulonephritis.

heme *n*. an iron-containing compound (a *porphyrin) that combines with the protein globin to form *hemoglobin, found in the red blood cells.

hemeralopia *n*. *see* day blindness.

hemi- *prefix denoting* (in medicine) the right or left half of the body. Example: *hemianesthesia* (anesthesia of one side of the body).

hemiachromatopsia *n*. loss of color appreciation in one half of the visual field.

hemianopia *n*. absence of half of the normal field of vision. The most common type is *homonymous hemianopia*, in which the same half (right or left) is lost in both eyes. Sometimes the inner halves of the visual field are lost in both eyes, producing a *binasal hemianopia*, while in others the outer halves are lost, producing a *bitemporal hemianopia*. Very rarely both upper halves or both lower halves are lost, producing an *altitudinal hemianopia*.

hemiarthroplasty *n*. replacement of the end of a bone on one side of a joint with a prosthesis (*see* arthroplasty). It is the treatment for some fractures of the hip and shoulder.

hemiballismus *n*. a violent involuntary movement usually restricted to one arm and primarily involving the proximal muscles. It is a symptom of disease of the *basal ganglia.

hemicolectomy *n*. surgical removal of about half the *colon (large intestine), usually the right section (*right hemicolectomy*) with subsequent joining of the *ileum to the transverse colon. This is performed for disease of the terminal part of the ileum (such as *Crohn's disease) or of the cecum or ascending colon (such as cancer or Crohn's disease).

hemicrania *n*. **1.** a headache affecting only one side of the head, usually *migraine. **2.** absence of half of the skull in a developing fetus.

hemihypertrophy *n*. a condition in which one side of the body is larger than the other. It is often benign but can be associated with *nephroblastoma.

hemimelia *n.* congenital absence or gross shortening (aplasia) of the distal portion of the arms or legs. Sometimes only one of the two bones of the distal arm (radius and ulna) or leg (tibia and fibula) may be affected. *See also* ectromelia.

hemin *n.* a chemical derivative of hemoglobin formed by removal of the protein part of the molecule, oxidation of the iron atom, and combination with an acid to form a salt (*compare* hematin). *Chlorohemin* forms characteristic crystals, the identification of which provides the basis of a chemical test for blood stains.

hemiparesis *n. see* hemiplegia.

hemiplegia (hemiparesis) *n.* paralysis of one side of the body. Movements of the face and arm are often more severely affected than those of the leg. It is caused by disease affecting the opposite (contralateral) hemisphere of the brain.

hemisacralization *n.* fusion of the fifth lumbar vertebra to one side only of the sacrum. *See* sacralization.

hemisphere *n.* one of the two halves of the *cerebrum, not in fact hemispherical but more nearly quarter-spherical.

hemizygous *adj.* describing genes that are carried on an unpaired chromosome, for example the genes on the X chromosome in humans. —**hemizygote** *n.*

hemlock *n.* the plant *Conium maculatum*, found in Britain and central Europe. It is a source of the poisonous alkaloid *coniine.

hemo- *prefix. see* hem-.

hemochromatosis (bronze diabetes, iron-storage disease) *n.* a hereditary disorder in which there is excessive absorption and storage of iron. This leads to damage and functional impairment of many organs, including the liver, pancreas, and endocrine glands. The main features are a bronze color of the skin, diabetes, and liver failure. It is inherited as an autosomal *recessive trait in people of northern European descent and is due to mutations in the hemochromatosis gene (*HFE*) in the majority of cases. Iron may be removed from the body by blood letting or an iron *chelating agent may be administered. *Compare* hemosiderosis.

hemoconcentration *n.* an increase in the proportion of red blood cells relative to the plasma, brought about by a decrease in the volume of plasma or an increase in the concentration of red blood cells in the circulating blood (*see* polycythemia). Hemoconcentration may occur in any condition in which there is a severe loss of water from the body. *Compare* hemodilution.

hemocytometer *n.* a special glass chamber of known volume into which diluted blood is introduced. The numbers of the various blood cells present are then counted visually, through a microscope. Hemocytometers have been largely replaced by electronic cell counters.

hemodialysis *n.* a technique of removing waste materials or poisons from the blood using the principle of *dialysis. Hemodialysis is performed on patients whose kidneys have ceased to function; the process takes place in an *artificial kidney*, or *dialyzer*. Blood taken from an artery is circulated through the dialyzer on one side of a semipermeable membrane, while a solution of similar electrolytic composition to the patient's blood circulates on the other side. Water and waste products from the patient's blood filter through the membrane, whose pores are too small to allow passage of blood cells and proteins. The purified blood is then returned to the patient's body through a vein.

hemodilution *n.* a decrease in the proportion of red blood cells relative to the plasma, brought about by an increase in the total volume of plasma. This may occur in a variety of conditions, including pregnancy and enlargement of the spleen (*see* hypersplenism). *Compare* hemoconcentration.

hemoglobin *n.* a substance contained within the red blood cells (*erythrocytes) and responsible for their color, composed of the pigment *heme linked to the protein *globin. Hemoglobin has the unique property of combining reversibly with oxygen and is the medium by which oxygen is transported within the body. It takes up oxygen as blood passes through the lungs and releases it as blood passes through the tissues. Blood normally contains 12–18 g/dl of hemoglobin. *See also* myohemoglobin, oxyhemoglobin.

hemoglobinometer *n.* an instrument for determining the concentration of hemoglobin in a sample of blood, which is a measure of its oxygen-carrying ability.

hemoglobinopathy *n.* any of a group of inherited diseases, including *thalassemia and *sickle-cell disease, in which there is an abnormality in the production of hemoglobin.

hemoglobinuria *n.* the presence in the urine of free hemoglobin. Hemoglobinuria occurs if hemoglobin, released from disintegrating red blood cells, cannot be taken up rapidly enough by blood proteins. The condition sometimes follows strenuous exercise. It is also associated with certain infectious diseases (such as blackwater fever), ingestion of certain chemicals (such as arsenic), and injury.

hemogram *n.* the results of a routine blood test, including an estimate of the blood hemoglobin level, the *packed cell volume, and the numbers of red and white blood cells (*see* blood count). Any abnormalities seen in microscopic examination of the blood are also noted.

hemolysin *n.* a substance capable of bringing about destruction of red blood cells (*hemolysis). It may be an antibody or a bacterial toxin.

hemolysis *n.* the destruction of red blood cells (*erythrocytes). Within the body, hemolysis may result from defects within the red cells or from poisoning, infection, or the action of antibodies; it may occur in mismatched blood transfusions. It usually leads to anemia. Hemolysis of blood specimens may result from unsatisfactory collection or storage or be brought about intentionally as part of an analytical procedure (*see* laking).

hemolytic *adj.* causing, associated with, or resulting from destruction of red blood cells (*erythrocytes). For example, a *hemolytic antibody* is one that causes destruction of red cells, and *hemolytic anemias* result from red-cell destruction (*see* anemia).

hemolytic disease of the newborn the condition resulting from destruction (hemolysis) of the red blood cells of the fetus by antibodies in the mother's blood passing through the placenta. This most commonly happens when the red blood cells of the fetus are Rh positive (i.e. they have the *rhesus factor) but the mother's red cells are Rh negative. The fetal cells are therefore incompatible in her circulation and evoke the production of antibodies. This may result in very severe anemia of the fetus, leading to heart failure with edema (*hydrops fetalis) or still-

birth. When the anemia is less severe the fetus may reach term in good condition, but the accumulation of the bile pigment bilirubin from the destroyed cells causes severe jaundice after birth, which may require *exchange transfusion. If untreated, it may cause serious brain damage (*see* kernicterus).

A blood test early in pregnancy enables the detection of antibodies in the mother's blood and the adoption of various precautions for the infant's safety. Some cases of predictably very severe hemolytic disease have been successfully treated by intrauterine transfusion. The incidence of the disease has been greatly reduced by preventing the formation of antibodies in a Rh negative mother. If at birth or after abortion the baby's blood is found to be incompatible with the mother's (i.e. Rh positive), she is given an injection of Rh antibody (anti-D immunoglobulin). This rapidly destroys any Rh positive fetal cells in the mother's blood so that they do not remain long enough in her circulation to stimulate antibody production (which could affect her next pregnancy).

hemolytic uremic syndrome a condition in which sudden rapid destruction of red blood cells (*see* hemolysis) causes acute renal failure due partly to obstruction of small arteries in the kidneys. The hemolysis also causes a reduction in the number of platelets, which can lead to severe hemorrhage. The syndrome may occur as a result of septicemia, following a respiratory or gastrointestinal infection (especially by pathogenic *Escherichia coli*), eclamptic convulsions in pregnancy (*see* eclampsia), or as a reaction to certain drugs. There may also be small sporadic outbreaks of the condition without any obvious cause.

hemopericardium *n.* the presence of blood within the membranous sac (pericardium) surrounding the heart, which may result from injury, tumors, rupture of the heart (e.g. following myocardial infarction), or a leaking aneurysm. The heart is compressed (*see* cardiac tamponade) and the circulation impaired; a large fall in blood pressure and cardiac arrest may result. Surgical drainage of the blood may be life saving.

hemoperitoneum *n.* the presence of blood in the peritoneal cavity, between the lining of the abdomen or pelvis and the membrane covering the organs within.

hemophilia *n.* either of two hereditary disorders in which the blood clots very slowly, due to a deficiency of either of two *coagulation factors: *hemophilia A*, due to deficiency of Factor VIII (antihemophilic factor); or *hemophilia B*, due to deficiency of Factor IX (Christmas factor). The patient may experience prolonged bleeding following any injury or wound, and in severe cases there is spontaneous bleeding into muscles and joints. Bleeding in hemophilia may be treated by recombinant DNA-derived Factor VIII or plasma Factor VIII concentrate. Alternatively, concentrated preparations of Factor VIII or Factor IX, obtained by freezing fresh plasma, may be administered (*see* cryoprecipitate). Heat-treated concentrate, which kills the hepatitis and AIDS viruses, is now available for home treatment. Home treatment has greatly improved the life and health of the hemophiliac because bleeding can be stopped before damage is done to other tissues, especially joints. Hemophilia is controlled by a *sex-linked gene, which means that it is almost exclusively restricted to males: women carry the disease – and pass it on to their sons – without being affected themselves. The genes encoding Factors VIII and IX have been used in gene therapy trials for hemophilia. —**hemophiliac** *n.*

hemophthalmia *n.* bleeding into the *vitreous humor of the eye; vitreous hemorrhage.

hemopneumothorax (pneumohemothorax) *n.* the presence of both blood and air in the pleural cavity, usually as a result of injury. Both must be drained out to allow the lung to expand normally. *See also* hemothorax.

hemopoiesis (hematopoiesis) *n.* the process of production of blood cells and platelets, which continues throughout life, replacing aged cells (which are removed from the circulation). In healthy adults, hemopoiesis is confined to the *bone marrow, but during embryonic life and in early infancy, as well as in certain diseases, it may occur in sites other than the bone marrow (*extramedullary hemopoiesis*). *See also* erythropoiesis, leukopoiesis, thrombopoiesis. —**hemopoietic** *adj.*

hemopoietic stem cell the cell from which all classes of blood cells are derived. It cannot be identified microscopically, but can be defined by the presence of a combination of cell-surface proteins. It can be demonstrated by *tissue culture of the blood-forming tissue of the bone marrow, as well as by growth of human hemopoietic cells in immunodeficient mice strains, such as nonobese diabetic/severe combined immunodeficient (NOD/SCID). *See also* hemopoiesis.

hemoptysis *n.* the coughing up of blood. This symptom should always be taken seriously, however small the amount. In some patients the cause is not serious; in others it is never found, but it should always be reported to a doctor.

hemorrhage (bleeding) *n.* the escape of blood from a ruptured blood vessel, externally or internally. Arterial blood is bright red and emerges in spurts, venous blood is dark red and flows steadily, while damage to minor vessels may produce only an oozing. Rupture of a major blood vessel such as the femoral artery can lead to the loss of several liters of blood in a few minutes, resulting in *shock, collapse, and death, if untreated. *See also* hematemesis, hematuria, hemoptysis.

hemorrhagic *adj.* associated with or resulting from blood loss (*see* hemorrhage). For example, *hemorrhagic anemia* is due to blood loss (*see* anemia).

hemorrhagic disease of the newborn a temporary disturbance in blood clotting caused by *vitamin K deficiency and affecting infants on the second to fourth day of life. It varies in severity from mild gastrointestinal bleeding to profuse bleeding into many organs, including the brain. It is more common in breast-fed and preterm infants. The condition can be prevented by giving all babies vitamin K, either by injection or orally, shortly after birth. Medical name: **melena neonatorum**.

hemorrhoidectomy *n.* the surgical operation for removing *hemorrhoids, which are tied and then excised. Possible complications are bleeding or, later, anal stricture (narrowing). The operation is usually performed only for second- or third-degree hemorrhoids that have not responded to simple measures.

hemorrhoids (piles) *pl. n.* enlarged veins in

the wall of the anus (*internal hemorrhoids*), usually a consequence of prolonged constipation or, occasionally, diarrhea. They most commonly occur at three main points equidistant around the circumference of the anus. Uncomplicated hemorrhoids are seldom painful; pain is usually caused by an anal *fissure. The main symptom is bleeding, and in *first-degree hemorrhoids*, which never appear at the anus, bleeding at the end of defecation is the only symptom. *Second-degree hemorrhoids* protrude beyond the anus as an uncomfortable swelling but return spontaneously; *third-degree hemorrhoids* remain outside the anus and need to be returned by pressure.

First- and second-degree hemorrhoids may respond to bowel regulation using a high-fiber diet with fecal softening agents. If bleeding persists, an irritant fluid (a sclerosing agent) may be injected around the swollen veins to make them shrivel up. Forceful dilation of the anus under general anesthesia is also effective, as is infrared coagulation. Third-degree hemorrhoids often require surgery (*see* hemorrhoidectomy), especially if they become *strangulated (as this produces severe pain and further enlargement).

External hemorrhoids are either prolapsed internal hemorrhoids or – more often – *perianal hematomas or the residual skin tags remaining after a perianal hematoma has healed.

hemosalpinx *n. see* hematosalpinx.

hemosiderin *n.* an iron-storage compound found mainly in the cells of the *macrophage-*monocyte system in the marrow, in *Kupffer's cells of the liver, and in the spleen. It contains around 30% iron by weight.

hemosiderosis *n.* the accumulation of iron in various tissues, usually in the form of *hemosiderin and usually without tissue damage.

hemostasis *n.* the arrest of bleeding, involving the physiological processes of *blood coagulation and the contraction of damaged blood vessels. The term is also applied to various surgical procedures (for example the application of *ligatures, lasers, or *diathermy to cut vessels) used to stop bleeding.

hemostatic (styptic) *n.* an agent that stops or prevents hemorrhage; for example,

*phytonadione. Hemostatics are used to control bleeding due to various causes and may be used in treating bleeding disorders, such as hemophilia.

hemothorax *n.* blood in the pleural cavity, usually due to injury. If the blood is not drained dense fibrous *adhesions occur between the pleural surfaces, which can impair the normal movement of the lung. The blood may also become infected (*see* empyema).

hemozoin *n.* an iron-containing pigment present in the organisms that cause malaria (*Plasmodium* species).

hemp *n. see* cannabis.

Henle's loop the part of a kidney tubule that forms a loop extending toward the center of the kidney. It is surrounded by blood capillaries, which absorb water and selected soluble substances back into the bloodstream. [F. G. J. Henle (1809–85), German anatomist]

Henoch-Schönlein purpura *see* Schönlein-Henoch purpura.

henry *n.* the *SI unit of inductance, equal to the inductance of a closed circuit with a magnetic flux of 1 weber per ampere of current. Symbol: H.

Hensen's node (primitive knot) the rounded front end of the embryonic *primitive streak. [V. Hensen (1835–1924), German pathologist]

heparin *n.* an *anticoagulant produced in liver cells, some white blood cells, and certain other sites, which acts by inhibiting the action of the enzyme *thrombin in the final stage of *blood coagulation. An extracted purified form of heparin is widely used for the prevention of blood coagulation both in patients with thrombosis and similar conditions and in blood collected for examination. The drug is usually administered by injection and the most important side effect is bleeding. *See also* low molecular weight heparin.

hepat- (hepato-) *prefix denoting* the liver. Examples: *hepatopexy* (surgical fixation of); *hepatorenal* (relating to the liver and kidney).

hepatalgia *n.* pain in or over the liver. It is caused by liver inflammation (especially an abscess) or swelling (as in cardiac failure or *steatosis).

hepatectomy *n.* the operation of removing the liver. *Partial hepatectomy* is the removal of one or more lobes of the liver;

it may be carried out after severe injury or to remove a tumor localized in one part of the liver.

hepatic *adj.* relating to the liver.

hepatic duct *see* bile duct.

hepatic encephalopathy (portosystemic encephalopathy) a condition in which brain function is impaired by the presence of toxic substances, absorbed from the colon, which are normally removed or detoxified by the liver. It occurs when the liver is severely damaged (as in cirrhosis) or bypassed. Symptoms include drowsiness, confusion, difficulty in performing tasks (e.g. writing), and coma. Treatment consists of stopping protein intake and giving antibiotics (to prevent bacterial production of toxins) and enemas and cathartics (to remove colonic toxins); lactulose is administered for chronic disease.

hepatic flexure the bend in the *colon, just underneath the liver, where the ascending colon joins the transverse colon.

hepaticostomy *n.* a surgical operation in which a temporary or permanent opening is made into the main duct carrying bile from the liver.

hepatic vein one of several short veins originating within the lobes of the liver as small branches, which unite to form larger veins that lead directly to the inferior vena cava, draining blood from the liver.

hepatitis *n.* inflammation of the liver caused by viruses, toxic substances, or immunological abnormalities. *Infectious hepatitis* is caused by viruses, several types of which have been isolated as specific causes of the disease and can be detected by blood tests, and includes hepatitis A, hepatitis B, hepatitis C, hepatitis D, and hepatitis E. Other viral causes of hepatitis include the *Epstein-Barr virus. *See also* Entamoeba.

Hepatitis A (epidemic hepatitis) is transmitted by food or drink contaminated by a carrier or patient and commonly occurs where sanitation is poor. After an incubation period of 15–40 days, the patient develops fever and sickness. Yellow discoloration of the skin (*see* jaundice) appears about a week later and persists for up to three weeks. The patient may be infectious throughout this period. Serious complications are unusual and an attack often confers immunity. Injection of *gamma globulin provides temporary protection.

Hepatitis B (formerly known as serum hepatitis) is transmitted by infected blood or blood products contaminating hypodermic needles, blood transfusions, or tattooing needles, by sexual contact, or by contact with any other body fluid (e.g. milk, sweat); it often occurs in drug addicts. Symptoms, which develop suddenly after an incubation period of 1–6 months, include headache, fever, chills, general weakness, and jaundice. Most patients make a gradual recovery but the mortality rate is 5–20%. A vaccine is available.

Hepatitis C (formerly known as non-A, non-B hepatitis) has a mode of transmission similar to that of hepatitis B; symptoms include fatigue, sore bones, and dryness of the eyes. *Hepatitis D* is a defective virus and occurs only with or after infection with hepatitis B. Patients with D virus usually have severe chronic hepatitis. *Hepatitis E* is transmitted by infected food or drink and can cause acute hepatitis. It often occurs in epidemics in places with poor sanitation.

Chronic hepatitis continues for months or years, eventually leading to *cirrhosis (*see also* hepatoma). It may be caused by persistent infection with a hepatitis virus (usually hepatitis B, C, or D), which may respond to treatment with *interferon, or by *autoimmune disease, treated by *corticosteroids or *immunosuppressant therapy.

hepatization *n.* the conversion of lung tissue, which normally holds air, into a solid liverlike mass during the course of acute lobar pneumonia.

hepato- *prefix. see* hepat-.

hepatoblastoma *n.* a malignant tumor of the liver occurring in children, made up of embryonic liver cells. It is often confined to one lobe of the liver; such cases may be treated by partial *hepatectomy.

hepatocellular *adj.* relating to or affecting the cells of the liver.

hepatocyte *n.* the principal cell type in the *liver: a large cell with many metabolic functions, including synthesis, storage, detoxification, and bile production.

hepatoma (hepatocellular carcinoma) *n.* a malignant tumor of the liver, originating in mature liver cells. In Western countries it is rare in normal livers, but often develops in patients with cirrhosis, particularly after hepatitis B or C infection. In Africa and other tropical countries it is frequent, possible causes including fungi (see aflatoxin) and other ingested toxins. Hepatomas often synthesize *alpha-fetoprotein, which circulates in the blood and is a useful indicator of these tumors.

The term hepatoma is often, though incorrectly, used to include malignant tumors arising in the bile duct (see cholangiocarcinoma).

hepatomegaly n. enlargement of the liver to such an extent that it can be felt below the rib margin. This may be due to congestion (as in heart failure), inflammation, infiltration (e.g. by fat), or tumor.

hepatotoxic adj. damaging or destroying liver cells. Drugs such as *acetaminophen and *phenacemide can cause liver damage at high doses or with prolonged use.

hept- (hepta-) prefix denoting seven.

HER2 human epidermal growth factor receptor 2: a protein occurring in excessive amounts on the surface of tumor cells in highly malignant forms of breast cancer. It acts as a receptor for epidermal *growth factor, which influences the growth and proliferation of the tumor.

hereditary adj. transmitted from parents to their offspring; inherited.

heredity n. the process that causes the biological similarity between parents and their offspring. *Genetics is the study of heredity.

heredo- prefix denoting heredity.

hermaphrodite n. an individual in which both male and female sex organs are present or in which the sex organs contain both ovarian and testicular cells. Human hermaphrodites are very rare. —**hermaphroditism** n.

hernia n. the protrusion of an organ or tissue out of the body cavity in which it normally lies. An inguinal hernia (or rupture) occurs in the lower abdomen; a sac of peritoneum, containing fat or part of the bowel, bulges through a weak part (inguinal canal) of the abdominal wall. It may result from physical straining or coughing. A sliding hernia is an inguinal hernia that has an element of descent ("slide") of related structures alongside the sac. A scrotal hernia is an inguinal hernia so large that it passes into the

scrotum; a femoral hernia is similar to an inguinal hernia but protrudes at the top of the thigh, through the point at which the femoral artery passes from the abdomen to the thigh. A diaphragmatic hernia is the protrusion of an abdominal organ through the diaphragm into the chest cavity; the most common type is the hiatus hernia, in which the stomach passes partly or completely into the chest cavity through the hole (hiatus) for the esophagus (gullet). This may be associated with *gastroesophageal reflux. An umbilical hernia (exomphalos) is the protrusion of abdominal organs into the umbilical cord because of a fault in embryonic development. It is present at birth and can be treated surgically.

Hernias may be complicated by becoming impossible to return to their normal site (irreducible); swollen and fixed within their sac (incarcerated); or cut off from their blood supply, becoming painful and eventually gangrenous (strangulated). The best treatment for hernias, especially if they are painful, is surgical repair (see hernioplasty).

hernio- prefix denoting a hernia.

hernioplasty n. the surgical operation to repair a hernia, in which the abnormal opening is sewn up and/or the weakness strengthened with suture material. The recommended techniques for repair include a layered suture repair or the insertion of a mesh of polypropylene.

herniorrhaphy n. surgical repair of a hernia. It can be performed through a *laparoscope. See also herniotomy.

herniotomy n. excision of a hernial sac: the first stage of the surgical repair of a hernia. In infants and young muscular subjects it is all that is needed to cure the hernia.

heroin (diacetylmorphine) n. a white crystalline powder derived from *morphine but with a shorter duration of action. Like morphine it is a powerful narcotic analgesic whose continued use leads to *dependence. Its use in medicine is illegal in the United States.

herpangina n. an acute viral infectious disease of sudden onset that causes fever, blisters, and ulceration of the soft palate and tonsillar area. It generally occurs in epidemics in infants and children and lasts 2–5 days.

herpes n. inflammation of the skin or mucous membranes that is caused by *herpesviruses and characterized by collections of small blisters. There are two types of *herpes simplex virus* (*HSV*): type I causes the common *cold sore*, usually present on or around the lips; type II is mainly associated with *genital herpes* and is sexually transmitted. However, types I and II can both cause either genital herpes or cold sores, depending on the site of initial infection. HSV blisters are contagious through skin-to-skin contact and are recurrent in some people. HSV can also affect the conjunctiva (*see also* dendritic ulcer).

Herpes zoster (*shingles*) is caused by the varicella-zoster virus, which also causes chickenpox. Following an attack of chickenpox, the virus lies dormant in the dorsal root ganglia of the spinal cord. Later, under one of a number of influences, the virus migrates down the sensory nerve to affect one or more *dermatomes on the skin in a band causing the characteristic shingles rash. One side of the face or an eye (*ophthalmic zoster*) may be involved. Shingles may be chronically painful (*postherpetic neuralgia*), especially in the elderly. *See also* Ramsay Hunt syndrome.

Treatment of all forms of herpes is with an appropriate preparation of *acyclovir or related antiviral drugs; shingles may require potent analgesics.

herpesvirus *n.* one of a group of DNA-containing viruses causing latent infections in humans and animals. The herpesviruses are the causative agents of *herpes and chickenpox. The group also includes the *cytomegalovirus and *Epstein-Barr virus. *Herpesvirus simiae* (*virus B*) causes an infection in monkeys similar to herpes simplex, but when transmitted to humans it can produce fatal encephalitis.

hertz *n.* the *SI unit of frequency, equal to one cycle per second. Symbol: Hz.

hesitation *n.* a *lower urinary tract symptom in which there is a delay between being ready to pass urine and the actual flow of urine.

Herxheimer reaction *see* Jarisch-Herxheimer reaction.

heter- (hetero-) *prefix denoting* difference; dissimilarity.

heterochromatin *n.* chromosome material (*see* chromatin) that stains most deeply

when the cell is not dividing. It is thought not to represent major genes but may be involved in controlling these genes, and also in controlling mitosis and development. *Compare* euchromatin.

heterochromia *n.* color difference in the iris of the eye, which is usually congenital but is occasionally secondary to inflammation of the iris (as in *Fuchs' heterochromic cyclitis). In *heterochromia iridis* one iris differs in color from the other; in *heterochromia iridum* one part of the iris differs in color from the rest.

heterogametic *adj.* describing the sex that produces two different kinds of gamete, which carry different *sex chromosomes, and that therefore determines the sex of the offspring. In humans men are the heterogametic sex: the sperm cells carry either an X or a Y chromosome. *Compare* homogametic.

heterogeneity *n.* (in oncology) variability or differences in the properties of cells within a tumor.

heterograft *n. see* xenograft.

heterophoria *n.* a tendency to squint. Under normal circumstances both the eyes work together and look at the same point simultaneously, but if one eye is covered it will move out of alignment with the object the other eye is still viewing. When the cover is removed, the eye immediately returns to its normal position. Most people have a small degree of the type of heterophoria known as *exophoria*, in which the covered eye turns outward, away from the nose (*compare* esophoria). Heterophoria often produces eyestrain because of the unconscious effort required to keep the two eyes coordinated. *See also* strabismus.

Heterophyes *n.* a genus of small parasitic *flukes occurring in Egypt and the Far East. Adult flukes of the species *H. heterophyes* live in the small intestine of humans and other fish-eating animals; in humans the flukes can produce serious symptoms (*see* heterophyiasis). The fluke has two intermediate hosts, a snail and a mullet fish.

heterophyiasis *n.* an infestation of the small intestine with the parasitic fluke *Heterophyes heterophyes*. Humans become infected on eating raw or salted fish that contains the larval stage of the fluke. The presence of adult flukes may provoke symptoms of abdominal pain and diarrhea; if the eggs reach the brain, spinal cord, and heart (via the bloodstream), they produce serious lesions. *Anthelmintics are used in treatment of the condition.

heteropsia *n.* different vision in each eye.

heterosexuality *n.* the pattern of sexuality in which sexual behavior and thinking are directed toward people of the opposite sex. It includes both normal and deviant forms of sexual activity. —**heterosexual** *adj., n.*

heterosis *n.* hybrid vigor: the increased sturdiness, resistance to disease, etc., of individuals whose parents are of different races or species compared both with their parents and with the offspring of genetically similar parents.

heterotopia (heterotopy) *n.* the displacement of an organ or part of the body from its normal position.

heterotrophic (organotrophic) *adj.* describing organisms (known as heterotrophs) that ingest complex organic compounds in order to synthesize their own organic materials. Most are *chemoheterotrophic*, i.e. they use the organic compounds as an energy source. This group includes the majority of bacteria and all animals and fungi. *Compare* autotrophic.

heterotropia *n. see* strabismus.

heterozygous *adj.* describing an individual in whom the members of a pair of genes determining a particular characteristic are dissimilar. *See* allele. *Compare* homozygous. —**heterozygote** *n.*

hex- (hexa-) *prefix denoting* six.

hexacanth *n. see* oncosphere.

hexachlorophene *n.* a disinfectant similar to *phenol, used in soaps and creams. Its use is regulated by the FDA because of the neurotoxic effects it might produce when absorbed into the body. Trade name: **pHisoHex**.

hexachromia *n.* the ability to distinguish only six of the seven colors of the spectrum, the exception being indigo. Most people cannot distinguish indigo from blue or violet.

hexamine *n. see* methenamine.

hexokinase *n.* an enzyme that catalyzes the conversion of glucose to glucose-6-phosphate. This is the first stage of *glycolysis.

hexosamine *n.* the amino derivative of a *hexose sugar. The two most important hexosamines are *glucosamine and galactosamine.

hexose *n.* a simple sugar with six carbon atoms. Hexose sugars are the sugars most frequently found in food. The most important hexose is *glucose.

HHS *see* Department of Health and Human Services.

5-HIAA *see* 5-hydroxyindoleacetic acid.

hiatus *n.* an opening or aperture. For example, the diaphragm contains hiatuses for the esophagus and aorta.

hiatus hernia *see* hernia.

Hib vaccine a vaccine that gives protection against the bacterium *Haemophilus influenzae* type B (Hib), which causes *meningitis, *epiglottitis, and joint infections. The vaccine is given with the triple DPT vaccine during the first year of life.

hiccup (hiccough) *n.* abrupt involuntary lowering of the diaphragm and closure of the sound-producing folds at the upper end of the trachea, producing a characteristic sound as the breath is drawn in. Hiccups, which usually occur repeatedly, may be caused by indigestion or more serious disorders, such as alcoholism. Medical name: **singultus**.

Hickman catheter a fine plastic cannula usually inserted into the subclavian vein in the neck to allow administration of drugs and to obtain repeated blood samples. The catheter is tunneled for several centimeters beneath the skin in order to prevent infection entering the bloodstream. It is used most frequently in patients who are receiving long-term chemotherapy. [R. O. Hickman (20th century), US surgeon]

hidr- (hidro-) *prefix denoting* sweat. Example: *hidropoiesis* (formation of).

hidradenitis (hidrosadenitis) *n.* inflammation of the sweat glands, usually occurring when the glands become blocked. This may occur in the armpit, around the nipple or umbilicus, or in the groin. *Hidradenitis suppurativa* is characterized by deep abscesses in the armpits, groin, and anogenital regions. Formerly believed to be an apocrine sweat gland disorder, it is now regarded as part of the *follicular occlusion tetrad. It is three times more common in women and may be under androgen control. Treatment is with long-term antibiotics, antiandrogens, or occasionally surgery.

hidrosis n. **1.** the excretion of sweat. **2.** excessive sweating.

hidrotic n. an agent that causes sweating. *Parasympathomimetic drugs are hidrotics.

hilar cell tumor an androgen-producing tumor of the ovary found in older women and often resulting in *virilization. Such tumors are so called as they tend to occur around the area of the ovary where the blood vessels enter (the hilum). They are usually small and are treated by surgical removal, with resolution of most of the symptoms.

Hill-Burton Act a 1946 amendment to the US Public Health Service Act authorizing grants to states for construction of hospitals and public-health centers. Funds are provided for states to study existing hospital and health-center facilities and to survey the need for additional facilities. The federal government may pay up to two-thirds of the construction costs of new facilities, depending upon such factors as the relative need and economic status of the area. The law also authorizes the US Surgeon General's office to establish standards for constructing and equipping hospitals built with Hill-Burton funds, for determining the number and distribution of public-health centers, the number of beds to be allocated for specific health problems (such as tuberculosis or mental illness), and the number of general hospital beds needed to provide adequate hospital services – a number that ranges from 4.5 to 5.5 per thousand population depending upon the population density of the area.

hilum n. (pl. **hila**) a hollow situated on the surface of an organ, such as the ovary, kidney, or spleen, at which structures such as blood vessels, nerve fibers, and ducts enter or leave it.

hindbrain (rhombencephalon) n. the part of the *brain comprising the cerebellum, pons, and medulla oblongata. The pons and medulla contain the nuclei of many of the cranial nerves, which issue from their surfaces, and the reticular formation. The fluid-filled cavity in the midline is the fourth *ventricle.

hindgut n. the back part of the embryonic gut, which gives rise to part of the large

intestine, the rectum, bladder, and urinary ducts. *See also* cloaca.

hindquarter amputation an operation involving removal of an entire leg and part or all of the pelvis associated with it. It is usually performed for soft tissue or bone sarcomas arising from the upper thigh, hip, or buttock. *Compare* forequarter amputation.

hinge joint *see* ginglymus.

hip n. the region of the body where the thigh bone (femur) articulates with the *pelvis: the region on each side of the pelvis.

hip bone (innominate bone) a bone formed by the fusion of the ilium, ischium, and pubis. It articulates with the femur by the *acetabulum* of the ilium, a deep socket into which the head of the femur fits (*see* hip joint). Between the pubis and ischium, below and slightly in front of the acetabulum, is a large opening – the *obturator foramen*. The right and left hip bones form part of the *pelvis.

hip girdle *see* pelvic girdle.

hip joint the ball-and-socket joint (*see* enarthrosis) between the head of the femur and the acetabulum (socket) of the ilium (*see* hip bone). It is a common site of osteoarthritis and rheumatoid arthritis, which is often treated surgically (by *hip replacement). *See also* congenital dislocation of the hip.

Hippelates n. a genus of small flies. The adults of *H. pallipes* are suspected of transmitting *yaws in the West Indies. Other species of *Hippelates* may be involved in the transmission of organisms causing conjunctivitis.

hippocampal formation a curved band of cortex lying within each cerebral hemisphere: in evolutionary terms one of the brain's most primitive parts. It forms a portion of the *limbic system and is involved in the complex physical aspects of behavior governed by emotion and instinct.

hippocampus n. a curved elevation in the floor of the lateral *ventricle of the brain. It contains complex foldings of cortical tissue and is involved, with other connections of the *hippocampal formation, in the workings of the *limbic system. —**hippocampal** adj.

Hippocratic oath the oath taken by a doctor that binds him to observe the code of behavior and practice followed by the Greek physician Hippocrates (460–370 BC), called the "Father of Medicine," and the students of the medical school in Cos where he taught.

hippus n. abnormal rhythmical variations in the size of the pupils, independent of the intensity of the light falling on the eyes. It is occasionally seen in various diseases of the nervous system.

hip replacement a surgical procedure developed for replacing a diseased hip joint with a prosthesis. A plastic or metal cup forms the socket, and the head of the femur is replaced by a metal ball on a stem placed inside the femur. There are many types of prosthesis, which can be fixed to the bone with or without cement. See also arthroplasty.

Hirschsprung's disease a congenital condition in which the rectum and sometimes part of the lower colon have failed to develop a normal nerve network. The affected portion does not expand or conduct the contents of the bowel, which accumulate in and distend the upper colon. Symptoms, which are usually apparent in the first weeks of life, are abdominal pain and swelling and severe or complete constipation. Diagnosis is by X-ray and by microscopic examination of samples of the bowel wall, which shows the absence of nerve cells. Treatment is by surgery to remove the affected segment and join the remaining (normal) colon to the anus. See also megacolon. [H. Hirschsprung (1830–1916), Danish physician]

hirsutism n. the presence of coarse pigmented hair on the face, chest, upper back, or abdomen in a female due to excessive androgen production (*hyperandrogenism). See also virilization.

hirudin n. an *anticoagulant present in the salivary glands of leeches and in certain snake venoms, that prevents *blood coagulation by inhibiting the action of the enzyme *thrombin.

hist- (histio-, histo-) prefix denoting tissue.

histaminase n. an enzyme, widely distributed in the body, that is responsible for the inactivation of histamine.

histamine n. a compound derived from the amino acid histidine. It is found in nearly all tissues of the body, associated mainly with the *mast cells. Histamine has pronounced pharmacologic activity, causing dilation of blood vessels and contraction of smooth muscle (for example, in the lungs). It is an important mediator of inflammation and is released in large amounts after skin damage (such as that due to animal venoms and toxins), producing a characteristic skin reaction (consisting of flushing, a flare, and a wheal). Histamine is also released in anaphylactic reactions and allergic conditions, including asthma, and gives rise to some of the symptoms of these conditions. See also anaphylaxis, antihistamine.

histamine acid phosphate a derivative of *histamine used to test for acid secretion in the stomach in conditions involving abnormal gastric secretion, such as *Zollinger-Ellison syndrome. It is administered by injection and can cause headache, wheezing, rapid heartbeat, disturbed vision, and digestive upsets.

histidine n. an *amino acid from which *histamine is derived.

histiocyte n. a fixed *macrophage, i.e. one that is stationary within connective tissue.

histiocytoma n. a tumor containing *macrophages or *histiocytes, large cells with the ability to engulf foreign matter and bacteria. See also fibrosarcoma (malignant fibrous histiocytoma).

histiocytosis n. any of a group of diseases in which there are abnormalities in certain large phagocytic cells (*histiocytes) due to: (1) biochemical defects, such as abnormal storage of fats (as in *Gaucher's disease); (2) inflammatory disorders (as in *Langerhans cell histiocytosis, which includes disorders previously called histiocytosis X); or (3) malignant proliferation of histiocytes.

histochemistry n. the study of the identification and distribution of chemical compounds within and between cells, by means of stains, indicators, and light and electron microscopy. —**histochemical** adj.

histocompatibility n. the form of *compatibility that depends on tissue components, mainly specific glycoprotein antigens in cell membranes. A high degree of histocompatibility is necessary for a tissue graft or organ transplant to be successful. —**histocompatible** adj.

histogenesis n. the formation of tissues.

histogram n. a form of statistical graph in

which values are plotted in the form of rectangles on a chart; a bar chart.

histoid *adj.* **1.** resembling normal tissue. **2.** composed of one type of tissue.

histological grade a classification of the *differentiation of a tumor, most typically applied to breast tumors.

histology *n.* the study of the structure of tissues by means of special staining techniques combined with light and electron microscopy. —**histological** *adj.*

histone *n.* a simple protein that combines with a nucleic acid to form a *nucleoprotein.

Histoplasma *n.* a genus of parasitic yeast-like fungi. The species *H. capsulatum* causes the respiratory infection *histoplasmosis.

histoplasmin *n.* a preparation of antigenic material from a culture of the fungus *Histoplasma capsulatum*, used to test for exposure to the disease *histoplasmosis. After a subcutaneous injection there is a skin reaction if the test is positive.

histoplasmosis *n.* an infection caused by inhaling spores of the fungus *Histoplasma capsulatum*. The primary pulmonary form usually produces no symptoms or harmful effects and is recognized retrospectively by X-rays and positive *histoplasmin skin testing. Occasionally, progressive histoplasmosis, which resembles tuberculosis, develops. The fungus may spread via the bloodstream to attack other organs, such as the liver, spleen, lymph nodes, or intestine. Symptomatic disease is treated with intravenous amphotericin B. The spores are found in soil contaminated by feces, especially from chickens and bats. The disease is endemic in the northern and central US, Argentina, Brazil, Venezuela, and parts of Africa.

histotoxic *adj.* poisonous to tissues: applied to certain substances and conditions.

HIV (human immunodeficiency virus) a *retrovirus responsible for *AIDS. There are two types, HIV-1 and HIV-2; the latter is most common in Africa. *See also* HTLV.

hives *n. see* urticaria.

HLA system human leukocyte antigen system: a series of four gene families (termed A, B, C, and D) that code for polymorphic proteins expressed on the surface of most nucleated cells. Individuals inherit from each parent one gene (or set of genes) for each subdivision of the HLA system. If two individuals have identical HLA types, they are said to be histocompatible. Successful tissue transplantation requires a minimum number of HLA differences between donor and recipient tissues.

HMG-CoA *see* hydroxymethylglutaryl coenzyme A reductase.

HMO *see* Health Maintenance Organization.

hobnail liver the liver of a patient with cirrhosis, which has a knobbly appearance caused by regenerating nodules separated by bands of fibrous tissue.

Hodgkin's disease a malignant disease of lymphatic tissues – a form of *lymphoma – usually characterized by painless enlargement of one or more groups of lymph nodes in the neck, armpits, groin, chest, or abdomen; the spleen, liver, bone marrow, and bones may also be involved. Apart from the enlarging nodes, there may also be weight loss, fever, profuse sweating at night, and itching (known as *B symptoms*). Hodgkin's disease is distinguished from other forms of lymphoma by the presence of large binucleate cells (*Reed-Sternberg cells*) in the lymph nodes. Treatment depends on the extent of disease and may include radiotherapy, drug therapy, surgery, or a combination of these. Drugs used in the treatment of the disease include nitrogen mustard, vincristine, procarbazine, prednisone, chlorambucil, and vinblastine. Many patients can be cured; in the early stages of the disease this may be in the order of 85% or more. [T. Hodgkin (1798–1866), British physician]

holistic *adj.* describing an approach to patient care in which the physical, mental, and social factors in the patient's condition are taken into account, rather than just the diagnosed disease. The term is applied to a range of orthodox and unorthodox methods of treatment. *See also* complementary medicine.

Holmes-Adie syndrome *see* Adie's syndrome.

holo- *prefix denoting* complete or entire.

holocrine *adj.* describing a gland or type of secretion in which the entire cell disintegrates when the product is released.

Home Health Agency an organization authorized by the Medicare amendment to the US Social Security Act to provide skilled nursing and other therapeutic services to patients in their homes. The Visiting Nurse Association is an example of a federally authorized Home Health Agency. Under terms of the law, a Home Health Agency may be reimbursed with federal funds for home care services provided for a Medicare or Medicaid patient.

home health aide a specially trained therapist who works with public health nurses and other health professionals in providing care to patients at home. The patients receiving such care generally are medically indigent persons with a chronic illness.

homeo- *prefix denoting* similar; like.

homeopathic *adj.* **1.** of or relating to *homeopathy. **2.** infinitesimally small, as applied to the dose of a drug.

homeopathy *n.* a system of medicine based on the theory that "like cures like." The patient is treated with an extremely small dose of a substance that in larger doses would normally cause or aggravate symptoms of his or her condition. The system was founded by Samuel Hahnemann (1755–1843) at the end of the 18th century and is followed by a minority of doctors. *See also* complementary medicine. —**homeopathist** *n.*

homeostasis *n.* the physiological process by which the internal systems of the body (e.g. blood pressure, body temperature, *acid-base balance) are maintained at equilibrium, despite variations in the external conditions. —**homeostatic** *adj.*

homeothermic *adj.* warm-blooded: capable of maintaining a constant body temperature independently of, and despite variations in, the temperature of the surroundings. Mammals (including humans) and birds are homeothermic. *Compare* poikilothermic. —**homeothermy** *n.*

homo- *prefix denoting* the same or common.

homocysteine *n.* a sulfur-containing amino acid that is an intermediate in the synthesis of *cysteine. A deficiency in the enzyme cystathionine synthetase results in elevated levels in the blood of homocysteine and homocystine (an oxidized form of homocysteine), resulting in el-

evated urinary levels (*see* homocystinuria). It is becoming increasingly recognized that elevated concentrations of homocysteine in the blood are a risk factor for vascular disease independent of diabetes, hypertension, elevated levels of cholesterol in the blood, and smoking.

homocystinuria *n.* an *inborn error of metabolism, inherited as an autosomal *recessive trait, caused by an enzyme deficiency resulting in an excess of *homocysteine in the blood and the presence of homocystine (an oxidized form of homocysteine) in the urine. Clinically affected individuals are mentally retarded, excessively tall with long fingers (due to overgrowth of bones), generally have loose ligaments (which may result in dislocation of the lens), and have a tendency to form blood clots in the veins and arteries, leading to stroke. Treatment is by diet, which may allow for normal development if the disease is recognized early enough, and high-dose vitamin B_6 therapy.

homogametic *adj.* describing the sex that produces only one kind of gamete, which carries the same *sex chromosome, and that therefore does not determine the sex of the offspring. In humans women are the homogametic sex: each egg cell carries an X chromosome. *Compare* heterogametic.

homogenize *vb.* to reduce material to a uniform consistency, e.g. by crushing and mixing. Organs and tissues are homogenized to determine their overall content of a particular enzyme or other substance. —**homogenization** *n.*

homogentisic acid a product formed during the metabolism of the amino acids phenylalanine and tyrosine. In normal individuals homogentisic acid is oxidized by the enzyme *homogentisic acid oxidase*. In rare cases this enzyme is lacking and a condition known as *alkaptonuria, in which large amounts of homogentisic acid are excreted in the urine, results.

homograft *n. see* allograft.

homolateral *adj. see* ipsilateral.

homologous *adj.* **1.** (in anatomy) describing organs or parts that have the same basic structure and evolutionary origin, but not necessarily the same function or superficial structure. *Compare* analogous. **2.** (in genetics) describing a pair of chromosomes of similar shape and size and having identical gene loci. One member of the pair is derived from the mother; the other from the father.

homonymous *adj.* describing a visual defect in which the visual field to one side of the body is restricted in both eyes (*see* hemianopia).

homosexuality *n.* a pattern of sexuality in which sexual behavior and thinking are directed toward people of the same sex (*see also* lesbianism). *Counseling can benefit people who are concerned about their sexual orientation. —**homosexual** *adj.*, *n.*

homozygous *adj.* describing an individual in whom the members of a pair of genes determining a particular characteristic are identical. *See* allele. *Compare* heterozygous. —**homozygote** *n.*

homunculus *n.* **1.** (**manikin**) a dwarf with no deformity or abnormality other than small size. **2.** (**manikin**) a small jointed anatomical model of a man. **3.** (in early biological theory) a miniature human being thought to be contained within each of the reproductive cells.

honeycomb lung the honeycomb pattern seen on X-ray at the later stages of chronic lung conditions, in which the lungs become less elastic and more fibrotic. Once the honeycomb appearance is visible on the X-ray, the lungs are likely to progress to respiratory failure.

hook *n.* a surgical instrument with a bent or curved tip, used to hold, lift, or retract tissue at operation.

hookworm *n.* either of two nematode worms, *Necator americanus* or *Ancylostoma duodenale*, which live as parasites in the intestine of humans. Both species, also known as the New and Old World hookworms, respectively, are of great medical importance (*see* hookworm disease).

hookworm disease a condition resulting from an infestation of the small intestine by hookworms. Hookworm larvae live in the soil and infect humans by penetrating the skin. The worms travel to the lungs in the bloodstream and from there pass via the windpipe and gullet to the small intestine. Heavy hookworm infections may cause considerable damage to the wall of the intestine, leading to a serious loss of blood; this, in conjunction with malnutrition, can provoke

severe anemia. Symptoms include abdominal pain, diarrhea, debility, and mental inertia. The disease occurs throughout the tropics and subtropics and is prevalent in areas of poor personal hygiene and inadequate sanitation. Mebendazole and pyrantel pamoate are used in treatment.

hordeolum *n. see* stye.

hormone *n.* a substance that is produced in one part of the body (by an *endocrine gland, such as the thyroid, adrenal, or pituitary), passes into the bloodstream, and is carried to other (distant) organs or tissues, where it acts to modify their structure or function. Examples of hormones are corticosteroids (from the adrenal cortex), growth hormone (from the pituitary gland), and androgens (from the testes).

hormone-binding globulins a family of plasma proteins whose function is to bind free hormone molecules to varying degrees and thus reduce their function. Alterations in levels of the binding globulins, for example during pregnancy or ill health, can result in variations in assays of hormone levels in individuals. Examples include *thyroid-binding globulin*, *sex hormone-binding globulin*, and *corticosteroid-binding globulin*.

hormone replacement therapy (HRT) the use of female hormones for the relief of symptoms resulting from cessation of ovarian function, either at the time of the natural *menopause or following surgical removal of the ovaries. Estrogenic hormones may be prescribed orally, transdermally, or by subcutaneous implant. The combination of progestogen with estrogen is preferred if the woman has retained her uterus, since administration of estrogen alone might cause overstimulation of the endometrium, resulting in uterine bleeding, or it may even cause cancer. HRT is effective against *vasomotor symptoms (e.g. hot flashes) and genitourinary atrophy (causing vaginal dryness); there is usually also an improvement in psychological well-being. It is most efficacious in preventing these conditions if prescribed as soon as the earliest symptoms of the menopause are detected. Long-term use of HRT may be associated with increased risk of breast cancer, dementia, heart disease, stroke, and blood clots in the legs and lungs and is therefore no longer recommended for the prevention of osteoporosis.

horn *n.* (in anatomy) a process, outgrowth, or extension of an organ or other structure. It is often paired. In the spinal cord crescent-shaped areas of gray matter (seen in cross-section) are known as the dorsal and ventral horns.

Horner's syndrome a group of symptoms that are due to a disorder of the sympathetic nerves in the brainstem or cervical (neck) region. The syndrome consists of a constricted pupil, drooping of the upper eyelid (*ptosis), and an absence of sweating over the affected side of the face. [J. F. Horner (1831–86), Swiss ophthalmologist]

horseshoe kidney an anatomic variation in kidney development whereby the lower poles of both kidneys are joined. This usually causes no trouble but it may be associated with impaired drainage of urine from the kidney by the ureters, which cross in front of the united lower segment.

hospice *n.* an institution that specializes in the care of terminally ill patients, especially those with cancer, emphasizing special concern for death with dignity and using narcotic drugs in carefully controlled doses for the relief of pain.

hospital *n.* an institution providing medical or psychiatric care and treatment for patients. Such care may be residential (inpatient), including the care of patients for a whole day and their return home at night (*day hospital*). Outpatient services include consultation with designated specialists by prior appointment, X-rays, laboratory tests, physiotherapy, and accident and emergency services for those requiring urgent care.

A *county hospital* is one operated by a county government. County hospitals are found in many rural and urban areas of the US, where they may provide health care for both paying and indigent patients. They may be managed or supervised by elected officials or citizens appointed to a board. In some urban areas, a hospital may be operated jointly by representatives of city and county governments. *Community hospitals* are organized primarily to provide adequate medical care for persons living in specific geographic areas. They are usually operated by independent nonprofit corporations with membership open to any interested citizen and governed by a board of trustees elected by the members. Administrative and medical personnel manage the day-to-day functions of the hospital. A *cooperative hospital* is operated primarily for the use of members of a group medical practice. Some larger hospitals have resources that are more highly specialized, to meet the needs of a wider population, often providing training for medical students (*teaching* or *university hospitals*) and for postgraduate education and research.

hospital fatality ratio *see* case fatality ratio.

hospital infection *see* nosocomial infection.

host *n.* an animal or plant in or upon which a *parasite lives. An *intermediate host* is one in which the parasite passes its larval or asexual stages; a *definitive host* is one in which the parasite develops to its sexual stage.

hot flash a reddening of the skin, especially of the face and/or the neck, that can occur in some emotional disorders and during the *menopause. *See also* hormone replacement therapy, vasomotor symptoms.

Hounsfield unit the numerical unit assigned electronically to each *pixel in a *computed tomography (CT) image according to its X-ray density. The fixed points on the scale are arbitrarily assigned as –1000 for air and 0 for water. The CT image is viewed in a "window." The range of Hounsfield units displayed (window width) and the center point of the range of interest (window level) can be varied by the radiologist in order to observe specific tissues (*see* windowing). The unit was named after Sir Godfrey Hounsfield (1919–), who developed CT scanning in the 1950s. Symbol: HU.

hourglass stomach a deformity of the stomach in which it is constricted by fibrosis caused by a chronic peptic ulcer, producing an upper and a lower cavity separated by a narrow channel. *Tea-pot* and *handbag* are other stomach shapes associated with a chronic peptic ulcer.

housemaid's knee a fluid-filled swelling of the bursa in front of the kneecap, often resulting from frequent kneeling. Treatment – and prevention – is by avoidance of kneeling. Medical name: **prepatellar bursitis.** *See also* bursitis.

HPV *see* human papillomavirus.

H₂-receptor antagonist *see* antihistamine.

H₂ receptors *see* antihistamine.

HRT *see* hormone replacement therapy.

HSA *see* Health Systems Agency.

5-HT 5-hydroxytryptamine (*see* serotonin).

5HT₁ agonist any one of a class of drugs that stimulate *serotonin receptors and are effective in the treatment of *migraine by rapidly reversing the dilation of blood vessels in the head that causes the migraine headache. The group includes *almotriptan* (Axert), *naratriptan* (Amerge), *sumatriptan, and *zolmitriptan* (Zomig).

HTLV (human T-cell lymphotropic virus, human T-cell leukemia/lymphoma virus) a family of viruses that includes the *AIDS virus, HTLV-III (or HIV). HTLV-I causes lymphoma.

human chorionic gonadotropin (hCG) *see* chorionic gonadotropin.

human chorionic somatomammotropin *see* human placental lactogen.

Human Genome Project a massive international research project to map the entire sequence of genes on all the human chromosomes. The human genome comprises some 3000 million nucleotide base pairs (*see* DNA) forming about 30,000 genes, distributed between 23 pairs of chromosomes. The sequence of these bases, along the length of each chromosome, is currently being determined in several centers in different parts of the world; the final version of the sequence was published in 2003. The Human Genome Project is by far the most ambitious biologic research program of all time. Beginning in 1988, it was scheduled to last for 15 years. Knowledge of the entire human genome will be of incalculable value to medicine and human biology. It has already resulted in the identification of genes associated with many hereditary disorders and revealed the existence of a genetic basis or component for many other diseases not previously known to have one. Theoretically, this would enable the development of drugs to alleviate conditions caused by deficiency of specific proteins and the large-scale genetic screening of

populations known to be susceptible to particular disorders.

human immunodeficiency virus *see* HIV.

human leukocyte antigen system *see* HLA system.

human papillomavirus (HPV) a virus – a member of the *papovavirus group – that causes warts, including genital warts. There are over 50 strains of HPV: certain strains are considered to be causative factors in the development of anal and genital cancers, especially cervical cancer, but additional factors are necessary before the cells become malignant. HPV is one of the most common sexually transmitted infections. In women the presence of HPV may be detected on colposcopic examination, although techniques using DNA amplification (*see* polymerase chain reaction) give more accurate results and suggest that up to 40% of a normal, apparently healthy, female population may harbor these viruses. In women with an abnormal cervical smear, the DNA test is found to be positive in a much higher percentage and is therefore a useful indicator of a high risk of developing cancer of the cervix.

human placental lactogen (human chorionic somatomammotropin) a protein hormone of 190 amino acids produced by the placenta during most but not all pregnancies. Despite its name it does not appear to have a role in lactation and its exact function remains obscure. It does, however, seem to contribute to the development of diabetes in some pregnancies.

humectant 1. *n.* a substance that is used for moistening. **2.** *adj.* causing moistening.

humerus *n.* the bone of the arm (see illustration). The *head* of the humerus articulates with the *scapula at the shoulder joint. At the lower end of the shaft, the *trochlea* articulates with the *ulna and part of the radius of the forearm. The radius also articulates with a rounded protuberance (*capitulum*) close to the trochlea. Depressions (*fossae*) at the front and back of the humerus accommodate the ulna and radius when the arm is flexed or straightened.

humor *n.* a body fluid. *See* aqueous humor, vitreous humor.

humoral *adj.* circulating in the bloodstream; humoral *immunity requires circulating antibodies.

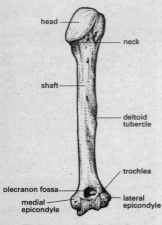

The humerus (posterior surface)

Labels: head, neck, shaft, deltoid tubercle, trochlea, olecranon fossa, medial epicondyle, lateral epicondyle

Hunner's ulcer *see* interstitial cystitis. [G. L. Hunner (1868–1957), US urologist]

Hunter's syndrome a hereditary disorder caused by deficiency of an enzyme that results in the accumulation of protein–carbohydrate complexes and fats in the cells of the body (*see* mucopolysaccharidosis). This leads to mental retardation, enlargement of the liver and spleen, and prominent coarse facial features (*gargoylism*). The disease is *sex-linked, being restricted to males, although females can be *carriers. Medical name: **mucopolysaccharidosis type II**. [C. H. Hunter (1872–1955), US physician]

Huntington's disease (Huntington's chorea) a hereditary disease caused by a defect in a single gene that is inherited as a *dominant characteristic, tending to appear in half of the children of parents with this condition. Symptoms, which begin to appear in early middle age, include unsteady gait and jerky involuntary movements (*see* chorea) accompanied by behavioral changes and progressive dementia. The defective gene, which is located on chromosome 4, has now been identified, and *genetic screening is possible for those at risk. [G. Huntington (1850–1916), US physician]

Hurler's syndrome a hereditary disorder caused by deficiency of an enzyme that results in the accumulation of protein–carbohydrate complexes and fats in the cells of the body (*see* mucopolysaccharidosis). This leads to severe mental retardation, enlargement of the liver and spleen, heart defects, deformities of the bones, and coarsening and thickening of facial features (*gargoylism*). A bone marrow transplant offers the only hope of treatment. Medical name: **mucopolysaccharidosis type I**. [G. Hurler (1889–1965), Austrian pediatrician]

Hürthle cell tumor a malignant tumor of the thyroid gland that arises from *Hürthle cells*, large eosinophilic cells occasionally occurring in the gland. This carcinoma is not as common as *papillary, follicular*, or *anaplastic* thyroid carcinomas. [K. W. Hürthle (1860–1945), German histologist]

Hutchinson's teeth narrowed and notched permanent incisor teeth: a sign of congenital *syphilis. [J. Hutchinson (1828–1913), British surgeon]

hyal- (hyalo-) *prefix denoting* **1.** glassy; transparent. **2.** hyalin. **3.** the vitreous humor of the eye.

hyalin *n.* a clear glassy material produced as the result of degeneration in certain tissues, particularly connective tissue and epithelial cells.

hyaline cartilage the most common type of *cartilage: a bluish-white elastic material with a matrix of chondroitin sulfate in which fine collagen fibrils are embedded.

hyaline membrane disease *see* respiratory distress syndrome.

hyalitis *n.* inflammation of the *vitreous humor of the eye. *See also* asteroid hyalosis.

hyaloid artery a fetal artery lying in the *hyaloid canal of the eye and supplying the lens.

hyaloid canal a channel within the vitreous humor of the *eye. It extends from the center of the optic disk, where it communicates with the lymph spaces of the optic nerve, to the posterior wall of the lens.

hyaloid membrane the transparent membrane that surrounds the *vitreous humor of the eye, separating it from the retina.

hyaluronic acid an acid *mucopolysaccharide that acts as the binding and protective agent of the ground substance of connective tissue. It is also present in the synovial fluid around joints and in the vitreous and aqueous humors of the eye.

hyaluronidase n. an enzyme that depolymerizes *hyaluronic acid and therefore increases the permeability of connective tissue. Hyaluronidase is found in the testes, in semen, and in other tissues.

hybrid n. the offspring of a cross between two genetically unlike individuals. A hybrid, whose parents are usually of different species or varieties, is often sterile.

HYCOSY (hysterosalpingo-contrast sonography) an outpatient technique that tests for blocked fallopian tubes. Using *transvaginal ultrasonography and an echo contrast medium, flow along the tubes can be reliably visualized. See also Doppler ultrasonography.

hydantoin n. any of a group of anticonvulsants used in the management of almost all forms of epilepsy. The most common hydantoins in current use are *phenytoin and *ethotoin.

hydatid n. a bladderlike cyst formed in various human tissues following the growth of the larval stage of an *Echinococcus tapeworm. E. granulosus produces a single large fluid-filled cyst, called unilocular hydatid, which gives rise internally to smaller daughter cysts. The entire hydatid is bound by a fibrous capsule. E. multilocularis forms aggregates of many smaller cysts with a jellylike matrix, called an alveolar hydatid, and enlarges by budding off external daughter cysts. Alveolar hydatids are not delimited by fibrous capsules and produce malignant tumors, which invade and destroy human tissues. See also hydatid disease.

hydatid disease (hydatidosis, echinococciasis, echinococcosis) a condition resulting from the presence in the liver, lungs, or brain of *hydatid cysts. The cysts of Echinococcus multilocularis form malignant tumors; those of E. granulosus exert pressure as they grow and thereby damage surrounding tissues. The presence of hydatids in the brain may result in blindness and epilepsy, and the rupture of any cyst can cause severe allergic reactions, including fever and *urticaria. Treatment may necessitate surgical removal of the cysts. Spread of hydatid disease, particularly common in sheep-raising countries, can be prevented by the deworming of dogs.

hydatidiform mole (hydatid mole, vesicular mole) a collection of fluid-filled sacs that develop when the membrane (chorion) surrounding the embryo degenerates in early pregnancy. These sacs give the placenta the appearance of a bunch of grapes. The embryo dies, the uterus enlarges, and there is a discharge of pinkish liquid and cysts from the vagina. A malignant condition may subsequently develop (see chorionepithelioma).

hydatidosis n. see hydatid disease.

hydr- (hydro-) prefix denoting water or a watery fluid.

hydragogue n. an agent that produces a watery discharge, particularly a laxative that produces watery stools.

hydralazine n. a *vasodilator drug used, usually in conjunction with *diuretics, to treat hypertension. It is given by mouth or injection; side effects, including rapid heart rate, headache, faintness, and digestive upsets, can occur, especially at high doses. Trade name: **Apresoline**.

hydramnios (hydramnio) n. the presence of an abnormally large amount of *amniotic fluid surrounding the fetus from about the 20th week of pregnancy. The uterus becomes swollen, which causes breathlessness, excess fluid in the body tissues, and other symptoms in the woman, and there may be a difficult birth. Most cases of hydramnios are associated with twin pregnancies or with fetal abnormalities, e.g. *anencephaly. The diagnosis is confirmed by ultrasound scan.

hydrargyria n. see mercurialism.

hydrarthrosis n. swelling at a joint caused by excessive synovial fluid. The condition usually involves the knees and may be recurrent. Often no cause is apparent; in some cases rheumatoid arthritis develops later.

hydremia n. the presence in the blood of more than the normal proportion of water.

hydroa (hidroa) n. an eruption of small blisters accompanied by intense itching, occurring (usually in preadolescent boys) on skin surfaces exposed to sunlight. Hydroa is a severe form of light-sensitive dermatitis, described as *polymorphic light eruptions*.

hydrocalycosis *n.* *see* caliectasis.

hydrocele *n.* the accumulation of watery liquid in a sac, usually the sac surrounding the testes. This condition is characterized by painless enlargement of the scrotum; it is treated surgically, by drainage of the fluid or removal of the sac.

hydrocephalus *n.* an abnormal increase in the amount of cerebrospinal fluid within the ventricles of the brain. In childhood, before the sutures of the skull have fused, hydrocephalus makes the head enlarge. In adults, because of the unyielding nature of the skull, hydrocephalus raises the intracranial pressure with consequent drowsiness and vomiting. Hydrocephalus may be caused by obstruction to the outflow of cerebrospinal fluid from the ventricles or a failure of its reabsorption into the cerebral sinuses. *Spina bifida is commonly associated with hydrocephalus in childhood. Treatment involves treating the underlying cause and, if necessary, diverting the excess cerebrospinal fluid into the abdominal cavity, where it is absorbed. This is achieved by tunneling a thin tube from the ventricles to the abdomen (a *ventriculo-peritoneal shunt*) or atrium (*ventriculo-atrial shunt*).

hydrochloric acid a strong acid present, in a very dilute form, in gastric juice. The secretion of excess hydrochloric acid by the stomach results in the condition *hyperchlorhydria.

hydrochlorothiazide *n.* a thiazide *diuretic used to treat fluid retention (edema) and high blood pressure. It is administered by mouth, and side effects can include digestive upsets, skin reactions, and dizziness. Trade names: **Esidrex**, **Hydro-DIURIL**, **Oretic**.

hydrocodone *n.* an opioid *analgesic and *antitussive used for the relief of moderate to severe pain (*Vicodin*, *Lortab*, *Norco*, *Zydone*) and for the suppression of coughing (*Hycodan*, *Hycomine*, *Hycotuss*). It is administered orally; common side effects include drowsiness, sedation, nausea and vomiting, and constipation.

hydrocortisone a pharmaceutical preparation of the steroid hormone *cortisol (*see also* corticosteroid). Hydrocortisone is used to treat adrenal failure (*Addison's disease) and inflammatory, allergic, and rheumatic conditions (including rheumatoid arthritis, colitis, and eczema). It may be given by mouth, by injection, or in the form of a cream, ointment, or eye or ear drops. Possible side effects of hydrocortisone therapy include peptic ulcers, bone and muscle damage, suppression of growth in children, and the signs of *Cushing's syndrome. Trade names: **Ansul-HC**, **Cortizone**, **Hydrocortone**, **Locoid**, **Pramosone**, **Proctocort**.

hydrocyanic acid (prussic acid) an intensely poisonous volatile acid that can cause death within a minute if inhaled. It smells of bitter almonds. *See* cyanide.

hydroflumethiazide *n.* a *diuretic used to treat fluid retention (edema) and high blood pressure. It is administered by mouth and may cause skin reactions, digestive upsets, dizziness, and weakness. Trade names: **Diucardin**, **Saluron**.

hydrogen *n.* a colorless odorless tasteless gas that is highly inflammable and explosive when mixed with air. It is the lightest element, occurs only sparsely in pure form, and is found in water and almost all organic compounds. Hydrogen is essential in the metabolic interaction of acids, bases, and salts within the body, in maintaining the fluid balance necessary for human survival, and in the process of *hydrolysis, by which compounds are split into simpler substances. Symbol: H.

hydrogenase *n.* an enzyme that catalyzes the addition of hydrogen to a compound in reduction reactions.

hydrogen bond a weak electrostatic bond formed by linking a hydrogen atom between two electronegative atoms (e.g. nitrogen or oxygen). The large number of hydrogen bonds in proteins and nucleic acids are responsible for maintaining the stable molecular structure of these compounds.

hydrogen peroxide a colorless liquid used as a disinfectant for cleansing wounds and, diluted, as a deodorant mouthwash or as ear drops for removing wax. Strong solutions irritate the skin.

hydrolase *n.* an enzyme that catalyzes the hydrolysis of compounds. Examples are the *peptidases.

hydrolysis *n.* the decomposition of a compound by the addition of water, the hydroxyl group (–OH) being incorporated into one component and the hydrogen atom (H) into the other.

hydroma *n. see* hygroma.

hydromorphone an opioid *analgesic used to treat moderate to severe pain. It is administered orally, by rectal suppository, or by injection. Common side effects include drowsiness, sedation, nausea and vomiting, and constipation. Trade name: **Dilaudid**.

hydromyelia *n.* a dilation of the central canal of the spinal cord (which is a continuation of the ventricular system of the brain). It has been suggested that the canal is distended by a rise in the pressure of the ventricular cerebrospinal fluid caused by a blockage to its normal outflow to the surface of the brain. The patient's symptoms are those of *syringomyelia. The condition is diagnosed by computed tomography or magnetic resonance imaging and treated surgically.

hydronephrosis *n.* distension and dilation of the pelvis of the kidney. This is due to an obstruction to the free flow of urine from the kidney. An obstruction at or below the neck of the bladder will cause hydronephrosis of both kidneys. The term *primary pelvic hydronephrosis* is used when the obstruction, usually functional, is at the junction of the renal pelvis and ureter. Surgical relief by *pyeloplasty is advisable to avoid the back pressure atrophy of the kidney and the complications of infection and stone formation. —**hydronephrotic** *adj.*

hydropericarditis *n. see* hydropericardium.

hydropericardium *n.* accumulation of a clear serous fluid within the membranous sac surrounding the heart. It occurs in many cases of *pericarditis (*hydropericarditis*). If the heart is compressed, the fluid is withdrawn (aspirated) via a needle inserted into the pericardial sac through the chest wall (*pericardiocentesis*). *See also* hydropneumopericardium.

hydroperitoneum *n. see* ascites.

hydrophobia *n. see* rabies.

hydrophthalmos *n. see* buphthalmos.

hydropneumopericardium *n.* the presence of air and clear fluid within the pericardial sac around the heart, which is most commonly due to entry of air during pericardiocentesis (*see* hydropericar-

dium). The presence of air does not affect the management of the patient.

hydropneumoperitoneum *n.* the presence of fluid and gas in the peritoneal cavity. This may be due either to the introduction of air through an instrument being used to remove the fluid, because a perforation in the digestive tract has allowed the escape of fluid and gas, or due to gas-forming bacteria growing in the peritoneal fluid.

hydropneumothorax (pneumohydrothorax) *n.* the presence of air and fluid in the pleural cavity. If the patient is shaken the fluid makes a splashing sound (called a *succussion splash*). An *effusion of serous fluid commonly complicates a *pneumothorax, and must be drained.

hydrops *n.* an abnormal accumulation of fluid in body tissues or cavities. For example, *corneal hydrops* is the sudden painful accumulation of fluid in the cornea seen in *keratoconus. It results in a sudden reduction of vision. *See also* hydrops fetalis.

hydrops fetalis severe edema that develops before birth. The excess fluid collects in the body cavities, particularly in the peritoneal cavity (*see* ascites) and the pleural cavity. There are several causes for this, but the most common is severe anemia associated with *hemolytic disease of the newborn. It can occur with a twin-to-twin transfusion. Other causes are congenital heart disease, kidney disease, and lung disease. Treatment can be undertaken before birth with intrauterine blood transfusions to the fetus; without treatment the mortality is high. Antenatal ultrasound scanning enables early recognition of hydrops fetalis.

hydrosalpinx *n.* the accumulation of watery fluid in one of the *fallopian tubes, which becomes swollen.

hydrostatic accouchement the management of normal labor with the mother partially immersed in a water bath.

hydrotherapy *n.* the use of water in the treatment of disorders, now restricted in orthodox medicine to exercises in remedial swimming pools for the rehabilitation of arthritic or partially paralyzed patients.

hydrothorax *n.* fluid in the pleural cavity. *See also* hydropneumothorax.

hydrotubation *n.* the introduction of a fluid (usually a dye) through the cervix of the uterus under pressure to allow visualization, by *laparoscopy, of the passage of the dye through the fallopian tubes. It is used to test whether or not the tubes are blocked in the investigation of infertility. *See also* HYCOSY.

hydroureter *n.* an accumulation of urine in one of the tubes (ureters) leading from the kidneys to the bladder. The ureter becomes swollen and the condition usually results from obstruction of the ureter by a stone or a misplaced artery.

hydroxocobalamine *n.* a cobalt-containing drug administered by injection to treat conditions involving vitamin B_{12} deficiency, such as pernicious anemia. Trade name: **alphaRedisol**.

hydroxyamphetamine *n.* a *sympathomimetic drug used in solution or sprays for the relief of nasal symptoms such as congestion, inflammation, and sinusitis. It is also used to dilate the pupil of the eye for eye examinations. Side effects can include headache, nausea, vomiting, and palpitations.

hydroxyapatite *n.* **1.** the crystalline component of bones and teeth, consisting of a complex form of calcium phosphate. **2.** a biocompatible ceramic material that is a synthetic form of natural hydroxyapatite. Some joint replacement prostheses are coated with a form of synthetic hydroxyapatite, which encourages bone to grow on to the implant. The material is also used in some forms of middle-ear surgery.

hydroxychloroquine *n.* a drug similar to *chloroquine, used mainly to treat malaria, lupus erythematosus, and rheumatoid arthritis. Side effects such as skin reactions, hair loss, and digestive upsets may occur and prolonged use can lead to eye damage. Trade name: **Plaquenil**.

5-hydroxyindoleacetic acid (5-HIAA) a metabolite of *serotonin, the most common secretion product of carcinoid tumors (*see* argentaffinoma). Measured over 24 hours in the urine, this is the most reliable screening test for such tumors.

hydroxymethylglutaryl coenzyme A reductase (HMG–CoA reductase) an enzyme that catalyzes the conversion of HMG–CoA to mevalonate, which is an early and rate-limiting step in the biosynthesis of cholesterol. *Statins that inhibit this enzyme are therefore used in the treatment of hypercholesterolemia.

hydroxyprogesterone *n.* a synthetic female sex hormone (*see* progestogen) administered by injection to prevent miscarriage and to treat menstrual disorders. There may be pain at the injection site, and progestogens taken by mouth are often preferred. Trade name: **Gesterol LA 250, Hylutin, Prodrox**.

hydroxyproline *n.* a compound, similar in structure to the *amino acids, found only in *collagen.

5-hydroxytryptamine *n. see* serotonin.

hydroxyurea *n.* a drug that prevents cell growth and is used to treat melanoma and some types of leukemia. It is administered by mouth. Hydroxyurea may lower the white cell content of the blood due to its effects on the bone marrow. Trade name: **Hydrea**.

hydroxyzine *n.* an *antihistamine drug with sedative properties, used to relieve anxiety, tension, and agitation and to treat nausea and vomiting. It is administered by mouth, injection, and in a syrup. Hydroxyzine may cause drowsiness, headache, dry mouth, and itching. Trade names: **Atarax, Vistaril**.

hygiene *n.* the science of health and the study of ways of preserving it, particularly by promoting cleanliness.

hygr- (hygro-) *prefix denoting* moisture.

hygroma (hydroma) *n.* a type of cyst. It may develop from a *lymphangioma (*cystic hygroma*) or from the liquified remains of a subdural *hematoma (*subdural hygroma*).

hygrometer *n.* an instrument for measuring the relative humidity of the atmosphere, i.e. the ratio of the moisture in the air to the moisture it would contain if it were saturated at the same temperature and pressure.

hymen *n.* the membrane that covers the opening of the vagina at birth but usually perforates spontaneously before puberty. If the initial opening is small, it may tear, with slight loss of blood, at the first occasion of sexual intercourse.

Hymenolepis *n.* a genus of small widely distributed parasitic tapeworms. The dwarf tapeworm, *H. nana*, only 40 mm in length, lives in the human intestine. Fleas can be important vectors of this species, and children in close contact with flea-infested dogs are particularly prone to infection. *H. diminuta* is a common parasite of rodents; humans occasionally become infected on swallowing stored cereals contaminated with insect pests – the intermediate hosts for this parasite. Symptoms of abdominal pain, diarrhea, loss of appetite, and headache are obvious only in heavy infections of either species. Treatment involves a course of *anthelmintics.

hymenotomy *n.* incision of the hymen at the entrance to the vagina. This operation may be performed on a young girl if the membrane completely closes the vagina and thus impedes the flow of menstrual blood. It is also carried out to relieve dyspareunia (painful intercourse).

hyo- *prefix denoting* the hyoid bone. Example: *hyoglossal* (relating to the hyoid bone and tongue).

hyoglossus *n.* a muscle that serves to depress the tongue. It has its origin on the hyoid bone.

hyoid bone a small isolated U-shaped bone in the neck, below and supporting the tongue. It is held in position by muscles and ligaments between it and the styloid process of the temporal bone.

hyoscine *n. see* scopolamine.

hyoscyamine *n.* a drug with similar activity to *scopolamine, used, often in mixtures, to treat muscle spasm. It is administered by mouth. Trade names: **Anaspaz**, **Levsin**, **Levsinex**.

hyp- (hypo-) *prefix denoting* **1.** deficiency, lack, or small size. Example: *hypognathous* (having a small lower jaw). **2.** (in anatomy) below; beneath. Example: *hypoglossal* (under the tongue).

hypalgesia *n.* an abnormally low sensitivity to pain.

Hypaque *n.* trade name for diatrizoate sodium, used as a water-soluble contrast medium in radiology of the urinary tract.

hyper- *prefix denoting* **1.** excessive; abnormally increased. **2.** (in anatomy) above.

hyperactive child syndrome *see* attention-deficit/hyperactivity disorder.

hyperacusis *n.* abnormally acute hearing or painful sensitivity to sounds.

hyperadrenalism *n.* overactivity of the adrenal glands. *See* Cushing's syndrome.

hyperalgesia *n.* an abnormal state of increased sensitivity to painful stimuli.

hyperandrogenism *n.* excessive secretion of androgen in women. It is associated with *hirsutism, acne, sparse or infrequent menstruation (oligomenorrhea), *metrorrhagia, absent or infrequent ovulation, infertility, endometrial *hyperplasia, *hyperlipidemia, *hyperglycemia, and hypertension; all these conditions may be the result of mutations in specific genes. *See also* virilization.

hyperbaric *adj.* at a pressure greater than atmospheric pressure.

hyperbaric oxygenation a technique for exposing a patient to oxygen at high pressure. It is used to treat carbon monoxide poisoning, gas gangrene, *compressed air illness, and acute breathing difficulties. It is also used in some cases during heart surgery.

hyperbilirubinemia *n.* excessive amounts of the *bile pigment bilirubin in the blood, which can lead to jaundice, anorexia, and malaise, and in the newborn to *kernicterus. The condition is usually associated with liver disease or biliary obstruction, but may also be due to excessive red blood cell destruction, as occurs in hemolytic anemia. *See also* Crigler-Najjar syndrome, Gilbert's syndrome.

hypercalcemia *n.* the presence in the blood of an abnormally high concentration of calcium. *Idiopathic hypercalcemia* is a congenital condition associated with mental retardation and heart defects. Hypercalcemia can also be caused by excessive ingestion of vitamin D, overactivity of the *parathyroid glands, and malignant disease. *Compare* hypocalcemia.

hypercalciuria (hypercalcinuria) *n.* the presence in the urine of an abnormally high concentration of calcium.

hypercapnia (hypercarbia) *n.* the presence in the blood of an abnormally high concentration of carbon dioxide.

hyperchloremia *n.* the presence in the blood of an abnormally high concentration of chloride.

hyperchlorhydria *n.* a greater than normal secretion of hydrochloric acid by the stomach, usually associated with a *duodenal ulcer. Extremely high levels of acid secretion are found in the *Zollinger-Ellison syndrome.

hypercholesterolemia *n. see* cholesterol.

hyperchromatism *n.* the property of the nuclei of certain cells (for example, those of tumors) to stain more deeply than normal. —**hyperchromatic** *adj.*

hyperdactylism (polydactylism) *n.* the condition of having more than the normal number of fingers or toes. The extra digits are commonly undersized (rudimentary) and are usually removed surgically shortly after birth.

hyperdynamia *n.* excessive activity of muscles.

hyperemesis *n.* severe vomiting. *Hyperemesis gravidarum* affects pregnant women: the stomach contents and bile are vomited, and the acidity of the arterial blood increases. If the vomiting is allowed to continue for a long time, marked dehydration and liver disease may develop. If rest, restriction of liquid intake, controlled diet, and drugs aimed at stopping the vomiting fail to cure the condition, it may be necessary to terminate the pregnancy. *Hyperemesis lactentium* is vomiting by babies at the breast-feeding stage.

hyperemia *n.* the presence of excess blood in the vessels supplying a part of the body. In *active hyperemia (arterial hyperemia)* the arterioles are relaxed and there is an increased blood flow. In *passive hyperemia* the blood flow from the affected part is obstructed.

hyperesthesia *n.* excessive sensibility, especially of the skin.

hyperextension *n.* excessive and forceful extension of a limb or joint beyond the normal limits, usually as part of an orthopedic procedure to correct deformity.

hyperglycemia *n.* an excess of glucose in the bloodstream. It may occur in a variety of diseases, most notably in *diabetes mellitus, due to insufficient insulin in the blood and excessive intake of carbohydrates. Untreated it may progress to diabetic coma.

hypergraphia *n.* a style of writing characterized by excessive verbosity, pedantic insistence on much nonessential detail, and obsessive inclusiveness that is a feature of the type of personality disturbance frequently associated with severe epilepsy. People manifesting hypergraphia will seldom accept that they have a communication problem.

hyperhidrosis (hyperidrosis) *n.* excessive sweating, which may occur in certain diseases, such as fevers or thyrotoxicosis, or following the use of certain drugs. More commonly, however, there is no underlying cause for this condition. There are many successful treatments, including anticholinergic drugs, injections of *botulinum toxin, and selective surgical *sympathectomy.

hyperinsulinism *n.* **1.** excessive secretion of the hormone insulin by the islet cells of the pancreas. **2.** metabolic disturbance due to administration of too much insulin.

hyperkalemia *n.* the presence in the blood of an abnormally high concentration of *potassium, usually due to failure of the kidneys to excrete the potassium. *See also* electrolyte.

hyperkeratosis *n.* thickening of the outer horny layer of the skin. It may occur as an inherited disorder, affecting the palms and soles. *See also* ichthyosis.

hyperkinesia *n.* a state of overactive restlessness in children. —**hyperkinetic** *adj.*

hyperkinetic syndrome *see* attention-deficit/hyperactivity disorder.

hyperlipidemia *n.* the presence in the blood of an abnormally high concentration of *cholesterol and/or triglycerides in the form of *lipoproteins, which predisposes to *atherosclerosis and coronary heart disease.

hyperlipoproteinemia *n.* the presence in the blood of abnormally high concentrations of *lipoproteins due to faulty lipoprotein metabolism.

hypermetropia *n. see* hyperopia.

hypermotility *n.* excessive movement or activity, especially of the stomach or intestine.

hypernatremia *n.* the presence in the blood of an abnormally high concentration of *sodium. *See also* electrolyte.

hypernephroma (Grawitz tumor, renal cell carcinoma) *n.* a malignant tumor of kidney cells, so called because it is said to resemble part of the adrenal gland and at one time was thought to originate from this site. It may be present for some years before giving rise to symptoms, which include fever, loin pain and swelling, and blood in the urine. Treatment is by surgery, but tumors are apt to recur locally or spread via the bloodstream and can often be seen growing along the renal vein. Secondary growths from a renal cell carcinoma in the lung have a characteristic "cannonball" appearance. These tumors are relatively insensitive to radiotherapy and cytotoxic drugs, but some respond to such hormones as progestogens. *Immunotherapy using such agents as *interferon and *interleukin 2 has shown promise in this disease.

hyperopia (hypermetropia, farsightedness) *n.* the condition in which parallel light rays are brought to a focus behind the retina when the *accommodation is relaxed (see illustration). Moderate degrees of hyperopia may not cause blurred vision in children and young adults because of their ability to accommodate, but for older people and those with greater degrees of hyperopia near vision is more blurred than distance vision. Normal vision can be restored by wearing glasses with convex lenses. *Compare* emmetropia, myopia.

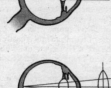

focusing point is beyond the retina

Uncorrected

Corrected

convex lens converges light rays falling on the eye

Hyperopia (farsightedness)

hyperosmia *n.* an abnormally acute sense of smell.

hyperosmolar nonketotic diabetic coma a coma induced by very poorly controlled *diabetes mellitus in which the blood-sugar levels have become markedly high with severe dehydration but no excessive *ketone production or acidosis. It is most common in elderly patients with type 2 diabetes and has a mortality of around 30%.

hyperostosis *n.* excessive enlargement of

the outer layer of a bone. The condition is harmless and is usually recognized as an incidental finding on X-ray. It commonly affects the frontal bone of the skull (*hyperostosis frontalis*). *Infantile cortical hyperostosis* (or *Caffey's disease*) affects infants under six months. There is swelling of the long bones, jaw, and shoulder blade, with pain and a fever. The condition settles spontaneously.

hyperparathyroidism *n.* overactivity of the parathyroid glands. Treatment is by surgery. *See* von Recklinghausen's disease.

hyperpiesia *n.* see hypertension.

hyperplasia *n.* the increased production and growth of normal cells in a tissue or organ. The affected part becomes larger but retains its normal form, as in *benign prostatic hyperplasia. During pregnancy the breasts grow in this manner. *See also* endometrial hyperplasia. *Compare* hypertrophy, neoplasia.

hyperpnea *n.* an increase in the rate of breathing that is proportional to an increase in metabolism, as, for example, during exercise. Usually it is an abnormal condition caused by disease. *Compare* hyperventilation.

hyperpraxia *n.* excessive motor activity, such as is seen in *mania and *attention-deficit/hyperactivity disorder.

hyperpyrexia *n.* a rise in body temperature above 106°F (41.1°C). *See* fever.

hypersensitive *adj.* prone to respond abnormally to the presence of a particular antigen, which may cause a variety of tissue reactions ranging from *serum sickness to an allergy (such as hay fever) or, at the severest, to anaphylactic shock (*see* anaphylaxis). It is thought that when the normal antigen-antibody defense reaction is followed by tissue damage this may be due to an abnormality in the working of the *complement system. *See also* allergy, immunity. —**hypersensitivity** *n.*

hypersomnia *n.* sleep lasting for exceptionally long periods, as occurs in some cases of brain inflammation.

hypersplenism *n.* a decrease in the numbers of red cells, white cells, and platelets in the blood resulting from destruction or pooling of these cells by an enlarged spleen. Hypersplenism may occur in any condition in which there is enlargement of the spleen (*see* splenomegaly).

hypersthenia n. an abnormally high degree of strength or physical tension in all or part of the body.

hypertension n. high *blood pressure, i.e. elevation of the arterial blood pressure above the normal range expected in a particular age group. Hypertension may be of unknown cause (*essential hypertension* or *hyperpiesia*). It may also result from kidney disease, including narrowing (stenosis) of the renal artery (*renal hypertension*), endocrine diseases (such as Cushing's disease or pheochromocytoma), or disease of the arteries (such as coarctation of the aorta), when it is known as *secondary* or *symptomatic hypertension*.

Complications that may arise from hypertension include atherosclerosis, heart failure, cerebral hemorrhage, and kidney failure, but treatment may prevent their development. Hypertension is symptomless until the symptoms of its complications develop. Some cases of hypertension may be cured by eradicating the cause. Most cases, however, depend upon long-term drug therapy to lower the blood pressure and maintain it within the normal range, although often a diet low in sodium and saturated fats and an adequate exercise program to maintain proper weight can control the condition. The drugs used include thiazide *diuretics, *beta blockers, *ACE inhibitors, *calcium antagonists, and *alpha blockers. Combinations of drugs may be needed to obtain optimum control. *See also* portal hypertension, pulmonary hypertension.

hyperthermia (hyperthermy) n. **1.** exceptionally high body temperature (about 41°C or above). *See* fever. **2.** treatment of disease by inducing fever. *Compare* hypothermia.

hyperthyroidism n. overactivity of the thyroid gland, either due to a tumor, overgrowth of the gland, or Graves' disease. *See* thyrotoxicosis.

hypertonia (hypertonicity) n. exceptionally high tension in muscles.

hypertonic adj. **1.** describing a solution that has a greater osmotic pressure than another solution. *See* osmosis. **2.** describing muscles that demonstrate an abnormal increase in *tonicity.

hypertrichosis n. excessive growth of hair (*see* hirsutism).

hypertrophy (hypertrophia) n. increase in the size of a tissue or organ brought about by the enlargement of its cells rather than by cell multiplication (as during normal growth and tumor formation). Muscles undergo this change in response to increased work. *Compare* hyperplasia.

hypertropia n. *see* strabismus.

hyperuricemia (lithemia) n. the presence in the blood of an abnormally high concentration of uric acid. *See* gout.

hyperuricuria (lithuria) n. the presence in the urine of an abnormally high concentration of uric acid.

hyperventilation n. breathing at an abnormally rapid rate at rest. This can be done deliberately and causes dizziness, tingling in the fingers, toes, and around the mouth, and eventually unconsciousness by lowering the carbon dioxide concentration in the blood. It occurs clinically with anxiety (*hyperventilation syndrome*), overventilation of patients on assisted ventilation, liver disease, fever, and septicemia.

hypervitaminosis n. the condition resulting from excessive consumption of vitamins. This is not serious in the case of water-soluble vitamins, when any intake in excess of requirements is easily excreted in the urine. However, fat-soluble vitamins A and D are toxic if taken in excessive amounts.

hypervolemia n. an increase in the volume of circulating blood.

hyphedonia n. a lower than normal capacity for achieving enjoyment.

hyphema n. bleeding into the chamber of the eye that lies in front of the iris.

hypn- (hypno-) prefix denoting **1.** sleep. **2.** hypnosis.

hypnagogic adj. *see* imagery.

hypnagogic hallucinations vivid and intense auditory or visual hallucinations occurring at the beginning or the end of sleep. They occur in 30–60% of patients with *narcolepsy.

hypnopompic adj. *see* imagery.

hypnosis n. a sleeplike state, artificially induced in a person by a *hypnotist*, in which the mind is more than usually receptive to suggestion and memories of past events – apparently forgotten – may be elicited by questioning. Hypnotic suggestion has been used for a variety of purposes in medicine, for example as a cure for addiction and in other forms of *psychotherapy.

hypnotic (soporific) n. a drug that produces sleep by depressing brain function. Hypnotics include benzodiazepines (such as *diazepam and *temazepam), *chloral hydrate, and *triazolam, and some sedative *antihistamines (e.g. *promethazine). Hypnotics are used for the short-term treatment of insomnia and sleep disturbances, especially in mental illnesses and in the elderly. They often cause hangover effects in the morning.

hypnotism n. the induction of *hypnosis.

hypo- prefix. see hyp-.

hypobaric adj. at a pressure lower than that of the atmosphere.

hypobulia n. mild deficiency of willpower. See abulia.

hypocalcemia n. the presence in the blood of an abnormally low concentration of calcium. See tetany. Compare hypercalcemia.

hypocapnia n. see acapnia.

hypochloremia n. the presence in the blood of an abnormally low concentration of chloride.

hypochlorhydria n. reduced secretion of hydrochloric acid by the stomach. See achlorhydria.

hypochondria n. preoccupation with the physical functioning of the body and with fancied ill health. It may amount to a handicapping neurosis and dominate a person's life. In the most severe form there are delusions of ill health, usually due to underlying *depression. When symptoms reach the level sufficient to be classified as a disorder, it is called hypochondriasis (in *DSM-IV) or hypochondriacal disorder (in ICD-10). Treatment with reassurance, *antidepressant drugs, and/or psychotherapy is usual, but the condition is often chronic. —**hypochondriac** adj., n.

hypochondrium n. the upper lateral portion of the *abdomen, situated beneath the lower ribs. —**hypochondriac** adj.

hypocretin n. a recently discovered neuropeptide that originates in the hypothalamus. Low levels of hypocretin in the cerebrospinal fluid are found in most patients with *narcolepsy and may also be found in patients who have suffered stroke, brain tumors, head injuries, and infections of the nervous system.

Hypoderma n. a genus of nonbloodsucking beelike insects – the warble flies – widely distributed in Europe, North America, and Asia. Cattle are the usual hosts for the parasitic maggots, but rare and accidental infections of humans have occurred (see myiasis), especially in farm workers. The maggots migrate beneath the skin surface, producing an inflamed linear lesion similar to that of *creeping eruption.

hypodermic adj. beneath the skin: usually applied to subcutaneous *injections. The term is also applied to the syringe used for such injections, and sometimes – loosely – to any injection.

hypodermoclysis n. the continuous infusion under the skin of saline or other medicated solution to clean away blood, pus, and foreign matter from a wound, or to replace water and salt lost during an illness or surgery.

hypodontia n. a reduction in the normal number of teeth through congenital absence.

hypoesthesia n. a condition in which the sense of touch is diminished; uncommonly this may be extended to include other forms of sensation.

hypofibrinogenemia (fibrinogenopenia) n. a deficiency of the clotting factor *fibrinogen in the blood, which results in an increased tendency to bleed. It may occur as an inherited disorder in which either production of fibrinogen is impaired or the fibrinogen produced does not function in the normal way (dysfibrinogenemia). Alternatively, it may be acquired. For example, it is the most common cause of blood coagulation failure during pregnancy, when the blood fibrinogen level falls below the normal pregnancy level of 4–6 g/l as a result of *disseminated intravascular coagulation (DIC). This usually occurs as a complication of severe *abruptio placentae, prolonged retention of a dead fetus, or amniotic fluid embolism.

hypogammaglobulinemia n. a deficiency of the protein *gamma globulin in the blood. This may occur in a variety of inherited disorders or as an acquired defect, as in chronic lymphocytic *leukemia (CLL). Since gamma globulin consists mainly of defensive antibodies (*immunoglobulins), hypogammaglobulinemia results in an increased susceptibility to infections.

hypogastrium *n.* that part of the central *abdomen situated below the region of the stomach. —**hypogastric** *adj.*

hypogeusia *n.* a condition in which the sense of taste is abnormally weak. *See also* hypoesthesia.

hypoglossal nerve the twelfth *cranial nerve (XII), which supplies the muscles of the tongue and is therefore responsible for the movements of talking and swallowing.

hypoglycemia *n.* a deficiency of glucose in the bloodstream, causing muscular weakness and incoordination, mental confusion, and sweating. If severe this may lead to *hypoglycemic coma*. Hypoglycemia most commonly occurs in *diabetes mellitus, as a result of insulin overdosage and insufficient intake of carbohydrates. It is treated by administration of glucose: by injection if the patient is in a coma, by mouth otherwise. *See also* reactive hypoglycemia. —**hypoglycemic** *adj.*

hypoglycemic unawareness a serious condition in which a diabetic patient loses the earliest warning signs of an approaching hypoglycemic episode. Patients thus may suffer a severe attack, with confusion, seizures, or even coma and death, because they fail to take the necessary measures to abort the episode. The condition is more common in long-standing diabetes and in those who experience many hypoglycemic episodes. It necessitates a temporary driving ban until awareness can be regained, usually by avoidance of further attacks for a period of time.

hypogonadism *n.* impaired function of the testes or ovaries, causing absence or impairment of the *secondary sexual characteristics.

hypohidrosis (hypoidrosis) *n. see* anhidrosis.

hypoinsulinism *n.* a deficiency of insulin due either to inadequate secretion of the hormone by the pancreas or to inadequate treatment of diabetes mellitus.

hypokalemia *n.* the presence of abnormally low levels of potassium in the blood: occurs in dehydration. *See* electrolyte.

hypomania *n.* a mild degree of *mania. Elated mood leads to faulty judgment; behavior lacks the usual social restraints

and the sexual drive is increased; speech is rapid and animated; the individual is energetic but not persistent and tends to be irritable. The abnormality is not so great as in mania and the patient may appear normal and "a bit of a character" to those who do not know him (*see* elation, euphoria). Treatment follows the same principles as for mania, and it may be difficult to prevent an individual from damaging his own interests with extravagant behavior. —**hypomanic** *adj., n.*

hypomenorrhea *n.* the release of an abnormally small quantity of blood at menstruation. The duration of bleeding may be normal or less than normal.

hyponatremia *n.* the presence in the blood of an abnormally low concentration of *sodium: occurs in dehydration. *See* electrolyte.

hypoparathyroidism *n.* subnormal activity of the parathyroid glands, causing a fall in the blood concentration of calcium and muscular spasms (*see* tetany).

hypopharynx *n. see* laryngopharynx, pharynx.

hypophysectomy *n.* the surgical removal or destruction of the pituitary gland (hypophysis) in the brain. The operation may be conducted by opening the skull or by inserting special needles that produce a very low temperature (*see* cryosurgery). Radiotherapy (e.g. by insertion of needles of radioactive *yttrium-90) can also be used to destroy parts of the pituitary.

hypophysis *n. see* pituitary gland.

hypophysitis *n.* a rare condition of inflammation of the *pituitary gland (hypophysis). The main cause is an infiltration by lymphocytes, most commonly during or just after pregnancy. This usually presents as a mass lesion of the pituitary with visual-field loss and headache or with anterior *hypopituitarism, which may be total or just involve particular hormone systems. Around 50% of cases are associated with other autoimmune endocrine diseases, and antipituitary antibodies have been identified.

hypopiesis *n.* abnormally reduced blood pressure in the absence of organic disease (*see* hypotension).

hypopituitarism *n.* subnormal activity of the pituitary gland, causing *dwarfism in childhood and a syndrome of impaired sexual function, pallor, and premature aging in adult life (*see* Simmond's disease).

hypoplasia *n.* underdevelopment of an organ or tissue. *Dental hypoplasia* is the defective formation of parts of a tooth due to illnesses such as measles or starvation while the tooth is being formed. It is marked by transverse lines of brown defective enamel, which define the date of the illness. —**hypoplastic** *adj.*

hypoplastic left heart a congenital heart disorder in which the left side of the heart, particularly the left ventricle, is underdeveloped. The first part of the aorta may also be abnormal. Affected babies usually develop severe heart failure within the first few days of life. The diagnosis can be confirmed on *echocardiography. Prognosis is generally very poor – most babies die within the first few weeks – but milder cases may be amenable to surgery. It is the most common cause of death in the neonatal period due to heart disease.

hypoplastic leukemia a stage of *leukemia in which there is a decrease in the number of white cells, red cells, and platelets in the blood and reduced *hemopoiesis in the bone marrow.

hypopnea *n.* a decrease in breathing rate, which indicates that the body is attempting to compensate for metabolic disturbances due to disease in nonrespiratory organs by retaining acid in the form of carbon dioxide. In *sleep apnea there is a reduction in the nasal airflow to less than 50% of normal, but more than 30% (*see* apnea), for more than 10 seconds.

hypopraxia *n.* **1.** a condition of diminished and enfeebled activity. **2.** a lack of interest in, or a disinclination for, activity; listlessness.

hypoproteinemia *n.* a decrease in the quantity of protein in the blood. It may result from malnutrition, impaired protein production (as in liver disease), or increased loss of protein from the body (as in the *nephrotic syndrome). It results in swelling (*edema), because of the accumulation of fluid in the tissues, and increased susceptibility to infections. *See also* hypogammaglobulinemia.

hypoprothrombinemia *n.* a deficiency of the clotting factor *prothrombin in the blood, which results in an increased ten-

dency to bleed. The condition may occur as an inherited defect or as the result of liver disease, vitamin K deficiency, or anticoagulant treatment.

hypopyon *n.* pus in the chamber of the eye that lies in front of the iris.

hyposensitive *adj.* tending to be less than normally responsive to the presence of antigenic material. *Compare* hypersensitive. —**hyposensitivity** *n.*

hyposensitization *n. see* desensitization.

hyposmia *n.* a condition in which the sense of smell is exceptionally weak. *See also* anosmia.

hypospadias *n.* a congenital abnormality in which the opening of the *urethra is on the underside of the penis: either on the glans penis (*glandular hypospadias*), at the junction of the glans with the shaft (*coronal hypospadias*), or on the shaft itself (*penile hypospadias*). All varieties can be treated surgically, and neither micturition nor sexual function need be impaired.

hypostasis *n.* accumulation of fluid or blood in a dependent part of the body, under the influence of gravity, in cases of poor circulation. Hypostatic congestion of the lung bases may be seen in debilitated patients who are confined to bed. It predisposes to pneumonia (hypostatic pneumonia) but may be prevented by careful nursing and physiotherapy. A similar condition affects the dependent parts of the body after death. —**hypostatic** *adj.*

hyposthenia *n.* a state of physical weakness or abnormally low muscular tension.

hyposthenuria *n.* the secretion of urine of low specific gravity. The inability to concentrate the urine occurs in patients at the final stage of chronic renal failure.

hypotension *n.* a condition in which the arterial *blood pressure is abnormally low. It occurs after excessive fluid loss (e.g. through diarrhea, burns, or vomiting) or following severe blood loss (hemorrhage) from any cause. Other causes include myocardial infarction, pulmonary embolism, severe infections, allergic reactions, arrhythmias, acute abdominal conditions (e.g. pancreatitis), Addison's disease, and drugs (e.g. an overdose of the drugs used to treat hypertension).

Some people experience a temporary fall in blood pressure when rising from a horizontal position (*orthostatic hypotension*). Temporary hypotension may result in a simple faint (syncope). The patient becomes light-headed, sweats, and may develop impaired consciousness. In severe cases peripheral circulatory failure (cardiogenic shock) may develop, with unrecordable blood pressure, weak pulses, and suppression of urine production. The patient is placed flat, with legs elevated, and given oxygen. Fluid and blood are replaced by an intravenous infusion as required. Specific treatment of the cause should be provided (e.g. corticosteroids in Addison's disease).

hypothalamus *n.* the region of the forebrain in the floor of the third ventricle, linked with the thalamus above and the *pituitary gland below (see brain). It contains several important centers controlling body temperature, thirst, hunger and eating, water balance, and sexual function. It is also closely connected with emotional activity and sleep and functions as a center for the integration of hormonal and autonomic nervous activity through its control of pituitary secretions (*see* neuroendocrine system, pituitary gland). —**hypothalamic** *adj.*

hypothenar *adj.* describing or relating to the fleshy prominent part of the palm of the hand below the little finger. *Compare* thenar.

hypothermia *n.* **1.** accidental reduction of body temperature below the normal range in the absence of protective reflex actions, such as shivering. Often insidious in onset, it is particularly liable to occur in babies and the elderly if they are living in poorly heated homes and have inadequate clothing. **2.** deliberate lowering of body temperature for therapeutic purposes. This may be done during surgery, in order to reduce the patient's requirement for oxygen.

hypothymia *n.* a diminished intensity of emotional response. It is a feature of *asthenic personalities, of some chronic schizophrenics, and of some depressives.

hypothyroidism *n.* subnormal activity of the thyroid gland. If present at birth and untreated it leads to *cretinism. In adult life it causes mental and physical slowing, undue sensitivity to cold, slowing of the pulse, weight gain, and coarsening of the skin (*myxedema*). The condition can

be treated by administration of thyroxine.

hypotonia *n.* a state of reduced tension in muscle.

hypotonic *adj.* **1.** describing a solution that has a lower osmotic pressure than another solution. *See* osmosis. **2.** describing muscles that demonstrate diminished *tonicity.

hypotony *n.* a very low intraocular pressure, usually as a result of trauma or surgery to the eye.

hypotrichosis *n.* a condition in which less hair develops than normal.

hypotropia *n. see* strabismus.

hypoventilation *n.* breathing at an abnormally shallow and slow rate, which results in an increased amount of carbon dioxide in the blood. *Alveolar hypoventilation* may be primary, which is very rare, or secondary, which can be due to destructive lesions of the brain or to an acquired blunting of respiratory drive arising from failure of the respiratory pump.

hypovitaminosis *n.* a deficiency of a vitamin caused either through lack of the vitamin in the diet or from an inability to absorb or utilize it.

hypovolemia (oligemia) *n.* a decrease in the volume of circulating blood. *See* shock.

hypoxemia *n.* reduction of the oxygen concentration in the arterial blood, recognized clinically by the presence of central and peripheral *cyanosis. When the partial pressure of oxygen (PO_2) falls below 8.0 kPa (60 mmHg), the condition is defined as respiratory failure.

hypoxia *n.* a deficiency of oxygen in the tissues. *See also* anoxia, hypoxemia.

hypsarrhythmia *n.* an abnormal and chaotic pattern of brain activity, demonstrated by *electroencephalography, that is usually associated with *infantile spasms.

hyster- (hystero-) *prefix denoting* **1.** the uterus. **2.** hysteria.

hysterectomy *n.* the surgical removal of the uterus, either through an incision in the abdominal wall or through the vagina. *Subtotal hysterectomy* (now rarely performed) involves removing the body of the uterus but leaving the cervix. The operation is performed for cancerous conditions affecting the uterus and for nonmalignant conditions (e.g. fibroids) in which there is excessive menstrual bleeding. Although pregnancy is no longer possible, hysterectomy does not affect sexual desire or activity.

ysteria *n.* **1.** formerly, a neurosis characterized by emotional instability, repression, dissociation, some physical symptoms (*see* hysterical), and vulnerability to suggestion. Two types were recognized: *conversion hysteria*, now known as *conversion disorder; and *dissociative hysteria*, comprising a group of conditions now generally regarded as *dissociative disorders. *See also* neurosis. **2.** a state of great emotional excitement.

ysterical *adj.* **1.** formerly, describing a symptom that is not due to organic disease, is produced unconsciously, and from which the individual derives some gain. What were known as hysterical symptoms are characteristic of *conversion disorder. **2.** describing a kind of *personality disorder characterized by instability and shallowness of feelings and by superficiality and a tendency to manipulate in personal relationships.

ysterosalpingography *n.* see uterosalpingography.

ysterosalpingosonography *n.* visualization of the fallopian tubes by means of an ultrasound beam, usually directed via a vaginal probe, after a contrast medium has been passed through them via the cervix. *See also* transvaginal ultrasonography.

ysteroscope (uteroscope) *n.* a tubular instrument with a light source for observing the interior of the uterus. *See also* endoscope.

ysterotomy *n.* incision of the uterus through the abdominal wall to remove a fetus before the 24th week of pregnancy; after this time, the operation is called *cesarean section. It is now rarely performed, having been replaced by use of drugs that induce abortion.

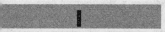

asis *suffix denoting* a diseased condition. Example: *leishmaniasis* (disease caused by *Leishmania* species).

atro- *prefix denoting* **1.** medicine. **2.** doctors.

iatrogenic *adj.* describing a condition that has resulted from treatment, as either an unforeseen or inevitable side effect.

IBD *see* inflammatory bowel disease.

IBS *see* irritable bowel syndrome.

ibuprofen *n.* an anti-inflammatory drug (*see* NSAID) used in the treatment of arthritic conditions, headaches, and primary dysmenorrhea. It is administered by mouth and sometimes causes skin rashes and digestive upsets. Trade names: **Advil**, **Haltran**, **Medipren**, **Motrin**, **Nuprin**, **PediaProfen**.

ibutilide *n.* an *antiarrhythmic drug used to treat atrial *fibrillation and atrial flutter. It is administered by intravenous injection; side effects include nausea and *ventricular tachycardia. Trade name: **Corvert**.

ICD *see* International Classification of Diseases.

ichor *n.* a watery material oozing from wounds or ulcers.

ichthyosis *n.* a group of genetically determined skin conditions (*see* genodermatosis) in which the skin is dry, rough, and scaly because of a defect in *keratinization (the scaly condition of the skin is reflected in the name of this disorder, which is derived from the Greek word for fish). Ichthyosis may be caused by a variety of genetic defects in skin shedding; the pattern of scaling varies according to the underlying defect. Ichthyosis varies in severity from slight skin dryness to a severe condition in which an infant is born, usually dead, with skin like armor plate. The most common form, *ichthyosis vulgaris*, is inherited as an autosomal *dominant and occurs in 1 in 300 of the population. *Lamellar ichthyosis* is a very rare condition in which the skin, particularly on the palms and soles, is thickened and lizardlike. Treatment for the mild forms of ichthyosis is with emollients, such as petrolatum or mineral oil. The more serious forms are treated with antibiotics or retinoids. *See also* xeroderma.

ICSH interstitial-cell-stimulating hormone: *see* luteinizing hormone.

ICSI (intracytoplasmic sperm injection) a technique of assisted conception in cases of male infertility caused by inability of the spermatozoa to penetrate the barriers surrounding the ovum, in which a single spermatozoon is injected into the cytoplasm of an ovum in vitro. The fertilized ovum is then implanted into the uterus.

icterus n. see jaundice.

ictus n. a stroke or any sudden attack. The term is often used for an epileptic seizure, stressing the suddenness of its onset.

ICU see intensive care unit.

id n. (in psychoanalysis) a part of the unconscious mind governed by the instinctive forces of *libido and the death wish. These violent forces seek immediate release in action or in symbolic form. The id is therefore said to be governed by the pleasure principle and not by the demands of reality or of logic. In the course of individual development some of the functions of the id are taken over by the *ego.

-id suffix denoting relationship or resemblance to. Example: spermatid (a stage of sperm formation).

ideation n. the process of thinking or of having *imagery or ideas.

identical twins see twins.

identification n. (in psychological development) the process of adopting other people's characteristics more or less permanently. Identification with a parent is important in personality formation, and it has been especially implicated in the development of a moral sense and of an appropriate sex role.

ideo- prefix denoting 1. the mind or mental activity. 2. ideas.

ideomotor adj. describing or relating to a motor action that is evoked by an idea. Ideomotor apraxia is the inability to translate the idea of a complex behavior into action.

idio- prefix denoting peculiarity to the individual.

idiocy n. a profound degree of *mental retardation in which the affected individual can do nothing for himself and cannot speak. The term is now obsolete, but roughly corresponds to an *intelligence quotient of less than 20. There are usually associated physical handicaps and there is always physical damage of the brain.

idiopathic adj. denoting a disease or condition the cause of which is not known or that arises spontaneously. —**idiopathy** n.

idiopathic facial pain a *neuralgia that has

no known cause and is typified by pain in the face that does not fit the distribution of nerves. It is often stress-related, and in many cases appears to be associated with defective metabolism of *tyramine.

idiopathic membranous nephropathy a kidney disease characterized by thickening of the basement membrane of the glomerular wall, although there is increased permeability to protein. The course of the disease is variable, but it is generally slowly progressive. It is a common cause of the *nephrotic syndrome in adults. Treatment is with steroids and immunosuppressant agents.

idiopathic thrombocytopenic purpura (ITP) an *autoimmune disease in which platelets are destroyed, leading to spontaneous bruising (see purpura). Acute ITP is a relatively mild disease of children, who usually recover without treatment. A chronic form of the disease, typically affecting adults, is more serious, requiring treatment with corticosteroids or, if there is no response, with splenectomy. If both fail, immunosuppressant drugs may be effective. Platelet concentrates are used for life-threatening bleeding. See also purpura.

idiosyncrasy n. an unusual and unexpected sensitivity exhibited by an individual to a particular drug or food. Drug idiosyncrasy commonly takes the form of undue susceptibility or hypersensitivity, so that the standard dose causes an excessive effect; the normal effect is produced by a small fraction of the standard dose. —**idiosyncratic** adj.

idiot savant an individual whose overall functioning is at the level of *mental retardation but who has one or more special intellectual abilities that are advanced to a high level. Musical ability, calculating ability, and rote memory are examples of abilities that may be highly developed. Many such individuals have *autism.

idiotype n. the structural features of an antibody that distinguish one antigen-binding site from another.

idioventricular adj. affecting or peculiar to the ventricles of the heart. The term is most often used to describe the very slow beat of the ventricles under the influence of their own natural subsidiary pacemaker (idioventricular rhythm).

idoxuridine *n.* an iodine-containing drug that inhibits the growth of viruses and is used to treat the eye condition *herpes simplex keratitis. It is administered in eye drops or ointment and may cause irritation and stinging on application. Trade names: **Herplex, Stoxil**.

ifosfamide *n.* a *cytotoxic drug (an *alkylating agent) used in the treatment of malignant disease, especially sarcomas, lymphomas, and germ cell testicular cancer. It is administered intravenously by injection or infusion. Side effects include nausea, vomiting, alopecia, and hemorrhagic cystitis; concomitant administration of *mesna is recommended to prevent cystitis. It is an orphan drug. Trade name: **Ifex**.

Ig *see* immunoglobulin.

IgA nephropathy *see* Berger's disease.

IGF insulin-like growth factor, which includes IGF-I and IGF-II. *See* growth factor, somatomedin.

IHS *see* Indian Health Service.

IGT impaired glucose tolerance (*see* glucose tolerance test).

IL-2 *see* interleukin.

ile- (ileo-) *prefix denoting* the ileum. Examples: *ileocecal* (relating to the ileum and cecum); *ileocolic* (relating to the ileum and colon).

ileal conduit a segment of small intestine (ileum) used to convey urine from the ureters to the exterior into an appliance (*see also* urinary diversion). The ureters are implanted into an isolated segment of bowel, usually ileum but sometimes sigmoid colon, one end of which is brought through the abdominal wall to the skin surface. This end forms a spout, or *stoma*, which projects into a suitable urinary appliance. The ureters themselves cannot be used for this purpose because they tend to narrow and retract if brought through the skin. The operation is performed if the bladder has to be removed or bypassed; for example, because of cancer.

ileal pouch (perineal pouch) a reservoir made from loops of ileum to replace a surgically removed rectum, avoiding the need for a permanent *ileostomy.

ileectomy *n.* surgical removal of the ileum (a section of the small intestine) or part of the ileum.

ileitis *n.* inflammation of the ileum (a section of the small intestine). It may be caused by *Crohn's disease, tuberculosis, the bacterium *Yersinia enterocolitica*, or typhoid or it may occur in association with ulcerative *colitis (when it is known as *backwash ileitis*).

ileocecal valve a valve at the junction of the small and large intestines consisting of two membranous folds that close to prevent the backflow of cecum and colon contents to the ileum.

ileocolitis *n.* inflammation of the ileum and the colon (small and large intestines). The most common causes are *Crohn's disease and tuberculosis.

ileocolostomy *n.* a surgical operation in which the ileum is joined to some part of the colon. It is usually performed when the right side of the colon has been removed or if it is desired to bypass either the terminal part of the ileum or right side of the colon.

ileocystoplasty *n. see* cystoplasty.

ileoproctostomy (ileorectal anastomosis) *n.* a surgical operation in which the ileum is joined to the rectum, usually after surgical removal of the colon (*see* colectomy).

ileostomy *n.* a surgical operation in which the ileum is brought through the abdominal wall to create an artificial opening (*stoma*) through which the intestinal contents can discharge, thus bypassing the colon. Various types of bag may be worn to collect the effluent. The operation is usually performed in association with *colectomy; or to allow the colon to rest and heal in cases of colitis; or following injury or surgery to the colon. It can be used as an alternative to *colostomy.

ileum *n.* the lowest of the three portions of the small *intestine. It runs from the jejunum to the *ileocecal valve. —**ileal**, **ileac** *adj.*

ileus *n.* intestinal obstruction, usually obstruction of the ileum. *Paralytic* or *adynamic ileus* is functional obstruction of the ileum due to loss of intestinal movement (peristalsis), which may be caused by abdominal surgery (*see* laparotomy), spinal injuries, deficiency of potassium in the blood (hypokalemia), or peritonitis. Treatment consists of intravenous administration of fluid and nutrients and removal of excess stomach secretions by tube until peristalsis returns. If possible, the underlying condition is treated. Mechanical obstruction of the ileum may be caused by a gallstone entering the bowel through a fistula or widened bile duct (*gallstone ileus*); thickened *meconium in newborn babies with *cystic fibrosis (*meconium ileus*); or intestinal worms, usually the pinworm *Enterobius vermicularis* (*verminous ileus*).

ili- (ilio-) *prefix denoting* the ilium.

iliac arteries the arteries that supply most of the blood to the lower limbs and pelvic region. The right and left *common iliac arteries* form the terminal branches of the abdominal aorta. Each branches into the *external iliac artery* and the smaller *internal iliac artery*.

iliacus *n.* a flat triangular muscle situated in the area of the groin. This muscle acts in conjunction with the *psoas muscle to flex the thigh.

iliac veins the veins draining most of the blood from the lower limbs and pelvic region. The right and left *common iliac veins* unite to form the inferior vena cava. They are each formed by the union of the *internal* and *external iliac veins*.

iliopsoas *n.* a composite muscle made up of the *iliacus and *psoas muscles, which have a common tendon.

ilium *n.* the haunch bone: a wide bone forming the upper part of each side of the *hip bone (*see also* pelvis). There is a concave depression (*iliac fossa*) on the inside of the pelvis; the right iliac fossa provides space for the vermiform appendix. —**iliac** *adj.*

illness *n.* any condition that deviates significantly from the normal healthy state, in which the physical, mental, emotional, social, or intellectual condition and functions of a person are greatly impaired or diminished. *See also* disease, disorder, malingering.

illusion *n.* a false perception due to misinterpretation of the stimuli arising from an object. For example, a patient may misinterpret the conversation of others as the voices of enemies conspiring to destroy him. Illusions can occur in quite normal people, but they are usually spontaneously corrected. They may also occur in almost any psychiatric syndrome, especially *depression. *Compare* hallucination.

Optical illusions are perceptions that do not agree with the actual object in the external world. They are produced by de-

ceptive qualities of the stimulus and are in no way pathological.

image intensifier an electronic device that provides a TV image from an X-ray source. The X-rays strike a fluorescent screen, giving off electrons, which are accelerated using an electron lens before striking a second fluorescent screen, which is usually attached to a video camera. The acceleration of the electrons amplifies the signal from the original image, giving a brighter picture, so that the radiation dose can be reduced. Images can be taken from the camera to be observed in real time on a video monitor or, using a brief higher-dose exposure, to provide a more detailed static image (*see* digital spot imaging).

imagery *n.* the production of vivid mental representations by the normal processes of thought. *Hypnagogic imagery* occurs just before falling asleep, and the images are often very distinct. *Hypnopompic imagery* occurs in the state between sleep and full wakefulness. Like hypnagogic imagery, the experiences may be very vivid. *Eidetic imagery*, more common in children than adults, is the production of images of exceptional clarity, which may be recalled long after being first experienced.

imaging *n.* (in radiology) the production of images of organs or tissues using a range of techniques. These images are used by physicians in diagnosis and in monitoring the effects of treatment. They can also be used to guide *interventional radiology techniques. *See also* computed tomography, magnetic resonance imaging, positron emission tomography, SPECT scanning, ultrasonography.

imago *n.* (in psychoanalysis) the internal unconscious representation of an important person in the individual's life, particularly a parent.

imatinib *n.* a *cytotoxic drug that works by inhibiting protein-tyrosine kinase, an enzyme that is active in some leukemia cells. Imatinib is used in the treatment of adults with chronic *myeloid leukemia in which the Philadelphia chromosome is present. It is indicated if interferon-alfa treatment fails or if the disease is in a highly active phase. It is also indicated for the treatment of malignant gastrointestinal stromal tumors (GIST). The most common side effects are intestinal upset, fluid retention, and muscle pain and cramps. Trade name: **Gleevec**.

imbecility n. a moderate to severe degree of *mental retardation that falls short of *idiocy. The term is now obsolete, but roughly corresponds to an *intelligence quotient of between 20 and 50. It is almost always caused by physical damage to the brain, and affected individuals usually require help and supervision throughout their lives.

imidazole n. any of a group of chemically related antifungal drugs that are also effective against a wide range of bacteria; some (e.g. *thiabendazole and *mebendazole) are also used as anthelmintics. This group includes *econazole, *clotrimazole, *ketoconazole, and *miconazole. They are administered by mouth or externally as creams.

imipramine n. a drug administered by mouth or injection to treat depression (see antidepressant). Its effects may be slow to develop; common side effects include dry mouth, blurred vision, constipation, sweating, and rapid heartbeat. Trade name: **Tofranil**.

imitation n. acting in the same way as another person, either temporarily or permanently. This is one of the mechanisms of *identification. It can be used in therapy (see modeling).

immersion foot see trench foot.

immobilization n. the procedure of making a normally movable part of the body, such as a joint, immovable. This helps an infected, diseased, or injured tissue (bone, joint, or muscle) to heal. Immobilization may be temporary (for example, by means of a plaster of Paris cast on a limb) or it may be permanent. Permanent immobilization of a joint is achieved by *arthrodesis.

immugen n. a complete *antigen. It can induce an immune response and combine with antibodies.

immune adj. protected against a particular infection by the presence of specific antibodies against the organisms concerned. See immunity.

immune response the response of the *immune system to antigens. There are two types of immune response produced by two populations of *lymphocytes. B lymphocytes (or B cells) are responsible for humoral immunity, producing free antibodies that circulate in the blood-

stream; and T lymphocytes (or T cells) are responsible for cell-mediated immunity (see cytotoxic T cell, helper T cell, killer cell, suppressor T cell).

immune system a network of body cells that protect against infectious agents. It is responsible for the production of *antibodies or such substances as *cytokines, which neutralize infectious agents. The primary *lymphoid tissues are the thymus and the bone marrow; the secondary lymphoid tissues are the lymph nodes and lymphoid aggregates (spleen, tonsils, gastrointestinal lymph tissue, and Peyer's patches).

immunity n. the body's ability to resist infection, afforded by the presence of circulating *antibodies and white blood cells. Healthy individuals protect themselves by means of physical barriers, phagocytic cells, *natural killer cells, and various blood-borne molecules. All of these mechanisms are present prior to exposure to infectious agents and are part of natural (or innate) immunity. Antibodies are synthesized specifically to deal with the antigens associated with different diseases as they are encountered. Active immunity arises when the body's own cells produce, and remain able to produce, appropriate antibodies following an attack of a disease or deliberate stimulation (see immunization). Passive immunity, which is only short-lived, is provided by injecting ready-made antibodies in *antiserum taken from another person or animal already immune. Babies have passive immunity, conferred by antibodies from the maternal blood and *colostrum, to common diseases for several weeks after birth. See also immune response.

immunization n. the production of *immunity by artificial means. Passive immunity, which is temporary, may be conferred by the injection of an *antiserum, but the production of active immunity calls for the use of treated antigens, to stimulate the body to produce its own antibodies: this is the procedure of *vaccination (also called inoculation). The material used for immunization (the *vaccine) may consist of live bacteria or viruses so treated that they are harmless while remaining antigenic or completely dead organisms or their products (e.g. toxins) chemically or physically altered to produce the same effect.

immuno- *prefix denoting* immunity or immunological response.

immunoassay *n.* any of various techniques for determining the levels of antigen and antibody in a tissue. *See also* immunoelectrophoresis, immunofluorescence, radioimmunoassay.

immunocompromised *adj.* describing patients in whom the immune response is reduced or defective due to *immunosuppression. Such patients are vulnerable to opportunistic infections.

immunodeficiency *n.* deficiency in the *immune response. This can be acquired, as in *AIDS, but there are many varieties of primary immunodeficiency occurring as inherited disorders characterized by *hypogammaglobulinemia or defects in T-cell function, or both.

immunodiffusion *n.* a technique for identifying *immunoglobulins. It is based on the formation of a visible *precipitin reaction, usually on a gel medium, that results from an antigen-antibody combination.

immunoelectrophoresis *n.* a technique for identifying antigenic fractions in a serum. The components of the serum are separated by *electrophoresis and allowed to diffuse through agar gel toward a particular antiserum. Where the antibody meets its antigen, a band of precipitation occurs. *See also* precipitin.

immunofluorescence *n.* a technique for observing the amount and/or distribution of antibody or antigen in a tissue section. The antibodies are labeled (directly or indirectly) with a fluorescent dye (e.g. fluorescein) and applied to the tissue, which is observed through an ultraviolet microscope. In *direct immunofluorescence* the antibody is labeled before being applied to the tissue. In *indirect immunofluorescence* the antibody is labeled after it has bound to the antigen, by means of fluorescein-labeled anti-immunoglobulin serum. —**immunofluorescent** *adj.*

immunogenicity *n.* the property that enables a substance to provoke an immune response, including foreignness (*see* antigen), size, route of entry into the body, dose, number and length of exposures to the antigen, and host genetic make-up.

immunoglobulin (Ig) *n.* one of a group of structurally related proteins (*gamma globulins) that act as antibodies. Five classes of immunoglobulins with different functions are distinguished – IgA, IgD, IgE, IgG, and IgM, IgG being the most prevalent and IgG, IgA, and IgM being the most important. They can be separated by *immunoelectrophoresis. *See* antibody.

immunological tolerance a failure of the body to distinguish between materials that are "self," and therefore to be tolerated, and those that are "not self," against which an *immune response is produced. Tolerance results from the interaction of antigens with lymphocytes under conditions in which the lymphocytes are not activated but rendered unresponsive.

immunology *n.* the study of *immunity and all of the phenomena connected with the defense mechanisms of the body. —**immunological** *adj.*

immunosuppressant *n.* a drug, such as *azathioprine, *tacrolimus, or *cyclophosphamide, that reduces the body's resistance to infection and other foreign bodies by suppressing the immune system. Immunosuppressants are used to maintain the survival of organ and tissue transplants and to treat various *autoimmune diseases, including rheumatoid arthritis. *Cyclosporine is the immunosuppressant usually used in organ transplant recipients. Because immunity is lowered during treatment with immunosuppressants, there is an increased susceptibility to infection and certain types of cancer.

immunosuppression *n.* suppression of the *immune response, usually by disease (e.g. AIDS) or by drugs (e.g. steroids, azathioprine, cyclosporine).

immunotherapy *n.* the prevention or treatment of disease using agents that may modify the immune response. It is a largely experimental approach, which has been studied most widely in the treatment of leukemias (especially hairy-cell leukemia), melanoma, and hypernephroma. *See* biological response modifier.

immunotoxin *n.* one of a new class of drugs undergoing clinical trials for the treatment of leukemia. Immunotoxins combine *monoclonal antibodies, which can specifically target cancerous cells, with a highly toxic compound (such as *ricin) that inactivates the cells' *ribosomes and thus inhibits protein synthesis. Because the toxin does not attack the whole cell only small amounts are required.

immunotransfusion *n.* the transfusion of an *antiserum to treat or give temporary protection against a disease.

impacted *adj.* firmly wedged. An *impacted tooth* (usually a wisdom tooth) is one that cannot erupt into a normal position because it is obstructed by other tissues. *Impacted feces* are so hard and dry that they cannot pass through the anus without special measures being taken (*see* constipation). An *impacted fracture* is one in which the bone ends are driven into each other. —**impaction** *n.*

impaired glucose tolerance (IGT) *see* glucose tolerance test.

impairment *n. see* handicap.

impalpable *adj.* describing a structure within the body that cannot be detected (or that can be detected only with difficulty) by feeling with the hand.

impedance plethysmography a noninvasive method of detecting changes in blood volume in the leg. Blood flow in the lower leg is stopped for a few minutes while calf electrodes measure the volume increase. When flow is resumed, the blood flow is decreased and the change in electrical resistance (impedance) is recorded.

imperforate *adj.* lacking an opening. Occasionally girls at puberty are found to have an *imperforate hymen* (a fold of membrane close to the vaginal orifice), which impedes the flow of menstrual blood.

imperforate anus (proctatresia) partial or complete obstruction of the anus: a condition, discovered at birth, due to failure of the anus to develop normally in the embryo. There are several different types of imperforate anus, including *developmental anal stenosis, persistent anal membrane,* and *covered anus* (due to fused genital folds). If the anal canal fails to develop, the rectum ends blindly above the muscles of the perineum. Most mild cases of imperforate anus can be treated by a simple operation. If the defect is extensive, a temporary opening is made in the colon (*see* colostomy), with later surgical reconstruction of the rectum and anus.

impetigo *n.* a bacterial skin infection usually caused by staphylococci, although occasionally by streptococci. Impetigo is particularly common in babies and children, occurring mainly on the face and limbs. The infection, which spreads quickly over the body, starts as a red patch and develops into small pustules that join together, forming crusty yellow sores. Impetigo is very contagious, especially in communities of children, being readily spread by contact and via towels and facecloths. The condition usually responds to treatment with antibiotics, applied locally, within 7 to 10 days. Impetigo of the newborn is rare today but an outbreak may spread rapidly in a nursery.

implant *n.* **1.** a drug (such as a subcutaneous hormone implant), a prosthesis (such as an artificial hip, an *intraocular lens implant* (*see* cataract), a *breast implant, a *cochlear implant, or an *artificial heart implant), or a radioactive source (such as radium needles) that is put into the body. **2.** (in dentistry) a rigid structure that is embedded in bone or under its periosteum to provide support for replacement teeth on a *denture or a *bridge. Recent types (*osseointegrated implants*) consist of a number of special metal inserts (often titanium), placed in the jawbone, onto which an artificial tooth superstructure is subsequently bolted. Osseointegrated implants are also used to retain facial *prostheses. *See also* osseointegration.

implantable hearing aid a form of hearing aid in which a small electrical vibrator is surgically attached to the auditory *ossicles. An external device with a microphone and an electronic processing unit passes information to the implanted device using radio-frequency waves. The external part is located behind the pinna and is powered by batteries. Trade name: **Soundbridge** (Vibrant Soundbridge).

implantation *n.* **1.** (**nidation**) the attachment of the early embryo to the lining of the uterus, which occurs at the *blastocyst stage of development, six to eight days after ovulation. The site of implantation determines the position of the placenta. **2.** the placing of a substance (e.g.

a drug) or an object (e.g. an artificial pacemaker) within a tissue. **3.** the surgical replacement of damaged tissue with healthy tissue (*see* transplantation).

implosion *n. see* flooding.

impotence *n.* inability in a man to have sexual intercourse. Impotence may be *erectile*, in which the penis does not become firm enough to enter the vagina, or *ejaculatory*, in which penetration occurs but there is no ejaculation of semen (orgasm). Either kind of impotence may be due to a physical disease, such as diabetes (*organic*), or to a psychological or emotional problem (*psychogenic*). Treatment is by means of a penile *prosthesis or drugs, administered by injection (*see* alprostadil) or orally (*see* sildenafil).

impregnate *vb.* **1.** to fertilize; to inseminate and make pregnant. **2.** to saturate or mix with another substance.

impression *n.* (in dentistry) an elastic mold made of the teeth and surrounding soft tissues or of a toothless jaw. A soft impression material is placed over the teeth or jaw and sets within several minutes. After removal from the mouth a plaster model is made; on this are constructed *restorations of teeth, *dentures, or *orthodontic appliances.

imprinting *n.* (in animal behavior) a rapid and irreversible form of learning that takes place in some animals during the first hours of life. Animals attach themselves in this way to members of their own species, but if they are exposed to creatures of a different species during this short period, they become attached to this species instead.

impulse *n.* (in neurology) *see* nerve impulse.

IMR *see* infant mortality rate.

in- (im-) *prefix denoting* **1.** not. **2.** in; within; into.

inactivate *vb.* to destroy the biological action of a substance, such a enzyme or virus, by chemical or physical means, as in the application of heat. *See also* deactivation. —**inactivation,** *n.*

inanition *n.* a condition of exhaustion caused by lack of nutrients in the blood. This may arise through starvation, malnutrition, or intestinal disease.

inappetence *n.* lack of desire, usually for food.

in articulo mortis Latin: at the moment of death.

inborn error of metabolism any one of a group of inherited conditions in which there is a disturbance in either the structure, synthesis, function, or transport of protein molecules. There are over 1500 inborn errors of metabolism; examples are *phenylketonuria, *homocystinuria, and *hypogammaglobulinemia.

inbreeding *n.* the production of offspring by parents who are closely related; for example, who are first cousins or siblings. The amount of inbreeding in a population is largely controlled by culture and tradition. *Compare* outbreeding.

incarcerated *adj.* confined or constricted so as to be immovable: applied particularly to a type of *hernia.

incidence rate a measure of morbidity based on the number of new episodes of illness arising in a population over an estimated period. It can be expressed in terms of sick persons or episodes per 1000 individuals at risk. *Compare* prevalence rate.

incidentaloma *n.* a growth found incidentally on (usually) an adrenal gland during CT or MRI scanning of the abdomen or thorax for other clinical reasons. These growths are rarely significant, particularly if small, but they do pose a clinical dilemma for the investigating clinician.

incision *n.* **1.** the surgical cutting of soft tissues, such as skin or muscle, with a knife or scalpel. **2.** the cut so made.

incisor *n.* any of the four front teeth in each jaw, two on each side of the midline. *See also* dentition.

incisure *n.* (in anatomy) a notch, small hollow, or depression.

inclusion bodies particles occurring in the nucleus and cytoplasm of cells usually as a result of virus infection. Their presence can sometimes be used to diagnose such an infection.

inclusion conjunctivitis a sexually transmitted disease caused by *Chlamydia trachomatis*. It can be transmitted to infants at birth, with the disease clinically apparent 5–13 days after birth. Diagnosis is by cell culture. Treatment in the newborn is with topical erythromycin, and in adults with oral tetracycline or doxycycline for three weeks.

incompatibility *n. see* compatibility.

incompetence *n.* impaired function of the

valves of the heart or veins, which allows backward leakage of blood. *See* aortic regurgitation, mitral incompetence, varicose veins.

incontinence *n.* **1.** the inappropriate involuntary passage of urine, resulting in wetting. *Stress incontinence* is the leak of urine on coughing and straining. It is common in women in whom the muscles of the pelvic floor are weakened after childbirth. *Genuine stress incontinence (GSI)* is incontinence in women for which a physical (as opposed to a psychological) cause can be identified. *Overflow incontinence* is leakage from a full bladder, which occurs most commonly in elderly men with bladder outflow obstruction or in patients with neurological conditions affecting bladder control. *Urge incontinence* is leakage of urine that accompanies an intense desire to urinate with failure of restraint. *See also* enuresis. **2.** an inability to control bowel movements (*fecal incontinence*).

incoordination *n.* (in neurology) an impairment in the performance of precise movements. These are dependent upon the normal function of the whole nervous system, and incoordination may result from a disorder in any part of it. *See* apraxia, ataxia, dyssynergia.

incubation *n.* **1.** the process of development of an egg or a culture of bacteria. **2.** the care of a premature baby in an *incubator.

incubation period (latent period) 1. the interval between exposure to an infection and the appearance of the first symptoms. **2.** (in bacteriology) the period of development of a bacterial culture.

incubator *n.* a transparent apparatus for keeping premature babies in controlled conditions and protecting them from infection. Other forms of incubator are used for cultivating bacteria in Petri dishes and for hatching eggs.

incus *n.* a small anvil-shaped bone in the middle *ear that articulates with the malleus and the stapes. *See* ossicle.

IND *see* investigational new drug.

indapamide *n.* a drug used for the treatment of high blood pressure (hypertension) and edema associated with congestive heart failure. It is administered by mouth; common side effects include headache, dizziness, and fatigue. Trade name: **Lozol**.

Index Medicus *see* MEDLARS.

Indian Health Service (IHS) an agency of HHS responsible for providing health care to American Indians and native Alaskans. The IHS operates 63 health centers, 36 hospitals, 44 clinics, and 5 residential treatment centers utilized by more than 1.6 million American Indians and Alaska natives.

indican *n.* a compound excreted in the urine as a detoxification product of *indoxyl. Indican is formed by the conjugation of indoxyl with sulfuric acid and potassium on the decomposition of tryptophan.

indicanuria *n.* the presence in the urine of an abnormally high concentration of *indican. This may be a sign that the intestine is obstructed.

indication *n.* (in medicine) a strong reason for believing that a particular course of action is desirable. In a wounded patient, the loss of blood, which would lead to circulatory collapse, is an indication for blood transfusion. *Compare* contraindication.

indigestion *n. see* dyspepsia.

indinavir *n. see* protease inhibitor.

indocyanine green angiography *see* angiography.

indole *n.* a derivative of the amino acid tryptophan, excreted in the urine and feces. Abnormal patterns of urinary indole excretion are found in some mentally retarded patients.

indolent *adj.* describing a disease process that is failing to heal or has persisted. The term is applied particularly to ulcers of skin or mucous membrane.

indomethacin *n.* an anti-inflammatory drug (*see* NSAID) used in the treatment of arthritic conditions. It is also used to close the patent ductus arteriosus in premature infants. It is administered by mouth in a suspension, or in suppositories; common side effects are headache, dizziness, and digestive upsets. Trade name: **Indocin**.

indoxyl *n.* an alcohol derived from *indole by bacterial action. It is excreted in the urine as *indican.

induction *n.* **1.** (in obstetrics) the starting of labor by artificial means. *Medical induction* is carried out by administering such drugs as *prostaglandins or *oxytocin, which stimulate uterine contractions. *Surgical induction* is performed by *amniotomy (artificial rupture of membranes), usually supplemented by oxytocic drugs. Induction of labor is carried out if the well-being or life of mother or child is threatened by continuance of the pregnancy. **2.** (in anesthesia) initiation of *anesthesia. General anesthesia is usually induced by the intravenous injection of rapid short-acting narcotic drugs, e.g. thiopental. **3.** (in embryology) the process by which a chemical released from one part of an embryo causes another part to develop in a particular way. Also called: **evocation.**

induration *n.* abnormal hardening of a tissue or organ. *See also* sclerosis.

indusium *n.* a thin layer of gray matter covering the upper surface of the *corpus callosum between the two cerebral hemispheres of the brain.

industrial disease *see* occupational disease.

inertia *n.* (in physiology) sluggishness or absence of activity in certain smooth muscles. In *uterine inertia* the muscular wall of the uterus fails to contract adequately during labor, making the process excessively long. This inertia may be present from the start of labor or it may develop because of exhaustion following strong contractions.

in extremis Latin: at the point of death.

infant *n.* a child incapable of any form of independence from its caregivers: a child under one year of age, especially a premature or newborn child. Some extend infancy to two years of age.

infantile *adj.* **1.** denoting conditions occurring in adults that are recognizable in childhood, e.g. poliomyelitis (*infantile paralysis*) and *infantile scurvy*. **2.** of, relating to, or affecting infants.

infantile spasms (salaam attacks) a form of epilepsy caused by serious congenital or acquired brain disease, usually beginning under the age of six months. The spasms are involuntary flexing movements of the arms, legs, neck, and trunk; each spasm lasts 1–3 seconds and is associated with flushing of the face, and runs of spasms occur over a period of several minutes. They may occur many times in one day. The baby fails to respond to human contact and development is profoundly slowed. An EEG pattern of *hypsarrhythmia is usual and diagnostic. Diagnosis may be delayed as spasms are sometimes confused with colic. Immediate recognition and treatment with antiepileptic medication, corticosteroids, or ACTH offers a chance of arresting the disease, but outcome depends primarily on the nature of the underlying brain abnormality.

infantilism *n.* persistence of childlike physical or psychological characteristics into adult life.

infant mortality rate (IMR) the number of deaths of infants under one year of age per 1000 live births in a given year. Included in the IMR are the *neonatal mortality rate* (calculated from deaths occurring in the first four weeks of life) and *postneonatal mortality rate* (from deaths in the remainder of the first year). Neonatal deaths are further subdivided into *early* (first week) and *late* (second, third, and fourth weeks). In prosperous countries neonatal deaths account for about two-thirds of infant mortalities, the majority being in the first week (usually due to prematurity and related problems). The IMR is usually regarded more as a measure of social affluence than a measure of the quality of antenatal and/or obstetric care; the latter is more truly reflected in the *perinatal mortality rate* (the number of deaths after 24 weeks of gestation, including stillbirths, and during the first week of life per 1000 total births). *See also* stillbirth.

infarct *n. see* infarction.

infarction *n.* the death of part or the whole of an organ that occurs when the artery carrying its blood supply is obstructed by a blood clot (thrombus) or an *embolus. For example, *myocardial infarction, affecting the muscle of the heart, follows coronary thrombosis. A small localized area of dead tissue produced as a result of an inadequate blood supply is known as an *infarct*.

infection *n.* invasion of the body by harmful organisms (pathogens), such as bacteria, fungi, protozoa, rickettsiae, or viruses. The infective agent may be transmitted by a patient or *carrier in airborne droplets expelled during coughing and sneezing or by direct contact, such as kissing or sexual intercourse (*see* sexually transmitted disease); by animal or insect *vectors; by ingestion of contaminated food or drink; or from an infected mother to the fetus during pregnancy or birth. Pathogenic organisms present in soil, organisms from animal intermediate hosts, or those living as *commensals on the body can also cause infections. Organisms may invade via a wound or bite or through mucous membranes. After an *incubation period symptoms appear, usually consisting of either localized inflammation and pain or more remote effects. Treatment with antibiotics is usually effective against most infections but there are few specific treatments for many of the common viral infections, including the common cold (see antiviral drug, interferon).

infectious disease see communicable disease.

infectious mononucleosis see glandular fever.

inferior adj. (in anatomy) lower in the body in relation to another structure or surface.

inferior dental block a type of injection to anesthetize the inferior *dental nerve. Inferior dental block is routinely performed to allow dental procedures to be carried out on the lower teeth on one side of the mouth.

inferior dental canal a bony canal in the *mandible on each side. It carries the inferior *dental nerve and vessels and for part of its length its outline is visible on a radiograph.

inferiority complex 1. an unconscious and extreme exaggeration of feelings of insignificance or inferiority, which is shown by behavior that is defensive or compensatory (such as aggression). **2.** (in psychoanalysis) a *complex resulting from the conflict between Oedipal wishes (see Oedipus complex) and the reality of the child's lack of power. This gives rise to repressed feelings of personal inferiority.

infertility n. inability in a woman to conceive or in a man to induce conception. Female infertility may be due to failure to ovulate, to obstruction of the *fallopian tubes, or to disease of the lining of the uterus (endometrium). Possible treatments (depending on the cause) include administration of such drugs as *clomiphene, *menotropin, and *LHRH analogues, surgery (*salpingostomy, *salpingolysis) to restore patency to blocked fallopian tubes, *gamete intrafallopian transfer (GIFT), and *in vitro fertilization. Causes of male infertility include decreased numbers or motility of spermatozoa (see oligospermia) and total absence of sperm (see azoospermia). See also andrology, sterility.

infestation n. the presence of animal parasites either on the skin (for example, ticks) or inside the body (for example, tapeworms).

infibulation n. see (female) circumcision.

infiltration n. **1.** the abnormal entry of a substance (infiltrate) into a cell, tissue, or organ. Examples of infiltrates are blood cells, cancer cells, fat, starch, or calcium and magnesium salts. **2.** the injection of a local anesthetic solution into the tissues to cause local *anesthesia. Infiltration anesthesia is routinely used to anesthetize upper teeth to allow dental procedures to be carried out.

inflammation n. the body's response to injury, which may be acute or chronic. Acute inflammation is the immediate defensive reaction of tissue to any injury, which may be caused by infection, chemicals, or physical agents. It involves pain, heat, redness, swelling, and loss of function of the affected part. Blood vessels near the site of injury are dilated, so that blood flow is locally increased. White blood cells enter the tissue and begin to engulf bacteria and other foreign particles. Similar cells from the tissues remove and consume the dead cells, sometimes with the production of pus, enabling the process of healing to commence. In certain circumstances healing does not occur and chronic inflammation ensues.

inflammatory bowel disease (IBD) any of a group of inflammatory conditions of the intestine that include (among others) *ulcerative colitis and *Crohn's disease.

infliximab n. a *monoclonal antibody used to treat severe cases of Crohn's disease and rheumatoid arthritis that have failed to respond to treatment with corticosteroids or immunosuppressants and antirheumatic drugs, respectively. It acts as an immunosuppressant by inhibiting the *tumor necrosis factor TNF-α. It is administered by infusion. Trade name: **Remicade.**

influenza (grippe) n. a highly contagious virus infection that affects the respiratory system. The viruses are transmitted in droplets expelled through coughing and sneezing. Symptoms commence after an incubation period of 1–4 days and include headache, fever, loss of appetite, weakness, and general aches and pains. They may continue for about a week. With bed rest and aspirin most patients recover, but a few may go on to develop pneumonia, either a primary influenzal viral pneumonia or a secondary bacterial pneumonia. Either of these may result in death from hemorrhage within the lungs. The main bacterial organisms that are responsible for secondary infection are *Streptococcus pneumoniae, Haemophilus influenzae*, and *Staphylococcus aureus*, against which appropriate antibiotic therapy must be given. An influenzal infection provides later protection only against the specific strain of virus concerned; the same holds true for immunization.

informed consent a legal requirement that physicians or researchers inform a patient undergoing surgery or invasive tests or a subject involved in a clinical trial of the nature, risks, and probable outcome of the treatment or research. The patient signs an agreement stating that he or she has been informed and accepts the treatment, surgery, or research protocol. Without informed consent, the physician or researcher is violating the patient's rights, regardless of whether the treatment is appropriate and successful.

infra- *prefix denoting* below.

infrared radiation the band of electromagnetic radiation that is longer in wavelength than the red of the visible spectrum. Infrared radiation is responsible for the transmission of radiant heat. It may be used in physiotherapy to warm tissues, reduce pain, and improve circulation, but it is not as effective as *diathermy for deep structures. Special photographic film sensitive to infrared radiation is used in *thermography.

infundibulum *n.* any funnel-shaped channel or passage, particularly the hollow conical stalk that extends downward from the hypothalamus and is continuous with the posterior lobe of the pituitary gland.

infusion *n.* **1.** the slow injection of a substance (e.g. saline or dextrose), usually into a vein (*intravenous infusion*). This is a common method for replacing water,

electrolytes, and blood products and is also used for the continuous administration of drugs (e.g. antibiotics, painkillers) or *nutrition. *See also* drip. **2.** the process whereby the active principles are extracted from plant material by steeping it in water that has been heated to boiling point (as in the making of tea). **3.** the solution produced by this process.

ingesta *pl. n.* food and drink that is introduced into the alimentary canal through the mouth.

ingestion *n.* **1.** the process by which food is taken into the alimentary canal. It involves chewing and swallowing. **2.** the process by which a phagocytic cell takes in solid material, such as bacteria.

ingravescent *adj.* gradually increasing in severity.

ingrown nail downward curving of the sides of a toenail, usually the big toenail, which causes chafing of the skin alongside the nail resulting in inflammation around the base of the nail. It is caused by faulty trimming of the toenails or pressure from a tight-fitting shoe.

inguinal *adj.* relating to or affecting the region of the groin (inguen).

inguinal canal either of a pair of openings that connect the abdominal cavity with the scrotum in the male fetus. The inguinal canals provide a route for the descent of the testes into the scrotum, after which they normally become obliterated.

inguinal hernia *see* hernia.

inguinal ligament (Poupart's ligament) a ligament in the groin that extends from the anterior superior iliac spine to the pubic tubercle. It is part of the *aponeurosis of the external oblique muscle of the abdomen.

inhalation *n.* **1.** (*or* **inspiration**) the act of breathing air into the lungs through the mouth or nose. *See* breathing. **2.** a gas, vapor, or aerosol breathed in for the treatment of conditions of the respiratory tract. —**inhaler** *n.*

inheritance *n.* **1.** the acquisition or expression of traits or conditions by transmission of genetic material from parents to offspring. **2.** the total genetic makeup of a fertilized ovum. *See also* gene, dominant, recessive.

inhibition *n.* **1.** (in physiology) the prevention or reduction of the functioning of an organ, muscle, etc., by the action of certain nerve impulses. **2.** (in psychoanalysis) an inner command that prevents one from doing something forbidden. Some inhibitions are essential for social adjustment, but excessive inhibitions can severely restrict one's life. **3.** (in psychology) a tendency not to carry out a specific action, produced each time the action is carried out.

inhibitor *n.* a substance that prevents the occurrence of a given process or reaction. *See also* MAO inhibitor.

inion *n.* a point located on the projection of the occipital bone that can be felt at the base of the skull.

initiation *n.* (in oncology) the first step in the development of cancer (*see* carcinogenesis).

initiator *n.* (in oncogenesis) a substance that induces an irreversible change in a cell's DNA that can result in a cancer. An example is dimethylbenzanthracene. *Compare* promoter.

injection *n.* introduction into the body of drugs or other fluids by means of a syringe, usually drugs that would be destroyed by the digestive processes if taken by mouth. Common routes for injection are into the skin (*intracutaneous* or *intradermal*); below the skin (*subcutaneous*), e.g. for insulin; into a muscle (*intramuscular*), for drugs that are slowly absorbed; and into a vein (*intravenous*), for drugs to be rapidly absorbed. **En-emas* are also regarded as injections.

injury scoring system (injury severity scale) a system used, particularly in **triage*, for grading the severity of an injury. *See also* abbreviated injury scale.

inlay *n.* **1.** a substance or piece of tissue inserted in a tissue to replace a defect. For example, a bone graft may be inlaid into an area of missing or damaged bone, or an aortic prosthesis placed using an inlay technique within an aneurysm. **2.** (in dentistry) a rigid restoration inserted into a tapered cavity in a tooth. It is held in place with a cement **lute*. Cast gold has been the most widely used material, but porcelain and composite resin are also used.

inlet *n.* an aperture providing the entrance to a cavity, such as that of the pelvis.

INN International Nonproprietary Name: the generic name, selected by the World Health Organization, of any pharmaceutical preparation. INNs, which are chosen according to standards established by WHO, are in the public domain and recognized and used throughout the world. The lists of these names are published in *WHO Drug Information. See also* USAN, USP.

innate *adj.* describing a condition or characteristic that is present in an individual at birth and is inherited from his parents. *See also* congenital, hereditary.

inner ear *see* labyrinth.

innervation *n.* the nerve supply to an area or organ of the body, which can carry either motor impulses to the structure or sensory impulses away from it toward the brain.

innocent *adj.* (of a tumor) benign; not malignant.

innominate artery *see* brachiocephalic artery.

innominate bone *see* hip bone.

innominate vein *see* brachiocephalic vein.

ino- *prefix denoting* **1.** fibrous tissue. **2.** muscle.

inoculation *n.* the introduction of a small quantity of material, such as a vaccine, in the process of **immunization*: a more general name for **vaccination*.

inoculum *n.* any material that is used for inoculation.

inorganic *adj.* **1.** not formed by living organisms. **2.** describing any compound that does not contain carbon. *Compare* organic.

inosine pranobex a drug that may increase the efficiency of the immune system by increasing the number of T lymphocytes and enhancing the activity of natural killer cells. Some early trials in HIV-positive people suggest that the drug could delay progression to AIDS. However, conclusive evidence is insufficient and more clinical evaluation is needed. The drug is not approved for sale in the US but is sold in Europe and other countries as a treatment for a number of viral diseases, including herpes, influenza A, and viral hepatitis.

inositol *n.* a compound similar to a hexose sugar that is a constituent of some cell phospholipids. Inositol is present in many foods, in particular in the bran of cereal grain. It is sometimes classified as a vitamin but it can be synthesized by most animals and there is no evidence that it is an essential nutrient in humans.

inositol triphosphate (IP$_3$) a short-lived biochemical *second messenger formed from *phospholipid in the cell membrane when a chemical messenger (e.g. a hormone or serotonin) binds to receptors on the cell surface. Inositol triphosphate triggers the rapid release of calcium into the cell fluid, which initiates various cellular processes, such as smooth muscle contraction and the release of glucose, histamine, etc. Inositol triphosphate exists for only a few seconds before being converted to inositol by the action of a sequence of enzymes.

inotropic *adj.* affecting the contraction of heart muscle. Drugs such as *dobutamine and *enoximone have positive inotropic action, stimulating heart muscle contractions and causing the heart rate to increase. *Beta blockers, such as *propranolol, have negative inotropic action, reducing heart muscle contractions and causing the heart rate to decrease.

inpatient *n.* a patient who is admitted to a bed in a hospital and remains there for a period of time for treatment, examination, or observation. *Compare* outpatient.

inquest *n.* an official judicial enquiry into the cause of a person's death: carried out when the death is sudden or takes place under suspicious circumstances. The results of medical and legal investigations that have been carried out are considered by a medical examiner sitting with or without a jury, and made publicly known. *See also* autopsy.

insanity *n.* a degree of mental illness in which the affected individual is not responsible for his actions or is not capable of entering into a legal contract. The term is used in legal rather than medical contexts.

insect *n.* a member of a large group of mainly land-dwelling *arthropods. The body of the adult is divided into a head, thorax, and abdomen. The head bears a single pair of sensory antennae; the thorax bears three pairs of legs and, in most insects, wings (these are absent in some parasitic groups, such as lice and fleas). Some insects are of medical importance. Various bloodsucking insects transmit tropical diseases, for example the female *Anopheles* mosquito transmits malaria and the tsetse fly transmits sleeping sickness. The bites of lice can cause intense irritation and, secondarily, bacterial infection. The organisms causing diarrhea and dysentery can be deposited on food from the bodies of flies. *See also* myiasis.

insecticide *n.* a preparation used to kill destructive or disease-carrying insects. Ideally, an insecticide should have no toxic effects when ingested by humans or animals, but modern powerful compounds have inherent dangers and have caused fatalities. Some insect powders contain organic phosphorus compounds and fluorides; when ingested accidentally they may damage the nervous system. The use of such compounds is generally under strict control. *See also* DDT, dieldrin.

insemination *n.* introduction of semen into the vagina. *See also* artificial insemination, intrauterine insemination.

insertion *n.* (in anatomy) the point of attachment of a muscle (e.g. to a bone) that is relatively movable when the muscle contracts. *Compare* origin.

insidious *adj.* describing a condition, disease, or symptom that is gradual or subtle in development. Often a condition, such as glaucoma or hypertension, can develop insidiously over a period of time with symptoms that are not detected until a disease state is fully established.

insight *n.* (in psychology) knowledge of oneself. The term is applied particularly to a patient's recognition that he has psychological problems; in this sense absence of insight is a feature of psychosis. The term is also applied to the patient's accuracy of understanding the development of his personality and his problems; in this sense insight is enhanced by psychotherapy.

insolation *n.* exposure to the sun's rays. *See also* heatstroke.

insomnia *n.* inability to fall asleep or to remain asleep for an adequate length of time, so that tiredness is virtually permanent. Insomnia may be associated with disease, particularly if there are painful symptoms, but is more often caused by worry.

inspiration *n. see* inhalation.

inspissated *adj.* (of secretions, etc.) thickened or dried by evaporation or dehydration.

instillation *n.* **1.** the application of liquid medication drop by drop, as into the eye.

2. the medication, such as eye drops, applied in this way.

instinct n. **1.** a complex pattern of behavior innately determined, which is characteristic of all individuals of the same species. The behavior is released and modified by environmental stimuli, but its pattern is relatively uniform and predetermined. **2.** an innate drive that urges the individual toward a particular goal (for example, *libido in psychoanalytic psychology).

institutionalization n. a condition produced by long-term residence in an unstimulating impersonal institution (such as some mental hospitals and orphanages). The individual adapts to the behavior characteristic of the institution to such an extent that he is handicapped in other environments. The features often include apathy, dependence, and a lack of personal responsibility. Some symptoms, such as *stereotypy, are more common in the institutionalized.

insufficiency n. inability of an organ or part, such as the heart or kidney, to carry out its normal function.

insufflation n. the act of blowing gas or a powder, such as a medication, into a body cavity.

insula n. an area of the *cerebral cortex that is overlapped by the sides of the deep lateral sulcus (cleft) in each hemisphere of the brain.

insulin n. a protein hormone, produced in the pancreas by the beta cells of the *islets of Langerhans, that is important for regulating the amount of sugar (glucose) in the blood. Insulin secretion is stimulated by a high concentration of blood sugar. Lack of this hormone gives rise to *diabetes mellitus, in which large amounts of sugar are present in the blood and urine. This condition may be treated successfully by insulin injections (*see* analogue insulins, isophane insulins, insulin pen, continuous insulin infusion pump). Several kinds of insulin are available, including pork, beef, and a semisynthetic human insulin. Trade names: **Humulin, Iletin, Novolin, Velosulin.**

insulinase n. an enzyme, found in such tissues as the liver and kidney, that is responsible for the normal breakdown of insulin in the body.

insulinoma n. an insulin-producing tumor of the beta cells in the *islets of Langer-

hans of the pancreas. Symptoms can include sweating, faintness, episodic loss of consciousness, and other features of *hypoglycemia (*see* Whipple's triad). Single tumors can be removed surgically. Multiple very small tumors that are scattered throughout the pancreas cannot be treated by surgery but do respond to drugs that inhibit the beta cells, including *diazoxide.

insulin pen a penlike device designed to inject a measured dose of insulin. The dose can be "dialed up" and then safely injected from a 3-ml cartridge contained within. The pen can be capped off and easily stored in a pocket or small bag; some types are disposable, while others can be refilled.

insulin shock a condition in which excess insulin in the body decreases the amount of glucose in the blood (hypoglycemia). If not treated with glucose or glucagon, coma and death can occur.

insulin stress test an important but potentially dangerous test of anterior pituitary function involving the deliberate induction of a hypoglycemic episode with injected insulin and the subsequent measurement of plasma cortisol and growth hormone at regular intervals over the next three hours. The stress of the hypoglycemia should induce a rise in the levels of these hormones unless the anterior pituitary or the adrenal glands are diseased. The test can induce epileptic seizures or angina in those with a predisposition and should not be performed in susceptible individuals. It is often combined with the thyrotropin-releasing hormone (TRH) test and the gonadotropin-releasing hormone (GnRH) test in what is known as the *triple test*.

insult n. an injury or physical trauma.

integration n. the blending together of the *nerve impulses that arrive through the thousands of synapses at a nerve cell body. Impulses from some synapses cause *excitation, and from others *inhibition; the overall pattern decides whether an individual nerve cell is activated to transmit a message or not.

integrative medicine *see* complementary medicine.

integrin n. any of a class of proteins that act as cell-adhesion receptors and mediate intracellular-to-extracellular and cell-to-cell interactions.

integument *n.* **1.** the skin. **2.** a membrane or layer of tissue covering any organ of the body.

intelligence quotient (IQ) an index of intellectual development. In childhood and adult life it represents intellectual ability relative to the rest of the population; in children it can also represent rate of development (*mental age as a percentage of chronological age). Most *intelligence tests are constructed so that the resulting intelligence quotients in the general population have a *mean of about 100 and a *standard deviation of about 15.

intelligence test a standardized assessment procedure for the determination of intellectual ability. The score produced is usually expressed as an *intelligence quotient. Most tests present a series of different kinds of problems to be solved. The best known are the Wechsler Adult Intelligence Scale (WAIS), the Wechsler Intelligence Scale for Children (WISC), and the Stanford–Binet Intelligence Scale. Scores on intelligence tests are used for such purposes as the diagnosis of *mental retardation and the assessment of intellectual deterioration.

intensive care unit (ICU) a section of a hospital providing specialized care to seriously ill patients. Sophisticated monitoring and treatment equipment is available to the multidisciplinary staff. Some units are specialized for the care of a select group; neonatal, cardiac, and surgical intensive care units are examples.

intention *n.* a process of healing. Healing by *first intention* is the natural healing of a wound or surgical incision when the edges are brought together under aseptic conditions and *granulation tissue forms. In healing by *second intention* the wound edges are separated and the cavity is filled with granulation tissue over which epithelial tissue grows from the wound edges. In healing by *third intention* the wound ulcerates, granulations are slow to form, and a scar forms at the wound site.

intention tremor *see* tremor.

inter- *prefix denoting* between. Examples: *intercostal* (between the ribs); *interosseous* (between bones), *intertrochanteric* (between the trochanters).

intercalated *adj.* describing structures, tis-

sues, etc., that are inserted or situated between other structures.

intercellular *adj.* situated or occurring between cells.

intercostal muscles muscles that occupy the spaces between the ribs and are responsible for controlling some of the movements of the ribs. The superficial *external intercostals* lift the ribs during inspiration; the deep *internal intercostals* draw the ribs together during expiration.

intercurrent *adj.* going on at the same time: applied to an infection contracted by a patient who already has an infection or other disease.

interferon *n.* a *glycoprotein substance that is produced by cells infected with a virus and has the ability to inhibit viral growth (*see also* cytokines). Interferon is active against many different viruses, but particular interferons are effective only in the species that produces them. There are three types of human interferons: *alpha* (from white blood cells), *beta* (from fibroblasts), and *gamma* (from lymphocytes). Human interferon can now be produced in bacterial host cells by *genetic engineering for clinical use. *Interferon alfa* (Intron A, Rolferon A, Alferon N) is used in treating hepatitis B and C, hairy-cell leukemia, Kaposi's sarcoma, and certain other forms of cancer; *peginterferon alfa* (Pegasys, PEG-Intron) is used for hepatitis C; and *interferon beta* (Avonex, Betaseron, Rebif) for multiple sclerosis. Side effects, including flulike symptoms, lethargy, and depression, may be severe.

interkinesis *n.* **1.** the resting stage between the two divisions of *meiosis. **2.** *see* interphase.

interlabial gap the vertical distance between the upper and lower lips that is present when the lips are relaxed.

interleukin *n.* any of a family of proteins that control aspects of hemopoiesis and the immune response (*see also* cytokines). Many interleukins are currently characterized. *Interleukin 2 (IL-2)* stimulates T lymphocytes to become *natural killer cells, active against cancer cells, and is being investigated for the treatment of cancer: recombinant interleukin 2 (*aldesleukin*, Proleukin), administered by subcutaneous injection, can be of benefit in the treatment of *hypernephroma (renal-cell carcinoma) and skin cancer that has spread to other parts of the body.

intermittency *n.* a *lower urinary tract symptom in which the flow of urine is not continuous but stops and starts.

intermittent claudication *see* claudication.

intermittent fever a fever that rises, subsides, then returns again. *See* malaria.

intermittent pneumatic compression a technique to prevent thrombosis in bedridden patients. It uses an inflatable device that squeezes the calf when it inflates, preventing pools of blood forming behind the valves in the veins, thus mimicking the effects of walking.

intermittent self-catheterization (ISC) a procedure in which the patient periodically passes a disposable catheter through the urethra into the bladder for the purpose of emptying it of urine. It is increasingly used in the management of patients of both sexes (including children) with chronic *retention and large residual urine volumes, often due to a *neuropathic bladder. ISC may prevent back pressure and dilation of the upper urinary tract with consequent infection and incontinence.

intern *n.* a medical or dental graduate, serving in a hospital, who assists and receives instruction from a *resident in preparation for being licensed to practice medicine or dentistry.

International Classification of Diseases (ICD) a list of all known diseases and syndromes, including mental and behavioral disorders, published by the *World Health Organization every ten years (approximately). Over the years the classification has moved from being disease-orientated to include a wider framework of illness and other health problems. The latest version, *ICD-10*, was published in 1992 and employs alphanumeric coding. It is used in many countries as the principal means of classifying both mortality and morbidity experience and allows comparison of morbidity and mortality rates both nationally and internationally. In the US, a modified classification, the *International Classification of Diseases, Clinical Modification* (*ICD-9-CM*), provides additional data required by clinicians, research workers, and medical record librarians or inpatient, outpatient, and community programs. A parallel list, the *International Classification of Impairments, Disabilities and Handicaps* (*ICIDH*), has also been compiled and is being used experimentally. *See also* handicap.

International Prostate Symptom Score (IPSS) a self-administered questionnaire completed by men with *lower urinary tract symptoms that gives a numerical score (on a scale of 0 to 35) to indicate the severity of their symptoms.

interneuron *n.* a neuron in the central nervous system that acts as a link between the different neurons in a *reflex arc. It usually possesses numerous branching processes (dendrites) that make possible extensive and complex circuits and pathways within the brain and spinal cord.

internode *n.* the length of *axon covered with a myelin sheath. Internodes are separated by nodes of Ranvier, where the sheath is absent.

interobserver error (in statistical surveys) *see* validity.

interoceptor *n.* any *receptor organ composed of sensory nerve cells that respond to and monitor changes within the body, such as the stretching of muscles or the acidity of the blood.

interparietal bone (inca bone, incarial bone) the bone lying between the *parietal bones, at the back of the skull.

interpeduncular *adj.* situated between the peduncles of the cerebrum or cerebellum in the brain.

interphase (interkinesis) *n.* the period when a cell is not undergoing division (mitosis), during which activities such as DNA synthesis occur.

intersex *n.* an individual who shows anatomical characteristics of both sexes. *See also* hermaphrodite, pseudohermaphroditism. —**intersexuality** *n.*

interstice *n.* a small space in a tissue or between parts of the body. —**interstitial** *adj.*

interstitial cells (Leydig cells) the cells interspersed between the seminiferous tubules of the *testis. They secrete *androgens in response to stimulation by *luteinizing hormone from the anterior pituitary gland.

interstitial-cell-stimulating hormone *see* luteinizing hormone.

interstitial cystitis a chronic nonbacterial inflammation of the bladder accompanied by an urgent desire to urinate frequently and bladder pain; it is often associated with an ulcer in the bladder wall (*Hunner's ulcer*). The cause is unknown and *contracture of the bladder eventually occurs. Treatment is by distension of the bladder under spinal or epidural anesthetic, instillation of anti-inflammatory solutions into the bladder, and administration of steroids or *NSAIDs. Bladder enhancement or augmentation (*see* cystoplasty) may be required for a contracted bladder.

intertrigo *n.* superficial inflammation (dermatitis) of two skin surfaces that are in contact, such as between the thighs or under the breasts, particularly in obese people. The dermatitis is caused by friction, warmth, moisture, and sweat and in many cases is aggravated by infection, especially with *Candida*. —**intertriginous** *adj.*

interventional radiology the performance of therapeutic or diagnostic procedures under the control of an appropriate imaging technique. Guidance is commonly by X-ray fluoroscopy, ultrasound, or computed tomography, and recently also by magnetic resonance imaging. Procedures commonly performed include the placing of vascular catheters, drainage of fluid collections or abscesses, stenting of obstructions to the gastrointestinal tract or blood vessels, embolization, cryotherapy, and radiofrequency ablation. Imaging is also used in many forms of *minimally invasive surgery, including *angioplasty, visualization of obstructions in the bile ducts (*see* [percutaneous] cholangiography), and the removal of kidney stones (*see* percutaneous nephrolithotomy).

intervention study a comparison of the outcome between two or more groups of patients that are deliberately subjected to different regimens (usually of treatment but sometimes of a preventive measure, such as vaccination). Wherever possible those entering the trial should be allocated to their respective groups by means of random numbers, and one such group (*controls*) should have no active treatment (*randomized controlled trial*). Ideally neither the patient nor the person assessing the outcome should be aware of which therapy is allocated to which patient (*blind trial*), nor should the doctor responsible for treatment (*double-blind trial*), and groups should exchange treatment after a prearranged period (*crossover trial*).

intervertebral disk the flexible plate of fibrocartilage that connects any two adjacent vertebrae in the backbone. At birth the central part of the disk – the *nucleus pulposus* – consists of a gelatinous substance, which becomes replaced by cartilage with age. The intervertebral disks account for one quarter of the total length of the backbone; they act as shock absorbers, protecting the brain and spinal cord from the impact produced by running and other movements. *See also* prolapsed intervertebral disk.

intestinal flora bacteria normally present in the intestinal tract. Some are responsible for the synthesis of *vitamin K. By producing a highly acidic environment in the intestine they may also prevent infection by pathogenic bacteria that cannot tolerate such conditions.

intestinal juice *see* succus entericus.

intestinal obstruction blockage of the intestine producing symptoms of vomiting, distension, and abdominal pain; failure to pass flatus or feces (complete constipation) is usual. The causes may be acute (e.g. hernia) or chronic (e.g. tumors, Crohn's disease). Conservative management is by nasogastric suction and replacement of water and electrolytes, but most cases require surgical cure by removing the underlying cause.

intestine (bowel, gut) *n.* the part of the *alimentary canal that extends from the stomach to the anus. It is divided into two main parts – the small intestine and the large intestine. The *small intestine* is divided into the *duodenum, *jejunum, and *ileum. It is here that most of the processes of digestion and absorption of food take place. The surface area of the inside of the small intestine is increased by the presence of fingerlike projections called *villi* (see illustration). Glands in the mucous layer of the intestine secrete digestive enzymes and mucus. The *large intestine* consists of the *cecum, vermiform *appendix, *colon, and *rectum. It is largely concerned with the absorption of water from the material passed from the small intestine. The contents of the intestines are propelled forward by means of rhythmic muscular contractions (*see* peristalsis). —**intestinal** *adj.*

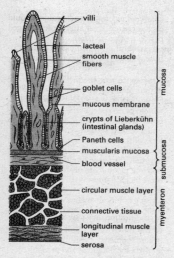

villi
lacteal
smooth muscle fibers
goblet cells
mucous membrane
crypts of Lieberkühn (intestinal glands)
Paneth cells
muscularis mucosa
blood vessel
circular muscle layer
connective tissue
longitudinal muscle layer
serosa

mucosa
submucosa
myenteron

Longitudinal section through the ileum

intima (tunica intima) *n.* **1.** the inner layer of the wall of an *artery or *vein. It is composed of a lining of endothelial cells and an elastic membrane. **2.** the inner layer of various other organs or parts.

intolerance *n.* the inability of a patient to tolerate a particular drug, manifested by various adverse reactions.

intoxication *n.* the symptoms of poisoning due to ingestion of any toxic material, including alcohol, drugs, and heavy metals.

intra- *prefix denoting* inside; within. Examples: *intralobular* (within a lobule); *intraosseous* (within the bone marrow); *intrauterine* (within the uterus).

intracellular *adj.* situated or occurring inside a cell or cells.

intracranial *adj.* within the skull.

intracytoplasmic sperm injection *see* ICSI.

intradermal *adj.* within the skin. An *intradermal injection* is made into the skin.

intramuscular *adj.* within a muscle. An *intramuscular injection* is made into a muscle.

intraobserver error (in statistical surveys) *see* validity.

intraocular *adj.* of or relating to the area within the eyeball. An *intraocular lens*

implant is a plastic lens placed inside the eye after *cataract extraction to replace the natural lens.

intraosseous needle a wide-bore needle for insertion directly into the bone marrow of (usually) the tibia in children, used only in emergencies when no means of intravenous access can be gained. An intraosseous needle enables fluids and drugs to be given rapidly to the patient. They are only for use with an unconscious patient and must be removed when alternative access is obtained.

intrastromal keratomileusis an operation to correct severe degrees of myopia (nearsightedness). A disk of corneal tissue (from the *stroma of the cornea) is removed, frozen, and remodeled on a lathe, then replaced into the cornea to alter its curvature and thus reduce the myopia. *Excimer laser treatment, which is easier to perform, is also now being used for treating severe myopia (*see* LASIK, LASEK).

intrathecal *adj.* **1.** within the *meninges of the spinal cord. An *intrathecal injection* is made into the meninges. **2.** within a sheath, e.g. a nerve sheath.

intrauterine device *see* IUD.

intrauterine growth retardation (IUGR) the condition resulting in the birth of a baby whose birth weight is abnormally low in relation to its gestational age (i.e. *small for dates*). Causes include maternal disease (e.g. infection, malnutrition, high blood pressure, smoking, and alcoholism), poor socioeconomic conditions, multiple pregnancy (e.g. twins), and fetal disease. It may be associated with *preterm birth.

intrauterine insemination (IUI) a procedure for assisting conception in cases of male infertility caused by inability of the spermatozoa to penetrate the cervical mucus or the barriers surrounding the ovum. The spermatozoa, which may be chemically treated in vitro to improve their motility and *acrosome reaction, are injected into the uterus through the vagina.

intravenous (IV) *adj.* into or within a vein. An *intravenous injection* is made into a vein. *See* infusion, injection.

intravenous feeding *see* nutrition.

intravenous urogram (IVU) a succession of X-ray images of the urinary tract following the injection into a vein of a *contrast medium; this was formerly called an *intravenous pyelogram* (*IVP*). The medium is concentrated and excreted by the kidneys, and the IVU reveals details of the kidneys, the ureters, and subsequently the bladder. An IVU tests kidney function and reveals the presence of stones, tumors, or dilation, which may be caused by obstruction, in the urinary tract. *See also* pyelography.

intraversion *n. see* introversion.

intra vitam Latin: during life.

intravitreal *adj.* within the vitreous humor.

intrinsic factor a glycoprotein secreted in the stomach. The secretion of intrinsic factor is necessary for the absorption of *vitamin B₁₂; a failure of secretion of intrinsic factor leads to a deficiency of the vitamin and the condition of *pernicious anemia.

intrinsic muscle a muscle that is contained entirely within the organ or part it acts on. For example, there are intrinsic muscles of the tongue, whose contractions change the shape of the tongue.

intro- *prefix denoting* in; into.

introitus *n.* (in anatomy) an entrance into a hollow organ or cavity.

introjection *n.* (in psychoanalysis) the process of adopting, or of believing that one possesses, the qualities of another person. This can be a form of *defense mechanism. *See also* identification.

intromission *n.* the introduction of one organ or part into another, e.g. the penis into the vagina.

introversion *n.* **1.** an enduring personality trait characterized by interest in the self rather than the outside world. People high in introversion (*introverts*), as measured by questionnaires and psychological tests, tend to have a small circle of friends, like to persist in activities once they have started, and are highly susceptible to permanent *conditioning. Introversion was first described by Carl Jung as a tendency to distancing oneself from others, to philosophical interests, and to reserved defensive reactions. *Compare* extroversion. **2.** a turning inward of a hollow organ (such as the uterus) on itself.

introvert *n. see* introversion.

intubation *n.* the introduction of a tube into part of the body for the purpose of diagnosis or treatment. Thus, *gastric intubation* may be performed to remove a sample of the stomach contents for analysis or to administer drugs directly into the stomach. In *endotracheal intubation* a tube is inserted through the mouth into the trachea to maintain an airway in an unconscious or anesthetized patient.

intumescence *n.* a swelling or an increase in the volume of an organ.

intussusception *n.* the telescoping (*invagination*) of one part of the bowel into another: most common in young children under the age of four years. As the contents of the intestine are pushed onward by muscular contraction more and more intestine is dragged into the invaginating portion, resulting in obstruction. Symptoms include intermittent colic or pain, screaming and pallor, vomiting, and the passing of bloody mucus with the stools; if the condition does not receive prompt surgical treatment, shock from gangrene of the bowel may result. A barium or other *contrast medium enema may confirm the diagnosis and in many cases may relieve the intussusception.

inulin *n.* a carbohydrate with a high molecular weight, used in a test of kidney function called *inulin clearance*. Inulin is filtered from the bloodstream by the kidneys. By injecting it into the blood and measuring the amount that appears in the urine over a given period, it is possible to calculate how much filtrate the kidneys are producing in a given time.

inunction *n.* the rubbing in with the fingers of an ointment or liniment.

invagination *n.* **1.** the infolding of the wall of a solid structure to form a cavity. It occurs in some stages of embryonic development. **2.** *see* intussusception.

invasion *n.* the spread of *cancer into neighboring normal structures; it is one of the cardinal features of malignancy.

inversion *n.* **1.** the turning inward or inside-out of a part or organ: often applied to the state of the uterus after childbirth when its upper part is pulled through the cervical canal. **2.** a chromosome mutation in which a block of genes within a chromosome are in reverse order, due to that section of the chromosome becoming inverted. The centromere may be included in the inverted segment (*pericentric inversion*) or not (*paracentric inversion*).

invertebrate 1. *n.* an animal without a

backbone. The following are invertebrate groups of medical importance: *insects, *ticks, *nematodes, *flukes, *protozoans, and *tapeworms. **2.** *adj.* not possessing a backbone.

investigational new drug (IND) a drug that has not yet been approved by the *Food and Drug Administration for marketing to the general population but is available for use in experiments to test its safety and effectiveness.

in vitro Latin: describing biological phenomena that are made to occur outside the living body (traditionally in a test tube).

in vitro fertilization (IVF) fertilization of an ovum outside the body, the resultant *zygote being incubated to the *blastocyst stage and then implanted in the uterus. The technique, pioneered in Britain, resulted in 1978 in the birth of the first *test-tube baby*. It is undertaken when a woman has blocked fallopian tubes or some other impediment to the union of sperm and ovum in the reproductive tract. The mother-to-be is given hormone therapy causing a number of ova to mature at the same time (*see* superovulation). Several of them are then removed from the ovary through a laparoscope. The ova are mixed with sperm from her partner and incubated in a culture medium until the blastocyst is formed. The blastocyst is then implanted in the mother's uterus and the pregnancy allowed to continue normally.

in vivo Latin: describing biological phenomena that occur or are observed occurring within the bodies of living organisms.

involucrum *n.* a growth of new bone, formed from the *periosteum, that sometimes surrounds a mass of infected and dead bone in osteomyelitis.

involuntary muscle muscle that is not under conscious control, such as the muscle of the gut, stomach, blood vessels, and heart. *See also* cardiac muscle, smooth muscle.

involution *n.* **1.** the shrinking of the uterus to its normal size after childbirth. **2.** atrophy of an organ in old age.

involutional melancholia a severe *depression, usually psychotic, appearing for the first time in the involutional period of middle life (approximately 40–55 for women, 50–65 for men). Such an illness classically has characteristic features, including agitation; delusions of ill health, poverty, sin, and sometimes of the nonexistence of the world; and preoccupations with death and loss. However, the features are not always classic, and most authorities do not regard the condition as a clinical entity separate from depressive psychosis. *See* manic-depressive psychosis.

iodine *n.* an element required in small amounts for healthy growth and development. An adult body contains about 30 mg of iodine, mostly concentrated in the thyroid gland: this gland requires iodine to synthesize *thyroid hormones. A deficiency of iodine leads to *goiter. The daily requirement of iodine in an adult is thought to be about 150 µg per day; dietary sources of iodine are sea food and vegetables grown in soil containing iodide and also iodized table salt. Iodine is used in the diagnosis and treatment of diseases of the thyroid gland (*see* Lugol's iodine, radioactive iodine therapy) and also as an antiseptic and skin disinfectant (in the form of *povidone-iodine*). Water-soluble contrast media used in X-ray examinations are organic chemicals containing iodine, which is radiopaque due to its high atomic weight. Symbol: I.

iodipamide *n.* a *radiopaque compound containing iodine, used as a *contrast medium in radiography for intravenous *cholangiography and *cholecystography. Trade name: **Cholografin**.

iodism *n.* iodine poisoning. The main features are a characteristic staining of the mouth and odor on the breath. Vomited material may be yellowish or bluish. There is pain and burning in the throat, intense thirst, and diarrhea, with dizziness, weakness, and convulsions. Emergency treatment includes administration of starch or flour in water and lavage with sodium thiosulfate solution.

iodohippurate sodium a radiopaque compound used as a contrast medium in radiology of the urinary tract. Labeled with radioiodine, it can be used to measure renal function. Trade name: **Hippuran I 131.**

iodopyracet (diodone) *n.* a *radiopaque medium containing iodine, used for imaging the urinary tract and any abnormalities that may be present (*see* pyelography).

iodoquinol *n.* an antiseptic used to treat bowel infections and dysentery caused by ameba. It is administered by mouth or as pessaries and occasionally causes irritation of the digestive system, headache, itching, and boils. Trade names: **Diquinol, Yodoquinol, Yodoxin**.

ion *n.* an atom or group of atoms that has lost one or more electrons, making it electrically charged and therefore more chemically active. *See* anion, cation, electrolyte, ionization.

ionization *n.* the process of producing *ions. Some molecules ionize in solution (*see* electrolyte). Ions can also be produced when ionizing radiation dislodges one or more electrons from an atom or molecule. This can be harmful to DNA in cells, resulting in tumors or genetic defects.

iontophoresis *n.* the technique of introducing through the skin, by means of an electric current, charged particles of a drug, so that it reaches a deep site. The method has been used to transfer salicylate ions through the skin in the treatment of deep rheumatic pain. *See also* cataphoresis.

iopanoic acid *n.* a *radiopaque compound containing iodine and used in radiography to outline the gallbladder (*see* cholecystography). Given by mouth, the iopanoic acid is concentrated in the bile by the liver and thus shows up the gallbladder clearly during X-ray examination. Trade name: **Telepaque**.

iophendylate *n.* a *radiopaque compound containing iodine that is sometimes used in radiography to show up the spinal canal (*see* myelography). It is injected through a *lumbar puncture needle.

IOUS *intra*operative *ultrasound examination (*see* ultrasonography).

IP₃ *see* inositol triphosphate.

ipecac (ipecacuanha) *n.* a plant extract used in small doses, usually in the form of tinctures and syrups, as an *expectorant to relieve coughing and to induce vomiting. Ipecac irritates the digestive system, and high doses may cause severe digestive upsets.

ipratropium *n.* an *anticholinergic drug used as a bronchodilator in the treatment of chronic reversible airways obstruction (*see* bronchospasm). It is administered by inhalation; side effects include cough, nausea, palpitations, and headache. Trade name: **Atrovent**.

ipsilateral (homolateral) *adj.* on or affecting the same side of the body: applied particularly to paralysis (or other symptoms) occurring on the same side of the body as the brain lesion that caused them. *Compare* contralateral.

IPSS *see* International Prostate Symptom Score.

IQ *see* intelligence quotient.

irbesartan *n. see* angiotensin II antagonist.

irid- (irido-) *prefix denoting* the iris.

iridectomy *n.* an operation on the eye in which a part of the iris is removed.

iridencleisis *n.* an operation for *glaucoma in which a small incision is made into the eye, beneath the *conjunctiva and close to the cornea, and part of the iris is drawn into it. The iris acts like a wick and keeps the incision open for the drainage of fluid from the front chamber of the eye to the tissue beneath the conjunctiva.

iridocyclitis *n.* inflammation of the iris and ciliary body of the eye. *See* uveitis.

iridodialysis *n.* a tear, caused by injury to the eye, in the attachment of the iris to the ciliary body. Usually a dark crescentic gap is seen at the edge of the iris where the tear has occurred, and the pupil pulls away from the site of the tear.

iridodonesis *n.* tremulousness of the iris when the eye is moved. It is due to absence of support from the lens, against which the iris normally lies, and occurs when the lens is absent or dislocated from its normal position.

iridoplegia *n.* paralysis of the iris, which is usually associated with *cycloplegia and results from injury, inflammation, or the use of pupil-dilating eye drops. In the case of injury, the pupil is usually larger than normal and moves little, if at all, in response to light and drugs.

iridotomy *n.* an operation on the eye in which an incision is made in the iris using a knife or *YAG laser.

irinotecan *n. see* topoisomerase inhibitor.

iris *n.* the part of the eye that regulates the amount of light that enters. It forms a colored muscular diaphragm across the front of the lens; light enters through a central opening, the *pupil*. A ring of muscle around the margin contracts in bright light, causing the pupil to become smaller (*see* pupillary reflex). In dim light a set of radiating muscles contract and the constricting muscles relax, increasing the size of the pupil. The outer margin of the iris is attached to the *ciliary body.

iris bombé an abnormal condition of the eye in which the iris bulges forward toward the cornea. It is due to pressure from the aqueous humor behind the iris when its passage through the pupil to the anterior chamber of the eye is blocked (*pupil-block glaucoma*).

iritis *n.* inflammation of the iris. *See* uveitis.

iron *n.* an element essential to life. The body of an adult contains on average 4 g of iron, over half of which is contained in *hemoglobin in the red blood cells, the rest being distributed between *myohemoglobin in muscles, *cytochromes, and iron stores in the form of *ferritin and *hemosiderin. Iron is an essential component in the transfer of oxygen in the body. The absorption and loss of iron is very finely controlled. A good dietary source is meat, particularly liver. The recommended daily intake of iron is 10 mg per day for men and 12 mg per day for women during their reproductive life. A deficiency of iron may lead to *anemia. Symbol: Fe.
Many preparations of iron are used to treat iron-deficiency anemia. These include preparations taken by mouth, such as *ferrous sulfate, and those administered by injection, such as *iron dextran.

iron dextran a drug containing *iron and *dextran, administered by intramuscular or intravenous injection to treat iron-deficiency anemia. Side effects can include pain at the site of injection, rapid beating of the heart, and allergic reactions. Trade names: **DexFerrum, InFeD.**

iron lung *see* respirator.

iron-storage disease *see* hemochromatosis.

irradiation *n.* **1.** exposure of the body's tissues to ionizing radiation (*see* ionization). The source may be background radiation, diagnostic X-rays, *radiotherapy, or nuclear accidents. **2.** exposure of a substance or object to ionizing radiation. Irradiation of food with gamma rays, which kill bacteria, is a technique used in food preservation.

irreducible *adj.* unable to be replaced in a normal position: applied particularly to a type of *hernia.

irrigation *n.* the process of washing out a wound or hollow organ with a continuous flow of water or medicated solution. Techniques are available for washing out the entire intestinal tract (*whole-gut irrigation*) as a prelude to surgery on the lower intestine.

irritability *n.* (in physiology) the property of certain kinds of tissue that enables them to respond in a specific way to outside stimuli. Irritability is shown by nerve cells, which can generate and transmit electrical impulses when stimulated appropriately, and by muscle cells, which contract when stimulated by nerve impulses.

irritable bowel syndrome (IBS, spastic colon, mucous colitis) a common condition in which recurrent abdominal pain with constipation and/or diarrhea continues for years without any general deterioration in health. There is no detectable structural disease; the symptoms are caused by abnormal muscular contractions in the intestine and heightened sensitivity to such stimuli as stretching or distension. The cause is unknown, but the condition is often associated with stress or anxiety and may follow severe infection of the intestine. Tests may be needed to rule out organic disease. Treatment is based on removing anxiety (psychotherapy), dietary adjustment and fecal softening agents, and drugs to reduce spasm or diminish pain sensitivity.

irritant *n.* any material that causes irritation of a tissue, ranging from nettles (causing pain and swelling) to tear gas (causing watering of the eyes). Chronic irritation by various chemicals can give rise to *dermatitis.

ISC *see* intermittent self-catheterization.

isch- (ischo-) *prefix denoting* suppression or deficiency.

ischemia *n.* an inadequate flow of blood to a part of the body, caused by constriction or blockage of the blood vessels supplying it. Ischemia of heart muscle produces *angina pectoris. Ischemia of the calf muscles of the legs on exercise (causing intermittent *claudication) or at rest (producing rest pain) is common in elderly subjects with atherosclerosis of the vessels at or distal to the point where the aorta divides into the iliac arteries. —**ischemic** adj.

ischi- (ischio-) prefix denoting the ischium.

ischiorectal abscess an abscess in the space between the sheet of muscle that assists in control of the rectum (levator ani) and the pelvic bone. It may occur spontaneously, but is often secondary to an anal fissure, thrombosed *hemorrhoids, or other disease of the anus. Symptoms are severe throbbing pain near the anus with swelling and fever; it may cause an anal *fistula. Pus is drained from the abscess by surgical incision.

ischium n. a bone forming the lower part of each side of the *hip bone (see also pelvis). —**ischiac, ischial** adj.

ischuria n. retention or suppression of the urine. See anuria, retention.

island n. (in anatomy) an area of tissue or group of cells clearly differentiated from surrounding tissues.

islet n. (in anatomy) a small group of cells that is structurally distinct from the cells surrounding it.

islet cell transplantation a new technique still under evaluation for curing type 1 *diabetes mellitus, which involves the injection of donated cells from the pancreatic *islets of Langerhans into the liver, where it is hoped they will seed and survive. The transplanted cells then take over insulin production from the recipient's diseased pancreas.

islets of Langerhans small groups of endocrine cells, scattered through the material of the *pancreas. There are three main histological types of cells: alpha (α) cells, which secrete *glucagon; beta (β) cells, which produce *insulin; and delta (δ) cells, which release *somatostatin and *pancreatic polypeptide. [P. Langerhans (1847–88), German physician and anatomist]

iso- prefix denoting equality, uniformity, or similarity.

isoagglutinin (isohemagglutinin) n. one of the antibodies occurring naturally in the plasma that causes *agglutination of red blood cells of a different group.

isoagglutinogen n. one of the *antigens naturally occurring on the surface of red blood cells that is attacked by an isoagglutinin in blood plasma of a different group, so causing *agglutination.

isoantibody n. an *antibody produced by an individual that reacts against the components of foreign tissues from another individual of the same species.

isoantigen n. an antigen that produces an *immune response when transferred to an individual of the same species who is not genetically similar, as in a blood transfusion or tissue graft. Thus, the antigens of the *HLA system are isoantigens, as are the agglutinogens of the different *blood groups.

isodactylism n. a congenital defect in which all the fingers are the same length.

isohemagglutinin n. see isoagglutinin.

isoimmunization n. the development of antibodies (isoantibodies) within an individual against antigens from another individual of the same species.

isolation n. **1.** the separation of a person with an infectious disease from noninfected people. See also quarantine. **2.** (in surgery) the separation of a structure from surrounding structures by the use of instruments.

isoleucine n. an *essential amino acid. See also amino acid.

isomerase n. any one of a group of enzymes that catalyze the conversion of one *isomer of a compound into another.

isomers pl. n. two or more compounds that have the same molecular weight and formula but different molecular structures, that is, the atoms are linked in different ways. In stereoisomers the linkages between the atoms in the compounds are the same but the atoms have different configurations, as in optical isomers (or enantiomers), in which the molecules are mirror images of each other. —**isomerism** n.

isometheptene n. a *sympathomimetic drug used in the treatment of migraine in combination with dichloralphenazone and *acetaminophen (as Midrin). It is administered by mouth. Possible side effects include dizziness and skin rash.

isometric exercises (isometrics) a system of exercises based on the principle of isometric contraction of muscles. This occurs when the fibers are called upon to contract and do work, but despite an increase in tension do not shorten in length. It can be induced in muscles that are used when a limb is made to pull or push against something that does not move. The exercises increase fitness and build muscle. *See also* exercise.

isometropia *n.* an equal power of *refraction in both eyes.

isomorphism *n.* the condition of two or more objects being alike in shape or structure. It can exist at any structural level, from molecules to whole organisms. —**isomorphic, isomorphous** *adj.*

isoniazid (isonicotinic acid hydrazide) *n.* a drug used in the treatment of *tuberculosis, usually taken by mouth. Because tuberculosis bacteria soon become resistant to isoniazid, it is usually given in conjunction with other antibiotics. Occasional side effects include digestive disturbances and dry mouth; high doses or prolonged treatment may cause inflammation of the nerves, which can be countered by administering pyridoxine (vitamin B_6). Trade names: **Laniazid, Nydrazid**.

isophane insulins a group of insulins in which the insulin molecules are combined with *protamine molecules to slow down their rate of absorption from the injection site. The insulin is released steadily from the skin into the bloodstream to stabilize blood sugar over a longer time period. Mixtures of isophane and fast-acting insulins are also available.

isoproterenol *n.* a *sympathomimetic drug used to dilate the air passages in asthma and other bronchial conditions. It also stimulates the heart and is used to treat some heart conditions involving reduced heart activity. It is administered by inhalation, by mouth or by injection. Side effects such as increased heart rate, palpitations, chest pain, dizziness, and fainting may occur. Trade names: **Isuprel, Medihaler-Iso**.

isosorbide *n.* a drug used for the long-term treatment of stable angina and acute angina in patients unable to take nitroglycerin. It acts by relaxing the smooth muscle of both arteries and veins, thus causing dilation (*see* vasodilator). It is administered by mouth; side effects are rare, but include headache, hypotension, nausea and vomiting, and skin rash. Trade names: **Ismo, Imdur, Isordil, Sorbitrate**.

isosthenuria *n.* inability of the kidneys to produce either a concentrated or a dilute urine. This occurs in the final stages of renal failure.

isotonic *adj.* **1.** describing solutions that have the same osmotic pressure. *See* osmosis. **2.** describing muscles that have equal *tonicity. *See also* exercise.

isotope *n.* any one of the different forms of an element, possessing the same number of protons (positively charged particles) in the nucleus, and thus the same atomic number, but different numbers of neutrons. Isotopes therefore have different atomic weights. Radioactive isotopes decay into other isotopes or elements, emitting alpha, beta, or gamma radiation. Some radioactive isotopes may be produced artificially by bombarding elements with neutrons. These are known as *nuclides* and are used extensively in *radiotherapy for the treatment of cancer.

isotretinoin *n.* a drug related to vitamin A (*see* retinoid) and used in the treatment of severe cystic acne that has failed to respond to other treatment. It is administered by mouth or topically. Possible side effects include dry skin, nose bleeds, eyelid and lip inflammation, muscle, joint, and abdominal pains, diarrhea, and some disturbances of vision. It cannot be used during pregnancy. Trade names: **Accutane, Isotrex**.

isotropic *adj.* (in *computed tomography or *magnetic resonance imaging) denoting the acquisition of data when the slice thickness is similar in size to that of an individual *pixel, i.e. the *voxel is a cube. Computerized reconstruction in any plane will not suffer any loss of detail. The concept is particularly applicable for *multislice CT scanning, in which slice thickness of less than 1 mm is used.

isoxsuprine *n.* a drug that dilates blood vessels and is used to improve blood flow in such conditions as cerebrovascular disease and arteriosclerosis and to inhibit contractions in premature labor. It is administered by mouth or injection and rarely it may cause flushing, increased heart rate, dizziness, and nausea. Trade name: **Vasodilan**.

isozyme (isoenzyme) *n.* a physically distinct form of a given enzyme. Isozymes catalyze the same type of reaction but have slight physical and immunological differences. Isozymes of dehydrogenases, oxidases, transaminases, phosphatases, and proteolytic enzymes are known to exist.

isthmus *n.* a constricted or narrowed part of an organ or tissue, such as the band of thyroid tissue connecting the two lobes of the thyroid gland.

itch *n.* local discomfort or irritation of the skin, prompting scratching or rubbing of the affected area. *See* pruritus.

-itis *suffix denoting* inflammation of an organ, tissue, etc. Examples: *arthritis* (of a joint); *peritonitis* (of the peritoneum).

ITP *see* idiopathic thrombocytopenic purpura.

itraconazole *n.* an antifungal drug that is administered by mouth or intravenous infusion to treat a wide variety of fungal infections, including candidiasis and ringworm. Side effects include nausea and abdominal pain. Trade name: **Sporanox**.

IUD (intrauterine device) a plastic or metal coil, spiral, or other shape, about 25 mm long, that is inserted into the cavity of the uterus to prevent conception. Its exact mode of action is unknown but it is thought to interfere with implantation of the embryo. Early IUDs (such as the *Lippes loop*) were made of plastic; later variants (such as the *Gravigard*) are covered with copper, which slowly dissolves and augments the contraceptive action. Devices such as the *Progestasert* release small amounts of a contraceptive hormone drug. About one-third of women fitted with an IUD find the side effects (heavy menstrual bleeding or back pain) unacceptable, but most have no complaints. The unwanted pregnancy rate is about 2 per 100 woman-years. If pregnancy should occur there is normally no need to remove the device (it may, however, become detached spontaneously). *See also* postcoital contraception.

IUGR *see* intrauterine growth retardation.

IUI *see* intrauterine insemination.

IV *see* intravenous.

ivermectin *n.* an *anthelmintic drug used in the treatment of *onchocerciasis and *strongyloidiasis. It is administered by mouth and acts by killing the immature forms (*microfilariae) of the parasite. Side effects, which are mild, include itching and swollen lymph nodes. It is an orphan drug. Trade name: **Stromectol**.

IVF *see* in vitro fertilization.

IVU *see* intravenous urogram.

Ixodes *n.* a genus of widely distributed parasitic ticks. Several species are responsible for transmitting *Lyme disease, *tularemia, Queensland tick typhus, and Russian spring-summer encephalitis. The bite of a few species can give rise to a serious paralysis, caused by a toxin in the tick's saliva.

ixodiasis *n.* any disease caused by the presence of *ticks.

Ixodidae *n.* a family of *ticks.

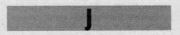

jacksonian epilepsy *see* epilepsy. [J. H. Jackson (1835–1911), British neurologist]

Jacquemier's sign a bluish or purplish coloration of the vagina: a possible indication of pregnancy. [J. M. Jacquemier (1806–79), French obstetrician]

jactitation *n.* restless tossing and turning of a person with a severe disease, frequently one with a high temperature.

Jaeger test types a card with text printed in type of different sizes, used for testing acuity of near vision. [E. R. Jaeger von Jastthal (1818–84), Austrian ophthalmologist]

jamais vu one of the manifestations of temporal lobe *epilepsy, in which there is a sudden feeling of unfamiliarity with everyday surroundings. *See also* déjà vu.

Janeway lesion a red spot on the palms of the hands or soles of the feet caused by a bacterial infection of the heart (*see* endocarditis). [E. G. Janeway (1841–1911), US physician]

Jarisch-Herxheimer reaction (Herxheimer reaction) exacerbation of the symptoms of syphilis that may occur on starting antibiotic therapy for the disease. The effect is transient and requires no treatment. [A. Jarisch (1850–1902), Austrian dermatologist; K. Herxheimer (1861–1944), German dermatologist]

jaundice *n.* a yellowing of the skin or whites of the eyes, indicating excess bilirubin (a bile pigment) in the blood. Jaundice is classified into three types. *Obstructive jaundice* occurs when bile made in the liver fails to reach the intestine due to obstruction of the *bile ducts (e.g. by gallstones) or to *cholestasis.

The urine is dark, the feces pale, and the patient may itch. *Hepatocellular jaundice* is due to disease of the liver cells, such as *hepatitis, when the liver is unable to utilize the bilirubin, which accumulates in the blood. The urine may be dark but the feces retain their color. *Hemolytic jaundice* occurs when there is excessive destruction of red cells in the blood (*see* hemolysis). Urine and feces retain their normal color. Medical name: **icterus**.

jaw *n.* either the *maxilla (upper jaw) or the *mandible (lower jaw). The jaws form the framework of the mouth and provide attachment for the teeth.

jaw thrust a maneuver for opening the airway of an unconscious patient. The palms of the hands are placed on the cheeks with the fingers hooked under the angles of the jaw so that the jaw can be pulled upward to separate the tongue from the back of the pharynx. The tongue often falls onto the back of the pharynx in unconsciousness, causing obstruction to the airway. This method is particularly useful when spinal injury is suspected and movement of the neck is undesirable. This is an alternative to the *head-tilt, chin-lift technique.

jejun- (jejuno-) *prefix denoting* the jejunum.

jejunal biopsy removal of a piece of the lining (mucosa) of the middle section of the small intestine. This can be done by a surgical operation but is usually performed by a gastroduodenoscope or a special metal capsule, swallowed by the patient. When the capsule is in the *jejunum a small knife within it is triggered by suction on an attached tube, cutting off a small piece of mucosa. The specimen may be examined microscopically to assist in the diagnosis of *celiac disease, *Whipple's disease, or intestinal infections, or its enzyme content may be measured chemically to detect, for example, *lactase deficiency.

jejunal ulcer *see* peptic ulcer, Zollinger-Ellison syndrome.

jejunectomy *n.* surgical removal of the jejunum or part of the jejunum.

jejunoileostomy *n.* an operation in which the jejunum is joined to the *ileum when either the end of the jejunum or the beginning of the ileum has been removed or is to be bypassed. It is usually performed for intestinal disease (e.g. Crohn's disease). It was formerly used to treat obesity but has been abandoned because of serious side effects.

jejunostomy *n.* a surgical operation in which the jejunum is brought through the abdominal wall and opened. It can enable the insertion of a catheter into the jejunum for short-term infusion of nutrients or other substances.

jejunotomy *n.* a surgical incision into the jejunum in order to inspect the interior or remove something from within it.

jejunum *n.* the middle part of the small *intestine. It comprises about two-fifths of the whole small intestine and connects the duodenum to the ileum. —**jejunal** *adj.*

jerk *n.* the sudden contraction of a muscle in response to a nerve impulse. The *knee jerk* (*see* patellar reflex) is the reflex kicking movement produced by contraction of the quadriceps muscle of the thigh after it has been stretched by tapping the tendon below the knee. Eliciting this and other jerks, such as the ankle and elbow jerks, is a means of testing the nerve pathways, via the spinal cord, which are involved in *reflexes.

jet lag the temporary decline in physical and psychological well-being experienced by travelers who have rapidly crossed several time zones. Jet lag is due to the lack of synchronization of internal body systems, such as the sleep-wake cycle and the body temperature cycle.

jigger *n. see* Tunga.

jock itch a fungal infection of the skin that chiefly affects the groin but may spread to the thighs and buttocks. It is caused by *dermatophyte fungi, usually *Trichophyton rubrum*, *T. interdigitale*, and *Epidermophyton floccosum*. Medical name: **tinea cruris**. *See also* ringworm.

Jod-Basedow phenomenon a collection of symptoms that includes skin rash, conjunctivitis, salivary gland inflammation, and hyperthyroidism due to the intake of high doses of iodine (German *Jod*, hence the name). [K. A. von Basedow (1799–1854), German physician]

joint *n.* the point at which two or more bones are connected. The opposing surfaces of the bones are lined with cartilaginous, fibrous, or soft (synovial) tissue. The three main classes of joint are *diarthrosis (freely movable), *amphiarthrosis (slightly movable), and *synarthrosis (immovable).

joule n. the *SI unit of work or energy, equal to the work done when the point of application of a force of 1 newton is displaced through a distance of 1 meter in the direction of the force. In electrical terms the joule is the work done per second when a current of 1 ampere flows through a resistance of 1 ohm. Symbol: J. See also calorie.

jugular adj. relating to or supplying the neck or throat.

jugular vein any one of several veins in the neck. The *internal jugular* is a very large paired vein running vertically down the side of the neck and draining blood from the brain, face, and neck. It ends behind the sternoclavicular joint, where it joins the subclavian vein. The *external jugular* is a smaller paired vein running superficially down the neck to the subclavian vein and draining blood from the face, scalp, and neck. Its tributary, the *anterior jugular*, runs down the front of the neck.

jugum n. (in anatomy) a ridge or furrow that connects two parts of a bone.

jumper's knee (patellar tendinitis) a form of *tendinitis that occurs in athletes and dancers. Repeated sudden contracture of the quadriceps muscle at take-off causes inflammation of the attachment of the patellar tendon to the lower end of the patella. Treatment is rest, physiotherapy, and anti-inflammatory medication.

junction n. (in anatomy) the point at which two different tissues or structures are in contact. See also neuromuscular junction.

juvenile polyp see polyp.

juvenile rheumatoid arthritis a condition of children beginning before 16 years of age in which heat, pain, swelling, and stiffness of joints occurs. Generally, the larger joints are involved, interfering with growth and development. Treatment consists of adequate rest and diet, exercise, and anti-inflammatory drugs. Complete remission often occurs. See also Still's disease.

juxta- prefix denoting proximity to. Example: *juxta-articular* (near a joint).

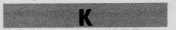

K

Kahn reaction a test for syphilis, in which antibodies specific to the disease are detected in a sample of the patient's blood by means of a *precipitin reaction. The test is not as reliable as other presently available tests. [R. L. Kahn (20th century), US bacteriologist]

kala-azar (visceral leishmaniasis, Dumdum fever) n. a tropical disease caused by the parasitic protozoan *Leishmania donovani*. The parasite, which is transmitted to humans by *sandflies, invades the cells of the lymphatic system, spleen, and bone marrow. Symptoms include enlargement and subsequent lesions of the liver and spleen; anemia; a low *leukocyte count; weight loss; and irregular fevers. The disease occurs in Asia, South America, the Mediterranean area, and Africa. Drugs containing antimony, or *pentamidine, are used in the treatment of this potentially fatal disease.

kallidin n. a naturally occurring polypeptide consisting of ten amino acids. Kallidin is a powerful vasodilator and causes contraction of smooth muscle; it is formed in the blood under certain conditions. See kinin.

kallikrein n. one of a group of enzymes found in the blood and body fluids that act on certain plasma globulins to produce bradykinin and kallidin. See kinin.

Kallmann's syndrome a familial condition that is the most common form of isolated *gonadotropin deficiency; it is combined with underdevelopment of the olfactory lobes, causing *anosmia. The syndrome is caused by a gene *deletion on the short arm of the X chromosome. Patients often present with delayed puberty. There is an association with *ichthyosis, mental retardation, obesity, renal and skeletal abnormalities, and undescended testes, but these features are very variable. [F. J. Kallmann (1897–1965), US geneticist]

kanamycin n. an *antibiotic used to treat a wide range of bacterial infections. It is administered mainly by injection but is given orally for infections of the intestine and by inhalation for respiratory infections. Mild side effects sometimes occur, including skin rashes, fever, headache, nausea, vomiting, and tingling sensations. Trade name: **Kantrex**.

kaolin *n.* a white clay that contains aluminum and silicon and is purified and powdered for use as an adsorbent. It is taken by mouth to treat the diarrhea and vomiting due to food poisoning and other digestive disorders. Kaolin is also used in dusting powders and poultices.

Kaposi's sarcoma a malignant tumor arising from blood vessels in the skin and appearing as purple to dark brown plaques or nodules. It is common in Africa but rare in the Western world, except in patients with *AIDS. The tumor evolves slowly; radiotherapy is the treatment of choice for localized lesions but chemotherapy may be of value in metastatic disease. [M. Kaposi (1837–1902), Austrian dermatologist]

Kartagener's syndrome a hereditary condition in which the heart and other internal organs lie on the opposite side of the body to the norm (i.e. the heart lies on the right; *see* dextrocardia); it is associated with chronic sinusitis and bronchiectasis. [M. Kartagener (1897–1975), German physician]

kary- (karyo-) *prefix denoting* a cell nucleus.

karyokinesis *n.* division of the nucleus of a cell, which occurs during cell division before division of the cytoplasm (*cytokinesis*). *See* mitosis.

karyolysis *n.* the breakdown of the cell nucleus in mitosis.

karyoplasm *n. see* nucleoplasm.

karyosome *n.* the dense mass of *chromatin found in the cell nucleus, which is composed mainly of chromosomes.

karyotype 1. *n.* the *chromosome set of an individual or species described in terms of both the number and structure of the chromosomes. **2.** *n.* the representation of the chromosome set in a diagram. **3.** *vb.* to determine the karyotype of a cell, as by microscopic examination.

katathermometer (psychrometer) *n.* a thermometer that is used to measure the cooling power of the air surrounding it, having its bulb covered with water-moistened material. The instrument is brought to a steady temperature of 100°F and then exposed to the air. The time taken for the temperature recorded by the thermometer to fall to 95°F gives an index of the air's cooling power.

Kawasaki disease (mucocutaneous lymph node syndrome) a condition of infants and children less than five years old characterized by lymph-node enlargement, fever, intermittent abdominal pain, rash on the trunk, edema, mucus membrane changes, and peeling of the palms and soles of the feet. The cause is unknown and there is no specific therapy, although cardiac and other complications can be treated. The disease can last for more than 12 weeks and can recur. Treatment is with aspirin, and *gamma globulin has recently been shown to reduce the risk of coronary artery disease. [T. Kawasaki (20th century), Japanese physician]

Kayser-Fleischer ring a brownish-yellow ring in the outer rim of the cornea of the eye. It is a deposit of copper granules and is diagnostic of *Wilson's disease. When well developed it can be seen by unaided observation, but faint Kayser-Fleischer rings may only be detected by specialized ophthalmological examination. [B. Kayser (1869–1954), German ophthalmologist; B. Fleischer (1848–1904), German physician]

K cell *see* killer cell.

Kegel exercises (pelvic-floor exercises) isometric exercises involving contraction of the pelvic-floor muscles for preventing stress incontinence, improving sexual response, and diminishing discomfort during pregnancy. These exercises lead to a cure in 50–80% of patients with stress incontinence. [A. H. Kegel (20th century), US gynecologist]

Kehr's sign pain in the left shoulder caused by irritation of the undersurface of the diaphragm by blood leaking from a ruptured spleen. The pain impulses are referred along the *phrenic nerve. [H. Kehr (1862–1913), German surgeon]

Kell antigens a group of antigens that may or may not be present on the surface of red blood cells, forming the basis of a *blood group. This group is important in blood transfusion reactions. [Mrs Kell (20th century), patient in whom they were first demonstrated]

Keller's operation a common operation for *bunions associated with displacement of the big toe toward the others (hallux valgus) or *hallux rigidus. It involves excision of the base of the first (proximal) phalanx of the big toe; the gap thus created fills with fibrous tissue. The toe will be slightly shorter and floppy. [W. L. Keller (1874–1959), US surgeon]

keloid (cheloid) *n.* an overgrowth of fibrous scar tissue following trauma to the skin. It does not resolve spontaneously but may be flattened by applied pressure or with injections of potent corticosteroids. Formation of keloid is particularly common at certain sites, such as the breastbone or ear lobe; surgical excision of benign (nonmalignant) lesions from such sites is therefore best avoided. *See also* scar.

kelvin *n.* the *SI unit of temperature, formally defined as the fraction 1/273.16 of the temperature of the triple point of water. A temperature in kelvins is equal to a Celsius temperature plus 273.15°C. Symbol: K.

Kemp echoes *see* otoacoustic emissions.

kerat- (kerato-) *prefix denoting* **1.** the cornea. Example: *keratopathy* (disease of). **2.** horny tissue, especially of the skin.

keratalgia *n.* pain arising from the cornea.

keratectasia *n.* bulging of the cornea at the site of scar tissue (which is thinner than normal corneal tissue).

keratectomy *n.* an operation in which a part of the cornea is removed, usually a superficial layer. This procedure is now frequently done by an *excimer laser, either to correct refractive errors (myopia, hyperopia), by reshaping the surface of the cornea (*photorefractive keratectomy*; PRK), or to remove diseased corneal tissue (*phototherapeutic keratectomy*). *See also* automated lamellar keratectomy.

keratin *n.* one of a family of proteins that are the major constituents of the nails, hair, and the outermost layers of the skin. The cytoplasm of epithelial cells, including *keratinocytes, contains a network of keratin filaments.

keratinization (cornification) *n.* the process by which cells become horny due to the deposition of *keratin within them. It occurs in the *epidermis of the skin and associated structures (hair, nails, etc.), where the cells become flattened, lose their nuclei, and are filled with keratin as they approach the surface.

keratinocyte *n.* a type of cell that makes up 95% of the cells of the epidermis. Keratinocytes migrate from the deeper layers of the epidermis and are finally shed from the surface of the skin.

keratitis *n.* inflammation of the *cornea of the eye. The eye waters and is very painful and vision is blurred. It may be due to physical or chemical agents (abrasions, exposure to dust, chemicals, ultraviolet light, etc.) or it may result from infection. In *disciform keratitis* a disk-shaped patch of edema and inflammation develops in the cornea, usually as an immune response to viral infection, commonly herpes simplex virus. *Filamentary keratitis* is associated with small mucoid deposits of epithelial filaments on the surface of the cornea, which come off to leave small corneal erosions that cause severe pain until they heal. Keratitis not due to infection usually responds to keeping the eyes covered until the corneal surface has healed; infections often require specific drug treatment, e.g. with antibiotics. *See also* microbial keratitis.

keratoacanthoma (molluscum sebaceum) *n.* a firm nodule, appearing singly on the skin and growing to around 2 cm across in about six weeks, and gradually disappearing during the next few months. Men are affected more often than women, commonly between the ages of 50 and 70 years. Keratoacanthomas occur on the nose, face, hands, and fingers and sometimes on the scalp or neck. The cause is not known. Although the nodules disappear spontaneously they may leave an unsightly scar, therefore treatment by curettage, cautery, or excision may be required.

keratocele (descemetocele) *n.* outward bulging of the base of a deep ulcer of the cornea. The deep layer of the cornea (Descemet's membrane) is elastic and relatively resistant to perforation; it therefore bulges when the overlying cornea has been destroyed.

keratoconjunctivitis *n.* combined inflammation of the cornea and conjunctiva of the eye. *Keratoconjunctivitis sicca* is dryness of the cornea and conjunctiva due to deficiency production of tears. It may be associated with systemic disorders, such as *Sjögren's syndrome, systemic lupus, systemic sclerosis, and sarcoidosis.

keratoconus *n.* conical cornea: an abnormal condition of the eye in which the cornea, instead of having a regular curvature, comes to a rounded apex toward its center. The "cone" tends to become sharper over a period of years.

keratoderma *n.* a horny thickening of the skin. In *keratoderma blennorrhagica* thick horny skin lesions occur on the palms, soles, toes, nails, and penis, a condition often seen in *Reiter's syndrome.

keratoglobus (megalocornea) *n.* a congenital disorder of the eye in which the whole cornea bulges forward in a regular curve. *Compare* keratoconus.

keratoma *n.* see keratosis.

keratomalacia *n.* a progressive nutritional disease of the eye due to vitamin A deficiency. The cornea softens and may become perforated. This condition is very serious and blindness is usually inevitable. *See also* xerophthalmia.

keratome *n.* any instrument designed for cutting the cornea. The simplest type has a flat triangular blade attached at its base to a handle, the other two sides being very sharp and tapering to a point. Power-driven keratomes have oscillating or rotating blades. An automated keratome is used in *automated lamellar keratectomy.

keratometer (ophthalmometer) *n.* an instrument for measuring the radius of curvature of the cornea. It is used for assessing the degree of abnormal curvature of the cornea in *astigmatism. Usually the vertical and horizontal curvatures are measured. All keratometers work on the principle that the size of the image of an object reflected from a convex mirror (in this case, the cornea) depends on the curvature of the mirror. The steeper the curve, the smaller the image. —**keratometry** *n.*

keratomileusis *n.* see intrastromal keratomileusis, LASIK (laser in situ keratomileusis), LASEK (laser in situ epithelial keratomileusis).

keratopathy *n.* any disorder relating to the cornea. *See* band keratopathy, bullous keratopathy.

keratoplasty (corneal graft) *n.* an eye operation in which any diseased parts of the cornea are replaced by clear corneal tissue from a donor. All layers of the cornea may be replaced (*penetrating keratoplasty*) or only some of its superficial layers, the deeper layer remaining (*lamellar keratoplasty*). In the latter case the thickness of the replacement cornea is correspondingly reduced. Lamellar keratoplasty has the advantage over penetrating keratoplasty of not requiring the eye to be opened, and therefore the risk of infection is greatly reduced.

keratoprosthesis *n.* an optically clear prosthesis that is implanted into the cornea to replace an area that has become opaque. Due to its poor success rate, it is used only as a last resort in an attempt to restore some sight to patients with severe disease and dry eyes when corneal transplantation (*see* keratoplasty) is certain to fail.

keratoscope (Placido's disk) *n.* an instrument for detecting abnormal curvature of the cornea. It consists of a black disk, about 20 cm in diameter, marked with concentric white rings. The examiner looks through a small lens in the center at the reflection of the rings in the patient's cornea. A normal cornea will reflect regular concentric images of the rings; a cornea that is abnormally curved (for example in *keratoconus) or scarred reflects distorted rings. Modern keratoscopes can print out a contour map of the corneal surface.

keratosis (keratoma) *n.* any horny growth of the skin. There are two common types. *Actinic* (or *solar*) *keratosis* is a well-defined red or skin-colored warty growth, usually occurring in middle or old age in fair-skinned people, caused by overexposure to the sun. The spots may become malignant. *Seborrheic keratoses* (or *basal-cell papillomas*), less correctly known as *seborrheic warts*, never become malignant. They are superficial yellowish spots, occurring especially on the trunk in middle age, that slowly darken and become warty over the years.

keratotomy *n.* an incision into the cornea. *See* arcuate keratotomy, radial keratotomy.

keratouveitis *n.* inflammation involving both the cornea (*see* keratitis) and the uvea (*see* uveitis).

kerion *n.* an uncommon and severe form of *ringworm of the scalp consisting of a painful inflamed mass. It is caused by a type of ringworm fungus that usually infects animal species.

kernicterus *n.* staining and subsequent

damage of the brain by bile pigment (bilirubin), which may occur in severe cases of *hemolytic disease of the newborn. Immature brain cells in the *basal ganglia are affected, and as brain development proceeds a pattern of *cerebral palsy emerges at about six months, with uncoordinated movements, deafness, disturbed vision, and feeding and speech difficulties.

Kernig's sign a symptom of *meningitis in which the hamstring muscles in the legs are so stiff that the patient is unable to extend the legs at the knee when the thighs are held at a right angle to the body. [V. Kernig (1840–1917), Russian physician]

Kernohan's phenomenon (or syndrome) *hemiplegia that is *ipsilateral to the brain lesion that caused it, due to pressure of the lesion (which is often a hematoma) on surrounding structures in the brain. [J. W. K. Kernohan (20th century), US pathologist]

ketamine n. a drug used to produce anesthesia when skeletal muscle relaxation is not required. It is administered by injection. Side effects include increased blood pressure and pulse rate, seizure-like movements, and reaction at the injection site. Trade name: **Ketalar**.

ketoacidosis n. a life-threatening condition in which an increase in acid content and of ketones is present in the tissues and fluids of the body, such as occurs in diabetes. Symptoms include nausea and vomiting, abdominal tenderness, confusion or coma, air hunger, acetone odor of breath, extreme thirst, and weight loss.

ketoconazole n. a drug used in the treatment of a variety of fungal diseases, including *candidiasis, *histoplasmosis, paracoccidioidomycosis, and *blastomycosis. It is taken by mouth; side effects include dizziness, drowsiness, nausea, and vomiting. Trade name: **Nizoral**.

ketogenesis n. the production of *ketone bodies. These are normal products of lipid metabolism and can be used to provide energy. The condition of *ketosis can occur when excess ketone bodies are produced.

ketogenic diet a diet that promotes the formation of *ketone bodies in the tissues. A ketogenic diet is one in which

the principal energy source is fat rather than carbohydrate.

ketone n. any member of a group of organic compounds consisting of a carbonyl group (=CO) flanked by two alkyl groups. The ketones acetoacetic acid, acetone, and β-hydroxybutyrate (known as *ketone* or *acetone bodies*) are produced during the metabolism of fats. *See also* ketosis.

ketonemia n. the presence in the blood of *ketone bodies.

ketonuria (acetonuria) n. the presence in the urine of *ketone (acetone) bodies. This may occur in diabetes mellitus, starvation, or after persistent vomiting and results from the partial oxidation of fats. Ketone bodies may be detected by adding a few drops of 5% sodium nitroprusside solution and a solution of ammonia to the urine; the gradual development of a purplish-red color indicates their presence.

ketoprofen n. an anti-inflammatory drug (*see* NSAID) administered by mouth to treat various arthritic and rheumatic diseases and primary *dysmenorrhea. Side effects are rare, but indigestion sometimes occurs. Trade name: **Orudis**.

ketose n. a simple sugar that terminates with a keto group (–C=O); for example, *fructose.

ketosis n. raised levels of *ketone bodies in the body tissues. Ketone bodies are normal products of fat metabolism and can be oxidized to produce energy. Elevated levels arise when there is an imbalance in fat metabolism, such as occurs in diabetes mellitus or starvation. Ketosis may result in severe *acidosis. *See also* ketonuria.

khat (qat, kat) n. the leaves of the shrub *Catha edulis*, which contain a stimulant. In Yemen these leaves are wrapped around betel nuts and chewed: this habit is associated with the development of oral *leukoplakia.

kidney n. either of the pair of organs responsible for the excretion of nitrogenous wastes, principally urea, from the blood (see illustration). The kidneys are situated at the back of the abdomen, below the diaphragm, one on each side of the spine; they are supplied with blood by the renal arteries. Each kidney is enclosed in a fibrous capsule and is composed of an outer *cortex* and an

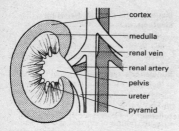

Section through a kidney

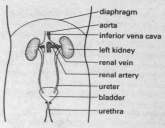

Position of the kidneys

inner *medulla*. The active units of the kidney are the *nephrons, within the cortex and medulla, which filter the blood under pressure and then reabsorb water and selected substances back into the blood. The *urine thus formed is conducted from the nephrons via the renal tubules into the *renal pelvis* and from there to the ureter, which leads to the bladder. *See also* hemodialysis, horseshoe kidney, renal function tests.

Kienböck's disease necrosis of the *lunate bone of the wrist, caused by interruption of its blood supply (*see* osteochondritis). It usually follows chronic stress to the bone or injury (often trivial) and presents with pain and stiffness of the wrist. Treatment is rest, but some cases require surgical shortening of the radius or *fusion of the wrist. [R. Kienböck (1871–1953), Austrian radiologist]

killer cell (K cell) a small lymphocyte without T or B cell markers that acts as an effector cell in antibody-dependent cell-mediated cytotoxicity. K cells recognize antibodies on target cells and lyse those cells by direct cell-to-cell contact that does not require *complement. *See also* natural killer cell.

Kiesselbach's plexus a collection of capillaries in the mucosa at the anterior part of the nasal septum. *Nosebleeds frequently have their origin from this plexus. *See* Little's area. [W. Kiesselbach (1839–1902), German laryngologist]

kilo- *prefix denoting* a thousand.

kilocalorie *n.* one thousand calories. *See* calorie.

kilogram *n.* the *SI unit of mass equal to 1000 grams and defined in terms of the international prototype (a cylinder of platinum-iridium alloy) kept at Sèvres, near Paris. Symbol: kg.

kin- (kine-) *prefix denoting* movement.

kinanesthesia *n.* inability to sense the positions and movements of parts of the body, with consequent disordered physical activity.

kinase *n.* **1.** an agent that can convert the inactive form of an enzyme (*see* proenzyme) to the active form. **2.** an enzyme that catalyzes the transfer of phosphate groups. An example is *phosphofructokinase.

kinematics *n.* the study of motion and the forces required to produce it. This includes the different forces at work during the movement of a single part of the body, and more complex movements such as running and climbing.

kineplasty *n.* a method of amputation in which the muscles and tendons of the affected limb are arranged so that they can be integrated with a specially made artificial replacement. This enables direct movement of the artificial hand or limb by the muscles.

kinesiology *n.* the study of the motion of the human body, including the anatomy, physiology, and mechanics of the active and passive structures involved.

-kinesis *suffix denoting* movement.

kinesthesia *n.* the sense that enables the brain to be constantly aware of the position and movement of muscles in different parts of the body. This is achieved by means of *proprioceptors, which send impulses from muscles, joints, and tendons. Without this sense, coordinated movement would be impossible with the eyes closed.

kinesthesiometer *n.* an instrument for measuring a patient's awareness of the muscular and joint movements of his own body: used during the investigation of nervous and muscular disorders and certain forms of brain damage.

kinetics *n.* the study of the forces that produce, modify, or stop the motion of the body and of the rate of change involved. Kinetics includes the study of the rates of chemical and enzyme-catalyzed reactions within the body.

kinetochore *n. see* centromere.

kinin *n.* one of a group of naturally occurring polypeptides that are powerful *vasodilators, which lower blood pressure, and cause contraction of smooth muscle. The kinins *bradykinin* and *kallidin* are formed in the blood by the action of proteolytic enzymes (*kallikreins*) on certain plasma globulins (*kininogens*). Kinins are not normally present in the blood but are formed under certain conditions; for example, when tissue is damaged or when there are changes in the pH and temperature of the blood. They are thought to play a role in inflammatory response.

kiss of life *see* mouth-to-mouth respiration.

Klebsiella *n.* a genus of gram-negative rod-like nonmotile mostly lactose-fermenting bacteria found in the respiratory, intestinal, and urogenital tracts of animals and humans. The species *K. oxytoca* is associated with human urinary infections; *K. pneumoniae* is associated with pneumonia and other respiratory infections. The species *K. rhinoscleromatis* causes *rhinoscleroma, a chronic infection of the nose and pharynx.

Klebs-Loeffler bacillus *see* Corynebacterium. [T. Klebs (1834–1913) and F. A. J. Loeffler (1852–1915), German bacteriologists]

Kleine-Levin syndrome a rare episodic disorder characterized by periods (usually of a few days or weeks) in which patients grossly overeat, sleep for most of the day and night, and may become more dependent or aggressive than normal. Between episodes patients are usually unaffected. It usually resolves spontaneously after early adult life. Symptomatic treatment with drugs, such as *amphetamines, is sometimes helpful. [W. Kleine (20th century), German neuropsychiatrist; M. Levin (20th century), US neurologist]

klepto- *prefix denoting* stealing.

kleptomania *n.* a pathologically strong impulse to steal, often in the absence of any desire for the stolen object or objects. It is sometimes associated with *depression.

Klinefelter's syndrome a genetic disorder in which there are three sex chromosomes, XXY, rather than the normal XX or XY. Affected individuals are male, but are tall and thin, with small testes, failure of normal sperm production (azoospermia), enlargement of the breasts (gynecomastia), and absence of facial and body hair. [H. F. Klinefelter (1912–), US physician]

Klumpke's paralysis a partial paralysis of the arm caused by injury to a baby's *brachial plexus during birth. This may result from an obstetric maneuver in which the arm is raised at the shoulder to an extreme degree, which damages the lower cervical (neck) and upper thoracic (chest) nerve roots of the spinal cord. It results in weakness and wasting of the muscles of the hand. [A. Klumpke (1859–1927), French neurologist]

K-nail *n. see* Küntscher nail.

kneading *n. see* petrissage.

knee *n.* the hinge joint (*see* ginglymus) between the end of the femur, the top of the tibia, and the back of the *patella (kneecap). It is commonly involved in *sports injuries (such as a torn meniscus or ligament) and is a common site of osteoarthritis and rheumatoid arthritis; it can be replaced by an artificial joint (*see also* arthroplasty).

knee-elbow position the buttocks-up position commonly assumed by patients undergoing anorectal examinations.

knight's-move thought a form of thought disorder, characteristic of *schizophrenia, in which the *associations of ideas are bizarre and tortuous.

knock knee abnormal in-curving of the legs, resulting in a gap between the feet when the knees are in contact. In severe cases there is stress on the knee, ankle, and foot joints, resulting eventually in degenerative arthritis. The condition may be corrected by *osteotomy. Medical name: **genu valgum.**

Kobberling-Dunnigan syndrome *see* lipodystrophy.

Kocher maneuver a method for *reduction of a dislocated shoulder by manipulation. [E. T. Kocher (1841–1917), Swiss surgeon]

Koch's bacillus *see* Mycobacterium. [R. Koch (1843–1910), German bacteriologist]

Koebner phenomenon (isomorphic response) a phenomenon that occurs in skin diseases, especially psoriasis and lichen planus, in which the characteristic lesions of the disease appear in linear form in response to such trauma as cuts, burns, or scratches. [H. Koebner (1834–1904), German dermatologist]

Koeppe nodule a type of nodule occurring in the iris at the pupil margin in both granulomatous and nongranulomatous *uveitis. [L. Koeppe (20th century), German ophthalmologist]

Köhler's disease inflammation of the *navicular bone of the foot (*see* osteochondritis). It occurs in children, causing pain and limping, and is treated by strapping the foot and by resting. [A. Köhler (1874–1947), German physician]

koilonychia *n.* the development of thin (brittle) concave (spoon-shaped) nails, a common disorder that can occur with anemia due to iron deficiency, although the cause is not known. Treatment is by treating any underlying disease.

Koplik's spots small red spots with bluish-white centers that often appear on the mucous membranes of the mouth in *measles. [H. Koplik (1858–1927), US physician]

koro *n.* a state of acute anxiety, seen particularly in certain cultures (such as that of the Chinese of SE Asia), characterized by a sudden belief that the penis is shrinking into the abdomen and will disappear. The sufferer is convinced that disappearance of the penis means death. It often occurs in epidemics. Occasionally women have a similar belief that their breasts are disappearing into their body. Koro is usually treated with tranquilizing drugs and reassurance.

Korsakoff's syndrome (Korsakoff's psychosis) an organic disorder affecting the brain that results in a memory defect in which new information fails to be learned although events from the past are still recalled, *disorientation for time and place occurs, and there is a tendency to invent material to fill memory blanks (*see* confabulation). The most common cause of the condition is alcoholism, es-

pecially when this has led to deficiency of thiamine (vitamin B_1). Large doses of thiamine are given as treatment. The condition often becomes chronic. [S. S. Korsakoff (1854–1900), Russian neurologist]

Krabbe's disease *see* leukodystrophy. [K. H. Krabbe (1885–1961), Danish neurologist]

K-ras *n.* a gene that mutates to form an important *oncogene for the causation of human lung and colon cancer.

kraurosis *n.* shrinking of a body part, usually the vulva in elderly women (*kraurosis vulvae*).

Krebs cycle (citric acid cycle) a complex cycle of enzyme-catalyzed reactions, occurring within the cells of all living animals, in which acetate, in the presence of oxygen, is broken down to produce energy in the form of *ATP (via the *electron transport chain) and carbon dioxide. The cycle is the final step in the oxidation of carbohydrates, fats, and proteins; some of the intermediary products of the cycle are used in the synthesis of amino acids. [Sir H. A. Krebs (1900–81), British biochemist]

Krukenberg's spindle a vertical spindle-shaped deposit of brownish-red pigment on the inner surface of the cornea (corneal endothelium), appearing in cases of pigment dispersion syndrome. [F. E. Krukenberg (1871–1946), German pathologist]

Krukenberg tumor a rapidly developing malignant growth in one or (more often) both ovaries. The tumor usually arises following the development of a similar growth in the stomach or intestine. [F. E. Krukenberg]

krypton-81m *n.* a radioactive gas that is the shortest-lived isotope in medical use (half-life, 13 seconds). It can be used to investigate the *ventilation of the lungs. The patient breathes a small quantity of the gas, the arrival of which in different parts of the lungs is recorded by means of a *gamma camera. This is often performed as part of *ventilation-perfusion scanning to look for pulmonary emboli. *See also* rubidium-81.

KUB X-ray an abdominal plain X-ray film that is longer than normal to enable it to include the *k*idneys, *u*reters, and the entire *b*ladder.

Küntscher nail (K-nail) a metal rod that is

inserted down the middle of the femur (thigh bone) to stabilize a transverse fracture of the shaft. [G. Küntscher (1902–72), German orthopedic surgeon]

Kupffer's cells phagocytic cells that line the sinusoids of the *liver (see macrophage). They are particularly concerned with the formation of *bile and are often seen to contain fragments of red blood cells and pigment granules derived from the breakdown of hemoglobin. [K. W. von Kupffer (1829–1902), German anatomist]

kuru (trembling disease) *n.* a disease that affects only members of the Fore tribe of New Guinea. It involves a progressive degeneration of the nerve cells of the central nervous system, particularly in the region of the brain that controls movement. Muscular control becomes defective and shiverlike tremors occur in the trunk, limbs, and head. Kuru affects mainly women and children and usually proves fatal within 9–12 months. It is thought to be caused by a *prion and transmitted by cannibalism. *See also* spongiform encephalopathy.

Kussmaul breathing the slow deep respiration associated with acidosis. [A. Kussmaul (1822–1902), German physician]

Kveim test a test used for the diagnosis of *sarcoidosis. Tissue from a lymph node of a person with the disease is injected intradermally; the development of a granuloma at the injection site indicates that the subject has sarcoidosis. [M. A. Kveim (20th century), Norwegian physician]

kwashiorkor *n.* a form of malnutrition due to a diet deficient in protein and energy-producing foods, common among certain African tribes. Kwashiorkor develops when, after prolonged breast feeding, the child is weaned onto an inadequate traditional family diet. The diet is such that it is physically impossible for the child to ingest the required quantity in order to obtain sufficient protein and energy. Kwashiorkor is most common in children between the ages of one and three years. The symptoms are *edema, loss of appetite, diarrhea, general discomfort, and apathy; the child fails to thrive and there is usually associated gastrointestinal infection.

Kyasanur Forest disease a tropical disease, common in southern India, caused by a virus transmitted to humans through the bite of the forest-dwelling tick *Haemaphysalis spinigera*. Symptoms include fever, headache, muscular pains, vomiting, conjunctivitis, exhaustion, bleeding of nose and gums, and, subsequently, internal bleeding and the *necrosis of various tissues. General therapy, in the absence of specific treatment, involves relief of dehydration and loss of blood; analgesics are given to alleviate pain.

kymograph *n.* an instrument for recording the flow and varying pressure of the blood within blood vessels. —**kymography** *n.*

kypho- *prefix denoting* a hump.

kyphos *n.* a sharply localized convex angulation of the spine, resulting in the appearance of a lump (the deformity of the traditional hunchback). The deformity is due to collapse of the anterior part of a vertebra, usually caused by osteoporosis, a secondary malignant deposit, or tuberculosis.

kyphoscoliosis *n.* abnormal curvature of the spine both forward and sideways: *kyphosis combined with *scoliosis. The deformity may occur during growth for no apparent reason (*idiopathic kyphoscoliosis*) or may result from any of several diseases involving the vertebrae and spinal muscles. Special braces can reduce the extent of the deformity if this is mild. Severe deformity requires surgical correction by *fusion of the spine.

kyphosis *n.* excessive outward curvature of the spine, causing hunching of the back and marked convexity when viewed from the side. A *mobile kyphosis* may be caused by bad posture or muscle weakness or may develop to compensate for another condition, such as deformity of the hip. A *fixed kyphosis* may result from collapse of the vertebrae (as in senile *osteoporosis), from *osteochondritis in the young, or from ankylosing *spondylitis. Lesser degrees of fixed kyphosis may be balanced by *lordosis (inward curvature) in another part of the spine. Treatment depends on the cause and may include physiotherapy, bracing, and spinal *osteotomy in severe cases. *See also* kyphos, kyphoscoliosis.

L

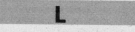

labeling index the proportion of cells in a sample of tissue that are producing DNA. Cells that are synthesizing DNA take up tritiated thymidine, which shows up on an autoradiograph (*see* autoradiography) of the sample.

labetalol *n.* a combined alpha- and beta-blocking drug, sometimes found to be more effective in the treatment of high blood pressure than beta blockers. It is administered by mouth or intravenous infusion. Possible side effects include faintness on standing up, scalp tingling, and difficulty with urination and ejaculation. Trade names: **Normodyne**, **Trandate**.

labia *pl. n. see* labium.

labial *adj.* **1.** relating to the lips or to a labium. **2.** designating the surface of a tooth adjacent to the lips.

labio- *prefix denoting* the lip(s).

labiomancy *n.* lipreading.

labioplasty (cheiloplasty) *n.* surgical repair of injury or deformity of the lips (*cleft lip).

labium *n.* (*pl.* **labia**) a lip-shaped structure, especially either of the two pairs of skin folds that enclose the *vulva. The larger outer pair are known as the *labia majora* and the smaller inner pair, the *labia minora*.

labor *n.* the sequence of actions by which a baby and the afterbirth (placenta) are expelled from the uterus at childbirth. The process usually starts spontaneously about 280 days after conception, but it may be started by artificial means (*see* induction). In the first stage the muscular wall of the uterus begins contracting while the muscle fibers of the cervix relax so that the cervix expands. A portion of the membranous sac (amnion) surrounding the baby is pushed into the opening and ruptures under the pressure, releasing *amniotic fluid to the exterior. In the second stage the baby's head appears at the cervix and the contractions of the uterus strengthen. The passage of the infant through the vagina is assisted by contractions of the abdominal muscles and conscious pushing by the mother. When the top of the baby's head appears at the vaginal opening, the whole infant is eased clear of the vagina, and the umbilical cord is cut. If the emergence of the head is impeded, an incision may be made in the surrounding tissue (*see* episiotomy). In the final stage the placenta and membranes are pushed out by the continuing contraction of the uterus, which eventually returns to its unexpanded state. The average duration of labor is about 12 hours in first pregnancies and about 8 hours in subsequent pregnancies. Labor pains can be reduced by previous training of the abdominal muscles and by the use of drugs (*accelerated labor*). *See also* cesarean section.

labor cost-push theory an explanation for increasing costs of health care based on the argument that the major factors are rising income and lower productivity among persons employed in the health industry. *Compare* demand-pull theory.

labrum *n.* (*pl.* **labra**) a lip or liplike structure; occurring, for example, around the margins of the articulating socket (acetabulum) of the hip bone.

labyrinth (inner ear) *n.* a convoluted system of cavities and ducts comprising the organs of hearing and balance. The *membranous labyrinth* is a series of interconnected membranous canals and chambers consisting of the *semicircular canals, *utricle, and *saccule (concerned with balance) and the central cavity of the *cochlea (concerned with hearing). (See illustration.) It is filled with a fluid – endolymph. The *bony labyrinth* is the system of the bony canals and chambers that surround the membranous labyrinth. It is embedded in the petrous part of the *temporal bone and is filled with fluid (*perilymph*).

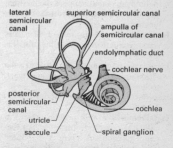

Membranous labyrinth of the right ear

labyrinthectomy *n.* a surgical procedure to ablate (*see* ablation) the structures of the *labyrinth, usually performed for cases of severe Ménière's disease.

labyrinthitis (otitis interna) *n.* inflammation of the inner ear (labyrinth). *See* otitis.

laceration *n.* a tear in the flesh producing a wound with irregular edges.

lacertus *n.* a band of fibers or a tendonlike structure.

lacrimal apparatus the structures that produce and drain away fluid from the eye (see illustration). The *lacrimal gland* secretes *tears, which drain away through small openings (*puncta*) at the inner corner of the eye into two *lacrimal canaliculi*. From there the tears pass into the nasal cavity via the *lacrimal sac* and the *nasolacrimal duct.

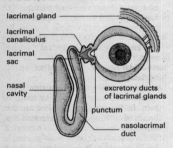

lacrimal gland

lacrimal canaliculus

lacrimal sac

nasal cavity

excretory ducts of lacrimal glands

punctum

nasolacrimal duct

The lacrimal apparatus

lacrimal bone the smallest bone of the face: either of a pair of rectangular bones that contribute to the orbits. *See* skull.

lacrimal nerve a branch of the *ophthalmic nerve that supplies the lacrimal gland (*see* lacrimal apparatus) and conjunctiva.

lacrimation *n.* the production of excess tears; crying. *See also* lacrimal apparatus.

lacrimator *n.* an agent that irritates the eyes, causing excessive secretion of tears, such as Mace.

lact- (lacti-, lacto-) *prefix denoting* **1.** milk. **2.** lactic acid.

lactalbumin *n.* a milk protein present in milk at a lower concentration than *casein. Unlike casein, it is not precipitated from milk under acid conditions; it is

therefore a constituent of cheese made from whey rather than curd.

lactase *n.* an enzyme, secreted by the glands of the small intestine, that converts *lactose (milk sugar) into glucose and galactose during digestion.

lactated Ringer's solution *see* Hartmann's solution.

lactation *n.* the secretion of milk by the *mammary glands of the breasts, which usually begins at the end of pregnancy. A fluid called *colostrum is secreted before the milk is produced; both secretions are released in response to the sucking action of the infant on the nipple. Lactation is controlled by hormones (*see* prolactin, oxytocin); it stops when the baby is no longer fed at the breast.

lacteal *n.* a blind-ended lymphatic vessel that extends into a villus of the small *intestine. Digested fats are absorbed into the lacteals.

lactic acid a compound that forms in the cells as the end product of glucose metabolism in the absence of oxygen (*see* glycolysis). During strenuous exercise pyruvic acid is reduced to lactic acid, which may accumulate in the muscles and cause cramps. Lactic acid (owing to its low pH) is an important food preservative. The lactic acid produced by the fermentation of milk is responsible for the preservation and flavor of cheese, yogurt, and other fermented milk products.

lactic acidosis excessive plasma acidity due to an accumulation of lactic acid. This may be caused by a variety of illnesses, including heart failure or severe dehydration. It can also be caused by the accumulation of *biguanide drugs used for treating type 2 *diabetes mellitus, particularly when kidney failure is present. Biguanides (*see* metformin) should therefore not be used to treat patients who also have kidney disease or heart failure or who are dehydrated.

lactiferous *adj.* transporting or secreting milk, as the *lactiferous ducts* of the breast.

lactifuge *n.* a drug that reduces the secretion of milk. Some estrogenic drugs, such as *chlorotrianisene and *dienestrol, have this effect and are used to suppress milk production in mothers not breast-feeding.

Lactobacillus *n.* a genus of gram-positive

nonmotile rodlike bacteria capable of growth in acid media and of producing lactic acid from the fermentation of carbohydrates. They are found in fermenting animal and plant products, especially dairy products, and in the alimentary tract and vagina. They are responsible for the souring of milk. The species *L. acidophilus* is found in milk and is associated with dental caries. It occurs in very high numbers in the feces of breast- or bottle-fed infants.

lactogenic hormone *see* prolactin.

lactose *n.* a sugar, consisting of one molecule of glucose and one of galactose, found only in milk. Lactose is split into its constituent sugars by the enzyme *lactase, which is secreted in the small intestine. This enzyme is missing or is of low activity in certain people of some Eastern and African races. This leads to the inability to absorb lactose, known as *lactose intolerance*.

lactosuria *n.* the presence of milk sugar (*lactose) in the urine. This often occurs during pregnancy and breast-feeding or if the milk flow is suppressed.

lactulose *n.* a disaccharide sugar that acts as a gentle but effective *laxative. It is administered by mouth but is not absorbed or broken down, remaining intact until it reaches the colon. There it is split by bacteria into simpler sugars that help to retain water, thereby softening the stools. Trade names: **Cephulac, Chronulac, Duphalac**.

lacuna *n.* (*pl.* **lacunae**) (in anatomy) a small cavity or depression; for example, one of the spaces in compact bone in which a bone cell lies.

laetrile *n.* a cyanide-containing compound extracted from apricot pits. It has been used, despite the lack of evidence for its therapeutic value, in *complementary medicine in the treatment of various forms of cancer.

lagena *n.* the closed end of the spiral *cochlea. This term is more commonly used to describe the structure homologous to the cochlea in primitive vertebrates.

lagophthalmos *n.* any condition in which the eye does not close completely. It may lead to corneal damage from undue exposure.

laking *n.* the physical or chemical treatment of blood to abolish the structure of the red cells and thus form a homogeneous solution. Laking is an important preliminary step in the analysis of hemoglobin or enzymes present in red cells.

-lalia *suffix denoting* a condition involving speech.

lallation (lalling) *n.* **1.** unintelligible speechlike babbling, as heard from infants. **2.** the immature substitution of one consonant for another (e.g. *l* for *r*).

Lamaze method a psychophysical technique of preparing a pregnant woman for labor and natural childbirth. Designed to minimize the pain of labor, the method involves classes that include instruction about the anatomy and physiology of pregnancy and delivery, exercises to strengthen and control the abdominal muscles and those of the birth canal, and techniques of breathing and relaxation to ease delivery. [F. Lamaze (1890–1957), French obstetrician]

lambda *n.* the point on the skull at which the lambdoidal and sagittal *sutures meet.

lambdoidal suture *see* suture (def. 1).

lambliasis *n. see* giardiasis.

lamella *n.* (*pl.* **lamellae**) **1.** a thin layer, membrane, scale, or platelike tissue or part. In *bone tissue, lamellae are thin bands of calcified matrix arranged concentrically around a Haversian canal. **2.** a thin gelatinous medicated disk used to apply drugs to the eye. The disk is placed on the eyeball; the gelatinous material dissolves and the drug is absorbed.

lamina *n.* (*pl.* **laminae**) a thin membrane or layer of tissue.

laminectomy (rachiotomy) *n.* surgical cutting into the backbone to obtain access to the spinal cord. The surgeon excises the rear part (the posterior arch) of one or more vertebrae. The operation is performed to remove tumors, to treat injuries to the spine, such as prolapsed intervertebral (slipped) disk (in which the affected disk is removed), or to relieve pressure on a spinal nerve.

lamivudine *n.* a reverse transcriptase inhibitor (*see* reverse transcriptase).

lamotrigine *n.* an anticonvulsant drug that is used in the control of epilepsy and generalized seizures related to Lennox-Gastaut syndrome. It is administered by mouth. Possible side effects include nausea, headache, double vision, dizziness, *ataxia, and skin rashes. Trade name: **Lamictal**.

lanatoside *n.* a drug similar to *digitalis, used in the treatment of heart failure. It is administered by mouth or injection. High doses may cause loss of appetite, nausea, vomiting, headache, disturbed vision, and abnormal heart activity.

Lancefield classification a classification of the *Streptococcus* bacteria based on the presence or absence of antigenic carbohydrate on the cell surface. Species are classified into the groups A–S. Most species causing disease in humans belong to groups A, B, and D. [R. C. Lancefield (1895–1981), US bacteriologist]

lancet *n.* a broad two-edged surgical knife with a sharp point.

lancinating *adj.* describing a sharp stabbing or cutting pain.

Landau reflex a reflex seen in normal babies from three months until one year, when it disappears. If the baby is held horizontally, face down, it will straighten its legs and back and try to lift up its head. The presence of this reflex beyond one year may be suggestive of a developmental disorder.

Landau-Kleffner syndrome epileptic *aphasia of childhood in which there is a progressive deterioration in expressive and receptive language abilities accompanied by epileptiform discharges in a generally temporal pattern, although generalized, bilateral, or multifocal discharges may also occur. [L. Landau (1848–1920), German gynecologist]

Landouzy-Dejerine dystrophy (or atrophy) *see* muscular dystrophy. [L. T. J. Landouzy (1845–1917), French physician; J. J. Dejerine (1849–1917), French neurologist]

Landry's paralysis a rapidly progressive form of the *Guillain-Barré syndrome. [J. B. O. Landry (1826–65), French physician]

Lange curve an obsolete method of detecting excess globulins in the protein of the cerebrospinal fluid. It was useful in the diagnosis of neurosyphilis and multiple sclerosis but has been superseded by more specific tests. [Described in 1912 by F. A. Lange, German physician]

Langerhans cell histiocytosis overgrowth of cells of the *reticuloendothelial system. This includes disorders previously

known as *histiocytosis X*, including *eosinophilic granuloma*, *Hand-Schüller-Christian disease*, and *Letterer-Siwe disease*. [P. Langerhans (1847–88), German physician and anatomist]

Langer's lines normal permanent skin creases. Incisions parallel to Langer's lines heal well and are less visible. [C. R. von E. Langer (1819–87), Austrian anatomist]

lanreotide *n.* a somatostatin analogue (*see* somatostatin).

lansoprazole *n. see* proton-pump inhibitor.

lanugo *n.* fine hair covering the body and limbs of the human fetus. It is most profuse at about the 28th week of gestation and is shed around 40 weeks.

laparo- *prefix denoting* the loins or abdomen.

laparoscope (peritoneoscope) *n.* a surgical instrument (a type of *endoscope) comprising an illuminated viewing tube generally connected to a camera, with the image viewed on a video screen. It is inserted through the abdominal wall to enable the surgeon to view the organs in the abdomen (*see* laparoscopy). It can be used as a means to allow surgical procedures to be carried out with special instruments without using a surgical incision.

laparoscopy (peritoneoscopy, abdominoscopy) *n.* examination of the abdominal structures (which are contained within the peritoneum) by means of an illuminated tubular instrument (*laparoscope). This is passed through a small incision in the wall of the abdomen after injecting carbon dioxide into the abdominal cavity (pneumoperitoneum). In addition to being a diagnostic aid, it is used when taking a biopsy, aspirating cysts, and dividing adhesions. Surgery, including *cholecystectomy, *colectomy, *fundoplication, *hemicolectomy, and the occlusion of fallopian tubes for sterilization, can also be performed through a laparoscope, using either a laser or diathermy to control bleeding (*see also* minimally invasive surgery). The laparoscope is also used for collecting ova for *in vitro fertilization and in performing gynecological operations using a laser (*laser laparoscopy*). —**laparoscopic** *adj.*

laparotomy *n.* a surgical incision into the abdominal cavity. The operation is done to examine the abdominal organs as a help to diagnosis; for example, to establish the spread of a tumor (*exploratory laparotomy*) or as a prelude to major surgery.

lardaceous *adj.* resembling lard: often applied to tissue infiltrated with the starch-like substance amyloid (*see* amyloidosis).

larva *n.* (*pl.* **larvae**) the preadult or immature stage hatching from the egg of some animal groups, e.g. insects and nematodes, which may be markedly different from the sexually mature adult and have a totally different way of life. For example, the larvae of some flies are parasites of animals and cause disease whereas the adults are free-living. —**larval** *adj.*

larva migrans *see* creeping eruption.

laryng- (laryngo-) *prefix denoting* the larynx.

laryngeal mask an airway tube with an elliptical inflatable cuff at one end for insertion into the mouth of a patient requiring artificial ventilation. It is designed to fit snugly in the patient's throat over the top of the laryngeal opening. While it is relatively easy to insert and allows delivery of effective artificial ventilation, it does not provide the absolute protection of the airway from vomitus afforded by an endotracheal tube (*see* intubation).

laryngeal reflex a cough produced by irritating the larynx.

laryngeal stroboscopy a method of studying the movements of the vocal cords of the *larynx by using stroboscopic light (controlled intermittent flashes) to slow or freeze the movement.

laryngectomy *n.* surgical removal of the whole or a part of the larynx, as in the treatment of laryngeal carcinoma. Postoperatively the patient breathes through a *tracheostomy. Speech is lost following the operation but can be restored by teaching the patient to swallow air and then expel it in a controlled fashion. Alternatively, a battery-powered vibrating device can be held in the mouth or underneath the chin to produce speech (*see* electrolarynx). Speech can also be facilitated by a one-way valve surgically implanted between the tracheostomy and the upper esophagus, allowing the patient to divert air into the throat. *Partial laryngectomy* conserves part of the larynx and allows patients to breathe and

speak normally. However, it is only suitable for a few patients with small tumors.

laryngismus *n.* closure of the vocal cords by sudden contraction of the laryngeal muscles, followed by a noisy indrawing of breath. It occurs in young children and was in the past associated with low-calcium rickets. Now it occurs when the larynx has been irritated following administration of an anesthetic, when a foreign body has lodged in the larynx, or in *croup.

laryngitis *n.* inflammation of the larynx and vocal cords, due to infection by bacteria or viruses or irritation by gases, chemicals, etc. The cords lose their vibrance (owing to swelling) and the voice becomes husky or is lost completely; breathing is harsh and difficult (*see* stridor); and the cough is painful and honking. Obstruction of the airways may occasionally be serious, especially in children (*see* croup). The patient should rest the voice and remain in a warm moisture-laden atmosphere; steam inhalations for 15–20 minutes every 2–3 hours are traditionally beneficial. The patient should avoid cold air or fog and smoking.

laryngocele *n.* a developmental defect in which an air sac communicates with the larynx. The sac forms a swelling in the neck that dilates on coughing or straining. The condition is usually congenital but is also noted in such people as glassblowers, who have chronically raised intralaryngeal pressure.

laryngofissure *n.* a surgical operation to open the larynx, enabling access for further procedures. *See also* laryngotomy.

laryngology *n.* the study of diseases of the larynx and vocal cords.

laryngomalacia *n.* a condition characterized by paroxysmal attacks of breathing difficulty and *stridor. It occurs in small children and is caused by flaccidity of the structure of the larynx. It usually resolves spontaneously by the age of two years.

laryngopharynx *n.* the part of the pharynx that lies below the hyoid bone.

laryngoscope *n.* an instrument consisting of a handle and a curved blade, fitted with a light, for moving the tongue and epiglottis aside in order to inspect the larynx. It is used to aid insertion of an endotracheal tube (*see* intubation) or for simple examination.

laryngoscopy *n.* examination of the larynx. This may be done indirectly using a small mirror or directly using a *laryngoscope.

laryngospasm *n.* involuntary closure of the larynx, obstructing the flow of air to the lungs. It usually occurs as part of an allergic reaction, such as *angioedema.

laryngotomy *n.* surgical incision of the larynx. *Inferior laryngotomy*, in which an incision is made in the cricothyroid membrane beneath the larynx, is a life-saving operation when there is obstruction to breathing at or above the larynx. *See* tracheostomy.

laryngotracheobronchitis *n.* a severe and almost exclusively viral infection of the respiratory tract, especially of young children, in whom there may be a dangerous degree of obstruction either at the larynx (*see* croup) or main air passages (bronchi) due to the thickness and stickiness of the fluid (exudate) produced by the inflamed tissues. Symptoms normally start at night. Treatment is supportive until the condition resolves naturally. In mild and moderate cases the child may benefit from being kept in a humid atmosphere (e.g. a steamy room). Nebulized medications and oxygen can help in more severe cases. In extreme cases endotracheal *intubation may be necessary. The condition may recur.

larynx *n.* the organ responsible for the production of vocal sounds, also serving as an air passage conveying air from the pharynx to the lungs. It is situated in the front of the neck, above the trachea. It is made up of a framework of nine cartilages (see illustration) – the epiglottis, thyroid, cricoid, arytenoid (two), corniculate (two), and cuneiform (two) – bound together by ligaments and muscles and lined with mucous membrane. Within are a pair of *vocal cords, which function in the production of the voice. —**laryngeal** *adj.*

LASEK *la*ser in *si*tu epithelial *k*eratomileusis: a technique of laser refractive eye surgery used to correct both nearsightedness (myopia) and farsightedness (hyperopia). The surface of the corneal epithelium is raised using a dilute solution of alcohol instead of a keratome, the cornea is reshaped using an *excimer laser, and the epithelium is then replaced. *Compare* LASIK.

laser *n.* a device that produces a very thin beam of light in which high energies are concentrated (the word derives from *l*ight *a*mplification by *s*timulated *e*mission of *r*adiation). In surgery, lasers can be used to operate on small areas of abnormality without damaging delicate surrounding tissue. For example, lasers are used in surgery of the retina, to unblock coronary arteries narrowed by atheroma, and to remove certain types of birthmark (*see* nevus). Different types of laser are used in eye surgery for operations on the cornea, lens capsule, and retina (*see* argon laser, diode laser, excimer laser, YAG laser). Lasers are also used in the treatment of *cervical intraepithelial neoplasia and in a specialized form (the *Nd:YAG laser*) for *endometrial ablation.

laser-assisted uvulopalatoplasty (LAUP) laser surgery to the palate, used in the treatment of obstructive *sleep apnea.

laser Doppler flowmeter an instrument for measuring blood flow through tissue (e.g. skin) utilizing a laser beam.

laser laparoscopy *see* laparoscopy.

laser palatoplasty *see* palatoplasty.

LASIK *la*ser in *si*tu *k*eratomileusis: a type of laser refractive eye surgery used to correct both *myopia (nearsightedness) and *hyperopia (farsightedness). A thin corneal flap (epithelium and stroma) is raised using a keratome, the cornea is reshaped using an *excimer laser, and

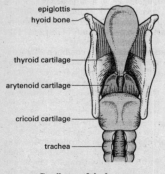

epiglottis
hyoid bone

thyroid cartilage

arytenoid cartilage

cricoid cartilage

trachea

Cartilages of the larynx

the flap is then replaced. *Compare* intrastromal keratomileusis, LASEK.

Lasix *n. see* furosemide.

Lassa fever a serious virus disease confined to Central West Africa. After an incubation period of 3–21 days, headache, high fever, and severe muscular pains develop; difficulty in swallowing often arises. Death from kidney or heart failure occurs in over 50% of cases. Treatment with plasma from recovered patients is the best therapy, and the causative virus is susceptible to ribavirin.

latah *n.* a pattern of behavior seen especially in certain cultures, such as that of Malaysia. After a psychological shock, the affected individual becomes very anxious and very suggestible and shows excessive obedience and pathological imitation of the actions of another person (echopraxia).

latanoprost *n.* a *prostaglandin drug (an analogue of PGF_2) that both increases the drainage of aqueous humor from the eye and reduces the production of aqueous humor. It is used topically as a treatment for glaucoma. Trade name: **Xalatan**.

latent period (in neurology) the pause of a few milliseconds between the time that a nerve impulse reaches a muscle fiber and the time that the fiber starts to contract.

lateral *adj.* **1.** situated at or relating to the side of an organ or organism. **2.** (in anatomy) relating to the region or parts of the body that are furthest from the *median plane. **3.** (in radiology) in the *sagittal plane.

lathyrism *n.* a disease, characterized by muscular weakness and paralysis, found among people whose staple diet consists mostly of large quantites of *Lathyrus sativus*, a kind of chick pea, and/or vetches and pulses related to it. Except in mild cases, complete recovery does not occur, despite administration of an adequate diet and physiotherapy.

laudanum *n.* a hydroalcoholic solution containing 1% morphine, prepared from macerated raw opium. It was formerly widely used as a narcotic analgesic, taken by mouth.

laughing gas *see* nitrous oxide.

LAUP *see* laser-assisted uvulopalatoplasty.

Laurence-Moon-Biedl syndrome an autosomal *recessive condition involving obesity, short stature, mental retardation, *retinitis pigmentosa, and, more variably, gonad failure. [J. Z. Laurence (1830–74), British ophthalmologist; R. C. Moon (1844–1914), US ophthalmologist; A. Biedl (1869–1933), Austrian physician]

lavage *n.* washing out a body cavity, such as the colon or stomach, with water or a medicated solution. In cases of bowel obstruction the washing out can be done during the operation (*on-table lavage*). *See also* bronchoalveolar lavage, diagnostic peritoneal lavage.

laxative (cathartic, purgative) *n.* a drug used to stimulate or increase the frequency of bowel evacuation, or to encourage a softer or bulkier stool. The common laxatives are the stimulants (castor oil, *bisacodyl, *senna and its derivatives); osmotic laxatives (*lactulose, magnesium sulfate and other mineral salts); and *methylcellulose and other bulking agents.

lazy eye *see* amblyopia.

LBC *see* liquid-based cytology.

LD_{50} the dose of a toxic compound that causes death in 50% of a group of experimental animals to which it is administered: used as a measure of the toxicity of drugs.

LDL low-density lipoprotein. *See* lipoprotein.

L-dopa *n. see* levodopa.

LE *see* lupus erythematosus.

lead¹ *n.* a soft bluish-gray metallic element that forms several poisonous compounds. Acute lead poisoning, which may follow inhalation of lead fumes or dust, causes abdominal pains, vomiting, and diarrhea, with paralysis and convulsions and sometimes *encephalitis. In chronic poisoning a characteristic bluish marking of the gums ("lead line") is seen and the peripheral nerves are affected; there is also anemia. Treatment is with *edetate disodium. The use of lead in paints is now strictly controlled. Symbol: Pb.

lead² *n.* a portion of an electrocardiographic record that is obtained from a single electrode or a combination of electrodes placed on a particular part of the body (*see* electrocardiogram, electrocardiography). In the conventional ECG, 12 leads are recorded. Each lead represents the electrical activity of the heart as "viewed" from a different position on the body surface and may help to localize myocardial damage.

learning difficulty *see* mental handicap.

learning disability any one of a diverse group of disorders manifested by significant difficulties in the acquisition and use of speaking, listening, reading, writing, reasoning, or mathematical abilities or social skills, caused by dysfunction of the central nervous system. *See also* mental handicap, attention-deficit/hyperactivity disorder.

leather-bottle stomach *see* linitis plastica.

Leber's congenital amaurosis a hereditary disease (inherited as an autosomal *recessive inherited condition) causing severe visual loss in infants. The back of the eye appears to be normal when examined with an *ophthalmoscope, but marked abnormalities are found on the ERG (*see* electroretinography). [T. Leber (1840–1917), German ophthalmologist]

Leber's optic atrophy a rare hereditary disorder, affecting young males, that is characterized by rapid loss of central vision due to neuroretinal degeneration.

lecithin *n.* one of a group of *phospholipids that are important constituents of cell membranes and are involved in the metabolism of fat by the liver. An example is *phosphatidylcholine*. Lecithins are present in the *surfactant that occurs in fetal lung tissue. The *lecithin-sphingomyelin ratio (LS ratio)* is used as a measure of fetal lung maturity; an LS ratio below 2 indicates a higher risk of *respiratory distress syndrome (RDS). In such cases cortisone may be given to stimulate fetal lung maturity and hence reduce the risk of RDS in the newborn.

lecithinase *n.* an enzyme from the small intestine that breaks *lecithin down into glycerol, fatty acids, phosphoric acid, and choline.

leech *n.* a type of worm that possesses suckers at both ends of its body. Leeches occur in tropical forests and grasslands and in water. Certain parasitic species suck blood from animals and humans, and their bites cause irritation and, occasionally, infection. Rarely, leeches are taken in with foul drinking water and pass from the mouth to the nose, where

they provoke headache and nose bleeds. A leech can be detached from its host by applying salt; calamine lotion eases the irritation of the bites. Formerly widely used for bloodletting, the medicinal leech (*Hirudo medicinalis*) may now be used following microsurgery (e.g. to replace a severed finger) to restore patency to blocked or collapsed blood vessels and thus encourage the growth of new capillaries. The anticoagulants in the saliva of this and other species are being investigated for the treatment and prevention of thrombosis. *See also* hirudin.

leflunomide *n.* an *immunosuppressant drug used to treat rheumatoid arthritis that has not responded to methotrexate or other antirheumatic drugs. Leflunomide is administered by mouth and side effects, including blood disorders caused by impairment of bone-marrow function, may be severe. Trade name: **Arava**.

Le Fort classification a classification of fractures involving the *maxilla (upper jaw) and *orbit. Type I involves the maxilla only, type II the anterior orbit, and type III the posterior orbit. [R. Le Fort (19th century), French surgeon]

leg *n.* technically, that part of the lower limb between the knee and the ankle, as distinguished from the thigh; the term is commonly used to denote the entire lower limb. Medical name: **crus**.

Legg-Calvé-Perthes disease (Perthes disease, pseudocoxalgia) necrosis of the head of the femur (thigh bone) due to interruption of its blood supply (*see* osteochondritis). Of unknown cause, it occurs most commonly in boys between the ages of five and ten and causes aching and a limp. The head of the femur can collapse and become deformed, resulting in a short leg and restricted hip movement. Affected boys are kept under observation and their activities are restricted; surgery may be required in more severe cases. [A. T. Legg (1874–1939), US surgeon; J. Calvé (1875–1954), French orthopedist; G. C. Perthes (1869–1927), German surgeon]

legionnaires' disease an infection of the lungs caused by the bacterium *Legionella pneumophila*, named after an outbreak at the American Legion convention in Pennsylvania in 1976. *Legionella* organisms are widely found in water; outbreaks of the disease have been associated with defective central heating, air conditioning, and other ventilating systems. Symptoms appear after an incubation period of 2–10 days: malaise and muscle pain are succeeded by a fever, dry cough, chest pain, and breathlessness. X-ray of the lungs shows patchy consolidation. Erythromycin provides the most effective therapy.

Leigh syndrome a rare metabolic disorder that affects movement and development. Affected children are initially normal but lose coordination and balance as the disease progresses. There is no known cure at present. *See also* mitochondrial disorders. [D. Leigh (1915–), British psychiatrist]

leio- *prefix denoting* smoothness. Example: *leiodermia* (abnormal smoothness of the skin).

leiomyoma *n.* a benign tumor of smooth muscle. Such tumors occur most commonly in the uterus (*see* fibroid) but can also arise in the digestive tract, walls of blood vessels, etc. They may undergo malignant change (*see* leiomyosarcoma).

leiomyosarcoma *n.* a malignant tumor of smooth muscle, most commonly found in the uterus, stomach, small bowel, and at the base of the bladder. It is the second most common *sarcoma of soft tissues. This tumor is rare in children, occurring most commonly in the bladder, prostate, and stomach.

Leishman-Donovan body *see* Leishmania. [Sir W. B. Leishman (1865–1926); British surgeon; C. Donovan (1863–1951), Irish physician]

Leishmania *n.* a genus of parasitic flagellate protozoans, several species of which cause disease in humans (*see* leishmaniasis). The parasite assumes a different form in each of its two hosts. In humans, especially in patients with *kala-azar, it is a small rounded structure, with no flagellum, called a *Leishman-Donovan body*, which is found within the cells of the lymphatic system, spleen, and bone marrow. In the insect carrier it is long and flagellated.

leishmaniasis *n.* a disease, common in the tropics and subtropics, caused by parasitic protozoans of the genus *Leishmania*, which are transmitted by the bite of sandflies. There are two principal forms of the disease: *visceral leishmaniasis*, in which the cells of various internal organs are affected (*see* kala-azar); and *cutaneous leishmaniasis*, which affects the tissues of the skin. Cutaneous leishmaniasis itself has several different forms, depending on the region in which it occurs and the species of *Leishmania* involved. In Asia it is common in the form of *oriental sore. In America there are several forms of leishmaniasis (*see* chiclero's ulcer, espundia). Leishmaniasis is treated with drugs containing antimony.

lemniscus *n.* a ribbonlike tract of nerve tissue conveying information from the spinal cord and brainstem upward through the midbrain to the higher centers. On each side a *medial lemniscus* acts as a pathway from the spinal cord, whereas an outer *lateral lemniscus* commences higher up and is mainly concerned with hearing.

Lennox-Gastaut syndrome a condition of the brain of unknown cause that results in epileptic seizures. It occurs in children, usually between two and eight years of age, but sometimes during adolescence. *Mental retardation is associated with radiologic signs of cerebral atrophy and a diffuse slow spike and wave pattern on electroencephalography. [W. G. Lennox (1884–1960), US neurologist; J. P. Gastaut (1915–), French biologist]

lens *n.* **1.** (in anatomy) the transparent crystalline structure situated behind the pupil of the eye and enclosed in a thin transparent *capsule*. It helps to refract incoming light and focus it onto the *retina. *See also* accommodation. **2.** (in optics) a piece of glass shaped to refract rays of light in a particular direction. *Convex lenses* converge the light, and *concave lenses* diverge it; they are worn to correct faulty eyesight. *See also* bifocal lens, contact lenses, trifocal lenses.

lens implantation *see* cataract.

lenticonus *n.* a condition in which the central part of the front surface of the lens of the eye (or sometimes, the back) has a much steeper curvature than normal and bulges forward in a blunted cone. It is usually congenital.

lenticular nucleus (lentiform nucleus) *see* basal ganglia.

lentigo *n.* (*pl.* **lentigines**) a flat dark brown spot found mainly in the elderly on skin exposed to light. Lentigines have increased numbers of *melanocytes in the basal layer of the epidermis (freckles, by contrast, do not show an increase in these cells). In *lentigo maligna* (or *Hutchinson's lentigo*), which occurs on the cheeks of the elderly, the spot is larger than 2 cm in diameter and has variable pigmentation; it is a precursor of malignant *melanoma that has not spread deeply. Diagnosis is by biopsy and treatment is by surgery, *cryosurgery, or radiation.

leontiasis *n.* overgrowth of the skull bones, said to resemble the appearance of a lion's head: a rare feature of untreated *Paget's disease. Medical name: **leontiasis ossea**.

lepra reaction an aggravation of lumps on the skin caused by *leprosy, accompanied by fever and malaise.

leproma *n.* a lump on the skin characteristic of *leprosy.

lepromin *n.* a chemical prepared from lumps on the skin caused by lepromatous *leprosy.

leprosy (Hansen's disease) *n.* a chronic disease, caused by the bacterium *Mycobacterium leprae*, that affects the skin, mucous membranes, and nerves. It is confined mainly to the tropics and is transmitted by direct contact. After an incubation period of 1–30 years, symptoms develop gradually and mainly involve the skin and nerves. *Lepromatous (multibacillary) leprosy* is a contagious steadily progressive form of the disease characterized by the development of widely distributed lumps on the skin, thickening of the skin and nerves, and in serious cases by severe numbness of the skin, muscle weakness, and paralysis leading to disfigurement and deformity. Tuberculosis is a common complication. *Tuberculoid leprosy* is a benign, often self-limiting, form of leprosy causing discoloration and disfiguration of patches of skin (sparsely distributed) associated with localized numbness. *Indeterminate leprosy* is a form of the disease in which skin manifestations represent a combination of the two main types: tuberculoid and indeterminate leprosy are known as *paucibacillary leprosy*. Like tuberculosis, leprosy should be treated with a combination of antibacterial drugs, to overcome the problem of resistance developing to a single drug. A combination of rifampicin and dapsone for six months is used to treat paucibacillary leprosy and these drugs with the addition of clofazimine for multibacillary leprosy, this *multidrug therapy* to be continued for two years. Reconstructive surgery can repair some of the damage caused by the disease. A vaccine is being developed and tested.

lept- (lepto-) *prefix denoting* **1.** slender; thin. **2.** small. **3.** mild; slight.

leptin *n.* a protein, produced by white *fat cells in adipose tissue, that is involved in controlling the amount of white adipose tissue laid down in the body. It acts on the brain, possibly as a signal to regulate appetite or energy expenditure. Mutations in the *ob* gene, which codes for leptin, are responsible for some cases of *obesity.

leptocyte *n.* a red blood cell (*erythrocyte) that is abnormally thin. *See* target cell.

leptomeninges *pl. n.* the inner two of three membranes (*meninges) that envelop the brain and spinal cord: the arachnoid and pia mater.

leptomeningitis *n.* inflammation of the inner membranes (the *arachnoid and *pia mater) of the brain and spinal cord. *See also* meningitis.

leptophonia *n.* weakness of the voice.

Leptospira *n.* a genus of spirochete bacteria, commonly bearing hooked ends. They are not visible with ordinary light microscopy and are best seen using dark-ground microscopy. The parasitic species *L. icterohaemorrhagiae* is the main causative agent of *leptospirosis (Weil's disease), but many closely related species cause similar symptoms.

leptospirosis (Weil's disease) *n.* an infectious disease, caused by bacteria of the genus *Leptospira* (especially *L. icterohaemorrhagiae*), that occurs in rodents, dogs, and other mammals and may be transmitted to people whose work brings them into contact with these animals. The disease begins with a high fever and headache and may affect the liver (causing jaundice) or meninges (resulting in meningitis); in some cases the kidneys are involved (resulting in renal failure). Treatment is with penicillin or tetracycline.

leptotene *n.* the first stage in the first prophase of *meiosis, in which the chromosomes become visible as single long threads.

leresis *n*. rambling speech, immature both in syntax and pronunciation. It is a feature of dementia.

Leriche's syndrome a condition in males characterized by absence of penile erection combined with absence of pulses in the femoral arteries and wasting of the buttock muscles. It is caused by occlusion of the abdominal aorta and iliac arteries. [R. Leriche (1879–1956), French surgeon]

lesbianism *n*. female *homosexuality: a pattern of sexuality in which a woman is sexually attracted to, or engages in sexual behavior with, another woman. —**lesbian** *adj.*, *n*.

Lesch-Nyhan disease a *sex-linked hereditary disease caused by an enzyme deficiency resulting in overproduction of uric acid. Affected boys are mentally retarded and have *spasticity and gouty arthritis. They also have a compulsion for self-mutilation. [M. Lesch (1939–) and W. L. Nyhan Jr. (1926–), US physicians]

lesion *n*. a zone of tissue with impaired function as a result of damage by disease or wounding. Apart from direct physical injury, examples of primary lesions include abscesses, ulcers, tumors; secondary lesions (such as crusts and scars) are derived from primary ones.

lethal gene a gene that, under certain conditions, causes the death of the individual carrying it. Lethal genes are usually *recessive: an individual will die only if both his parents carry the gene. If only one parent is affected, the lethal effects of the gene will be masked by the dominant *allele inherited from the normal parent.

lethargy *n*. mental and physical sluggishness: a degree of inactivity and unresponsiveness approaching or verging on the unconscious. The condition results from disease (such as sleeping sickness) or hypnosis.

letrozole *n*. see aromatase inhibitor.

Letterer-Siwe disease see Langerhans cell histiocytosis. [E. Letterer (20th century) and S. A. Siwe (1897–1966), German physicians]

leucine *n*. an *essential amino acid. See also amino acid.

leucovorin *n*. see folinic acid.

leuk- (leuko-, leuc-, leuco-) *prefix denoting* **1.** lack of color; white. **2.** leukocytes.

leukemia *n*. any of a group of malignant diseases in which the bone marrow and other blood-forming organs produce increased numbers of certain types of white blood cells (*leukocytes). Overproduction of these white cells, which are immature or abnormal forms, suppresses the production of normal white cells, red cells, and platelets. This leads to increased susceptibility to infection (due to *neutropenia), *anemia, and bleeding (due to *thrombocytopenia). Other symptoms include enlargement of the spleen, liver, and lymph nodes.

Leukemias are classified into *acute* or *chronic* varieties, depending on the rate of progression of the disease. They are also classified according to the type of white cell that is proliferating abnormally; for example *acute lymphoblastic leukemia* (see lymphoblast), *acute myeloblastic leukemia* (see myeloblast), *chronic lymphocytic leukemia* (see lymphocyte), *monocytic leukemia* (see monocyte), and *hairy-cell leukemia* (see hairy cell). (*See also* myeloid leukemia.) Leukemias are treated with *cytotoxic drugs or *monoclonal antibodies, which suppress the production of the abnormal cells, or occasionally with radiotherapy.

leukocidin *n*. a bacterial *exotoxin that selectively destroys white blood cells (leukocytes).

leukocyte (white blood cell) *n*. any blood cell that contains a nucleus. In health there are three major subdivisions: *granulocytes, *lymphocytes, and *monocytes, which are involved in protecting the body against foreign substances and in antibody production. In disease, a variety of other types may appear in the blood, most notably immature forms of the normal red or white blood cells.

leukocytosis *n*. an increase in the number of white blood cells (leukocytes) in the blood. See basophilia, eosinophilia, lymphocytosis, monocytosis.

leukocytospermia *n*. the presence of excess white blood cells (leukocytes) in the semen (more than 1 million/ml). It has an adverse effect on fertility.

leukoderma *n*. loss of pigment in areas of the skin, resulting in the appearance of white patches or bands. *Compare* vitiligo.

leukodystrophy *n.* any one of a group of metabolic diseases in infants and children involving the white matter of the brain. Most of them are inherited disorders related to a defect in lipid metabolism (such as *Krabbe's disease* and *Pelizaeus-Merzbacher disease*), characterized by progressive cerebral deterioration and mental retardation and the pathologic absence or degeneration of the myelin of the central and perpheral nervous systems. *Prenatal diagnosis of these diseases can be made by *amniocentesis.

leukolysin *n.* see lysin.

leukoma *n.* a white opacity in the cornea. Most leukomas result from scarring after corneal inflammation or ulceration. Congenital types may be associated with other abnormalities of the eye.

leukonychia *n.* white discoloration of the nails, which may be total or partial. The cause is unknown.

leukopenia *n.* a reduction in the number of white blood cells (leukocytes) in the blood. *See* eosinopenia, lymphopenia, neutropenia.

leukoplakia *n.* thickened white patches on mucous membranes, such as the mouth lining or vulva, due to an overgrowth of the tissues. It is not a specific disease and is present in about 1% of the elderly. Occasionally leukoplakia can become malignant, *Hairy leukoplakia*, with a shaggy or hairy appearance, is a marker of AIDS. *See also* khat.

leukopoiesis *n.* the process of the production of white blood cells (leukocytes), which normally occurs in the blood-forming tissue of the *bone marrow. *See also* granulopoiesis, hemopoiesis, lymphopoiesis, monoblast.

leukorrhea *n.* a whitish or yellowish discharge of mucus from the vaginal opening. It may occur normally, the quantity increasing before and after menstruation. An abnormally large discharge may indicate infection of the lower reproductive tract, e.g. by the protozoan *Trichomonas vaginalis* (*see* vaginitis).

leukosis *n.* the abnormal proliferation of leukocyte-forming tissue, which is the basis of *leukemia.

leukotaxine *n.* a chemical, present in inflammatory exudates, that attracts white blood cells (leukocytes) and increases the permeability of blood capillaries. It is probably produced by injured cells.

leukotomy *n.* the surgical operation of interrupting the pathways of white nerve fibers within the brain: it is the most common procedure in *psychosurgery. In the original form, *prefrontal leukotomy* (*lobotomy*), the operation involved cutting through the nerve fibers connecting the *frontal lobe with the *thalamus and the association fibers of the frontal lobe. This was often successful in reducing severe emotional tension but had serious side effects, and the procedure has now been abandoned.

Modern procedures use *stereotaxy and make selective lesions in smaller areas of the brain. Side effects are uncommon and the operation is occasionally used for intractable pain, severe depression, obsessional neurosis, and chronic anxiety, where very severe emotional tension has not been relieved by other treatments.

leukotriene *n.* one of a class of powerful chemical agents synthesized from arachidonic acid by mast cells, basophils, macrophages, and various other tissues. Leukotrienes are involved in inflammatory reactions and the immune response: they increase the permeability of small blood vessels, cause contraction of smooth muscle, and attract neutrophils to the site of an infection.

leukotriene receptor antagonist one of a class of drugs that prevent the action of *leukotrienes by blocking their receptors on cell membranes, such as those in the airways. These drugs are used in the treatment of asthma for their effects in relaxing the smooth muscle of the airways and in reducing inflammation in the bronchial linings. Examples are *montelukast* (Singulair) and *zafirlukast* (Accolate), both of which are administered by mouth.

leuprolide *n.* an *LHRH analogue used in the treatment of advanced carcinoma of the prostate, endometriosis, uterine fibroids, and precocious puberty in children. The drug is administered by injection; side effects include general pain, hot flushes, and edema. Leuprolide is also available as an implant (*Viadur*) for the palliative treatment of advanced prostate cancer. Trade names: **Eligard**, **Lupron**.

levamisole *n.* an antineoplastic adjunct that stimulates the immune system by increasing T-cell responsiveness and encouraging the activity of *phagocytes. It is used with fluorouracil for the treatment of colon cancer. Levamisole is administered by mouth; possible side effects include joint pain and interference with blood-cell production, which limit its use. Trade name: **Ergamisol**.

levator *n.* **1.** a surgical instrument used for raising displaced bone fragments in a depressed fracture of the skull. **2.** any muscle that lifts the structure into which it is inserted; for example, the *levator scapulis* helps to lift the shoulder blade.

levo- *prefix denoting* **1.** the left side. **2.** (in chemistry) levorotation.

levobunolol *n.* a *beta blocker used as eye drops in the treatment of *glaucoma; side effects may include local stinging and burning. Trade names: **AKBeta**, **Betagan**.

levocardia *n.* the normal position of the heart, in which its apex is directed toward the left. *Compare* dextrocardia.

levodopa (L-dopa) *n.* a naturally occurring amino acid administered by mouth to treat *parkinsonism. Common side effects are nausea, vomiting, loss of appetite, and involuntary facial movements; high doses may cause weakness, faintness, and dizziness. Trade names: **Dopar**, **Larodopa**, **Sinemet**.

levodopa test a test of the ability of the pituitary to secrete growth hormone, in which levodopa is administered by mouth and plasma levels of growth hormone are subsequently measured (they should peak within the following hour). It is a safer alternative to the *insulin stress test but does not give information on cortisol production, which it is usually more clinically important to know.

levonorgestrel *n.* a synthetic female sex hormone – a *progestogen – used as a contraceptive, either in combination with an estrogen or as a progestogen-only preparation. Side effects include breakthrough bleeding, headache, and nervousness. Trade names: **Alesse**, **Levlen**, **Nordette**.

levorphanol *n.* a narcotic analgesic, similar to *morphine, used to relieve severe pain. It is administered by mouth or in-

jection and may cause nausea, vomiting, loss of appetite, constipation, and confusion. Dependence may develop. Trade name: **Levo-Dromoran**.

levothyroxine *n.* a hormone used in the treatment of hypothyroidism. It is administered by mouth, intramuscularly, or intravenously; side effects are rare but include nervousness, palpitations, and weight loss. Trade names: **Levothroid**, **Levoxine**, **Synthroid**.

levulosuria *n. see* fructosuria.

Lewy bodies *see* cortical Lewy body disease. [F. H. Lewy (1885–1950), German neurologist]

Leydig cells *see* interstitial cells. [F. von Leydig (1821–1908), German anatomist]

Leydig tumor a tumor of the *interstitial (Leydig) cells of the testis. Such tumors often secrete testosterone, which in prepubertal boys causes *virilization.

LH *see* luteinizing hormone.

Lhermitte's sign a tingling shocklike sensation passing down the arms or trunk when the neck is flexed. It is a nonspecific indication of disease in the cervical (neck) region of the spinal cord, generally seen in patients with multiple sclerosis, cervical *spondylosis, and deficiency of vitamin B_{12}. [J. Lhermitte (1877–1959), French neurologist]

LHRH analogue any one of a group of analogues of *luteinizing hormone-releasing hormone*, which stimulates the release of *luteinizing hormone (LH) from the pituitary gland. LHRH analogues are more powerful than the naturally occurring hormone, initially increasing the secretion of LH by the pituitary: this acts to block the hormone receptors and to inhibit the release of further LH. LHRH analogues, which are also known as *GnRH analogues* (see gonadotropin-releasing hormone), are effective in the treatment of endometriosis; administered by depot injection or nasal spray, they ensure ovarian suppression. They are also used to shrink fibroids and in the treatment of some types of infertility. Two LHRH analogues, *goserelin and *leuprolide, are increasingly being used in the treatment of advanced prostate cancer. Both are given subcutaneously in depot form into the abdominal wall at one- or three-monthly intervals. After causing an initial rise in plasma testosterone for approximately ten days, the level then falls to the same low level as that achieved by castration. Because the initial flare in testosterone may cause an acute enlargement of the cancer, *antiandrogens are given at the same time. *See also* buserelin, gonadorelin.

libido *n.* the sexual drive: the term is often used to refer to the intensity of sexual desires. In psychoanalytic theory, the libido (like the death instinct) is one of the fundamental sources of energy for all mental life. The normal course of development (*see* psychosexual development) can be altered by fixation at one level and by regression.

Librium *n. see* chlordiazepoxide.

lice *pl. n. see* louse, pediculosis.

lichen *n.* any of several types of skin disease in which round hard lesions occur close together. For example, *lichen planus* is an inflammatory, extremely itchy, condition in which wide flat mauve pimples are found mainly on the forearms, neck, on the inside of the wrists, and between the thighs. It may occur in the mouth and often causes symptomless white patches; occasionally it forms painful erosions. Trauma, such as a scratch, may induce a linear form of the disease (*see* Koebner phenomenon). *Lichen sclerosus* is a chronic skin disease affecting the anogenital area, especially in women, characterized by sheets of thin ivory-white skin. In 20% of patients other skin areas are also affected. *See also* neurodermatitis (lichen simplex chronicus).

lichenification *n.* thickening of the epidermis of the skin with exaggeration of the normal creases. The cause is abnormal scratching or rubbing of the skin.

lichenoid *adj.* describing any skin disease that resembles *lichen.

lidocaine *n.* a widely used local *anesthetic administered by injection for minor surgery and dental procedures. It can also be applied directly to the eye, throat, and mouth because it is absorbed through mucous membranes. Lidocaine topical systems are used to relieve pain and discomfort, especially associated with *herpes zoster virus infection. Lidocaine is also injected to treat conditions involving abnormal heart rhythm, particularly myocardial infarction. When used as a local anesthetic, side

effects are rare. Trade names: **DermaFlex, Lidocaine, Lidoderm, Xylocaine**.

Lieberkühn's glands (crypts of Lieberkühn) simple tubular glands in the mucous membrane of the *intestine. In the small intestine they lie between the villi. They are lined with columnar *epithelium in which various types of secretory cells are found. In the large intestine Lieberkühn's glands are longer and contain more mucus-secreting cells. [J. N. Lieberkühn (1711–56), German anatomist]

lien *n. see* spleen.

lien- (lieno-) *prefix denoting* the spleen. Example: *lienopathy* (disease of).

lientery *n.* diarrhea with the passage of undigested food in the feces. This may indicate simply rapid transit of food through the digestive tract or some form of *malabsorption.

life table an actuarial presentation of the ages at which a group of males and/or females will die and from which mean *life expectancy* at any age can be estimated, based on the assumption that mortality patterns current at the time of preparation of the table will continue to apply.

ligament *n.* **1.** a tough band of white fibrous connective tissue that links two bones together at a joint. Ligaments are inelastic but flexible; they both strengthen the joint and limit its movements to certain directions. **2.** a sheet of peritoneum that supports or links together abdominal organs.

ligand *n.* a molecule that binds to another molecule, as in antigen–antibody and hormone–receptor bondings.

ligation *n.* the application of a *ligature.

ligature *n.* any material – for example, nylon, silk, catgut, or wire – that is tied firmly round a blood vessel to stop it bleeding or around the base of a structure (such as the *pedicle of a growth) to constrict it.

light adaptation reflex changes in the eye to enable vision either in normal light after being in darkness or in very bright light after being in normal light. The pupil contracts (*see* pupillary reflex) and the pigment in the *rods is bleached. *Compare* dark adaptation.

lightening *n.* the sensation experienced, usually after the 36th week of gestation, by many pregnant women, particularly those carrying their first child, as the head of the fetus turns down toward the vagina. This reduces the pressure on the diaphragm and the woman notices that it is easier to breathe. *Compare* engagement.

light reflex *see* pupillary reflex.

limbic system a complex system of nerve pathways and networks in the brain, involving several different nuclei, that is involved in the expression of instinct and mood in activities of the endocrine and motor systems of the body. Among the brain regions involved are the *amygdala, *hippocampal formation, and *hypothalamus. The activities of the body that are governed are those concerned with self-preservation (e.g. searching for food, fighting) and preservation of the species (e.g. reproduction and the care of offspring), the expression of fear, rage, and pleasure, and the establishment of memory patterns. *See also* reticular activating system.

limb lengthening an orthopedic procedure for increasing the length of a limb (usually the leg). An *external fixator is attached to the bone. This can be a circular frame surrounding the bone, which was invented by the Russian surgeon Ilizarov, or a bar down one side of the limb. The bone is divided, and the gap produced is slowly widened by moving the two ends of the frame apart; if a bar fixator is used, its body has a screw thread that is turned to increase the distance between the two ends. New bone is produced in the widening gap as the bone is stretched (*see* callotasis). Limb lengthening is undertaken when there is inequality in the length of the legs; for example, following trauma or resulting from paralysis in childhood. Both legs can be lengthened to increase the height of a person of excessively short stature.

limbus *n.* (in anatomy) an edge or border; for example, the *limbus sclerae* is the junction of the cornea and sclera of the eye.

limen *n.* (in anatomy) a border or boundary. The *limen nasi* is the boundary between the bony and cartilaginous parts of the nasal cavity.

liminal *adj.* (in physiology) relating to the threshold of perception.

limosis *n.* abnormal hunger or an excessive desire for food.

linac *n. see* linear accelerator.

lincomycin *n.* an *antibiotic used to treat infections caused by a narrow range of bacteria, particularly in patients unable to take penicillin. It is administered by mouth or injection and occasionally causes colitis, nausea, and stomach pains. Trade names: **Lincocin, Lincorex.**

linctus *n.* a syrupy liquid medicine, particularly one used in the treatment of irritating coughs.

lindane (gamma benzene hexachloride) a drug used in creams, lotions, solutions, or shampoos to treat infestations caused by scabies, mites, and lice (including head lice). Mild skin reactions occasionally occur.

Lindau's tumor *see* hemangioblastoma. [A. Lindau (1892–1958), Swedish pathologist]

linea *n.* (*pl.* **lineae**) (in anatomy) a line, narrow streak, or stripe. The *linea alba* is a tendinous line, extending from the xiphoid process to the pubic symphysis, where the flat abdominal muscles are attached.

linear accelerator (linac) a machine that accelerates particles to produce high-energy radiation, used in the treatment of malignant disease.

linezolid *n.* a member of a new class of antibiotics – the *oxazolidinones* – that are active against gram-positive bacteria, including *MRSA. Linezolid is used to treat pneumonia and soft-tissue infections caused by these organisms. It is administered by mouth or intravenous infusion; the most common side effects are headache, a metallic taste in the mouth, diarrhea, and nausea. Trade name: **Zyvox.**

lingual *adj.* relating to, situated close to, or resembling the tongue (lingua). The lingual surface of a tooth is the surface adjacent to the tongue.

lingula *n.* **1.** the thin forward-projecting portion of the anterior lobe of the cerebellum, in the midline. **2.** a small section of the upper lobe of the left lung, extending downward in front of the heart. **3.** a bony spur on the inside of the mandible, above the angle of the jaw. **4.** a small backward-pointing projection on each side of the sphenoid bone.

liniment *n.* a medicinal preparation that is rubbed onto the skin or applied on a surgical dressing. Liniments often contain camphor.

lining *n.* (in dentistry) a protective layer placed in a prepared tooth cavity before a restoration is inserted.

linitis plastica (leather-bottle stomach) diffuse infiltration of the stomach submucosa with malignant tissue, producing rigidity and narrowing. Diagnosis by endoscopy may be difficult but radiological changes are more marked.

linkage *n.* (in genetics) the situation in which two or more genes lie close to each other on a chromosome and are therefore very likely to be inherited together. The farther two genes are apart, the more likely they are to be separated by *crossing over during meiosis.

linoleic acid *see* essential fatty acid.

linolenic acid *see* essential fatty acid.

lint *n.* a material used in surgical dressings, made of scraped linen or a cotton substitute. It is usually fluffy on one side and smooth on the other.

liothyronine *n.* a preparation of the hormone *triiodothyronine, produced by the thyroid gland, that is used to treat conditions of thyroid deficiency. It is administered by mouth or injection and has a rapid but short-lived effect. Trade names: **Cytomel, Triostat**.

liotrix *n.* a synthetic combination thyroid preparation used in the treatment of hypothyroid conditions. The drug is administered orally and the most serious side effects include nervousness, increased heart rate, insomnia, and fever. Trade names: **Euthroid, Thyrolar**.

lip *n.* either of the two structures that surround the mouth. The *vermilion marks the transition from the mucosa in the mouth to the skin. The lips participate in eating, speech, nonverbal communication, and sensory feedback.

lip- (lipo-) *prefix denoting* **1.** fat. **2.** lipid.

lipase (steapsin) *n.* an enzyme, produced by the pancreas and the glands of the small intestine, that breaks down fats into glycerol and fatty acids during digestion.

lipemia *n.* the presence in the blood of an abnormally large amount of fat.

lipid *n.* one of a group of naturally occurring compounds that are soluble in solvents such as chloroform or alcohol, but insoluble in water. Lipids are important dietary constituents, not only because of their high energy value, but also because certain vitamins and essential fatty acids are associated with them. The group includes *fats, *steroids, *phospholipids, and *glycolipids.

lipidosis (lipoidosis) *n.* (*pl.* **-ses**) any disorder of lipid metabolism within the cells of the body. The *brain lipidoses* (*see* Gaucher's disease, Hunter's syndrome, Hurler's syndrome, Tay-Sachs disease) are inborn defects causing the accumulation of lipids within the brain.

lipoatrophy *n.* an immune reaction to insulin injections close to the site of injection, resulting in localized hollowing of the fat tissue, which is unsightly. It is rarely seen with more modern, highly purified, insulins.

lipochondrodystrophy *n.* multiple congenital defects affecting lipid (fat) metabolism, cartilage and bone, skin, and the major internal organs, leading to mental retardation, dwarfism, and deformities of the bones.

lipochrome *n.* a pigment that is soluble in fat and therefore gives color to fatty materials. An example is *carotene, the pigment responsible for the color of egg yolks, carrots, and butter.

lipodystrophy *n.* **1.** any disturbance of fat metabolism or of the distribution of fat in the body. In *insulin lipodystrophy*, sometimes occurring in diabetics, it disappears from the areas at which insulin is injected. **2.** a group of conditions resulting in the loss of fat tissue from part or all of the body. It may be congenital or acquired later in life. Congenital lipodystrophies include the *Kobberling-Dunnigan syndrome*, an autosomal *dominant condition more common in women, who lose fat tissue from their limbs and lower bodies and often also suffer with *polycystic ovary syndrome. Another condition is *Beradinelli-Seip syndrome*, which is autosomal *recessive and involves more generalized fat-tissue loss. Acquired forms usually follow an acute illness in childhood and may involve all or part of the body.

lipofuscin *n.* a brownish pigment staining with certain fat stains. It is most common in the cells of heart muscle, nerves, and liver and is normally contained within the *lysosomes.

lipogenesis *n.* the process by which glucose and other substances, derived from carbohydrate in the diet, are converted to *fatty acids in the body.

lipogranulomatosis *n.* an abnormality of lipid metabolism causing deposition of yellowish nodules in the skin.

lipohypertrophy *n.* a local buildup of fat tissue near the site of repeated insulin injections, which is both unsightly and tends to alter the rate of absorption of further injections into the body. It is caused by the local action of the insulin, which (among other things) promotes fat storage.

lipoic acid a sulfur-containing compound that can be readily interconverted to and from its reduced form, *dihydrolipoic acid*. Lipoic acid functions in carbohydrate metabolism as one of the *coenzymes in the oxidative decarboxylation of pyruvate and other α-keto acids.

lipoidosis *n. see* lipidosis.

lipolysis *n.* the process by which lipids, particularly triglycerides in fat, are broken down into their constituent fatty acids in the body by the enzyme *lipase. —**lipolytic** *adj.*

lipoma *n.* (*pl.* **lipomas** or **lipomata**) a common benign tumor composed of well-differentiated fat cells.

lipomatosis *n.* **1.** the presence of an abnormally large amount of fat in the tissues. **2.** the presence in the tissues of multiple *lipomas.

lipopolysaccharide *n.* a complex molecule containing both a lipid component and a polysaccharide component. Lipopolysaccharides are constituents of the cell walls of gram-negative bacteria and are important in determining the antigenic properties of these bacteria.

lipoprotein *n.* one of a group of compounds, found in blood plasma and lymph, each consisting of a protein (*see* apolipoprotein) combined with a lipid (which may be *cholesterol, a triglyceride, or a phospholipid). Lipoproteins are important for the transport of lipids in the blood and lymph. Cholesterol is transported in the bloodstream in the form of *low-density lipoproteins* (*LDLs*). Cholesterol is removed from the bloodstream by means of special LDL receptors, which are inserted into the membranes of cells and bind the LDLs. LDLs are then taken into the cell. Other forms of lipoprotein are *high-density lipoprotein* (*HDL*), which transports cholesterol from the tissues to the liver, and *very low-density lipoprotein* (*VLDL*), which is the precursor of LDL.

liposarcoma *n.* a rare malignant tumor of fat cells. Liposarcoma is most commonly found in the thigh and is rare under the age of 30 years. There are four main histological types: *well-differentiated, myxoid, pleomorphic,* and *round-cell liposarcomas.* Treatment is usually by surgery.

liposome *n.* a microscopic spherical membrane-enclosed vesicle or sac (20–30 nm in diameter) made artificially in the laboratory by the addition of an aqueous solution to a phospholipid gel. The membrane resembles a cell membrane and the whole vesicle is similar to a cell organelle. Liposomes can be incorporated into living cells and are used to transport relatively toxic drugs into cancer cells, where they can exert their maximum effects. For example, liposomes containing *methotrexate or *doxorubicin can be injected into the patient's blood. The cancerous organ is at a temperature higher than normal body temperature, so that when the liposome passes through the tumor's blood vessels the membrane melts and the drug is released. Liposomes are also undergoing clinical trials as vehicles in *gene therapy for cystic fibrosis.

liposuction *n.* a technique for removing unwanted collections of subcutaneous fat by using a powerful suction tube passed through the skin at different locations.

lipotropic *adj.* describing a substance that promotes the transport of fatty acids from the liver to the tissues or accelerates the utilization of fat in the liver itself. An example of such a substance is the amino acid methionine.

lipotropin *n.* a hormonelike substance from the anterior pituitary gland that stimulates the transfer of fat from the body stores to the bloodstream.

lipping *n.* overgrowth of bone as seen in X-rays near a joint margin. This is a characteristic sign of degenerative or inflammatory joint disease and occurs most frequently and prominently in osteoarthrosis. *See also* osteophyte.

lipuria *n.* the presence of fat or oil droplets in the urine.

liquid-based cytology (LBC) a new technology intended to improve the detection of cytologic abnormalities, which has been heralded as a way forward for cervical screening. It includes liquid-based thin-layer cytology (ThinPrep, AutoCyte), computerized rescreening (PAPNET), and algorithm-based computer rescreening (AutoPap). LBC provides uniformly well-fixed preparations that are free of inflammatory exudate and blood and seem easier to screen than conventional smears.

liquor *n.* (in pharmacy) any solution, usually an aqueous solution.

Lisch nodules well-defined dome-shaped pigmented nodules (*see* hamartoma) projecting from the *iris. They are found in patients with *tuberous sclerosis and *neurofibromatosis. [K. Lisch (1907-99), Austrian ophthalmologist]

lisinopril *n.* a drug used in the treatment of high blood pressure (hypertension). It inhibits the action of angiotensin, which leads to decreased vasopressor (blood-vessel constricting) activity and to decreased aldosterone secretion. It is administered by mouth; the most common side effects are dizziness, headache, fatigue, cough, and diarrhea. Trade names: **Prinivil, Zestril.**

lissencephaly *n. see* agyria.

Listeria *n.* a genus of gram-positive aerobic motile rodlike bacteria that are parasites of warm-blooded animals. The single species, *L. monocytogenes*, infects many domestic and wild animals. If it is transmitted to humans, by eating infected animals or animal products, it may cause disease (*listeriosis*), especially in the frail, ranging from influenza-like symptoms to *meningoencephalitis. In pregnant women it may cause termination of the pregnancy or damage the fetus.

liter *n.* a unit of volume equal to the volume occupied by 1 kilogram of pure water at 4°C and 760 mmHg pressure. In *SI units the liter is treated as a special name for the cubic decimeter, but is not used when a high degree of accuracy is required (1 liter = 1.0000028 dm³). For approximate purposes 1 liter is assumed to be equal to 1000 cubic centimeters (cc), therefore 1 milliliter (ml) is often taken to be equal to 1 cc. This practice is now deprecated.

lith- (litho-) *prefix denoting* a calculus

(stone). Example: *lithogenesis* (formation of).

-lith *suffix denoting* a calculus (stone). Example: *fecalith* (a stony mass of feces).

lithagogue *n.* an agent that promotes the removal of stones (calculi), such as kidney stones in the urine or gallstones from the gallbladder.

lithemia *n. see* hyperuricemia.

lithiasis *n.* formation of stones (*see* calculus) in an internal organ, such as the gallbladder (*see* gallstone), urinary system, pancreas, or appendix.

lithium (lithium carbonate) *n.* a drug given by mouth to prevent manic-depressive psychosis or to treat mania. Side effects include tremor, weakness, nausea, thirst, and excessive urination. Thyroid function can be interfered with, and changes in the kidney can appear after long-term treatment. Excessive doses can cause an *encephalopathy and even death. The levels of lithium in the blood are therefore usually checked during long-term therapy. Trade names: **Eskalith, Lithane, Lithobid, Lithonate, Lithotabs.**

litholapaxy (lithotripsy) *n.* the operation of crushing a stone in the bladder, using an instrument called a *lithotrite.* The small fragments of stone can then be removed by irrigation and suction.

lithonephrotomy *n.* surgical removal of a stone from the kidney. *See* nephrolithotomy, pyelolithotomy.

lithopedion *n.* a fetus that has died in the uterus or abdominal cavity and has become calcified.

lithotomy *n.* the surgical removal of a stone (calculus) from the urinary tract. *See* nephrolithotomy, pyelolithotomy, ureterolithotomy.

lithotripsy *n.* **1.** the destruction of calculi (stones) by the application of shock waves. In *extracorporeal shock-wave lithotripsy (ESWL),* used for destroying calculi in the upper urinary tract and gallstones, the shock waves are generated and transmitted by an external power source. The specialized machine (a *lithotripter*) consists of a sophisticated radiological system to localize the stone accurately by biplanar X-ray or ultrasound and a shock head or transducer to produce and focus the energy source. The prototype machines required the patient to be anesthetized and immersed in a water bath for treatment, but the modern machines require neither water bath nor general anesthesia. In *electrohydraulic lithotripsy (EHL)*, used for destroying urinary calculi, an electrically generated shock wave is transmitted to the stone by a contact probe delivered via a *nephroscope or *ureteroscope. **2.** *see* litholapaxy.

lithotrite *n.* a surgical instrument used for crushing a stone in the bladder. *See* litholapaxy.

lithotrophic *adj. see* autotrophic.

lithuresis *n.* the passage of small stones or *gravel in the urine.

lithuria *n. see* hyperuricuria.

litmus *n.* a blue dye that is used to determine *pH. Acid substances or solutions turn blue litmus red; alkaline substances or solutions do not cause a color change in the litmus.

Little's area the anterior region of the nasal septum (*see* nose). It has a rich capillary supply, called *Kiesselbach's plexus, and is a common site from which *nosebleeds arise. [J. L. Little (1836–85), US surgeon]

Little's disease a form of *cerebral palsy involving both sides of the body and affecting the legs more severely than the arms. [W. J. Little (1810–94), British surgeon]

Litzmann's obliquity *see* asynclitism. [K. C. T. Litzmann (1815–90), German obstetrician]

livedo *n.* a discolored area or spot on the skin, often caused by local congestion of the circulation.

liver *n.* the largest gland of the body, weighing 1200–1600 g. Situated in the top right portion of the abdominal cavity, the liver is divided by fissures (*fossae*) into four lobes: the *right* (the largest lobe), *left, quadrate,* and *caudate lobes.* It is connected to the diaphragm and abdominal walls by five ligaments: the membranous *falciform* (which separates the right and left lobes), *coronary,* and *right* and *left triangular ligaments* and the fibrous *round ligament,* which is derived from the embryonic umbilical vein. Venous blood containing digested food is brought to the liver in the *hepatic portal vein* (*see* portal system). Branches of this vein pass in between the lobules and terminate in the *sinusoids* (see illustration). Oxygenated blood is supplied in the *hepatic artery.* The blood leaves the

liver via a central vein in each lobule, which drains into the *hepatic vein. The liver is supplied by parasympathetic nerve fibers from the vagus nerve, and by sympathetic fibers from the solar plexus. The liver has a number of important functions. It synthesizes *bile, which drains into the *gallbladder before being released into the duodenum. The liver is an important site of metabolism of carbohydrates, proteins, and fats. It regulates the amount of blood sugar, converting excess glucose to *glycogen; it removes excess amino acids by breaking them down into ammonia and finally *urea; and it stores and metabolizes fats. The liver also synthesizes *fibrinogen and *prothrombin (essential blood-clotting substances) and *heparin, an anticoagulant. It forms red blood cells in the fetus and is the site of production of plasma proteins. It has an important role in the detoxification of poisonous substances and it breaks down worn out red cells and other unwanted substances, such as excess estrogen in the male (*see also* Kupffer's cells). The liver is also the site of *vitamin A synthesis; this vitamin is stored in the liver, together with vitamins B_{12}, D, and K.

The liver is the site of many important diseases, including *hepatitis, *cirrho-

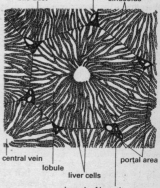

branch of hepatic portal vein

bile duct   sinusoids

central vein

lobule

liver cells

portal area

branch of hepatic artery

The microscopic structure of the liver

sis, amebic *dysentery, *hydatid disease, and *hepatomas.

liver spot a local brown discoloration on the skin known medically as senile *lentigo. The term is sometimes also used for *chloasma and some medical sources also apply the term to *pityriasis versicolor.

livid *adj.* denoting a bluish color of the skin, such as that produced locally by a bruise or of the general complexion in *cyanosis.

living will a statement signed by a person that outlines the degree of life-saving treatment desired in case of incapacitation. It enables terminally ill patients to refuse resuscitation in the event of cardiac arrest. *See* advance directive.

Loa *n.* a genus of parasitic nematode worms (*see* filaria). The adult eye worm, *L. loa*, lives within the tissues beneath the skin, where it causes inflammation and swelling (*see* loiasis). The motile embryos, present in the blood during the day, may be taken up by bloodsucking *Chrysops* flies. Here they develop into infective larvae, ready for transmission to a new human host.

lobe *n.* a major division of an organ or part of an organ, especially one having a rounded form and often separated from other lobes by fissures or bands of connective tissue. Organs that are divided into lobes include the brain, liver, and lung. —**lobar** *adj.*

lobectomy *n.* the surgical removal of a lobe of an organ or gland, such as the lung, thyroid, or brain. Lobectomy of the lung may be performed for cancer or other disease of the lung; in some cases the operation can be done through an endoscope.

lobeline *n.* a drug administered by injection to stimulate breathing or given by mouth as a smoking deterrent. Side effects can include nausea, vomiting, coughing, headache, tremors, and dizziness.

lobotomy (prefrontal leukotomy) *n. see* leukotomy.

lobule *n.* a subdivision of a part or organ that can be distinguished from the whole by boundaries, such as septa, that are visible with or without a microscope. For example, the *lobule of the liver* is a structural and functional unit seen in cross-section under a microscope as a

column of cells drained by a central vein and bounded by a branch of the portal vein. The *lung lobule* is a practical subdivision of the lung tissue seen macroscopically in lung slices as outlined by incomplete septa of fibrous tissue. It is made up of three to five lung *acini.

lochia *n.* the material eliminated from the uterus through the vagina after the completion of labor. The first discharge, *lochia rubra* (*lochia cruenta*), consists largely of blood. This is followed by *lochia serosa*, a brownish mixture of blood and mucus, and finally *lochia alba* (*lochia purulenta*), a yellowish or whitish discharge containing microorganisms and cell fragments. Each stage may last for several days. —**lochial** *adj.*

locked-in syndrome *see* persistent vegetative state.

lockjaw *n. see* tetanus.

locomotor ataxia *see* tabes dorsalis.

loculus *n.* (in anatomy) a small space or cavity.

locum tenens a doctor who stands in temporarily for a colleague who is absent or ill and looks after the patients in his practice. Often shortened to **locum.**

locus *n.* **1.** (in anatomy) a region or site. The *locus caeruleus* is a small pigmented region in the floor of the fourth ventricle of the brain. **2.** (in genetics) the region of a chromosome occupied by a particular gene.

log- (logo-) *prefix denoting* words; speech.

logopedics *n.* the scientific study of defects and disabilities of speech and of the methods used to treat them; speech therapy.

logorrhea *n.* a rapid flow of voluble speech, often with incoherence, such as is encountered in *mania.

-logy (-ology) *suffix denoting* field of study. Example: *cytology* (study of cells).

loiasis *n.* a disease, occurring in West and Central Africa, caused by the eye worm *Loa loa*. The adult worms live and migrate within the skin tissues, causing the appearance of transitory *calabar* swellings. These are probably an allergic reaction to the worms' waste products, and they sometimes lead to fever and itching. Worms often migrate across the eyeball just beneath the conjunctiva, where they cause irritation and congestion. Loiasis is treated with appropriate anthelmintics, such as *diethylcarbamazine.

loin n. the region of the back and side of the body between the lowest rib and the pelvis.

lomefloxacin n. a *quinolone drug used in the treatment of infections caused by a broad spectrum of microorganisms. It is administered by mouth; side effects include nausea, headache, and dizziness. Trade name: **Maxaquin**.

lomustine n. an *alkylating agent used in the treatment of a variety of malignant diseases, such as brain tumors and Hodgkin's disease. It is administered orally; side effects include loss of appetite, fatigue, weakness, fever, and dizziness. Trade name: **CeeNU**.

longitudinal study see cohort study.

loop n. **1.** a bend in a tubular organ, e.g. *Henle's loop in a kidney tubule. **2.** one of the patterns of dermal ridges in *fingerprints.

loperamide n. a drug used in the treatment of nonspecific diarrhea and that associated with inflammatory bowel disease. It acts by reducing *peristalsis of the digestive tract and is administered by mouth; side effects are rare, but include abdominal distension, drowsiness, and skin rash. Trade name: **Imodium**.

lopinavir n. see protease inhibitor.

loracarbef n. a *beta-lactam antibiotic used in infections of the respiratory tract, skin and skin structures, and urinary tract. It is administered by mouth; side effects include diarrhea, nausea, and vomiting. Trade name: **Lorabid**.

lorazepam n. a *benzodiazepine with *anxiolytic and sedative effects used to relieve moderate or severe anxiety and tension and to treat insomnia. It is administered by mouth and may cause drowsiness, dizziness, blurred vision, and nausea. Trade name: **Ativan**.

loratidine n. see antihistamine.

lordosis n. inward curvature of the spine. A certain degree of lordosis is normal in the lumbar and cervical regions of the spine: loss of this is a sign of ankylosing *spondylitis. Exaggerated lordosis may occur in adolescence, through faulty posture, or as a result of disease affecting the vertebrae and spinal muscles. Compare kyphosis.

losartan n. see angiotensin II antagonist.

lotion n. a medicinal solution for washing or bathing the external parts of the body. Lotions usually have a cooling, soothing, or antiseptic action.

Lou Gehrig's disease amyotrophic lateral *sclerosis. See also motor neuron disease. [Lou Gehrig (1903–41), US baseball player who suffered from it]

loupe n. a small magnifying hand lens used for examining the front part of the eye. It is usually used with a pocket light to provide illumination. In modern practice a slit-lamp microscope is used.

louse n. (pl. **lice**) a small wingless insect that is an external parasite of humans. Lice attach themselves to hair and clothing using their well-developed legs and claws. Their flattened leathery bodies are resistant to crushing and their mouthparts are adapted for sucking blood. Lice thrive in overcrowded and unhygienic conditions: they can infest humans (see pediculosis) and they may transmit disease. See also Pediculus, Phthirus.

lovastatin n. a drug used to lower *cholesterol levels in the blood in patients with primary hypercholesterolemia. It is administered by mouth; side effects include headache, skin rash, and abdominal pain. Trade name: **Mevacor**.

Løvset's maneuver rotation and traction of the trunk of the fetus during a breech birth to facilitate delivery of the arms and the shoulders. [J. Løvset (20th century), Norwegian obstetrician]

low-density lipoprotein (LDL) see lipoprotein.

lower urinary tract symptoms (LUTS) symptoms occurring during urine storage, voiding, or immediately after. These include *frequency, *urgency, *nocturia, *incontinence, *hesitation, *intermittency, *terminal dribble, *dysuria, and *postmicturition dribble. These symptoms used to be known as prostatism. Sometimes they are due to *benign prostatic hyperplasia, but they may be due to *detrusor overactivity, excessive drinking, diuresis due to poorly controlled diabetes, or a urethral stricture.

low molecular weight heparin a type of *heparin that is more readily absorbed and requires less frequent administration than standard heparin preparations used as anticoagulant therapy to prevent deep-vein thrombosis following surgery or during kidney dialysis. It also produces less risk of bleeding. Preparations in use include *dalteparin and *enoxaparin*.

loxapine *n.* an *antipsychotic drug used in the treatment of schizophrenia. It is administered orally or by injection. Side effects include drowsiness, extrapyramidal reactions (such as *parkinsonism, writhing and other abnormal body movements), dry mouth, insomnia, and hypersensitivity reactions. Trade name: **Loxitane.**

lozenge *n.* a medicated tablet containing sugar. Lozenges should dissolve slowly in the mouth so that the medication is applied to the mouth and throat.

LSD *see* lysergic acid diethylamide.

lubb-dupp *n.* a representation of the normal heart sounds as heard through the stethoscope. Lubb (the first heart sound) coincides with closure of the mitral and tricuspid valves; dupp (the second heart sound) is due to closure of the aortic and pulmonary valves.

lucid interval temporary recovery of consciousness after a blow to the head, before relapse into coma. It is a sign of intracranial arterial bleeding.

Ludwig's angina severe inflammation caused by infection of both sides of the floor of the mouth, resulting in massive swelling of the neck. If untreated, it may obstruct the airways, necessitating tracheostomy. [W. F. von Ludwig (1770–1865), German surgeon]

lues *n.* a serious infectious disease such as syphilis.

Lugol's iodine a solution of 5% iodine and 10% potassium iodide, used in the treatment of thyrotoxicosis in emergencies, such as *thyroid storm, or when surgery cannot wait for more conventional treatments. For its mode of action it utilizes the abnormal *Wolff-Chaikoff effect, seen in cases of thyroiditis. [J. G. A. Lugol (1786–1851), French physician]

lumbago *n.* low backache, of any cause or description. Severe lumbago, of sudden onset while bending or lifting, can be due either to a slipped disk or to a strained muscle or ligament. When associated with *sciatica it is often due to a slipped disk.

lumbar *adj.* relating to the loin.

lumbar puncture a procedure performed under local anesthesia in which cerebrospinal fluid is withdrawn by means of a hollow needle inserted into the *subarachnoid space in the region of the lower back (usually between the third and fourth lumbar vertebrae). The fluid thus obtained is examined for diagnostic purposes. The procedure is usually without risk to the patient, but in patients with raised intracranial pressure it may be hazardous. CT and MRI scanning prior to lumbar puncture have greatly reduced the risk of performing the test in patients with unsuspected raised intracranial pressure. *See also* Queckenstedt test.

lumbar triangle a weak area in the abdomen bounded by the iliac crest (below), the external oblique muscle (in front), and the erector spinae muscle (behind). It can be the site of a *lumbar hernia*.

lumbar vertebrae the five bones of the *backbone that are situated between the thoracic vertebrae and the sacrum, in the lower part of the back. They are the largest of the unfused vertebrae and have stout processes for attachment of the strong muscles of the lower back. *See also* vertebra.

lumbo- *prefix denoting* the loin; lumbar region.

lumbosacral *adj.* relating to part of the spine composed of the lumbar vertebrae and the sacrum.

lumen *n.* **1.** the space within a tubular or saclike part, such as a blood vessel, the intestine, or the stomach. **2.** the *SI unit of luminous flux, equal to the amount of light emitted per second in unit solid angle of 1 steradian by a point source of 1 candela. Symbol: lm.

luminescence *n.* the emission of light from a substance after it has been irradiated. *Fluorescence is a type of luminescence. This phenomenon is used in a *fluoroscope, a *gamma camera, an X-ray *cassette, and some types of *dosimeter.

lumpectomy *n.* an operation for breast cancer in which the tumor mass and surrounding breast tissue are removed. Muscles, skin, and nodes are left intact. The procedure, usually followed by radiation, is indicated for patients with a tumor less than 2 cm in diameter and who have no metastases to local lymph nodes or to distant organs. *Compare* mastectomy.

lunate bone a bone of the wrist (*see* car-

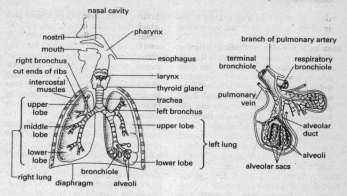

The lungs and main air passages, with details of the alveoli

pus). It articulates with the capitate and hamate bones in front, with the radius behind, and with the triquetral and scaphoid at the sides.

lung *n.* one of the pair of organs of *respiration, situated in the chest cavity on either side of the heart and enclosed by a serous membrane (*see* pleura). The lungs are fibrous elastic sacs that are expanded and compressed by movements of the rib cage and diaphragm during *breathing. They communicate with the atmosphere through the *trachea, which opens into the pharynx. The trachea divides into two bronchi (*see* bronchus), which enter the lungs and branch into *bronchioles. These divide further and terminate in minute air sacs (*see* alveolus), the sites of gaseous exchange. (See illustration.) Atmospheric oxygen is absorbed and carbon dioxide from the blood of the pulmonary capillaries is released into the lungs; in each case down a concentration gradient (*see* pulmonary circulation). The total capacity of the lungs in an adult male is about 5.5 liters, but during normal breathing only about 500 ml of air is exchanged (*see also* residual volume). Other functions of the lung include water evaporation: an important factor in the fluid balance and heat regulation of the body.

lung cancer cancer arising in the epithelium of the air passages (*bronchial cancer*) or lung. It is a very common form of cancer and is strongly associated with cigarette smoking and exposure to industrial air pollutants (including asbestos). There are often no symptoms in the early stages of the disease, when diagnosis is made on X-ray examination. Treatment includes surgical removal of the affected lobe or lung (up to 20% of cases are suitable for surgery), radiotherapy, and chemotherapy.

lunula *n.* the whitish crescent-shaped area at the base of a *nail.

lupus *n.* any of several chronic skin diseases. *See* lupus erythematosus, lupus verrucosus, lupus vulgaris.

lupus erythematosus (LE) a chronic inflammatory disease of connective tissue, affecting the skin and various internal organs (*systemic LE, SLE*). Typically, there is a red scaly rash on the face, affecting the nose and cheeks; arthritis; and progressive damage to the kidneys. Often the heart, lungs, and brain are also affected by progressive attacks of inflammation followed by the formation of scar tissue (fibrosis). In a milder form of the disease, known as *discoid LE (DLE)*, only the skin is affected. LE is an *autoimmune disease and can be diagnosed by the presence of abnormal antibodies in the bloodstream. The disease is treated with corticosteroids or immunosuppressant drugs.

lupus verrucosus a rare tuberculous infection of the skin – commonly the arm or hand – typified by warty lesions. It occurs in those who have been reinfected with tuberculosis.

lupus vulgaris tuberculous infection of the skin, usually due to direct inoculation of the tuberculosis bacillus into the skin. It is no longer common. This type of lupus often starts in childhood, with dark red patches on the nose or cheek. Unless treated, lupus vulgaris spreads, ulcerates, and causes extensive scarring. Treatment is with antituberculous drugs.

lute *n.* (in dentistry) a thin layer of cement inserted into the minute space between a prepared tooth and a crown or inlay to hold it permanently in place.

lutein *n.* **1.** *see* xanthophyll. **2.** the yellow pigment of the corpus luteum.

luteinizing hormone (LH) a hormone (*see* gonadotropin), synthesized and released by the anterior pituitary gland, that stimulates ovulation, *corpus luteum formation, progesterone synthesis by the ovary (*see also* menstrual cycle), and androgen synthesis by the interstitial cells of the testes. Also called: **interstitial-cell-stimulating hormone (ICSH)**. *See also* LHRH analogue.

luteo- *prefix denoting* **1.** yellow. **2.** the corpus luteum.

luteotropin (luteotropic hormone) *n. see* prolactin.

LUTS *see* lower urinary tract symptoms.

lux *n.* the *SI unit of intensity of illumination, equal to 1 lumen per square meter. This unit was formerly called the meter candle. Symbol: lx.

luxation *n. see* dislocation.

lyase *n.* one of a group of enzymes that catalyze the linking of groups by double bonds.

lycanthropy *n.* a very rare symptom of mental disorder in which an individual believes that he is or that he can change into a wolf.

Lyell's disease *see* staphylococcal scalded skin syndrome. [A. Lyell (20th century), British dermatologist]

Lyme disease a disease caused by a spirochete, *Borrelia burgdorferi*, and transmitted by certain ticks of the genus *Ixodes*. It was originally described in the town of Lyme, Connecticut. Following a 3–32-day incubation period, a slowly extending red rash develops in approximately 75% of cases; intermittent systemic symptoms include fever, malaise, headache, neck stiffness, and muscle and joint pains. Later, 60% of patients have intermittent attacks of arthritis, especially of the knees, each attack lasting months and recurring over several years. The spirochete has been identified in synovium and synovial fluid. Neurological and cardiac involvement occurs in a smaller percentage of cases. Treatment is with tetracycline or penicillin.

lymph *n.* the fluid present within the vessels of the *lymphatic system. It consists of the fluid that bathes the tissues, which is derived from the blood and is drained by the lymphatic vessels. Lymph passes through a series of filters (*lymph nodes) and is ultimately returned to the bloodstream via the *thoracic duct. It is similar in composition to plasma, but contains less protein and some cells, mainly *lymphocytes.

lymphaden- (lymphadeno-) *prefix denoting* lymph node(s).

lymphadenectomy *n.* surgical removal of lymph nodes, an operation commonly performed when a cancer has invaded nodes in the drainage area of an organ infiltrated by a malignant growth.

lymphadenitis *n.* inflammation of lymph nodes, which become swollen, painful, and tender. Some cases may be chronic (e.g. tuberculous lymphadenitis) but most are acute and localized adjacent to an area of infection. The most commonly affected lymph nodes are those in the neck, in association with tonsillitis. The lymph nodes help to contain and combat the infection. Occasionally, generalized lymphadenitis occurs as a result of virus infections. The treatment is that of the cause.

lymphadenoma *n.* an obsolete term for *lymphoma.

lymphagogue *n.* an agent that stimulates the secretion of lymph.

lymphangi- (lymphangio-) *prefix denoting* a lymphatic vessel.

lymphangiectasis *n.* dilation of the lymphatic vessels, which is usually congenital and produces enlargement of various parts of the body (e.g. the leg in Milroy's disease). It may also be caused by obstruction of the lymphatic vessels. *See* lymphedema.

lymphangiography *n.* X-ray examination of the lymphatic vessels and lymph nodes after a contrast medium has been injected into them (*see* angiography). Its main uses are in the investigation of the extent and spread of cancer of the lymphatic system and in the investigation of lymphedema. Alternatively, the lymphatic system can be imaged using a gamma camera following the injection of a radioactive tracer. This examination has now largely been replaced by other *cross-sectional imaging techniques.

lymphangioma *n.* a localized collection of distended lymphatic vessels, which may result in a large cyst in the neck or armpit (*cystic hygroma*). This can be removed surgically.

lymphangiosarcoma *n.* a rare malignant tumor of the lymphatic vessels. It is most commonly seen in the chronically swollen (edematous) arms of women who have had a mastectomy for breast cancer and may be induced by radiation.

lymphangitis *n.* inflammation of the lymphatic vessels, which can be seen most commonly as red streaks in the skin adjacent to a focus of streptococcal infection. Occasionally, a more chronic form results in *lymphedema. The infected part is rested and the infection can be eliminated by an antibiotic.

lymphatic 1. *n.* a lymphatic vessel. *See* lymphatic system. **2.** *adj.* relating to or transporting lymph.

lymphatic system a network of vessels that conveys electrolytes, water, proteins, etc. – in the form of *lymph – from the tissue fluids to the bloodstream (see illustration). It consists of fine blind-ended lymphatic capillaries, which unite to form lymphatic vessels. At various points along the lymphatic vessels are *lymph nodes. Lymph drains into the capillaries and passes into the lymphatic vessels, which have valves to prevent backflow of lymph. The lymphatics lead to two large channels – the *thoracic duct* and the *right lymphatic duct* – which return the lymph to the bloodstream via the brachiocephalic veins.

lymphedema *n.* an accumulation of lymph in the tissues, producing swelling: the legs are most often affected. It may be due to a congenital abnormality of the lymphatic vessels (as in *Milroy's disease*, congenital lymphedema of the legs) or result from obstruction of the lymphatic vessels by a tumor, parasites, inflamma-

tion, or injury. Treatment consists of elastic support, by stockings or bandages, and diuretic drugs. A variety of surgical procedures have been devised but with little success.

lymph node one of a number of small swellings found at intervals along the lymphatic system. Groups of nodes are found in many parts of the body; for example, in the groin and armpit and behind the ear. They are composed of lymphoid tissue and act as filters for the lymph, preventing foreign particles from entering the bloodstream; they also produce lymphocytes.

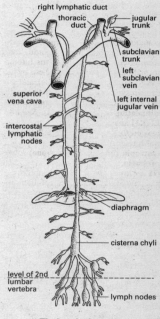

right lymphatic duct
thoracic duct
jugular trunk
subclavian trunk
left subclavian vein
left internal jugular vein
superior vena cava
intercostal lymphatic nodes
diaphragm
cisterna chyli
level of 2nd lumbar vertebra
lymph nodes

The lymphatic system

lympho- *prefix denoting* lymph or the lymphatic system.

lymphoblast *n.* an abnormal cell present in the blood and blood-forming organs in a type of leukemia (*lymphoblastic leukemia*). It has a large nucleus with very scanty cytoplasm and is thought to be the precursor of the lymphocyte. —**lymphoblastic** adj.

lymphocele n. a cystic mass of lymph in the tissues, which follows injury to, or operations upon, lymph nodes or ducts.

lymphocyte n. a variety of white blood cell (leukocyte), present also in the lymph nodes, spleen, thymus gland, intestinal wall, and bone marrow. With *Romanovsky stains, lymphocytes are seen to have dense nuclei with clear pale-blue cytoplasm. Lymphocytes with scanty cytoplasm are *small lymphocytes*; those with abundant cytoplasm are *large lymphocytes*. There are normally $1.5-4.0 \times 10^9$ lymphocytes per liter of blood. They are involved in *immunity and can be subdivided into *B lymphocytes* (or *B cells*), which produce circulating antibodies, and *T lymphocytes* (or *T cells*), which are primarily responsible for cell-mediated immunity. T lymphocytes can differentiate into *helper T cells, *cytotoxic T cells, or *suppressor T cells (*see also* killer cell). There is an increase in the number of lymphocytes in the blood and bone marrow in chronic lymphocytic *leukemia. —**lymphocytic** adj.

lymphocytopenia n. see lymphopenia.

lymphocytosis n. an increase in the number of *lymphocytes in the blood. Lymphocytosis may occur in a wide variety of diseases, including chronic lymphocytic *leukemia and infections due to viruses.

lymphogranuloma venereum a sexually transmitted disease that is caused by *Chlamydia* and is most common in tropical regions. An initial lesion on the genitals is followed by swelling and inflammation of the lymph nodes in the groin; the lymph vessels in the genital region may become blocked, causing thickening of the skin of that area. Early treatment with sulfonamides or tetracyclines is usually effective.

lymphography n. see lymphangiography.

lymphoid tissue a tissue responsible for the production of lymphocytes and antibodies. It occurs as discrete organs, in the form of the lymph nodes, tonsils, thymus, and spleen, and also as diffuse groups of cells not separated from surrounding tissue. *See also* immune system.

lymphokine n. a substance produced by lymphocytes that has effects on other cells involved in the immune system (*see* cytokines). An example is *interleukin-2 (IL-2).

lymphoma n. any malignant tumor of lymph nodes, including *Hodgkin's disease and *non-Hodgkin's lymphomas*. There is a broad spectrum of malignancy, with prognosis ranging from a few months to many years. The patient usually shows evidence of multiple enlarged lymph nodes and may have constitutional symptoms such as weight loss, fever, and sweating (the so-called "B symptoms"). Disease is usually widespread, but in some cases is confined to a single area, such as the tonsil. Treatment is with drugs such as chlorambucil or combinations of cyclophosphamide, vincristine, and prednisone, sometimes with the addition of doxorubicin and/or bleomycin; response to these drugs is often dramatic. Localized disease may be treated with radiotherapy followed by drugs. Patients with non-Hodgkin's lymphoma who do not respond to chemotherapy may be considered for a bone-marrow transplant.

lymphopenia (lymphocytopenia) n. a decrease in the number of *lymphocytes in the blood, which may occur in a wide variety of diseases.

lymphopoiesis n. the process of the production of *lymphocytes, which occurs in the *bone marrow as well as in the lymph nodes, spleen, thymus gland, and intestinal wall. The precursor cell from which lymphocytes are derived is thought to be the *lymphoblast.

lymphorrhagia n. the escape of the lymph from lymphatic vessels that have been injured.

lymphosarcoma n. a former term for non-Hodgkin's *lymphoma.

lymphuria n. the presence in the urine of lymph.

Lyon hypothesis the hypothesis that gene dosage imbalance between males and females, because of the presence of two X chromosomes in females (XX) as opposed to only one in males (XY), is compensated for by random inactivation of one of the X chromosomes in the somatic cells of females. The inactivated X chromosome becomes the Barr body (*see* sex chromatin). [M. F. Lyon (1925–), British geneticist]

lypressin n. an antidiuretic and vasoconstrictor drug used in the treatment of diabetes insipidus to decrease urinary loss. It is administered by intranasal spray. Adverse reactions, which are infrequent and mild, include nasal congestion and irritation, nausea, cramping, and angina in patients with vascular disease. Trade name: **Diapid.**

lys- (lysi-, lyso-) *prefix denoting* lysis; dissolution.

lysergic acid diethylamide (LSD) a *psychedelic drug that is also a *hallucinogen. It was formerly used to aid treatment of psychological disorders. Side effects include digestive upsets, dizziness, tingling, anxiety, sweating, dilated pupils, muscle incoordination, and tremor. Alterations in sight, hearing, and other senses occur, psychotic effects, depression, and confusion are common, and tolerance to the drug develops rapidly. Because of these toxic effects, LSD is no longer used clincally.

lysin *n.* a specific *complement-fixing antibody that is capable of bringing about the destruction (lysis) of whole cells. Names are given to varieties of lysin with different targets; for example, *hemolysin* attacks red blood cells; *leukolysin*, white cells; and a *bacteriolysin*, bacterial cells.

lysine *n.* an *essential amino acid. *See also* amino acid.

lysis *n.* the destruction of cells through damage or rupture of the plasma membrane, allowing escape of the cell contents. *See also* autolysis, lysozyme.

-lysis *suffix denoting* **1.** lysis; dissolution. **2.** remission of symptoms.

lysogenic *adj.* producing *lysis.

lysogeny *n.* an interaction between a *bacteriophage and its host in which a latent form of the phage (*prophage*) exists within the bacterial cell, which is not destroyed. Under certain conditions (e.g. irradiation of the bacterium) the phage can develop into an active form, which reproduces itself and eventually destroys the bacterial cell.

lysosome *n.* a particle in the cytoplasm of cells that contains enzymes responsible for breaking down substances in the cell and is bounded by a single membrane. Lysosomes are especially abundant in liver and kidney cells. Foreign particles (e.g. bacteria) taken into the cell are broken down by the enzymes of the lysosomes. When the cell dies, these enzymes

are released to break down the cell's components.

lysozyme *n.* an enzyme found in tears and egg white. It catalyzes the destruction of the cell walls of certain bacteria. Bacterial cells that are attacked by lysozyme are said to have been *lysed*.

lytic *adj.* **1.** pertaining to *lysis or a *lysin. **2.** producing lysis.

M

maceration *n.* **1.** the softening of a solid by leaving it immersed in a liquid. **2.** (in obstetrics) the natural breakdown of a dead fetus within the uterus.

Macleod's syndrome (Swyer-James syndrome) pulmonary *emphysema affecting only one lung and beginning in childhood or in adolescence; it occurs secondarily to necrotizing bronchitis, probably caused by a virus. [W. M. Macleod (1911–77), British physician]

macr- (macro-) *prefix denoting* large size. Example: *macrencephaly* (abnormally enlarged brain).

macrocephaly (megalocephaly) *n.* abnormal largeness of the head in relation to the rest of the body. *Compare* microcephaly.

macrocheilia *n.* hypertrophy of the lips: a congenital condition in which the lips are abnormally large. *Compare* microcheilia.

macrocyte (megalocyte) *n.* an abnormally large red blood cell (*erythrocyte), seen in certain anemias. *See also* macrocytosis. —**macrocytic** *adj.*

macrocytosis *n.* the presence of abnormally large red cells (*macrocytes*) in the blood. Macrocytosis is a feature of certain anemias (*macrocytic anemias*), including those due to deficiency of vitamin B_{12} or folic acid, and also of anemias in which there is an increase in the rate of red cell production.

macrodactyly *n.* abnormally large size of one or more of the fingers or toes.

macrodontia *n.* a condition in which the teeth are unusually large.

macrogamete *n.* the nonmotile female sex cell of the malarial parasite (*Plasmodium*) and other protozoa. The macrogamete is similar to the ovum of higher animal groups and larger than the male sex cell (*see* microgamete).

macrogametocyte *n.* a cell that undergoes meiosis to form mature female sex cells (macrogametes) of the malarial parasite (*see* Plasmodium). Macrogametocytes are found in the blood of humans but must be ingested by a mosquito before developing into macrogametes.

macrogenitosoma *n.* excessive bodily growth with marked enlargement of the genitalia. *Macrogenitosoma precox* is a variant occurring in early childhood.

macroglia *n.* one of the two basic classes of *glia (the non-nervous cells of the central nervous system), divided into *astrocytes and *oligodendrocytes. *Compare* microglia.

macroglobulin *n.* **1. (immunoglobulin M, IgM)** a protein of the globulin series that is present in the blood and functions as an antibody, forming an effective first-line defense against bacteria in the bloodstream. *See also* immunoglobulin. **2.** an abnormal form of IgM (*see* paraprotein) produced by *lymphoma cells or in other plasma-cell disorders, such as multiple *myeloma.

macroglobulinemia *n.* the presence in the blood of excessive amounts of macroglobulin, produced by malignant proliferation of the lymphocytes in certain *lymphomas.

macroglossia *n.* an abnormally large tongue. It may be due to a congenital defect, such as thyroid deficiency (cretinism); to infiltration of the tongue with *amyloid or a tumor; or to obstruction of the lymph vessels.

macrognathia *n.* a condition in which one or both jaws are unusually large.

macromelia *n.* abnormally large size of the arms or legs. *Compare* micromelia.

macronormoblast *n.* an abnormal form of any of the cells (*normoblasts) that form a series of precursors of red blood cells. Macronormoblasts are unusually large but have normal nuclei (*compare* megaloblast); they are seen in certain anemias in which red cell production is impaired.

macronutrient *n.* any essential nutrient required in relatively large quantities for the normal physiological processes of the body. These substances include the major elements, such as oxygen, hydrogen, carbon, calcium, chloride, potassium, phosphorus, magnesium, and sulfur. *Compare* micronutrient.

macrophage (clasmatocyte) *n.* a large scavenger cell (a *phagocyte) present in connective tissue and many major organs and tissues, including the bone marrow, spleen, *lymph nodes, liver (*see* Kupffer's cells), and the central nervous system (*see* microglia). Macrophages are closely related to *monocytes. *Fixed macrophages (histiocytes)* are stationary within connective tissue; *free macrophages* wander between cells and aggregate at focal sites of infection, where they remove bacteria or other foreign bodies from blood or tissues. *See also* reticuloendothelial system.

macropsia *n.* a condition in which objects appear visually larger than they really are. It is usually due to disease of the retina affecting the *macula but may also occur in spasm of *accommodation.

macroscopic *adj.* visible to the naked eye. *Compare* microscopic.

macrosomia *n.* abnormally large size. In *fetal macrosomia* a large baby is associated with poorly controlled maternal diabetes. The increased size is due to excessive production of fetal insulin and thence to increased deposition of glycogen in the fetus.

macrotia *n.* a congenital deformity of the external ear in which the *pinna is larger than normal.

macula *n.* (*pl.* **maculae**) a small anatomical area that is distinguishable from the surrounding tissue. The *macula lutea* is the yellow spot on the retina at the back of the eye, which surrounds the greatest concentration of cones (*see* fovea). Maculae occur in the saccule and the utricle of the inner ear (see illustration). Tilting of the head causes the otoliths to bend

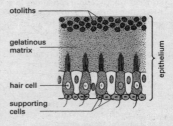

A macula of the inner ear

the hair cells, which send impulses to the brain via the vestibular nerve. *See also* labyrinth. —**macular** *adj.*

macular degeneration a group of conditions affecting the *macula lutea of the eye, resulting in a reduction or loss of central vision. *Age-related macular degeneration* (*AMD*, *ARMD*) is the most common cause of blindness in the elderly. Two types are commonly recognized. *Atrophic* (or *dry*) *AMD* results from chronic choroidal ischemia: small blood vessels of the choroid, which lies beneath the retina, become constricted, reducing the blood supply to the macula. This gives rise to degenerative changes in the retinal pigment epithelium (RPE; *see* retina), clinically recognized by macular pigmentation and the deposition of *drusen. *Wet AMD* is associated with the growth of abnormal new blood vessels under the retina, derived from the choroid (*see* [choroidal] neovascularization). These can leak fluid and blood into the RPE, which further reduces macular function. Laser surgery (*see* photocoagulation) can halt the degenerative process. *See also* vitelliform degeneration.

macule *n.* a flat circumscribed area of skin or an area of altered skin color (e.g. a freckle). *Compare* papule.

maculopapular *adj.* describing a rash that consists of both *macules and *papules.

maculopathy *n.* any abnormality of the *macula of the eye. For example, *bull's-eye maculopathy* describes the appearance of the macula in some toxic conditions (e.g. chloroquine toxicity) and in some hereditary disorders of the macula. *See also* epiretinal membrane (cellophane maculopathy).

madarosis *n.* **1.** a congenital deficiency of the eyelashes and eyebrows, which are sometimes absent altogether. **2.** a deficiency of the eyelashes alone, caused by chronic *blepharitis.

mad cow disease a colloquial name for bovine *spongiform encephalopathy.

Maddox rod a transparent rod that is used to change a point source of light into a linear streak, used in testing visual fusion. [E. E. Maddox (1860–1933), British ophthalmologist]

Madelung's disease the presence of multiple lipomas around the head and neck. [O. Madelung (1846–1926), German surgeon]

Madopar *n.* see benserazide.

Madura foot an infection of the tissues and bones of the foot producing chronic inflammation (mycetoma), occurring in the tropics. It is caused by various filamentous fungi (e.g. *Madurella*) and certain bacteria of the genera *Nocardia* and *Streptomyces*. Medical name: **maduromycosis**.

Madurella *n.* a genus of widely distributed fungi. The species *M. grisea* and *M. mycetomi* cause the tropical infection *Madura foot.

maduromycosis *n.* see Madura foot.

MAG3 *m*ercaptoacetyltriglycine: a *tracer used in nuclear medicine, during *renography, when labeled with technetium-99m. This agent is both filtered and excreted by the kidneys and gives similar results to *pentetic acid with a lower dose of ionizing radiation. It enables the function and drainage of each kidney to be assessed.

magenta *n.* see fuchsin.

maggot *n.* the wormlike larva of a fly, which occasionally infests human tissues (*see* myiasis). Formerly maggots were, in some cases, allowed to feed on dead and rotting tissues and so assist in the cleaning and healing of serious wounds. Interest in this ancient practice has revived in light of the growing resistance of bacteria to antibiotics: encouraging results were obtained in a recent clinical trial in which maggots were applied to refractory leg ulcers in patients unfit for surgery.

magic bullet a colloquial name for any drug treatment that is designed to target diseased tissue without adversely affecting healthy tissue. The term has been used especially in reference to new treatments for cancer.

Magill's forceps long angled forceps for use with a *laryngoscope in removing foreign bodies from the mouth and throat of an unconscious patient. [Sir I. V. Magill (1888–1975), British anesthetist]

magnesium *n.* a metallic element essential to life. The body of an average adult contains about 25 g of magnesium, concentrated mostly in the bones. Magnesium is necessary for the proper functioning of muscle and nervous tissue. It is required as a *cofactor for approximately 90 enzymes. A good source of magnesium is green leafy vegetables. Symbol: Mg.

magnesium carbonate a weak *antacid used to relieve indigestion, heartburn, and also pain due to stomach and duodenal ulcers. It is usually given with other compounds in mixtures, powders, and tablets.

magnesium hydroxide a magnesium salt used as an osmotic *laxative and in combination with other compounds as an *antacid. Trade names: **Maalox**, **Milk of Magnesia**, **Mylanta**, **Rolaids**.

magnesium sulfate a magnesium salt given in mixtures or enemas to treat constipation (*see* laxative). It is also administered by injection to treat magnesium deficiency and for the treatment of *preeclampsia and preterm labor. Side effects include flushing, nausea, and hypothermia.

magnesium trisilicate a compound of magnesium with antacid and absorbent properties, used in the treatment of heartburn and other digestive disorders. Trade name: **Gaviscon**.

magnetic resonance imaging (MRI) a diagnostic technique based on analysis of the absorption and transmission of high-frequency radio waves by the hydrogen in water molecules and other components of tissues when placed in a strong magnetic field (*see* nuclear magnetic resonance). Using modern high-speed computers, this analysis can be used to "map out" the variation in tissue signals in any plane and thus produce images of the tissues in most parts of the body. MRI can be used for the noninvasive diagnosis and treatment planning of a wide range of diseases, including cancer, and is increasingly used to guide interventional radiological procedures. It has the advantage that it does not use potentially harmful ionizing radiation, such as X-rays. However, MRI should not be undertaken in patients with pacemakers, metal clips, or metal heart valves because the strong magnetic field may cause damage. *See* interventional radiology, minimally invasive surgery.

magnetic resonance spectroscopy (MRS) a diagnostic technique that utilizes the phenomenon of *nuclear magnetic resonance to obtain a biochemical profile of

tissues by exciting elements other than hydrogen in water and other body components. It is particularly useful for biochemical analysis of tissues in the living body. The technique is still largely at the research level.

MAI complex a group of bacteria comprising *Mycobacterium avium* and *M. intracellulare*, which are responsible for *opportunistic infections of the lung. *See* Mycobacterium.

mal *n.* illness or disease.

mal- *prefix denoting* disease, disorder, or abnormality.

malabsorption *n.* a state in which absorption of one or more substances by the small intestine is reduced. It commonly affects fat (causing *steatorrhea), vitamins (such as B_{12}, folic acid, vitamin D, and vitamin K), *electrolytes (such as calcium, potassium), iron, and amino acids. Symptoms (depending on the substances involved) include weight loss, diarrhea, anemia, swelling (edema), and vitamin deficiencies. The most common causes are *celiac disease, *pancreatitis, *cystic fibrosis, *blind loop syndrome, or surgical removal of a length of small intestine.

malacia *n.* abnormal softening of a part, organ, or tissue, such as bone (*see* osteomalacia).

-malacia *suffix denoting* abnormal softening of a tissue. Example: *keratomalacia* (of the cornea).

maladie de Roger (Roger's disease) a form of congenital heart disease in which there is a small *ventricular septal defect. It usually causes no symptoms. [H. L. Roger (1809–91), French physician]

maladjustment *n.* **1.** failure of a body part, such as a muscle or tendon, to assume a correct position for proper functioning. **2.** (in psychiatry) failure of a person to fit into his physical and social environment, marked by irritability, depression, and anxiety.

malaise *n.* a general feeling of being unwell. The feeling may be accompanied by identifiable physical discomfort and may indicate the presence of disease.

malar bone *see* zygomatic bone.

malaria (ague, marsh fever, periodic fever, paludism) *n.* an infectious disease due to the presence of parasitic protozoa of the genus *Plasmodium* (*P. falciparum*, *P. malariae*, *P. ovale*, or *P. vivax*) within the red blood cells. The disease is transmitted by the *Anopheles* mosquito and is confined mainly to tropical and subtropical areas.

Parasites in the blood of an infected person are taken into the stomach of the mosquito as it feeds. Here they multiply and then invade the salivary glands. When the mosquito bites an individual, parasites are injected into the bloodstream and migrate to the liver and other organs, where they multiply. After an incubation period varying from 12 days (*P. falciparum*) to 10 months (some varieties of *P. vivax*), parasites return to the bloodstream and invade the red blood cells. Rapid multiplication of the parasites results in destruction of the red cells and the release of more parasites capable of infecting other red cells. This causes a short bout of shivering, fever, and sweating, and the loss of healthy red cells results in anemia. When the next batch of parasites is released symptoms reappear. The interval between fever attacks varies in different types of malaria: in *quartan malaria* (or *fever*), caused by *P. malariae*, it is three days; in *tertian malaria* (*P. ovale* or *P. vivax*) two days; and in *malignant tertian* (or *quotidian*) *malaria* (*P. falciparum*) – the most severe kind – from a few hours to two days (*see also* blackwater fever). Preventive and curative treatment relies on such drugs as *chloroquine, *quinacrine, and *pyrimethamine.

Malassezia *n.* a genus of fungi, formerly named *Pityrosporum*, producing superficial infections of the skin. *See* pityriasis.

malathion *n.* an organophosphorous insecticide used to treat head and pubic lice and scabies. It is applied externally in the form of a lotion; possible side effects are skin irritation and allergic reactions. Trade name: **Ovide**.

malformation *n.* any variation from the normal physical structure, due either to congenital or developmental defects or to disease or injury.

malignant *adj.* **1.** describing a tumor that invades and destroys the tissue in which it originates and can spread to other sites in the body via the bloodstream and lymphatic system. If untreated such tumors cause progressive deterioration and death. *See* cancer. **2.** describing any

disorder that becomes life-threatening if untreated (e.g. *malignant hypertension*). *Compare* benign.

malignant melanoma *see* melanoma.

malingering *n.* pretending to be ill, usually in order to avoid work or gain attention. Neck and low back pain are the most common complaints. It may be a sign of mental disorder (*see also* Münchausen's syndrome).

malleolus *n.* either of the two protuberances on each side of the ankle: the *lateral malleolus* at the lower end of the *fibula or the *medial malleolus* at the lower end of the *tibia.

mallet finger a condition in which a condition in which a finger (usually the index finger) is bent downward at the tip, due to *avulsion of the long extensor tendon from the bone. Treatment is to hold the tip of the finger straight with a splint for at least six weeks.

malleus *n.* a hammer-shaped bone in the middle *ear that articulates with the incus and is attached to the eardrum. *See* ossicle.

Mallory bodies large irregular masses located in the hepatocytes of the liver. They are found in patients with alcoholic hepatitis, Wilson's disease, primary biliary cirrhosis, severe obesity, and hepatocellular carcinoma. [F. B. Mallory (1862–1941), US pathologist]

Mallory's triple stain a histological stain consisting of water-soluble aniline blue or methyl blue, orange G, and oxalic acid. Before the stain is applied, the tissue is mordanted, then treated with acid fuchsin and phosphomolybdic acid. Nuclei stain red, muscle stains red to orange, nervous tissue stains lilac, collagen stains dark blue, and mucus and connective tissue become blue. [F. B. Mallory]

Mallory-Weiss syndrome tearing of the tissues around the junction of the esophagus (gullet) and stomach as a result of violent vomiting or straining to vomit. It is associated with *hematemesis and perforation of the esophagus. [G. K. Mallory (1926–), US pathologist; S. Weiss (1899–1942), US physician]

malnutrition *n.* the condition caused by an improper balance between what an individual eats and what he requires to maintain health. This can result from eating too little (*subnutrition* or *starva-

tion) but may also imply dietary excess or an incorrect balance of basic foodstuffs such as protein, fat, and carbohydrate. A deficiency (or excess) of one or more minerals, vitamins, or other essential ingredients may arise from *malabsorption of digested food or metabolic malfunction of one or more parts of the body as well as from an unbalanced diet.

malocclusion *n.* a condition in which there is an abnormal arrangement of the teeth, either within one jaw or in one jaw in relation to the other. If severe, it may require *orthognathic surgery.

Malpighian body the part of a *nephron comprising the blood capillaries of the glomerulus and its surrounding Bowman's capsule. [M. Malpighi (1628–94), Italian anatomist]

Malpighian layer the stratum germinativum: one of the layers of the *epidermis.

malposition *n.* (in obstetrics) an abnormal position of the fetal head when this is the presenting part in labor. The head is in such a position that the diameter of the skull in relation to the pelvic opening is greater than normal. This is likely to result in a prolonged and complicated labor.

malpractice *n.* professional misconduct: treatment falling short of the standards of skill and care that can reasonably be expected from a qualified medical practitioner.

malpresentation *n.* the condition in which the presenting part of the fetus (see presentation) is other than the head. Malpresentation is likely to complicate labor and may necessitate delivery by *cesarean section.

malt *n.* a mixture of carbohydrates, predominantly maltose, produced by the breakdown of starch contained in barley or wheat grains. The cereal grain is allowed to germinate and the malt is extracted with hot water. Malt is used for brewing and distilling; it has been used as a source of nutrients in wasting diseases.

MALT mucosa-associated lymphoid tissue: an important part of the peripheral lymphoid system with special features of immune cell production. It is associated with the digestive tract and is concentrated in such areas as the *tonsils and *Peyer's patches.

Malta fever *see* brucellosis.

maltase *n.* an enzyme, present in saliva and pancreatic juice, that converts maltose into glucose during digestion.

maltose *n.* a sugar consisting of two molecules of glucose. Maltose is formed from the digestion of starch and glycogen and is found in germinating cereal seeds.

malunion *n.* *union of a fracture in which the bone ends are poorly aligned. Arthritis of adjoining joints may develop as a complication later. *Osteotomy may be needed to correct the deformity and prevent the complication.

mamilla *n.* *see* nipple.

mamillary bodies two paired rounded swellings in the floor of the *hypothalamus, immediately behind the pituitary gland.

mamma *n.* *see* breast.

mammary gland the milk-producing gland of female mammals. *See* breast.

mammography *n.* X-ray examination of the female breast. Using low-energy X-rays, fine details of breast tissue can be visualized, particularly the presence of calcification or soft tissue masses enabling the early diagnosis of breast cancer. *See also* radiography, thermography.

mammoplasty *n.* plastic surgery of the breasts, in order to alter their shape or increase or decrease their size. In the case of sagging breasts skin and glandular tissue are removed and the remaining breast tissue is fixed in the normal position. After a mastectomy, or when the breasts are too small, a *prosthesis (*see* breast implant) may be inserted to improve the contour.

mammothermography *n.* the technique of examining the breasts for the presence of abnormalities by *thermography.

managed care a system that integrates the financing and delivery of medical care by means of contracts with physicians and with hospitals. Physicians and hospitals agree to provide comprehensive health care services, assure quality control, and provide incentives for patients to use their services. Providers of managed care are called *Health Maintenance Organizations or *Preferred Provider Organizations.

Manchester operation *see* Donald-Fothergill operation.

mancinism n. the condition of being left-handed.

mandible n. the lower jawbone. It consists of a horseshoe-shaped *body*, the upper surface of which bears the lower teeth (*see* alveolus, def. 2), and two vertical parts (*rami*). Each ramus divides into a *condyle* and a *coronoid process*. The condyle articulates with the temporal bone of the cranium to form the *temporomandibular joint* (a hinge joint). *See also* maxilla, skull. —**mandibular** adj

mandibular advancement splint (MAS) an orthodontic device used to advance the mandible to improve the airway in the pharynx during sleep in the treatment of obstructive *sleep apnea.

manganese n. a grayish metallic element, the oxide of which, when inhaled by miners in underventilated mines, causes brain damage and symptoms very similar to those of *parkinsonism. Minute quantities of the element are required by the body (*see* trace element). Symbol: Mn.

mania n. a state of mind characterized by excessive cheerfulness and increased activity. The mood is euphoric and changes rapidly to irritability. Thought and speech are rapid to the point of incoherence and the connections between ideas may be impossible to follow. Behavior is overactive, extravagant, overbearing, and sometimes violent. Judgment is impaired, and therefore the person may damage his own interests. There may be grandiose delusions. Treatment is usually with drugs such as lithium or phenothiazines. Hospital admission is frequently necessary. *See also* affective disorder, manic-depressive psychosis. —**manic** adj.

-mania suffix denoting obsession, compulsion, or exaggerated feeling for. Example: *pyromania* (for starting fires).

manic-depressive psychosis (bipolar disorder) a severe mental illness causing repeated episodes of *depression, *mania, or both. These episodes can be precipitated by upsetting events but are out of proportion to these causes. Sometimes chronic depression or chronic mania can result. The disease is genetically inherited but full expression can be altered by environmental factors. Treatment is with *phenothiazine drugs for mania and with *antidepressant drugs or, in severe cases, *electroconvulsive therapy for depression. *Lithium can prevent or reduce the frequency and severity of attacks, and the person is usually well in the intervals between them.

manikin n. see homunculus.

manipulation n. the use of the hands to produce a desired movement or therapeutic effect in part of the patient's body. Physiotherapists and osteopaths use manipulation to restore normal working to stiff joints.

mannitol n. a *diuretic administered by intravenous infusion to supplement other diuretics in the treatment of fluid retention (edema), to treat some kidney disorders, to relieve pressure in brain injuries, and also in the emergency treatment of glaucoma. Headache, chest pain, chills, fever, and dry mouth may occur following injection. Trade names: **Osmitrol, Resectisol**.

Mann-Whitney U test see significance.

manometer n. a device for measuring pressure in a liquid or gas. A manometer often consists of a U-tube containing mercury, water, or other liquid, open at one end and exposed to the fluid under pressure at the other end. The pressure can be read directly from a graduated scale. *See also* sphygmomanometer.

manometry n. measurement of pressures within organs of the body. The technique is used to record changes within fluid-filled chambers (e.g. cerebral ventricles) or to indicate muscular activity in motile tubes, such as the esophagus, rectum, or bile duct.

mantle adj. see treatment field.

Mantoux test see tuberculin. [C. Mantoux (1877–1947), French physician]

manubrium n. (pl. **manubria**) **1.** the upper section of the breastbone (*see* sternum). It articulates with the clavicles and the first costal cartilage; the second costal cartilage articulates at the junction between the manubrium and body of the sternum. **2.** the handlelike part of the *malleus (an ear ossicle), attached to the eardrum. —**manubrial** adj.

MAO see monoamine oxidase.

MAO inhibitor a drug that prevents the activity of the enzyme *monoamine oxidase (MAO) in brain tissue and therefore affects mood. MAO inhibitors include isocarboxazid, *phenelzine, and *tranylcypromine. They are *antidepressants, whose use is now restricted because of the severity of their side effects. These include interactions with other drugs (e.g. ephedrine, amphetamine) and foods containing *tyramine (e.g. cheese) to produce a sudden increase in blood pressure.

maple syrup urine disease (aminoacidopathy) an inborn defect of amino acid metabolism causing an excess of valine, leucine, isoleucine, and alloisoleucine in the urine, which has an odor like maple syrup. Treatment is dietary in mild cases, otherwise peritoneal *dialysis or *hemodialysis are effective. If untreated, it leads to mental retardation and death in infancy.

mapping *n.* (in genetics) the process of locating the relative positions of *genes on *chromosomes. *See also* Human Genome Project.

maprotiline *n.* a drug used to treat all types of depression, including that associated with anxiety (*see* antidepressant). It is administered by mouth and may cause drowsiness, dizziness, and tremor. Trade name: **Ludiomil**.

marasmus *n.* severe wasting in infants, when body weight is below 60% of that expected for age. The infant looks "old," pallid, apathetic, lacks skin fat, and has thin sparse hair and subnormal temperature. The condition may be due to *malabsorption, wrong feeding, metabolic disorders, repeated vomiting, diarrhea, severe disease of the heart, lungs, kidneys, or urinary tract, or chronic bacterial or parasitic disease (especially in tropical climates). Maternal rejection of an infant may cause marasmus through undereating. Acute infection may precipitate death. Treatment depends on the underlying cause, but initially very gentle nursing and the provision of nourishment and fluids by gradual steps is appropriate for all.

marble-bone disease *see* osteopetrosis.

Marburg disease (green monkey disease) a virus disease of vervet (green) monkeys transmitted to humans by contact (usually in laboratories) with blood or tissues from an infected animal. It was first described in Marburg, Germany. Symptoms include fever, malaise, severe headache, vomiting, diarrhea and bleeding from mucous membranes in the mouth and elsewhere. Treatment with

antiserum and measures to reduce the bleeding are sometimes effective.

march fracture a fracture through the neck of the second or third metatarsal bone, associated with excessive walking.

Marcus Gunn's jaw-winking syndrome a congenital condition characterized by drooping (*ptosis) of one eyelid. On opening or moving the mouth, the droopy lid elevates momentarily, resembling a wink. It is believed to be due to an abnormal innervation of the levator muscle by the trigeminal nerve. [R. Marcus Gunn (1850–1909), British ophthalmologist]

Marfan's syndrome an inherited disorder of connective tissue characterized by excessive height, abnormally long and slender fingers and toes (*arachnodactyly*), heart defects, and partial dislocation of the lenses of the eyes. [B. J. A. Marfan (1858–1942), French physician]

marijuana (marihuana) *n. see* cannabis.

Marion's disease obstruction of the outlet of the bladder caused by enlargement of the muscle cells in the neck of the bladder. [J. B. C. G. Marion (1869–1960), French surgeon]

Marjolin's ulcer a carcinoma that develops at the edge of a chronic ulcer of the skin, usually a venous *ulcer in the ankle region. [J. N. Marjolin (1780–1850), French surgeon]

marrow *n. see* bone marrow.

marsupialization *n.* an operative technique for curing a cyst. The cyst is opened, its contents removed, and the edges then stitched to the skin incision. The wound is kept open until it has healed by *granulation.

MAS *see* mandibular advancement splint.

masculinization *n.* development of excess body and facial hair, deepening of the voice, and increase in muscle bulk (secondary male sexual characteristics) in a female due to a hormone disorder or to hormone therapy. *See also* virilism, virilization.

masochism *n.* sexual pleasure derived from the experience of pain. The word is sometimes used loosely for all forms of behavior that lead to pain or humiliation. *See* sexual deviation. —**masochist** *n.* —**masochistic** *adj.*

massage *n.* manipulation of the soft tissues of the body with the hands. Massage is used to improve circulation, reduce edema, prevent *adhesions in tissues after injury, reduce muscular spasm, and improve the tone of muscles. *See also* effleurage, petrissage, tapotement.

masseter *n.* a thick muscle in the cheek extending from the zygomatic arch to the outer corner of the mandible. It is important for mastication and acts by closing the jaws.

mast- (masto-) *prefix denoting* the breast.

mastalgia *n.* pain in the breast.

mast cell a large cell in *connective tissue with many coarse cytoplasmic granules. These granules contain the chemicals *heparin, *histamine, and *serotonin, which are released during inflammation and allergic responses.

mastectomy *n.* surgical removal of a breast. *Simple mastectomy*, performed for extensive but not necessarily invasive tumors, involves removal of the breast; the skin and if possible the nipple may be retained and a prosthesis (*see* breast implant) may be inserted under the skin to give the appearance of normality. When breast cancer has spread to involve the lymph nodes, *radical mastectomy* may be performed. This classically involves removal of the breast with the skin and underlying pectoral muscles together with all the lymphatic tissue of the armpit. This treatment may be followed up with radiotherapy and/or chemotherapy. In modern surgical practice a modified radical mastectomy, preserving the pectoral muscles, is more usual than the classical technique. *See also* lumpectomy.

mastication *n.* the process of chewing food.

mastitis *n.* inflammation of the breast, usually caused by bacterial infection through damaged nipples. It most often occurs as acute *puerperal mastitis*, which develops during the period of breastfeeding, about a month after childbirth, and sometimes involves the discharge of pus. Chronic *cystic mastitis* has a different cause and does not involve inflammation. The breast feels lumpy due to the presence of cysts, and the condition is thought to be caused by hormone imbalance.

mastoid *n.* the *mastoid process of the temporal bone. *See also* mastoiditis.

mastoidectomy *n.* an operation to remove some or all of the air cells in the bone behind the ear (the *mastoid process of the temporal bone) when they have become infected (*see* mastoiditis) or invaded by *cholesteatoma. *See also* atticotomy.

mastoiditis *n.* inflammation of the *mastoid process behind the ear and of the air space (*mastoid antrum*) connecting it to the cavity of the middle ear. It is usually caused by bacterial infection that spreads from the middle ear: *see* (acute) otitis (media). Usually the infection responds to antibiotics, but surgery (*see* mastoidectomy) may be required in severe cases.

mastoid process a nipple-shaped process on the *temporal bone that extends downward and forward behind the ear canal and is the point of attachment of several neck muscles. It contains many air spaces (*mastoid cells*), which communicate with the cavity of the middle ear via an air-filled channel, the *mastoid antrum*. This provides a possible route for the spread of infection from the middle ear (*see* mastoiditis).

masturbation *n.* physical self-stimulation of the external genital organs in order to produce sexual pleasure, which may result in orgasm.

matched pair study *see* case control study.

materia medica the study of drugs used in medicine and dentistry, including *pharmacognosy, *pharmacy, *pharmacology, and therapeutics.

maternal mortality rate the number of deaths due to complications of pregnancy, childbirth, and the puerperium expressed as a proportion of all births (i.e. including *stillbirths). Formerly, the rate was expressed per 1000 births but with the low levels currently reported it is customary to use a base of a 100,000 births.

matrix *n.* **1.** (in histology) the substance of a tissue or organ in which more specialized structures are embedded; for example, the ground substance of connective tissue. **2.** (in radiology) the division of an image into rows and columns with equally sized elements (*pixels). The final image is completed by assigning a density to each of these elements. Increasing the number of pixels in the matrix improves the resolution of the final image. A typical value could be 256 rows × 256 columns.

matrix band a flexible strip that is placed round a tooth to restore a wall, thus simplifying insertion of a dental filling.

maturation n. the process of attaining full development. The term is applied particularly to the development of mature germ cells (ova and sperm).

maturity-onset diabetes of the young (MODY) a rare form of *diabetes mellitus caused by a number of identified genetic disorders and resulting in type 2 diabetes in people under 25 years old. Insulin is not required to treat the condition.

maxilla n. (pl. **maxillae**) loosely, the upper jaw, which bears the upper teeth. Strictly, the maxilla is one of a pair of bones that partly forms the upper jaw, the outer walls of the maxillary sinus, and the floor of the orbit. See also mandible, skull. —**maxillary** adj.

maxillary sinus see paranasal sinuses.

maxillofacial adj. describing or relating to the region of the face, jaws, and related structures.

maxwell n. a unit of magnetic flux equal to a flux of 1 gauss per square centimeter. It is equal to 10^{-8} webers.

Mayer-Rokitansky-Küster-Hauser syndrome a congenital absence of the vagina with varying degrees of development of the uterus, often associated with skeletal abnormalities. Fertility is often reduced but can sometimes be restored by surgery. [K. W. Mayer (1795–1868), German gynecologist; K. von Rokitansky (1804–78), Austrian pathologist; H. Küster and G. A. Hauser (20th century), German gynecologists]

Mayo operation an overlapping repair of an umbilical hernia. [W. J. Mayo (1861–1939), US surgeon]

mazindol n. a drug that reduces the appetite and is used in the treatment of obesity. Masindol is administered by mouth and may cause constipation, dry mouth, and insomnia. Trade names: **Mazanor, Sanorex.**

McArdle's disease an *inborn error of metabolism in which a deficiency of the enzyme myophosphorylase prevents the breakdown of glycogen to lactate in exercising muscle. This results in fatigue, pain, and cramps in exercising muscles. The only treatment is avoidance of sustained or excessive exercise. Medical name: **glycogen storage disease, type V** (or **type 5**) **glycogenesis**. [B. McArdle (20th century), British biochemist]

McBurney's point the point on the abdomen that overlies the anatomical position of the appendix and is the site of maximum tenderness in acute appendicitis. It lies one-third of the way along a line drawn from the anterior superior iliac spine (the projecting part of the hipbone) to the umbilicus. [C. McBurney (1845–1913), US surgeon]

McCormick toy test a hearing test used in preschool children in which the child must discriminate between similar speech sounds. The test consists of 14 toys that are paired because their names rhyme or sound similar; for example, tree and key, plane and plate. Having first identified all the objects, the child is then asked in a quiet voice to indicate a particular toy (e.g. Can you find the key?).

McCune-Albright syndrome *fibrous dysplasia of long bones coupled with *café au lait spots and precocious puberty, occurring in both males and females. [D. J. McCune (1902–76), US pediatrician; F. Albright (1900–69), US physician]

MCU micturating cystourethrogram. See urethrography.

ME myalgic encephalomyelitis. See chronic fatigue syndrome.

mean (arithmetic mean) n. the average of a group of observations calculated by adding their values and dividing by the number in the group. When one or more observations are substantially different from the rest, which can influence the arithmetic mean unduly, it is preferable to use the geometric mean (a similar calculation based on the logarithmic values of the observations) or – more commonly – the median (the middle observation of the series arranged in ascending order). A further method of obtaining an average value of a group is to identify the mode – the observation (or group of observations when these occur as a continuous quantitative *variable) that occurs most often in the series.

measles n. a highly infectious virus disease that tends to appear in epidemics every 2–3 years and mainly affects children. After an incubation period of 8–15 days, symptoms resembling those of a cold develop accompanied by a high fever. Small red spots with white centers (Ko-

plik's spots) may appear on the inside of the cheeks. On the third to fifth day, a blotchy slightly elevated pink rash develops, first behind the ears then on the face and elsewhere; it lasts 3–5 days. The patient is infectious throughout this period. In most cases the symptoms soon subside but patients are susceptible to pneumonia and middle ear infections. Complete recovery may take 2–4 weeks. Severe complications include encephalitis (one in 1000 cases) and *subacute sclerosing panencephalitis. Measles is a common cause of childhood mortality in malnourished children, particularly in the developing world. Vaccination against measles provides effective immunity (*see* MMR vaccine). Medical names: **rubeola, morbilli.**

meat- (meato-) *prefix denoting* a meatus. Example: *meatotomy* (incision into the urethral meatus).

meatus *n.* (in anatomy) a passage or opening. The *external auditory meatus* is the passage leading from the pinna of the outer *ear to the eardrum. A *nasal meatus* is one of three groovelike parts of the nasal cavity beneath each of the nasal conchae. The *urethral meatus* is the external opening of the urethra.

mebendazole *n.* an *anthelmintic drug used to treat roundworms, hookworms, pinworms, and whipworms. Side effects may include stomach upsets. Trade name: **Vermox.**

mecamylamine *n.* a drug used for the management of moderate to severe essential hypertension. It is administered by mouth and may cause dizziness, blurred vision, digestive upsets, and dry mouth. Trade name: **Inversine.**

mechanoreceptor *n.* a group of cells that respond to mechanical distortion, such as that caused by stretching or compressing a tissue, by generating a nerve impulse in a sensory nerve (*see* receptor). Touch receptors, *proprioceptors, and the receptors for hearing and balance all belong to this class.

mechanotherapy *n.* the use of mechanical equipment during physiotherapy to produce regularly repeated movements in part of the body. This is done to improve the functioning of muscles and joints.

mechlorethamine *n.* a drug used to treat various types of cancer, including Hodgkin's disease and some types of leukemia. It is administered by injection; common side effects include nausea and vomiting, and the drug may damage the bone marrow, causing serious blood disorders. Trade name: **Mustargen.**

Meckel's cartilage a cartilaginous bar in the fetus around which the *mandible develops. Part of Meckel's cartilage develops into the malleus (an ear ossicle) in the adult. [J. F. Meckel, the Younger (1781–1833), German anatomist]

Meckel's diverticulum *see* diverticulum.

meclizine *n.* an *antihistamine drug used mainly to prevent and treat nausea and vomiting, particularly in motion sickness, and also to relieve allergic reactions. It is administered by mouth. Trade names: **Antivert, Bonine, Dramamine.**

meclofenamate *n.* a nonsteroidal anti-inflammatory drug (*see* NSAID) used in the treatment of rheumatoid arthritis and osteoarthritis. It is given by mouth; common side effects include diarrhea, skin rash, and headache. Trade name: **Meclomen.**

meconism *n.* poisoning from the effects of eating or smoking *opium or the products derived from it, especially *morphine.

meconium *n.* the first stools of a newborn baby, which are sticky and dark green and composed of cellular debris, mucus, and bile pigments. The presence of meconium in the amniotic fluid during labor indicates fetal distress. Meconium examination is used as the basis of a newborn screening test for *cystic fibrosis. *See also* (meconium) ileus, (meconium) peritonitis.

meconium aspiration a condition occurring during childbirth in which the baby inhales meconium into the lungs during delivery. This can cause plugs in the airways and the baby may become short of oxygen (hypoxic). Treatment is to assist breathing if necessary, with physiotherapy and antibiotics.

media (tunica media) *n.* **1.** the middle layer of the wall of a *vein or *artery. It is the thickest of the three layers, being composed of elastic fibers and smooth muscle fibers in alternating layers. **2.** the middle layer of various other organs or parts.

medial *adj.* relating to or situated in the central region of an organ, tissue, or the body.

median *adj.* **1.** (in anatomy) situated in or toward the plane that divides the body into right and left halves. **2.** (in statistics) *see* mean.

mediastinitis *n.* inflammation of the midline partition of the chest cavity (mediastinum), usually complicating a rupture of the esophagus (gullet). *Sclerosing mediastinitis* often leads to *fibrosis, which may cause compression of other structures in the thorax, such as the superior vena cava, the bronchial tree, or the esophagus.

mediastinoscopy *n.* examination of the *mediastinum, usually by means of an endoscope inserted through a small incision in the neck region. It can be used to assess the spread of intrathoracic tumors and for lymph node biopsy.

mediastinum *n.* the space in the thorax (chest cavity) between the two pleural sacs. The mediastinum contains the heart, aorta, trachea, esophagus, and thymus gland and is divided into anterior, middle, posterior, and superior regions.

Medicaid a program of health-care services made available to medically indigent and other needy persons, regardless of age, under terms of a 1965 amendment to the US *Social Security Act. Medicaid funds are alloted as federal matching payments that vary, according to the state's per capita income, from 50% to as much as 83% of the cost of administrative and therapeutic services. Medicaid programs cover five basic services: inpatient hospital services, outpatient hospital services, other laboratory and X-ray services, skilled nursing home services, and physician services. Each participating state also is required to provide family-planning services and a program for screening children for physical defects and chronic conditions. States may include a variety of other health-care services on an optional basis. *See also* National Health Insurance.

medical *adj.* **1.** of or relating to medicine, the diagnosis, treatment and prevention of disease. **2.** of or relating to conditions that require the attention of a physician rather than a surgeon. For example, a *medical ward* of a hospital accommodates patients with such conditions.

medical audit a process by which doctors systematically review the procedures used for diagnosis, care, and treatment, examining how associated resources are used and investigating the effect care has on the outcome and quality of life for the patient. When this process is undertaken by doctors, nurses, and other health-care professionals, it is referred to as *clinical audit*.

medical committee a group of doctors on the staff of a hospital who give medical viewpoints on affairs concerned with overall policies on patient care, resource allocation, and the running of the hospital. Representatives of other hospital professions (nursing, administration, planning, and residents) are usually in attendance.

Medic Alert an international nonprofit organization founded in the US in 1947 that maintains a database of medical information for more than four million members worldwide that is available only to authorized personnel through a 24-hour emergency response center. Members wear the Medic Alert emblem on a bracelet or pendant that is quickly recognized by emergency response and law enforcement personnel.

medical examiner the official who presides at an inquest; formerly known as a *coroner*.

medical jurisprudence the study or practice of the legal aspects of medicine. *See* forensic medicine.

medical social worker a person with some medical training, employed to assist patients with problems that may arise through illness, such as domestic problems and obtaining assistance from state or federal agencies.

Medicare a national program of health insurance for persons who are 65 and older, disabled, or who have permanent kidney failure. The program, which was authorized under terms of a 1965 amendment to the US *Social Security Act, consists of two parts: hospital insurance, which provides coverage for inpatient hospital services, skilled nursing facilities, home health services, and hospice care; and medical insurance, which helps pay for the cost of physician services, outpatient hospital services, medical equipment and supplies, and other preventive services, such as cancer screening tests. Various supplemental insurance policies, managed care plans, and private fee-for-service plans are available to provide additional benefits not covered by Medicare. *See also* National Health Insurance.

medicated *adj.* containing a medicinal drug: applied to lotions, soaps, sweets, etc. Medicated dressings are applied to wounds to prevent infection and allow normal healing.

medication *n.* **1.** a substance administered by mouth, applied to the body, or introduced into the body for the purpose of treatment. *See also* premedication. **2.** treatment of a patient using drugs.

medicine *n.* **1.** the science or practice of the diagnosis, treatment, and prevention of disease. **2.** the science or practice of nonsurgical methods of treating disease. **3.** any drug or preparation used for the treatment or prevention of disease, particularly one that is taken by mouth.

medicochirurgical *adj.* of or describing matters that are related to both medicine and surgery. A medicochirurgical disorder is one that calls for treatment by both a physician and a surgeon.

medicolegal *adj.* relating to the legal aspects of the practice of medicine. There has been rapid expansion of the branch of the law relating to medicine due to the increasing number of court actions for accidents and injuries, many of them seeking compensation for negligence by doctors or hospitals.

meditation *n.* the process of intentionally focusing attention and awareness on a specific thought or image in order to eliminate external stimuli, reduce stress, and achieve a state of calmness and relaxation for both body and mind. It is one of the techniques used in *complementary medicine.

Mediterranean fever 1. *see* brucellosis. **2.** *see* polyserositis.

medium *n.* **1.** any substance, usually a broth, agar, or gelatin, used for the *culture of microorganisms or tissue cells. An *assay medium* is used to determine the concentration of a growth factor or chemical by measuring the amount of growth it produces in a particular microorganism; all other nutrients are present in amounts adequate for growth. **2.** *see* contrast medium.

MEDLARS *Medical Literature Analysis and Retrieval System*: a computerized bibliographic literature retrieval system of the National Library of Medicine, which is part of the *National Institutes of Health. The system consists of more than 40 databases and databanks containing references to medical articles in professional journals and books published since 1966. The databases are accessible through the Internet and are the source from which the *Index Medicus*, a monthly listing of published medical articles, is compiled. *See also* MEDLINE.

MEDLINE *MEDLARS on Line*: a computerized bibliographic database of the National Library of Medicine, the online segment of *MEDLARS. It references biomedical journal articles published since 1966 and is accessible through the library's PubMed Internet site.

medroxyprogesterone *n.* a synthetic female sex hormone (*see* progestogen) used to treat menstrual disorders (including amenorrhea and endometriosis) and certain cancers and (in combination with an estrogen) in *oral contraceptives and in *hormone replacement therapy. It is administered by mouth or injection. It is also used as a long-term contraceptive administered by *depot injection. Side effects include headache, fatigue, and backache. Trade names: **Curretab, Cycrin, Depo-Provera, Prempro, Provera**.

medulla *n.* **1.** the inner region of any organ or tissue when it is distinguishable from the outer region (the cortex), particularly the inner part of the kidney, adrenal glands, or lymph nodes. **2.** *see* medulla oblongata. **3.** the *myelin layer of certain nerve fibers. —**medullary** *adj.*

medulla oblongata (myelencephalon) the extension within the skull of the upper end of the spinal cord, forming the lowest part of the *brainstem. Besides forming the major pathway for nerve impulses entering and leaving the skull, the medulla contains centers that are responsible for the regulation of the heart and blood vessels, respiration, salivation, and swallowing. *Cranial nerves VI–XII leave the brain in this region.

medullary carcinoma (encephaloid) a soft tumor of the epithelium, containing little or no fibrous tissue, whose consistency was thought to resemble that of bone marrow; common sites include the breast and thyroid gland. *Medullary carcinoma of the thyroid* has associations with tumors of other organs (multiple endocrine neoplasia; *see* MENS) and is often familial: it arises from the *C cells of the thyroid and produces calcitonin, which can often be used as a *tumor marker.

medulloblastoma *n.* a malignant brain tumor (*see* cerebral tumor) that occurs during childhood. It is derived from cells that have the apparent potential to mature into neurons and develops in the cerebellum, the part of the brain that is predominantly involved in the control of balance. The flow of cerebrospinal fluid (CSF) may become obstructed, causing *hydrocephalus. Symptoms include headaches, dizziness, and unsteadiness. Treatment involves surgery to remove most of the tumor and restore CSF flow, followed by radiotherapy directed using *stereotactic localization. Medulloblastoma is the second most common form of cancer of childhood (after leukemia); recent advances have improved the survival rate so that 40% of affected children live for more than five years.

mefenamic acid an anti-inflammatory drug (*see* NSAID) used to treat headache, toothache, rheumatic pain, and primary *dysmenorrhea. It is administered by mouth; side effects include digestive upsets, drowsiness, and skin rashes. Trade name: **Ponstel**.

mefloquine *n.* a drug used in the prevention and treatment of malaria that is resistant to other drugs. It is administered by mouth; side effects include nausea and vomiting, dizziness, fatigue, and psychological disturbances, and the drug should not be taken during pregnancy, by psychiatric patients, or with beta blockers. Trade name: **Lariam**.

mega- *prefix denoting* **1.** large size, or abnormal enlargement or distension. Example: *megacecum* (of the cecum). **2.** a million. Example: *megavolt* (a million volts).

megacolon *n.* dilation, and sometimes lengthening, of the colon. It is caused by obstruction of the colon, *Hirschsprung's disease, or long-standing constipation, or it may develop as a complication of ulcerative *colitis (*toxic megacolon*).

megakaryoblast *n.* a cell that gives rise to the platelet-forming cell *megakaryocyte, found in the blood-forming tissue of the bone marrow. It is derived from a *hemopoietic stem cell and matures via an intermediate stage (called a *promegakaryocyte*) into a megakaryocyte.

megakaryocyte *n.* a cell in the bone marrow that produces *platelets. It is large (35–160 μm in diameter), with an irregular multilobed nucleus, and with *Romanovsky stains its abundant cytoplasm appears pale blue with fine reddish granules. *See also* thrombopoiesis.

megal- (megalo-) *prefix denoting* abnormal enlargement. Example: *megalomelia* (of limbs).

megaloblast *n.* an abnormal form of any of the cells that are precursors of red blood cells (*see* erythroblast). Megaloblasts are unusually large and their nuclei fail to mature in the normal way; they are seen in the bone marrow in certain anemias (*megaloblastic anemias*) due to deficiency of vitamin B_{12} or folic acid. —**megaloblastic** *adj.*

megalocephaly *n.* **1.** *see* macrocephaly. **2.** overgrowth and distortion of skull bones (*see* leontiasis).

megalocyte *n. see* macrocyte.

megalomania *n.* delusions of grandeur, such as being God, royalty, etc. It may be a feature of a schizophrenic or manic illness or of cerebral syphilis.

megaloureter (megaureter) *n.* gross dilation of the *ureter. This occurs above the site of a long-standing obstruction in the ureter, which blocks the free flow of urine from the kidney. A common cause of megaloureter is reflux of urine from the bladder into the ureters (*see* vesicoureteric reflux), but some of the most striking examples are found in so-called *idiopathic megaloureter*. In this condition, which may affect one or both ureters, there is a segment of normal ureter of varying length at the extreme lower end of the bladder, above which the ureter is enormously dilated. Both reflux and idiopathic megaloureter progress to urinary infection and/or renal impairment. Treatment is by corrective surgery.

-megaly *suffix denoting* abnormal enlargement. Example: *splenomegaly* (of the spleen).

megestrol *n.* a synthetic female sex hormone (*see* progestogen) that is used in the treatment of metastatic breast cancer and metastatic endometrial carcinoma. It is administered by mouth; side effects include weight gain, breakthrough bleeding, and nausea and vomiting. Trade name: **Megace**.

meglitinides *pl. n.* a group of *oral hypoglycemic drugs, including *repaglinide* (Prandin) and *nateglinide* (Starlix), used for treating type 2 *diabetes mellitus. They act by stimulating insulin release from the pancreas and should be taken before each meal.

meibomian cyst *n. see* chalazion.

meibomian glands (tarsal glands) small sebaceous glands that lie under the conjunctiva of the eyelids.

meibomianitis *n.* inflammation of the *meibomian glands of the eyelids.

Meige's syndrome an abnormality of muscle tone causing symmetrical spasms of the facial muscles, which produce lip retraction and uncontrolled jaw opening and closing and which may involve the eyes. [H. Meige (1866–1940), French physician]

Meigs' syndrome the rare combination of a benign ovarian *fibroma with *ascites and a right-sided pleural effusion. [J. V. Meigs (1892–1963), US gynecologist]

meiosis (reduction division) *n.* a type of cell division that produces four daughter cells, each having half the number of chromosomes of the original cell. It occurs before the formation of sperm and ova and the normal (*diploid) number of chromosomes is restored after fertilization. Meiosis also produces genetic variation in the daughter cells, brought about by the process of *crossing over. Meiosis consists of two successive divisions, each divided into four stages (*see* prophase, metaphase, anaphase, telophase). (See illustration.) *Compare* mitosis. —**meiotic** *adj.*

Meissner's plexus (submucous plexus) a fine network of parasympathetic nerve fibers in the wall of the alimentary canal, supplying the muscles and mucous membrane. [G. Meissner (1829–1905), German physiologist]

melan- (melano-) *prefix denoting* **1.** black coloration. **2.** melanin. Example: *melanemia* (presence in the blood of melanin).

melancholia *n. see* depression, involutional melancholia.

melanin *n.* a dark-brown to black pigment

occurring in the hair, the skin, and in the iris and choroid layer of the eyes. Melanin is contained within special cells (*chromatophores* or *melanophores*) and is produced by the metabolism of the amino acid tyrosine. Production of

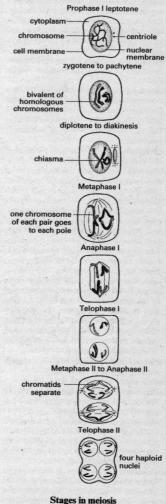

Stages in meiosis

melanin by *melanocytes* in the epidermis of the skin is increased by the action of sunlight (producing tanning), which protects the underlying skin layers from the sun's radiation.

melanism (melanosis) *n.* an unusually pronounced darkening of body tissues as a result of excessive production of the pigment *melanin. For example, melanism may affect the hair, the skin (after sunburn, during pregnancy, or in *Addison's disease), or the eye.

melanocyte *n.* a cell within the epidermis of skin that produces the pigment *melanin.

melanocyte-stimulating hormone (MSH) a hormone synthesized and released by the pituitary gland. In amphibians MSH brings about color changes in the skin but its physiological role in humans is uncertain.

melanoderma *n.* an abnormal increase in the skin pigment (*melanin).

melanoma (malignant melanoma) *n.* a highly malignant tumor of melanin-forming cells, the *melanocytes. Such tumors usually occur in the skin (excessive exposure to sunlight is a contributory factor) but are also found in the eye and the mucous membranes. They may contain melanin or be free of pigment (*amelanotic melanomas*). Spread of this cancer to other parts of the body, especially to the lymph nodes and liver, is common. In these cases melanin or its precursors (*melanogens*) may be excreted in the urine and the whole of the skin may be deeply pigmented. The prognosis is inversely related to the thickness of the tumor; almost all patients with tumors less than 0.76 mm survive following surgical excision.

melanonychia *n.* blackening of the nails with the pigment *melanin.

melanophore *n. see* melanin.

melanoplakia *n.* pigmented areas of *melanin in the mucous membrane lining the inside of the cheeks.

melanosis *n.* **1.** *see* melanism. **2.** a disorder in the body's production of the pigment melanin. **3.** *cachexia associated with the spread of the skin cancer *melanoma. —**melanotic** *adj.*

melanuria *n.* the presence of dark pigment in the urine. This may be caused by the presence of melanin or its precursors, in some cases of *melanoma; it may alter-

natively be caused by metabolic disease, such as *porphyria.

MELAS mitochondrial encephalopathy lactic acidosis and strokelike episodes: a rare metabolic disorder, usually inherited from the mother, that results in short stature and high levels of lactic acid in the blood (*see* lactic acidosis). Affected individuals are usually diagnosed in late childhood and early adult life. *See also* mitochondrial disorders.

melasma *n. see* chloasma.

melatonin *n.* a hormone produced by the *pineal body in darkness but not in bright light. Melatonin receptors in the brain, in a nucleus immediately above the *optic chiasm, react to this hormone and synchronize the nucleus to the 24-hour day/night rhythm, thus informing the brain when it is day and when it is night. Melatonin is a derivative of *serotonin, with which it works to regulate the sleep cycle, and is being used experimentally to treat jet lag, *SAD, and insomnia in shift workers and the elderly.

melena *n.* black tarry feces due to the presence of partly digested blood from higher up the digestive tract. Melena is not apparent unless at least 500 ml of blood has entered the intestine. It often occurs after vomiting blood (*see* hematemesis), having the same causes, but may be due to disease in the small intestine or upper colon, such as carcinoma or *angiodysplasia. *See also* hemorrhagic disease of the newborn (melena neonatorum).

melioidosis *n.* a disease of wild rodents caused by the bacterium *Pseudomonas pseudomallei*. It can be transmitted to humans, possibly by rat fleas, causing pneumonia, multiple abscesses, and septicemia. It is often fatal.

Melkersson-Rosenthal syndrome a rare disorder characterized by the occurrence together of facial paralysis, enlargement of the glottis, and swollen lips, which is due to lymphatic *stasis and the consequent build-up of protein in the facial tissues. [E. Melkersson (1898–1932), Swedish physician; C. Rosenthal (20th century), German neurologist]

melomelus *n.* a fetus with one or more pairs of supernumerary limbs.

melphalan *n.* a drug used to treat various types of cancer, particularly multiple myeloma but also including tumors of the breast and ovaries and Hodgkin's disease. It is administered by mouth or injection. Side effects include digestive upsets, mouth ulcers, *amenorrhea, and temporary hair loss. Trade name: **Alkeran**.

membrane *n.* **1.** a thin layer of tissue surrounding the whole or part of an organ or tissue lining a cavity, or separating adjacent structures or cavities. *See also* basement membrane, mucous membrane, serous membrane. **2.** the lipoprotein envelope that surrounds a cell (*plasma* or *cell membrane*). —**membranous** *adj.*

membrane bone a bone that develops in connective tissue by direct *ossification, without cartilage being formed first. The bones of the face and skull are membrane bones.

membranous labyrinth *see* labyrinth.

memory *n.* the mental faculty that receives, stores, and retrieves previously learned knowledge and all information regarding previously experienced sensations, impressions, ideas, and concepts. In short-term memory (STM) data and stimuli are stored briefly, unless reinforced, and deterioration occurs rapidly, sometimes within a few seconds or minutes (*see* Alzheimer's disease, dementia). Long-term memory (LTM) is considered the permanent storehouse of information and experience.

MEN multiple endocrine neoplasia. *See* MENS.

men- (meno-) *prefix denoting* menstruation.

menadione *n.* a synthetic form of *vitamin K that is used in the treatment of blood clotting disorders, especially those associated with hepatic and renal diseases and malabsorption syndromes. It is administered orally or by injection.

menarche *n.* the start of the menstrual periods and other physical and mental changes associated with puberty. The menarche occurs when the reproductive organs become functionally active and may take place at any time between 10 and 18 years of age. *Compare* gonadarche.

mendelism *n.* the theory of inheritance based on *Mendel's laws.

Mendel's laws rules of inheritance based on the breeding experiments of the Austrian monk Gregor Mendel (1822–84), which showed that the inheritance of characteristics is controlled by particles now known as *genes. In modern terms they are as follows. (1) Each body (somatic) cell of an individual carries two factors (genes) for every characteristic and each gamete carries only one. It is now known that the genes are arranged on chromosomes, which are present in pairs in somatic cells and separate during gamete formation by the process of *meiosis. (2) Each pair of factors segregates independently of all other pairs at meiosis, so that the gametes show all possible combinations of factors. This law applies only to genes on different chromosomes; those on the same chromosome are affected by *linkage. *See also* dominant, recessive.

Mendelson's syndrome inhalation of regurgitated stomach contents by an anesthetized patient, which may result in death from anoxia or cause extensive lung damage or pulmonary *edema with severe *bronchospasm. This is a well-recognized hazard of general anesthesia in obstetrics, and may be prevented by giving gastric acid inhibitors (e.g. *cimetidine, *ranitidine) or sodium citrate before inducing anesthesia. [C. L. Mendelson (1913–), US obstetrician]

Ménétrier's disease a disorder in which gross enlargement (*see* hypertrophy) of the cells of the mucous membrane lining the stomach is associated with anemia. [P. Ménétrier (1859–1935), French physician]

Ménière's disease (Ménière's syndrome) a disease of the inner ear characterized by episodes of deafness, buzzing in the ears (*tinnitus), and *vertigo. Typically, the attacks are preceded by a sensation of fullness in the ear. Symptoms last for several hours and between attacks the affected ear may return to normal, although hearing does tend to deteriorate gradually with repeated attacks. It is thought to be caused by the build-up of fluid in the inner ear. Drug treatments include *prochlorperazine to reduce vertigo in acute attacks and *betahistine as prophylactic treatment. Ototoxic drugs, such as *gentamicin, can be injected through the eardrum into the middle ear to reduce activity in the inner ear. Surgical procedures used include decompression or drainage of the *endolymphatic sac, *vestibular nerve section, and *labyrinthectomy. Medical name: **endolymphatic hydrops**. [P. Ménière (1799–1862), French physician]

mening- (meningo-) *prefix denoting* the meninges.

meninges *pl. n.* (*sing.* **meninx**) the three connective tissue membranes that line the skull and vertebral canal and enclose the brain and spinal cord (see illustration). The outermost layer – the *dura mater (pachymeninx) – is inelastic, tough, and thicker than the middle layer (the *arachnoid mater) and the innermost layer (the *pia mater). The inner two membranes are together called the *leptomeninges*; between them circulates the *cerebrospinal fluid.

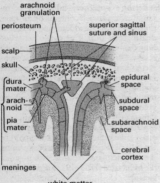

Section through the skull and brain to show meninges

meningioma *n.* a tumor arising from the fibrous coverings of the brain and spinal cord (*meninges). It is usually slow growing and produces symptoms by pressure on the underlying nervous tissue. In the brain the tumor may cause focal *epilepsy and gradually progressive neurological disability. In the spinal cord it may cause paraplegia and *Brown-Séquard's syndrome. Some meningiomas may behave in a malignant fashion and can invade neighboring tissues. Treatment of the majority of cases is by surgical removal if the tumor is accessible; some tumors may also require additional radiotherapy. Some patients have been known to have symptoms for as long as 30 years before the tumor has been discovered.

meningism *n.* stiffness of the neck mimicking that found in meningitis but without actual inflammation of the meninges. It is most common in childhood and is usually a symptom of chest infection or inflammation in the upper respiratory tract. Examination of the *cerebrospinal fluid reveals no abnormalities.

meningitis *n.* an inflammation of the *meninges due to infection by viruses, bacteria, or fungi. Meningitis causes an intense headache, fever, loss of appetite, intolerance to light and sound, rigidity of muscles, especially those in the neck (*see also* Kernig's sign), and in severe cases convulsions, vomiting, and delirium leading to death. The most important causes of bacterial meningitis are *Haemophilus influenzae* (especially in young children); two strains of *Neisseria meningitidis* (the meningococcus), B and C; and *Streptococcus pneumoniae* (*pneumococcal meningitis*). Immunization against *Haemophilus* meningitis is routine (*see* Hib vaccine), and a vaccine for meningitis C is now available but is not routinely used in the US; there is currently no vaccine available for meningitis B. In *meningococcal meningitis* (meningitis B and C, previously known as *cerebrospinal fever* and *spotted fever*) the symptoms appear suddenly and the bacteria can cause widespread meningococcal infection, which can culminate in *meningococcal septicemia*, with its characteristic hemorrhagic purple rash anywhere on the body. Unless rapidly diagnosed and treated, death can occur within a few hours.

Bacterial meningitis is treated with large doses of antibiotics administered as soon as possible after diagnosis. With the exception of herpes simplex *encephalitis (which is treated with acyclovir), viral meningitis does not respond to drugs but normally has a relatively benign prognosis. *See also* leptomeningitis, pachymeningitis.

meningocele *n. see* neural tube defects.

meningococcemia *n.* the presence of meningococci (bacteria of the species *Neisseria meningitidis*) in the bloodstream. *See* meningitis.

meningococcus n. (pl. **meningococci**) the bacterium *Neisseria meningitidis*, which can cause a serious form of septicemia and is a common cause of *meningitis. —**meningococcal** adj.

meningoencephalitis n. inflammation of the brain and its membranous coverings (the meninges) caused by bacterial, viral, or fungal infection. The disease may also involve the spinal cord, producing *myelitis with paralysis of both legs, sometimes called *meningomyelitis*.

meningoencephalocele n. see neural tube defects.

meningomyelitis n. see meningoencephalitis.

meningomyelocele n. see neural tube defects.

meningovascular adj. relating to or affecting the meninges covering the brain and spinal cord and the blood vessels that penetrate them to supply the underlying neural tissues. The term is used to describe tertiary syphilitic infection of the nervous system.

meninx n. **1.** the thin layer of mesoderm that surrounds the brain of the embryo. It gives rise to most of the skull and the membranes (meninges) that surround the brain. *See also* chondrocranium. **2.** see meninges.

meniscectomy n. surgical removal of a cartilage (meniscus) in the knee. This is carried out when the meniscus has been torn or is diseased, to relieve pain and "locking" of the knee joint. The operation can now be performed through an *arthroscope.

meniscus n. (in anatomy) a crescent-shaped structure, such as the fibrocartilaginous disk that divides the cavity of a synovial joint.

Menkes kinky-hair syndrome a genetic disorder characterized by severe mental retardation, seizures, poor vision, sparse colorless kinky hair; and chubby red cheeks. There is no treatment and affected infants usually die before the age of three. [J. H. Menkes (1928–), US neurologist]

menopause (climacteric) n. the time in a woman's life when the ovaries cease to produce an egg cell every four weeks and therefore menstruation ceases. The menopause can occur at any age between the middle thirties and the middle fifties, most commonly between 45 and 55. Natural menopause can only be established in retrospect after 12 consecutive months of *amenorrhea. Around the time of the menopause (the *perimenopause*) there are marked changes in the menstrual cycle. Menstruation may decrease gradually in successive periods or the intervals between periods may lengthen; alternatively there may be a sudden and complete stoppage of the periods. At the time of the menopause, there is a change in the balance of sex hormones in the body, which sometimes leads to hot flashes and other *vasomotor symptoms, palpitations, and dryness of the mucous membrane lining the vagina. Some women may also experience emotional disturbances. Some of these symptoms may be alleviated by *hormone replacement therapy. The term "menopause" is also used to refer to the postmenopausal period. —**menopausal** adj.

menorrhagia (epimenorrhagia) n. abnormally heavy bleeding at menstruation, which may or may not be associated with abnormally long periods. Menorrhagia may associated with hormonal imbalance (in which case it is described as *dysfunctional uterine bleeding*), pelvic inflammatory disease, tumors (especially fibroids) in the pelvic cavity, endometriosis, or the presence of an IUD. In some cases no obvious disease can be demonstrated.

menotropin n. a fertility drug consisting of gonadotropic hormones, extracted from the urine of postmenopausal women, used to induce ovulation and pregnancy in infertile women. The drug is administered by intramuscular injection. Adverse reactions include enlargement of the ovary accompanied by abdominal distention and pain, *hemoperitoneum, multiple pregnancy, and possible birth defects. Trade names: **Humegon, Pergonal.**

MENS multiple endocrine neoplasia syndromes: a group of syndromes characterized by combinations of symptoms and signs caused by tumors and/or hyperplasia of more than one endocrine gland. The tumors may involve the pituitary, thyroid, parathyroid, and adrenal glands and the pancreas, but some combinations predominate and are designated as type I (*Wermer's syn-*

drome), type IIA (*Sipple's syndrome*), and type IIB. Type I involves the parathyroid, pituitary, and pancreas, whereas type IIA involves the thyroid medullary cells, the adrenal medulla (*pheochromocytoma), and the parathyroids. Type IIB is similar to IIA, but patients tend to resemble people with *Marfan's syndrome and have multiple *neuromas on their mucous membranes. *See also* APUD cells.

menses *n.* **1.** the blood and other materials discharged from the uterus at menstruation. **2.** *see* menstruation.

menstrual cycle the periodic sequence of events in sexually mature nonpregnant women by which an egg cell (ovum) is released from the ovary at four-week intervals until the change of life (*see* menopause). The stages of the menstrual cycle are shown in the diagram. An ovum develops within a *graafian follicle in the ovary. When mature, it bursts from the follicle and travels along the fallopian tube to the uterus. A temporary endocrine gland – the corpus luteum – develops in the ruptured follicle and secretes the hormone *progesterone, which causes the lining of the uterus (*endometrium) to become thicker and richly supplied with blood in preparation for pregnancy. If the ovum is not fertilized the cycle continues: the corpus luteum shrinks and the endometrium is shed at *menstruation. If fertilization does take place, the fertilized ovum becomes attached to the endometrium and the corpus luteum continues to secrete progesterone, that is, pregnancy begins.

menstruation *n.* the discharge of blood and fragments of *endometrium from the vagina at intervals of about one month in women of child-bearing age (*see* menarche, menopause). Menstruation is that stage of the *menstrual cycle during which the endometrium, which is thickened in readiness to receive a fertilized egg cell (ovum), is shed if fertilization has not occurred. The normal duration of discharge varies from three to seven days. In *anovular menstruation*, discharge takes place without previous release of an egg cell from the ovary. *Vicarious menstruation* is bleeding from a mucous membrane other than the endometrium when normal menstruation is due. *Retrograde menstruation* is the backflow of blood and endometrial cells through the fallopian tubes (*see* endometriosis). *See also* amenorrhea, dysmenorrhea, epimenorrhea, hypomenorrhea, menorrhagia, oligomenorrhea.

mental[1] *adj.* relating to or affecting the mind.

mental[2] *adj.* relating to the chin.

mental age a measure of the intellectual level at which an individual functions; for example, someone described as having a mental age of 6 years would be functioning at the level of an average 6-year-old child. This measure has largely been replaced by a comparison of the functioning of persons of the same age group (*see* intelligence quotient, intelligence test).

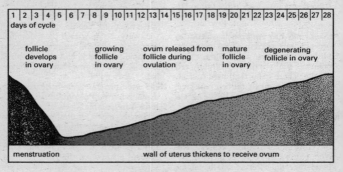

| 1 | 2 | 3 | 4 | 5 | 6 | 7 | 8 | 9 | 10 | 11 | 12 | 13 | 14 | 15 | 16 | 17 | 18 | 19 | 20 | 21 | 22 | 23 | 24 | 25 | 26 | 27 | 28 |

days of cycle

follicle develops in ovary

growing follicle in ovary

ovum released from follicle during ovulation

mature follicle in ovary

degenerating follicle in ovary

menstruation

wall of uterus thickens to receive ovum

The menstrual cycle

mental deficiency *see* mental retardation.

mental handicap delayed or incomplete intellectual development combined with some form of social malfunction, such as educational or occupational failure or inability to look after oneself. Good education alters the course of the handicap, for which the term *learning disability* (or *difficulty*) is now widely used. *See also* mental retardation.

mental illness a disorder of one or more of the functions of the mind (such as emotion, perception, memory, or thought), which causes suffering to the patient or others. If the sole problem is that the individual's behavior as a whole is out of line with society's expectations, then the term "illness" is not appropriate. Mental illness should be distinguished from *mental retardation, in which an individual has a general failure of development of the normal intellectual capacities. Mental illness is broadly divided into *psychosis, in which the capacity for appreciating reality is lost, and *neurosis, in which such capacity is retained.

mental impairment (mostly in legal usage) the condition of significant or severe impairment of intellectual and social functioning associated with abnormally aggressive or seriously irresponsible behavior.

mental retardation the state of those whose intellectual powers have failed to develop to such an extent that they are in need of care and protection and require special education. It is also known as *mental deficiency* and *mental handicap. The handicap may be classified according to the *intelligence quotient (IQ) as mild (IQ 50–70), moderate to severe (IQ 20–50), and profound (IQ less than 20). Mildly handicapped people often make a good adjustment to life after special help with education. The moderately and severely handicapped usually need much more help and most are permanently dependent on other people, while the profoundly handicapped usually need constant attention. There are very many causes of mental retardation, including *Down's syndrome, inherited metabolic disorders, brain injury, and gross psychological deprivation; some are preventable or treatable. Early therapy to improve motor and verbal skills

has allowed increasing numbers of people with mental retardation to remain in the community and become moderately self-sufficient.

mento- *prefix denoting* the chin.

mentum *n.* the chin.

meperidine *n.* a potent *analgesic drug with mild sedative action, used to relieve moderate or severe pain. It is administered by mouth or injection; side effects may include nausea, dizziness, and dry mouth, and *dependence may occur with prolonged use. Trade name: **Demerol**.

mephenytoin *n.* an *anticonvulsant drug used to prevent or reduce the severity of seizures in *epilepsy. It is administered by mouth; common side effects are drowsiness, dizziness, and nausea. Trade name: **Mesantoin**.

meprobamate *n.* a drug used to relieve anxiety and nervous tension (*see* anxiolytic). It is administered by mouth; side effects include digestive upsets, headache, and drowsiness. Trade names: **Equanil, Meprospan, Miltown**.

meralgia paresthetica painful tingling and numbness that is felt over the outer surface of the thigh when the lateral cutaneous nerve is trapped as it passes through the fibrous and muscular tissues of the groin.

mercaptoacetyltriglycine *n. see* MAG3.

mercaptopurine *n.* a drug that prevents the growth of cancer cells and is administered by mouth, chiefly in the treatment of some types of leukemia (*see* antimetabolite). It commonly reduces the numbers of white blood cells; mouth ulcers and digestive upsets may also occur. Trade name: **Purinethol**.

mercurialism (hydrargyria) *n.* mercury poisoning. Metallic mercury is absorbed through the skin and alimentary canal, and its vapor is taken in through the lungs. Acute poisoning causes vomiting, severe abdominal pains, bloody diarrhea, and kidney damage, with failure to produce urine. Treatment is with *dimercaprol. Chronic poisoning causes mouth ulceration, loose teeth, loss of appetite, and intestinal and renal disturbances, with anemia and nervous irritability. Treatment is removing the patient from further exposure.

mercury *n.* a silvery metallic element that is liquid at room temperature. Its toxicity has caused a decline in the use of its compounds in medicine during the 20th century; mercurial compounds were formerly used in the treatment of syphilis and as purgatives, teething pastes and powders, fungicides, and antiparasitic agents. Mercury is widely used in dentistry as a component of *amalgam fillings; when the mercury is combined with the filling alloy, it is nontoxic. Symbol: Hg. *See also* mercurialism, pink disease.

merocrine (eccrine) *adj.* describing a type of *secretion in which the glandular cells remain intact during the process of secretion.

merozoite *n.* a stage in the life cycle of the malaria parasite (*Plasmodium*). Many merozoites are formed during the asexual division of the schizont (*see* schizogony). The released merozoites may invade new red blood cells or new liver cells and continue the asexual phase with the production of yet more merozoites, effectively spreading the infection. Alternatively, merozoites invade red blood cells and begin the sexual cycle with the formation of male and female sex cells (*see* microgametocyte, macrogametocyte).

mes- (meso-) *prefix denoting* middle or medial.

mesaortitis *n.* inflammation of the middle layer (media) of the wall of the aorta, generally the result of late syphilis. Aneurysm formation may result. The infection can be eradicated with penicillin.

mesarteritis *n.* inflammation of the middle layer (media) of an artery, which is often combined with inflammation in all layers of the artery wall. It is seen in syphilis, polyarteritis, temporal *arteritis, and Buerger's disease.

mescaline *n.* an alkaloid present in *mescal buttons* (the dried tops of the Mexican cactus *Lophophora williamsii*) that produces inebriation and vivid colorful hallucinations when ingested.

mesencephalon *n. see* midbrain.

mesenchyme *n.* the undifferentiated tissue of the early embryo that forms almost entirely from *mesoderm. It is loosely organized and the individual cells migrate to different parts of the body where they form most of the skeletal and connective tissue, the blood and blood system, and the visceral (smooth) muscles.

mesentery *n.* a double layer of *peritoneum attaching the stomach, small intestine, pancreas, spleen, and other abdominal organs to the posterior wall of the abdomen. It contains blood and lymph vessels and nerves supplying these organs. —**mesenteric** *adj.*

mesial *adj.* **1.** medial. **2.** relating to or situated in the *median line or plane. **3.** designating the surface of a tooth toward the midline of the jaw.

mesiodens *n.* an extra tooth that may occur in the midline of the palate, between the central incisors, and may interfere with their eruption.

mesmerism *n.* *hypnosis based on the ideas of the 18th-century physician Franz Mesmer, sometimes using magnets and a variety of other equipment.

mesna *n.* a drug administered intravenously by injection or infusion to prevent the toxic effect of the drugs *ifosfamide and *cyclophosphamide on the bladder. It binds with the toxic metabolite acrolein in the urine. It is an orphan drug. Trade name: **Mesnex**.

mesoappendix *n.* the *mesentery of the appendix.

mesocolon *n.* the fold of peritoneum by which the colon is fixed to the posterior abdominal wall. Usually only the *transverse* and *sigmoid mesocolons* persist in the adult, attached to the transverse and sigmoid colon, respectively.

mesoderm *n.* the middle *germ layer of the early embryo. It gives rise to cartilage, muscle, bone, blood, kidneys, gonads and their ducts, and connective tissue. It separates into two layers – an outer *somatic* and an inner *splanchnic mesoderm*, separated by a cavity (*celom*) that becomes the body cavity. The dorsal somatic mesoderm becomes segmented into a number of *somites. *See also* mesenchyme. —**mesodermal** *adj.*

mesometrium *n.* the broad ligament of the uterus: a sheet of connective tissue that carries blood vessels to the uterus and attaches it to the abdominal wall.

mesomorphic *adj.* describing a *body type that has a well-developed skeletal and muscular structure and a sturdy upright posture. *Compare* ectomorphic, endomorphic. —**mesomorph** *n.* —**mesomorphy** *n.*

mesonephros (wolffian body) *n.* the second area of kidney tissue to develop in the embryo. Its excretory function only lasts for a very brief period before it degenerates. However, parts of it become incorporated into the male reproductive structures. Its duct – the *mesonephric* (or *wolffian*) *duct* – persists in males as the epididymis and vas deferens, which conduct sperm from the testis. —**mesonephric** *adj.*

mesophilic *adj.* describing organisms, especially bacteria, that grow best at temperatures of about 25–45°C. *Compare* psychrophilic, thermophilic.

mesoridazine besylate an *antipsychotic drug used in the treatment of schizophrenia, psychoneurotic conditions, behavioral problems associated with mental deficiency and chronic brain syndrome, and alcohol dependence. The drug is administered either orally or intramuscularly. Side effects include drowsiness, hypotension, tremor, and hypersensitivity reactions. Because the drug can cause life-threatening irregular heartbeats, it should only be used in patients who have not responded to other antipsychotic medications. Trade name: **Serentil.**

mesosalpinx *n.* a fold of peritoneum that surrounds the fallopian tubes. It is the upper part of the broad ligament that surrounds the uterus.

mesosome *n.* a structure occurring in some bacterial cells, formed by infolding of the cell membrane. Mesosomes are associated with the DNA and play a part in cell division.

mesotendon *n.* the delicate connective tissue membrane that surrounds a tendon.

mesothelioma *n.* a tumor of the pleura, peritoneum, or pericardium. The occurrence of pleural mesothelioma has a strong association with exposure to asbestos dust (*see* asbestosis), and workers in the asbestos industry who develop such tumors are entitled to industrial compensation. In other cases, however, there is no history of direct asbestos exposure, but the patients had been exposed to asbestos via the clothes of relatives who had had direct contact with asbestos, or they themselves has lived close to an asbestos factory. There is no curative treatment for the disease, but good results have occasionally been obtained from radical surgery for limited disease, from radiotherapy, and more recently from chemotherapy.

mesothelium *n.* the single layer of cells that lines *serous membranes. It is derived from embryonic mesoderm. *Compare* epithelium.

mesovarium *n.* the *mesentery of the ovaries.

messenger RNA a type of RNA that carries the information of the *genetic code of the DNA from the cell nucleus to the ribosomes, where the code is translated into protein. *See* transcription, translation.

mestranol *n.* a synthetic female sex hormone that is one of the most commonly used estrogens in *oral contraceptive pills and as hormone replacement therapy.

met- (meta-) *prefix denoting* **1.** distal to; beyond; behind. **2.** change; transformation.

metabolic syndrome (syndrome X) a common combination of conditions, including insulin resistance with type 2 diabetes, obesity with fat distribution mainly around the waist, high blood pressure, hypercholesterolemia, and early atherosclerosis, that increase the risk of developing heart disease, stroke, and diabetes.

metabolism *n.* **1.** the sum of all the chemical and physical changes that take place within the body and enable its continued growth and functioning. Metabolism involves the breakdown of complex organic constituents of the body with the liberation of energy, which is required for other processes (*see* catabolism) and the building up of complex substances, which form the material of the tissues and organs, from simple ones (*see* anabolism). *See also* basal metabolism. **2.** the sum of the biochemical changes undergone by a particular constituent of the body; for example, protein metabolism. —**metabolic** *adj.*

metabolite *n.* a substance that takes part in the process of *metabolism. Metabolites are either produced during metabolism or are constituents of food taken into the body.

metacarpal 1. *adj.* relating to the bones of the hand (*metacarpus). **2.** *n.* any of the bones forming the metacarpus.

metacarpus *n.* the five bones of the hand that connect the *carpus (wrist) to the *phalanges (digits).

metacentric *n.* a chromosome in which the

centromere is at or near the center of the chromosome. —**metacentric** *adj*.

metacercaria *n.* (*pl.* **metacercariae**) a mature form of the *cercaria larva of a fluke. Liver fluke metacercariae are enveloped by thin cysts and develop on various kinds of vegetation.

metachromasia (metachromatism) *n.* **1.** the property of a dye of staining certain tissues or cells a colour that is different from that of the stain itself. **2.** the variation in color produced in certain tissue elements that are stained with the same dye. **3.** the abnormal coloration of a tissue that is produced by a particular stain. —**metachromatic** *adj*.

Metagonimus *n.* a genus of small flukes, usually less than 3 mm in length, common as parasites of dogs and cats in the Far East, N. Siberia, and the Balkan States. Adult flukes of *M. yokogawai* occasionally infect the duodenum of humans if undercooked fish (the intermediate host) is eaten. They may cause inflammation and some ulceration of the intestinal lining, which produces a mild diarrhea. Flukes can be easily removed with tetrachloroethylene.

metamorphopsia *n.* a visual disturbance in which objects appear distorted. It is usually due to a disorder of the retina affecting the *macula (the most sensitive part).

metamyelocyte *n.* an immature *granulocyte (a type of white blood cell), having a kidney-shaped nucleus (*compare* myelocyte) and cytoplasm containing neutrophil, eosinophil, or basophil granules. It is normally found in the blood-forming tissue of the bone marrow but may appear in the blood in a wide variety of diseases, including acute infections and chronic *myeloid leukemia. *See also* granulopoiesis.

metanephros *n.* the excretory organ of the fetus, which develops into the kidney and is formed from the rear portion of the *nephrogenic cord. It does not become functional until birth, since urea is transferred across the placenta to the mother.

metaphase *n.* the second stage of *mitosis and of each division of *meiosis, in which the chromosomes line up at the center of the *spindle, with their centromeres attached to the spindle fibers.

metaphysis *n.* the growing portion of a long bone that lies between the *epiphyses (the ends) and the *diaphysis (the shaft).

metaplasia *n.* an abnormal change in the nature of a tissue. For instance, columnar epithelium lining the bronchi may be converted to squamous epithelium (*squamous metaplasia*): this may be an early sign of malignant change. *Myeloid metaplasia* is the development of bone marrow elements, normally found only within the marrow cavities of the bones, in organs such as the spleen and liver. This may occur after bone marrow failure.

metaproterenol *n.* a bronchodilator used in the treatment of bronchial asthma and reversible *bronchospasm, which may occur associated with bronchitis and emphysema. It is administered by mouth and as an inhalant; common side effects are nervousness, tachycardia, tremor, and nausea. Trade name: **Alupent**.

metaraminol *n.* a *sympathomimetic drug that stimulates alpha receptors and is used as a *vasoconstrictor to treat severe *hypotension occurring with spinal anesthesia. It is administered by injection. Trade name: **Aramine**.

metastasis *n.* the distant spread of malignant tumor from its site of origin. This occurs by three main routes: (1) through the bloodstream; (2) through the lymphatic system; (3) across body cavities, e.g. through the peritoneum. Highly malignant tumors have a greater potential for metastasis. Individual tumors may spread by one or all of the above routes, although *carcinoma is said classically to metastasize via the lymphatic system and *sarcoma via the bloodstream. —**metastatic** *adj*.

metastasize *vb.* (of a malignant tumor) to spread by *metastasis.

metatarsal 1. *adj.* relating to the bones of the foot (*metatarsus). **2.** *n.* any of the bones forming the metatarsus.

metatarsalgia *n.* aching pain in the metatarsal bones of the foot. Repeated injury, arthritis, and deformities of the foot are common causes, and corrective footwear and insoles may be prescribed.

metatarsus *n.* the five bones of the foot that connect the *tarsus (ankle) to the *phalanges (toes).

metathalamus *n.* a part of the *thalamus consisting of two nuclei through which impulses pass from the eyes and ears to be distributed to the cerebral cortex.

metencephalon n. part of the hindbrain, formed by the pons and the cerebellum and continuous below with the medulla oblongata. *See* brain.

meteorism n. *see* tympanites.

meter n. the *SI unit of length that is equal to 39.37 inches. It is formally defined as the length of the path traveled by light in vacuum during a time interval of 1/299 792 458 of a second. Symbol: m.

-meter *suffix denoting* an instrument for measuring. Example: *perimeter* (instrument for measuring the field of vision).

metformin n. a *biguanide drug that reduces blood sugar levels and is used to treat noninsulin-dependent *diabetes. It is administered by mouth and may cause loss of appetite and minor digestive upsets; it should not be used in patients with kidney disease, in whom it may cause *lactic acidosis. Trade name: **Glucophage**. *See also* oral hypoglycemic drug.

methadone n. a potent narcotic *analgesic drug administered by mouth or injection to relieve severe pain and as a linctus to suppress coughs. It is also used to treat heroin addiction and as maintenance therapy. Digestive upsets, drowsiness, and dizziness may occur, and prolonged use may lead to dependence. Trade names: **Dolophine, Methadose.**

methamphetamine n. a drug of the *amphetamine group. Methamphetamine chloride is administered by mouth to treat *attention-deficit/hyperactivity disorder; it has been used as a short-term adjunct in a regimen of weight reduction, but is no longer recommended for this purpose. Abuse of this drug may lead to dependence. Trade name: **Desoxyn.**

methanol n. *see* methyl alcohol.

methemalbumin n. a chemical complex composed of the pigment portion of hemoglobin (*heme*) and the plasma protein *albumin. It is formed in the blood in such conditions as *blackwater fever, in which red blood cells are destroyed and free hemoglobin is released into the plasma. In such conditions methemalbumin can be detected in both the blood and urine.

methemoglobin n. a substance that is formed when the iron atoms of the

blood pigment *hemoglobin have been oxidized from the ferrous to the ferric form (*compare* oxyhemoglobin). Methemoglobin cannot bind molecular oxygen and therefore cannot transport oxygen around the body. The presence of methemoglobin in the blood (*methemoglobinemia*) may result from ingestion of oxidizing drugs or from an inherited abnormality of the hemoglobin molecule. Symptoms include fatigue, headache, dizziness, and *cyanosis.

methenamine (hexamine) n. an *antiseptic with a wide range of antibacterial activity, used to treat infections and inflammation of the urinary tract, such as cystitis. Methenamine is administered by mouth. High doses may cause irritation of the stomach or bladder. Trade names: **Hiprex, Mandelamine, Urex.**

methicillin n. a semisynthetic penicillin that was originally used to treat infections by penicillin-resistant staphylococci. It has been superseded for this purpose by *cloxacillin sodium but continues to be used to test the drug sensitivity of staphylococci. *Methicillin-resistant staphylococci (MRS)* can be responsible for increasing rates of infection in hospitals. Until recently, such infections have responded to *vancomycin, but strains of bacilli have started to emerge that are resistant to both methicillin and vancomycin, giving rise to infections that are very difficult to treat. Trade name: **Staphcillin.** *See also* superinfection.

methimazole n. a drug that reduces thyroid activity, used to treat *thyrotoxicosis and to prepare patients for surgical removal of the thyroid gland. It is administered by mouth or injection; side effects include rashes, digestive upsets, and headache. Trade names: **Tapazole, Thiamazole.**

methionine n. a sulfur-containing *essential amino acid. *See also* amino acid.

methixene n. a drug with effects similar to those of *atropine, used to control the tremors and other symptoms in parkinsonism and to relieve spasm of smooth muscle in digestive disorders. It is administered by mouth; side effects can include dry mouth, disturbed vision, flushing, and dizziness.

methohexital n. an ultrashort-acting barbiturate anesthetic used for short surgical procedures and for induction of a hypnotic state. The drug is administered intravenously; side effects include respiratory depression, hypotension, headache, nausea, abdominal pain, and skin rash. Trade name: **Brevital**.

methotrexate n. a drug that interferes with cell growth and is used to treat various types of cancer, including leukemia and breast cancer (see antimetabolite), and for the management of severe rheumatoid arthritis in patients who do not respond to or tolerate other antirheumatic agents. It is administered by mouth or injection; common side effects include mouth sores, digestive upsets, skin rashes, and hair loss. Trade names: **Amethopterin, Rheumatrex, Trexall**.

methotrimeprazine n. a tranquilizing, sedative, and analgesic drug used to treat anxiety, tension, and agitation and to relieve moderate or severe pain. It is administered by intramuscular injection; common side effects are drowsiness and weakness. Trade name: **Levoprome**.

methoxamine n. a *sympathomimetic drug that causes blood vessels to constrict and thus raises blood pressure. It is administered by injection to maintain blood pressure during surgical operations. High doses may cause headache and vomiting. Trade name: **Vasoxyl**.

methoxyphenamine n. a *sympathomimetic drug used to treat asthma and other allergic conditions, such as rhinitis, and added to cough mixtures. It is administered by mouth and may cause nausea, dizziness, and dry mouth.

methyclothiazid n. a thiazide *diuretic used in the treatment of high blood pressure (*hypertension) and *edema associated with congestive heart failure, cirrhosis, other drug therapy, and kidney dysfunction. It prevents reabsorption of sodium, chloride, and, to a lesser extent, potassium. It is administered by mouth; side effects include loss of appetite, dizziness, and hypotension. Trade names: **Aquatensen, Enduron**.

methyl alcohol (methanol) wood alcohol: an alcohol that is oxidized in the body much more slowly than ethyl alcohol and forms poisonous products. As little as 10 ml of pure methyl alcohol can produce permanent blindness, and 100 ml is likely to be fatal. The breakdown product formaldehyde is responsible for damage to the eyes; it is itself converted to formic acid, which causes acidosis and death from respiratory failure. See also methylated spirits.

methylated spirits a mixture consisting mainly of ethyl alcohol with *methyl alcohol and petroleum hydrocarbons. The addition of pyridine gives it an objectionable smell, and the dye methyl violet is added to make it recognizable as unfit to drink. It is used as a solvent, cleaning fluid, and fuel.

methylcellulose n. a compound that absorbs water and is used as a bulk *laxative to treat constipation, to control diarrhea, and in patients with a *colostomy. It is administered by mouth and usually has no side effects. Trade name: **Citrucel**.

methyldopa n. a drug that acts on receptors in the brain to reduce blood pressure (see sympatholytic). Methyldopa is administered by mouth or injection, and drowsiness commonly occurs during the first days of treatment. Trade name: **Aldomet**.

methylene blue a blue dye used to stain bacterial cells for microscopic examination.

methylergonovine n. a drug that stimulates contractions of the uterus. It is used in childbirth to control bleeding following delivery and to help the uterus return to normal. It is administered by mouth or injection and may cause headache and vertigo. Trade names: **Methergine, Methylergometrine**.

methyl green a basic dye used for coloring the stainable part of the cell nucleus (chromatin) and – with pyronine – for the differential staining of RNA and DNA, which give a red and a green color, respectively.

methylphenidate n. a drug related to the *amphetamines that stimulates the central nervous system. It is used to treat attention-deficit/hyperactivity disorder in children, and to overcome lethargy associated with drug treatment. It is administered by mouth; side effects such as nervousness and insomnia may occur. Trade names: **Concerta, Metadate, Ritalin**.

methylprednisolone n. a glucocorticoid (see corticosteroid) used in the treatment of inflammatory conditions, such as rheumatoid arthritis, rheumatic fever, and allergic states, and for adrenocortical insufficiency. It is administered by mouth, intravenously, and intramuscularly; side effects include *electrolyte imbalance, muscle weakness, and abdominal distension. Trade names: **AmethaPred, depMedalone, Depo-Medrol, Medrol, Solu-Medrol**.

methyl salicylate oil of wintergreen: a liquid with *counterirritant and *analgesic properties, applied to the skin to relieve pain in lumbago, sciatica, and rheumatic conditions.

methyltestosterone *n.* a synthetic male sex hormone (*see* androgen) administered by mouth to treat sexual underdevelopment in men. It is also used to suppress lactation, to treat menstrual and menopausal disorders, and to treat breast cancer in women. Side effects are those of *testosterone. Trade names: **Estratest, Testred**.

methyl violet (gentian violet) a dye used mainly for staining protozoa.

methysergide *n.* a drug used to prevent severe migraine attacks and to control diarrhea associated with tumors in the digestive system. It is administered by mouth; common side effects are digestive upsets, dizziness, and drowsiness. Trade name: **Sansert**.

metoclopramide *n.* a *dopamine receptor antagonist that speeds up digestion. It is used to treat nausea, vomiting, indigestion, heartburn, and flatulence. It is administered by mouth or injection; high doses may cause drowsiness and muscle spasms. Trade names: **Maxolon, Octamide, Reglan**.

metolazone *n.* a *diuretic used to treat fluid retention (edema) and high blood pressure. It is administered by mouth; side effects include headache, loss of appetite, and digestive upsets, and blood potassium levels may be reduced. Trade names: **Mykrox, Zoroxolyn**.

metoprolol *n.* a drug that controls the activity of the heart (*see* beta blocker) and is used to treat high blood pressure and angina. It is administered by mouth; the most common side effects are tiredness and digestive upsets. Trade names: **Lopressor, Toprol XL**.

metr- (metro-) *prefix denoting* the uterus.

metric system a decimal system of measurement based on the *meter as the unit of length, the *liter as the unit of volume,

and the *gram as the unit of weight. It is the universal system for scientific and medical use. *See also* SI units.

metritis *n.* inflammation of the uterus. *See also* endometritis, myometritis.

metronidazole *n.* a drug used to treat infections of the urinary, genital, and digestive systems (such as trichomoniasis, amebiasis, and giardiasis) and acute ulcerative gingivitis, and to control rosacea. It is administered by mouth, by injection, or in suppositories; side effects include digestive upsets, drowsiness, headache, and an unpleasant metallic taste in the mouth. Trade names: **Flagyl, MetroGel, Metro I.V., Protostat**.

metropathia hemorrhagica irregular episodes of bleeding from the uterus, without previous ovulation, due to excessive estrogenic activity. It is associated with *endometrial hyperplasia and usually with follicular cysts of the ovary.

metroptosis *n.* *prolapse of the uterus.

metrorrhagia *n.* bleeding from the uterus other than the normal menstrual periods. It may indicate serious disease and should always be investigated.

-metry *suffix denoting* measuring or measurement.

metyrapone *n.* a drug that interferes with the production of the hormones *cortisol and *aldosterone and is used in the treatment of *Cushing's syndrome. It is administered by mouth. Side effects may include nausea, vomiting, low blood pressure, and allergic reactions. Trade name: **Metopirone**.

mexiletine *n.* an *antiarrhythmic drug used in the treatment or prevention of severe heart irregularity arising in the lower chambers (ventricles). It is administered by mouth. Possible side effects include nausea and vomiting, dizziness, tremor, and double vision. Trade name: **Mexitil**.

mg *symbol for* milligram.

MHC major histocompatibility complex: a series of genes located on chromosome 6 that code for antigens, including the HLA antigens (*see* HLA system), that are important in the determination of histocompatibility.

MIBG *meta*iodobenzylguanidine: a radioactive *tracer, labeled with iodine-123 or iodine-131, which binds to adrenergic nerve tissue. With the aid of a gamma camera, it can be used to detect the presence of a range of adrenergic tumors, including *neuroblastoma and *pheochromocytoma.

micelle *n.* one of the microscopic particles into which the products of fat digestion (i.e. fatty acids and monoglycerides), present in the intestinal tract, are dispersed by the action of *bile salts. Fatty material in this finely dispersed form is more easily absorbed by the small intestine.

miconazole *n.* a drug used to treat fungal infections, such as *ringworm of the scalp, body, and feet, fungal meningitis, coccidioidomycosis, and candidiasis. It is administered by intravenous injection, intravaginally, and topically; side effects include itching, skin rash, and nausea and vomiting. Trade names: **Micatin, Monistat, Zeasorb-AF**.

micr- (micro-) *prefix denoting* **1.** small size. **2.** one millionth part.

microaerophilic *adj.* describing microorganisms that grow best at very low oxygen concentrations (i.e. below the atmospheric level).

microalbuminuria *n.* the presence of albumin in the urine at levels that are higher than normal but lower than those detected by standard screening methods. The measured cut-offs are 30–300 mg/24 hours. Microalbuminuria is an important risk factor for the development of cardiac disease among diabetics. Its presence can be reversed by medication and careful control of blood pressure.

microaneurysm *n.* a minute localized swelling of a capillary wall, which is found in the retina of patients with diabetic *retinopathy. It is recognized as a small red dot when the interior of the eye is examined with an *ophthalmoscope.

microangiopathy *n.* damage to the walls of the smallest blood vessels. It may result from a variety of diseases, including diabetes mellitus, connective tissue diseases, infections, and cancer. Common manifestations of microangiopathy are kidney failure, hemolysis (damage to red blood cells), and purpura (bleeding into the skin). The treatment is that of the underlying cause.

microbe *n. see* microorganism.

microbial keratitis infection of the eye caused by wearing contact lenses. The infecting organisms are usually gram-

negative; *Pseudomonas* is a common cause. Contamination occurs when the contact lens equipment and solutions are handled improperly. Treatment is with topical cefazolin and tobramycin.

microbiology *n.* the science of *microorganisms. Microbiology in relation to medicine is concerned mainly with the isolation and identification of the microorganisms that cause disease. —**microbiological** *adj.* —**microbiologist** *n.*

microblepharon (microblepharism) *n.* the condition of having abnormally small eyelids.

microbubbles *pl. n.* (in radiology) an ultrasound *contrast medium consisting of small bubbles containing gas that are introduced into the vascular system or the fallopian tubes in order to enhance ultrasound images.

microcephaly *n.* abnormal smallness of the head in relation to the size of the rest of the body: a congenital condition in which the brain is not fully developed. *Compare* macrocephaly.

microcheilia *n.* abnormally small size of the lips. *Compare* macrocheilia.

Micrococcus *n.* a genus of spherical grampositive bacteria occurring in colonies. They are saprophytes or parasites. The species *M. tetragenus* (formerly *Gaffkya tetragena*) is normally a harmless parasite in humans but it can become pathogenic, causing arthritis, endocarditis, meningitis, or abscesses in tissues. It occurs in groups of four.

microcyte *n.* an abnormally small red blood cell (*erythrocyte). *See also* microcytosis. —**microcytic** *adj.*

microcytosis *n.* the presence of abnormally small red cells (*microcytes*) in the blood. Microcytosis is a feature of *microcytic anemias*, which include iron-deficiency anemias, certain *hemoglobinopathies, anemias associated with chronic infections, etc.

microdactyly *n.* abnormal smallness or shortness of the fingers.

microdiskectomy *n.* surgical removal of all or part of a *prolapsed intervertebral disk using an *operating microscope, a very short incision, and very fine instruments that can be inserted between the individual vertebrae of the backbone. The procedure is used to relieve pressure on spinal nerve roots or on the spinal cord caused by protrusion of the pulpy matter of the disk (*nucleus pulposus*). This is a form of *minimally invasive surgery.

microdissection *n.* the process of dissecting minute structures under the microscope. Miniature surgical instruments, such as knives made of glass, are manipulated by means of geared connections that reduce the relatively coarse movements of the operator's fingers into microscopic movements. Using this technique, it is possible to dissect the nuclei of cells and even to separate individual chromosomes. *See also* microsurgery.

microdontia *n.* a condition in which the teeth are unusually small.

microelectrode *n.* an extremely fine wire used as an electrode to measure the electrical activity in small areas of tissue. Microelectrodes can be used for recording the electrical changes that occur in the membranes of cells, such as those of nerve and muscle.

microfilaria *n.* (*pl.* **microfilariae**) the motile embryo of certain nematodes (*see* filaria). The slender microfilariae, 150–300 μm in length, are commonly found in the circulating blood or lymph of patients with an infection of any of the filarial worms, e.g. *Wuchereria*. They mature into larvae, which are infective, within the body of a bloodsucking insect, such as a mosquito.

microgamete *n.* the motile flagellate male sex cell of the malarial parasite (*Plasmodium*) and other protozoa. The microgamete is similar to the sperm cell of higher animal groups and smaller than the female sex cell (*see* macrogamete).

microgametocyte *n.* a cell that undergoes meiosis to form 6–8 mature male sex cells (microgametes) of the malarial parasite (*see* Plasmodium). Microgametocytes are found in the blood of humans but must be ingested by a mosquito before developing into microgametes.

microglia *n.* one of the two basic classes of *glia (the non-nervous cells of the central nervous system), having a mainly scavenging function (*see* macrophage). *Compare* macroglia.

microglossia *n.* abnormally small size of the tongue.

micrognathia *n.* a condition in which one or both jaws are unusually small.

microgram *n.* one millionth of a gram. Symbol: μg.

micrograph (photomicrograph) *n.* a photograph of an object viewed through a microscope. An *electron micrograph* is photographed through an electron microscope; a *light micrograph* through a light microscope.

microgyria *n.* a developmental disorder of the brain in which the folds (convolutions) in its surface are small and its surface layer (cortex) is structurally abnormal. It is associated with mental and physical retardation.

microhematocrit *n.* a measurement of the proportion of red blood cells in a volume of circulating blood. It is determined by taking a sample of the patient's blood in a fine tube and spinning it in a centrifuge until settling is complete. *See* packed cell volume.

micromanipulation *n.* the manipulation of extremely small structures under the microscope, as in *microdissection, or *microsurgery.

micromelia *n.* abnormally small size of the arms or legs. *Compare* macromelia.

micrometastasis *n.* a secondary tumor that is undetectable by clinical examination or diagnostic tests but is visible under the microscope.

micrometer[1] *n.* an instrument for making extremely fine measurements of thickness or length, often relying upon the movement of a screw thread and the principle of the *vernier.

micrometer[2] *n.* one millionth of a meter (10^{-6} m). Symbol: μm.

micronutrient *n.* any essential dietary substance, such as any of the *vitamins or *trace elements, that is required only in minute quantities for the normal physiological processes of the body. *Compare* macronutrient.

microorganism (microbe) *n.* any organism too small to be visible to the naked eye. Microorganisms include *bacteria, some *fungi, *mycoplasmas, *protozoa, *rickettsiae, and *viruses.

microphotograph *n.* **1.** a photograph reduced to microscopic proportions. **2.** (loosely) a *photomicrograph.

microphthalmos (nanophthalmos) *n.* a congenitally small eye, usually associated with a small eye socket.

micropipette *n.* an extremely fine tube from which minute volumes of liquid can be delivered. It can also be used to draw up minute quantities of liquid for examination. Using a micropipette, it is possible to add or take away material from individual cells under the microscope.

micropsia *n.* a condition in which objects appear smaller than they really are. It is usually due to disease of the retina affecting the *macula but may occur in paralysis of *accommodation.

microscope *n.* an instrument for producing a greatly magnified image of an object, which may be so small as to be invisible to the naked eye. *Light* or *optical microscopes* use light as a radiation source for viewing the specimen and combinations of lenses to magnify the image, usually an *objective and an *eyepiece. *See also* electron microscope, operating microscope, ultramicroscope. —**microscopical** *adj.* —**microscopy** *n.*

microscopic *adj.* **1.** too small to be seen clearly without the use of a microscope. **2.** of, relating to, or using a microscope.

microsome *n.* a small particle consisting of a piece of *endoplasmic reticulum with ribosomes attached. Microsomes are formed when homogenized cells are centrifuged. —**microsomal** *adj.*

Microsporum *n.* a genus of fungi causing *ringworm. *See also* dermatophyte.

microsurgery *n.* the branch of surgery in which extremely intricate operations are performed through highly refined *operating microscopes using miniaturized precision instruments (forceps, scissors, needles, etc.). The technique enables surgery of previously inaccessible parts of the eye, inner ear, spinal cord, and brain (e.g. for the removal of tumors and repair of cerebral aneurysms), as well as the reattachment of amputated fingers and limbs (necessitating the suturing of minute nerves and blood vessels) and the reversal of vasectomies.

microsurgical epididymal sperm aspiration the removal of spermatozoa from the epididymis by needle *aspiration. This procedure, performed under anesthetic, may be undertaken to assist conception in cases in which the normal passage of sperm from the testis is obstructed, for example, by blockage (through infection) of the ducts or by vasectomy. The extracted sperm are subjected to special treatment to select the strongest and most motile; these are then chemically treated to activate them and used for *in vitro fertilization.

microtia *n.* a congenital deformity of the external ear in which the *pinna is small or absent. The ear canal may also be absent, giving a conductive *deafness. Microtia may be associated with other congenital deformities.

microtome *n.* an instrument for cutting extremely thin slices of material that can be examined under a microscope. The material is usually embedded in a suitable medium, such as paraffin wax. A common type of microtome is a steel knife.

microvascular *adj.* involving small vessels. The term is often applied to techniques of *microsurgery for reuniting small blood vessels (the same techniques are applied frequently to nerve suture).

microvillus *n.* (*pl.* **microvilli**) one of a number of microscopic hairlike structures (about 5 μm long) projecting from the surface of epithelial cells (*see* epithelium). They serve to increase the surface area of the cell and are seen on absorptive and secretory cells. In some regions (particularly the intestinal tract) microvilli form a dense covering on the free surface of the cells: this is called a *brush border*.

microwave therapy a form of *diathermy using electromagnetic waves of extremely short wavelength. In a modern apparatus the electric currents induced in the tissues have frequencies of up to 25,000 million cycles per second.

micturating cystourethrogram (MCU) *see* urethrography.

micturition *n. see* urination.

midazolam *n.* a *benzodiazepine drug used as a sedative for minor surgery, as a premedication, and to induce general anesthesia. It is administered by injection. Possible side effects include headache, dizziness, and difficulty in breathing. Trade name: **Versed**.

midbrain (mesencephalon) *n.* the small portion of the *brainstem, excluding the pons and the medulla, that joins the hindbrain to the forebrain.

middle ear (tympanic cavity) the part of the *ear that consists of an air-filled space within the petrous part of the temporal bone. It is lined with mucous membrane and is connected to the pharynx by the *eustachian tube and to the outer ear by the eardrum (*tympanic membrane). Within the middle ear are three bones – the auditory *ossicles – which transmit sound vibrations from the outer ear to the inner ear (see labyrinth).

midgut n. the middle portion of the embryonic gut, which gives rise to most of the small intestine and part of the large intestine. Early in development it is connected with the *yolk sac outside the embryo via the *umbilicus.

midstream specimen of urine (MSU) a specimen of urine that is subjected to examination for the presence of microorganisms. In order to obtain a specimen that is free of contamination, the periurethral area is cleansed and the patient is requested to discard the initial flow of urine before collecting the specimen in a sterile container.

midwifery n. the profession of providing assistance and medical care to women who are undergoing labor and childbirth. See also obstetrics. —**midwife** n.

mifepristone (RU-486) n. a drug used to produce an abortion within the first trimester of pregnancy: it acts by blocking the action of *progesterone, which is essential for maintaining pregnancy. It is taken by mouth, usually in conjunction with *misoprostol. Side effects include faintness, headache, and vaginal bleeding. Trade name: **Mifeprex**.

migraine n. a condition resulting from spasm and subsequent overdilation of certain arteries in the brain, which causes a recurrent throbbing headache that characteristically affects one side of the head. There is sometimes forewarning of an attack (an aura) consisting of visual disturbances or tingling and/or weakness of the limbs, which clears up as the headache develops. It is often accompanied by prostration, nausea, vomiting, and *photophobia. Stress, food and food preservatives, bright lights, and smoking can trigger migraine. It occurs more often in women. Effective preventive therapies now exist and drugs known as *5HT₁ agonists (e.g. *sumatriptan, zolmitriptan, naratriptan) may be used to treat acute attacks. See also cluster headache.

Mikulicz's disease an abnormal swelling of the lacrimal and salivary glands, with narrowing of the corners of the eyes,

conjunctivitis, and dryness of the mouth, resulting from infiltration with *lymphoid tissue. It is associated with a variety of diseases, including leukemia, lupus erythematosus, lymphoma, and tuberculosis. [J. von Mikulicz Radecki (1850–1905), Polish surgeon]

miliaria n. see prickly heat.

miliary adj. describing or characterized by very small nodules or lesions, resembling millet seed.

miliary tuberculosis acute generalized *tuberculosis characterized by lesions in affected organs, which resemble millet seeds.

milium (whitehead) n. (pl. milia) a white nodule in the skin, particularly on the face. Up to 4 mm in diameter, milia are small *keratin cysts occurring just beneath the outer layer (epidermis) of the skin. Milia are commonly seen in newborn babies around the nose; they disappear without active treatment. In adults they may be lifted out with a needle or removed by an abrasive sponge.

milk n. the liquid food secreted by female mammals from the mammary gland. It is the sole source of food for the young of most mammals at the start of life. Milk is a complete food in that it has most of the nutrients necessary for life: protein, carbohydrate, fat, minerals, and vitamins. The composition of milk varies very much from mammal to mammal. Cows' milk contains nearly all the essential nutrients but is comparatively deficient in vitamins C and D. Human milk contains more sugar (lactose) and less protein than cows' milk.

milk rash a spotty red facial rash that is common during the first few months of life; it disappears without treatment.

milk teeth Colloquial. the deciduous teeth of young children. See dentition.

Miller-Deiker syndrome a chromosomal abnormality resulting in a characteristic facial appearance and the absence of the grooves on the surface of the brain (see agyria). Affected individuals are severely mentally retarded.

milli- prefix denoting one thousandth part.

milliampere n. one thousandth of an ampere (10^{-3} A). Symbol: mA.

milligram n. one thousandth of a gram. Symbol: mg.

milliliter n. one thousandth of a liter. Symbol: ml.

millimeter n. one thousandth of a meter (10^{-3} m). Symbol: mm.

Milroy's disease see lymphedema. [W. F. Milroy (1855–1942), US physician]

Minamata disease a form of mercury poisoning (from ingesting methyl mercury in contaminated fish) that caused 43 deaths in the Japanese coastal town of Minamata during 1953–56. The source of mercury was traced to an effluent containing mercuric sulfate from a local polyvinylchloride factory. Symptoms include numbness, difficulty in controlling the limbs, and impaired speech and hearing.

mineralocorticoid n. see corticosteroid.

minim n. a unit of volume used in pharmacy, equivalent to one sixtieth part of a fluid *dram.

minimal bacterial concentration the lowest concentration of antibiotic that on subculture fails to show growth or results in a 99.9% decrease of the initial inoculum.

minimally invasive surgery surgical intervention involving the least possible physical trauma to the patient, particularly surgery performed using an operating laparoscope or other endoscope (see laparoscopy) passed through a tiny incision. Several types of abdominal surgery, including gallbladder removal (see cholecystectomy) and extracorporeal shock-wave *lithotripsy for stones in the urinary or bile drainage system, are commonly performed in this way. Such methods usually allow the patient to resume normal activity much sooner than would be possible after more conventional procedures. See also interventional radiology.

minitracheostomy n. temporary *tracheostomy using a needle or fine-bore tube inserted through the skin.

minocycline n. a semisynthetic tetracycline antibiotic active against a wide range of bacteria and against rickettsial infections, mycoplasmal pneumonia, or relapsing fever. It is administered by mouth, by intravenous injection, or topically; side effects include skin rash, loss of appetite, and dizziness. Trade names: **Arestin, Minocin.**

minoxidil n. a peripheral vasodilator used in the treatment of high blood pressure (hypertension) when other drugs are not effective. It is administered by mouth in conjunction with a *diuretic; side effects include electrocardiographic changes, transient edema, and abnormal hair growth. The last adverse effect has led to its use in the treatment of male pattern baldness. Trade names: **Loniten, Rogaine.**

mio- prefix denoting **1.** reduction or diminution. **2.** rudimentary.

miosis (myosis) n. constriction of the pupil. This occurs normally in bright light, but persistent miosis is most commonly caused by certain types of eye drops used to treat glaucoma. See also miotic. Compare mydriasis.

miotic n. a drug that causes the pupil of the eye to contract. Miotics, such as *physostigmine and *pilocarpine, are used to counteract the dilation of the pupil caused by drugs such as ephedrine and phenylephrine and to reduce the pressure in the eye in the treatment of glaucoma.

miracidium n. (pl. **miracidia**) the first-stage larva of a parasitic *fluke. Miracidia hatch from eggs released into water with the host's excreta. They have *cilia and swim about until they reach a snail. The miracidia then bore into the snail's soft tissues and there continue their development as *sporocysts.

miscarriage n. see abortion.

miso- prefix denoting hatred. Example: misopedia (of children).

misophonia n. dislike of or aversion to sound. See hyperacusis, phonophobia.

misoprostol n. a synthetic *prostaglandin drug that is used to prevent gastric ulcers in patients taking nonsteroidal antiinflammatory drugs, including aspirin. Misoprostol is also used in combination with *mifepristone to end an early pregnancy. It is administered by mouth; side effects include diarrhea, abdominal pain, and headache. Trade name: **Cytotec.**

missed case a person with an infection in whom the symptoms and signs are so minimal that either there is no request for medical assistance or the doctor fails to make the diagnosis. The patient usually has partial immunity to the disease, but since the infecting organisms (pathogens) are of normal virulence, nonimmune contacts can be affected with the full manifestations of the illness. The period of infectivity is confined to the shortened duration of the illness (in contrast to a *carrier, in whom the pathogen is present without necessarily causing any ill effect). Alternatively the subject has had the disease but retains some of the pathogens (e.g. in the throat or bowel) and so acts as a continuing reservoir of infection.

mite *n.* a free-living or parasitic arthropod belonging to a group (Acarina) that also includes the *ticks. Most mites are small, averaging 1 mm or less in length. A mite has no antennae or wings, and its body is not divided into a distinct head, thorax, and abdomen. Medically important mites include the many species causing dermatitis (e.g. *Dermatophagoides*) and the harvest mite (*see* Trombicula), which transmits scrub typhus.

mitochondrial disorders a group of inherited conditions transmitted through mitochondrial DNA (*see* mitochondrion), which can affect any organ and can present at any age. Most of these conditions are very rare; examples of those that are less rare include *Leigh syndrome, congenital *lactic acidosis, *MELAS, and Pearson syndrome.

mitochondrion (chondriosome) *n.* (*pl.* **mitochondria**) a structure, occurring in varying numbers in the cytoplasm of every cell, that is the site of the cell's energy production. Mitochondria contain *ATP and the enzymes involved in the cell's metabolic activities, and also their own DNA; mitochondrial genes (which in humans encode 13 proteins) are inherited through the female line. Each mitochondrion is bounded by a double membrane, the inner being folded inward to form projections (*cristae*). —**mitochondrial** *adj.*

mitogen *n.* any substance that can cause cells to begin division (*mitosis).

mitomycin *n.* an *anthracycline antibiotic that inhibits the growth of cancer cells. It causes severe marrow suppression but is of use in the treatment of cancers of the stomach, pancreas, and breast. Trade name: **Mutamycin.**

mitosis *n.* a type of cell division in which a single cell produces two genetically identical daughter cells. It is the way in which new body cells are produced for both growth and repair. Division of the nucleus (*karyokinesis*) takes place in four stages (*see* prophase, metaphase, anaphase, telophase) and is followed by di-

vision of the cytoplasm (*cytokinesis*) to form two daughter cells (see illustration). *Compare* meiosis. —**mitotic** *adj.*

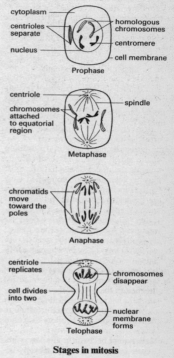

Stages in mitosis

mitotane *n.* a cytotoxic drug used in the palliative treatment of inoperable carcinoma of the adrenal cortex. It is administered orally; side effects include gastrointestinal disturbances, lethargy, sleepiness, dizziness, and adrenal insufficiency. Trade name: **Lysodren.**

mitotic index the proportion of cells in a tissue that are dividing at a given time.

mitoxantrone *n.* a *cytotoxic drug used for treating secondary progressive multiple sclerosis and, in combination with other drugs, in the treatment of certain cancers, including breast cancer, leukemia, and lymphomas. Side effects include fever, nausea and vomiting, and gastrointestinal bleeding. Trade name: **Novantrone**.

mitral incompetence failure of the *mitral valve to close, allowing a reflux of blood from the left ventricle of the heart to the left atrium. It most often results from scarring of the mitral valve by rheumatic fever, but it can also develop as a complication of myocardial infarction or cardiomyopathies. It may occur as a congenital defect. Its manifestations include breathlessness, atrial *fibrillation, embolism, enlargement of the left ventricle, and a systolic *murmur. Mild cases are symptomless and require no treatment, but in severe cases the affected valve should be replaced with an artificial one (*mitral prosthesis*).

mitral stenosis narrowing of the opening of the mitral valve: a result of chronic scarring that follows rheumatic fever. It may be seen alone or combined with *mitral incompetence. The symptoms are similar to those of mitral incompetence except that the patient has a diastolic *murmur. Mild cases need no treatment, but severe cases are treated surgically by reopening the stenosis (*mitral valvotomy*) or by inserting an artificial valve (*mitral prosthesis*).

mitral valve (bicuspid valve) a valve in the heart consisting of two flaps (cusps) attached to the walls at the opening between the left atrium and left ventricle. It allows blood to pass from the atrium to the ventricle, but prevents any backward flow.

mittelschmerz *n.* pain in the lower abdomen experienced about midway between successive menstrual periods, i.e. when the egg cell is being released from the ovary. *See also* menstrual cycle.

mixed connective tissue disease a disease with features in common with systemic *lupus erythematosus, *polymyositis, and *scleroderma. Some authorities dispute its status as a separate entity.

ml *symbol for* milliliter.

MLC (MLR) mixed lymphocyte culture (or reaction): a test in which lymphocytes from prospective donor and recipient are cultured together in a test tube to assess the suitability of transplanting organs or bone marrow cells.

MLD minimal lethal dose: the smallest quantity of a toxic compound that is recorded as having caused death. *See also* LD$_{50}$.

MLR *see* MLC.

mm *symbol for* millimeter.

mmHg a unit of pressure equal to 1 millimeter of mercury. 1 mmHg = 133.3224 pascals.

MMR vaccine a combined vaccine against *m*easles, *m*umps, and German measles (*r*ubella). It is now recommended that this vaccine is given to all children between 12 and 15 months old. Specific contraindications include immunosuppression, allergy to neomycin, and anaphylactic reaction to eggs. Links between the vaccine and autism and Crohn's disease have been suggested, but these are as yet unsubstantiated.

MND *see* motor neuron disease.

Mobitz type I and type II types of abnormality on an *electrocardiogram (ECG) tracing that indicate forms of *heart block, in which the communication between the upper and lower chambers of the heart is impaired. [W. Mobitz (20th century), German cardiologist]

moclobemide *n.* an antidepressant drug that reversibly inhibits the enzyme monoamine oxidase. The adverse effects of existing *MAO inhibitors, which include severe reactions when cheese or other tyramine-containing foods are eaten by patients taking them, are less likely with reversible inhibitors. Trade name: **Manerix**.

modality *n.* **1.** a form of sensation, such as smell, hearing, tasting, or detecting temperature. Differences in modality are not due to differences in the structure of the nerves concerned, but to differences in the working of the sensory receptors and the areas of the brain that receive the messages. **2.** one form of therapy as opposed to another, such as the modality of physiotherapy contrasted with that of radiotherapy.

mode *n. see* mean.

modeling *n.* a technique used in *behavior modification, whereby an individual learns a behavior by observing someone else doing it. Together with *prompting, it is useful for introducing new behaviors to the individual.

modiolus *n.* the conical central pillar of the *cochlea in the inner ear.

MODS *see* multiple organ dysfunction syndrome.

MODY *see* maturity-onset diabetes of the young.

Mohs chemosurgery a technique in which zinc chloride fixative is applied to a skin tumor, resulting in removal of the obvious tumor mass. A saucer-shaped piece of tissue surrounding the area of involvement is then excised and checked to ensure that all of the tumor was removed. The technique is used generally for removal of basal cell and squamous cell carcinomas. [F. E. Mohs (20th century), US surgeon]

molar *n.* in the permanent *dentition, the sixth, seventh, or eighth tooth from the midline on each side in each jaw (*see also* wisdom tooth). Permanent molars do not replace deciduous teeth. In the deciduous dentition, molars are the fourth and fifth teeth from the midline on each side in each jaw.

molarity *n.* the strength of a solution, expressed as the weight of dissolved substance in grams per liter divided by its molecular weight, i.e. the number of moles per liter. Molarity is indicated as 0.1 M, 1 M, 2 M, etc.

molar solution a solution in which the number of grams of dissolved substance per liter equals its molecular weight, i.e. a solution of molarity 1 M.

mold *n.* any multicellular filamentous fungus that commonly forms a rough furry coating on decaying matter.

molding *n.* the changing of the shape of an infant's head during labor, brought about by the pressures to which it is subjected when passing through the birth canal.

mole¹ *n.* the *SI unit of amount of substance, equal to the amount of substance that contains as many elementary units as there are atoms in 0.012 kilograms of carbon-12. The elementary units, which must be specified, may be atoms, molecules, ions, electrons, etc., or a specified group of such entities. One mole of a compound has a mass equal to its molecular weight expressed in grams. Symbol: mol.

mole² *n.* **1.** a nonmalignant collection of pigmented cells in the skin. Moles are rare in infancy, increase in numbers during childhood and especially in adolescence, but decline in numbers in old age. They vary widely in appearance, being flat or raised, smooth or hairy. Changes in the shape, color, etc., of moles in adult life should be investigated because this may be an early sign of malignant *melanoma. Medical name: **pigmented nevus**. *See also* atypical mole syndrome. **2.** a mass or tumor formed in the uterus as a result of degeneration or abnormal development of a fertilized ovum. *See* hydatidiform mole.

molecular biology the study of the molecules that are associated with living organisms, especially proteins and nucleic acids.

molluscum *n.* any of several skin diseases typified by the development of soft rounded tumors. Commonly, the term is used for *molluscum contagiosum*, a poxvirus disease that produces small rounded pearllike swellings with craters containing broken-down matter. The condition is transmitted by direct contact, often venereal. After several months, the lesions may disappear spontaneously; otherwise treatment is by freezing, removal with a *curet, *electrocautery, or by instilling carbolic acid locally. *See also* keratoacanthoma (molluscum sebaceum).

Molteno implant a device used in the surgical treatment of some types of glaucoma to control intraocular pressure by allowing fluid to drain from the anterior chamber into the subconjunctival space.

mon- (mono-) *prefix denoting* one, single, or alone.

Mongolian blue spots blue-black pigmented areas seen at the base of the back and on the buttocks of babies. They are more common in dark-skinned babies and usually fade during the first year of life. The spots are sometimes mistaken for bruising.

mongolism *n. see* Down's syndrome.

Monilia *n.* the former name of the genus of yeasts now known as *Candida*.

moniliasis *n.* an obsolete name for *candidiasis.

monoamine oxidase (MAO) an enzyme that catalyzes the oxidation of a large variety of monoamines, including epinephrine, norepinephrine, serotonin, and tyramine. Monoamine oxidase is found in most tissues, particularly the liver and nervous system. Drugs that act as inhibitors of this enzyme are widely used in the treatment of depression (*see* MAO inhibitor).

monoarthritis n. see arthritis.

monoblast n. the earliest identifiable cell that gives rise to a *monocyte. It is probably identical with the *myeloblast and matures via an intermediate stage (*promonocyte*). It is normally found in the blood-forming tissue of the *bone marrow but may appear in the blood in certain diseases, most notably in acute monoblastic *leukemia.

monochromat n. a person who is completely color blind. There are two types. The *rod monochromat* appears to have totally defective *cones: there is very poor visual acuity as well as the inability to discriminate colors. The *cone monochromat* has normal visual acuity: the cones appear to respond normally to light but to be completely unable to discriminate colors. It is possible in this case that the defect does not lie in the cones themselves but in the integration of the nerve impulses as they pass from the cones to the brain. Both types of color blindness are probably inherited.

monochromatic adj. denoting radiation, especially light, of the same frequency or wavelength.

monoclonal antibody an antibody produced artificially from a cell *clone and therefore consisting of a single type of immunoglobulin. Monoclonal antibodies are produced by fusing antibody-forming lymphocytes from mouse spleen with mouse myeloma cells. The resulting hybrid cells multiply rapidly (like cancer cells) and produce the same antibody as their parent lymphocytes. Monoclonal antibodies can be used for treating various disorders, including some malignant tumors (e.g. brain tumors, breast cancer, lymphoma, and leukemia), which can be targeted by these antibodies (known colloquially as "magic bullets"). See also abciximab, alemtuzumab, gemtuzumab ozogamicin, infliximab, palivizumab, rituximab, trastuzumab.

monocular adj. relating to or used by one eye only. Compare binocular.

monocyte n. a variety of white blood cell, 16–20 μm in diameter, with a kidney-shaped nucleus and grayish-blue cytoplasm (when treated with *Romanovsky stains). Its function is the ingestion of foreign particles, such as bacteria and tissue debris. There are normally 0.2–0.8 × 10^9 monocytes per liter of blood. —**monocytic** adj.

monocytosis n. an increase in the number of *monocytes in the blood. Monocytosis occurs in a variety of diseases, including monocytic *leukemia and infections due to some bacteria and protozoa.

monodactylism n. the congenital absence of all but one digit on each hand and foot.

monoiodotyrosine n. an iodine-containing substance produced in the thyroid gland from which the *thyroid hormones are derived.

monomania n. the state in which a particular delusion or set of delusions is present in an otherwise normal person. See also paranoia.

mononeuritis n. disease affecting a single peripheral nerve. Entrapment of the nerve or interference with its blood supply are the most common causes. *Mononeuritis multiplex* is the separate involvement of two or more nerves. Compare peripheral neuropathy.

mononucleosis n. the condition in which the blood contains an abnormally high number of mononuclear leukocytes (*monocytes and *lymphocytes). See glandular fever (infectious mononucleosis).

monophobia n. an extreme fear of being alone.

monophyletic adj. describing a number of individuals, species, etc., that have evolved from a single ancestral group. Compare polyphyletic.

monoplegia n. paralysis of only one limb. —**monoplegic** adj.

monoploid adj. see haploid.

monorchism n. absence of one testis. This is usually due to failure of one testicle to descend into the scrotum before birth. The term is sometimes used for the condition in which one testicle has been removed surgically or destroyed by injury or disease. If the single testis is normal, no adverse effects result from the absence of the other.

monosaccharide n. a simple sugar having the general formula $(CH_2O)_n$. Monosaccharides may have between three and nine carbon atoms, but the most common number is five or six. Monosaccharides are classified according to the number of carbon atoms they possess. Thus, *trioses* have three carbon atoms, *tetroses* four, *pentoses* five, and *hexoses* six. The most abundant monosaccharide is glucose (a hexose).

monosomy *n.* a condition in which there is one chromosome missing from the normal (*diploid) set. *Compare* trisomy. —**monosomic** *adj.*

monozygotic twins *see* twins.

mons *n.* (in anatomy) a rounded eminence. The *mons pubis* is the mound of fatty tissue lying over the pubic symphysis.

montelukast *n. see* leukotriene receptor antagonist.

Mooren's ulcer a severe ulceration at the periphery of the cornea, characterized by an overhanging advancing edge and vascularization of the ulcer bed. It is usually very painful, progressive, and difficult to control. [A. Mooren (1829–99), German ophthalmologist]

MOPP *m*echlorethamine (Mustargen), *O*ncovin (vincristine), *p*rocarbazine (Matulane), and *p*rednisone: a combination chemotherapy drug regimen that is used in cancer treatment, specifically for *Hodgkin's disease.

Moraxella *n.* a genus of short rodlike gramnegative aerobic bacteria, usually occurring in pairs. They exist as parasites in many warm-blooded animals. The species *M. lacunata* causes conjunctivitis.

morbid *adj.* diseased or abnormal; pathological.

morbidity *n.* the state of being diseased. The *morbidity rate* is the number of cases of a disease found to occur in a stated number of the population, usually given as cases per 100,000 or per million (the number may be smaller for common diseases). Annual figures for morbidity rate give the incidence of the disease, which is the number of new cases reported in the year. *See also* incidence rate, prevalence rate.

morbilli *n. see* measles.

morbilliform *adj.* describing a skin rash resembling that of measles.

morbus *n.* disease. The term is usually used as part of the medical name of a specific disease.

mordant *n.* (in microscopy) a substance, such as alum or phenol, used to fix a *stain in a tissue.

moribund *adj.* dying.

moricizine *n.* a drug administered by mouth to treat life-threatening irregularity of the heartbeat (*arrhythmia). Possible side effects include worsening of the arrhythmia and heart failure, and it is used only in cases in which these risks are thought to be justified. Trade name: **Ethmozine**.

morning sickness nausea and vomiting during early pregnancy. In some women the symptoms disappear if a small amount of food is eaten before rising in the morning. *See also* hyperemesis. Medical name: **nausea gravidarum**.

Moro reflex (startle reflex) a primitive reflex seen in newborn babies in response to the stimulus of a sudden noise or movement: the baby will fling its arms and legs wide and will appear to stiffen; the arms and legs are then drawn back into flexion. The Moro reflex should disappear spontaneously by four months. Its presence beyond this age is suggestive of an underlying neurological disorder, such as cerebral palsy. [E. Moro (1874–1951), German pediatrician]

morphea *n.* a localized form of *scleroderma that is characterized by firm ivory-colored waxy plaques in the skin without any internal sclerosis. The plaques may often disappear spontaneously but resolution is slow.

morphine *n.* a potent analgesic and *narcotic drug used mainly to relieve severe and persistent pain. It is administered by mouth, injection, or suppository; common side effects are loss of appetite, nausea, constipation, and confusion. Morphine causes feelings of euphoria; *tolerance develops rapidly and *dependence may occur. Trade names: **Astramorph, Duramorph, Roxanol, MS Contin, MSIR**.

morpho- *prefix denoting* form or structure.

morphogenesis *n.* the development of form and structure of the body and its parts.

morphology *n. see* anatomy.

-morphous *suffix denoting* form or structure (of a specified kind).

Morquio-Brailsford disease a defect of *mucopolysaccharide metabolism (*see* inborn error of metabolism) causes dwarfism with a *kyphosis, a short neck, *knock knee, and an angulated sternum in affected children. Intelligence is normal. Medical name: **mucopolysaccharidosis IV**. [L. Morquio (1865–1935),

Uruguayan physician; J. F. Brailsford (1888–1961), British radiologist]

mortality (mortality rate) *n.* the incidence of death in the population in a given period. The *annual mortality rate* is the number of registered deaths in a year, multiplied by 1000 and divided by the population at the middle of the year. *See also* infant mortality rate, maternal mortality rate.

mortification *n. see* necrosis.

Morton's neuralgia (Morton's foot, metatarsalgia, or **toe)** a painful condition of the foot, around the metatarsal bones, caused by compression of the plantar nerve. It is commonly seen in athletes, often due to overuse during training. [T. G. Morton (1835–1903), US surgeon]

morula *n.* an early stage of embryonic development formed by *cleavage of the fertilized ovum. It consists of a solid ball of cells and is an intermediate stage between the zygote and *blastocyst.

mosaicism *n.* a condition in which the cells of an individual do not all contain identical chromosomes; there may be two or more genetically different populations of cells. Often, one of the cell populations is normal and the other carries a chromosome defect such as *Down's syndrome or *Turner's syndrome. In affected individuals the chromosome defect is usually not fully expressed. —**mosaic** *adj.*

mosquito *n.* a small winged bloodsucking insect belonging to a large group – the *Diptera (two-winged flies). Its mouthparts are formed into a long proboscis for piercing the skin and sucking blood. Female mosquitoes transmit the parasites responsible for several major infectious diseases, such as *malaria. *See* Anopheles, Aëdes, Culex.

motile *adj.* being able to move spontaneously, without external aid: usually applied to a *microorganism or a cell (e.g. a sperm cell).

motion sickness (travel sickness) nausea, vomiting, and headache caused by motion during travel by sea, road, or air. The symptoms are due to overstimulation of the balance organs in the inner ear by repeated small changes in the position of the body and are aggravated by movements of the horizon. Sedative

antihistamine drugs (*see* antiemetic) are effective in preventing motion sickness.

motor cortex the region of the *cerebral cortex that is responsible for initiating nerve impulses that bring about voluntary activity in the muscles of the body. It is possible to map out the cortex to show which of its areas is responsible for which particular part of the body. The motor cortex of the left cerebral hemisphere is responsible for muscular activity in the right side of the body.

motor nerve one of the nerves that carries impulses outward from the central nervous system to bring about activity in a muscle or gland. *Compare* sensory nerve.

motor neuron one of the units (*neurons) that goes to make up the nerve pathway between the brain and an effector organ, such as a skeletal muscle. An *upper motor neuron* has a cell body in the brain and an axon that extends into the spinal cord, where it ends in synapses. It is thus entirely within the central nervous system. A *lower motor neuron*, on the other hand, has a cell body in the spinal cord or brainstem and an axon that extends outward in a cranial or spinal motor nerve to reach an effector.

motor neuron disease (MND) a progressive degenerative disease of the motor system occurring in middle age and causing muscle weakness and wasting. It primarily affects the cells of the anterior horn of the spinal cord, the motor nuclei in the brainstem, and the corticospinal fibers. There are three clinically distinct forms: *amyotrophic lateral sclerosis* (*ALS, Lou Gehrig's disease*), *progressive muscular atrophy*, and *progressive bulbar palsy*. Some forms of MND are familial (inherited). The drug riluzole has been used for the treatment of MND with upper motor neuron involvement, but its benefits are limited. Extensive supportive therapy may help maintain patients' independence and function.

mountain sickness *see* altitude sickness.

mouth *n.* **1.** the oral cavity: the anterior opening of the digestive tract, bound by the lips and containing the tongue and teeth. **2.** any opening or orifice. Medical name: **os.**

mouth-to-mouth respiration a form of *artificial respiration, performed mouth-to-mouth, by blowing air into the victim's lungs to inflate them and then allowing exhalation to occur automatically. It is commonly known as the *kiss of life*. The operator should aim to produce roughly 20 cycles of respiration per minute, or more for a younger victim.

mouthwash *n.* an aqueous solution with antiseptic, astringent, or deodorizing properties used for rinsing of the mouth and teeth. Mouthwashes are used to prevent dental *caries (*see also* chlorhexidine, fluoride) and to treat mild throat infections.

mouthwash test a simple noninvasive procedure that enables the detection of *carriers for single gene defects, e.g. *cystic fibrosis. Epithelial cells from the buccal cavity are obtained from a saline mouthwash: from these it is possible to isolate DNA, which is amplified by the *polymerase chain reaction to enable gene analysis.

moxibustion *n.* a form of treatment favored in Japan, in which cones of sunflower pith or down from the leaves of the plant *Artemisia moxa* are stuck to the skin and ignited. The heat produced by the smoldering cones acts as a counterirritant and is reputed to cure a variety of disorders.

MRI *see* magnetic resonance imaging.

MRS *see* magnetic resonance spectroscopy.

MRSA methicillin- (or multiple-)resistant *Staphylococcus aureus*: an increasingly common dangerous bacterium that is resistant to many antibiotics and is responsible for outbreaks of infection in hospitals. *See* methicillin.

MS *see* multiple sclerosis.

MSA *see* multiple system atrophy.

MSH *see* melanocyte-stimulating hormone.

MSU *see* midstream specimen of urine.

mucilage *n.* (in pharmacy) a thick aqueous solution of a gum used as a lubricant in skin preparations (*see also* glycerin), for the production of pills, and for the suspension of insoluble substances. The most important mucilages are of acacia, tragacanth, and starch.

mucin *n.* the principal constituent of *mucus. Mucin is a *glycoprotein.

muco- *prefix denoting* **1.** mucus. **2.** mucous membrane.

mucocele *n.* a space or organ distended with mucus. For example, it may occur in the gallbladder when the exit duct becomes obstructed so that the mucus secretions are retained and dilate the cavity of the organ. A mucocele in the soft tissues arising from a salivary gland occurs when the duct is blocked or ruptured.

mucociliary transport the process by which cilia (*see* cilium) move a thin film of *mucus from the upper and lower respiratory tracts toward the digestive tract. Particles of dust and microorganisms are trapped on the mucus and thereby removed from the respiratory tract.

mucolipidosis *n.* any of a group of metabolic disorders in which there is an accumulation of *mucopolysaccharides and lipids in the tissues but, unlike the *mucopolysaccharidoses, not an excess in the urine.

mucolytic *n.* an agent, such as carbocysteine, tyloxapol, or dornase alfa (*see* DNase), that dissolves or breaks down mucus. Mucolytics are used to treat chest conditions involving excessive or thickened mucus secretions.

mucopolysaccharide *n.* one of a group of complex carbohydrates functioning mainly as structural components in connective tissue. Mucopolysaccharide molecules are usually built up of two repeating sugar units, one of which is an amino sugar. An example of a mucopolysaccharide is *chondroitin sulfate, occurring in cartilage.

mucopolysaccharidosis *n.* any one of a group of several rare genetic diseases that are *inborn errors of metabolism in which the storage of complex carbohydrates is disordered. The two most common are *Hunter's syndrome and *Hurler's syndrome.

mucoprotein *n.* one of a group of proteins found in the *globulin fraction of blood plasma. Mucoproteins are globulins combined with a carbohydrate group (an amino sugar). They are similar to *glycoproteins but contain a greater proportion of carbohydrate.

mucopurulent *adj.* containing mucus and pus. *See* mucopus.

mucopus *n.* a mixture of *mucus and *pus.

Mucor *n.* a genus of mold fungi commonly seen on dead and decaying organic matter. They can be pathogenic in humans (*see* phycomycosis).

mucormycosis *n. see* phycomycosis.

mucosa *n. see* mucous membrane. —**mucosal** *adj.*

mucous membrane (mucosa) the moist membrane lining many tubular structures and cavities, including the nasal sinuses, respiratory tract, gastrointestinal tract, and biliary and pancreatic systems. The surface of the mouth is lined by mucous membrane, the nature of which varies according to its site. The mucous membrane consists of a surface layer of *epithelium, which contains glands secreting *mucus, with underlying layers of connective tissue (lamina propria) and muscularis mucosae, which forms the inner boundary of the mucous membrane.

mucoviscidosis *n. see* cystic fibrosis.

mucus *n.* a viscous fluid secreted by *mucous membranes. Mucus acts as a protective barrier over the membranes, a lubricant, and a carrier of enzymes. It consists chiefly of *glycoproteins, particularly *mucin*. —**mucous** *adj.*

MUGA scan (multiple-gated acquisition scan) a technique used in *nuclear medicine for studying the left-ventricular function and wall motion of the heart. The patient's red cells are labeled with radioactive technetium-99m. A gamma camera, connected to an ECG, collects information over a prolonged period for each phase of heart movement (*ECG gating*) to form an image of the blood pool within the heart at specific points in the cardiac cycle. Tomographic reconstructions can be made to give cross-sectional images of the heart in different phases of the cardiac cycle, using reconstruction *algorithms comparable to CT scanning (*see* SPECT scanning).

Müllerian duct *see* paramesonephric duct. [J. P. Müller (1801–58), German physiologist]

multifactorial *adj.* describing a condition believed to have resulted from the interaction of genetic factors, usually polygenes, with an environmental factor or factors. Many disorders, e.g. spina bifida and anencephaly, are thought to be multifactorial.

multifocal lenses lenses in which the power (*see* diopter) of the lower part gradually increases toward the lower edge. There is no dividing line on the lens as there is between the upper and lower segments of *bifocal lenses. The wearer can see clearly at any distance by lowering or raising his eyes.

multigravida *n.* a woman who has been pregnant at least twice.

multi-organ failure the terminal stage of serious illness.

multipara *n.* a woman who has given birth to a live child after each of at least two pregnancies.

multiple-gated acquisition scan *see* MUGA scan.

multiple organ dysfunction syndrome (MODS) a common cause of death following severe injury, overwhelming infection, or immune deficiency states.

multiple personality disorder a psychiatric disorder in which the affected person has two or more distinct, and often contrasting, personalities. As each personality assumes dominance, it determines attitudes and behavior and usually appears to be unaware of the other personality (or personalities). Transition is sudden and the mental states of the different personalities are normal. The condition is thought to be a late result of child abuse. Treatment is by psychotherapy.

multiple sclerosis (MS, disseminated sclerosis) a chronic disease of the nervous system affecting young and middle-aged adults. The *myelin sheaths surrounding nerves in the brain and spinal cord are damaged, which affects the function of the nerves involved. The course of the illness is usually characterized by recurrent relapses followed by remissions, but a small proportion of patients run a chronic progressive course. The disease affects different parts of the brain and spinal cord, resulting in typically scattered symptoms. These include unsteady gait and shaky movements of the limbs (ataxia), abnormal movements of the eyes (e.g. *nystagmus and internuclear *ophthalmoplegia), defects in speech pronunciation (dysarthria), spastic weakness, and *optic neuritis. The underlying cause of the nerve damage remains unknown. Steroid treatment may be used in an acute relapse, and beta-*interferon therapy reduces the relapse rate in some patients.

multiple system atrophy (MSA) a condition that results from degeneration of brain cells in the *basal ganglia (resulting in *parkinsonism), the *cerebellum, and the *pyramidal system and degeneration of cells in the *autonomic nervous system.

multislice CT scanning a development of

*spiral CT scanning using more than one array of detectors at the same time in a modified spiral CT scanner. Patients can be scanned more quickly and with thinner cuts, enabling greater detail to be achieved. This is particularly valuable for obtaining three-dimensional reconstructions of tissues and bones. In the future, detector arrays are likely to be replaced by a single flat plate similar to that used for *digital radiography. *See* isotropic.

multivariate analysis *see* correlation.

mummification *n.* **1.** the conversion of dead tissue into a hard shrunken mass, chiefly by dehydration. **2.** (in dentistry) the application of a fixative to the dental pulp to prevent decomposition.

mumps *n.* a common virus infection mainly affecting school-age children. Symptoms appear 2–3 weeks after exposure: fever, headache, and vomiting may precede a typical swelling of the *parotid salivary glands. The gland on one side of the face often swells up days before the other but sometimes only one side is affected. The symptoms usually vanish within three days, the patient remaining infectious until the swelling has completely disappeared, but the infection may spread to other salivary glands and to the pancreas, brain (causing aseptic meningitis), and testicles (after puberty mumps affecting the testicles can cause sterility). Vaccination against mumps provides effective immunity (*see* MMR vaccine). Medical name: **infectious parotitis**.

Münchausen's syndrome a mental disorder in which the patient persistently tries to obtain hospital treatment, especially surgery, for an illness that is nonexistent: an extreme form of malingering. The disease may be described in vivid detail, and in some cases injury may be deliberately self-inflicted in an attempt to give the appearance of authenticity to the claims being made. In *Münchausen's syndrome by proxy*, the patient inflicts harm on others (often children) in order to attract medical attention. [Baron von Munchausen, a fictional character who told exaggerated stories]

murmur *n.* a noise, heard with the aid of a stethoscope, that is generated by turbulent blood flow within the heart or blood vessels. Turbulent flow is produced by damaged valves, *septal defects, narrowed arteries, or arteriovenous communications. Heart murmurs can also be heard in normal individuals, especially those who have hyperactive circulation, and frequently in normal children (*innocent murmurs*). Murmurs are classified as *systolic* or *diastolic* (heard in ventricular *systole or *diastole, respectively); *continuous murmurs* are heard throughout systole and diastole. *See also* bruit.

Murphy's sign a sign of inflammation of the gallbladder: continuous pressure over the gallbladder while the patient is taking a deep breath will cause a catch in the breath at the point of maximum inhalation. [J. B. Murphy (1857–1916), US surgeon]

muscae volitantes black spots seen floating before the eyes, usually due to the presence of opaque specks in the vitreous humor as it becomes more fluid with age.

muscle *n.* a tissue whose cells have the abil-

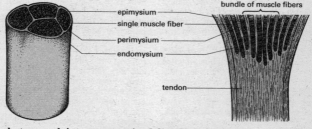

A voluntary muscle in transverse section (left) and in longitudinal section at its junction with a tendon (right)

ity to contract, producing movement or force (see illustration). Muscles possess mechanisms for converting energy derived from chemical reactions into mechanical energy. The major functions of muscles are to produce movements of the body, to maintain the position of the body against the force of gravity, to produce movements of structures inside the body, and to alter pressures or tensions of structures in the body. There are three types of muscle: *striated muscle, attached to the skeleton; *smooth muscle, which is found in such tissues as the stomach, intestinal tract, and blood vessels; and *cardiac muscle, which forms the walls of the heart.

muscle relaxant an agent that reduces tension in voluntary muscles. Drugs such as *baclofen, *dantrolene, and *diazepam are used to relieve skeletal muscular spasms in various spastic conditions, parkinsonism, and tetanus. Other drugs, e.g. *gallamine and *succinylcholine, paralyze voluntary muscles and are used in addition to anesthetics to relax the muscles during surgical operations.

muscle spindle a specialized receptor, sensitive to stretch, that is embedded between and parallel to the fibers of striated muscles. These receptors are important for coordinated muscular movement. *See also* stretch receptor.

muscular dystrophy a group of muscle diseases, marked by weakness and wasting of selected muscles, in which there is a recognizable pattern of inheritance. The affected muscle fibers degenerate and are replaced by fatty tissue. The muscular dystrophies are classified according to the patient's age at onset, distribution of the weakness, the progression of the disease, and the mode of inheritance. Isolated cases may occur as a result of gene mutation. Confirmation of the diagnosis is based upon *electromyography and muscle biopsy.

The most common form is *Duchenne's muscular dystrophy*, which is inherited as a sex-linked recessive character and is nearly always restricted to boys. It usually begins before the age of four years, with selective weakness and wasting of the muscles of the pelvic girdle and back. The child has a waddling gait and *lordosis of the lumbar spine. The calf muscles – and later the shoulders and upper

limbs – often become firm and bulky. A similar but less severe form with later onset is *Becker muscular dystrophy*, in which affected males develop an increase in muscle size followed by weakness and wasting. It usually starts between the ages of 5 and 15; 25 years after onset most patients are wheelchair-bound. Although most men become severely disabled, life expectancy is close to normal. *Facioscapulohumeral muscular dystrophy* (*Landouzy-Dejerine dystrophy*) is a relatively benign autosomal dominant form characterized by weakness of the muscles of the face, shoulder girdles, and arms, usually beginning in early adolescence. The condition progresses slowly and life expectancy is normal. Although these diseases cannot be cured, physiotherapy and orthopedic measures can relieve the disability. The identification of the gene abnormality raises the possibility of *gene therapy for these conditions. *See also* dystrophia myotonica (myotonic dystrophy).

muscularis *n.* a muscular layer of the wall of a hollow organ (such as the stomach) or a tubular structure (such as the intestine or ureter). The *muscularis mucosae* is the muscular layer of a mucous membrane complex, especially that of the stomach or intestine.

muscular rheumatism any aching pain in the muscles and joints. Commonly the symptoms are due to *fibrositis, wear and tear of the joints (*osteoarthritis), or to inflammation of the muscles associated with abnormal immune reactions (*polymyalgia rheumatica).

musculo- *prefix denoting* muscle.

musculocutaneous nerve a nerve of the *brachial plexus that supplies some muscles of the arm and the skin of the lateral part of the forearm.

mushroom *n.* the aerial fruiting (spore-producing) body of various fungi. Edible species include the field and cultivated mushrooms (*Agaricus campestris* and *A. bisporus*), the chanterelle (*Cantherellus cibarius*), and the parasol (*Lepiota procera*). However, great care must be taken in identifying edible fungi. Many species are poisonous, especially the death cap and panther cap (*see* Amanita).

mutagen *n.* an external agent that, when applied to cells or organisms, can increase the rate of *mutation. Mutagens usually only increase the number of mutants formed and do not cause mutations that are not found under natural conditions. Several kinds of radiation, many chemicals, and some viruses can act as mutagens. *Compare* antimutagen.

mutant *n.* **1.** an individual in which a mutation has occurred, especially when the effect of the mutation is visible. **2.** a characteristic showing the effects of a mutation. —**mutant** *adj.*

mutation *n.* a change in the genetic material (*DNA) of a cell, or the change this causes in a characteristic of the individual, which is not caused by normal genetic processes. In a *point* (or *gene*) *mutation* there is a change in a single gene; in a *chromosome mutation* there is a change in the structure or number of the chromosomes. All mutations are rare events and may occur spontaneously or be caused by external agents (*mutagens). If a mutation occurs in developing sex cells (gametes), it may be inherited. Mutations in any other cells (*somatic mutations*) are not inherited.

mutism *n.* inability or refusal to speak; dumbness. Innate speechlessness most commonly occurs in those who have been totally deaf since birth (*deafmutism*). Inability to speak may result from brain damage (*see* aphasia). It may also be caused by depression or psychological trauma, in which case the patient either does not speak at all or speaks only to particular persons or in particular situations. This latter condition is called *elective mutism*.

Treatment of mutism due to psychological causes is increasingly by behavioral means, such as *prompting: people that the patient does not address are gradually introduced into the situation where the patient does speak. This may be done either alone or in combination with more traditional psychotherapy. —**mute** *adj.*, *n.*

mutualism *n.* the intimate but not necessarily obligatory association between two different species of organism in which there is mutual aid and benefit. *Compare* symbiosis.

my- (myo-) *prefix denoting* muscle.

myalgia *n.* pain in the muscles.

myalgic encephalomyelitis (ME) *see* chronic fatigue syndrome.

myasthenia gravis a chronic disease marked by abnormal fatiguability and weakness of selected muscles, which is relieved by rest and steroids. The degree of fatigue is so extreme that these muscles are temporarily paralyzed. The muscles initially affected are those around the eyes, mouth, and throat, resulting in drooping of the upper eyelids (*ptosis), double vision, *dysarthria, and *dysphagia. Myasthenia gravis is an *autoimmune disease in which the body's own antibodies bind to cholinergic receptors on muscle cells, which impairs the ability of the neurotransmitter acetylcholine to induce muscular contraction. It chiefly affects adolescents and young adults (usually women) and adults over 40 years of age. Treatment with *anticholinesterase drugs and surgical removal of the thymus in younger patients (under the age of 45 years) lessen the severity of the symptoms. Steroid therapy or plasma exchange may be used to treat the more severely affected patients.

myc- (myco-, mycet(o)-) *prefix denoting* a fungus.

mycelium *n.* (*pl.* **mycelia**) the tangled mass of fine branching threads that make up the feeding and growing part of a *fungus.

mycetoma *n.* a chronic inflammation of tissues caused by a fungus. *See* Madura foot.

Mycobacterium *n.* a genus of rodlike grampositive aerobic bacteria that can form filamentous branching structures. Some species are pathogenic to animals and humans: *M. leprae* (*Hansen's bacillus*) causes *leprosy; *M. tuberculosis* (*Koch's bacillus*) causes *tuberculosis. *M. bovis* causes tuberculosis in cattle but can also infect the lungs, joints, and intestines of humans. *M. paratuberculosis*, which causes Johne's disease in cattle, can also be transmitted in milk and is suspected of being a cause of Crohn's disease.

M. tuberculosis is by far the most common species responsible for infections of the lung. Other mycobacteria that infect the lung are variously described as atypical, anonymous, or *opportunistic – the favored term since they usually require preexisting lung damage or a defect in the patient's immunity before they can give rise to infection. The opportunistic mycobacteria that most commonly cause lung infections are *M. kansacii, M. xenopi, M. malmoense,* and a group known as the *MAI complex* (*M. avium, M. intracellulare*). Infections caused by all these organisms can mimic pulmonary tuberculosis but are much more difficult to treat since they are resistant to many of the antituberculosis drugs. The MAI organisms are particularly likely to cause superimposed infection in cases of AIDS.

mycology *n.* the science of fungi. *See also* microbiology. —**mycologist** *n.*

mycoplasma *n.* one of a group of minute nonmotile microorganisms that lack a rigid cell wall and hence display a variety of forms. They are regarded by most authorities as primitive bacteria. The group includes some species that cause severe respiratory disease in cattle, sheep, and goats; one of these, *Mycoplasma pneumoniae,* causes *atypical pneumonia in humans. The group also includes the so-called *pleuropneumonia-like organisms* (*PPLO*).

mycosis *n.* any disease caused by a fungus, including actinomycosis, aspergillosis, cryptococcosis, rhinosporidiosis, ringworm, and sporotrichosis.

mycosis fungoides a disease that is a variety of *reticulosis confined to the skin, with plaques and later nodules infiltrated with T-lymphocytes. It progresses slowly and can be treated initially with topical corticosteroids, later with *PUVA and electron-beam therapy; chemotherapy is not helpful.

mydriasis *n.* widening of the pupil, which occurs normally in dim light. The most common cause of prolonged mydriasis is drug therapy (*see* mydriatic) or injury to the eye. *See also* cycloplegia. *Compare* miosis.

mydriatic *n.* a drug that causes the pupil of the eye to dilate. Examples are *atropine, *cyclopentolate, and *phenylephrine. Mydriatics are used to aid examination of the eye and to treat some eye inflammations such as iritis and cyclitis.

myectomy *n.* a surgical operation to remove part of a muscle.

myel- (myelo-) *prefix denoting* **1.** the spinal cord. **2.** bone marrow. **3.** myelin.

myelencephalon *n. see* medulla oblongata.

myelin *n.* a complex material formed of protein and *phospholipid that is laid

down as a sheath around the *axons of certain neurons, known as *myelinated* (or *medullated*) *nerve fibers.* The material is produced and laid down in concentric layers by *Schwann cells at regular intervals along the nerve fiber (see illustrations). Myelinated nerves conduct impulses more rapidly than nonmyelinated nerves.

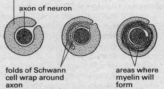

Formation of a myelin sheath

myelinated (medullated) nerve fiber any nerve fiber that has a sheath of *myelin surrounding and insulating its axon.

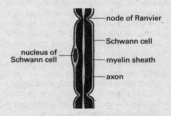

Longitudinal section through a myelinated nerve fiber

myelination *n.* the process in which *myelin is laid down as an insulating layer around the axons of certain nerves. Myelination of nerve tracts in the central nervous system is completed by the second year of life.

myelitis *n.* **1.** an inflammatory disease of the spinal cord. The most usual kind (*transverse myelitis*) most often occurs during the development of multiple sclerosis, but it is sometimes a manifestation of *encephalomyelitis, when it can occur as an isolated attack. The inflammation spreads more or less completely across the tissue of the spinal cord, resulting in a loss of its normal function to transmit nerve impulses up and down. It is as though the spinal cord had been severed: paralysis and numbness affect the legs and trunk below the level of the diseased tissue. **2.** inflammation of the bone marrow. *See* osteomyelitis.

myeloblast *n.* the earliest identifiable cell that gives rise to a *granulocyte, having a large nucleus and scanty cytoplasm. It is normally found in the blood-forming tissue of the bone marrow, but it may appear in the blood in a variety of diseases, most notably in acute myeloblastic *leukemia. *See also* granulopoiesis. —**myeloblastic** *adj.*

myelocele *n. see* neural tube defects.

myelocyte *n.* an immature form of *granulocyte having an oval nucleus (*compare* metamyelocyte) and eosinophil, neutrophil, or basophil granules in its cytoplasm (*compare* promyelocyte). It is normally found in the blood-forming tissue of the bone marrow, but may appear in the blood in a variety of diseases, including infections, infiltrations of the bone marrow, and certain leukemias. *See also* granulopoiesis.

myelofibrosis *n.* a chronic but progressive disease characterized by *fibrosis of the bone marrow, which leads to anemia and the presence of immature red and white blood cells in the circulation. Other features include enlargement of the spleen and the presence of blood-forming (myeloid) tissue in abnormal sites, such as the spleen and liver (extramedullary hemopoiesis). Its cause is unknown.

myelography *n.* a specialized method of X-ray examination to demonstrate the spinal canal that involves injection of a radiopaque contrast medium into the subarachnoid space. The X-rays obtained are called *myelograms*. It is of importance in the recognition of tumors of the spinal cord and other conditions compressing the cord or the nerve roots. The former use of oil-based dyes in myelography was an occasional cause of *arachnoiditis. This complication is now avoided by the use of water-soluble contrast media. Myelography is now often combined with simultaneous CT scanning.

myeloid *adj.* **1.** like, derived from, or relating to bone marrow. **2.** resembling a

*myelocyte. **3.** relating to the spinal cord.

myeloid leukemia a variety of *leukemia in which the type of blood cell that proliferates abnormally originates in the blood-forming (myeloid) tissue of the bone marrow. Myeloid leukemias may be acute or chronic and may involve any one of the cells produced by the marrow. Blood cells in patients with chronic myeloid leukemia contain a reciprocal *translocation between chromosomes 9 and 22 (*see* Philadelphia chromosome). Molecular characterization of the translocation has led to the development of a specific drug to block the effects of this abnormality (*see* imatinib).

myeloid tissue a tissue in the *bone marrow in which the various classes of blood cells are produced. *See also* hemopoiesis.

myeloma (multiple myeloma, myelomatosis) *n.* a malignant disease of the bone marrow, characterized by two or more of the following criteria: (1) the presence of an excess of abnormal malignant plasma cells in the bone marrow; (2) typical lytic deposits in the bones on X-ray, giving the appearance of holes; (3) the presence in the serum of an abnormal gamma globulin, usually IgG (an immunoglobulin; *see* paraprotein). *Bence-Jones protein may also be found in the serum or urine. The patient may complain of tiredness due to anemia and of bone pain and may develop pathological fractures. Treatment of myeloma is usually with such drugs as melphalan or cyclophosphamide, with local radiotherapy to particular areas of pain. *See also* plasmacytoma.

myelomalacia *n.* softening of the tissues of the spinal cord, most often caused by an impaired blood supply.

myelomatosis *n. see* myeloma.

myelomeningocele *n. see* neural tube defects.

myelosuppression *n.* a reduction in blood-cell production by the bone marrow. It commonly occurs after chemotherapy and may result in anemia, infection, and abnormal bleeding (*see* thrombocytopenia, neutropenia). —**myelosuppressive** *adj.*

myenteric reflex a reflex action of the intestine in which a physical stimulus causes the intestine to contract above and relax below the point of stimulation.

myenteron *n.* the muscular layer of the *intestine, consisting of a layer of circular muscle inside a layer of longitudinal muscle. These muscles are used in *peristalsis. —**myenteric** *adj.*

myiasis *n.* an infestation of a living organ or tissue by maggots. The flies normally breed in decaying animal and vegetable matter; myiasis therefore generally occurs only in regions of poor hygiene, and in most cases the infestations are accidental. Various genera may infect humans. *Gasterophilus*, *Hypoderma*, *Dermatobia*, and *Cordylobia* affect the skin; *Fannia* invades the alimentary canal and the urinary system; *Phormia* and *Wohlfahrtia* infest open wounds and ulcers; *Oestrus* attacks the eyes; and *Cochliomyia* invades the nasal passages. Treatment of external myiases involves the destruction and removal of maggots followed by the application of antibiotics to wounds and lesions.

mylohyoid *n.* a muscle in the floor of the mouth, attached at one end to the mandible and at the other to the hyoid bone.

myo- *prefix. see* my-.

myoblast *n.* a cell that develops into a muscle fiber. —**myoblastic** *adj.*

myocardial infarction death of a segment of heart muscle, which follows interruption of its blood supply (*see* coronary thrombosis). Myocardial infarction is usually confined to the left ventricle. The patient experiences a "heart attack": sudden severe chest pain, which may spread to the arms and throat. The main danger is that of ventricular *fibrillation, which accounts for most of the fatalities. Other *arrhythmias are also frequent; *ectopic beats in the ventricle are especially important as they predispose to ventricular fibrillation. Other complications include heart failure, rupture of the heart, phlebothrombosis, pulmonary embolism, pericarditis, shock, mitral incompetence, and perforation of the septum between the ventricles.
The best results from the management of patients with myocardial infarction follow mobile and hospital-based coronary care with facilities for the early detection, prevention, and treatment of arrhythmias and *cardiac arrest. Most survivors of myocardial infarction are able to return to a full and active life, including those who have been successfully resuscitated from cardiac arrest.

myocarditis *n.* acute or chronic inflammation of the heart muscle. It may be seen alone or as part of pancarditis (*see* endomyocarditis).

myocardium *n.* the middle of the three layers forming the wall of the heart (*see also* endocardium, epicardium). It is composed of *cardiac muscle and forms the greater part of the heart wall, being thicker in the ventricles than in the atria. —**myocardial** *adj.*

myoclonus *n.* a sudden spasm of the muscles. Occasional *myoclonic jerks* occur between seizures in patients with idiopathic *epilepsy, and myoclonus is a major feature of some progressive neurological illnesses with extensive degeneration of brain cells (including the *spongiform encephalopathies). Myoclonic jerks on falling asleep (*nocturnal myoclonus*) may occur in normal individuals. —**myoclonic** *adj.*

myocyte *n.* a muscle cell.

myodynia *n.* pain in the muscles.

myoepithelium *n.* a tissue consisting of cells of epithelial origin having a contractile cytoplasm. Myoepithelial cells play an important role in moving the secretion of substances into ducts.

myofibril *n.* one of numerous contractile filaments found within the cytoplasm of *striated muscle cells. When viewed under a microscope, myofibrils show alternating bands of high and low refractive index, which give striated muscle its characteristic appearance.

myogenic *adj.* originating in muscle: applied to the inherent rhythmicity of contraction of some muscles (e.g. cardiac muscle), which does not depend on neural influences.

myoglobin *n. see* myohemoglobin.

myoglobinuria *n. see* myohemoglobinuria.

myogram *n.* a recording of the activity of a muscle. *See* electromyography.

myograph *n.* an instrument for recording the activity of muscular tissues. *See* electromyography.

myohemoglobin (myoglobin) *n.* an iron-containing protein, resembling *hemoglobin, found in muscle cells. Like hemoglobin it contains a heme group which binds reversibly with oxygen, and so acts as an oxygen reservoir within the muscle fibers.

myohemoglobinuria (myoglobinuria) *n.* the presence in the urine of the pigment myohemoglobin.

myokymia *n.* prominent quivering of a few muscle fibers, not associated with any other abnormal features. It is a benign condition. *See also* fasciculation.

myology *n.* the study of the structure, function, and diseases of the muscles.

myoma *n.* a benign tumor of muscle. It may originate in smooth muscle (*see* leiomyoma) or in striated muscle (*see* rhabdomyoma).

myomectomy *n.* an operation in which benign tumors (fibroids) are removed from the muscular wall of the uterus.

myometritis *n.* inflammation of the muscular wall (myometrium) of the uterus.

myometrium *n.* the muscular tissue of the uterus, which surrounds the *endometrium. It is composed of smooth muscle that undergoes small regular spontaneous contractions. The frequency and amplitude of these contractions alter in response to the hormones *estrogen, *progesterone, and *oxytocin, which are present at particular stages of the menstrual cycle and pregnancy.

myoneural junction *see* neuromuscular junction.

myopathy *n.* any disease of the muscles. The myopathies are usually subdivided into those that are inherited (*see* muscular dystrophy) and those that are acquired. The acquired myopathies include *polymyositis and muscular diseases complicating endocrine disorders or carcinoma. All are typified by weakness and wasting of the muscles, which may be associated with pain and tenderness.

myopia (nearsightedness) *n.* the condition in which parallel light rays are brought to a focus in front of the retina (see illustration). Distant objects are blurred and cannot be made sharp by *accommodation. The condition is corrected by wearing glasses with concave lenses and can now be treated by surgery (*see* excimer laser, intrastromal keratomileusis, LASEK, LASIK, radial keratotomy). *Compare* emmetropia, hyperopia. —**myopic** *adj.*

myoplasm *n. see* sarcoplasm.

myoplasty *n.* the plastic surgery of muscle,

in which part of a muscle is partly detached and used to repair tissue defects or deformities in the vicinity of the muscle. It is frequently used in *flap surgery and anal operations (*anoplasty).

myosarcoma *n.* a malignant tumor of muscle. *See also* leiomyosarcoma, rhabdomyosarcoma.

myosin *n.* the most abundant protein in muscle fibrils, having the important properties of elasticity and contractility. With actin, it comprises the principal contractile element of muscles. *See* striated muscle.

myosis *n. see* miosis.

myositis *n.* any of a group of muscle diseases in which inflammation and degenerative changes occur. *Polymyositis is the most commonly occurring example, but myositis may be found in relation to systemic *connective tissue diseases and a minority are caused by bacterial or parasitic infections.

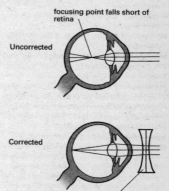

focusing point falls short of retina

Uncorrected

Corrected

concave lens diverges light rays falling on the eye

Myopia (nearsightedness)

myositis ossificans the formation of bone tissue in a muscle that occurs after dislocations or fractures, especially around the elbow. It is initially painful and swollen, and the joint then becomes very stiff, surrounded by a mass of new bone.

myotactic *adj.* relating to the sense of touch in muscles.

myotatic reflex *see* stretch reflex.

myotome *n.* that part of the segmented

mesoderm in the early embryo that gives rise to all the skeletal muscle of the body. Visceral (smooth) muscles develop from unsegmented mesoderm (*see* mesenchyme). *See also* somite.

myotomy *n.* the dissection or surgical division of a muscle. For example, *cardiomyotomy* is division of the *sphincter muscle of the gastroesophageal junction (*see* achalasia).

myotonia *n.* a disorder of the muscle fibers that results in abnormally prolonged contractions. The patient has difficulty in relaxing a movement (e.g. his grip) after any vigorous effort. It is a feature of a hereditary condition starting in infancy or early childhood (*myotonia congenita*) and of a form of muscular dystrophy (*dystrophia myotonica*).

myotonic *adj.* **1.** relating to muscle tone. **2.** relating to or characterized by *myotonia.

myotonus *n.* **1.** a tonic muscular spasm. **2.** muscle tone.

myringa *n.* the eardrum (*see* tympanic membrane).

myringitis *n.* inflammation of the eardrum. *See* otitis.

myringoplasty (tympanoplasty) *n.* surgical repair of a perforated eardrum by grafting.

myringotomy (tympanotomy) *n.* incision of the eardrum to create an artificial opening, which allows drainage of fluid from an inflamed middle ear (*otitis media).

myx- (myxo-) *prefix denoting* mucus.

myxedema *n.* **1.** a dry firm waxy swelling of the skin and subcutaneous tissues found in patients with underactive thyroid glands (*see* hypothyroidism). **2.** the clinical syndrome due to hypothyroidism in adult life, including coarsening of the skin, intolerance to cold, weight gain, and mental dullness. The symptoms are reversed with thyroxine treatment. *Compare* cretinism.

myxedema coma a life-threatening condition due to severe *hypothyroidism, which is often precipitated by an acute event, such as surgery, prolonged exposure to cold, infection, trauma, other severe illness, or sedative drugs. It manifests as hypothermia, slowing of the heart rate with a reduction in blood pressure and sometimes heart failure, pleural and peritoneal effusions, urinary retention, and a gradually reduced conscious state resulting in coma. Blood tests show hypothyroidism, *hyponatremia, hypercholesterolemia, retention of carbon dioxide, and anemia. Treatment is with intravenous *thyroxine at a high dosage until the patient wakes up, when tablets can be administered. Support on a ventilator and intravenous fluids may be needed. Active slow rewarming should be undertaken.

myxofibroma *n.* a benign tumor of fibrous tissue that contains myxomatous elements (*see* myxoma) or has undergone mucoid degeneration.

myxoid cyst a small cyst containing a thick sticky fluid. It develops over the end joint of a finger or toe and should not be cut out, because the cyst is usually in communication with the underlying joint.

myxoma *n.* a benign gelatinous tumor of connective tissue. *Atrial myxoma* is a tumor of the heart, usually of the left side, arising from the septum dividing the two upper chambers. Symptoms may include fever, lassitude, joint pains, and sudden loss of consciousness caused by obstruction of the blood flow. The tumor may be wrongly diagnosed as stenosis of the mitral valve because it can produce a similar murmur. Treatment is by surgical removal. —**myxomatous** *adj.*

myxosarcoma *n.* a *sarcoma containing mucoid material. It is doubtful whether this represents a true entity and it may be simply a variant of other sarcomas, such as a *liposarcoma or a *fibrosarcoma.

myxovirus *n.* a member of a group of RNA-containing viruses that are associated with various diseases in animals and humans. The *orthomyxoviruses* cause diseases of the respiratory tract, most notably influenza. The related *paramyxoviruses* include the *respiratory syncytial virus (RSV) and the agents causing measles, mumps, and parainfluenza.

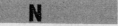

N

nabilone *n.* a drug related to cannabis, used to control severe nausea and vomiting caused by anticancer drugs, when this has not responded to other antiemetics. Administered by mouth, it can cause drowsiness, vertigo, dry mouth, mood changes, and hallucinations. Trade name: **Cesamet**.

nabothian follicle (nabothian cyst, nabothian gland) one of a number of cysts on the cervix of the uterus near its opening to the vagina. The sacs, which contain a thick liquid, form when the ducts of the glands in the cervix are blocked by a new growth of surface cells (epithelium) over an area damaged through infection.

NAD (nicotinamide adenine dinucleotide) a *coenzyme that acts as a hydrogen acceptor in oxidation-reduction reactions, particularly in the *electron transport chain in cellular respiration. NAD and the closely related coenzyme *NADP (nicotinamide adenine dinucleotide phosphate)* are derived from niacin; they are reduced to *NADH* and *NADPH*, respectively.

nadolol *n.* a beta blocker used in the treatment of angina pectoris and high blood pressure (hypertension). It is administered by mouth; side effects include decreased heart rate, dizziness, and low blood pressure. Trade names: **Corgard**, **Nadolol**.

NADP (nicotinamide adenine dinucleotide phosphate) *see* NAD.

Naegleria *n.* a genus of *amebas that normally live in damp soil or mud. *Naegleria* species can, however, live as parasites in humans and are believed to have caused some rare, but fatal, infections of the brain.

nafcillin *n.* a semisynthetic penicillin used in the treatment of severe infections that are caused by penicillinase-producing staphylococci. The drug is administered orally, by infusion, or by intramuscular injection. Side effects include nausea, vomiting, and hypersensitivity reactions. Trade names: **Nallpen, Unipen**.

Naga sore *see* tropical ulcer.

Nägele's obliquity *see* asynclitism. [F. K. Nägele (1777–1851), German obstetrician]

Nägele's rule a method used to estimate the probable date of the onset of labor: nine months and seven days are added to the date of the first day of the last menstrual period. A correction is required if the woman does not have 28-day menstrual cycles. [F. K. Nägele]

nail *n.* a horny structure, composed of keratin, formed from the epidermis on the dorsal surface of each finger and toe (see illustration). The exposed part of the nail is the *body*, behind which is the *root*. The whitish crescent-shaped area at the base of the body is called the *lunula*. Growth of the nail occurs at the end of the nail root by division of the germinative layer of the underlying *epidermis (which forms part of the *matrix*). The growing nail slides forward over the *nail bed*. The fold of skin that lies above the root is the *nail fold*; folds of skin on either side of the nail are the *nail walls*. The epidermis of the nail fold that lies next to the nail root is called the *eponychium* (forming the "cuticle" at the base of the nail). Anatomical name: **unguis**.

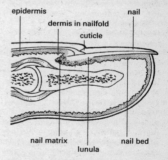

Longitudinal section through the fingertip and nail

nalidixic acid a quinolone antibiotic active against various bacteria and used to treat urinary infections. It is administered by mouth; common side effects are nausea, vomiting, and skin reactions. Trade name: **NegGram**.

nalorphine *n.* a drug that reduces the effects of morphine and similar narcotic drugs and is used to stimulate breathing and restore consciousness after an overdose of these drugs. It is administered by injection and, given alone, may depress breathing and cause drowsiness or restlessness. Trade name: **Nalline**.

naloxone *n.* a drug that is a specific antidote to morphine and similar narcotic drugs. It is administered by intravenous or subcutaneous injection. As it is short-acting, repeated doses may be necessary. Trade name: **Narcan**.

naltrexone *n.* a narcotic antagonist drug that is used in the maintenance treatment of heroin- and other opiate-dependent patients. It is administered by mouth. Possible side effects include abdominal cramps, nausea and vomiting, sleep difficulties, and dizziness. Trade name: **ReVia**.

nandrolone *n.* a synthetic male sex hormone with *anabolic effects. It is administered by injection in the treatment of aplastic *anemia and high doses may cause signs of *virilization in women. Trade names: **Deca-Durabolin**, **Hybolin Decanoate**, **Kabolin**.

nano- *prefix denoting* **1.** extremely small size. **2.** one billionth part (10^{-9}).

nanometer *n.* one billionth of a meter (10^{-9} m). One nanometer is equal to 10 angstrom. Symbol: nm.

nanophthalmos *n. see* microphthalmos.

naphazoline *n.* a drug that constricts small blood vessels and is used to relieve congestion in rhinitis and sinusitis and in the eye. It is administered as eye and nasal drops and may cause slight irritation. Trade names: **Albalon**, **Allerest**, **Comfort Eye Drops**, **Degest-2**, **Naphcon**, **Vasoclear**, **Vasocon**.

naprapathy *n.* a system of medicine based on the belief that a great many diseases are attributable to displacement of ligaments, tendons, and other connective tissues and that cure can be brought about only by manipulation to correct these displacements.

naproxen *n.* an analgesic drug that also reduces inflammation and fever (*see* NSAID). It is used to treat rheumatoid arthritis, ankylosing spondylitis, and gout. It is administered by mouth; side effects may include digestive upsets and rashes. Trade names: **Aleve**, **Anaprox**, **Naprelan**, **Naprosyn**.

naratriptan *n. see* $5HT_1$ agonist.

narcissism *n.* an excessive involvement with oneself and one's self-importance. In Freudian terms it is a state in which the *ego has taken itself as a love object. Some degree of narcissism is present in most individuals, but when it is shown to an extreme degree it may be a symptom of schizophrenia, personality disorder, and other conditions. —**narcissistic** *adj.*

narco- *prefix denoting* narcosis; stupor.

narcolepsy *n.* an extreme tendency to fall asleep, often in quiet surroundings or when engaged in monotonous activities, but also in such hazardous situations as when driving. The patient can be woken easily and is immediately alert. Narcolepsy is often associated with *cataplexy, *sleep paralysis, and *hypnagogic hallucinations. One in 2000 individuals may be affected. It has recently been found that narcolepsy is strongly associated with reduced levels of *hypocretin in the cerebrospinal fluid. —**narcoleptic** *adj., n.*

narcosis *n.* a state of diminished consciousness or complete unconsciousness caused by the use of *narcotic drugs, which have a depressant action on the nervous system. The body's normal reactions to stimuli are diminished and the body may become sedated or completely anesthetized.

narcotic *n.* a drug that induces stupor and insensibility and relieves pain. The term is used particularly for *morphine and other derivatives of opium (*see* opiate) but is also applied to other drugs that depress brain function (e.g. general anesthetics and hypnotics). In legal terms a narcotic is any addictive drug subject to illegal use. Narcotics (i.e. morphine and morphinelike drugs) have been largely replaced as sleeping drugs because of their ability to cause *dependence and tolerance; they are still used for relief of severe pain (*see* analgesic).

nares *pl. n.* (*sing.* **naris**) openings of the nose. The two *external* (or *anterior*) *nares* are the nostrils, leading from the nasal cavity to the outside. The two *internal* (or *posterior*) *nares* (*choanae*) are the openings leading from the nasal cavity into the pharynx.

nasal bone either of a pair of narrow oblong bones that together form the bridge and root of the nose. *See* skull.

nasal cavity the space inside the nose that lies between the floor of the cranium and the roof of the mouth. It is divided into two halves by a septum: each half communicates with the outside via the nostrils and with the nasopharynx through the posterior nares.

nasal concha (turbinate bone) any of three thin scroll-like bones that form the sides of the *nasal cavity. The *superior* and *middle nasal conchae* are part of the *ethmoid bone; the *inferior nasal conchae* are a separate pair of bones of the face. *See* skull.

nasion *n.* the point on the bridge of the nose at the center of the suture between the nasal and frontal bones.

naso- *prefix denoting* the nose.

nasogastric tube a tube passed through the nose into the stomach, used to aspirate fluid from, or introduce material into, the stomach (*see* Ryle's tube).

nasolacrimal *adj.* relating to the nose and the lacrimal (tear-producing) apparatus.

nasolacrimal duct the duct that passes through the hole (*nasolacrimal canal*) in the palatine bone of the skull. It drains the tears away from the *lacrimal apparatus into the inferior meatus of the nose.

nasopharyngeal airway a curved tube to be slotted down one nostril of an unconscious patient, to sit behind the tongue, to create a patent airway. *See also* oropharyngeal airway.

nasopharynx (postnasal space, rhinopharynx) *n.* the part of the *pharynx that lies above the level of the junction of the hard and soft palates. It connects the *nasal cavity to the *oropharynx. —**nasopharyngeal** *adj.*

nateglinide *n. see* meglitinides.

nates *pl. n.* the buttocks. —**natal** *adj.*

National Health Insurance (NHI) a plan for providing health services to all members of the population, regardless of ability to pay, using funds collected by the government through taxation or other means to finance the system. The concept originated in Germany in the mid 19th century, and some form of government-sponsored health-care delivery had been adopted by most industrialized nations of the world by the 1970s. In the US, a true form of National Health Insurance has not been established but a series of segmented health-care programs are operated by the *Department of Health and Human Services. They include *Medicare, financed primarily through social security taxes to make medical care available to all persons 65 years of age and older regardless of income, and *Medicaid, which is financed by general taxation to provide medical care for persons considered too poor to pay for services of physicians and hospitals.

National Health Service (in Britain) a comprehensive service offering therapeutic and preventive medical and surgical care, including the prescription and dispensing of medicines, glasses, and medical and dental appliances. Government funds pay for the services of doctors, nurses, and other professionals, as well as residential costs in NHS hospitals, and meet a substantial part of the cost of the medicines and appliances. Legislation enacted in 1946 was implemented in 1948 and the services were subjected to substantial reorganization in 1974 and again in 1982, 1991, and 1999. In England overall responsibility is vested in the Secretary of State for Health assisted by a comprehensive department.

National Institutes of Health (NIH) an agency of the Public Health Service division of the US Department of Health and Human Services that is devoted to research on the diseases of mankind. It is composed of 27 separate institutes, each concerned with a specific disease or specialty, such as the National Institute of Child Health and Human Development, the National Heart, Lung, and Blood Institute, and the National Cancer Institute. Each institute conducts research and also funds research at other centers. Patients accepted into designated research studies are treated free of charge in a modern hospital at the National Institutes of Health center in Bethesda, Maryland. The National Library of Medicine is also part of the NIH complex.

natriuresis *n.* the excretion of sodium in the urine: a normal phenomenon. However, the term usually applies to sodium excretion greater than normal.

natriuretic *n.* an agent that promotes the excretion of sodium salts in the urine. Most *diuretics are natriuretics.

natural killer cell (NK cell) a type of *lymphocyte that is able to kill virus-infected cells and cancerous cells and mediates rejection of bone-marrow grafts. NK cells are a part of natural (or innate) *immunity. Their function is regulated by a balance between activating receptors, which recognize proteins on cancerous or virus-infected cells, and inhibitory receptors specific for certain molecules encoded by the *HLA system.

naturopathy *n.* a system of medicine that relies upon the use of only "natural" substances for the treatment of disease, rather than drugs. Herbs, food grown without artificial fertilizers and prepared without the use of preservatives or coloring material, pure water, sunlight, and fresh air are all used in an effort to rid the body of "unnatural" substances, which are said to be at the root of most illnesses.

nausea *n.* the feeling that one is about to vomit, as experienced in seasickness and in morning sickness of early pregnancy. Actual vomiting often occurs subsequently.

navel *n.* see umbilicus.

navicular bone a boat-shaped bone of the ankle (*see* tarsus) that articulates with the three cuneiform bones in front and with the talus behind.

nearsightedness *n.* see myopia.

nearthrosis *n.* see pseudarthrosis.

nebula *n.* a faint opacity of the cornea that remains after an ulcer has healed.

nebulizer *n.* an instrument used for applying a liquid in the form of a fine spray.

NEC *see* necrotizing enterocolitis.

Necator *n.* a genus of *hookworms that live in the small intestine. The human hookworm, *N. americanus*, occurs in tropical Africa, Central and South America, India, and the Pacific Islands. The worm possesses two pairs of sharp cutting plates inside its mouth cavity, which enable it to feed on the blood and tissues of the gut wall. *Compare* Ancylostoma.

necatoriasis *n.* an infestation of the small intestine by the parasitic hookworm *Necator americanus*. *See also* hookworm disease.

neck *n.* **1.** the part of the body that connects the head and the trunk. It is the region supported by the *cervical vertebrae. **2.** see cervix.

necro- *prefix denoting* death or dissolution.

necrobiosis *n.* a gradual process by which cells lose their function and die. *Necrobiosis lipoidica* is patchy degeneration of the skin, particularly the shins, causing areas of white scarring and thinning. It is most commonly seen in women and in diabetics.

necrology *n.* the study of the phenomena of death, involving determination of the moment of death and the different changes that occur in the tissues of the body after death.

necromania *n.* morbid desire for a dead body or bodies. This may be *necrophilism, but the attraction is sometimes not sexual. A bereaved person, for instance, who is not grieving normally, may occasionally treasure the body of a loved one.

necrophilism (necrophilia) *n.* sexual attraction to corpses. *See also* sexual deviation. —**necrophile** *n.*

necropsy *n.* see autopsy.

necrosis (mortification) *n.* the death of some or all of the cells in an organ or tissue, caused by disease, physical or chemical injury, or interference with the blood supply (*see* gangrene). *Caseous necrosis* occurs in pulmonary tuberculosis, the lung tissue becoming soft, dry, and cheeselike.

necrospermia *n.* the presence of either dead or motionless spermatozoa in the semen. *See* infertility.

necrotizing enterocolitis (NEC) a serious disease affecting the gastrointestinal tract during the first three weeks of life; it is much more common in *preterm births. The abdomen distends and blood and mucus appear in the stools; the bowel may perforate. Treatment is to rest the bowel and administer antibiotics. If the bowel becomes necrotic, surgery may be necessary. The cause is unknown but the disease may be the result of a reduced supply of oxygen to the bowel or infection.

necrotizing fasciitis bacterial infection of the layer of *fascia beneath the skin by *Streptococcus* Type A. There is tissue necrosis and toxin production causing shock and organ failure. Symptoms appear rapidly after initial infection; they include a rash with blistering and discoloration of the skin, pain and inflammation of the lymph nodes, fever, drowsiness, diarrhea, and vomiting. The elderly and those who have recently undergone surgery are particularly vulnerable to the infection, which requires prompt treatment with antibiotics (e.g. clindamycin) and excision of the involved tissue.

necrotomy *n.* **1.** the removal of a dead piece of bone (*see* sequestrum). **2.** dissection of a dead body.

nedocromil *n.* an anti-inflammatory drug used to prevent asthma attacks and to treat allergic conjunctivitis. It is administered by metered-dose aerosol inhaler or as eye drops; possible side effects include local irritation, nausea, and brief headaches. Trade names: **Alocril, Tilade.**

needle *n.* a slender sharp-pointed instrument used for a variety of purposes. Needles used for sewing up tissue during a surgical operation are of various designs, for specific operations, and are equipped with an eye for threading suture material or they have the suture material fused onto them (so-called *atraumatic needles*). Hollow needles are used to inject substances into the body (in hypodermic syringes), to obtain specimens of tissue (*see* biopsy, puncture), or to withdraw fluid from a cavity (*see* aspiration). *See also* stop needle.

needle-stick injury a common accidental injury to the fingers and hands of nurses and doctors by contaminated injection needles. It can result in transmitted infections (e.g. hepatitis, AIDS).

needling *n.* a form of *capsulotomy in which a sharp needle is used to make a hole in the capsule surrounding the lens of the eye. The technique has been replaced by the use of the *YAG laser.

negative feedback loops physiological loops for the control of hormone production by various glands. High levels of a circulating hormone act to reduce production of the releasing factors triggering its own production, i.e. they have a negative *feedback on these trigger factors. As circulating levels of the hormone fall, the negative feedback is reduced and the releasing factor starts to be produced again, allowing the hormone level to rise again.

negativism *n.* behavior that is the opposite of that suggested by others. In *active negativism* the individual does the opposite of what he is asked (for example, he screws his eyes up when asked to open them). This is uncommon in adult life and is usually associated with other features of *catatonia. In *passive negativism*

the person fails to cooperate (for example, he does not eat). This occurs in *schizophrenia and *depression.

Neisseria *n.* a genus of spherical gramnegative aerobic nonmotile bacteria characteristically grouped in pairs. They are parasites of animals, and some species are normal inhabitants of the respiratory tract of humans. The species *N. gonorrhoeae* (the *gonococcus*) causes *gonorrhea. Gonococci are found within pus cells of urethral and vaginal discharge; they can be cultured only on serum or blood agar. *N. meningitidis* (the *meningococcus*) causes meningococcal *meningitis. Meningococci are found within pus cells of infected cerebrospinal fluid and blood or in the nasal passages of carriers. They, too, can only be cultured on serum or blood agar.

nelfinavir *n. see* protease inhibitor.

Nelson's syndrome a condition in which an *ACTH-producing pituitary tumor develops after loss of negative *feedback following bilateral adrenalectomy, usually for *Cushing's syndrome. [D. H. Nelson (1925–), US physician]

nematode (roundworm) *n.* any one of a large group of worms having an unsegmented cylindrical body, tapering at both ends. This distinguishes nematodes from other *helminths. Nematodes occur either as free-living forms in the sea, fresh water, and soil or as parasites of plants, animals, and humans. *Hookworms and *pinworms infest the alimentary canal. *Filariae are found in the lymphatic tissues. The *guinea worm and *Onchocerca affect connective tissue. Some nematodes (e.g. pinworms) are transmitted from host to host by the ingestion of eggs; others (e.g. *Wuchereria*) by the bite of a bloodsucking insect.

neo- *prefix denoting* new or newly formed.

neoadjuvant chemotherapy chemotherapy given before treatment of the primary tumor with the aim of improving the results of surgery or radiotherapy and preventing the development of metastases. *Compare* adjuvant therapy.

neocerebellum *n.* the middle lobe of the *cerebellum, excluding the pyramid and uvula. In evolutionary terms it is the newest part, occurring only in mammals.

neologism *n.* (in psychiatry) the invention of words to which meanings are attached. It is common in childhood, but when it occurs in an adult it may be a symptom of a psychotic illness, such as *schizophrenia. It should be distinguished from *paraphasia, in which new meanings are attached to ordinary words.

neomycin n. an *aminoglycoside antibiotic administered orally in preoperative bowel preparation to prevent infection during surgery and topically to treat infections caused by a wide range of bacteria, mainly those affecting the skin, ears, and eyes. Topical neomycin is usually applied in creams or drops with other antibiotics. Trade names: **Mycifradin**, **Myciguent**.

neonatal mortality rate see infant mortality rate.

neonatal screening *screening tests carried out on newborn babies to detect diseases that appear in the neonatal period, such as phenylketonuria (see Guthrie test) and *cystic fibrosis (see meconium). If these diseases are detected early enough, treatment may be instigated before any irreversible damage occurs to the baby.

neonate n. an infant at any time during the first four weeks of life. The word is particularly applied to infants just born or in the first week of life. —**neonatal** adj.

neopallium n. an enlargement of the wall of each cerebral hemisphere of the brain. In evolutionary terms it is the newest part of the cerebrum, formed by the development of new pathways for sight and hearing in mammals.

neoplasia n. the formation of abnormal cells. See cervical intraepithelial neoplasia (CIN), MENS (multiple endocrine neoplasia syndromes, prostatic intraepithelial neoplasia (PIN). Compare hyperplasia.

neoplasm n. any new abnormal growth: any *benign or *malignant tumor. —**neoplastic** adj.

neosphincter n. a substituted muscle or an implant for an absent or ineffective sphincter (see artificial sphincter).

neostigmine n. an *anticholinesterase drug used mainly to diagnose and treat *myasthenia gravis and as an antidote to some *muscle-relaxant drugs, such as *tubocurarine. It is also used to treat some intestinal disorders and glaucoma. Neostigmine is administered by mouth,

injection, or in eye drops; side effects include digestive upsets and increased saliva flow. Trade name: **Prostigmin**.

neovascularization n. the abnormal formation of new and fragile blood vessels, usually in response to ischemia. In choroidal neovascularization, which occurs in such conditions as *macular degeneration and diabetic *retinopathy, abnormal vessels, derived from the *choroid, form a choroidal neovascular membrane in the space below the retinal pigment epithelium (see retina).

nephr- (nephro-) prefix denoting the kidney(s).

nephralgia n. pain in the kidney. The pain is felt in the loin and can be caused by a variety of kidney complaints.

nephrectomy n. surgical removal of a kidney. When performed for cancer of the kidney, the entire organ is removed together with its surrounding fat and the adjacent adrenal gland (radical nephrectomy). Removal of either the upper or lower pole of the kidney is termed partial nephrectomy.

nephritis (Bright's disease) n. inflammation of the kidney. Nephritis is a nonspecific term used to describe a condition resulting from a variety of causes. See glomerulonephritis.

nephroblastoma (Wilms' tumor) n. a malignant tumor of the kidney found in children, usually below the age of three and rarely over the age of eight. In some cases it involves both kidneys. The most obvious symptom is an abdominal swelling. Treatment is by *nephrectomy followed by chemotherapy. Considerable improvement in the results of treatment has occurred in recent years since the use of *cytotoxic drugs, such as *dactinomycin and *vincristine, as a routine. The number of children that survive at least five years after diagnosis is improving, being currently around 75%. In some children the tumor is associated with an abnormality of chromosome number 13; in these cases other features, such as absence of the iris in the eye (see aniridia) and *hemihypertrophy, are present (see WAGR syndrome).

nephrocalcinosis n. the presence of calcium deposits in the kidneys. This can be caused by excess calcium in the blood, as caused by overactivity of the parathyroid glands, or it may result from an underlying abnormality of the kidney. The cause of nephrocalcinosis must be detected by full biochemical, radiological, and urological investigation so that appropriate treatment can be undertaken.

nephrogenic cord either of the paired ridges of tissue that run along the dorsal surface of the abdominal cavity of the embryo. Parts of it develop into the kidney, ovary, or testis and their associated ducts. Intermediate stages of these developments are the *pronephros, *mesonephros, and *metanephros.

nephrolithiasis *n.* the presence of stones in the kidney (see calculus). Such stones can cause pain and blood in the urine, but they may produce no symptoms. Full investigation is undertaken to determine the underlying cause of stone formation. When stones are associated with urinary obstruction and infection, they usually require surgical removal (*see* nephrolithotomy, pyelolithotomy).

nephrolithotomy *n.* the surgical removal of a stone from the kidney by an incision into the kidney. It is normally performed in combination with an incision into the renal pelvis (*see* pyelolithotomy). *See also* percutaneous nephrolithotomy.

nephrology *n.* the branch of medicine concerned with the study, investigation, and management of diseases of the kidney. *See also* urology. —**nephrologist** *n.*

nephron *n.* the active unit of excretion in the kidney (see illustration). Blood, supplied by branches of the renal artery, is filtered through a knot of capillaries (*glomerulus*) into the cup-shaped *Bowman's capsule* so that water, nitrogenous waste, and many other substances (excluding colloids) pass into the *renal tubule*. Here, most of the substances are reabsorbed into the blood, the remaining fluid (*urine*) passing into the collecting duct, which drains into the *ureter.

nephropathy *n.* disease of the kidney. *See also* Berger's disease, diabetic nephropathy.

nephropexy *n.* an operation to fix a mobile kidney. The kidney is fixed to the twelfth rib and adjacent posterior abdominal wall to prevent descent of the kidney on standing (*see* nephroptosis).

nephroptosis *n.* abnormal descent of a kidney into the pelvis on standing, which may occur if it is excessively mobile (for

example, in thin women). If this is accompanied by pain and obstruction to free drainage of urine by the kidney, *nephropexy may be advised.

nephrosclerosis *n.* hardening of the arteries and arterioles of the kidneys. *Arteriolar nephrosclerosis* is associated with *hypertension.

nephroscope *n.* an instrument (*endoscope) used for examining the inside of the kidney (*nephroscopy*), usually passed into the renal pelvis through a track from the skin surface after needle *nephrostomy and dilation of the tract over a guide wire. The nephroscope allows the passage of instruments under direct vision to remove calculi (*see* percutaneous nephrolithotomy) or disintegrate them by ultrasound probes or electrohydraulic shock waves (*see* lithotripsy).

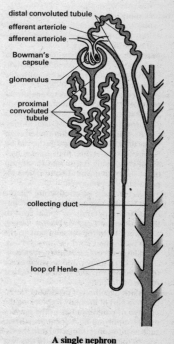

distal convoluted tubule
efferent arteriole
afferent arteriole
Bowman's capsule
glomerulus
proximal convoluted tubule
collecting duct
loop of Henle

A single nephron

nephrosis n. (in pathology) degenerative changes in the epithelium of the kidney tubules. The term is sometimes used loosely for the *nephrotic syndrome.

nephrostomy n. drainage of urine from the kidney by a tube (catheter) passing into the pelvis of the kidney via the skin surface. This is commonly used as a temporary procedure after operations on the kidney. Long-term urine drainage by nephrostomy may be complicated by the attendant problems of infection and obstruction of the catheter by debris. Nephrostomy also enables the passage of a *nephroscope.

nephrotic syndrome a condition in which there is great loss of protein in the urine, reduced levels of albumin in the blood, and generalized swelling of the tissues due to *edema. It can be caused by a variety of disorders, most usually *glomerulonephritis. Treatment is with corticosteroids.

nephrotomy n. surgical incision into the substance of the kidney. This is usually undertaken to remove a kidney stone (see nephrolithotomy).

nephrotoxic adj. liable to cause damage to the kidneys. Nephrotoxic drugs include *aminoglycoside antibiotics, sulfonamides, and gold compounds.

nephroureterectomy (ureteronephrectomy) n. surgical removal of a kidney together with its ureter. This operation is performed for cancer of the kidney pelvis or ureter. It is also undertaken when the kidney has been destroyed by *vesicoureteric reflux, to prevent subsequent continuing reflux into the stump of the ureter that would occur if the kidney alone were removed.

nerve n. a bundle of conducting *nerve fibers (see illustration) that transmits impulses from the brain or spinal cord to the muscles and glands (*motor nerves*) or inward from the sense organs to the brain and spinal cord (*sensory nerves*). Most large nerves are *mixed nerves*, containing both motor and sensory nerve fibers running to and from a particular region of the body.

nerve block a method of producing *anesthesia in part of the body by blocking the passage of pain impulses in the sensory nerves supplying it. A local anesthetic, such as lidocaine, is injected into the tissues in the region of a nerve. In this way anesthesia can be localized, so that minor operations can be performed without the necessity of giving a general anesthetic. A *ring block is a common technique used for anesthetizing a digit.

nerve cell see neuron.

nerve ending the final part (terminal) of one of the branches of a nerve fiber, where a *neuron makes contact either with another neuron at a synapse or with a muscle or gland cell at a neuromuscular or neuroglandular junction.

nerve entrapment syndrome any condition resulting from pressure on a nerve from surrounding structures. Examples include the *carpal tunnel syndrome and *meralgia paresthetica.

nerve fiber the long fine process that extends from the cell body of a *neuron and carries nerve impulses. Bundles of nerve fibers running together form a *nerve. Each fiber has a sheath, which in medullated nerve fibers is a relatively thick layer containing the fatty insulating material *myelin.

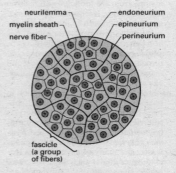

neurilemma — endoneurium
myelin sheath — epineurium
nerve fiber — perineurium
fascicle (a group of fibers)

Transverse section through a nerve

nerve gas any gas that disrupts the normal functioning of nerves and thus of the muscles they supply. There are two groups, the *G agents* and the *V agents*. The latter are more than 300 times as deadly as mustard gas: one inhalation can kill by paralyzing the respiratory muscles. V agents also act through the skin; therefore gas masks are ineffective protection against them.

nerve growth factor (NGF) a protein (see growth factor), consisting of two polypeptide chains, that is required for the development and longevity of some neurons, including those in the sympathetic nervous system and some central nervous system and sensory neurons. Nerve growth factor is necessary for axon growth and also for initiating new neuronal connections with other cells. The role of NGFs in preventing the degeneration of brain cells in Alzheimer's disease is being explored.

nerve impulse the electrical activity in the membrane of a *neuron that – by its rapid spread from one region to the next – is the means by which information is transmitted within the nervous system along the axons of the neurons. The membrane of a resting nerve is charged (*polarized*) because of the different concentrations of ions inside and outside the cell. When a nerve impulse is triggered, a wave of *depolarization spreads, and ions flow across the membrane (*see* action potential). Until the nerve has undergone *repolarization, no further nerve impulses can pass.

nerve regeneration the growth of new nerve tissue, which occurs at a very slow rate (1–2 mm per day) after a nerve has been severed and is often partially or totally incomplete. *Microsurgery has improved the results by facilitating primary repair in the immediate aftermath of injury. *See also* axonotmesis, neurotmesis.

nervous breakdown a popular term applied to a range of emotional crises varying from a brief attack of "hysterical" behavior to a major psychoneurotic illness with severe long-term effects on the life of the patient. The term is also sometimes used as a euphemism for a frank psychiatric illness, such as *schizophrenia.

nervous system the vast network of cells specialized to carry information (in the form of *nerve impulses) to and from all parts of the body in order to bring about bodily activity. The brain and spinal cord together form the *central nervous system; the rest of the nervous tissue is known as the *peripheral nervous system and includes the *autonomic nervous system, which is itself divided into the sympathetic and parasympathetic nervous systems. The basic functional unit of the nervous system is the *neuron (nerve cell).

Nesbit's operation an operation devised to surgically straighten a congenitally curved penis but now more frequently used to correct the penile curvature caused by *Peyronie's disease. [R. M. Nesbit (20th century), US surgeon]

nesidioblastosis *n.* a rare condition of childhood in which abnormal cells in the pancreas fail to mature properly and secrete a selection of hormones (including insulin) in an uncontrolled manner. This causes a variety of problems, including recurrent *hypoglycemia. It can sometimes be treated with medication; if this fails, surgical removal of a portion of the pancreas may be necessary.

nettle rash *see* urticaria.

neur- (neuro-) *prefix denoting* nerves or the nervous system.

neural arch *see* vertebra.

neural crest the two bands of ectodermal tissue that flank the *neural plate of the early embryo. Cells of the neural crest migrate throughout the embryo and develop into sensory nerve cells and peripheral nerve cells of the autonomic nervous system.

neuralgia *n.* a severe burning or stabbing pain often following the course of a nerve. *Postherpetic neuralgia* is an intense debilitating pain felt at the site of a previous attack of shingles. In *trigeminal neuralgia* (*tic douloureux*) there are brief paroxysms of searing pain felt in the distribution of one or more branches of the *trigeminal nerve in the face. Trigeminal neuralgia is managed principally by prescription of *carbamazepine. The facial pain of *migrainous neuralgia* (*cluster headache) lasts between 15 minutes and three hours and usually occurs in the early hours of the morning.

neural plate the strip of ectoderm lying along the central axis of the early embryo that forms the *neural tube and subsequently the central nervous system.

neural spine the spinous process situated on the neural arch of a *vertebra.

neural tube the embryological structure from which the brain and spinal cord develop. It is a hollow tube of ectodermal tissue formed when two edges of a groove in a plate of primitive neural tissue (*neural plate*) come together and fuse. Failure of normal fusion results in a number of congenital defects (*see* neural tube defects).

neural tube defects a group of congenital abnormalities caused by failure of the *neural tube to form normally. In *spina bifida the bony arches of the spine, which protect the spinal cord and its coverings (the meninges), fail to close. More severe defects of fusion of these bones result in increasingly serious neurological conditions. A *meningocele* is the protrusion of the meninges through the gap in the spine, the skin covering being vestigial. There is a constant risk of damage to the meninges, with resulting infection. Urgent surgical treatment to protect the meninges is required. In a *meningomyelocele* (*myelomeningocele* or *myelocele*) the spinal cord and the nerve roots are exposed, often adhering to the fine membrane that overlies them. There is a constant risk of infection and this condition is accompanied by paralysis and numbness of the legs and urinary incontinence. *Hydrocephalus and the *Arnold-Chiari malformation are usually present. A failure of fusion at the cranial end of the neural tube (*cranium bifidum*) gives rise to comparable disorders. The bone defect is most often in the occipital region of the skull but it may occur in the frontal or basal regions. A protrusion of the meninges alone is called a *cranial meningocele*. The terms *meningoencephalocele*, *encephalocele*, and *cephalocele* are used to indicate the protrusion of brain tissue through the skull defect. This is accompanied by severe mental and physical disorders.

neurapraxia *n.* temporary loss of nerve function resulting in tingling, numbness, and weakness. It is usually caused by compression of the nerve and there is no structural damage involved. Complete recovery occurs. *Compare* axonotmesis, neurotmesis.

neurasthenia *n.* a set of psychological and physical symptoms, including fatigue, irritability, headache, dizziness, anxiety, and intolerance of noise. It can be caused by organic damage, such as a head injury, or it can be due to neurosis. —**neurasthenic** *adj.*, *n.*

neurectasis *n.* the surgical procedure for stretching a peripheral nerve.

neurectomy *n.* the surgical removal of the whole or part of a nerve.

neurilemma (neurolemma) *n.* the sheath of the *axon of a nerve fiber. The neurilemma of a medullated fiber contains *myelin laid down by Schwann cells. —**neurilemmal** *adj.*

neurilemoma (neurinoma) *n.* a benign slow-growing tumor arising from the neurilemma of a nerve fiber.

neurinoma *n. see* neurilemoma.

neuritis *n.* a disease of the peripheral nerves showing the pathological changes of inflammation. The term is also used in a less precise sense as an alternative to *neuropathy. *See also* optic neuritis.

neuroanatomy *n.* the study of the structure of the nervous system, from the gross anatomy of the brain down to the microscopic details of neurons.

neurobiotaxis *n.* the predisposition of a nerve cell to move toward the source of its stimuli during development.

neuroblast *n.* any of the nerve cells of the embryo that give rise to functional nerve cells (neurons).

neuroblastoma *n.* a malignant tumor composed of embryonic nerve cells. It may originate in any part of the sympathetic nervous system, most commonly in the medulla of the adrenal gland, and secondary growths are often widespread in other organs and in bones. It occurs usually before three years of age, and males are more affected than females. Treatment is with surgery, radiotherapy, and chemotherapy.

neurocranium *n.* the part of the skull that encloses the brain.

neurodermatitis (lichen simplex chronicus) *n.* a skin disease in which localized areas itch persistently and, because of constant scratching, become thickened (*see* lichenification). Women are affected more than men and the cause is uncertain, although stress is a causative factor. Common sites are the back of the neck in women and the lower legs in men.

neuroendocrine system the system of dual control of certain activities of the body by means of both nerves and circulating hormones. The functioning of the autonomic nervous system is particularly closely linked to that of the pituitary and adrenal glands. The system can give rise to *neuroendocrine tumors*, which have special structural features and often produce active hormones. *See* neurohormone, neurosecretion.

neuroepithelioma *n.* a malignant tumor of

the retina of the eye. It is a form of *glioma and commonly spreads into the brain.

neuroepithelium *n.* a type of epithelium associated with organs of special sense. It contains sensory nerve endings and is found in the retina, the membranous labyrinth of the inner ear, the mucous membrane lining the nasal cavity, and the taste buds. —**neuroepithelial** *adj.*

neurofibril *n.* one of the microscopic threads of cytoplasm found in the cell body of a *neuron and also in the *axoplasm of peripheral nerves.

neurofibroma (Schwannoma) *n.* a benign tumor growing from the fibrous coverings of a peripheral nerve caused by abnormal proliferation of *Schwann cells: it is usually symptomless. When it develops from the sheath of a nerve root, it causes pain and may compress the spinal cord.

neurofibromatosis (von Recklinghausen's disease) *n.* a congenital disease, inherited as a *dominant characteristic, that is typified by numerous benign tumors growing from the fibrous coverings of nerves (*see* neurofibroma). Tumors may occur in the spinal canal, where they may press on the spinal cord. The tumors can be felt beneath the skin along the course of the nerves; they sometimes become malignant, giving rise to *neurofibrosarcomas*. Pigmented patches on the skin (*café au lait spots*) are commonly found. Neurofibromatosis is sometimes associated with *fibrous dysplasia and occasionally with the adrenal tumor *pheochromocytoma, acoustic *neuroma, *glioma, or *meningioma.

neurogenesis *n.* the growth and development of nerve cells.

neurogenic *adj.* **1.** caused by disease or dysfunction of the nervous system. **2.** arising in nervous tissue. **3.** caused by nerve stimulation.

neuroglia *n.* *see* glia.

neurohormone *n.* a hormone that is produced within specialized nerve cells and is secreted from the nerve endings into the circulation. Examples are the hormones oxytocin and vasopressin, produced within the nerve cells of the hypothalamus and released into the circulation in the posterior pituitary gland, and norepinephrine, released from

*chromaffin tissue in the adrenal medulla.

neurohumor *n.* a *neurohormone or a *neurotransmitter.

neurohypophysis *n.* the posterior lobe of the *pituitary gland.

neurolemma *n.* *see* neurilemma.

neurology *n.* the study of the structure, functioning, and diseases of the nervous system (including the brain, spinal cord, and all the peripheral nerves). —**neurological** *adj.* —**neurologist** *n.*

neuroma *n.* any tumor derived from cells of the nervous system. Such tumors are usually categorized more specifically (e.g. *neurofibroma, *neurilemoma). An *acoustic neuroma* is a slow-growing benign tumor of the sheath of the vestibular branch of the *vestibulocochlear nerve that arises in the auditory canal. It progresses to cause tinnitus and hearing loss.

neuromuscular junction (myoneural junction) the meeting point of a nerve fiber and the muscle fiber that it supplies. Between the enlarged end of the nerve fiber (*motor end-plate*) and the membrane of the muscle is a gap across which a *neurotransmitter must diffuse from the nerve to trigger contraction of the muscle.

neuromyelitis optica (Devic's disease) a condition that is closely related to multiple sclerosis. Typically there is a transverse *myelitis, producing paralysis and numbness of the legs and trunk below the inflamed spinal cord, and *optic (retrobulbar) neuritis affecting both optic nerves. The attacks of myelitis and optic neuritis may coincide or they may be separated by days or weeks. Recovery from the initial attack is often incomplete, but relapses appear to be less common than in conventional multiple sclerosis.

neuron (nerve cell) *n.* one of the basic functional units of the nervous system: a cell specialized to transmit electrical *nerve impulses and so carry information from one part of the body to another (see illustration). Each neuron has an enlarged portion, the *cell body* (*perikaryon*), containing the nucleus; from the body extend several processes (*dendrites*) through which impulses enter from their branches. A longer process, the nerve fiber (*see* axon), extends outward and carries impulses away from the cell body. This is normally un-branched except at the *nerve ending. The point of contact of one neuron with another is known as a *synapse.

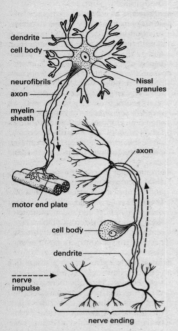

dendrite
cell body
neurofibrils
Nissl granules
axon
myelin sheath
axon
motor end plate
cell body
dendrite
nerve impulse
nerve ending

Types of neuron: motor (left) and sensory (right)

neuronophagia n. the process whereby damaged or degenerating nerve cells finally disintegrate and are removed by scavenger cells (*phagocytes).

neuronoplasty n. reconstructive surgery for damaged or severed peripheral nerves.

neuropathic bladder a malfunctioning bladder due to partial or complete interruption of its nerve supply. Causes include injury to the spinal cord, spina bifida, multiple sclerosis, and diabetic neuropathy.

neuropathy n. any disease of the peripheral nerves, usually causing weakness and numbness. In a *mononeuropathy* a single nerve is affected and the extent of the symptoms depends upon the distribution of that nerve. In a *polyneuropathy* (*see* peripheral neuropathy) many or all of the nerves are involved and the symptoms are most profound at the extremities of the limbs. *See also* diabetic neuropathy.

neurophysiology n. the study of the complex chemical and physical changes that are associated with the activity of the nervous system.

neuropil n. nerve tissue that is visible microscopically as a mass of interwoven and interconnected nerve endings, dendrites, and other neuron components, rather than an ordered array of axons.

neuropsychiatry n. the branch of medicine concerned with the psychiatric effects of disorders of neurological function or structure. Increasingly, the correlation is being drawn between demonstrable brain changes and the resulting effects on the mind. It is the function of the growing speciality of neuropsychiatry to investigate this relationship.

neuroretinitis n. combined inflammation of the optic nerve and the retina.

neurosecretion n. any substance produced within, and secreted by, a nerve cell. Important examples are the hormone-releasing factors produced by the cells of the *hypothalamus and released into blood vessels of the pituitary gland, on which they act.

neurosis n. (*pl.* **neuroses**) any long-term mental or behavioral disorder in which contact with reality is retained and the condition is recognized by the patient as abnormal. A neurosis essentially features anxiety or behavior exaggeratedly designed to avoid anxiety. Defense mechanisms against anxiety take various forms and may appear as phobias, obsessions, compulsions, or sexual dysfunctions. In a recent reclassification, the disorders formerly included under the neuroses have been renamed. In *DSM-IV the general term is now *anxiety disorder* (*see* anxiety); hysteria has become *conversion disorder; amnesia, fugue, multiple personality, and depersonalization are called *dissociative disorders; obsessional neurosis is now known as *obsessive–compulsive disorder* (see obsession); and depressive neurosis has become *dysthymic disorder* (see depression). Psychoanalysis has proved of little value in curing these conditions and Freud's speculations as to their origins are not now widely accepted outside Freudian schools of thought. Neurotic disorders are probably best regarded as being the result of inappropriate early programming. *Behavior therapy seems effective in some cases. —**neurotic** *adj.*

neurosurgery *n.* the surgical or operative treatment of diseases of the brain and spinal cord. This includes management of head injuries, the relief of raised intracranial pressure and compression of the spinal cord, eradication of infection, control of intracranial hemorrhage, and the diagnosis and treatment of tumors. The development of neurosurgery has been supported by advances in anesthetics, radiology, and scanning techniques.

neurosyphilis *n.* *syphilis affecting the nervous system.

neuroticism *n.* a dimension of personality derived from questionnaires and psychological tests. People with high scores in neuroticism are anxious and intense and more prone to develop neurosis.

neurotmesis *n.* the complete severance of a peripheral nerve, which is associated with degeneration of the nerve fibers distal to the point of severance and slow *nerve regeneration. *Compare* axonotmesis, neurapraxia.

neurotomy *n.* the surgical procedure of severing a nerve.

neurotoxic *adj.* poisonous or harmful to nerve cells.

neurotransmitter *n.* a chemical substance released from nerve endings to transmit impulses across *synapses to other nerves and across the minute gaps between the nerves and the muscles or glands that they supply. Outside the central nervous system the chief neurotransmitter is *acetylcholine; *norepinephrine is released by nerve endings of the sympathetic system. In the central nervous system, besides acetylcholine and norepinephrine, *dopamine, *serotonin, *gamma-aminobutyric acid, the amino acid glutamate, and several other substances act as transmitters.

neurotrophic *adj.* relating to the growth and nutrition of neural tissue in the body.

neurotropic *adj.* growing toward or having an affinity for neural tissue. The term may be applied to viruses, chemicals, or toxins.

neutropenia *n.* a decrease in the number of *neutrophils in the blood. Neutropenia may occur in a wide variety of diseases, including certain hereditary defects, aplastic *anemias, tumors of the bone marrow, *agranulocytosis, and acute leukemias. It may also occur after chemotherapy or radiotherapy and results in an increased susceptibility to infections.

neutrophil *n.* a variety of *granulocyte (a type of white blood cell) distinguished by a lobed nucleus and the presence in its cytoplasm of fine granules that stain purple with *Romanovsky stains. It is capable of ingesting and killing bacteria and provides an important defense against infection. There are normally $2.0–7.5 \times 10^9$ neutrophils per liter of blood.

nevirapine *n.* a *reverse transcriptase inhibitor of the human immunodeficiency virus type 1 (*HIV-1), indicated for the treatment of HIV-1 infection in combination with at least two other active antiretroviral agents when therapy is warranted. This combination of agents blocks the replication of HIV and prevents healthy T cells from becoming infected with the virus. Nevirapine is administered orally; common side effects include rash, muscle and joint aches, oral lesions, headache, excessive tiredness, vomiting and diarrhea. Trade name: **Viramune**.

nevus *n.* (*pl.* **nevi**) a birthmark: a clearly defined malformation of the skin, present at birth. There are many different types of nevi. Some are composed of small blood vessels (see hemangioma). These blood-vessel birthmarks include the *strawberry mark*, which usually disappears in early life, and the *port-wine stain*, which does not disappear and can now be treated by laser. Occasionally a port-wine stain may be associated with a malformation of blood vessels over the brain, for example in the Sturge-Weber syndrome (see angioma). A pale or white halo often develops around an ordinary pigmented nevus, especially on the trunk, forming a *halo nevus*. The pigmented nevus disappears over the course of a few months; this is followed by resolution of the pale area. A *blue nevus* is a small blue-gray papule appearing at birth or later in life, mainly on the extremities. Progression to malignant melanoma is very rare. A *nevus of Ota* (*oculodermal melanocytosis*) is a blue-gray pigmented area on the cheek, eyelid, or forehead; similar pigmentation is seen in the sclera of an eye. It is associated with melanomas of the uvea, orbit, and brain as well as with glaucoma of the affected eye. *See also* angioma, mole[2].

New Drug Application (NDA) a request to the Food and Drug Administration (FDA) for approval to market a drug that is not generally recognized as safe and effective for human use in interstate commerce. The Kefauver-Harris Amendment of 1962 requires that efficacy of new drugs must be proved before they can be prescribed by physicians, and in 1976 the law was extended to require that safety and efficacy of medical devices be demonstrated before they can be used in the treatment of disease or injury. The application must include data from clinical studies to prove that the drug is safe and effective and technical information on its chemistry, its pharmacology, its medical uses, and, if applicable, its microbiologic effects. How the drug is manufactured, processed, and packaged and the quality controls are also required. A typical review takes an average of two years; if no new studies or data are required, the review averages about 13 months. For some critical drugs, such as those for the treatment of AIDS, the process can be shortened.

newton *n.* the *SI unit of force, equal to the force required to impart to 1 kilogram an acceleration of 1 meter per second per second. Symbol: N.

Nexium *n. see* esomeprazole.

nexus *n.* (in anatomy) a connection or link.

NGF *see* nerve growth factor.

niacin (nicotinic acid) *n.* a B vitamin. Niacin is a derivative of pyridine and is interchangeable with its amide, *nicotinamide*. Both forms of the vitamin are equally active. Niacin is a component of the coenzymes *NAD (nicotinamide

adenine dinucleotide) and NADP, its phosphate. Niacin is required in the diet but can also be formed in small amounts in the body from the essential amino acid tryptophan. A deficiency of the vitamin leads to *pellagra. Good sources of niacin are meat, yeast extracts, and some cereals. Niacin is present in some cereals (e.g. corn) in a bound unavailable form. The adult recommended intake is 18 mg equivalent per day (1 mg equivalent is equal to 1 mg of available niacin or 60 mg tryptophan). It is used in the treatment of hypercholesterolemia.

nicardipine *n.* a *calcium antagonist used to treat long-term angina. It is administered by mouth. Possible side effects include nausea, chest pain, dizziness, headache, flushing, and palpitations. Trade name: **Cardene**.

niche *n.* (in anatomy) a recess or depression in a smooth surface.

niclosamide *n.* an *anthelmintic drug used to remove tapeworms. It is administered by mouth; unlike older treatments, it is free from serious side effects. Trade name: **Niclocide**.

nicorandil *n. see* potassium-channel activator.

nicotinamide *n.* a B vitamin: the amide of *niacin.

nicotinamide adenine dinucleotide *see* NAD.

nicotine *n.* a poisonous alkaloid derived from *tobacco, responsible for the dependence of regular smokers on cigarettes. In small doses nicotine has a stimulating effect on the autonomic nervous system, causing in regular smokers such effects as raised blood pressure and pulse rate and impaired appetite. Large doses cause paralysis of the autonomic ganglia. It is applied transdermally and used in chewing gum, nasal sprays, and inhalers as an aid to smoking cessation.

nicotinic acid *see* niacin.

nictitation *n.* exaggerated and frequent blinking or winking of the eyes.

nidation *n. see* implantation.

nidus *n.* a place in which bacteria have settled and multiplied because of particularly suitable conditions: a focus of infection.

nifedipine *n.* a *calcium antagonist used in the treatment of angina, high blood pressure (hypertension), and Raynaud's phenomenon. It is administered by mouth; side effects include dizziness, headache, and nausea. Trade names: **Adalat, Procardia**.

night blindness the inability to see in dim light or at night. It is due to a disorder of the cells in the retina that are responsible for vision in dim light (*see* rod), and can result from dietary deficiency of *vitamin A. If the vitamin deficiency continues, night blindness may progress to *xerophthalmia and *keratomalacia. Night blindness may be caused by other retinal diseases, e.g. *retinitis pigmentosa. *Congenital stationary night blindness* is characterized by poor night vision from early childhood that does not get worse. Medical name: **nyctalopia**. *Compare* day blindness.

night sweat copious sweating during sleep. Night sweats may be an early indication of such diseases as tuberculosis, AIDS, or Hodgkin's disease.

night terror the condition in which a child (usually aged 2–5 years), soon after falling asleep, starts screaming and appears terrified. The child cannot be comforted because he remains mentally inaccessible; the attack ceases when he wakes up fully and is never remembered. Attacks sometimes follow a stressful experience.

Nile blue an oxazine chloride, used for staining lipids and lipid pigments. *Nile blue A* (*Nile blue sulfate*), which stains fatty acids, changes from blue to purplish at pH 10–11.

nimodipine *n.* a *calcium antagonist used to prevent strokes in patients with subarachnoid hemorrhage. It is administered by mouth; side effects include reduced blood pressure, rash, and gastrointestinal symptoms. Trade name: **Nimotop**.

ninhydrin reaction a histochemical test for proteins, in which ninhydrin (triketohydrindene hydrate) is boiled with the test solution and gives a blue color in the presence of amino acids and proteins.

nipple (mamilla, papilla) *n.* the protuberance at the center of the *breast. In females the milk ducts open at the nipple.

Nissl granules collections of dark-staining material, containing RNA, seen in the cell bodies of neurons on microscopic examination. [F. Nissl (1860–1919), German neuropathologist]

nit *n.* the egg of a *louse. The eggs of head lice are firmly cemented to the hair, usually at the back of the head; those of body lice are fixed to the clothing. Nits, 0.8×0.3 mm, are visible as light white specks.

nitrates *pl. n.* a class of drugs used as coronary *vasodilators for the treatment and prevention of angina attacks. They include glyceryl trinitrate (*nitroglycerin), *isosorbide dinitrate, and isosorbide mononitrate.

nitric acid a strong corrosive mineral acid, HNO_3, the concentrated form of which is capable of producing severe burns of the skin. Swallowing the acid leads to intense burning pain and ulceration of the mouth and throat. Treatment is by immediate administration of alkaline solutions, followed by milk or olive oil.

nitric oxide an important member of the group of gaseous mediators, which – together with amine mediators (e.g. epinephrine, norepinephrine, histamine, acetylcholine) and lipid mediators (e.g. prostaglandins) – produce many physiological responses (e.g. smooth muscle relaxation). Nitric oxide is involved in the manifestations of sepsis and septic shock. The medical importance of nitric oxide is a growing area of interest. Formula: NO.

nitrofurantoin *n.* a drug used to treat bacterial infections of the urinary system. It is administered by mouth and may cause nausea, vomiting, and skin rashes. Trade names: **Furadantin, Macrobid, Macrodantin**.

nitrogen *n.* a gaseous element and a major constituent of air (79%). Nitrogen is an essential constituent of proteins and nucleic acids and is obtained by animals in the form of protein-containing foods (atmospheric nitrogen cannot be utilized directly). Nitrogenous waste is excreted as *urea. Liquid nitrogen is used to freeze some specimens for pathologic examination. Symbol: N.

nitrogen balance the relationship between the nitrogen taken into the body and that excreted, denoting the balance between the manufacture and breakdown of the body mass. A negative nitrogen balance, when excretion exceeds intake, is usual after injury or operations as the energy requirements of the body are met disproportionately from endogenous sources.

nitroglycerin (glyceryl trinitrate) a drug that dilates blood vessels and is used to prevent and treat angina (*see* vasodilator). It is administered by mouth, injection, sprays, ointments, and skin patches, and large doses may cause flushing, headache, and fainting. Trade names: **Deponit, Minitran, Nitro-Bid, Nitrodisc, Nitro-Dur, Nitrogard, Nitrol Ointment, Nitrolingual Spray, Nitrong, Nitrostat, Transderm-Nitro, Tridil.**

nitrosourea *n.* any of a group of *alkylating agents used in the chemotherapy of various cancers. They have severe toxic effects, primarily *myelosuppression. Among these drugs are *carmustine and *lomustine.

nitrous oxide a colorless gas used as an *anesthetic with good *analgesic properties. It is administered by inhalation, in conjunction with oxygen, and is used as a vehicle for potent anesthetic vapors, such as halothane. A mixture of oxygen and nitrous oxide provides effective analgesia for some dental procedures and in childbirth; such a state is known as *relative analgesia*. However, long-term exposure to the gas is toxic, so its use has been greatly limited. Nitrous oxide was formerly referred to as *laughing gas* because of its tendency to excite the patient when used alone.

nizatidine *n.* a histamine H_2-receptor antagonist (*see* antihistamine) used to treat duodenal ulcers and prevent their recurrence and to treat *gastroesophageal reflux disease. It is administered by mouth; side effects include headache, diarrhea, and rhinitis. Trade name: **Axid.**

NK cell *see* natural killer cell.

nm *symbol for* nanometer.

NMR *see* nuclear magnetic resonance.

Nocardia *n.* a genus of rodlike or filamentous gram-positive nonmotile bacteria found in the soil. As cultures age, filaments form branches, but these soon break up into rodlike or spherical cells. Three or more spores may form in each cell; these germinate to form filaments. Some species are pathogenic: *N. asteroides* causes *nocardiosis and *N. madurae* is associated with the disease *Madura foot.

nocardiosis *n.* a disease caused by bacteria

of the genus *Nocardia*, primarily affecting the lungs, skin, and brain, resulting in the formation of abscesses. Treatment involves antibiotics and sulfonamides.

noci- *prefix denoting* pain or injury.

nociceptive *adj.* describing nerve fibers, endings, or pathways that are concerned with the condition of pain.

nociceptor *n.* a *receptor that responds to the stimuli responsible for the sensation of pain. Nociceptors may be *interoceptors, responding to such stimuli as inflammation, or *exteroceptors, sensitive to heat, etc.

no-code *n. see* DNR (do not resuscitate).

noct- (nocti-) *prefix denoting* night.

noctambulation *n. see* somnambulism.

nocturia *n.* the passage of urine at night. In the absence of a high fluid intake, sleep is not normally interrupted by the need to pass urine. Nocturia usually occurs in elderly men or women. In younger men or women, less urine is made at night than during the day, but this rhythm is lost with age in both sexes. Men may have additional problems arising from *benign prostatic hyperplasia, but transurethral resection of the prostate often does not reduce nocturia.

node *n.* a small swelling or knot of tissue. *See* atrioventricular node, lymph node, sinoatrial node.

node of Ranvier one of the gaps that occurs at regular intervals in the *myelin sheath of medullated nerve fibers, between adjacent *Schwann cells.

nodule *n.* a small swelling or aggregation of cells.

noma *n.* a gangrenous infection of the mouth that spreads to involve the face. It is rare in civilized communities and is usually found in debilitated or malnourished individuals. Noma is a severe form of *ulcerative gingivitis.

noncompliance *n.* failure or refusal to adhere to a therapeutic regimen or treatment, especially medications or medical schedules and appointments, due to cultural or religious beliefs or other social, psychological, or physical reasons.

nondisjunction *n.* a condition in which pairs of homologous chromosomes fail to separate during meiosis or a chromosome fails to divide at *anaphase of mitosis or meiosis. It results in a cell with an abnormal number of chromosomes (*see* monosomy, trisomy).

non-Hodgkin's lymphoma *see* lymphoma.

noninvasive *adj.* **1.** denoting techniques of investigation or treatment that do not involve penetration of the skin by needles or knives. **2.** denoting tumors that do not spread into surrounding tissues (*see* benign).

Nonne's syndrome (cerebellar syndrome) *see* (cerebellar) ataxia. [M. Nonne (1861–1959), German neurologist]

nonsecretor *n.* a person in whose body fluids it is not possible to detect soluble forms of the A, B, or O agglutinogens that determine blood group. *Compare* secretor.

non-small-cell lung cancer any type of lung cancer except small-cell lung cancer (*see* oat cell). These cancers include *adenocarcinoma of the lung, large-cell carcinomas, and squamous cell carcinoma of the lung.

nonsteroidal anti-inflammatory drug *see* NSAID.

Noonan's syndrome an autosomal *dominant condition of males who have all or some of the physical features of *Turner's syndrome in females but normal sex chromosomes. It is often associated with a low testosterone level and sometimes with reduced sperm production. Other features include cardiovascular defects and most individuals with the condition have short stature and mild mental retardation. [J. Noonan (1921–), US pediatrician]

norepinephrine (noradrenaline) *n.* a hormone, closely related to *epinephrine and with similar actions, secreted by the medulla of the *adrenal gland and also released as a *neurotransmitter by sympathetic nerve endings. Among its many actions are constriction of small blood vessels leading to an increase in blood pressure, increased blood flow through the coronary arteries and a slowing of the heart rate, increase in the rate and depth of breathing, and relaxation of the smooth muscle in intestinal walls.

norethindrone *n.* a synthetic female sex hormone (*see* progestogen) administered by mouth to treat menstrual disorders, including amenorrhea. It is also used in oral contraceptives, often in combination with an estrogen. Trade names: **Micronor, Nor-Q.D**.

norfloxacin *n.* an antibacterial drug, a *quinolone, used in the treatment of urinary tract infections, sexually transmitted diseases, and conjunctivitis. It is administered by mouth and in eye drops; side effects include nausea, headache, dizziness, and fatigue. Trade names: **Chibroxin, Noroxin**.

norgestrel *n.* a *progestogen used either alone or in combination with an estrogen as an oral contraceptive. Common side effects include irregular menstrual periods, breast pain, headache, dizziness, and acne. Trade names: **Ovral, Ovrette**.

norma *n.* a view of the skull from one of several positions, from which it can be described or measured. For example the *norma lateralis* is a side view of the skull; the *norma verticalis* is the view of the top of the skull.

normalization *n.* (in psychiatry) the process of making the living conditions of people with *mental handicap as similar as possible to those of people who are not handicapped. This includes living outside institutions and encouragement to cope with work, pay, social life, sexuality, and civil rights.

normo- *prefix denoting* normality.

normoblast *n.* a nucleated cell that forms part of the series giving rise to the red blood cells and is normally found in the blood-forming tissue of the bone marrow. Normoblasts pass through three stages of maturation: *early* (or *basophilic*), *intermediate* (or *polychromatic*), and *late* (or *orthochromatic*) forms. *See also* erythroblast, erythropoiesis.

normocyte *n.* a red blood cell of normal size. A *normocytic anemia* is anemia characterized by the presence of such cells. —**normocytic** *adj.*

normotensive *adj.* describing the state in which arterial blood pressure is within the normal range. *Compare* hypertension, hypotension.

Northern blot analysis a technique for identifying a specific form of messenger RNA in cells. It uses a gene *probe known to match the RNA being sought. *Compare* Southern blot analysis, Western blot analysis.

nortriptyline *n.* a tricyclic *antidepressant drug used to relieve all types of depression. It is administered by mouth; side effects may include dry mouth and drowsiness. Trade names: **Aventyl, Pamelor**.

nose *n.* the organ of olfaction, which also acts as an air passage that warms, moistens, and filters the air on its way to the lungs. The *external nose* is a triangular projection in the front of the face that is composed of cartilage and covered with skin. It leads to the *nasal cavity* (*internal nose*), which is lined with mucous membrane containing olfactory cells and is divided into two chambers (*fossae*) by the *nasal septum*. The lateral wall of each chamber is formed by the three scroll-shaped *nasal conchae, below each of which is a groovelike passage (*meatus*). The *paranasal sinuses open into these meatuses.

nosebleed *n.* bleeding from the nose, which may be caused by physical injury or may be associated with fever from low-grade infections, high blood pressure, blood disorders, or tumors of the nose or sinuses. The blood often comes from a vessel just inside the nostril, in which case the flow may be stopped by applying pressure on the side of the nose or cauterizing the bleeding vessel. Otherwise gauze packing or specially designed inflatable balloons may be effective in controlling the loss of blood. Occasionally surgery is required to stop the flow of blood. *See also* Little's area, Kiesselbach's plexus. Medical name: **epistaxis**.

noso- *prefix denoting* disease.

nosocomial infection (hospital infection) an infection originating in a hospital. It may develop in a hospitalized patient without having been present or incubating at the time of admission, or it may be acquired in hospital but only appears after discharge. Causes include the altered immune systems of many patients, the presence of antibiotic-resistant bacteria (*see* MRSA), and hospital environments conducive to the growth of bacteria and other microorganisms; the term also includes infections developing among hospital staff.

nosology *n.* the naming and classification of diseases.

Nosopsyllus *n.* a genus of fleas. The common rat flea of temperate regions, *N. fasciatus*, will, in the absence of rats, bite humans and may therefore transmit plague or murine typhus from an infected rat population. The rat flea is also an intermediate host for the larval stage of two tapeworms, *Hymenolepis diminuta* and *H. nana*.

nostrils *n. see* nares.

notch *n.* (in anatomy) an indentation, especially one in a bone.

notifiable disease a disease that must be reported to the health authorities in order that speedy control and preventive action may be undertaken if necessary. In the US such diseases must be reported to the county, state, or federal health officials. Notifiable diseases include AIDS, anthrax, cholera, diphtheria, encephalitis/meningitis, food poisoning, hepatitis, infective jaundice, malaria, measles, poliomyelitis, tuberculosis, typhoid, sexually transmitted diseases, and whooping cough. The list varies for different countries, and some diseases are internationally notifiable through the *World Health Organization; these include cholera, plague, and yellow fever.

notochord *n.* a strip of mesodermal tissue that develops along the dorsal surface of the early embryo, beneath the *neural tube. It becomes almost entirely obliterated by the development of the vertebrae, persisting only as part of the intervertebral disks.

novobiocin *n.* an antibiotic administered by mouth or injection to treat certain infections resistant to other antibiotics. Side effects, including digestive upsets and rashes, occur frequently and for this reason other antibiotics are usually preferred. Trade name: **Albamycin**.

NSAID (nonsteroidal anti-inflammatory drug) any one of a large group of drugs used for pain relief, particularly in rheumatic disease associated with inflammation but also in dysmenorrhea and metastatic bone disease. NSAIDs act by inhibiting the *cyclo-oxygenase* enzymes (COX-1 and COX-2) responsible for controlling the formation of *prostaglandins, which are important mediators of inflammation. They include *aspirin, *ibuprofen, and *diclofenac. Adverse effects include gastric bleeding and ulceration. Some NSAIDs act by selectively inhibiting COX-2 and are therefore less likely to cause gastric side effects (*see* COX-2 inhibitor).

nucha *n.* the nape of the neck. —**nuchal** *adj.*

nuchal thickness scanning an ultrasound screening test performed during pregnancy at 10–14 weeks of gestation that looks specifically at the thickness of the skin at the back of the neck (the nuchal fold) of the fetus as an aid to the prenatal diagnosis of chromosomal defects. The thicker the nuchal fold, the higher the risk of the baby having a chromosomal defect. *See also* ultrasound marker.

nuclear cardiology the study and diagnosis of heart disease by the intravenous injection of different types of *radionuclide. The radionuclide emits gamma rays, enabling a gamma camera and computer to form an image of the heart. *See* MUGA scan, SPECT scanning, thallium scan.

nuclear magnetic resonance (NMR) the absorption and emission of high-frequency radio waves by the nuclei of certain elements when placed in a strong magnetic field. The strongest signal is obtained from hydrogen atoms, which are abundant in the water and organic molecules in the body. In clinical use for *magnetic resonance imaging, the signal is highly dependent on the concentration and mobility of water molecules within each tissue. NMR has important applications in noninvasive diagnostic techniques. *See also* magnetic resonance spectroscopy.

nuclear medicine the use of *radionuclides (especially *technetium-99m) as *tracers to study the structure and function of organs of the body. The radionuclide is attached to a compound suitable for the particular test and then injected, inhaled, or ingested. When concentrated in the organ under investigation, the tracer can be imaged using a *gamma camera, revealing the structure or demonstrating the function of the organ. Alternatively, blood or urine samples may be analyzed. *See also* nuclear cardiology.

nuclease *n.* an enzyme that catalyzes the breakdown of nucleic acids by cleaving the bonds between adjacent nucleotides. Examples are *ribonuclease*, which acts on RNA, and *deoxyribonuclease*, which acts on DNA.

nucleic acid either of two organic acids, *DNA or *RNA, present in the nucleus and in some cases the cytoplasm of all living cells. Their main functions are in heredity and protein synthesis.

nucleolus *n.* (*pl.* **nucleoli**) a dense spherical structure within the cell *nucleus that

disappears during cell division. The nucleolus contains *RNA for the synthesis of *ribosomes and plays an important part in RNA and protein synthesis.

nucleoplasm (karyoplasm) *n.* the protoplasm making up the nucleus of a cell.

nucleoprotein *n.* a compound that occurs in cells and consists of nucleic acid and protein tightly bound together. *Ribosomes are nucleoproteins containing RNA; *chromosomes are nucleoproteins containing DNA.

nucleoside *n.* a compound consisting of a nitrogen-containing base (a *purine or *pyrimidine) linked to a sugar. Examples are *adenosine, *guanosine, *cytidine, *thymidine, and *uracil.

nucleoside analogues *see* antiviral drug.

nucleotide *n.* a compound consisting of a nitrogen-containing base (a *purine or *pyrimidine) linked to a sugar and a phosphate group. Nucleic acids (DNA and RNA) are long chains of linked nucleotides (*polynucleotide* chains), which in DNA contain the purine bases adenine and guanine and the pyrimidines thymine and cytosine; in RNA, thymine is replaced by uracil.

nucleus *n.* **1.** the part of a *cell that contains the genetic material *DNA. The DNA, which is combined with protein, is normally dispersed throughout the nucleus as *chromatin. During cell division the chromatin becomes visible as *chromosomes. The nucleus also contains *RNA, most of which is located in the *nucleolus. The nucleus is separated from the cytoplasm by a double membrane, the *nuclear envelope*. **2.** an anatomically and functionally distinct mass of nerve cells within the brain or spinal cord.

nude mouse a mouse born without a thymus and therefore no T-lymphocytes. Human tumors will often grow in these mice. For unknown reasons these mice are also hairless, hence the name.

nuisance *n.* any noxious substance, accumulating in refuse or as dust or effluent, that is deemed to be injurious to health or offensive. It can also include dwellings, work premises, animals, and noise.

null hypothesis *see* significance.

nullipara *n.* a woman who has never given birth to an infant capable of survival.

numbness *n.* partial or total loss of feeling

or sensation in part or all of the body. *See also* anesthesia, neuropathy.

nurse *n.* a person trained and licensed in nursing matters and entrusted with the care of the sick and the carrying out of medical and surgical routines under the supervision of a doctor. In addition, the nurse is concerned with the patient's response to the problem, providing nurturing and protection in a way that promotes health. *Registered nurses* often specialize, as in anesthesiology or surgery, and *nurse practitioners* can provide expanded care and perform many of the duties of a physician, including prescribing medications. *Practical nurses*, on the other hand, are not nursing school graduates and can provide limited nursing care.

nutation *n.* the act of nodding the head.

nutrient *n.* a substance that must be consumed as part of the diet to provide a source of energy, material for growth, or substances that regulate growth or energy production. Nutrients include carbohydrates, fats, proteins, minerals, and vitamins. *See also* essential amino acid, essential fatty acid, trace element.

nutrition *n.* **1.** the study of food in relation to the physiological processes that depend on its absorption by the body (growth, energy production, repair of body tissues, etc.). The science of nutrition includes the study of diets and deficiency diseases. **2.** the intake of nutrients and their subsequent absorption and assimilation by the tissues. Patients who cannot be fed in a normal way can be given nutrients by tubes into the intestines (*enteral feeding*) or by infusion into a vein (*intravenous feeding*).

nux vomica the seed of the tree *Strychnos nux-vomica*, which contains the poisonous alkaloid *strychnine.

nyct- (nycto-) *prefix denoting* night or darkness.

nyctalopia *n. see* night blindness.

nyctohemeral *adj.* denoting a cyclical event occurring both in the day and the night. *Compare* circadian, ultradian.

nyctophilia *n.* an intense preference for the darkness and an avoidance of activity in daylight hours. This is sometimes a form of social *phobia.

nyctophobia *n.* extreme fear of the dark. It is common in children and can occur in normal adults.

nyctophonia *n.* speaking in the night but not in the daytime: a form of elective *mutism.

nylidrin hydrochloride a drug whose main action is to dilate blood vessels, particularly those in skeletal muscles. Administered orally, intramuscularly, and subcutaneously, it is used to increase the blood flow to muscle, especially in vascular disease due to spasm of the arteries. It may cause palpitations and stimulate gastric secretion. Trade name: **Arlidin**.

nymph *n.* **1.** an immature stage in the life history of certain insects, such as grasshoppers and *reduviid bugs. On emerging from the eggs, nymphs resemble the adult insects except that they are smaller, do not have fully developed wings, and are not sexually mature. **2.** the late larval stage of a tick.

nympho- *prefix denoting* **1.** the labia minora. **2.** female sexuality.

nymphomania *n.* an extreme degree of sexual promiscuity in a woman. *Compare* satyriasis. —**nymphomaniac** *adj., n.*

nystagmus *n.* rapid involuntary movements of the eyes that may be from side to side, up and down, or rotatory. Nystagmus may be congenital and associated with poor sight; it also occurs in disorders of the part of the brain responsible for eye movements and their coordination and in disorders of the organ of balance in the ear or the associated parts of the brain. *Optokinetic nystagmus* occurs in normal people when they try to look at a succession of objects moving quickly across their line of sight. Jerking eye movements sometimes occur in normal people when tired. These are called *nystagmoid jerks* and they do not imply disease.

nystatin *n.* an antibiotic active against fungi, used especially to treat yeast infections, such as candidiasis. It is applied as a cream for skin infections, by mouth for oral and intestinal infections, as pessaries or suppositories for vaginal or anal infections, or as eye drops for eye infections. Side effects include mild digestive upsets. Trade names: **Mycostatin**, **Nilstat**, **Nystex**.

OAE *see* otoacoustic emissions.

oat cell a cell type of carcinoma of the bronchus. Oat cells are small round or oval cells with darkly staining nuclei and scanty indistinct cytoplasm. Oat-cell carcinoma is usually related to smoking and accounts for about one quarter of bronchial carcinomas; it carries a poor prognosis. It is now increasingly known as *small-cell lung cancer* and can be cured in the early stages by chemotherapy and radiotherapy.

obesity *n.* the condition in which excess fat has accumulated in the body, mostly in the subcutaneous tissues. Clinical obesity is usually considered to be present when a person has a *body mass index of 30 or over. The accumulation of fat is caused by the consumption of more food than is required for producing enough energy for daily activities. However, recent evidence indicates that a genetic element is involved. Hunger and satiety appear to be controlled by peptide messengers, encoded by specific genes and acting on the brain; an example is *leptin. Obesity is the most common nutritional disorder of recent years to occur in Western societies: some patients may require surgical treatment to attain worthwhile weight reduction; drug treatments may also help (*see* orlistat, sibutramine). —**obese** *adj.*

obex *n.* the curved lower margin of the fourth *ventricle of the brain, between the medulla oblongata and the cerebellum.

objective *n.* (in microscopy) the lens or system of lenses in a light microscope that is nearest to the object under examination and farthest from the *eyepiece. In many microscopes interchangeable objectives with different powers of magnification are provided.

obligate *adj.* describing an organism that is restricted to one particular way of life; for example, an *obligate parasite* cannot exist without a host. *Compare* facultative.

observer error *see* validity.

obsession *n.* a recurrent thought, feeling, or action that is unpleasant and provokes anxiety but cannot be eliminated. Although an obsession dominates the person, he (or she) realizes its senselessness and struggles to expel it. The obsession may be a vivid image, a fear (for example, of contamination), a thought, or an impulse (for example, to wash the hands repetitively). It is a feature of *obsessive–compulsive disorder* (*see* neurosis) and sometimes of depression and organic states, such as encephalitis. It can be treated with behavior therapy and also with psychotherapy and anxiolytic drugs. *See also* anancastic. —**obsessional** *adj.*

obstetrics *n.* the branch of medical science concerned with the care of women during pregnancy, childbirth, and the period of about six weeks following the birth, when the reproductive organs are recovering. *Compare* gynecology. —**obstetric** *adj.* —**obstetrician** *n.*

obstipation *n.* severe or complete constipation.

obstructive airways disease *see* bronchospasm.

obstructive sleep apnea *see* sleep apnea.

obtund *vb.* to blunt or deaden sensitivity; for example, by the application of a local anesthetic, which reduces or causes complete loss of sensation in nearby nerves.

obturation *n.* obstruction of a body passage, usually by impaction of a foreign body, thickened secretions, or hard feces.

obturator *n.* **1.** *see* obturator muscle. **2.** a wire or rod within a cannula or hollow needle for piercing tissues or fitting aspirating needles. **3.** a removable form of denture that both closes a defect in the palate and also restores the dentition. The defect may be congenital, as in a cleft palate, or result from the removal of a tumor.

obturator foramen a large opening in the *hip bone, below and slightly in front of the acetabulum. *See also* pelvis.

obturator muscle either of two muscles that cover the outer surface of the anterior wall of the pelvis (the *obturator externus* and *obturator internus*) and are responsible for lateral rotation of the thigh and movements of the hip.

obtusion *n.* the weakening or blunting of normal sensations. This may be associated with disease.

occipital bone a saucer-shaped bone of the *skull that forms the back and part of the base of the cranium. At the base of the occipital are two *occipital condyles*: rounded surfaces that articulate with the first (atlas) vertebra of the spine. Between the condyles is the *foramen magnum*, the cavity through which the spinal cord passes.

occiput *n.* the back of the head. —**occipital** *adj.*

occlusal *adj.* (in dental anatomy) denoting or relating to the biting surface of a premolar or molar tooth.

occlusal rim the occlusal extension of a denture base to allow the recording of jaw relations in the construction of *dentures.

occlusion *n.* **1.** the closing or obstruction of a hollow organ or part. **2.** (in dentistry) the relation of the upper and lower teeth when they are in contact. Maximum contact between the teeth is known as *intercuspal* or *centric occlusion*. *See also* malocclusion.

occult *adj.* not apparent to the naked eye; not easily determined or detected. For example *occult blood* is blood present in such small quantities, for example in the feces, that it can only be detected microscopically or by chemical testing.

occupational disease any one of various specific diseases to which workers in certain occupations are particularly prone. *Industrial diseases*, associated with a particular industry or group of industries, fall within this category. Examples of such diseases include the various forms of *pneumoconiosis, which affect the lungs of workers continually exposed to dusty atmospheres; cataracts in glassblowers; decompression sickness in divers; poisoning from toxic metals in factory and other workers; and infectious diseases contracted from animals by farm workers. *See also* Workmen's Compensation Laws.

occupational mortality rates and causes of death in relation to different jobs or occupational and socioeconomic groups. Because some occupations have older incumbents than others (e.g. judges) allowance for age bias is made by comparing either *standardized mortality ratios* for those aged 15–64 years or related but less familiar indices, such as *comparative mortality figures* or *proportional mortality ratios*.

Occupational Safety and Health Administration (OSHA) a US government agency that is responsible for establishing standards for maintaining safe and healthful workplaces and for protection against exposure to hazardous materials and working conditions. OSHA also is responsible for enforcing regulations designed to protect the health of industrial workers, although state governments also may establish and enforce laws governing the health and safety of persons exposed to potentially hazardous working conditions. This agency generally coordinates its standards with recommendations of another federal agency, the National Institute of Occupational Safety and Health (NIOSH).

occupational therapy the treatment of physical and psychiatric conditions by encouraging patients to undertake specific selected activities that will help them to reach their maximum level of function and independence in all aspects of daily life. These activities are designed to make the best use of the patient's capabilities and are based on individual requirements. They range from printing, woodwork, and metalwork to pottery and other artistic and creative activities, household management, social skills (for psychiatric patients), and leisure activities (for geriatric patients). Occupational therapy also includes assessment for mechanical aids and adaptations in the home.

ochronosis *n.* the presence of brown-black pigment in the skin, cartilage, and other tissues due to the abnormal accumulation of homogentisic acid that occurs in the metabolic disease *alkaptonuria.

oct- (octa-, octi-, octo-) *prefix denoting* eight.

octreotide *n.* a somatostatin analogue (*see* somatostatin).

ocular *adj.* of or concerned with the eye or vision.

oculist *n.* a former term for an *ophthalmologist.

oculo- *prefix denoting* the eye.

oculogyric *adj.* causing or concerned with movements of the eye.

oculomotor *adj.* concerned with eye movements.

oculomotor nerve the third *cranial nerve (III), which is composed of motor fibers distributed to muscles in and around the eye. Fibers of the parasympathetic system are responsible for altering the size of the pupil and the lens of the eye. Fibers outside the eye run to the upper eyelid and to muscles that turn the eyeball in different directions.

oculonasal *adj.* concerned with the eye and nose.

oculoplastics *n.* a surgical specialty concerned with reconstructive and cosmetic surgery around the eye (including the orbit, eyelids, lacrimal apparatus, and other accessory structures).

oculoplethysmography *n.* measurement of the pressure inside the eyeball. A rising or above-normal pressure is an important indication of the presence of *glaucoma.

odont- (odonto-) *prefix denoting* a tooth. Example: *odontalgia* (toothache).

odontoblast *n.* a cell that forms dentine. Odontoblasts line the pulp and have small processes that extend into the dentine.

odontoid process a toothlike process from the upper surface of the axis vertebra. *See* cervical vertebrae.

odontology *n.* the study of the teeth.

odontoma *n.* an abnormal mass of calcified dental tissue, which usually represents a developmental abnormality. *Compare* hamartoma.

-odynia *suffix denoting* pain in (a specified part).

odynophagia *n.* a sensation of pain behind the sternum as food or fluid is swallowed; particularly, the burning sensation experienced by patients with *esophagitis when hot, spicy, or alcoholic liquid is swallowed.

Oedipus complex repressed sexual feelings of a child for its opposite-sexed parent, combined with rivalry toward the same-sexed parent: said, in Freudian psychoanalytical theory, to be a normal stage of development. The end of the Oedipus complex in children is marked by a loss of sexual feelings toward the opposite-sexed parent and an increase in identification with the same-sexed parent. Arrest of development at the Oedipal stage is said to be responsible for sexual deviations and other neurotic behavior.

Oesophagostomum *n.* a genus of parasitic nematodes occurring in Brazil, Africa, and Indonesia. It is a rare intestinal parasite of humans, producing symptoms of dysentery in cases of heavy infection.

The worms may also invade the tissues of the intestinal wall, giving rise to abscesses. The worms can be eliminated with anthelmintics.

Oestrus *n.* a genus of widely distributed nonbloodsucking flies, occurring wherever sheep and goats are raised. The parasitic larvae of *O. ovis,* the sheep nostril fly, may occasionally and accidentally infect humans. By means of large mouth hooks, it attaches itself to the conjunctiva of the eye, causing a painful *myiasis that may result in loss of sight. This is an occupational disease of shepherds. Larvae can be removed with forceps following anesthesia.

ofloxacin *n.* a *quinolone antibiotic used especially to treat infections of the urinary tract, lower respiratory tract, and sexually transmitted infections, as well as infections of the skin, eye, and ear canal. It is administered by mouth, injection, or as eye or ear drops; possible side effects include nausea, vomiting, headache, and skin rashes. Trade names: **Floxin, Floxin Otic, Ocuflox**.

ohm *n.* the *SI unit of electrical resistance, equal to the resistance between two points on a conductor when a constant potential difference of 1 volt applied between these points produces a current of 1 ampere. Symbol: Ω.

-oid *suffix denoting* like; resembling. Example: *pemphigoid* (condition resembling pemphigus).

ointment *n.* a greasy preparation, which may or may not contain medication, for use on skin or mucous membranes. Although less pleasant to use than the equivalent *cream, it is more effective since it forms an impermeable layer in the outer layer of the skin, reducing evaporation from the surface.

olanzapine *n. see* antipsychotic.

olecranon process the large process of the *ulna that projects behind the elbow joint.

oleic acid *see* fatty acid.

oleo- *prefix denoting* oil.

oleothorax *n.* the procedure of introducing a light oil into the *pleural cavity so that the lung is allowed to collapse. This was sometimes formerly undertaken to allow healing in a lung damaged by tuberculosis.

oleum *n.* (in pharmacy) an oil.

olfaction *n.* **1.** the sense of smell. **2.** the

process of smelling. Sensory cells in the mucous membrane that lines the nasal cavity are stimulated by the presence of chemical particles dissolved in the mucus. *See* nose. —**olfactory** *adj.*

olfactory nerve the first *cranial nerve (I): the special sensory nerve of smell. Fibers of the nerve run upward from smell receptors in the nasal mucosa high in the roof of the nose, through minute holes in the skull, join to form the olfactory tract, and pass back to reach the brain.

olig- (oligo-) *prefix denoting* **1.** few. **2.** a deficiency.

oligemia *n. see* hypovolemia.

oligoarthritis *n. see* arthritis.

oligodactylism *n.* the congenital absence of some of the fingers and toes.

oligodendrocyte *n.* one of the cells of the *glia, responsible for producing the *myelin sheaths of the neurons of the central nervous system and therefore equivalent to the *Schwann cells of the peripheral nerves.

oligodendroglioma *n.* a tumor of the central nervous system derived from a type of *glia (the supporting tissue) rather than from the nerve cells themselves. *See also* glioma.

oligodipsia *n.* a condition in which thirst is diminished or absent.

oligodontia *n.* the congenital absence of some of the teeth.

oligohydramnios *n.* a condition in which the amount of amniotic fluid bathing a fetus during pregnancy is abnormally small. It is usually associated with retarded fetal growth and may indicate serious fetal kidney abnormalities. *See* Potter's syndrome.

oligomenorrhea *n.* sparse or infrequent menstruation.

oligo-ovulation *n.* infrequent occurrence of ovulation.

oligospermia *n.* the presence of less than the normal number of spermatozoa in the semen. Normal semen produced on ejaculation usually contains more than 60 million sperm/ml, of which about 80% are motile and morphologically normal. In oligospermia, the sperm are reduced in number, usually have poor motility, and often include many bizarre and immature forms (*teratospermia*). Treatment is directed to any underlying cause (such as *varicocele). *See also* andrology, infertility.

oliguria *n.* the production of an abnormally small volume of urine. This may be a result of copious sweating associated with intense physical activity and/or hot weather. It can also be due to kidney disease, retention of water in the tissues (*see* edema), loss of blood, diarrhea, or poisoning.

olive (olivary body) *n.* a smooth oval swelling in the upper part of the medulla oblongata on each side of the brain. It contains a mass of nerve cells, mainly gray matter (*olivary nucleus*). —**olivary** *adj.*

Ollier's disease *see* dyschondroplasia. [L. L. X. E. Ollier (1830–1900), French surgeon]

-ology *suffix. see* -logy.

olsalazine *n.* a salicylate preparation used to treat mild ulcerative colitis. It is administered by mouth. Possible side effects include diarrhea, nausea, vomiting, headache, joint pain, and skin rashes. Trade name: **Dipentum**.

om- (omo-) *prefix denoting* the shoulder. Example: *omodynia* (pain in).

-oma *suffix denoting* a tumor. Examples: *hepatoma* (of the liver); *lymphoma* (of the lymph nodes).

omentectomy *n.* the removal of all or part of the omentum (the fold of peritoneum between the stomach and other abdominal organs).

omentopexy *n.* an operation in which the *omentum is attached to some other tissue, usually the abdominal wall (in order to improve blood flow through the liver) or the heart (to increase the blood supply to the heart).

omentum (epiploon) *n.* a double layer of *peritoneum attached to the stomach and linking it with other abdominal organs, such as the liver, spleen, and intestine. The *great omentum* is a highly folded portion of the omentum, rich in fatty tissue, that covers the intestines in an apronlike fashion. It acts as a heat insulator and prevents friction between abdominal organs. The *lesser omentum* links the stomach with the liver. —**omental** *adj.*

omeprazole *n.* a *proton-pump inhibitor that is used to treat gastric and duodenal ulcers, reflux *esophagitis, and the *Zollinger-Ellison syndrome. Omeprazole can be effective in cases that have failed to respond to H_2-receptor antagonists, such as *ranitidine. Administered by mouth, it is long-acting and need only be taken once a day. Possible side effects include nausea, diarrhea, headache, constipation, and skin rashes. Trade names: **Losec, Prilosec.**

Ommaya reservoir a device inserted into the ventricles of the brain to enable the repeated injection of drugs into the cerebrospinal fluid. It is used, for example, in the treatment of malignant meningitis, particularly in children with leukemia. It can also be used to allow aspiration of cystic gliomas.

omphal- (omphalo-) *prefix denoting* the navel or umbilical cord.

omphalitis *n.* inflammation of the navel, especially in newborn infants.

omphalocele *n.* an umbilical *hernia.

omphalus *n. see* umbilicus.

Onchocerca *n.* a genus of parasitic worms (*see* filaria) occurring in central Africa and central America. The adult worms are found in fibrous nodules within the connective tissues beneath the skin and their presence causes disease (*see* onchocerciasis). Various species of black fly, in which *Onchocerca* undergoes part of its development, transmit the infective larvae to humans.

onchocerciasis *n.* a tropical disease of the skin and underlying connective tissue caused by the parasitic worm *Onchocerca volvulus.* Fibrous nodular tumors grow around the adult worms in the skin; these may take several months to appear, and if secondary bacterial infection occurs they may degenerate into abscesses. The skin also becomes inflamed and itches. The migration of the larvae into the eye can cause total or partial blindness – the *river blindness* of Africa. Onchocerciasis occurs in Africa and Central and South America. The drugs *suramin, *diethylcarbamazine, and *ivermectin are used in treatment; if possible, the nodules are removed as and when they appear.

onco- *prefix denoting* **1.** a tumor. **2.** volume.

oncofetal antigen a protein normally produced only by fetal tissue but often produced by certain tumors. An example is *carcinoembryonic antigen (CEA), which has been used as a *tumor marker, especially in colorectal carcinomas.

oncogene *n.* a gene in viruses (*v-onc*) and mammalian cells (*c-onc*) that can cause cancer. It results from the mutation of a normal gene. An oncogene is capable of both initiation and continuation of malignant transformation of normal cells. It probably produces proteins (*growth factors) regulating cell division that, under certain conditions, become uncontrolled and may transform a normal cell to a malignant state.

oncogenesis *n.* the development of a new abnormal growth (a benign or malignant tumor).

oncogenic *adj.* describing a substance, organism, or environment that is known to be a causal factor in the production of a tumor. Some animal viruses are known to be oncogenic; others are suspected of being so in humans, including some *papovaviruses, *adenoviruses, *retroviruses, and *herpesviruses. *See also* carcinogen.

oncology *n.* the study and practice of treating tumors. It is often subdivided into medical, surgical, and radiation oncology. —**oncologist** *n.*

oncolysis *n.* the destruction of tumors and tumor cells. This may occur spontaneously or, more usually, in response to treatment with drugs or radiotherapy.

oncometer *n.* an instrument for measuring the volume of blood circulating in one of the limbs. *See* plethysmography.

oncosphere (hexacanth) *n.* the six-hooked larva of a *tapeworm. If ingested by a suitable intermediate host, such as a pig or an ox, the larva will use its hooks to penetrate the wall of the intestine. The larva subsequently migrates to the muscles, where it develops into a *cysticercus.

oncotic *adj.* **1.** characterized by a tumor or swelling. **2.** relating to an increase in volume or pressure.

oncotic pressure the pressure difference that exists between the osmotic pressure of blood and that of the lymph or tissue fluid. Oncotic pressure is important for regulating the flow of water between blood and tissue fluid. *See also* osmosis.

ondansetron *n.* a drug that is used to control severe nausea and vomiting, especially when it results from chemotherapy and radiotherapy. Ondansetron works by opposing the action of the neurotransmitter *serotonin (5-hydroxytryptamine). It is given orally or by injection; side effects include diarrhea, headache, and constipation. Trade name: **Zofran**.

oneir- (oneiro-) *prefix denoting* dreams or dreaming.

oneirism *n.* daydreaming. Obviously, this is a normal phenomenon, but in excess it may impair the ability to cope with life. This is a feature of *schizoid and *asthenic personalities.

onomatomania *n.* the repeated intrusion of a specific word or a name into a person's thoughts: a form of *obsession.

onomatopoiesis *n.* inventing words that reflect the sound made by the object or event to be described. It is one of the principles that guide some schizophrenics in the production of *neologisms.

ontogeny *n.* the history of the development of an individual from the fertilized egg to maturity.

onych- (onycho-) *prefix denoting* the nail(s).

onychia *n.* inflammation of the matrix of the *nail, which results in loss of the nail.

onychogryphosis *n.* gross thickening and hardening of the nail, which becomes elongated and deformed. The cause is unknown.

onycholysis *n.* separation or loosening of part or all of a nail from its bed. The condition may occur in *psoriasis and in fungus infections of the skin and nail bed; it may also be caused by drugs.

onychomadesis *n.* loss of the nails.

onychomycosis *n.* fungus infection of the nails, usually caused by *Epidermophyton* or *Candida*. The nails become white, opaque, thickened, and brittle. *See also* ringworm.

onychopathy (onychosis) *n.* any disease or deformity of the nails.

O'nyong-nyong fever (joint-breaker fever) an East African disease caused by an *arbovirus and transmitted to humans by mosquitoes of the genus *Anopheles*. The disease is similar to *dengue and symptoms include rigor, severe headache, an irritating rash, fever, and pains in the joints. The patient is given drugs to relieve the pain and fever.

oo- *prefix denoting* an egg; ovum.

oocyst *n.* a spherical structure, 50–60 μm in diameter, that develops from the zygote (*see* ookinete) of the malarial parasite (*Plasmodium*) on the outer wall of the mosquito's stomach. The oocyst steadily grows in size and its contents divide repeatedly to form *sporozoites, which are released into the body cavity of the mosquito when the oocyst bursts.

oocyte *n.* a cell in the ovary that undergoes *meiosis to form an ovum. *Primary oocytes* develop from *oogonia in the fetal ovary as they enter the early stages of meiosis. Only a fraction of the primary oocytes survive until puberty, and even fewer will be ovulated. At ovulation the first meiotic division is completed and a *secondary oocyte* and a *polar body* are formed. Fertilization stimulates the completion of the second meiotic division, which produces a second polar body and an ovum.

oocyte donation the transfer of oocytes from one woman to another. Possible recipients include women with primary or secondary ovarian failure or severe genetic disorders, and women in whom ovulation has been suppressed as an incidental result of drug treatment for another condition (e.g. cancer). Pregnancy rates are higher than with *in vitro fertilization.

oogenesis *n.* the process by which mature ova (egg cells) are produced in the ovary (see illustration). Primordial germ cells multiply to form *oogonia, which start their first meiotic division to become

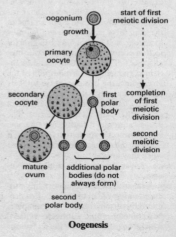

Oogenesis

*oocytes in the fetus. This division is not completed until each oocyte is ovulated. The second division is only completed on fertilization. Each meiotic division is unequal, so that one large ovum is produced with a much smaller polar body.

oogonium n. (pl. **oogonia**) a cell produced at an early stage in the formation of an ovum (egg cell). Primordial germ cells that have migrated to the embryonic ovary multiply to form numerous small oogonia. After the fifth month of pregnancy, they enter the early stages of the first meiotic division to form *oocytes. See also oogenesis.

ookinete n. the motile elongated *zygote of the malarial parasite (*Plasmodium), formed after fertilization of the *macrogamete. The ookinete bores through the lining of the mosquito's stomach and attaches itself to the outer wall, where it later forms an *oocyst.

oophor- (oophoro-) prefix denoting the ovary.

oophorectomy (ovariectomy) n. surgical removal of an ovary, performed, for example, when the ovary contains tumors or cysts or is otherwise diseased. See also ovariotomy.

oophoritis (ovaritis) n. inflammation of an ovary, either on the surface or within the organ. Oophoritis may be associated with infection of the fallopian tubes (see salpingitis) or the lower part of the abdominal cavity. Follicular oophoritis is inflammation of the ovarian (graafian) follicles. A bacterial infection usually responds to antibiotics.

oophoropexy n. the stitching of a displaced ovary to the wall of the pelvic cavity.

operant adj. describing a unit of behavior that is defined by its effect on the environment. See conditioning.

operating microscope a binocular microscope commonly used in microsurgery and in such operations as the removal of a blood clot from an artery (see endarterectomy). The field of operation is illuminated through the objective lens by a light source within the microscope (see illustration). Many models incorporate a beam splitter and a second set of eyepieces, to enable the surgeon's assistant to view the operation.

operculum n. (pl. **opercula**) **1.** a plug of mucus that blocks the cervical canal of the uterus in a pregnant woman. When the cervix begins to dilate at the start of labor, the operculum, slightly stained with blood, is discharged. **2.** (in embryology) a plug of fibrin and blood cells that develops over the site at which a developing fertilized ovum has become embedded in the wall of the uterus. **3.** (in neurology) one of the folded and overlapping regions of cerebral cortex that conceal the *insula on each side of the brain. **4.** (in dentistry) a flap of gingival tissue that overlies the crown of a partially erupted tooth.

operon n. a group of closely linked genes that regulate the production of enzymes. An operon is composed of one or more *structural genes*, which determine the nature of the enzymes made, and *operator* and *promoter genes*, which control the working of the structural genes. The operator is itself controlled by a *regulator gene*, which is not part of the operon.

ophthalm- (ophthalmo-) prefix denoting the eye.

ophthalmectomy n. an operation in which the eye is removed. See enucleation.

ophthalmia n. inflammation of the eye, particularly the conjunctiva (see conjunctivitis). *Sympathetic ophthalmia* is a granulomatous *uveitis affecting all parts of the uveal tract of both eyes that may develop after trauma or (more rarely) after eye surgery.

ophthalmia neonatorum a form of conjunctivitis occurring in newborn infants, who contract the disease as they pass through an infected birth canal. The two most common infections are gonorrhea and *Chlamydia* (see inclusion conjunctivitis); if untreated, the infection may cause permanent eye disease. Diagnosis should be confirmed on a culture swab, and treatment is with antibiotics.

ophthalmic adj. concerned with the eye.

ophthalmic nerve the smallest of the three branches of the *trigeminal nerve. It supplies sensory fibers to the eyeball, conjunctiva, and lacrimal gland, to a small region of the nasal mucous membrane, and to the skin of the nose, brows, and scalp.

ophthalmitis n. inflammation of the eye. See conjunctivitis, uveitis.

ophthalmodynamometry n. measurement of the blood pressure in the vessels of the retina of the eye. A small instrument is pressed against the eye until the vessels

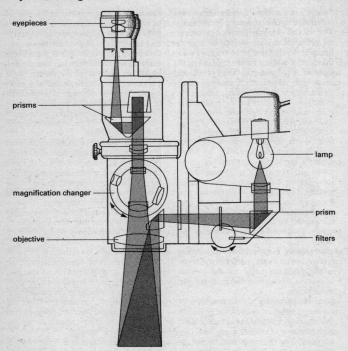

eyepieces

prisms

lamp

magnification changer

prism

objective

filters

An operating microscope

are seen (through an *ophthalmoscope) to collapse. The pressure recorded by the instrument reflects the pressure within the vessels of the retina. In certain disorders of the blood circulation to the eye, the pressure in the vessels is reduced and the vessels can be made to collapse by a pressure that is lower than normal.

ophthalmologist *n.* a doctor who specializes in the diagnosis and treatment of eye diseases.

ophthalmology *n.* the branch of medicine that is devoted to the study and treatment of eye diseases. —**ophthalmological** *adj.*

ophthalmometer *n. see* keratometer.

ophthalmoplegia *n.* paralysis of the muscles of the eye. *Internal ophthalmoplegia* affects the muscles inside the eye: the iris (which controls the size of the pupil) and

the ciliary muscle (which is responsible for *accommodation). *External ophthalmoplegia* affects the muscles that move the eye. *Chronic progressive external ophthalmoplegia* is a progressive disease of the extrinsic eye muscles leading to *ptosis and then paralysis of the muscles; eye movements become increasingly frozen in the primary position. Ophthalmoplegia may accompany *exophthalmos that is associated with thyrotoxicosis. *Internuclear ophthalmoplegia*, due to a lesion in the brainstem, is commonly seen in patients with multiple sclerosis or stroke.

ophthalmorrhexis *n.* rupture of the eyeball. This is usually due to a severe blow to the eye.

ophthalmoscope *n.* an instrument for examining the interior of the eye (see illustration). There are two types. The *direct ophthalmoscope* enables a fine beam of light to be directed into the eye and at the same time allows the examiner to see the spot where the beam falls inside the eye. Examiner and subject are very close together. In the *indirect ophthalmoscope* an image of the inside of the eye is formed between the subject and the examiner; it is this image that the examiner sees. The examiner and subject are almost an arm's length apart. A *scanning laser ophthalmoscope* uses a scanning camera, rather than a human observer, to view the inside of the eye. —**ophthalmoscopy** *n.*

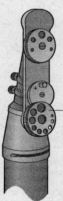
disk for changing lenses

An ophthalmoscope

ophthalmotomy *n.* the operation of making an incision in the eyeball.

ophthalmotonometer *n.* see tonometer.

-opia *suffix denoting* a defect of the eye or of vision. Example: *asthenopia* (eyestrain).

opiate *n.* strictly, one of a group of drugs derived from opium; however, the term is often used to include synthetic drugs with similar effects, in which case *opioid* is used synonymously. The group includes *apomorphine, *codeine, *morphine, and *papaverine. Opiates depress the central nervous system: they relieve pain, suppress coughing, and stimulate vomiting. The most important opiate – morphine – and its synthetic derivative

heroin are *narcotics, producing feelings of euphoria before inducing stupor. They are only used for severe pain since they may cause *dependence.

opisth- (opistho-) *prefix denoting* 1. dorsal; posterior. 2. backward.

opisthorchiasis *n.* a condition caused by the presence of the parasitic fluke *Opisthorchis in the bile ducts. The infection is acquired through eating raw or undercooked fish that contains the larval stage of the parasite. Heavy infections can lead to considerable damage of the tissues of the bile duct and liver, progressing in advanced cases to *cirrhosis. Symptoms may include loss of weight, abdominal pain, indigestion, and sometimes diarrhea. The disease, occurring in E Europe and the Far East, is treated with *chloroquine.

Opisthorchis *n.* a genus of parasitic flukes occurring in E Europe and parts of SE Asia. *O. felineus* is normally a parasite of fish-eating mammals but accidental infections of humans have occurred. The adult flukes, which live in the bile ducts, can cause *opisthorchiasis.

opisthotonos *n.* the position of the body in which the head, neck, and spine are arched backward. It is assumed involuntarily by patients with tetanus and strychnine poisoning.

opium *n.* an extract from the poppy *Papaver somniferum*, which has analgesic and narcotic action due to its content of *morphine. It has the same uses and side effects as morphine and prolonged use may lead to *dependence. *See also* opiate.

opponens *n.* one of a group of muscles in the hand that brings the digits opposite to other digits. For example, the *opponens pollicis* is the principal muscle causing opposition of the thumb.

opportunistic *adj.* denoting a disease that occurs when the patient's immune system is impaired by, for example, an infection, another disease, or drugs. The infecting organism, which is also described as opportunistic, rarely causes the disease in healthy persons. Opportunistic infections, such as *Pneumocystis carinii* pneumonia, and that caused by the MAI complex (*see* Mycobacterium), are common in persons with AIDS.

opposition *n.* (in anatomy) the position of the thumb in relation to the other fingers when it is moved toward the palm of the hand.

-opsia *suffix denoting* a condition of vision. Example: *erythropsia* (red vision).

opsoclonus (opsoclonia) *n.* a series of erratic eye movements in any direction, which is seen in people with disease of the cerebellum.

opsonic index a numerical measurement of the power of a person's serum to attack invading bacteria and prepare them for destruction by *phagocytes. It is measured by dividing the average number of bacteria in the blood per phagocyte in the presence of immune serum by the corresponding number in the presence of normal serum. A vaccine increases the opsonic index.

opsonin *n.* a serum *complement component that attaches itself to invading bacteria and apparently makes them more attractive to *phagocytes and thus more likely to be engulfed and destroyed.

opsonization *n.* the process by which opsonins render foreign organisms or particles more attractive to *phagocytes by attaching to their outer surfaces and changing their physical and chemical composition. Phagocytic leukocytes express receptors for these opsonins and thereby engulf and digest foreign organisms or particles.

opt-' (opto-) *prefix denoting* vision or the eye.

optic *adj.* concerned with the eye or vision.

optical activity the property possessed by some substances of rotating the plane of polarization of polarized light. A compound that rotates the plane to the left is described as *levorotatory* (or l-); one that rotates the plane to the right is described as *dextrorotatory* (or d-).

optic atrophy degeneration of the optic nerve. It may be secondary to disease within the eye or it may follow damage to the nerve itself resulting from injury or inflammation. It is visible as pallor of the optic nerve as viewed inside the eye with an ophthalmoscope.

optic chiasm (optic commissure) the X-shaped structure formed by the two optic nerves, which pass backward from the eyeballs to meet in the midline beneath the brain, near the pituitary gland (see illustration). Nerve fibers from the nasal side of the retina of each eye cross

over to join fibers from the lateral side of the retina of the opposite eye. The optic tracts resulting from the junction pass backward to the occipital lobes.

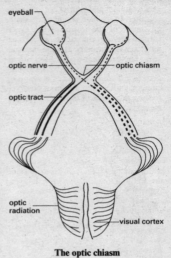

The optic chiasm

optic cup either of the paired cup-shaped outgrowths of the embryonic brain that form the retina and iris of the eyes.

optic disk (optic papilla) the start of the optic nerve, where nerve fibers from the rods and cones leave the eyeball. *See* blind spot.

optic foramen the groove in the top of the *orbit that contains the optic nerve and the ophthalmic artery.

optician (dispensing optician) *n.* a person who makes and fits glasses. *Compare* optometrist.

optic nerve the second *cranial nerve (II), which is responsible for vision. Each nerve contains about one million fibers that receive information from the rod and cone cells of the retina. It passes into the skull behind the eyeball to reach the *optic chiasm, after which the visual pathway continues to the cortex of the occipital lobe of the brain on each side.

optic neuritis inflammation of the optic nerve. It is classified as either *intraocular*, affecting that part of the nerve within the eyeball (*see* papillitis), or *retrobulbar*, affecting that part of the nerve behind the eyeball (*see* retrobulbar neuritis).

optokinetic (opticokinetic) *adj.* relating to the movements of the eye.

optometer (refractometer) *n.* an instrument for measuring the *refraction of the eye. An *autorefractor* calculates the required spectacle lens correction automatically. Because the design and use of optometers is very complex, errors of refraction are usually determined using a *retinoscope.

optometrist *n.* a person specialized in the examination, diagnosis, treatment, and management of disorders of the visual system and of the eye and associated structures as well as the diagnosis of related systemic conditions. Doctors of optometry are independent primary health care providers. *Compare* optician.

oral *adj.* **1.** relating to the mouth. **2.** taken by mouth: applied to medicines, etc.

oral cavity the mouth.

oral contraceptive the Pill: a preparation, consisting of one or more synthetic female sex hormones, taken by women to prevent conception. Most oral contraceptives are combined pills, consisting of an *estrogen, which blocks the normal process of ovulation, and a *progestogen, which acts on the pituitary gland to block the normal control of the menstrual cycle. Progestogens also alter the lining of the uterus and the viscosity of mucus in its outlet, the cervix, so that conception is less likely should ovulation occur. These pills are taken every day for three weeks and then stopped for a week, during which time menstruation occurs. Side effects may include headache, weight gain, nausea, skin changes, and depression. There is also a small risk that blood clots may form in the veins, especially those of the legs (which may lead to *pulmonary embolism), or that prolonged use of hormonal contraceptives may reduce fertility. The unwanted pregnancy rate is less than 1 per 100 woman-years. With progestogen-only pills (sometimes known as *minipills*) the unwanted pregnancy rate is slightly higher (1–2 per 100 woman-years) but there are fewer side effects (due to the absence of estrogen). Other hormonal contraceptives include injections and implants (*see* contraception). *See also* postcoital contraception.

oral hypoglycemic drug (oral antidiabetic drug) one of the group of drugs that reduce the level of glucose in the blood and are taken by mouth for the treatment of noninsulin-dependent (type 2) *diabetes mellitus. They include the *sulfonylurea group (e.g. *chlorpropamide, *glipizide, and *tolbutamide), *metformin (a biguanide), *alpha-glucosidase inhibitors, *meglitinides, and *thiazolidinediones.

oral rehabilitation the procedure of rebuilding a dentition that has been mutilated as a result of disease, wear, or trauma.

oral rehydration therapy the administration of an isotonic solution of various sodium salts, potassium chloride, glucose, and water to treat acute diarrhea, particularly in children. In developing countries it is the mainstay of treatment for cholera. Once the diarrhea has stopped, normal feeding is gradually resumed.

orbicularis *n.* either of two circular muscles of the face. The *orbicularis oris*, around the mouth, closes and compresses the lips. The *orbicularis oculi*, around each orbit, is responsible for closing the eye.

orbit *n.* the cavity in the skull that contains the eye. It is formed from parts of the frontal, sphenoid, zygomatic, lacrimal, ethmoid, palatine, and maxillary bones. —**orbital** *adj.*

orbitotomy *n.* a surgical incision into the bony orbit containing the eye.

orchi- (orchio-) *prefix denoting* the testis or testicle. Example: *orchioplasty* (plastic surgery of).

orchialgia *n.* pain in the testicle, often due to a *varicocele, *orchitis, or *torsion of the testis. The pain may also be caused by a hernia in the groin or the presence of a stone in the lower ureter.

orchidometer *n.* a calliper device used for measuring the size of the testicles. The *Prader orchidometer* consists of a collection of testicle-shaped beads of different sizes, each of known volume, for direct comparison to and sizing of the testicles. It enables the precise charting of testicular growth.

orchiectomy (orchidectomy) *n.* surgical removal of a testis, usually to treat germ-cell tumors of the testis, such as

*seminoma or *teratoma, which are malignant tumors of the testis. Removal of both testes (*castration) causes sterility and reduces levels of testosterone by 90%, which is an effective treatment for prostate cancer.

orchiopexy (orchidopexy) *n.* the operation of mobilizing an undescended testis in the groin and fixing it in the scrotum. The operation should be performed well before puberty to allow the testis every chance of normal development (*see* cryptorchidism).

orchiotomy (orchidotomy) *n.* an incision into the testis, usually done to obtain *biopsy material for histological examination, particularly in men with few or no sperm in their semen (*see* azoospermia, oligospermia).

orchitis *n.* inflammation of the testis. This causes pain, redness, and swelling of the scrotum, and may be associated with inflammation of the epididymis (*epididymo-orchitis*). The condition may affect one or both testes; it is usually caused by infection spreading down the vas deferens but can develop in mumps. Mumps orchitis affecting both testes may result in sterility. Treatment of epididymo-orchitis is by local support and administration of analgesics and antibiotics; mumps orchitis often responds to *corticosteroids.

orf *n.* a poxvirus infection of sheep and goats that can be transmitted to humans, causing a mild skin eruption on the fingers, hands, and forearms that resolves spontaneously.

organ *n.* a part of the body, composed of more than one tissue, that forms a structural unit responsible for a particular function (or functions). Examples are the heart, lungs, and liver.

organelle *n.* a structure within a cell that is specialized for a particular function. Examples of organelles are the nucleus, endoplasmic reticulum, Golgi apparatus, lysosomes, and mitochondria.

organic *adj.* **1.** relating to any or all of the organs of the body. **2.** describing chemical compounds containing carbon, found in all living systems. *Compare* inorganic.

organic disorder a disorder associated with changes in the structure of an organ or tissue. *Compare* functional disorder.

organism *n.* any living thing, which may

consist of a single cell (*see* microorganism) or a group of differentiated but interdependent cells.

organo- *prefix denoting* organ or organic. Examples: *organogenesis* (formation of); *organopathy* (disease of).

organ of Corti (spiral organ) the sense organ of the *cochlea of the inner ear, which converts sound signals into nerve impulses that are transmitted to the brain via the cochlear nerve. [A. Corti (1822–88), Italian anatomist]

organ of Jacobson (vomeronasal organ) a small blind sac in the wall of the nasal cavity. In humans it never develops properly and has no function, but in lower animals (e.g. snakes) it is one of the major organs of olfaction. [L. L. Jacobson (1783–1843), Danish anatomist]

organotherapy (Brown-Séquard's treatment) *n.* the treatment of disease with preparations made from animal endocrine organs or their extracts. Synthetic preparations are now frequently used instead of actual extracts of a gland.

organotrophic *adj. see* heterotrophic.

orgasm *n.* the climax of sexual excitement, which – in men – occurs simultaneously with *ejaculation. In women its occurrence is much more variable, being dependent upon a number of physiological and psychological factors.

oriental sore (Baghdad boil, Delhi boil, Aleppo boil) a skin disease, occurring in tropical and subtropical Africa and Asia, caused by the parasitic protozoan *Leishmania tropica* (*see* leishmaniasis). The disease commonly affects children and takes the form of a slow-healing open sore or ulcer, which sometimes becomes secondarily infected with bacteria. Antibiotics are administered to combat the infection.

orientation *n.* (in psychology) awareness of oneself in time, space, and place. Orientation may be disturbed in such conditions as organic brain disease, toxic drug states, and concussion.

orifice *n.* the opening to any body part or cavity.

origin *n.* (in anatomy) **1.** the point of attachment of a muscle that remains relatively fixed during contraction of the muscle. *Compare* insertion. **2.** the point at which a nerve or a blood vessel branches from a main nerve or blood vessel.

orlistat *n.* a drug that reduces the absorption of fat in the stomach and small intestine by inhibiting the action of pancreatic *lipases. It is administered by mouth to treat clinical *obesity. Side effects include the production of copious oily stools and flatulence. Trade name: **Xenical**.

ornithine *n.* an *amino acid produced in the liver as a by-product during the conversion of ammonia to *urea.

Ornithodoros (Ornithodorus) *n.* a genus of soft *ticks, a number of species of which are important in various parts of the world in the transmission of *relapsing fever.

ornithosis *n.* see psittacosis.

oro- *prefix denoting* the mouth.

oroantral fistula a connection between the mouth and the maxillary sinus (antrum) usually as a sequel to tooth extraction. It may resolve or require surgical closure.

oropharyngeal airway a curved tube designed to be placed in the mouth of an unconscious patient, behind the tongue, to create a patent airway. *See also* nasopharyngeal airway.

oropharynx *n.* the part of the *pharynx that lies between the level of the junction of the hard and soft palates above, the hyoid bone (which is situated near the upper portion of the epiglottis) below, and the arch of the soft palate in front. It contains the *tonsils and connects the oral cavity and *nasopharynx to the *laryngopharynx. —**oropharyngeal** *adj.*

Oroya fever see bartonellosis.

orphan drug a drug used for treating rare diseases, such as *Gilles de la Tourette syndrome and *Wilson's disease, that has no potential of recovering the cost of research, development, and distribution of the product for the drug manufacturer. Many of these pharmaceuticals are developed in other countries but are not available in the US until several years later. For such drugs, the 1983 Orphan Drug Act allows many *Food and Drug Administration requirements to be omitted. More than 200 orphan drugs are now available.

orphenadrine *n.* a drug that relieves spasm in muscle, used to treat all types of parkinsonism. It is administered by mouth or injection; side effects may include dry mouth, sight disturbances, and difficulty in urination. Trade names: **Disipal**, **Norflex**.

ortho- *prefix denoting* **1.** straight. Example: *orthograde* (having straight posture). **2.** normal. Example: *orthocrasia* (normal reaction to drugs).

orthochromatic *adj.* describing or relating to a tissue specimen that stains normally.

orthodontic appliance an appliance used to move teeth as part of orthodontic treatment. A *fixed appliance* is fitted to the teeth and used to perform complex tooth movements; it is used by dentists with specialist training (*orthodontists*). A *removable appliance* is a dental plate with appropriate retainers and springs to perform simple tooth movements; it is removed from the mouth for cleaning by the patient.

orthodontics *n.* the branch of dentistry concerned with the growth and development of the face and jaws and the treatment of irregularities of the teeth. *See* orthodontic appliance. —**orthodontic** *adj.*

orthognathic surgery surgical correction of severe *malocclusion, in which development of one or both jaws is abnormal, to improve facial appearance. It needs to be carried out in combination with orthodontic treatment and may involve surgery to one or both jaws.

orthokeratology *n.* the use of contact lenses designed to reshape the cornea in the treatment of refractive errors, such as myopia (nearsightedness).

orthopantomogram *n.* see pantomography.

orthopedics *n.* the science or practice of correcting deformities caused by disease of or damage to the bones and joints of the skeleton. This specialized branch of surgery may involve operation, manipulation, traction, *orthoses or *prostheses. —**orthopedic** *adj.*

orthophoria *n.* the condition of complete balance between the movements of the two eyes, so that perfect alignment is maintained even when one eye is covered. This theoretically normal state is in fact rarely seen, since most people have a slight tendency to squint (*see* heterophoria).

orthopnea *n.* breathlessness that prevents the patient from lying down, so that he has to sleep propped up in bed or sitting in a chair. —**orthopneic** *adj.*

orthoptics *n.* the practice of using nonsurgical methods, particularly eye exercises, to treat abnormalities of vision and of coordination of eye movements, most commonly strabismus (squint) and amblyopia. Orthoptics also includes the detection and measurement of the degree of such abnormalities. —**orthoptist** *n.*

orthoptoscope *n. see* amblyoscope.

orthosis *n. (pl.* **orthoses)** a surgical appliance that exerts external forces on part of the body to support joints or correct deformity. An example is a spinal brace.

orthostatic *adj.* relating to the upright position of the body: used when describing this posture or a condition caused by it. *Orthostatic hypotension,* for example, is low blood pressure found in some patients when they stand upright.

orthotics *n.* the science and practice of fitting surgical appliances to assist weakened joints.

Ortolani's sign *see* Barlow maneuver. [M. Ortolani (20th century), Italian orthopedic surgeon]

os[1] *n. (pl.* **ossa)** a bone.

os[2] *n. (pl.* **ora)** the mouth or a mouthlike part.

osche- (oscheo-) *prefix denoting* the scrotum. Example: *oscheocele* (a scrotal hernia).

oscilloscope *n.* a cathode-ray tube designed to display electronically a wave form corresponding to the electrical data fed into it. Oscilloscopes are used to provide a continuous record of many different measurements, such as the activity of the heart and brain. *See* electrocardiography, electroencephalography.

osculum *n.* (in anatomy) a small aperture.

Osgood-Schlatter disease inflammation and swelling at the site of insertion of the main quadriceps tendon at the top of the tibia, just below the knee (*see* apophysitis, osteochondritis). It is common in adolescence and results from excessive physical activity. Most cases resolve with time and rest. [R. B. Osgood (1873–1956), US orthopedist; C. Schlatter (1864–1934), Swiss surgeon]

OSHA *see* Occupational Safety and Health Administration.

-osis *suffix denoting* **1.** a diseased condition. Examples: *nephrosis* (of the kidney); *leptospirosis* (caused by *Leptospira* species). **2.** any condition. Example: *narcosis* (of stupor). **3.** an increase or excess. Examples: *polyposis* (of polyps); *leukocytosis* (of leukocytes).

osm- (osmo-) *prefix denoting* **1.** smell or odor. **2.** osmosis or osmotic pressure.

osmic acid *see* osmium tetroxide.

osmiophilic *adj.* describing a tissue that stains readily with osmium tetroxide.

osmium tetroxide (osmic acid) a colorless or faintly yellowish compound used to stain fats or as a *fixative in the preparation of tissues for microscopical study. Osmium tetroxide evaporates readily, the vapor having a toxic action on the eyes, skin, and respiratory tract.

osmolality *n.* the concentration of body fluids (e.g. plasma, urine) measured in terms of the amount of dissolved substances per unit mass of water. It is usually given in units of mol kg^{-1}.

osmole *n.* a unit of osmotic pressure equal to the molecular weight of a solute in grams divided by the number of ions or other particles into which it dissociates in solution.

osmoreceptor *n.* a *receptor in the *hypothalamus that monitors the concentration of blood. Should this increase abnormally, as in dehydration, the osmoreceptors send nerve impulses to the hypothalamus, which then increases the rate of release of *vasopressin from the posterior pituitary gland. Loss of water from the body in the urine is thus restricted until the blood concentration returns to normal.

osmosis *n.* the passage of a solvent from a less concentrated to a more concentrated solution through a *semipermeable membrane. This tends to equalize the concentrations of the two solutions. In living organisms the solvent is water and cell membranes function as semipermeable membranes, and the process of osmosis plays an important role in controlling the distribution of water. The *osmotic pressure* of a solution is the pressure by which water is drawn into it through the semipermeable membrane; the more concentrated the solution (i.e. the more solute molecules it contains), the greater its osmotic pressure. —**osmotic** *adj.*

osseointegration *n.* the process by which certain materials, such as titanium, may be introduced into living bone without producing a foreign-body reaction. This allows a very tight and strong joint between the two structures. Osseointegration is used, for example, to fix recently developed types of dental *implants and *bone-anchored hearing aids.

osseous *adj.* bony: applied to the bony parts of the inner ear (cochlea, semicircular canals, labyrinth).

ossicle *n.* a small bone. The *auditory ossicles* are three small bones (the incus, malleus, and stapes) in the middle *ear. They transmit sound from the outer ear to the labyrinth (inner ear).

ossification (osteogenesis) *n.* the formation of *bone, which takes place in three stages by the action of special cells (osteoblasts). A meshwork of collagen fibers is deposited in connective tissue, followed by the production of a cementing polysaccharide. Finally, the cement is impregnated with minute crystals of calcium salts. The osteoblasts become enclosed within the matrix as *osteocytes* (*bone cells*). In *intracartilaginous* (or *endochondral*) ossification the bone replaces cartilage. This process starts to occur soon after the end of the second month of embryonic life. *Intramembranous ossification* is the formation of a *membrane bone (e.g. a bone of the skull). This starts in the early embryo and is not complete at birth (*see* fontanelle).

ost- (oste-, osteo-) *prefix denoting* bone. Examples: *ostalgia* (pain in); *osteocarcinoma* (carcinoma of); *osteonecrosis* (death of); *osteoplasty* (plastic surgery of).

ostectomy *n.* the surgical removal of a bone or a piece of bone. *See also* osteotomy.

osteitis *n.* inflammation of bone, due to infection, damage, or metabolic disorder. *Osteitis fibrosa cystica* refers to the characteristic cystic changes that occur in bones during long-standing *hyperparathyroidism. *See also* Paget's disease (of bone; osteitis deformans).

osteo- *prefix. see* ost-.

osteoarthritis (osteoarthrosis) *n.* a degenerative disease of joints resulting from wear of the articular cartilage, which may lead to secondary changes in the underlying bone. It can be primary or it can occur secondarily to abnormal load to the joint or damage to the cartilage

from inflammation or trauma. The joints are painful and stiff with restricted movement. Osteoarthritis is recognized on X-ray by narrowing of the joint space (due to loss of cartilage) and the presence of *osteophytes, *osteosclerosis, and cysts in the bone. Treatment consists of aspirin and other analgesics, reduction of pressure across the joint (by weight loss and the use of a walking stick in osteoarthritis of the hip), and corrective and prosthetic surgery (*see* osteotomy, arthrodesis, arthroplasty).

osteoarthropathy *n.* any disease of the bone and cartilage adjoining a joint. *Hypertrophic osteoarthropathy* is characterized by the formation of new bony tissue and occurs as a complication of chronic diseases of the chest, including pulmonary abscess, mesothelioma, and lung cancer.

osteoarthrosis *n. see* osteoarthritis.

osteoarthrotomy *n.* surgical excision of the bone adjoining a joint.

osteoblast *n.* a cell, originating in the mesoderm of the embryo, that is responsible for the formation of *bone. *See also* ossification.

osteochondritis *n.* **1.** necrosis of a bone due to interruption of its blood supply, which causes it to fragment and collapse before undergoing revascularization. *See* Kienböck's disease, Köhler's disease, Legg-Calvé-Perthes disease. **2.** inflammation of an *apophysis from the pull of the attached tendon, usually occurring during the adolescent growth spurt. A fragment of bone may be avulsed (*see* avulsion), producing a lump. *See* Osgood-Schlatter disease, Sever's disease.

osteochondritis dissecans separation of a small fragment (or fragments) of bone and cartilage from the surface of a joint, most frequently the knee, with resulting pain, swelling, and limitation of movement. If the condition persists the fragment can be reattached or removed via an *arthrotomy or through an *arthroscope.

osteochondroma *n.* a bone tumor composed of cartilage-forming cells. It appears as a painless mass, usually at the end of a long bone, and is most common between the ages of 10 and 25 years. Because a small proportion of these tumors becomes malignant if untreated, they are excised.

osteochondrosis n. see osteochondritis.

osteoclasis (osteoclasia, osteoclasty) n. **1.** the deliberate breaking of a malformed or malunited bone, carried out by a surgeon in order to correct deformity. Remodeling of bone by *osteoclasts occurs, resulting in the healing of the fracture. **2.** dissolution of bone through disease (see osteolysis).

osteoclast n. **1.** a large multinucleate cell that resorbs calcified bone. Osteoclasts are only found when bone is being resorbed and may be seen in small depressions on the bone surface. **2.** a device for fracturing bone for therapeutic purposes.

osteoclastoma n. a rare tumor of bone, caused by proliferation of *osteoclast cells.

osteocyte n. a bone cell: an *osteoblast that has ceased activity and has become embedded in the bone matrix.

osteodystrophy n. any generalized bone disease resulting from a metabolic disorder. In renal osteodystrophy chronic kidney failure leads to diffuse bone changes resulting from osteomalacia, secondary hyperparathyroidism (excessive secretion of *parathyroid hormone), osteoporosis, and osteosclerosis. See also Albright's syndrome.

osteogenesis n. see ossification.

osteogenesis imperfecta (fragilitas ossium) a congenital disorder in which the bones are unusually brittle and fragile. No treatment is available, but the tendency to fracture sometimes diminishes at adolescence. There are four types, of varying severity, the worst being lethal at birth. The sclerae may be blue, and the teeth can be deformed.

osteogenic adj. arising in, derived from, or composed of any of the tissues that are concerned with the production of bone. An osteogenic sarcoma (see osteosarcoma) affects bone-producing cells.

osteology n. the study of the structure and function of bones and related structures.

osteolysis n. dissolution of bone through disease, commonly by infection or loss of the blood supply (ischemia) to the bone. In acro-osteolysis the terminal bones of the fingers or toes are affected: a common feature of some disorders involving blood vessels (including *Ray-naud's disease), *scleroderma, and systemic *lupus erythematosus.

osteoma n. a benign bone tumor. A cancellous osteoma (exostosis) is an outgrowth from the end of a long bone, usually rising to a point. A compact osteoma (ivory tumor) is usually harmless but may rarely compress surrounding structures, as within the skull. An osteoid osteoma is an overgrowth of bone-forming cells, usually causing pain in the middle of a long bone. Compact and osteoid osteomas are treated by surgical excision.

osteomalacia n. softening of the bones caused by a deficiency of *vitamin D, either from a poor diet or lack of sunshine or both. It is the adult counterpart of *rickets. Vitamin D is necessary for the uptake of calcium from food; the deficiency therefore leads to progressive decalcification of bony tissues, often causing bone pain. The condition may become irreversible if treatment with vitamin D is not given.

osteomyelitis n. inflammation of bone due to infection, which may remain localized or spread to the bone marrow and other tissues. Acute osteomyelitis occurs when bacteria enter the bone via the bloodstream and is more common in children. There is severe pain, tenderness, and redness over the involved bone, accompanied by general illness and high fever. Treatment is by antibiotics, and surgical drainage and curettage are often required. Chronic osteomyelitis may develop from partially treated acute osteomyelitis or after open fractures or surgery during which the bone is contaminated; tuberculosis is an occasional cause. Osteomyelitis can cause fracture and deformity of the bone.

osteopathy n. a system of diagnosis and treatment based on the theory that many diseases are associated with disorders of the musculoskeletal system. Diagnosis and treatment includes palpation, manipulation, and massage. Osteopathy provides relief for many disorders of bones and joints, especially those producing back pain. —**osteopath** n. —**osteopathic** adj.

osteopetrosis (Albers-Schönberg disease, marble-bone disease) n. a congenital abnormality in which bones become abnormally dense and brittle and tend to fracture. Affected bones appear unusually opaque on X-rays. In severe forms the bone marrow is obliterated, causing anemia and infections. Treatment is by bone marrow transplantation. *See also* osteosclerosis.

osteophyte *n.* a projection of bone, usually shaped like a rose thorn, that occurs at sites of cartilage degeneration or destruction near joints and intervertebral disks. Osteophyte formation is an X-ray sign of *osteoarthritis but is not a cause of symptoms in itself.

osteoporosis *n.* loss of bony tissue, resulting in bones that are brittle and liable to fracture. Infection, injury, and *synovitis can cause localized osteoporosis of adjacent bone. Generalized osteoporosis is common in the elderly, and in women often follows the menopause. It is also a feature of *Cushing's syndrome and prolonged steroid therapy. Osteoporosis can be detected by *quantitative digital radiography and by *DEXA scans. A calcium-rich diet and exercise are preventive, and *bisphosphonates and *raloxifene can be used to reduce further bone loss and prevent osteoporotic fractures.

osteosarcoma (osteogenic sarcoma) *n.* a highly malignant tumor arising from within a bone, usually in the *metaphysis of the long bones of the body and especially around the knee and the proximal end of the humerus. It is usually seen in children and adolescents but can occur in adults of all ages, occasionally in association with *Paget's disease of bone. In children the usual site for the tumor is the leg, particularly the femur. Secondary growths (metastases) are common, most frequently in the lungs (although other sites, such as the liver, may also be involved). The symptoms are usually pain and swelling at the site of the tumor and there is often a history of preceding trauma, although it is doubtful whether this contributes to the cause. Treatment of disease localized to the primary site was traditionally by amputation of the limb; limb-sparing surgery is now possible after *neoadjuvant chemotherapy, with replacement of the diseased bone by a metal prosthesis. Many centers also give *adjuvant therapy in an attempt to kill any residual microscopic tumor that might have already spread. Drugs used include doxorubicin, cisplatin, vincristine, cyclophosphamide, and methotrexate.

osteosclerosis *n.* an abnormal increase in the density of bone, as a result of poor blood supply, chronic infection, or tumor. The affected bone is more opaque to X-rays than normal bone. *See also* osteopetrosis.

osteotome *n.* a surgical chisel designed to cut bone (see illustration).

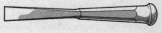

An osteotome

osteotomy *n.* a surgical operation to cut a bone into two parts, followed by realignment of the ends to allow healing. The operation is performed to reduce pain and disability in an arthritic joint, by changing the biomechanics of the joint, for cases in which conservative treatment has failed. Osteotomy of the jaws is performed to improve severe discrepancies in jaw relationships.

ostium *n.* (*pl.* **ostia**) (in anatomy) an opening. The *ostium abdominale* is the opening of the fallopian tube into the abdominal cavity.

ostomy *n.* a surgical procedure in which an artificial opening (*see* stoma) is made in the abdomen to enable the passage of urine from the bladder or intestinal contents from the bowel. *See also* colostomy, ileostomy.

-ostomy *suffix. see* -stomy.

ot- (oto-) *prefix denoting* the ear. Example: *ototomy* (surgical incision of).

otalgia *n.* pain in the ear. Apart from local causes it may be due to diseases of the jaw joints, neck, throat, or teeth or to a lesion of the geniculate ganglion of the facial nerve (*geniculate otalgia*) or to herpes zoster affecting the facial nerve (*Ramsay Hunt syndrome).

OTC drug *see* over-the-counter drug.

otic *adj.* relating to the ear.

otic capsule the cup-shaped cartilage in the head of an embryo that later develops into the bony *labyrinth of the ear.

otitis *n.* inflammation of the ear. Otitis externa is inflammation of the canal between the eardrum and the external opening of the ear (the external auditory meatus) and is often found in swimmers (*swimmer's ear*). *Myringitis* is inflammation of the eardrum, often due to viral infection. *Acute otitis media* is inflammation, usually due to viral or bacterial infection, of the middle ear (the chamber lying behind the eardrum and containing the three bony ossicles that conduct sound to the inner ear). Symptoms include severe pain and a high temperature; unless treated with antibiotics and sometimes by surgical drainage (*myringotomy), it may lead to conductive *deafness. *Secretory otitis media* (*glue ear*) is a chronic accumulation of fluid in the tympanic cavity, causing deafness. *Chronic suppurative otitis media* is inflammation of the middle ear associated with perforations of the eardrum and in some instances with *cholesteatoma. The treatment involves surgical repair of perforations (*see* myringoplasty) or removal of the air cells in the mastoid bone (*mastoidectomy). *Otitis interna* (*labyrinthitis*) is inflammation of the inner ear, causing the sudden onset of vomiting, vertigo, and loss of balance.

otoacoustic emissions (OAE, Kemp echoes) tiny sounds that emerge from the inner ear either simultaneously or shortly after the ear is exposed to an external sound. They are used as the basis for an objective test of hearing.

otoconium *n. see* otolith.

otocyst *n.* a small cavity in the mesoderm of the head of an embryo that later develops into the membranous *labyrinth of the ear.

otolaryngology *n.* the study of diseases of the ears and larynx.

otolith (otoconium) *n.* one of the small particles of calcium carbonate associated with a macula in the *saccule or *utricle of the inner ear.

otology *n.* the study of diseases of the ear.

-otomy *suffix. see* -tomy.

otomycosis *n.* a fungus infection of the ear, causing irritation and inflammation of the canal between the eardrum and the external opening of the ear (external auditory meatus). It is one of the causes of *otitis externa.

otoplasty *n.* surgical repair or reconstruction of the ears after injury or in the correction of a congenital defect (such as "bat ears").

otorhinolaryngology *n.* the study of ear, nose, and throat diseases (i.e. ENT disorders).

otorrhagia *n.* bleeding from the ear.

otorrhea *n.* any discharge from the ear, commonly a purulent discharge in chronic middle ear infection (*otitis media).

otosclerosis *n.* a disorder causing deafness in adult life. An overgrowth of the bone of the inner ear leads to the third ear ossicle (the stapes) becoming fixed to the fenestra ovalis, which separates the middle and inner ears, so that sounds cannot be conducted to the inner ear. *Deafness is progressive and may become very severe, but surgical treatment is highly effective (*see* fenestration, stapedectomy). Nonsurgical treatments include fluoride tablets and the provision of suitable *hearing aids.

otoscope (auriscope) *n.* an apparatus for examining the eardrum and the passage leading to it from the ear (external meatus). It consists of a funnel (speculum), a light, and lenses (see illustration).

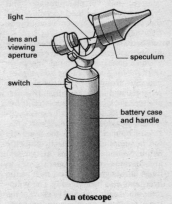

light
lens and viewing aperture
switch
speculum
battery case and handle

An otoscope

ototoxic *adj.* having a toxic effect on the organs of balance or hearing in the inner ear or on the vestibulocochlear nerve. Ototoxic drugs may be used in the treatment of *Ménière's disease.

ouabain *n.* a drug that stimulates the heart and is used in emergency treatment of heart failure and other heart conditions. It is administered by mouth or injection and has the same actions and side effects as *digitalis.

outbreeding n. the production of offspring by parents who are not closely related. *Compare* inbreeding.

outer ear the pinna and the external auditory meatus of the *ear.

out-of-the-body experience a form of *derealization in which there is a sensation of leaving one's body and visions of traveling through tunnels into light or of journeys on another plane of existence. It typically occurs after anesthesia or severe illness and is often attributed to *anoxia of the brain.

outpatient n. a patient who receives treatment at a hospital, either at a single attendance or at a series of attendances, but is not admitted to a bed in the hospital. Large hospitals have *clinics at which outpatients with various complaints can be given specialist treatment. *Compare* inpatient.

oval window see fenestra (ovalis).

ovari- (ovario-) *prefix denoting* the ovary.

ovarian cancer a malignant tumor of the ovary, usually a carcinoma. Ovarian cancer is not readily detected in the early stages of development, when the tumor is small and produces few symptoms. The incidence of the disease reaches a peak in postmenopausal women; treatment involves surgery and most cases also require combined chemotherapy and radiotherapy (*see also* paclitaxel). In an attempt to facilitate a better understanding of the disease, and hence an earlier diagnosis and treatment, the World Health Organization (WHO) published in 1992 a revised Histological Classification of Ovarian Neoplasms and Tumor-like Lesions. An ultrasound screening test for ovarian cancer is being developed.

ovarian cyst a fluid-filled sac, one or more of which may develop in the ovary. Although most ovarian cysts are not malignant, they may reach a very large size or become twisted on their stalks, cutting off their blood supply and producing severe pain and vomiting. In such cases the cysts are surgically removed. Ovarian cysts that do become malignant may not be recognized until the tumor has advanced to a stage where treatment may be unsuccessful in eradicating the cancer. Screening programs, based on ultrasound techniques, can assist with the early detection of ovarian cysts and tumors.

ovariectomy n. see oophorectomy.

ovariotomy n. literally, incision into an ovary. However, the term commonly refers to surgical removal of an ovary (*oophorectomy).

ovaritis n. see oophoritis.

ovary n. the main female reproductive organ, which produces ova (egg cells) and steroid hormones in a regular cycle (*see* menstrual cycle) in response to hormones (*gonadotropins) from the anterior pituitary gland. There are two ovaries, situated in the lower abdomen, one on each side of the uterus (*see* reproductive system). Each ovary contains numerous *follicles*, within which the ova develop (see illustration), but only a small proportion of them reach maturity (*see* graafian follicle, oogenesis). The follicles secrete *estrogen and small amounts of androgen. After ovulation a *corpus luteum forms at the site of the ruptured follicle and secretes progesterone. Estrogen and progesterone regulate the changes in the uterus throughout the menstrual cycle and pregnancy. —**ovarian** *adj.*

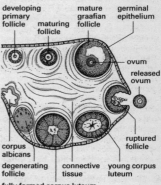

Section of the ovary showing ova in various stages of maturation

overbite n. the vertical overlap of the upper incisor teeth over the lower ones.

overcompensation n. (in psychology) the

situation in which a person tries to overcome a disability by making greater efforts than are required. This may result in the person becoming extremely efficient in what he (or she) is trying to achieve; alternatively, excessive overcompensation may be harmful to the person.

overjet *n.* the horizontal overlap of the upper incisor teeth in front of the lower ones.

overt *adj.* plainly to be seen or detected: applied to diseases with observable signs and symptoms, as opposed to those whose presence may not be suspected for years despite the fact that they cause insidious damage. An infectious disease becomes overt only at the end of an incubation period.

over-the-counter drug (OTC drug) a drug that may be purchased without a doctor's prescription. Current government policy is to extend the range of OTC drugs: a number have already been derestricted (e.g. ibuprofen) and this trend is expected to increase, which will place an additional advisory responsibility on pharmacists.

ovi- (ovo-) *prefix denoting* an egg; ovum.

oviduct *n. see* fallopian tube.

ovulation *n.* the process by which an ovum is released from a mature *graafian follicle. The fluid-filled follicle distends the surface of the ovary until a thin spot breaks down and the ovum floats out surrounded by a cluster of follicle cells (the cumulus oophoricus) and starts to travel down the fallopian tube to the uterus. Ovulation is stimulated by the secretion of *luteinizing hormone by the anterior pituitary gland.

ovum (egg cell) *n.* the mature female sex cell (*see* gamete). The term is often applied to the secondary *oocyte, although this is technically incorrect. The final stage of meiosis occurs only when the oocyte has been activated by fertilization.

oxacillin *n.* an antibiotic used to treat infections caused by a wide variety of bacteria. It is administered by mouth or injection; side effects include allergic reactions and digestive upsets. Trade name: **Bactocill**.

oxalic acid an extremely poisonous acid, $C_2H_2O_4$. It is a component of some bleaching powders and is found in many plants, including sorrel and the leaves of rhubarb and spinach. Oxalic acid is a powerful local irritant; when swallowed, it produces burning sensations in the mouth and throat, vomiting of blood, breathing difficulties, and circulatory collapse. Treatment is with calcium lactate or other calcium salts, lime water, or milk.

oxalosis *n.* an inborn defect of metabolism causing deposition of oxalate in the kidneys and elsewhere and eventually leading to renal failure.

oxaluria *n.* the presence in the urine of oxalic acid or oxalates, especially calcium oxalate. Excessive amounts of oxalates are excreted in *oxalosis.

oxazepam *n.* a *benzodiazepine drug used to relieve anxiety and tension and for the treatment of alcoholism. It is administered by mouth and commonly causes drowsiness. *See also* anxiolytic. Trade name: **Serax**.

oxidant *n.* (in biologic systems) a molecule that serves as an electron acceptor. In human disease oxidants are derived from normal intracellular processes and released by inflammatory cells. Oxidants are counteracted by *antioxidants, such as *beta-carotene.

oxidase *n. see* oxidoreductase.

oxidation *n.* **1.** a chemical reaction that increases the oxygen content of a substance, as by the addition of oxygen. **2.** a reaction in which a molecule loses electrons, catalyzed by *oxidoreductase enzymes.

oxidoreductase *n.* one of a group of enzymes that catalyze oxidation-reduction reactions. This class includes the enzymes formerly known either as *dehydrogenases* or as *oxidases*.

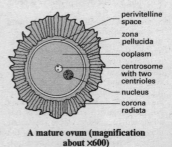

A mature ovum (magnification about ×600)

oximeter *n.* an instrument for measuring the proportion of oxygenated hemoglobin (oxyhemoglobin) in the blood.

oxolinic acid an antibacterial drug used to treat infections of the urinary system caused by gram-negative organisms. It is administered by mouth; side effects may include digestive upsets and disturbances of vision.

oxprenolol *n.* a drug that controls the activity of the heart (*see* beta blocker), used to treat angina, high blood pressure, and abnormal heart rhythm. It is administered by mouth or injection; side effects may include dizziness, drowsiness, headache, and digestive upsets.

oxtriphylline a drug used to dilate the air passages in asthma, emphysema, and chronic bronchitis. It is administered by mouth and can cause digestive upsets, headache, and nausea. Trade name: **Choledyl**.

oxybutynin *n.* an *anticholinergic drug administered orally to reduce frequency and urgency of passing urine associated with an unstable bladder or instability of the *detrusor muscle of the bladder wall. It acts by relaxing the bladder muscle. It is administered by mouth or transdermally; side effects include dry mouth, blurred vision, abnormal heartbeat, rash, and constipation. Trade names: **Ditropan, Oxytrol**.

oxycephaly (turricephaly) *n.* a deformity of the bones of the skull giving the head a pointed appearance. *See* craniosynostosis. —**oxycephalic** *adj.*

oxycodone *n.* an opioid *analgesic used to treat moderate to severe pain. It is administered orally; common side effects include drowsiness, dizziness, nausea, and constipation. Trade names: **Oxy-Contin, Percocet, Percodan, Roxicodone**.

oxygen *n.* an odorless colorless gas that makes up one-fifth of the atmosphere. Oxygen is essential to most forms of life in that it combines chemically with glucose (or some other fuel) to provide energy for metabolic processes. In humans oxygen is absorbed into the blood from air breathed into the lungs. Oxygen is administered therapeutically in various conditions in which the tissues are unable to obtain an adequate supply through the lungs (*see* oxygenator, [oxygen] tent). Symbol: O.

oxygenator *n.* a machine that oxygenates blood outside the body. It is used together with pumps to maintain the patient's circulation while he is undergoing open heart surgery (*see* heart-lung machine) or to improve the circulation of a patient with heart or lung disorders that lower the amount of blood oxygen.

oxygen deficit a physiological condition that exists in cells during periods of temporary oxygen shortage. During periods of violent exertion the body requires extra energy, which is obtained by the breakdown of glucose in the absence of oxygen, after the available oxygen has been used up. The breakdown products are acidic and cause muscle pain. The oxygen required to get rid of the breakdown products (called the oxygen deficit) must be made available after the exertion stops.

oxygen tent *see* tent.

oxyhemoglobin *n.* the bright-red substance formed when the pigment *hemoglobin in red blood cells combines reversibly with oxygen. Oxyhemoglobin is the form in which oxygen is transported from the lungs to the tissues, where the oxygen is released. *Compare* methemoglobin.

oxymetazoline *n.* a *sympathomimetic drug administered as a nasal spray to treat nasal congestion. Possible side effects include irritation of the nose, headache, fast pulse, and insomnia. Trade names: **Neo-Synephrine, Vicks Sinex**.

oxymetholone *n.* a synthetic male sex hormone with *anabolic effects. It is used for the treatment of anemia caused by deficiency of red cell production. It is administered by mouth; side effects include virilization in women, insomnia, and acne. Trade name: **Anadrol-50**.

oxymorphone *n.* an opioid *analgesic used to treat moderate to severe pain. It is administered by injection or as a rectal suppository. Common side effects include drowsiness, sedation, nausea, and constipation. Trade name: **Numorphan**.

oxyntic cells (parietal cells) cells of the *gastric glands that secrete hydrochloric acid in the fundic region of the stomach.

oxyphencyclimine *n.* a drug with actions similar to *atropine. Since it slows down the digestive processes, it is used to treat stomach and duodenal ulcers and other digestive disorders. It is administered by mouth; side effects include dry mouth, thirst, and disturbances of vision.

oxytetracycline n. an *antibiotic used to treat infections caused by a wide variety of bacteria. It is administered by mouth; side effects are those of the other *tetracyclines. Trade name: **Terramycin**.

oxytocic n. any agent that induces or accelerates labor by stimulating the muscles of the uterus to contract. *See also* oxytocin.

oxytocin n. a hormone, released by the pituitary gland, that causes increased contraction of the uterus during labor and stimulates the ejection of milk from the breasts. Oxytocin also may be given by injection to induce uterine contractions and to control or prevent hemorrhage after the birth. Trade names: **Pitocin, Syntocinon**.

oxyuriasis n. *see* enterobiasis.

Oxyuris n. *see* pinworm.

ozena n. a disorder of the nose in which the bones forming the sides of the nasal cavity become atrophied, with the production of an offensive discharge and crusts.

ozone n. a poisonous gas containing three oxygen atoms per molecule. Ozone is a very powerful oxidizing agent and is formed when oxygen or air is subjected to electric discharge. Ozone is found in the atmosphere at very high altitudes (the *ozone layer*) and is responsible for destroying a large proportion of the sun's ultraviolet radiation. Without this absorption by ozone the earth would be subjected to a lethal amount of ultraviolet radiation.

P

p53 n. a gene that mutates to form an important *oncogene for human *cancers. Recent trials of *gene therapy that involved replacing the oncogene with the normal version of the gene have had a limited success.

PABA *see* para-aminobenzoic acid.

pacchionian body *see* arachnoid villus. [A. Pacchioni (1665–1726), Italian anatomist]

pacemaker n. **1.** a device used to produce and maintain a normal heart rate in patients who have *heart block. The unit consists of a battery that stimulates the heart through an insulated electrode wire attached to the surface of the ventricle (*epicardial pacemaker*) or lying in contact with the lining of the heart (*endocardial pacemaker*). A pacemaker may be used as a temporary measure with an external battery or it may be permanent, when the whole apparatus is surgically implanted under the skin. Some pacemakers stimulate the heart at a fixed rate; others sense when the natural heart rate falls below a predetermined value and then stimulate the heart (*demand pacemaker*). **2.** the part of the heart that regulates the rate at which it beats: the *sinoatrial node.

pachy- *prefix denoting* **1.** thickening of a part or parts. **2.** the dura mater.

pachydactyly n. abnormal enlargement of the fingers and toes, occurring either as a congenital abnormality or as part of an acquired disease (such as *acromegaly).

pachyderma n. any abnormal thickening of the skin.

pachyglossia n. abnormal thickness of the tongue.

pachymeningitis n. inflammation of the dura mater, one of the membranes (meninges) covering the brain and spinal cord (*see* meningitis).

pachymeninx n. the *dura mater, outermost of the three meninges.

pachymeter n. an instrument that is used to measure the thickness of any object, especially a thin object, such as the cornea. —**pachymetry** n.

pachyonychia n. thickening of the nails. Rarely, this may occur as an inherited disease (*pachynychia congenita*), which is associated with other ectodermal abnormalities (*see* genodermatosis).

pachysomia n. thickening of parts of the body, which occurs in certain diseases.

pachytene n. the third stage of the first prophase of *meiosis, in which *crossing over begins.

pacinian corpuscles sensory receptors for touch in the skin, consisting of sensory nerve endings surrounded by capsules of membrane in "onion-skin" layers. They are especially sensitive to changes in pressure and so detect vibration particularly well. [F. Pacini (1812–83), Italian anatomist]

pack n. a pad of folded moistened material, such as cotton wool, applied to the body or inserted into a cavity.

packed cell volume (hematocrit) the volume of the red cells (erythrocytes) in blood, expressed as a fraction of the total volume of the blood. The packed cell volume is determined by centrifuging blood in a tube and measuring the height of the red cell column as a fraction of the total. Automated instruments calculate packed cell volume as the product of the erythrocyte count and the measured mean red cell volume (*mean corpuscular volume*; *MCV*).

paclitaxel *n.* a *cytotoxic drug formerly obtainable only from the bark of the Pacific yew tree but now synthesized and produced by biotechnological methods (*see* taxane). Administered by intravenous infusion, it is used to treat ovarian and breast cancers that are resistant to standard chemotherapy, Kaposi's sarcoma, and certain types of lung cancer. Side effects include numbness and tingling of the extremities, damage to bone marrow, and loss of hair. Trade name: **Taxol.**

PACS (picture archiving and communication system) an electronic system enabling the storage of digital images (*see* digital radiography, computerized radiography, computed tomography, digitization) on electronic media, for later retrieval and subsequent display on high-resolution monitors. Images are moved using a hospital computer network; thus they do not need to be printed on film, which reduces costs. Transport costs and delay are also largely eliminated. Images can be viewed at local or distant sites and can be seen simultaneously by more than one person. The system also allows the manipulation of images on screen.

pad *n.* cotton wool, foam rubber, or other material used to protect a part of the body from friction, bruising, or other unwanted contact.

Paget's disease 1. a chronic disease of bones, occurring in the elderly and most frequently affecting the skull, backbone, pelvis, and long bones. Affected bones become thickened and their structure disorganized: X-rays reveal patchy *sclerosis. There are often no symptoms, but pain, deformity, and fracture can occur; when the skull is affected, blindness and deafness can occur due to nerve compression. There is a very small (1%) risk

of malignant change (*osteosarcoma). Treatment is with *bisphosphonates or *calcitonin. Medical name: **osteitis deformans. 2.** a malignant condition of the nipple, resembling eczema in appearance, associated with underlying infiltrating cancer of the breast. *See also* breast cancer. **3.** an uncommon condition of the vulva or penis characterized by an epithelial lesion that histologically resembles the lesion of Paget's disease of the nipple. It may be associated with locally invasive *adenocarcinomas of the surrounding skin, as well as tumors at other sites. [Sir J. Paget (1814–99), British surgeon]

pain *n.* a localized or diffuse unpleasant sensation ranging from mild discomfort to agony or distress, associated with real or potential tissue damage, and caused by stimulation of the functionally specific sensory nerve endings. Pain may be mild to severe, chronic or acute, localized or *referred, and it is usually described by such terms as dull, burning, sharp, piercing, or throbbing. Pain is a response to impulses from the peripheral nerves in damaged tissue, which pass to nerves in the spinal cord, where they are subjected to a gate control. This gate modifies the subsequent passage of the impulses in accordance with descending controls from the brain. Because attention is a crucial component of pain, distraction can act as a basis for pain therapy. On the other hand, anxiety and depression focus the attention and exaggerate the pain. If the nerve pathways are damaged, the brain can increase the amplification in the pathway, maintaining the sensation as a protective mechanism. Pain serves as a protective device by inducing withdrawal from the source and thus avoiding greater damage, and it is a valuable aid in the diagnosis of many conditions and disorders. *Pain threshold* is the point at which a stimulus activates the nerve ending receptors and the sensation of pain is felt. Persons with a low threshold experience pain sooner than those with a higher threshold.

pain clinic a clinic that specializes in techniques of long-term pain relief, such as *transcutaneous electrical nerve stimulation (TENS). Pain clinics are usually directed by anesthetists.

paint *n.* (in pharmacy) a liquid preparation that is applied to the skin or mucous membranes. Paints usually contain antiseptics, astringents, caustics, or analgesics.

palate *n.* the roof of the mouth, which separates the mouth from the nasal cavity and consists of two portions. The *hard palate*, at the front of the mouth, is formed by processes of the maxillae and palatine bones and is covered by mucous membrane. The *soft palate*, further back, is a movable fold of mucous membrane that tapers at the back of the mouth to form a fleshy hanging flap of tissue – the *uvula*.

palatine bone either of a pair of approximately L-shaped bones of the face that contribute to the hard *palate, the nasal cavity, and the orbits. *See* skull.

palato- *prefix denoting* 1. the palate. 2. the palatine bone.

palatoplasty *n.* plastic surgery of the roof of the mouth, usually to correct cleft palate or other defects present at birth. *Laser palatoplasty* is carried out under local or general anesthesia to shorten and/or stiffen the palate in the treatment of snoring.

palatorrhaphy *n. see* staphylorrhaphy.

paleo- *prefix denoting* 1. ancient. 2. primitive.

paleocerebellum *n.* the anterior lobe of the cerebellum of the brain. In evolutionary terms it is one of the earliest parts of the hindbrain to develop in mammals.

paleopathology *n.* the study of the diseases of humans and other animals in prehistoric times, from examination of their bones or other remains. By examining the bones of specimens of Neanderthal man it has been discovered that spinal arthritis was a disease that existed at least 50,000 years ago.

paleostriatum *n. see* pallidum.

paleothalamus *n.* the anterior and central part of the *thalamus, older in evolutionary terms than the lateral part, the neothalamus, which is well developed in apes and humans.

pali- (**palin-**) *prefix denoting* repetition or recurrence.

palilalia *n.* a disorder of speech in which a word spoken by the individual is rapidly and involuntarily repeated. It is seen, with other tics, in the *Gilles de la Tourette syndrome. It is also encountered when encephalitis or other processes damage the *extrapyramidal system of the brain.

palindromic *adj.* relapsing: describing diseases or symptoms that recur or get worse.

palingraphia *n.* a disorder of writing in which syllables, words, or phrases are repeated. It is a feature of acquired brain disease, such as stroke.

paliphrasia *n.* repetition of phrases while speaking: a form of *stammering or a kind of *tic.

palivizumab *n.* a *monoclonal antibody used as an immunizing agent to prevent infection caused by *respiratory syncytial virus in young children and infants. It is administered by intramuscular injection; common side effects include skin rash, runny nose, and difficulty in breathing. Trade name: **Synagis.**

palliative *n.* a medicine that gives temporary relief from the symptoms of a disease but does not actually cure the disease. Palliatives are often used in the treatment of such diseases as cancer.

pallidotomy (**pallidectomy**) *n.* a neurosurgical operation to destroy or modify the effects of the globus pallidus (*see* basal ganglia). This operation was used for the relief of *parkinsonism and other conditions in which involuntary movements are prominent before the advent of modern drug therapies. The development of more accurate techniques to localize the globus pallidus has led to a revival in the use of the operation: in the modern form of pallidotomy, a lesion is made in the globus pallidus by stereotactic surgery (*see* stereotaxy).

pallidum (**paleostriatum**) *n.* one of the dense collections of gray matter, deep in each cerebral hemisphere, that go to make up the *basal ganglia.

pallium *n.* the outer wall of the cerebral hemisphere as it appears in the early stages of evolution of the mammalian brain. In the modern brain it corresponds to the *cerebral cortex.

pallor *n.* abnormal paleness of the skin, due to reduced blood flow or lack of normal pigments. Pallor may be associated with an indoor mode of life; it may also indicate shock, anemia, cancer, or other diseases.

palm *n.* the anterior, flexor surface of the

hand, extending from the wrist to the tip of the fingers.

palmitic acid *see* fatty acid.

palpation *n.* the process of examining part of the body by careful feeling with the hands and fingertips. Using palpation it is possible, in many cases, to distinguish between swellings that are solid and those that are cystic (*see* fluctuation). Palpation is also used to discover the presence of a fetus in the uterus (*see* ballottement).

palpebral *adj.* relating to the eyelid (palpebra).

palpitation *n.* an awareness of the heartbeat. This is normal with fear, emotion, or exertion. It may also be a symptom of neurosis, arrhythmias, heart disease, and overactivity of the circulation (as in thyrotoxicosis).

palsy *n.* paralysis. This archaic word is retained in compound terms, such as *Bell's palsy, *cerebral palsy, and *Todd's paralysis (*or* palsy).

paludism *n. see* malaria.

pamidronate *n. see* bisphosphonates.

pan- (pant[o]-) *prefix denoting* all; every: hence (in medicine) affecting all parts of an organ or the body; generalized.

panacea *n.* a medicine said to be a cure for all diseases and disorders, no matter what their nature. Unfortunately, panaceas do not exist, despite the claims of many patent medicine manufacturers.

pancarditis *n. see* endomyocarditis.

Pancoast syndrome pain and paralysis involving the lower branches of the brachial plexus due to infiltration by a malignant tumor of the apical region of the lung. *Horner's syndrome may also be present. [H. K. Pancoast (1875–1939), US radiologist]

pancreas *n.* a compound gland, about 15 cm long, that lies behind the stomach. One end lies in the curve of the duodenum; the other end touches the spleen. It is composed of clusters (*acini*) of cells that secrete *pancreatic juice. This contains a number of enzymes concerned in digestion. The juice drains into small ducts that open into the *pancreatic duct*. This unites with the common *bile duct and the secretions pass into the duodenum. Interspersed among the acini are the *islets of Langerhans – isolated groups of cells that secrete the hormones

*insulin and *glucagon into the bloodstream. —**pancreatic** *adj.*

pancreas divisum a congenital abnormality in which the pancreas develops in two parts draining separately into the duodenum, the small ventral pancreas through the main ampulla and the larger dorsal pancreas through an accessory papilla. In rare instances this is associated with recurrent abdominal pain, probably caused by inadequate drainage of the dorsal pancreas. Diagnosis is made by *ERCP.

pancreatectomy *n.* surgical removal of the pancreas. *Total pancreatectomy* (*Whipple's operation*) involves the entire gland and part of the duodenum. In *subtotal pancreatectomy* most of the gland is removed, usually leaving a small part close to the duodenum. In *partial pancreatectomy* only a portion of the gland is removed. The operations are performed for tumors in the gland or because of chronic or relapsing *pancreatitis. After total or subtotal pancreatectomy it is necessary to administer pancreatic enzymes with food to aid digestion and insulin injections to replace that normally secreted by the gland.

pancreatic juice the digestive juice secreted by the *pancreas. Its production is stimulated by hormones secreted by the duodenum, which in turn is stimulated by contact with food from the stomach. If the duodenum produces the hormone *secretin, the pancreatic juice contains a large amount of sodium bicarbonate, which neutralizes the acidity of the stomach contents. Another hormone (*see* cholecystokinin) stimulates the production of a juice that is rich in digestive enzymes, including trypsinogen and chymotrypsinogen (which are converted to *trypsin and *chymotrypsin in the duodenum), *amylase, *lipase, and *maltase.

pancreatic polypeptide a hormone released from the delta cells of the *islets of Langerhans of the pancreas in response to protein in the small intestine. Its actions are to inhibit pancreatic bicarbonate and protein enzyme secretion and to relax the gallbladder. It belongs to a family of similar hormones that have actions on appetite and food metabolism.

pancreatin *n.* an extract obtained from the

*pancreas, containing the pancreatic enzymes. Pancreatin is administered for conditions in which pancreatic secretion is deficient; for example, in pancreatitis.

pancreatitis *n.* inflammation of the pancreas. *Acute pancreatitis* is a sudden illness in which the patient experiences severe pain in the upper abdomen and back, with shock; its cause is not always discovered, but it may be associated with gallstones or alcoholism. It may be mistaken for a perforated peptic ulcer but differs from this condition in that the level of the enzyme *amylase in the blood is raised. The main complication is formation of a *pseudocyst. Treatment consists of intravenous feeding (no food or drink should be given by mouth), and *anticholinergic drugs. *Relapsing pancreatitis*, in which the above symptoms are recurrent and less severe, may be associated with gallstones or alcoholism; prevention is by removal of gallstones and avoidance of alcohol and fat. Operations may be done to improve drainage of the pancreatic duct. *Chronic pancreatitis* may produce symptoms similar to relapsing pancreatitis or may be painless; it leads to pancreatic failure causing *malabsorption and *diabetes mellitus. The pancreas often becomes calcified, producing visible shadowing on X-rays. The malabsorption is treated by a low-fat diet with pancreatic enzyme supplements, and the diabetes with insulin.

pancreatogram *n.* a radiographic image of the pancreatic ducts obtained by injecting a contrast medium into them by direct puncture under *ultrasound guidance, at the time of laparotomy or by *ERCP.

pancreatotomy *n.* surgical opening of the duct of the pancreas in order to inspect the duct, to join the duct to the intestine, or to inject contrast material in order to obtain X-ray pictures of the duct system.

pancreozymin *n. see* cholecystokinin.

pancuronium bromide a drug used to produce skeletal muscle relaxation, especially to arrest fetal movement when *magnetic resonance imaging studies are done. The drug is injected into the fetus intramuscularly under *ultrasound guidance. There is a small risk to the fetus from the needle puncture, but no side effects of the drug. As an adjunct to general anesthesia, it is injected intravenously. Side effects include increased heart rate, prolonged muscular paralysis, and *bronchospasm. Trade name: **Pavulon**.

pancytopenia *n.* a simultaneous decrease in the numbers of red cells (*anemia), white cells (*neutropenia), and platelets (*thrombocytopenia) in the blood. It occurs in a variety of disorders, including aplastic *anemias, *hypersplenism, and tumors of the bone marrow. It may also occur after chemotherapy or total body irradiation.

panda sign a sign of bilateral periorbital *hematoma associated with injury to the anterior cranial fossa, the front of the skull cavity that supports the frontal lobes of the brain. The name derives from its similarity in appearance to the black eye patches of a panda.

pandemic *n.* an *epidemic so widely spread that vast numbers of people in different countries are affected. The Black Death, the epidemic plague that ravaged Europe in the fourteenth century and killed over one third of the population, was a classic pandemic. AIDS is currently considered to be pandemic. —**pandemic** *adj.*

panic disorder a condition featuring recurrent brief episodes of acute distress, mental confusion, and fear of impending death. The heart beats rapidly, breathing is deep and fast, and sweating occurs. Overbreathing (hyperventilation) often makes the attack worse. These panic attacks usually occur about twice a week but may be more frequent and they are especially common in people with *agoraphobia. The condition tends to run in families and appears to be an organic disorder with a strong psychologic component. Treatment is with *antidepressant drugs. *Behavior therapy can also be helpful.

panmixis *n.* random mating within a population, i.e. when there is no selection of partners on religious, racial, social, or other grounds.

panniculitis *n.* inflammation of the layer of fat beneath the skin (*panniculus adiposus*), leading to multiple tender nodules in the thighs, trunk, and breasts. When there are other features, including fever and enlargement of the liver and spleen, the condition is known as the *Weber-Christian disease*.

panniculus *n.* a membranous sheet of tissue. For example, the *panniculus adiposus* is the fatty layer of tissue underlying the skin.

pannus *n.* invasion of the outer layers of the cornea of the eye by tissue containing many blood vessels, which grows in from the conjunctiva. It is seen as a response to inflammation of the cornea or conjunctiva, particularly in *trachoma.

panophthalmitis *n.* inflammation involving the whole of the interior of the eye.

Panstrongylus *n.* a genus of large blood-sucking bugs (*see* reduviid). *P. megistus* is important in transmitting *Chagas' disease to humans in Brazil.

pant- (panto-) *prefix. see* pan-.

pantaloon hernia a double sac comprising the sac of an indirect (external) and a direct (internal) inguinal *hernia on the same side.

pantomography *n.* a method of *tomography that provides a picture (*pantomogram* or *orthopantomogram*) of all the teeth of both jaws on a single film. It is obtained by an instrument called a *pantomograph*.

pantoprazole *n. see* proton-pump inhibitor.

pantothenic acid a B vitamin that is a constituent of *coenzyme A. It plays an important role in the transfer of acetyl groups in the body. Pantothenic acid is widely distributed in food and a deficiency is therefore unlikely to occur.

pantropic *adj.* describing a virus that can invade and affect many different tissues of the body, for example the nerves, skin, or liver, without showing a special affinity for any one of them.

papain *n.* a preparation that contains one or more protein-digesting enzymes. It is obtained from the papaya and is used as a digestant.

Papanicolaou test (Pap test) *see* cervical smear. [G. N. Papanicolaou (1883–1962), Greek physician, anatomist, and cytologist]

papaverine *n.* an alkaloid, derived from opium, that relaxes smooth muscle. It is administered by mouth or injection to treat muscle spasm in such conditions as colic. When injected into the corpora cavernosa of the penis, it causes tumescence and may produce an erection. It is

being increasingly used both diagnostically and therapeutically in the investigation and management of *impotence. It may cause abnormal heart rate. Trade names: **Pavabid, Pavased, Pavatine**.

papilla *n.* (*pl.* **papillae**) any small nipple-shaped protuberance. Several different kinds of papillae occur on the *tongue, in association with the taste buds. The *optic papilla* is an alternative name for the *optic disk.

papilledema *n.* swelling of the first part of the optic nerve (the optic disk or optic papilla).

papillitis *n.* inflammation of the first part of the optic nerve (the optic disk or optic papilla), i.e. where the nerve leaves the eyeball. *See* retrobulbar neuritis.

papilloma *n.* a benign nipple-like growth on the surface of skin or mucous membrane (for example, in the uterus or bladder). Papillomas, which develop from the *epidermis, are usually in the form of a conical, flattish, or stalked protuberance, 2–5 mm in diameter. *Warts are a type of papilloma. —**papillomatous** *adj.*

papillomatosis *n.* a condition in which many *papillomas grow on an area of skin or mucous membrane.

papillotomy *n.* the operation of cutting the *ampulla of Vater to widen its outlet in order to improve bile drainage and allow the passage of stones from the common bile duct. It is usually performed using a diathermy wire through a *duodenoscope following *ERCP.

papovavirus *n.* one of a group of small DNA-containing viruses producing tumors in animals (subgroup *polyomaviruses*) and in animals and humans (subgroup *papillomaviruses*). *See also* human papillomavirus.

pappataci fever *see* sandfly fever.

papule *n.* a small superficial raised abnormality or spot on the skin. It usually forms part of a rash, such as appears with chickenpox.

papulo- *prefix denoting* a papule or pimple.

papulosquamous *adj.* **1.** describing a rash that is both papular and scaly. **2.** denoting a group of skin diseases that have this characteristic, including *pityriasis rosea, seborrheic *dermatitis, *lichen planus, and *psoriasis.

para- *prefix denoting* **1.** beside or near. Example: *paranasal* (near the nasal cavity).

2. resembling. Example: *paradysentery* (a mild form of dysentery). **3.** abnormal. Example: *paralalia* (abnormal speech).

para-aminobenzoic acid (PABA) a naturally occurring drug used in lotions and creams to prevent sunburn.

para-aminosalicylic acid (PAS) a drug, chemically related to aspirin, used – in conjunction with isoniazid or streptomycin – to treat various types of tuberculosis. It is administered by mouth and commonly causes nausea, vomiting, diarrhea, and rashes.

paracentesis *n.* tapping: the process of drawing off fluid from a part of the body through a hollow needle or *cannula.

paracetamol *n. see* acetaminophen.

parachute reflex a reflex action of the body that develops by five to six months and never disappears. If the body is held by the waist face down and lowered, the arms and legs extend automatically.

Paracoccidioides *n.* a genus of yeastlike fungi causing infection of the skin and mucous membranes. The species *P. brasiliensis* causes a chronic skin disease, South American *blastomycosis.

paracrine *adj.* describing a hormone that is secreted by an endocrine gland and affects the function of nearby cells, rather than being transported distally by the blood or lymph.

paracusis *n.* any abnormality of hearing.

paradidymis *n.* the vestigial remains of part of the embryonic *mesonephros that are found near the testis of the adult. Some of the mesonephric collecting tubules persist as the functional *vasa efferentia but the rest degenerate almost completely. A similar vestigial structure (the *paroophoron*) is found in females.

paradox *n.* (in *family therapy) a surprising interpretation or suggestion made in the course of therapy in order to demonstrate the relationship between a psychological symptom and a system of family relationships. For example, a child might be told to go on stealing from his parents because their concern about the symptom is all that is keeping their marriage intact.

paradoxical breathing breathing movements in which the chest wall moves in on inspiration and out on expiration, in reverse of the normal movements. It may be seen in children with respiratory distress of any cause, which leads to indrawing of the intercostal spaces during inspiration. Patients with chronic airways obstruction also show indrawing of the lower ribs during inspiration, due to the distorted action of a depressed and flattened diaphragm. Crush injuries of the chest, with fractured ribs and sternum, can lead to a severe degree of paradoxical breathing.

paraffin *n.* one of a series of hydrocarbons derived from petroleum. *Paraffin wax* (*hard paraffin*), a whitish mixture of solid hydrocarbons melting at 45–60°C, is used in medicine mainly as a base for ointments; it is also used for *embedding specimens for microscopical study. *Liquid paraffin* is a mineral oil, which has been used as a laxative.

paraganglioma *n.* a benign tumor arising from *paraganglion cells. Such tumors can occur around the aorta, the carotid artery (carotid body tumor), and the cervical portion of the vagus nerve (*glomus tumor), as well as in the abdomen and the eye.

paraganglion *n.* one of the small oval masses of cells found in the walls of the ganglia of the sympathetic nervous system, near the spinal cord. They are *chromaffin cells, like those of the adrenal gland, and may secrete epinephrine.

parageusia (parageusis) *n.* abnormality of the sense of taste.

paragonimiasis (endemic hemoptysis) *n.* a tropical disease, occurring principally in the Far East, caused by the presence of the fluke *Paragonimus westermani* in the lungs. The infection is acquired by eating inadequately cooked shellfish, such as crayfish and crabs. Symptoms resemble those of chronic *bronchitis, including the coughing up of blood and difficulty in breathing (dyspnea). Paragonimiasis is treated with the drug *chloroquine.

Paragonimus *n.* a genus of large tropical parasitic *flukes that are particularly prevalent in the Far East. The adults of *P. westermani* live in the lungs of humans, where they cause destruction and bleeding of the tissues (*see* paragonimiasis). However, they may also be found in other organs of the body. Eggs are passed out in the sputum and the larvae undergo their development in two other hosts, a snail and a crab.

paragranuloma *n.* a former term for one of the types of *Hodgkin's disease. It is now known as *lymphocyte-predominant Hodgkin's disease* and has the best prognosis of all the types.

paragraphia *n.* a disorder of writing, involving the omission or transposition of letters or of whole words. The appearance of this in adult life is usually due to damage to the brain. In childhood it usually reflects a developmental delay in learning to write correctly.

parainfluenza viruses a group of large RNA-containing viruses that cause infections of the respiratory tract producing mild influenza-like symptoms. They are included in the paramyxovirus group (*see* myxovirus).

paraldehyde *n.* a *hypnotic and *anticonvulsant drug used to control insomnia, induce hypnotic states of sedation, and control seizures of *status epilepticus. It is administered orally, rectally, or by injection; side effects may include digestive upsets and, in large doses, prolonged unconsciousness. Trade name: **Paral**.

parallel track protocol a system that allows access to promising new investigational drugs for patients who have life-threatening diseases, particularly those with AIDS, who are unable to take standard therapies or are unable to participate in ongoing clinical trials. These studies are conducted in parallel with controlled clinical trials.

paralysis *n.* muscle impairment or loss of muscle function that varies in its extent, its severity, and the degree of *spasticity or flaccidity according to the nature of the underlying disease and its distribution in the brain, spinal cord, peripheral nerves, or muscles. *See* diplegia, hemiplegia, paraplegia, poliomyelitis. —**paralytic** *adj.*

paramedian *adj.* situated close to or beside the *median plane.

paramedical personnel (allied health personnel) health workers closely linked to the medical profession and working in conjunction with them. Such workers require expert knowledge and experience in certain fields, but no medical degree. Paramedical personnel in a hospital include the radiographers, physiotherapists, occupational therapists, and dietitians.

paramesonephric duct (Müllerian duct) either of the paired ducts that form adjacent to the mesonephric ducts (*see* mesonephros) in the embryo. In the female these ducts develop into the fallopian tubes, uterus, and part of the vagina. However, in the male they degenerate almost completely.

parameter *n.* (in medicine) a measurement of some factor, such as blood pressure, pulse rate, or hemoglobin level, that may have a bearing on the condition being investigated.

parametric test *see* significance.

parametritis (pelvic cellulitis) *n.* inflammation of the loose connective tissue and smooth muscle around the uterus (the parametrium). The condition may be associated with *puerperal infection.

parametrium *n.* the layer of connective tissue surrounding the uterus.

paramnesia *n.* a distorted memory, such as *confabulation or *déjà vu.

paramyoclonus multiplex a benign disorder of the nervous system that is characterized by brief, irregular twitchlike contractions of the muscles of the limbs and trunk.

paramyotonia congenita a rare constitutional disorder in which prolonged contraction of muscle fibers (*see* myotonia) develops when the patient is exposed to cold. This may be due to a disorder of potassium channels.

paramyxovirus *n. see* myxovirus.

paranasal sinuses the air-filled spaces, lined with mucous membrane, within some of the bones of the skull. They open into the nasal cavity, via the meatuses, and are named according to the bone in which they are situated. They

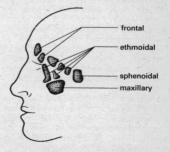

frontal
ethmoidal
sphenoidal
maxillary

Paranasal sinuses projected to the surface

comprise the *frontal sinuses* and the *maxillary sinuses* (one pair of each), the *ethmoid sinuses* (consisting of many spaces inside the ethmoid bone), and the two *sphenoid sinuses*. (See illustration.)

paraneoplastic syndrome signs or symptoms that may occur in a patient with cancer but are not due directly to local effects of the cancer cells. Removal of the cancer usually leads to resolution of the problem. An example is *myasthenia gravis secondary to a tumor of the thymus.

paranoia *n.* a mental disorder characterized by *delusions organized into a system, without hallucinations or other marked symptoms of mental illness. It is a rare chronic condition; most people with such delusions will in time develop signs of other mental illness.

The same term is sometimes used more loosely for a state of mind in which the individual has a strong belief that he is persecuted by others. His behavior is therefore suspicious and isolated. This can be a result of *personality disorder as well as mental illnesses causing *paranoid states.

paranoid *adj.* **1.** describing a mental state characterized by fixed and logically elaborated *delusions. There are many causes, including paranoid *schizophrenia, *manic-depressive psychosis, organic psychoses such as *alcoholism, *paraphrenia, and severe emotional stress. **2.** describing a personality distinguished by such traits as excessive sensitivity to rejection or accusation by other people, suspiciousness, hostility, and self-importance.

paraparesis *n.* weakness of both legs, resulting from disease of the nervous system.

paraphasia *n.* a disorder of language in which unintended syllables, words, or phrases are interpolated in the patient's speech. A severe degree of paraphasia results in speech that is a meaningless jumble of words and sounds, called *jargon aphasia*.

paraphilia *n.* any psychosexual disorder in which sexual activity or fantasies are expressed in ways that are usually socially unacceptable or prohibited, such as *exhibitionism, *fetishism, *pedophilia, *voyeurism, and *zoophilism.

paraphimosis *n.* retraction and constric-

tion of the foreskin behind the glans penis. This occurs in some patients with *phimosis on erection of the penis: the tight foreskin cannot be drawn back over the glans and becomes painful and swollen. Manual replacement of the foreskin can usually be achieved under local or general anesthesia, but *circumcision is required to prevent a recurrence.

paraphrenia *n.* a mental disorder characterized by systematic *delusions and prominent *hallucinations but without any other marked symptoms of mental illness. The only loss of contact with reality is in areas affected by the delusions and hallucinations. It is typically seen in the elderly and deaf. Some patients, if followed over a period of years, eventually show other symptoms of *schizophrenia. It is therefore debatable whether paraphrenia constitutes a separate entity.

paraplegia *n.* *paralysis of both legs, usually due to disease or injury of the spinal cord. It is often accompanied by loss of sensation below the level of the injury and disturbed bladder function. —**paraplegic** *adj., n.*

paraprotein *n.* an abnormal protein of the *immunoglobulin series. Paraproteins appear in malignant disease of the spleen, bone marrow, liver, etc. Examples of paraproteins include *myeloma globulins, *macroglobulin, and *Bence-Jones protein.

parapsoriasis *n.* a former term for the earliest phase of *mycosis fungoides.

parapsychology *n.* the study of *extrasensory perception, *psychokinesis, and other mental abilities that appear to defy natural law.

Paraquat *n. Trademark.* the chemical compound dimethyl dipyridilium, widely used as a weedkiller. When swallowed it exerts its most serious effects upon the lungs, the tissues of which it destroys after a few days. Paraquat poisoning is almost invariably fatal.

parasite *n.* any living thing that lives in (*see* endoparasite) or on (*see* ectoparasite) another living organism (*see* host). The parasite, which may spend all or only part of its existence with the host, obtains food and/or shelter from the host and contributes nothing to its welfare. Some parasites cause irritation and interfere with bodily functions; others destroy host tissues and release toxins into the body, thus injuring health and causing disease. Human parasites include fungi, bacteria, viruses, protozoa, and worms. *See also* commensal, symbiosis. —**parasitic** *adj.*

parasiticide *n.* an agent, such as *lindane, that destroys parasites (excluding bacteria and fungi). *See also* acaricide, anthelmintic, trypanocide.

parasitology *n.* the study and science of parasites.

parasternal *adj.* situated close to the sternum. The *parasternal line* is an imaginary vertical line parallel to and midway between the lateral margin of the sternum and the vertical line through the nipple.

parasuicide *n.* a self-injuring act (such as an overdose of sleeping tablets) that is not motivated by a genuine wish to die. It differs from attempted *suicide in being common in young people who are distressed but not seriously mentally ill. However, many people who have acted in this way go on to attempt, or even to achieve, suicide. Help in sorting out their difficulties should therefore be given.

parasympathetic nervous system one of the two divisions of the *autonomic nervous system, having fibers that leave the central nervous system from the brain and the lower portion of the spinal cord and are distributed to blood vessels, glands, and the majority of internal organs. The system works in balance with the *sympathetic nervous system, the actions of which it frequently opposes.

parasympatholytic *adj.* opposing the effects of the *parasympathetic nervous system. *Anticholinergic drugs have this effect by preventing acetylcholine from acting as a neurotransmitter.

parasympathomimetic *adj.* having the effect of stimulating the *parasympathetic nervous system. The actions of parasympathomimetic drugs are *cholinergic* (resembling those of *acetylcholine) and include stimulation of skeletal muscle, *vasodilation, depression of heart rate, increasing the tension of smooth muscle, increasing secretions (such as saliva), and constricting the pupil of the eye. They are used in the treatment of *myasthenia gravis (*see* anticholinesterase),

glaucóma (*see* miotic), and urinary retention (e.g. *carbachol, *bethanechol).

paratenon *n.* the tissue of a tendon sheath that fills up spaces around the tendon.

parathion *n.* an organic phosphorus compound, used as a pesticide, that causes poisoning when inhaled, ingested, or absorbed through the skin. Like several other organic phosphorus compounds, it attacks the enzyme *cholinesterase and causes excessive stimulation of the parasympathetic nervous system. The symptoms are headache, sweating, salivation, lacrimation, vomiting, diarrhea, and muscular spasms. Treatment is by administration of *atropine.

parathormone *n. see* parathyroid hormone.

parathyroidectomy *n.* surgical removal of the parathyroid glands, usually as part of the treatment of *hyperparathyroidism.

parathyroid glands two pairs of yellowish-brown *endocrine glands that are situated behind, or sometimes embedded within, the *thyroid gland. They are stimulated to produce *parathyroid hormone by a decrease in the amount of calcium in the blood.

parathyroid hormone (parathormone) a hormone, synthesized and released by the parathyroid glands, that controls the distribution of calcium and phosphate in the body. A high level of the hormone causes transfer of calcium from the bones to the blood; a deficiency lowers blood calcium levels, causing *tetany. This condition may be treated by injections of calcium gluconate. *Compare* calcitonin.

paratyphoid fever an infectious disease caused by the bacterium *Salmonella paratyphi A, B,* or *C.* Bacteria are spread in the feces of patients or carriers, and outbreaks occur as a result of poor sanitation or unhygienic food handling. After an incubation period of 1–10 days, symptoms, including diarrhea, mild fever, and a pink rash on the chest, appear and last for about a week. Treatment with chloramphenicol is effective. Vaccination with *TAB vaccine provides temporary immunity against paratyphoid A and B.

paregoric *n.* a preparation of powdered opium, anise oil, benzoic acid, camphor, diluted alcohol, and glycerin that reduces peristalsis and is used in the treatment of diarrhea and as an analgesic.

pareidolia n. misperception of random stimuli as real things or people, as when faces are vividly seen in the flames of a fire.

parenchyma n. the functional part of an organ, as opposed to the supporting tissue (*stroma*).

parenteral adj. administered by any way other than through the mouth: applied, for example, to the introduction of drugs or other agents into the body by injection.

paresis n. muscular weakness caused by disease of the nervous system. It implies a lesser degree of weakness than *paralysis, although the two words are often used interchangeably.

paresthesia n. a spontaneously occurring abnormal tingling sensation, sometimes described as *pins and needles*. The sensations may be symptoms of partial damage to a peripheral nerve, such as that caused by external pressure on the affected part, but can also result from damage to sensory fibers in the spinal cord. *Compare* dysesthesia.

paries n. (pl. **parietes**) **1.** the enveloping or surrounding part of an organ or other structure. **2.** the wall of a cavity.

parietal adj. **1.** of or relating to the inner walls of a body cavity, as opposed to the contents: applied particularly to the membranes lining a cavity (*see* peritoneum, pleura). **2.** of or relating to the parietal bone.

parietal bone either of a pair of bones forming the top and sides of the cranium. *See* skull.

parietal cells *see* oxyntic cells.

parietal lobe one of the major divisions of each cerebral hemisphere of the brain (*see* cerebrum), lying behind the frontal lobe, above the temporal lobe, and in front of the occipital lobe. It is thus beneath the crown of the skull. It contains the *sensory cortex and *association areas.

parity n. a term used to indicate the number of pregnancies a woman has had that have each resulted in the birth of an infant capable of survival. *See also* grand multiparity.

parkinsonism n. a clinical picture characterized by tremor, rigidity, slowness of movement, and postural instability. The first and most prominent symptom is tremor, which often affects one hand, spreading first to the leg on the same side and then to the other limbs. It is most pronounced in resting limbs, interfering with such actions as holding a cup. The patient has an expressionless face, an unmodulated voice, an increasing tendency to stoop, and a shuffling walk (a shuffling run is needed to maintain balance). Parkinsonism is a disease affecting the basal ganglia of the brain and associated with a deficiency of the neurotransmitter *dopamine. Sometimes a distinction is made between *Parkinson's disease*, a degenerative disorder associated with aging, and parkinsonism due to other causes (e.g. drugs). Drug-induced parkinsonism may complicate the use of psychoactive substances, including the phenothiazines, butyrophenones, and metoclopramide. Uncommonly it can be attributed to the late effects of *encephalitis or coal gas poisoning or to *Wilson's disease. Relief of the symptoms may be obtained with *anticholinergic drugs, dopamine-receptor agonists (*see* dopamine), *levodopa, *selegiline, and subcutaneous *apomorphine injections and infusions. New surgical treatments include stereotactic *pallidotomy and pallidal stimulation. The latter procedure involves placing an electronic stimulator in the globus pallidus that can be controlled by an external switch or control panel. [J. Parkinson (1755–1824), British physician]

paromomycin n. an antibiotic, active against intestinal bacteria and amebas, used to treat dysentery and gastroenteritis. Paromomycin is administered by mouth; side effects include stomach pains, itching, and heartburn. Trade name: **Humatin**.

paronychia n. inflammation and swelling of the skinfolds and tissues surrounding a fingernail or toenail. Chronic paronychia is usually caused by the fungus *Candida or it can occur in psoriasis. The condition occurs mainly in those who habitually engage in wet work, so that it is vital to keep the hands dry in order to control chronic paronychia. Acute paronychia is the result of bacterial infection with *Staphylococcus aureus*. *See also* felon.

paroophoron *n.* the vestigial remains of part of the mesonephric duct (*see* mesonephros) in the female, situated next to each ovary. It is associated with a similar structure, the *epoophoron*. Both are without known function.

parosmia *n.* any disorder of the sense of smell.

parotid gland one of a pair of *salivary glands situated in front of each ear. The openings of the parotid ducts (*Stensen's ducts*) are on the inner sides of the cheeks, opposite the second upper molar teeth.

parotitis *n.* inflammation of the parotid salivary glands. *See* mumps (infectious parotitis).

parous *adj.* having given birth to one or more live children.

paroxetine *n.* an antidepressant drug that acts by prolonging the action of the neurotransmitter serotonin (5-hydroxytryptamine) in the brain (*see* SSRI). It is taken by mouth; side effects may include dizziness, agitation, tremor, nausea, diarrhea, and drowsiness. Trade name: **Paxil**.

paroxysm *n.* **1.** a sudden violent attack, especially a spasm or convulsion. **2.** the abrupt worsening of symptoms or recurrence of disease. —**paroxysmal** *adj.*

parrot disease *see* psittacosis.

pars *n.* a specific part of an organ or other structure, such as any of parts of the pituitary gland.

parthenogenesis *n.* reproduction in which an organism develops from an unfertilized ovum. It is common in plants and occurs in some lower animals (e.g. aphids).

partial volume artifact an apparent decrease in the visibility of a structure in a *cross-sectional imaging technique, such as CT or MRI, when either the thickness of the object is much less than that of the slice being used to make the image, or when the object is only partially within the slice. *See* artifact.

parturition *n.* childbirth. *See* labor.

parvi- *prefix denoting* small size.

parvovirus *n.* any of the small single-stranded DNA viruses belonging to the family Parvoviridae, which infect mammals and birds. The species that infects humans, human parvovirus B19, causes aplastic crises in patients with hemolytic anemia or sickle-cell disease, *hydrops

fetalis, *erythema infectiosum, fetal death, and spontaneous abortion.

PAS *see* para-aminosalicylic acid.

pascal *n.* the *SI unit of pressure, equal to 1 newton per square meter. Symbol: Pa.

Paschen bodies particles that occur in the cells of skin rashes in patients with *cowpox; they are thought to be the virus particles. [E. Paschen (1860–1936), German pathologist]

passive movement movement not brought about by a patient's own efforts. Passive movements are induced by manipulation of the joints by a physiotherapist. They are useful in maintaining function when a patient has nerve or muscle disorders that prevent voluntary movement.

passive smoke the smoke from other people's cigarettes, cigars, and pipes that is inhaled by nonsmokers. Ongoing research continues to show that passive smoke can be injurious to nonsmokers, especially infants and young children, and can aggravate certain illnesses, especially respiratory conditions, and contribute to other serious diseases.

paste *n.* (in pharmacy) a medicinal preparation of a soft sticky consistency, which is applied externally.

Pasteurella *n.* a genus of small rodlike gram-negative bacteria that are parasites of animals and humans. The species *P. multocida* generally infects animals but may be transmitted to humans through bites or scratches.

pasteurization *n.* the treatment of milk by heating it to 65°C for 30 minutes, or to 72°C for 15 minutes, followed by rapid cooling, to kill such bacteria as those causing tuberculosis and typhoid fever.

pastille *n.* a medicinal preparation containing gelatin and glycerin, usually coated with sugar, that is dissolved in the mouth so that the medication is applied to the mouth or throat.

Patau syndrome a chromosome disorder in which there is an extra chromosome 13 (three instead of the usual two), causing abnormal brain development, severe mental retardation, and defects in the heart, kidney, and scalp. Affected individuals rarely survive. [K. Patau (20th century), US geneticist]

patch test a test to discover which allergen is responsible for contact *dermatitis in a patient. Very low concentrations of common allergens (and any substances suspected of causing the dermatitis in the individual patient) are applied under a patch on the back. The patches are removed after 48 hours and the underlying skin is examined then and again after a further 48 hours. A positive test will show an eczematous reaction.

patella *n.* the lens-shaped bone that forms the kneecap. It is situated in front of the knee joint in the tendon of the quadriceps muscle of the thigh. *See also* sesamoid bone.

patellar reflex the knee jerk, in which stretching the muscle at the front of the thigh by tapping its tendon below the knee cap causes a *reflex contraction of the muscle, so that the leg kicks. This is a test of the connection between the sensory nerves attached to stretch receptors in the muscle, the spinal cord, and the motor neurons running from the cord to the thigh muscle, all of which are involved in the reflex. Disease or damage may result in absence of the reflex.

patent ductus arteriosus *see* ductus arteriosus.

path- (patho-) *prefix denoting* disease. Example: *pathophobia* (morbid fear of).

pathogen *n.* a microorganism, such as a bacterium, that parasitizes animals (or plants) or humans and produces a disease.

pathogenic *adj.* capable of causing disease. The term is applied to a parasitic microorganism (especially a bacterium) in relation to its host. —**pathogenicity** *n.*

pathognomonic *adj.* describing a symptom or sign that is characteristic of or unique to a particular disease. The presence of such a sign or symptom allows positive diagnosis of the disease.

pathological *adj.* relating to or arising from disease. For example, a pathological *fracture is one associated with disease of the bone, such as tumors, infection, congenital bone defects, or osteoporosis.

pathology *n.* the study of disease processes with the aim of understanding their nature and causes. This is achieved by observing samples of blood, urine, feces, and diseased tissue obtained from the living patient or at autopsy, by the use of X-rays, and by many other techniques. (*See* biopsy.) *Clinical pathology* is the application of the knowledge gained to the treatment of patients. —**pathologist** *n.*

pathway *n.* **1.** (in neurology) the network of structures through which nerve impulses are transmitted from any part of the body to the spinal cord and brain or from the central nervous system to organs, muscles, and cells. **2.** (**metabolic pathway**) any sequence of reactions in a cell or organism that takes place in *anabolism or *catabolism. *See also* metabolism.

-pathy *suffix denoting* **1.** disease. Example: *nephropathy* (of the kidney). **2.** therapy. Example: *osteopathy* (by bone manipulation).

pauciarthritis *n. see* arthritis.

pavementation (pavementing) *n.* the sticking of white blood cells to the linings of blood vessels (capillaries) when inflammation occurs.

PCOS *see* polycystic ovary syndrome.

PCP *Pneumocystis carinii* pneumonia. *See* Pneumocystis.

PCR *see* polymerase chain reaction.

PCWP *see* pulmonary capillary wedge pressure.

PDGF platelet-derived growth factor (*see* growth factor).

peak expiratory flow rate (PEFR) the rate at which a person can expel air from the lungs: a reliable measure of lung reserves in tests of vital capacity.

peau d'orange a dimpled appearance of the skin over a breast tumor, resembling the surface of an orange. The skin is thickened and the openings of hair follicles and sweat glands are enlarged.

PECT positron emission computed tomography (*see* positron emission tomography).

pecten *n.* **1.** the middle section of the anal canal, below the anal valves (*see* anus). **2.** a sharp ridge on the upper branch of the pubis. —**pectineal** *adj.*

pectoral *adj.* relating to the chest.

pectoral girdle *see* shoulder girdle.

pectoral muscles the chest muscles (see illustration). The *pectoralis major* is a large fan-shaped muscle that works over the shoulder joint, drawing the arm forward across the chest and rotating it medially. Beneath it, the *pectoralis minor* depresses the shoulder and draws the scapula down toward the chest.

pectoriloquy *n.* abnormal transmission of the patient's voice sounds through the chest wall so that they can be clearly heard through a stethoscope. Whispered sounds (*whispering pectoriloquy*) can be heard over the lung of a patient with pneumonia.

pectus *n.* the chest or breast.

pectus carinatum *see* pigeon chest.

pectus excavatum *see* funnel chest.

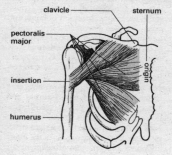

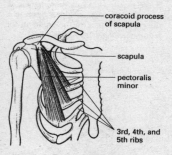

Pectoral muscles

ped- (pedo-) *prefix denoting* children.

pederasty *n.* *sodomy with a boy or a young man.

pediatric dentistry (pedodontics) the branch of dentistry concerned with the oral health care of children and adolescents.

pediatrics *n.* the general medicine of childhood. Handling the sick child requires a special approach at every age from birth (or preterm birth) to adolescence and also a proper understanding of parents. It also requires detailed knowledge of genetics, obstetrics, psychological development, management of handicaps at home and in school, and effects of social conditions on child health. *See also* Child Health Act. —**pediatrician** *n.*

pedicle *n.* **1.** the narrow neck of tissue connecting some tumors to the normal tissue from which they have developed. **2.** (in plastic surgery) a narrow folded tube of skin by means of which a piece of skin used for grafting remains attached to its original site. A pedicle graft is used when the recipient site is unsuited to take an independent skin graft (for example, because of poor blood supply). *See also* flap, skin graft. **3.** (in anatomy) any slender stemlike process.

pediculicide *n.* an agent that kills lice; for example *benzyl benzoate, *lindane, *malathion, or *permethrin.

Pediculoides *see* Pyemotes.

pediculosis *n.* an infestation of the body and/or scalp with lice, which causes intense itching; continued scratching by the patient may result in secondary bacterial infection of the skin. Untreated head lice (*see* Pediculus) can lead to a condition in which the hair becomes matted together by the exudate from weeping skin lesions; they are treated with *malathion and *permethrin lotions and by the use of a fine-toothed comb. Body lice are destroyed by dusting the body and clothes with *lindane. Pubic lice (*see* Phthirus), which are usually sexually transmitted, respond to the same treatment as head lice.

Pediculus *n.* a widely distributed genus of lice. There are two varieties of the species affecting humans: *P. humanus capitis*, the head louse; and *P. humanus corporis*, the body louse. The presence of these parasites can irritate the skin (*see* pediculosis), and in some parts of the world body lice are involved in transmitting *relapsing fever and *typhus.

pedigree *n.* (in genetics) a chart or graph that is used to analyze inheritance, especially an inherited trait or condition in a particular family. A person's ancestral line is diagrammed, using stylized symbols, usually plain and shaded or partially shaded squares and circles to indicate normal males and females, those affected by the trait or condition, and those who are carriers. *See also* genetic counseling, genetic screening.

pedodontics n. see pediatric dentistry.

pedometer n. a small portable device that records the number of paces walked, and thus the approximate distance covered. A pedometer is usually attached to the leg or hung at the belt.

pedophilia n. sexual attraction to children (of either sex). The condition is usually caused by psychological and social factors, which affect the development of sexuality. Pedophiles may seek treatment because of society's disapproval: *behavior therapy can be used, or the sexual drive can be reduced by drug treatment. —**pedophile** n. —**pedophilic** adj.

peduncle n. a narrow process or stalklike structure, serving as a support or a connection. For example, the middle cerebellar peduncle connects the pons and cerebellum in the brain.

PEFR see peak expiratory flow rate.

Pelizaeus-Merzbacher disease see leukodystrophy. [F. Pelizaeus (1850–1917) and L. Merzbacher (1879–1953), German physicians]

pellagra n. a nutritional disease due to a deficiency of *niacin (a B vitamin). Pellagra results from the consumption of a diet that is poor in either niacin or the amino acid tryptophan, from which niacin can be synthesized in the body. It is common in corn-eating communities. The symptoms of pellagra are scaly dermatitis on exposed surfaces, diarrhea, and depression.

pellicle n. a thin layer of skin, membrane, or any other substance.

pelvic-floor exercises see Kegel exercises.

pelvic girdle (hip girdle) the bony structure to which the bones of the lower limbs are attached. It consists of the right and left *hip bones.

pelvic inflammatory disease (PID) an acute or chronic condition in which the uterus, fallopian tubes, and ovaries are infected. The inflammation is the result of infection spreading from an adjacent infected organ (such as the appendix) or ascending from the vagina (as in the case of infection with *Chlamydia trachomatis); it may also result from a blood-borne infection, such as tuberculosis. The main feature is lower abdominal pain that may, at times, be severe. An acute infection may respond to treatment with antibiotics, but in the chronic state, when pelvic *adhesions have developed, surgical removal of the diseased tissue may be necessary. Blockage of the fallopian tubes is a common result of pelvic inflammatory disease and can lead to *ectopic pregnancy or infertility. Treatment is generally with multiple antibiotics.

pelvimetry n. the measurement of the four internal diameters of the pelvis (transverse, anteroposterior, left oblique, and right oblique). Pelvimetry helps in determining whether it will be possible for a fetus to be delivered in the normal way. Abnormality of any of the diameters may be an indication for cesarean section.

pelvis n. (pl. **pelves**) 1. the bony structure formed by the *hip bones, *sacrum, and *coccyx: the bony pelvis (see illustration). The hip bones are fused at the back to the sacrum to form a rigid structure that protects the organs of the lower abdomen and provides attachment for the bones and muscles of the lower limbs. 2. the lower part of the abdomen. 3. the cavity within the bony pelvis. 4. any structure shaped like a basin, e.g. the expanded part of the ureter in the kidney (renal pelvis). —**pelvic** adj.

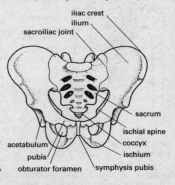

The male pelvis (ventral view)

pemoline n. a weak stimulant of the nervous system used to treat *attention-deficit/hyperactivity disorder in children. It is administered by mouth. Possible side effects include headache, irritability, dizziness, sweating, palpitations, loss of appetite, weight loss, and dry mouth. Trade name: Cylert.

pemphigoid (bullous pemphigoid) *n.* a chronic itchy blistering disorder of the elderly. The blisters most commonly occur on the limbs and persist for several days, unlike those of *pemphigus. Pemphigoid is an *autoimmune disease and responds to treatment with corticosteroids or immunosuppressant drugs. *Ocular pemphigoid* is a potentially blinding disease in which there is blistering and scarring of the conjunctiva, leading to dryness of the eye, and shortening of the fornices (the inferior and superior lines of reflection from the conjunctiva from the eyelid to the eyeball), due to adhesions to the eyelid.

pemphigus *n.* any of several distinctive *autoimmune diseases of the skin marked by successive outbreaks of blisters. There are several types; for example, *benign familial pemphigus*, which is a hereditary condition; and *pemphigus vulgaris*, a rare serious disease occurring in middle age and initially affecting the mucous membranes. Treatment is with steroids and immunosuppressant drugs. The term is often used alone to denote pemphigus vulgaris.

Pendred's syndrome goiter associated with congenital deafness due to deficiency of *peroxidase, an enzyme that is essential for the utilization of iodine. [V. Pendred (1869–1946), British physician]

penetrance *n.* the frequency with which the characteristic controlled by a gene is seen in the individuals possessing it. Complete penetrance occurs when the characteristic is seen in all individuals known to possess the gene. If a percentage of individuals with the gene do not show its effects, penetrance is incomplete. In this way a characteristic in a family may appear to skip a generation.

-penia *suffix denoting* lack or deficiency. Example: *neutropenia* (of neutrophils).

penicillamine *n.* a drug that binds metals and therefore aids their excretion (*see* chelating agent). It is used to treat *Wilson's disease, poisoning by metals such as lead, copper, and mercury, and severe rheumatoid arthritis. It is administered by mouth and commonly causes digestive upsets and allergic reactions. Trade names: **Cuprimine, Depen**.

penicillin *n.* a large group of natural and semisynthetic *beta-lactam antibiotics derived from species of the mold *Penicillium* and used to treat infections caused by a wide variety of bacteria. Penicillin first became available for treating bacterial infections in 1941. Since then several similar drugs have been prepared from *Penicillium* (*see* penicillin G benzathine, penicillin V), and a number of antibiotics have been derived from the penicillins (including *amoxicillin, *ampicillin, and *cloxacillin sodium); these antibacterials are called *semisynthetic penicillins. See also* ticarcillin.

penicillinase *n.* an enzyme, produced by some bacteria, that is capable of antagonizing the antibacterial action of *penicillin. Purified penicillinase, obtained from a strain of *Bacillus cereus*, may be used to treat reactions to penicillin. It is also used in diagnostic tests to isolate microorganisms from the blood of patients receiving penicillin.

penicillin G benzathine a long-acting antibiotic (*see* penicillin), given by intramuscular injection, that is slowly absorbed and effective against most gram-positive bacteria (streptococci, staphylococci, and pneumococci). Patients hypersensitive to the penicillins have allergic reactions. Trade name: **Bicillin,**

penicillin V an antibiotic (*see* penicillin), used to treat infections caused by a wide variety of microorganisms. It is administered by mouth and may cause diarrhea and allergic reactions. Trade names: **Beepen-VK, Betapen-VK, Ledercillin VK, Pen-Vee K, V-Cillin K, Veetids**.

Penicillium *n.* a genus of moldlike fungi that commonly grow on decaying fruit, bread, or cheese. The species *P. chrysogenum* is the major natural source of the antibiotic *penicillin. Some species of *Penicillium* are pathogenic to humans, causing diseases of the skin and respiratory tract.

penile prosthesis *see* prosthesis.

penis *n.* the male organ that carries the *urethra, through which urine and semen are discharged (see illustration). Urination can occur in the normal hanging position. Most of the organ is composed of erectile tissue (*see* corpus cavernosum, corpus spongiosum), which becomes filled with blood under conditions of sexual excitement so that the penis is erected. In this position it can act as a sexual organ, capable of entering the vagina and ejaculating semen. *See also* glans, prepuce.

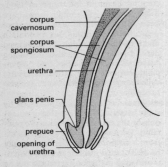

corpus cavernosum
corpus spongiosum
urethra
glans penis
prepuce
opening of urethra

The penis (median section)

pent- (penta-) *prefix denoting* five.

pentaerythritol *n.* a drug that dilates blood vessels and is used in the treatment of angina and other heart conditions. It is administered by mouth and may cause headache and indigestion. Trade name: **Peritrate**.

pentagastrin *n.* a synthetic hormone that has the same effects as *gastrin in stimulating the secretion of gastric juice from the stomach. It is injected to test for gastric secretion in the diagnosis of digestive disorders. Trade name: **Peptavlon**.

pentamidine *n.* a drug effective against protozoans and used in the treatment of *Pneumocystis carinii* pneumonia in AIDS patients, *trypanosomiasis, and *leishmaniasis. It is administered by injection or from an inhaler. Possible side effects include low blood pressure, heart irregularity, low blood sugar (hypoglycemia), low white blood count, and damage to the kidneys. Trade names: **NebuPent, Pentam 300**.

pentazocine *n.* a potent *analgesic drug used to relieve moderate or severe pain. It is administered by mouth, injection, or in suppositories; side effects include dizziness and digestive upsets. Trade names: **Fortral, Talwin Nx**.

pentetic acid (DTPA) diethylenetriamine pentaacetic acid, which when labeled

with *technetium-99m is used as a tracer to obtain *scintigrams of the kidney over a period of time, by means of a *gamma camera. Pentetic acid is filtered out of the blood by the kidneys and passes into the urine; it is used to show function and reflux. It is particularly useful in assessing obstruction to urinary drainage from the kidneys.

pentobarbital *n.* a *barbiturate drug used to relieve insomnia and agitation and also as an *anticonvulsant. It is administered by mouth, injection, or in suppositories. Side effects include rashes, digestive upsets, and lethargy, and prolonged use may lead to *dependence. Trade name: **Nembutal**.

pentose *n.* a simple sugar with five carbon atoms: for example, ribose and xylose.

pentostatin *n.* a *cytotoxic drug that is used in treating *hairy cell leukemia; it works by interfering with the action of the enzyme adenosine deaminase. Pentostatin is administered by intravenous injection; side effects, which may be severe, include *myelosuppression. Trade name: **Nipent**.

pentosuria *n.* an inborn defect of sugar metabolism causing abnormal excretion of pentose in the urine. There are no serious ill effects.

pentoxifylline *n.* a vasodilator drug used for the treatment of intermittent *claudication. It increases the flow of blood by decreasing its viscosity. It is administered by mouth; most common side effects are gastric upsets, nausea, dizziness, and headache. Trade name: **Trental**.

pepsin *n.* an enzyme in the stomach that begins the digestion of proteins by splitting them into peptones (*see* peptidase). It is produced by the action of hydrochloric acid on *pepsinogen*, which is secreted by the gastric glands. Once made, pepsin itself can act on pepsinogen to produce more pepsin.

pepsinogen *n. see* pepsin.

peptic *adj.* **1.** relating to pepsin. **2.** relating to digestion.

peptic ulcer a breach in the lining (mucosa) of the digestive tract produced by digestion of the mucosa by pepsin and acid. This may occur when pepsin and acid are present in abnormally high concentrations or when some other mechanism reduces the normal protective mechanisms of the mucosa; bile salts may play a part, especially in stomach ulcers. A peptic ulcer may be found in the esophagus (*esophageal ulcer*, associated with reflux *esophagitis); the stomach (*see* gastric ulcer); duodenum (*see* duodenal ulcer); jejunum (*jejunal ulcer*, usually in the *Zollinger-Ellison syndrome); in a Meckel's *diverticulum; and close to a *gastroenterostomy (*stomal ulcer*, *anastomotic ulcer*, *marginal ulcer*).

peptidase n. one of a group of digestive enzymes that splits proteins in the stomach and intestine into their constituent amino acids. The group is divided into *endopeptidases and *exopeptidases.

peptide n. a molecule consisting of two or more *amino acids linked by bonds between the amino group (–NH) and the carboxyl group (–CO). This bond is known as a *peptide bond. See also polypeptide.

peptone n. a large protein fragment produced by the action of enzymes on proteins in the first stages of protein digestion.

peptonuria n. the presence in the urine of *peptones, intermediate compounds formed during the digestion of proteins.

perception n. (in psychology) the process by which information about the world, received by the senses, is analyzed and made meaningful. Abnormalities of perception include *hallucinations, *illusions, and *agnosia.

percussion n. the technique of examining part of the body by tapping it with the fingers or an instrument (*plessor*) and sensing the resultant vibrations. With experience it is possible to detect the presence of abnormal solidification or enlargement in different organs and the presence of fluid, for example in the lungs.

percutaneous adj. through the skin: the term is often applied to the route of administration of drugs in ointments, etc., which are absorbed through the skin.

percutaneous epididymal sperm aspiration see PESA.

percutaneous nephrolithotomy a technique of removing stones from the kidney via a *nephroscope passed into the kidney through a track from the skin surface previously established by the presence of a catheter.

percutaneous transhepatic cholangiopancreatography a method for outlining the bile ducts and pancreatic ducts with radiopaque dyes, which are introduced by a catheter inserted into the ducts from the surface of the skin. See cholangiography.

perforation n. the creation of a hole in an organ, tissue, or tube (e.g. a *duodenal ulcer, colonic *diverticulitis, or stomach cancer), allowing the contents of the intestine to enter the peritoneal cavity, which causes acute inflammation (*peritonitis) with sudden severe abdominal pain and shock. Treatment is usually by surgical repair of the perforation, but conservative treatment with antibiotics may result in spontaneous healing. Perforation may also be caused accidentally by instruments – for example a gastroscope may perforate the stomach, a curette may perforate the uterus – or by injury, for example, to the eardrum.

perfusion n. **1.** the passage of fluid through a tissue, especially the passage of blood through the lung tissue to pick up oxygen from the air in the alveoli, which is brought there by *ventilation, and release carbon dioxide. If ventilation is impaired, deoxygenated venous blood is returned to the general circulation. If perfusion is impaired, insufficient gas exchange takes place. **2.** the deliberate introduction of fluid into a tissue, usually by injection into the blood vessels supplying the tissue.

perfusion scan a technique for demonstrating an abnormal blood supply to an organ by injecting a radioactive *tracer or *contrast medium. One of the most common uses, often in conjunction with ventilation scanning (*see* ventilation-perfusion scanning), is to detect obstruction of pulmonary arteries due to embolism by thrombus (*see* pulmonary embolism). Particles that are labeled with radioactive tracer are injected intravenously and become temporarily lodged in the capillaries in the lungs. Areas not being perfused show up as holes on the gamma-camera images. In *magnetic resonance imaging or *computed tomography, contrast medium is injected and a series of images is obtained. The rate of change of enhancement is an index of the blood supply to the area of interest. This technique can be used to study blood supply to the brain, heart, or kidneys (in particular), to help diagnose arterial strictures or blockages, or to tumors in which blood supply may be increased by abnormal vessels.

pergolide *n.* a drug that stimulates *dopamine receptors in the brain and is used in the treatment of *parkinsonism. It is administered by mouth. Possible side effects include confusion, hallucinations, sleepiness, heart irregularity, nausea, breathing difficulties, and double vision. Trade name: **Permax**.

peri- *prefix denoting* near, around, or enclosing. Examples: *pericardial* (around the heart); *peritonsillar* (around a tonsil).

periadenitis *n.* inflammation of tissues surrounding a gland.

perianal hematoma (external hemorrhoid) a small painful swelling beside the anus, occurring after a bout of straining to pass feces or coughing. Perianal hematomas are caused by the rupture of a small vein in the anus. They often heal spontaneously but occasionally rupture. Rarely, this is followed by abscess formation. If severe pain continues, surgical removal can be undertaken. *See also* hemorrhoids.

periapical *adj.* around an apex, particularly the apex of a tooth. The term is applied to bone surrounding the apex and to X-ray views of this area.

peri-arrest period the recognized period, either just before or just after a full *cardiac arrest, when the patient's condition is very unstable and care must be taken to prevent progression or regression into a full cardiac arrest.

periarteritis nodosa *see* polyarteritis nodosa.

periarthritis *n.* inflammation of tissues around a joint capsule, including tendons and *bursae. *Chronic periarthritis*, which may be spontaneous or follow an injury, is a common cause of pain and stiffness of the shoulder; it usually responds to local steroid injections or physiotherapy.

peribulbar *adj.* (in ophthalmology) denoting the area around the eye.

pericard- (pericardio-) *prefix denoting* the pericardium.

pericardiectomy (pericardectomy) *n.* sur-

gical removal of the membranous sac surrounding the heart (pericardium). It is used in the treatment of chronic constrictive pericarditis and chronic pericardial effusion (*see* pericarditis).

pericardiocentesis *n.* removal of excess fluid from within the sac (pericardium) surrounding the heart by means of needle *aspiration. *See* pericarditis, hydropericardium.

pericardiolysis *n.* the surgical separation of *adhesions between the heart and surrounding structures within the ribcage (*adherent pericardium*). The operation is now rarely used.

pericardiorrhaphy *n.* the repair of wounds in the membrane surrounding the heart (pericardium), such as those due to injury or surgery.

pericardiostomy *n.* an operation in which the membranous sac around the heart is opened and the fluid within drained via a tube. It is sometimes used in the treatment of septic pericarditis.

pericardiotomy (pericardotomy) *n.* surgical opening or puncture of the membranous sac (pericardium) around the heart. It is required to gain access to the heart in heart surgery and to remove excess fluid from within the pericardium.

pericarditis *n.* acute or chronic inflammation of the membranous sac (pericardium) that surrounds the heart. Pericarditis may be seen alone or as part of pancarditis (*see* endomyocarditis). It has numerous causes, including virus infections, uremia, and cancer. *Acute pericarditis* is characterized by fever, chest pain, and a pericardial friction rub. Fluid may accumulate within the pericardial sac (*pericardial effusion*). Rarely, chronic thickening of the pericardium (*chronic constrictive pericarditis*) develops. This interferes with activity of the heart and has many features in common with *heart failure, including edema, pleural effusions, ascites, and engorgement of the veins. Constrictive pericarditis most often results from tubercular infection.

The treatment of pericarditis is directed to the cause. Pericardial effusions may be aspirated by a needle inserted through the chest wall. Chronic constrictive pericarditis is treated by surgical removal of the pericardium (*pericardiectomy*).

pericardium *n.* the membrane surrounding

the heart, consisting of two portions. The outer *fibrous pericardium* completely encloses the heart and is attached to the large blood vessels emerging from the heart. The internal *serous pericardium* is a closed sac of *serous membrane: the inner visceral portion (*epicardium*) is closely attached to the muscular heart wall and the outer parietal portion lines the fibrous pericardium. Within the sac is a very small amount of fluid, which prevents friction when the two surfaces slide over one another as the heart beats. —**pericardial** *adj.*

pericardotomy *n. see* pericardiotomy.

perichondritis *n.* inflammation of cartilage and surrounding soft tissues, usually due to chronic infection. A common site is the external ear.

perichondrium *n.* the dense layer of fibrous connective tissue that covers the surface of *cartilage.

pericoronitis *n.* inflammation around the crown of a tooth, particularly a partially erupted third molar.

pericranium *n.* the *periosteum of the skull.

pericystitis *n.* inflammation in the tissues around the bladder, causing pain in the pelvis, fever, and symptoms of *cystitis. It usually results from infection in the fallopian tubes or uterus, but can occasionally arise from severe infection in a *diverticulum of the bladder itself. Treatment of pericystitis is directed to the underlying cause and usually involves antibiotic therapy. Pericystitis associated with a pelvic abscess clears when the abscess is surgically drained.

pericyte *n.* a type of cell surrounding the smallest blood vessels (terminal arterioles and venules and capillaries). Its function is uncertain.

periderm *n. see* epitrichium.

perifolliculitis *n.* inflammation around the hair follicles.

perihepatitis *n.* inflammation of the membrane covering the liver. It is usually associated with abnormalities of the liver (including liver abscess, cirrhosis, tuberculosis) or in chronic peritonitis.

perikaryon *n. see* cell body.

perilymph *n.* the fluid between the bony and membranous *labyrinths of the ear.

perimenopause *n.* the period of time around the *menopause in which marked changes in the menstrual cycle occur and estrogen levels begin to drop, usually accompanied by hot flashes, and in which no 12 consecutive months of amenorrhea have yet occurred. Some studies have shown that *hormone replacement therapy may be more effective, especially in preventing bone loss, if started during perimenopause.

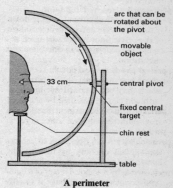

arc that can be rotated about the pivot

movable object

33 cm — central pivot

fixed central target

chin rest

table

A perimeter

perimeter *n.* an instrument for mapping the extent of the *visual field (see illustration). The patient looks steadily at a target in the center of the inner surface of the hemisphere. Objects are presented on this surface and the patient says if he sees them. The area of the visual field can be defined and any gaps in the field can be detected. There are several types of perimeter. In the *static perimeter* the movable object is replaced by a system of tiny lights, set in a black background, that can be flashed singly or in patterns. If the patient has a field defect, he will fail to see the lights that flash in the area of the defect. Modern visual field testing uses computer-assisted *automated perimeters* to map out and analyze visual fields and thus detect very subtle field defects (*computerized perimetry*). Automated perimeters are commonly used in the diagnosis and follow-up of glaucoma. —**perimetry** *n.*

perimetritis *n.* inflammation of the membrane on the outer surface of the uterus. The condition may be associated with *parametritis.

perimetrium n. the *peritoneum of the uterus.

perimysium n. the fibrous sheath that surrounds each bundle of *muscle fibers.

perinatal adj. relating to the period from about three months before to one month after birth.

perinatal mortality rate see infant mortality rate.

perindopril n. see ACE inhibitor.

perineal descent abnormal bulging down of the *perineum as a result of weakness of the pelvic floor muscles. It often accompanies problems with defecation and micturition.

perineal pouch see ileal pouch.

perineal tear an injury to the perineum, which may be sustained during childbirth and can be classified by degree of involvement of the perineal muscles, the anal sphincter complex, and the rectal mucosa.

perineoplasty n. an operation to enlarge the vaginal opening by incising the hymen and part of the perineum.

perineorrhaphy n. surgical repair of a damaged perineum. The damage is usually the result of a tear in the perineum sustained during childbirth.

perinephric abscess a collection of pus around the kidney, usually secondary to *pyonephrosis.

perinephritis n. inflammation of the tissues around the kidney. This is usually due to spread of infection from the kidney itself (see pyelonephritis, pyonephrosis). The patient has pain in the loins, fever, and bouts of shivering. Prompt treatment of the underlying renal infection is required to prevent progression to an abscess.

perineum n. the region of the body between the anus and the urethral opening, including both skin and underlying muscle. In females it is perforated by the vaginal opening. —**perineal** adj.

perineurium n. the sheath of connective tissue that surrounds individual bundles (fascicles) of nerve fibers within a large *nerve.

periodic acid–Schiff (PAS) reaction a test for the presence of glycoproteins, polysaccharides, certain mucopolysaccharides, glycolipids, and certain fatty acids in tissue sections. The tissue is treated with periodic acid, followed by *Schiff's reagent. A positive reaction is the development of a red or magenta coloration.

periodic fever see malaria.

periodontal adj. denoting or relating to the tissues surrounding the teeth.

periodontal abscess an abscess that arises in the periodontal tissues and is invariably an acute manifestation of periodontal disease.

periodontal disease disease of the tissues that support and attach the teeth, comprising the gums, periodontal membrane, and alveolar bone. It is caused by the metabolism of bacterial *plaque on the surfaces of the teeth adjacent to these tissues. Periodontal disease includes *gingivitis and the more advanced stage of *periodontitis*, which results in the formation of spaces between the gums and the teeth (*periodontal pockets*), the loss of some fibers that attach the tooth to the jaw, and the loss of bone. The disease is widespread and is the most common cause of tooth loss in older people. Poor oral hygiene is a major contributory factor, but the resistance of the patient has some influence; for example, the reduced resistance of AIDS patients may predispose to periodontal disease.

periodontal membrane (periodontal ligament) the ligament around a *tooth, by which it is attached to the bone.

periodontal pocket a space between the gingival tissues and tooth occurring in periodontitis. See periodontal disease.

periodontics n. the branch of dentistry concerned with the diagnosis, prevention, and treatment of *periodontal disease.

periodontium n. the tissues that support and attach the teeth: the gums (see gingiva), *periodontal membrane, alveolar bone, and *cementum.

periodontology n. the branch of dentistry concerned with the scientific study, in both health and disease, of the structure and function of the tissues that support and attach the teeth. See also periodontal disease, periodontics.

periorbital adj. 1. around the eye socket (*orbit). 2. relating to the periosteum within the orbit.

periosteum n. a layer of dense connective tissue that covers the surface of a bone except at the articular surfaces. The outer layer of the periosteum is extremely dense and contains a large number of blood vessels (*see also* osteoclast). The inner layer is more cellular in appearance and contains osteoblasts and fewer blood vessels. The periosteum provides attachment for muscles, tendons, and ligaments.

periostitis *n.* inflammation of the membrane surrounding a bone (*see* periosteum). *Acute periostitis* results from direct injury to the bone and is associated with a *hematoma, which may later become infected. The uncomplicated condition subsides quickly with rest and anti-inflammatory analgesics. *Chronic periostitis* sometimes follows but is more often due to an inflammatory disease, such as tuberculosis or syphilis, or to a chronic ulcer overlying the bone involved. Chronic periostitis causes thickening of the underlying bone, which is evident on X-ray.

peripheral nervous system all parts of the nervous system lying outside the central nervous system (brain and spinal cord). It includes the *cranial nerves and *spinal nerves and their branches, which link the receptors and effector organs with the brain and spinal cord. *See also* autonomic nervous system.

peripheral neuropathy (polyneuropathy, peripheral neuritis) any of a group of disorders affecting the sensory and/or motor nerves in the peripheral nervous system. They tend to start distally, in the fingers and toes, and progress proximally. Symptoms include pins and needles, stabbing pains and a numbness on the sensory side, and weakness of the muscles. The most common causes of peripheral neuropathy are diabetes, alcohol, certain drugs, and such infections as HIV; genetic causes of peripheral neuropathy include amyloidosis and *Charcot-Marie-Tooth disease. The diagnosis may be established by neurophysiological tests, blood tests, and occasionally a nerve biopsy.

periphlebitis *n.* inflammation of the tissues around a vein: seen as an extension of *phlebitis.

perisalpingitis *n.* inflammation of the peritoneal membrane on the outer surface of a fallopian tube.

perisplenitis *n.* inflammation of the external coverings of the spleen.

peristalsis *n.* a wavelike movement that progresses along some of the hollow

tubes of the body. It occurs involuntarily and is characteristic of tubes that possess circular and longitudinal muscles, such as the *intestines. It is induced by distension of the walls of the tube. Immediately behind the distension the circular muscle contracts. In front of the distension the circular muscle relaxes and the longitudinal muscle contracts, which pushes the contents of the tube forward. —**peristaltic** *adj.*

peritendineum *n.* the fibrous covering of a tendon.

peritendinitis *n. see* tenosynovitis.

peritomy *n.* an eye operation in which an incision of the conjunctiva is made in a complete circle around the cornea.

peritoneoscope *n. see* laparoscope.

peritoneum *n.* the *serous membrane of the abdominal cavity (see illustration). The *parietal peritoneum* lines the walls of the abdomen, and the *visceral peritoneum* covers the abdominal organs. *See also* mesentery, omentum. —**peritoneal** *adj.*

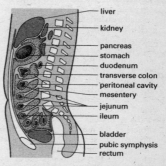

liver
kidney
pancreas
stomach
duodenum
transverse colon
peritoneal cavity
mesentery
jejunum
ileum
bladder
pubic symphysis
rectum

Sagittal section of the abdomen to show arrangement of the peritoneum

peritonitis *n.* inflammation of the *peritoneum. *Primary peritonitis* is caused by bacteria spread via the bloodstream: examples are *pneumococcal peritonitis* and *tuberculous peritonitis*. Symptoms are diffuse abdominal pain and swelling, with fever and weight loss. Fluid may accumulate in the peritoneal cavity (see ascites) or the infection may complicate existing ascites. *Secondary peritonitis* is due to perforation or rupture of an abdominal organ (for example, a duodenal ulcer or the vermiform appendix), allowing access of bacteria and irritant digestive juices to the peritoneum. This produces sudden severe abdominal pain, first at the site of rupture but becoming generalized. Shock develops, and the abdominal wall becomes rigid; X-ray examination may reveal gas within the peritoneal cavity. Treatment is usually by surgical repair of the perforation, but in some cases conservative treatment using antibiotics and intravenous fluid may be used. *Subphrenic abscess is a possible complication. *Meconium peritonitis* occurs in newborn infants as a result of a perforated intestine; it is initially a sterile contamination of the peritoneum.

peritonsillar abscess *see* quinsy.

peritrichous *adj.* describing bacteria in which the flagella cover the entire cell surface.

perityphlitis *n. Archaic.* inflammation of the tissues around the cecum. *See* typhlitis.

periureteritis *n.* inflammation of the tissues around a ureter. This is usually associated with inflammation of the ureter itself (*ureteritis) often behind an obstruction caused by a stone or stricture. Treatment is directed to relieving any obstruction of the ureter and controlling the infection with antibiotics.

PERLA pupils equal, react to light and accommodation: used in hospital notes.

perle *n.* a soft capsule containing medicine.

perlèche *n.* dryness and cracking of the corners of the mouth, sometimes with infection caused by such organisms as *Candida albicans*, staphylococci, or streptococci. Perlèche may be caused by persistent lip licking or by a vitamin-deficient diet.

permethrin *n.* a synthetic derivation of the naturally occurring insecticide pyrethrin that is applied externally to treat head lice, pubic lice, and scabies. It may cause itching. Trade names: **Elimite, Nix**.

pernicious *adj.* describing diseases that are highly dangerous or likely to result in death if untreated. *See also* pernicious anemia.

pernicious anemia a form of *anemia resulting from deficiency of *vitamin B_{12}. This in turn results either from failure to produce the substance (*intrinsic factor)

that facilitates absorption of B_{12} from the bowel or from dietary deficiency of the vitamin. Pernicious anemia is characterized by defective production of red blood cells and the presence of *megaloblasts in the bone marrow. In severe forms the nervous system is affected (*see* subacute combined degeneration of the cord). The condition is treated by injections of vitamin B_{12}.

pernio *n. see* chilblain.

perniosis *n.* any one of a group of conditions caused by the effect of persistent cold on individuals whose skin blood vessels are especially sensitive. The small arteries constrict and the capillaries dilate slowing the blood flow. The blood loses all its oxygen and fluid passes from the stagnant capillary blood into the tissues. The affected area becomes blue, swollen, and cold. Perniosis includes such conditions as *chilblains, *acrocyanosis, *erythrocyanosis, and *Raynaud's disease.

pero- *prefix denoting* deformity; defect. Example: *peromelia* (of the limbs).

peroneal *adj.* relating to or supplying the outer (fibular) side of the leg.

peroneus *n.* one of the muscles of the leg that arises from the fibula. The *peroneus longus* and *peroneus brevis* are situated at the side of the leg and inserted into the metatarsal bones of the foot. They help to turn the foot outward.

peroxidase *n.* an enzyme, found mainly in plants but also present in leukocytes and milk, that catalyzes the dehydrogenation (oxidation) of various substances in the presence of hydrogen peroxide (which acts as a hydrogen acceptor, being converted to water in the process).

peroxisome *n.* a small structure within a cell that is similar to a *lysosome but contains different enzymes, some of which may take part in reactions involving hydrogen peroxide.

perphenazine *n.* a phenothiazine *antipsychotic drug used to treat schizophrenia and mania, to relieve anxiety, tension, and agitation, and to prevent nausea and vomiting. It is administered by mouth; side effects are similar to those of *chlorpromazine. Trade name: **Trilafon**.

perseveration *n.* **1.** excessive persistence at a task that prevents the individual from turning his attention to new situations. It is a symptom of organic disease of the brain and sometimes of obsessional neurosis. **2.** the phenomenon in which an image continues to be perceived briefly in the absence of the object. This is a potentially serious neurological disorder.

persistent vegetative state the condition of living like a vegetable, without consciousness or the ability to initiate voluntary action, as a result of brain damage. People in the vegetative state may sometimes give the appearance of being awake and conscious, with open eyes. They may make random movements of the limbs or head and may pick or rub with the fingers, but there is no response to any form of communication and no reason to suppose that there is any awareness of the environment.

The vegetative state must be distinguished from apparently similar conditions, such as the psychiatric state of *catatonia, in which consciousness is retained and from which full recovery is possible, and the *locked-in syndrome*, resulting from damage to the brainstem, in which the patient is conscious but unable to speak or make any movement of any part of the body, except for blinking and upward eye movements, which permit signaling.

personality *n.* (in psychology) an enduring disposition to act and feel in particular ways that differentiate one individual from another. These patterns are sometimes conceptualized as different categories (*see* personality disorder) and sometimes as different dimensions (*see* extroversion, neuroticism).

personality disorder a deeply ingrained and maladjusted pattern of behavior, persisting through many years. It is usually manifested by the time the individual is an adolescent. The abnormality of behavior must be sufficiently severe that it causes suffering, either to the patient or to other people (or to both). Most forms of psychotherapy claim to be of therapeutic value, but the worth of any treatment remains debatable. *See* anancastic, antisocial personality disorder, avoidant, borderline, hysterical, paranoid, schizoid personality.

perspiration *n.* *sweat or the process of sweating. *Insensible perspiration* is sweat that evaporates immediately from the skin and is therefore not visible; *sensible*

perspiration is visible on the skin in the form of drops.

Perthes' disease *see* Legg-Calvé-Perthes disease.

pertussis *n.* *see* whooping cough.

perversion *n.* *see* sexual deviation.

pes *n.* (in anatomy) the foot or a part resembling a foot.

PESA (percutaneous epididymal sperm aspiration) a method of removing spermatozoa directly from the *epididymis, a new technique used in assisted conception. The sperm are then used to fertilize egg cells in vitro.

pes cavus *see* clawfoot.

pes planus *see* flatfoot.

pessary *n.* **1.** a plastic or metal device, often ring-shaped, that fits into the vagina and keeps the uterus in position: used to treat *prolapse. **2. (vaginal suppository)** a plug or cylinder of cocoa butter or other soft material containing a drug that is fitted into the vagina for the treatment of gynecological disorders (e.g. vaginitis) or for the induction of labor.

pesticide *n.* a chemical agent used to kill insects or other organisms harmful to crops and other cultivated plants. Some pesticides, such as *parathion and *dieldrin, have caused poisoning in human beings and livestock after accidental exposure.

PET *see* positron emission tomography.

petechia *n.* (*pl.* **petechiae**) a small round flat dark-red spot caused by bleeding into the skin or beneath the mucous membrane. Petechiae occur, for example, in the *purpuras.

petit mal *see* epilepsy.

Petri dish a flat shallow circular glass or plastic dish with a pillboxlike lid, used to hold solid agar or gelatin media for culturing bacteria. [J. R. Petri (1852–1921), German bacteriologist]

petrissage (malaxation) *n.* kneading: a form of *massage in which the skin is lifted up, pressed down and squeezed, and pinched and rolled. Alternate squeezing and relaxation of the tissues stimulates the local circulation and may have a pain-relieving effect in muscular disorders.

petrositis *n.* inflammation of the petrous part of the *temporal bone (which encloses the inner ear), usually due to an extension of *mastoiditis.

petrous bone *see* temporal bone.

Peutz-Jeghers syndrome a hereditary disorder in which the presence of multiple *polyps in the lining of the small intestine (intestinal *polyposis) is associated with pigmented areas (similar to freckles) around the lips, on the inside of the mouth, and on the palms and soles. The polyps may bleed, resulting in anemia, or may cause obstruction of the bowel. Half of those affected develop malignant tumors (not necessarily of the bowel). [J. L. A. Peutz (1886–1957), Dutch physician; H. J. Jeghers (1904–90), US physician]

-pexy *suffix denoting* surgical fixation. Example: *omentopexy* (of the omentum).

Peyer's patches oval masses of *lymphoid tissue on the mucous membrane lining the small intestine. [J. C. Peyer (1653–1712), Swiss anatomist]

Peyronie's disease a dense fibrous plaque in the penis, which can be felt in the erectile tissue as an irregular hard lump. The penis curves or angulates at this point on erection and pain often results. The cause is unknown. The penis can be straightened surgically by means of *Nesbit's operation*. [F. de la Peyronie (1678–1747), French surgeon]

pH a measure of the concentration of hydrogen ions in a solution, and therefore of its acidity or alkalinity. A pH of 7 indicates a neutral solution, a pH below 7 indicates acidity, and a pH in excess of 7 indicates alkalinity.

PHA *n. see* phytohemagglutinin.

phaco- *prefix denoting* the lens of the eye.

phacoemulsification *n.* the use of a high-frequency *ultrasound probe to break up a cataract so that it can be removed through a very small incision. This is now a popular method of performing cataract surgery.

phag- (phago-) *prefix denoting* 1. eating. 2. phagocytes.

phage *n. see* bacteriophage.

phagedena *n.* rapidly spreading ulceration with sloughing of dead skin. *See also* bedsore.

-phagia *suffix denoting* a condition involving eating.

phagocyte *n.* a cell that is able to engulf and digest bacteria, protozoa, cells and cell debris, and other small particles. Phagocytes include many white blood cells (*see* leukocyte) and *macrophages,

which play a major role in the body's defense mechanism. —**phagocytic** *adj.*

phagocytosis *n.* the engulfment and digestion of bacteria and other foreign particles by a cell (*see* phagocyte). *Compare* pinocytosis.

phakic *adj.* denoting the state in which the natural crystalline lens of the eye is still in place, as contrasted with aphakic (*see* aphakia) or pseudophakic (*see* pseudophakia).

phalangeal cells rows of supporting cells between the sensory hair cells of the organ of Corti (*see* cochlea).

phalangectomy *n.* surgical removal of one or more of the small bones (phalanges) in the fingers or toes.

phalanges *n.* (*sing.* **phalanx**) the bones of the fingers and toes (the digits). The first digit (the thumb or big toe) has two phalanges. Each of the remaining digits has three phalanges. —**phalangeal** *adj.*

phalangitis *n.* inflammation of a finger or toe, causing swelling and pain. The condition may be caused by infection of the soft tissues, tendon sheaths, bone, or joints or by some rheumatic diseases, such as *psoriatic arthritis. *See also* dactylitis.

phalanx *n. see* phalanges.

phalloplasty *n.* surgical reconstruction or repair of the penis. It is required to correct congenital deformity of the penis, as in *hypospadias or *epispadias, and sometimes also following injury to the penis with loss of skin.

phallus *n.* **1.** the embryonic penis, before the urethral duct has reached its final state of development. **2.** the penis.

phanero- *prefix denoting* visible; apparent.

phaneromania *n.* an excessively strong impulse to touch or rub parts of one's own body.

phantom limb the sensation that an arm or leg, or part of an arm or leg, is still attached to the body after it has been amputated. Pain may seem to come from the amputated part. This may arise because of stimulation of the amputation stump, which contains severed nerves that formerly carried messages from the removed portion, or may occur because the neural representation of the limb is still present in the brain and may become activated.

phantom pregnancy *see* pseudocyesis.

phantom tumor a swelling, in the abdomen or elsewhere, caused by local muscular contraction or the accumulation of gases, that mimics a swelling caused by a tumor or other structural change. The condition is usually associated with emotional disorder, and the "tumor" may disappear under anesthesia.

pharmaceutical *adj.* relating to pharmacy or drugs.

pharmacist *n.* a person who is qualified by examination and registered and authorized to dispense medicines.

pharmaco- *prefix denoting* drugs. Example: *pharmacophobia* (morbid fear of).

pharmacodynamics *n.* the interaction of drugs with cells. It includes such factors as the binding of drugs to cells, their uptake, and intracellular metabolism.

pharmacognosy *n.* the knowledge or study of pharmacologically active principles derived from plants.

pharmacokinetics *n.* the study of how drugs are handled within the body, including their absorption, distribution, metabolism, and excretion. It is concerned with such matters as how drug concentration in the body changes with time, how drugs pass across cell membranes, how often they should be given, what the effect of long-term administration may be, how drugs interact with each other, and how individual variations affect all these things.

pharmacology *n.* the science of the properties of drugs and their effects on the body. —**pharmacological** *adj.*

pharmacomania *n.* an abnormal desire to take medicines.

pharmacopeia *n.* a book containing a list of the drugs used in medicine, with details of their formulas, methods of preparation, dosages, standards of purity, etc.

pharmacy *n.* **1.** the preparation and dispensing of drugs. **2.** premises registered to dispense medicines and sell poisons.

pharyng- (pharyngo-) *prefix denoting* the pharynx. Example: *pharyngopathy* (disease of).

pharyngeal arch (branchial or **visceral arch)** any of the paired segmented ridges of tissue in each side of the throat of the early embryo that correspond to the gill arches of fish. Each arch contains a cartilage, a cranial nerve, and a blood vessel. Between each arch there is a *pharyngeal pouch.

pharyngeal cleft (branchial or **visceral cleft)** any of the paired segmented clefts in each side of the throat of the early embryo that correspond to the gills of fish. Soon after they have formed they close to form the *pharyngeal pouches, except for the first cleft, which persists as the external auditory meatus.

pharyngeal pouch (branchial or **visceral pouch)** any of the paired segmented pouches in the side of the throat of the early embryo. They give rise to the tympanic cavity, the parathyroid glands, the thymus, and probably the thyroid gland.

pharyngeal reflex *see* gag reflex.

pharyngectomy *n.* surgical removal of part of the pharynx.

pharyngismus *n.* spasmodic contraction of the muscles of the pharynx.

pharyngitis *n.* inflammation of the part of the throat behind the soft palate (pharynx). It produces *sore throat and is usually associated with *tonsillitis.

pharyngocele *n.* a pouch or cyst opening off the pharynx (*see* branchial cyst).

pharyngoscope *n.* an *endoscope for the examination of the pharynx.

pharynx *n.* a muscular tube, lined with mucous membrane, that extends from the beginning of the esophagus (gullet) up to the base of the skull. It is divided into the *nasopharynx, *oropharynx, and the *laryngopharynx (see illustration) and

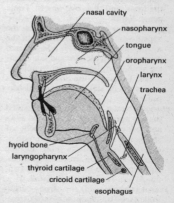

Longitudinal section of the pharynx

it communicates with the posterior *nares, *eustachian tube, the mouth, larynx, and esophagus. The pharynx acts as a passageway for food from the mouth to the esophagus, and as an air passage from the nasal cavity and mouth to the larynx. It also acts as a resonating chamber for the sounds produced in the larynx. —**pharyngeal** adj.

phenacemide n. an *anticonvulsant drug used in the treatment of severe epilepsy. It is administered by mouth; side effects include digestive upsets, fever, and rash. Mental changes and damage to liver, kidneys, and bone marrow may also occur. Trade name: **Phenurone**.

phenazopyridine n. an *analgesic drug used to relieve pain in inflammatory conditions of the bladder and urinary tract, such as cystitis and urethritis. It is administered by mouth and occasionally causes digestive upsets; in patients with kidney disease it may damage the red blood cells. Trade names: **Azo-Standard, Pyridium, Urogesic**.

phendimetrazine tartate a drug used as an appetite suppressant in the treatment of exogenous obesity. The drug is administered orally; side effects include central nervous system stimulation, elevated blood pressure, insomnia, and dry mouth. Trade name: **Prelu-2**.

phenelzine n. a drug used to relieve depression and anxiety (see MAO inhibitor). It is administered by mouth; side effects include dizziness, drowsiness, tiredness, and digestive upsets. Trade name: **Nardil**.

phenmetrazine n. a drug that reduces the appetite and was formerly used in the treatment of obesity. It is administered by mouth and its actions and side effects are similar to those of the *amphetamines. Prolonged use and large doses may cause mental depression and *dependence.

phenobarbital n. a *barbiturate drug used to treat insomnia and anxiety and as an anticonvulsant in the treatment of epilepsy. It is administered by mouth or injection; side effects may include drowsiness and skin sensitivity reactions, and dependence may result from continued use. Trade name: **Solfoton**.

phenol (carbolic acid) n. a strong *disinfectant used for cleansing wounds, treating inflammations of the mouth, throat, and ear, and as a preservative in injections. It is administered as solution, ointments, and lotions and is highly toxic if taken by mouth.

phenolphthalein n. a stimulant *laxative administered by mouth, usually given at night to act the following morning. Side effects may include stomach cramps. Trade names: **Evac-Q, Ex-Lax, Phenolax, Prulet**.

phenolsulfonphthalein n. a red dye administered by injection in a test for kidney function.

phenothiazines pl. n. a group of chemically related compounds with various pharmacological actions. Some (e.g. *chlorpromazine and *trifluoperazine) are *antipsychotic drugs; others (e.g. *piperazine) are anthelmintics.

phenotype n. **1.** the observable characteristics of an individual, which result from interaction between the genes he possesses (*genotype) and the environment. **2.** the expression in a person or on a cell of characteristics determined by genes that are not fully defined.

phenoxybenzamine n. a drug that dilates blood vessels (see alpha blocker). It is used to reduce high blood pressure in patients with *pheochromocytoma and to treat conditions involving poor circulation, such as Raynaud's disease and chilblains. It is administered by mouth and may cause dizziness and fast heartbeat. Trade name: **Dibenzyline**.

phensuximide n. an *anticonvulsant drug used to prevent or reduce absence seizures in epilepsy. It is administered by mouth; side effects may include dizziness, drowsiness, nausea, and loss of appetite. Trade name: **Milontin**.

phentermine n. a *sympathomimetic drug that suppresses the appetite and is used in the treatment of obesity. It is administered by mouth; side effects include dry mouth, nausea, and restlessness, and continued use produces *tolerance. Trade names: **Adipex-P, Fastin, Ionamin**.

phentolamine n. a drug that dilates blood vessels (see alpha blocker) and is used to reduce high blood pressure in patients with *pheochromocytoma and to treat conditions of poor circulation such as Raynaud's disease and chilblains. It is administered by mouth or injection; side effects include fast heartbeat and digestive upsets. Trade name: **Regitine**.

phenylalanine *n.* an *essential amino acid that is readily converted to tyrosine. Blockade of this metabolic pathway causes *phenylketonuria, which is associated with abnormally large amounts of phenylalanine and phenylpyruvic acid in the blood and retarded mental development.

phenylephrine *n.* a drug that constricts blood vessels (*see* sympathomimetic). It is given by injection to increase blood pressure, in a nasal spray to relieve nasal congestion, and in eye drops to dilate the pupils. Irritation may occur when applied. Trade names: **Alconefrin, Mydfrin, Neo-Synephrine.**

phenylketonuria (PKU) *n.* an inherited defect of protein metabolism (*see* inborn error of metabolism) causing an excess of the amino acid phenylalanine in the blood, which damages the nervous system and leads to severe mental retardation. Screening of newborn infants by testing a blood sample for phenylalanine (the *Guthrie test) enables the condition to be detected soon enough for dietary treatment to prevent any brain damage: the baby's diet contains proteins from which phenylalanine has been removed. The gene responsible for phenylketonuria is recessive, so that a child is affected only if both parents are carriers of the defective gene.

phenylpropanolamine *n.* a *sympathomimetic drug with actions similar to those of *ephedrine.

phenylthiourea (phenylthiocarbamide) *n.* a substance that tastes bitter to some individuals but is tasteless to others. Response to phenylthiourea appears to be controlled by a single pair of genes (*alleles): ability to taste it is *dominant to the inability to taste it.

phenytoin *n.* an *anticonvulsant drug used to control major and focal epileptic seizures. It is administered by mouth or injection; the side effects include gum hypertrophy, hirsutism, and skin rashes. Overdosage causes unsteadiness. Trade name: **Dilantin.**

pheochromocytoma *n.* a small vascular tumor of the inner region (medulla) of the adrenal gland. By its uncontrolled and irregular secretion of the hormones *epinephrine and *norepinephrine, the tumor causes raised blood pressure, increased heart rate, palpitations, and headache. *See also* dexamethasone.

phial *n.* a small glass bottle for storing medicines or poisons.

Philadelphia chromosome an abnormality of chromosome 22 in which portions of its long arm are missing, usually translocated to chromosome 9. The condition is seen in the marrow cells of patients with chronic *myeloid leukemia.

-philia *suffix denoting* morbid craving or attraction. Example: *nyctophilia* (for darkness).

phimosis *n.* narrowing of the opening of the foreskin, which cannot therefore be drawn back over the underlying glans penis. This predisposes to inflammation (*see* balanitis, balanoposthitis), which results in further narrowing. Treatment is by surgical removal of the foreskin (*circumcision).

phleb- (phlebo-) *prefix denoting* a vein or veins. Example: *phlebectopia* (abnormal position of).

phlebectomy *n.* the surgical removal of a vein (or part of a vein), sometimes performed for the treatment of varicose veins in the legs (*variectomy*).

phlebitis *n.* inflammation of the wall of a vein, which is most commonly seen in the legs as a complication of *varicose veins. A segment of vein becomes painful and tender and the surrounding skin feels hot and appears red. Thrombosis commonly develops (*see* thrombophlebitis). Treatment consists of elastic support together with drugs, such as phenylbutazone, to relieve the inflammation and pain. Anticoagulants are not used (*compare* phlebothrombosis). Phlebitis may also complicate sepsis (*see* pylephlebitis) or cancer, especially of the stomach, bronchus, or pancreas. In pancreatic cancer the phlebitis may affect a variety of veins (*thrombophlebitis migrans*).

phlebography *n. see* venography.

phlebolith *n.* a stonelike structure, usually found incidentally on abdominal X-ray, that results from deposition of calcium in a venous blood clot. It appears as a small round white opacity in the pelvic region. It does not produce symptoms and requires no treatment.

phlebosclerosis (venosclerosis) *n.* a rare degenerative condition, of unknown cause, that affects the leg veins of young men. The vein walls become thickened and feel like cords under the skin. It is not related to arteriosclerosis and needs no treatment.

phlebothrombosis *n.* obstruction of a vein by a blood clot, without preceding inflammation of its wall. It is most common within the deep veins of the calf of the leg – *deep vein thrombosis (DVT)* – (in contrast to *thrombophlebitis, which affects superficial leg veins). Prolonged immobility, heart failure, pregnancy, injury, and surgery predispose to thrombosis by encouraging sluggish blood flow. Many of these conditions are associated with changes in the clotting factors in the blood that increase the tendency to thrombosis; these changes also occur in some women taking oral contraceptives.

The affected leg may become swollen and tender. The main danger is that the clot may become detached and give rise to *pulmonary embolism. Regular leg exercises help to prevent deep vein thrombosis, and anticoagulant drugs (such as warfarin and heparin) are used in prevention and treatment. Large clots may be removed surgically in the operation of *thrombectomy* to relieve leg swelling.

Phlebotomus *n.* see sandfly.

phlebotomy (venesection) *n.* the surgical opening or puncture of a vein in order to remove blood (in the treatment of *polycythemia) or to infuse fluids, blood, or drugs in the treatment of many conditions. It may also be required for cardiac *catheterization and *angiocardiography.

phlegm *n.* mucus or sputum.

phlegmasia alba dolens see thrombophlebitis.

phlegmon *n.* inflammation of connective tissue, leading to ulceration.

phlyctena *n.* (*pl.* **phlyctenae**) a small pinkish-yellow nodule surrounded by a zone of dilated blood vessels that occurs in the conjunctiva or in the cornea. It develops into a small ulcer that heals without trace in the conjunctiva but produces some residual scarring in the cornea. Phlyctenae, which are prone to recur, are thought to be caused by a type of allergy to certain bacteria.

phobia *n.* a pathologically strong *fear of a particular event or thing. Avoiding the feared situation may severely restrict one's life and cause much suffering. The main kinds of phobia are *specific phobias* (isolated fears of particular things, such as sharp knives), *agoraphobia, *claustrophobia, *social phobias* of encountering people, and *animal phobias*, as of spiders, rats, or dogs (*see also* preparedness). Treatment is with behavior therapy, especially *desensitization, *graded self-exposure, and *flooding. *Psychotherapy and drug therapy are also useful.

-phobia *suffix denoting* morbid fear or dread.

phocomelia *n.* congenital absence of the upper arm and/or upper leg, the hands or feet or both being attached to the trunk by a short stump. The condition is extremely rare except as a side effect of the drug *thalidomide taken during early pregnancy.

phon *n.* a unit of loudness of sound. The intensity of a sound to be measured is compared by the human ear to a reference tone of 2×10^{-5} pascal sound pressure and 1000 hertz frequency. The intensity of the reference tone is increased until it appears to be equal in loudness to the sound being measured; the loudness of this sound in phons is then equal to the number of decibels by which the reference tone has had to be increased.

phon- (phono-) *prefix denoting* sound or voice.

phonasthenia *n.* weakness of the voice, especially when due to fatigue.

phonation *n.* the production of vocal sounds, particularly speech.

phoniatrics *n.* the study of the voice and its disorders.

phonocardiogram *n.* see electrocardiophonography. —**phonocardiography** *n.*

phonophobia *n.* excessive sensitivity to certain specific sounds. *see* hyperacusis, misophonia.

phonosurgery *n.* surgery performed on the larynx externally or endoscopically to improve or modify the quality of the voice.

-phoria *suffix denoting* (in ophthalmology) an abnormal deviation of the eyes or turning of the visual axis. Example: *heterophoria* (tendency to squint).

Phormia *n.* a genus of nonbloodsucking flies, commonly known as blowflies. The maggot of *P. regina* normally breeds in decaying meat but it has occasionally been found in suppurating wounds, giving rise to a type of *myiasis.

phosgene n. a poisonous gas developed during World War I. It is a choking agent, acting on the lungs to produce *edema, with consequent respiratory and cardiac failure.

phosphagen n. creatine phosphate (see creatine).

phosphatase n. one of a group of enzymes capable of catalyzing the hydrolysis of phosphoric acid esters. An example is glucose-6-phosphatase, which catalyzes the hydrolysis of glucose-6-phosphate to glucose and phosphate. Phosphatases are important in the absorption and metabolism of carbohydrates, nucleotides, and phospholipids and are essential in the calcification of bone. *Acid phosphatase* is present in kidney, semen, serum, and the prostate gland. *Alkaline phosphatase* occurs in teeth, developing bone, plasma, kidney, and intestine.

phosphatemia n. the presence of phosphates in the blood. Sodium, calcium, potassium, and magnesium phosphates are normal constituents.

phosphatidylcholine n. see lecithin.

phosphatidylserine n. a cephalin-like phospholipid containing the amino acid serine. It is found in brain tissue. *See also* cephalin.

phosphaturia (phosphuria) n. the presence of an abnormally high concentration of phosphates in the urine, making it cloudy. The condition may be associated with the formation of stones (calculi) in the kidneys or bladder.

phosphocreatine n. creatine phosphate (see creatine).

phosphofructokinase n. an enzyme that catalyzes the conversion of fructose-6-phosphate to fructose-1,6-diphosphate. This is an important reaction occurring during the process of *glycolysis.

phospholipid n. a *lipid containing a phosphate group as part of the molecule. Phospholipids are constituents of all tissues and organs, especially the brain. They are synthesized in the liver and small intestine and are involved in many of the body's metabolic processes. Examples are *cephalins, *lecithins, plasmalogens, and phosphatidylserine.

phosphonecrosis n. the destruction of tissues caused by excessive amounts of phosphorus in the system. The tissues likely to suffer in phosphorus poisoning are the liver, kidneys, muscles, bones, and the cardiovascular system.

phosphorus n. a nonmetallic element. Phosphorus compounds are major constituents in the tissues of both plants and animals. In humans, phosphorus is mostly concentrated in *bone. However, certain phosphorus-containing compounds – for example adenosine triphosphate (*ATP) and *creatine phosphate – play an important part in energy conversions and storage in the body. In a pure state, phosphorus is toxic. Symbol: P.

phosphorylase n. any enzyme that catalyzes the combination of an organic molecule (usually glucose) with a phosphate group (phosphorylation). Phosphorylase is found in the liver and kidney, where it is involved in the breakdown of glycogen to glucose-1-phosphate.

phosphuria n. see phosphaturia.

phot- (photo-) prefix denoting light.

photalgia n. pain in the eye caused by very bright light.

photoablation n. the use of light or lasers to destroy tissue.

photochemotherapy n. see photodynamic therapy, PUVA.

photocoagulation n. the destruction of tissue by heat released from the absorption of light shone on it. In eye disorders the technique is used to destroy diseased retinal tissue, occurring, for example, as a complication of diabetes (diabetic *retinopathy) and *macular degeneration; and to produce scarring between the retina and choroid, thus binding them together, in cases of *detached retina. Photocoagulation of the retina is usually done with an *argon or *diode laser.

Photocoagulation is also a method of arresting bleeding by causing coagulation, usually using an infrared light source.

photodermatitis n. a condition in which the skin becomes sensitized to a substance (certain antiseptics used in soaps may be a trigger) but only those parts of the skin subsequently exposed to light react by developing *dermatitis.

photodermatosis n. any of various skin diseases caused by exposure to light of varying wavelength (see photosensitivity). The facial prominences and the "V" of the neck are most commonly affected. The photodermatoses include certain *porphyrias, notably porphyria cutanea tarda, and polymorphic light eruption.

photodynamic therapy (PDT, photoradiation therapy, phototherapy, photochemotherapy) a treatment for some types of superficial cancers. A photosensitizing agent is injected into the bloodstream and remains in cancer cells for a longer time than in normal cells. Exposure to laser radiation produces an active form of oxygen that destroys the treated cancer cells. The laser radiation can be directed through a fiberoptic bronchoscope into the airways, through a gastroscope into the esophagus, or through a cystoscope into the bladder. PDT causes minimal damage to healthy tissue, but since it cannot pass through more than about 3 cm of tissue, it is restricted to treating tumors on or just under the skin or on the lining of internal organs. Photodynamic therapy makes the skin and eyes sensitive to light for six weeks or more after treatment.

photomicrograph *n.* an enlarged photographic record of an object taken through an optical or electron microscope. *Compare* microphotograph.

photomultiplier tube an electronic device that magnifies the light emitted from a *scintillator by accelerating electrons in a high-voltage field. The resulting signal can be used to display the scintillations on a TV screen. Such devices are commonly used in *gamma cameras.

photophobia *n.* an abnormal intolerance of light, in which exposure to light produces intense discomfort of the eyes with tight contraction of the eyelids and other reactions aimed at avoiding the light. In most cases the light simply aggravates already existing discomfort from eye disease. Photophobia may be associated with dilation of the pupils as a result of drug administration or with migraine, measles, German measles, or meningitis.

photophthalmia *n.* inflammation of the eye due to exposure to light. It is usually caused by the damaging effect of ultraviolet light on the cornea, for example in snow blindness.

photopic *adj.* relating to or describing conditions of bright illumination. For example, *photopic vision* is vision in bright light, in which the *cones of the retina are responsible for visual perception. —**photopia** *n.*

photopsia *n.* the sensation of flashes of light caused by irritation of the retina of the eye, usually due to inflammation or slight movements of the retina.

photoradiation *n.* see photodynamic therapy.

photorefractive keratectomy *see* keratectomy.

photoretinitis *n.* damage to the retina of the eye caused by looking at the sun without adequate protection for the eyes. The retina may be burned by the intense light focused on it; this affects the central part of the visual field, which may be permanently lost (*sun blindness*).

photosensitivity *n.* abnormal and severe reaction of the skin to sunlight. This characterizes certain skin diseases (*see* photodermatosis). Photosensitivity reactions may also occur in those taking such drugs as tetracyclines, phenothiazines, furosemide, amiodarone, and NSAIDs. In these cases the effect may resemble severe sunburn. —**photosensitive** *adj.*

photosynthesis *n.* the process whereby green plants and some bacteria manufacture carbohydrates from carbon dioxide and water, using energy absorbed from sunlight by the green pigment chlorophyll. In green plants this complex process may be summarized thus:

$$6CO_2 + 6H_2O \rightarrow C_6H_{12}O_6 + 6O_2$$

phototaxis *n.* movement of a cell or organism in response to a stimulus of light.

phototherapeutic keratectomy *see* keratectomy.

phototherapy *n.* **1.** the treatment of disorders, such as acne, herpes simplex, pressure sores, psoriasis, and neonatal hyperbilirubinemia, by exposure to light, especially ultraviolet light. The process may be used in combination with light-sensitive drugs (*see* PUVA). **2.** *see* photodynamic therapy.

phototoxicity *n.* damage caused by prolonged exposure to light; for example, *retinal phototoxicity* is damage to the retina of the eye as a result of prolonged exposure to light.

photuria *n.* the excretion of phosphorescent urine, which glows in the dark, due to the presence of certain phosphorus-containing compounds derived from phosphates.

phren- (phreno-) *prefix denoting* 1. the mind or brain. 2. the diaphragm. 3. the phrenic nerve.

-phrenia *suffix denoting* a condition of the mind. Example: *hebephrenia* (schizophrenia affecting young adults).

phrenic avulsion formerly, the surgical removal of a section of the *phrenic nerve, which paralyzes the diaphragm. The procedure was used as a means of resting a lung infected with tuberculosis but is now obsolete.

phrenic nerve the nerve that supplies the muscles of the diaphragm. On each side it arises in the neck from the third, fourth, and fifth cervical spinal roots and passes downward between the lungs and the heart to reach the diaphragm. Impulses through the nerves from the brain bring about the regular contractions of the diaphragm during breathing.

phrenology *n.* the study of the bumps on the outside of the skull in order to determine a person's character. It is based on the mistaken theory that the skull becomes modified over the different functional areas of the cortex of the brain.

phrygian cap a normal radiological appearance of the tip of the gallbladder, seen in a minority of cholecystograms (*see* cholecystography). Its name is derived from its resemblance to the characteristic Balkan headgear.

Phthirus *n.* a widely distributed genus of lice. The crab (or pubic) louse *P. pubis* is a common parasite of humans that lives permanently attached to the body hair, particularly that of the pubic or perianal regions but also on the eyelashes and the hairs in the armpits. Crab lice are not known to transmit disease but their bites can irritate the skin (*see* pediculosis). An infestation may be acquired during sexual intercourse or from hairs left on clothing, towels, and lavatory seats.

phthisis *n.* 1. any disease resulting in wasting of tissues. *Phthisis bulbi* is a shrunken eyeball that has lost its function due to disease or damage. 2. a former name for pulmonary *tuberculosis.

phycomycosis (mucormycosis, zygomycosis) *n.* a disease caused by parasitic fungi of the genera *Rhizopus*, *Absidia*, and *Mucor*. The disease affects the sinuses,

the central nervous system, the lungs, and the skin tissues. The fungi are able to grow within the blood vessels of the lungs and nervous tissue, thus causing blood clots that cut off the blood supply (*see* infarction). Treatment with the antibiotic *amphotericin B has proved to be effective.

phylogenesis *n.* the evolutionary history of a species or individual.

physi- (physio-) *prefix denoting* 1. physiology. 2. physical.

physical *adj.* (in medicine) relating to the body rather than to the mind. For example, a *physical sign* is one that a doctor can detect when examining a patient, such as abnormal dilation of the pupils or the absence of a knee-jerk reflex (*see also* functional disorder, organic disorder).

physical medicine a medical specialty originally devoted to the diagnosis and management of rheumatic diseases, but later extended to the *rehabilitation of patients with physical disabilities ranging from asthma and hand injuries to paraplegia and poliomyelitis.

physician *n.* a registered medical practitioner who specializes in the diagnosis and treatment of disease by other than surgical means. In the US the term is applied to any authorized medical practitioner. *See also* Doctor.

physiological solution one of a group of solutions used to maintain tissues in a viable state. These solutions contain specific concentrations of substances that are vital for normal tissue function (e.g. sodium, potassium, calcium, chloride, magnesium, bicarbonate, and phosphate ions, glucose, and oxygen). An example of such a solution is *Ringer's solution.

physiology *n.* the science of the functioning of living organisms and of their component parts. —**physiological** *adj.* —**physiologist** *n.*

physiotherapy *n.* the branch of treatment that uses physical methods to promote healing, including the use of light, infrared and ultraviolet rays, heat, electric current, ultrasound, massage, manipulation, hydrotherapy, and remedial exercise.

physis *n.* the part of a bone that is involved with growth or lengthening.

physo- *prefix denoting* air or gas.

physostigmine n. a *anticholinergic drug used mainly to constrict the pupil of the eye and to reduce pressure inside the eye in *glaucoma. It is administered by injection, in eye drops, or in an ointment; side effects include digestive upsets and salivation. Trade names: **Eserine Salicylate**, **Eserine Sulfate**, **Isopto Eserine**.

phyt- (phyto-) prefix denoting plants; of plant origin.

phytohemagglutinin (PHA) n. a plant-derived alkaloid that stimulates T lymphocytes to divide in the test tube.

phytonadione n. a form of *vitamin K occurring naturally in green plants but usually synthesized for use as an antidote to overdosage with anticoagulant drugs. It promotes the production of prothrombin, essential for the normal coagulation of blood. Trade names: **Aquamephyton**, **Konakion**, **Mephyton**.

phytophotodermatitis n. an eruption of large blisters occurring after exposure to light in people who have been in contact with certain plants, such as wild parsnip or cow parsley, to which they are sensitive. A particularly dramatic reaction occurs with giant hogweed (Heracleum mantegazzianum).

phytotherapy n. medical treatment based exclusively on plant extracts and products. Plants have provided a wide range of important drugs and current research into drugs from plants continues to be fruitful. Recent examples are the *taxanes. However, it is essential that any drugs derived directly from plants should be extracted, purified, assayed, and tested before being used as medication. The use of crude plant extracts as medicines can be dangerous because seemingly identical samples of the same plant may contain widely differing amounts of the active ingredient.

phytotoxin n. any poisonous substance (toxin) produced by a plant, such as any of the toxins produced by fungi of the genus *Amanita.

pia (pia mater) n. the innermost of the three *meninges surrounding the brain and spinal cord. The membrane is closely attached to the surface of the brain and spinal cord, faithfully following each fissure and sulcus. It contains numerous finely branching blood vessels that supply the nerve tissue within.

The subarachnoid space separates it from the arachnoid.

pian n. see yaws.

pica n. the indiscriminate eating of non-nutritious or harmful substances, such as clay, grass, stones, or clothing. It is common in early childhood but may also be found in mentally handicapped and psychotic patients. Although previously thought to be completely nonadaptive, some evidence suggests that some patients showing pica may have particular mineral deficiencies (such as iron deficiency).

Pick's disease a cause of *dementia, usually in middle-aged people. The damage is mainly in the frontal and temporal lobes of the brain, in contrast with the diffuse degeneration of *Alzheimer's disease. [A. Pick (1851–1924), Czech psychiatrist]

pico- prefix denoting one trillionth (10^{-12}).

picornavirus n. one of a group of small RNA-containing viruses (pico = small; hence pico-RNA-virus). The group includes *coxsackieviruses, *echoviruses, *polioviruses, and *rhinoviruses.

picric acid (trinitrophenol) a yellow crystalline solid used as a dye and as a tissue *fixative.

picture archiving and communication system see PACS.

PID 1. see pelvic inflammatory disease. **2.** see prolapsed intervertebral disk.

piebaldness n. a condition in which patches of the skin and hair lack pigmentation and appear white due to the absence of *melanocytes in those areas.

piedra n. a fungal disease of the hair in which the hair shafts carry hard masses of black or white fungus. The black fungus, Piedraia hortae, is found mainly in the tropics and the white varieties, Trichosporon species, in temperate regions.

Pierre Robin syndrome a congenital disease in which affected infants have a very small lower jawbone (mandible) and a cleft palate. They are susceptible to feeding and respiratory problems. [Pierre Robin (1867–1950), French dentist]

piezoelectric adj. denoting or relating to an electrically generated pulse or polarity that is caused by pressure.

pigeon chest forward protrusion of the breastbone resulting in deformity of the chest. The condition is painless and harmless. Medical name: **pectus carina-tum**.

pigeon toes an abnormal posture in which the toes are turned inward. It is often associated with *knock knee.

pigment *n.* a substance giving color to a tissue. Physiologically important pigments include the blood pigments (especially *hemoglobin), *bile pigments, and retinal pigment (*see* rhodopsin). The pigment *melanin occurs in the skin and in the iris of the eye. Important plant pigments include *chlorophyll and the *carotenoids.

pigmentation *n.* coloration produced in the body by the deposition of one pigment, especially in excessive amounts. Pigmentation may be produced by natural pigments, such as bile pigments (as in jaundice) or melanin, or by foreign material, such as lead or arsenic in chronic poisoning.

pigment epitheliopathy acute posterior multifocal placoid pigment epitheliopathy (APMPPE): an inflammatory disease of the retinal pigment epithelium (RPE; *see* retina), characterized by the presence of multiple cream-colored irregular lesions scattered in the posterior segment of the eye. The disease occurs in young adults and usually affects both eyes. Visual acuity usually recovers with time.

piles *n.* *see* hemorrhoids.

pili (fimbriae) *pl. n.* (*sing.* **pilus, fimbria**) hairlike processes present on the surface of certain bacteria. They are thought to be involved in adhesion of bacteria to other cells and in transfer of DNA during *conjugation.

pill *n.* **1.** a small tablet of variable size, shape, and color, sometimes coated with sugar, that contains one or more medicinal substances in solid form. It is taken by mouth. **2. the Pill** *see* oral contraceptive.

pillar *n.* (in anatomy) an elongated apparently supportive structure. For example, the *pillars of the fauces* are folds of mucous membrane on either side of the opening from the mouth to the pharynx.

pilo- *prefix denoting* hair. Example: *pilosis* (excessive development of).

pilocarpine *n.* a *parasympathomimetic drug used to constrict the pupil of the eye (*see* miotic) and to reduce the pressure inside the eye in glaucoma. It is ad-

ministered as eye drops and may cause digestive upsets and salivation if absorbed into the system. It is also administered orally to treat dryness of the mouth and throat caused by decreased salivation after radiation treatment for cancer of the head or neck or in patients with *Sjögren's syndrome. Trade names: **Absorbocarpine, Isopto Carpine, Pilagan, Piloptic, Salagen** (oral).

pilomotor nerves sympathetic nerves that supply muscle fibers in the skin, around the roots of hairs. Activity of the sympathetic nervous system causes the muscles to contract, raising the hairs and giving the "gooseflesh" effect of fear or cold.

pilonidal sinus a short tract leading from an opening in the skin in or near the cleft at the top of the buttocks and containing hairs. The sinus may be recurrently infected, leading to pain and the discharge of pus. Treatment is by surgical opening and cleaning of the sinus.

pilosebaceous *adj.* relating to the hair follicles and their associated sebaceous glands.

pilus *n.* a hair. *See also* pili.

pimel- (pimelo-) *prefix denoting* fat; fatty.

pimozide *n.* an *antipsychotic drug used to relieve hallucinations and delusions occurring in schizophrenia and to relieve tics caused by *Gilles de la Tourette syndrome. It is administered by mouth; side effects may include skin rashes, tremors, and abnormal movements. Trade name: **Orap.**

pimple *n.* a small inflamed swelling on the skin that contains pus. It may be the result of bacterial infection of a skin pore that has become obstructed with fatty secretions from the sebaceous glands. Pimples occurring in large numbers on the chest, back, and face are usually described as *acne, a common condition of adolescence.

PIN *see* prostatic intraepithelial neoplasia.

pincement *n.* one of the techniques used in massage, in which pinches of the patient's flesh are taken between finger and thumb and twisted or rolled before release. This is said to improve the tone of the skin, improve circulation, and alleviate underlying pain.

pindolol a *beta blocker used in the treatment of *hypertension, *angina pectoris, and other cardiac disorders. It is administered orally; common side effects include lightheadedness, heartburn, insomnia, gastrointestinal disturbances, and muscle or joint pain. Trade name: **Visken.**

pineal body (pineal gland) a pea-sized mass of tissue attached by a stalk to the posterior wall of the third ventricle of the brain, deep between the cerebral hemispheres at the back of the skull. It functions as a gland, secreting the hormone *melatonin. The gland becomes calcified as age progresses, providing a useful landmark in X-rays of the skull. Anatomical name: **epiphysis cerebri.**

pinguecula n. a degenerative change in the conjunctiva of the eye, seen most commonly in the elderly and in those who live in hot dry climates. Thickened yellow triangles develop on the conjunctiva at the inner and outer margins of the cornea.

pink disease a severe illness of children of teething age, marked by pink cold clammy hands and feet, heavy sweating, raised blood pressure, a rapid pulse, photophobia, loss of appetite, and insomnia. It has been suggested that the condition is an allergic reaction to mercury, since it used to occur when teething powders, lotions, and ointments containing mercury were used. Although there is no definite proof of this, the disease has virtually disappeared since all mercury-containing pediatric preparations have been banned. Medical names: **acrodynia, erythredema.**

pink eye *see* conjunctivitis.

pinna (auricle) n. the flap of skin and cartilage that projects from the head at the exterior opening of the external auditory meatus (see illustration). In humans the pinna is largely vestigial but it may be partly concerned with detecting the direction of sound sources.

pinocytosis n. the intake of small droplets of fluid by a cell by cytoplasmic engulfment. It occurs in many white blood cells and in certain kidney and liver cells. *Compare* phagocytosis.

pins and needles *see* paresthesia.

pinta n. a skin disease, prevalent in tropical America, that seems to affect only the dark-skinned races. It is caused by the *spirochete *Treponema carateum*, a microorganism similar to those causing *yaws and *syphilis. The disease is thought to be transmitted either by direct contact between individuals or by flies that carry the infective spirochetes on their bodies. Symptoms include thickening and eventual loss of pigment of the skin, particularly on the hands, wrists, feet, and ankles. Pinta is rarely disabling or fatal and is treated successfully with *penicillin.

pinworm (threadworm) n. a parasitic nematode worm of the genus *Enterobius* (*Oxyuris*), which lives in the upper part of the large intestine of humans. The threadlike female worm, some 12 mm long, is larger than the male; it emerges from the anus in the evening to deposit its eggs, and later dies. If the eggs are swallowed by humans and reach the intestine, they develop directly into adult worms. Pinworms cause *enterobiasis, a disease common in children throughout the world.

pioglitazone n. *see* thiazolidinediones.

piperazine n. a drug used to treat infestations by roundworms and pinworms. It is administered by mouth; side effects do not usually occur, but continued treatment at high doses may cause nausea, vomiting, headache, tingling sensations, and rashes. Trade name: **Entacyl.**

piriform fossae two pear-shaped depressions that lie on either side of the opening to the larynx.

piroxicam n. a nonsteroidal anti-inflammatory drug (*see* NSAID) used to relieve pain and stiffness in osteoarthritis, rheumatoid arthritis, gout, and ankylosing spondylitis. It is administered by mouth; side effects include dizziness, skin rash, and gastrointestinal symptoms. Trade name: **Feldene.**

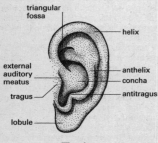

triangular fossa

helix

external auditory meatus

anthelix
concha
antitragus

tragus

lobule

The pinna

pisiform bone the smallest bone of the wrist (*carpus): a pea-shaped bone that articulates with the triquetral bone and, indirectly by cartilage, with the ulna.

pit *n.* (in anatomy) a hollow or depression, such as any of the depressions on the surface of an embryo marking the site of future organs.

pithiatism *n.* the treatment of certain disorders by persuading the patient that all is well. Symptoms that disappear in these circumstances are regarded as manifestations of psychological disturbance and are classified as conversion disorders.

pithing *n.* the laboratory procedure in which a part or the whole of the central nervous system of an experimental animal (such as a frog) is destroyed, usually by inserting a probe through the foramen magnum, in preparation for physiological or pharmacological experiments.

pitting *n.* the formation of depressed scars, as occurs on the skin following smallpox or acne. *Pitting edema* is swelling of the tissues due to excess fluid in which fingertip pressure leaves temporary indentations in the skin.

pituicyte *n.* a type of cell found in the posterior lobe of the pituitary gland, similar in appearance to an *astrocyte, with numerous fine branches that end in contact with the lining membrane of the blood channels in the gland.

pituitary apoplexy acute intrapituitary hemorrhage, usually into an existing tumor, presenting as severe headache and collapse. It is a medical emergency. Due to the sudden expansion in size of the gland with the hemorrhage, it is accompanied by lesions of the cranial nerves running close to the pituitary gland, causing paralysis of the muscles of the orbit and occasionally the face. Anterior pituitary insufficiency usually results, but posterior pituitary function survives. Surprisingly, pituitary function usually recovers.

pituitary gland (hypophysis) the master endocrine gland: a pea-sized body attached beneath the *hypothalamus in a bony cavity at the base of the skull. It has an anterior lobe (*adenohypophysis*), which secretes *thyroid-stimulating hormone, *ACTH (adrenocorticotropic hormone), *gonadotropins, *growth hormone, *prolactin, *lipotropin, and *melanocyte-stimulating hormone. The secretion of all these hormones is regulated by specific *releasing hormones*, which are produced in the hypothalamus (*see also* corticotropin-releasing hormone, gonadotropin-releasing hormone, thyrotropin-releasing hormone). The posterior lobe (*neurohypophysis*) secretes *vasopressin and *oxytocin, which are synthesized in the hypothalamus and transported to the pituitary, where they are stored before release.

pityriasis *n.* (originally) any of a group of skin diseases typified by the development of fine branlike scales. The term is now used only with a modifying adjective. *Pityriasis alba* is a common condition in children in which pale scaly patches occur on the face; it may be related to atopic *eczema. *Pityriasis rosea* is a common skin rash, believed to be viral in origin, that starts with a single patch (a *herald patch*) on the trunk and is followed by an eruption of oval pink scaly *macules. The spots are often aligned along the ribs. The rash clears completely in about eight weeks. *Pityriasis versicolor* is a common chronic infection of the skin caused by the fungus *Malassezia furfur*, which is a normal inhabitant of the scalp. In susceptible people it changes to a pathogenic form and produces a persistent depigmented scaly rash on the trunk. Treatment with *selenium sulfide shampoo or with oral itraconazole readily kills the organism but the skin may take months to regain its normal colour. *See also* dandruff (pityriasis capitis).

Pityrosporum *n.* a former name for *Malassezia*. *See* pityriasis.

pivot joint *see* trochoid joint.

pixel *n.* short for "picture element," the smallest individual component of an electronically produced image. Numerical values are ascribed to each pixel, which describe its position and relative intensity and/or color. A two-dimensional *matrix of pixels produces the final image.

PKU *see* phenylketonuria.

placebo *n.* a medicine that is ineffective but may help to relieve a condition because the patient has faith in its powers. New drugs are tested against placebos in clinical trials: the drug's effect is compared with the *placebo response*, which occurs even in the absence of any pharmacologically active substance in the placebo.

placenta *n.* an organ within the uterus by means of which the embryo is attached to the wall of the uterus. Its primary function is to provide the embryo with nourishment, eliminate its wastes, and exchange respiratory gases. This is accomplished by the close proximity of the maternal and fetal blood systems within the placenta. It also functions as a gland, secreting human *chorionic gonadotropin, *progesterone, and estrogens, which regulate the maintenance of pregnancy. *See also* afterbirth. —**placental** *adj.*

placenta previa a placenta situated wholly or partially in the lower and noncontractile part of the uterus. When this becomes elongated and stretched during the last few weeks of pregnancy, and the cervix becomes stretched either before or during labor, placental separation and hemorrhage will occur. The cause is unknown. In the more severe degrees of placenta previa, where the placenta is situated entirely before the presenting part of the fetus, delivery must be by cesarean section.

placentography *n.* *radiography of the pregnant uterus in order to determine the position of the *placenta, which has been superseded by the use of ultrasound (*see* ultrasonography).

placode *n.* any of the thickened areas of ectoderm in the embryo that will develop into nerve ganglia or the special sensory structures of the eye, ear, or nose.

plagiocephaly *n.* any distortion or lack of symmetry in the shape of the head, usually due to irregularity in the closure of the sutures between the bones of the skull.

plague *n.* **1.** any epidemic disease with a high death rate. **2.** an acute epidemic disease of rats and other wild rodents caused by the bacterium *Yersinia pestis*, which is transmitted to humans by rat fleas. *Bubonic plague*, the most common form of the disease, has an incubation period of 2–6 days. Headache, fever, weakness, aching limbs, and delirium develop and are followed by acute painful swellings of the lymph nodes (*see* bubo). In favorable cases the buboes burst after

about a week, releasing pus, and then heal. In other cases bleeding under the skin, producing black patches, can lead to ulcers, which may prove fatal (hence the former name *Black Death*). In the most serious cases bacteria enter the bloodstream (*septicemic plague*) or lungs (*pneumonic plague*); if untreated, these are nearly always fatal. Treatment with tetracycline, streptomycin, or chloramphenicol is effective; vaccination against the disease provides only partial protection.

plane *n.* a level or smooth surface, especially any of the hypothetical flat surfaces – orientated in various directions – used to divide the body; for example, the *coronal and *sagittal planes.

planoconcave *adj.* describing a structure, such as a lens, that is flat on one side and concave on the other.

planoconvex *adj.* describing a structure, such as a lens, that is flat on one side and convex on the other.

plantar *adj.* relating to the sole of the foot (*planta*). *See also* flexion.

plantar arch the arch in the sole of the foot formed by anastomosing branches of the plantar arteries.

plantar fasciitis (policeman's heel) inflammation of the point of attachment of the *fascia in the sole of the foot to the calcaneus (heel bone), causing pain and localized tenderness of the heel. Treatment is a pad under the heel, anti-inflammatory medication, or steroid injections.

plantar reflex a reflex obtained by drawing a bluntly pointed object along the outer border of the sole of the foot from the heel to the little toe. The normal *flexor response* is a bunching and downward movement of the toes. An upward movement of the big toe is called an *extensor response* (or *Babinski reflex*). In all persons over the age of 18 months this is a sensitive indication of damage to the *pyramidal system in the brain or spinal cord.

plantar wart a wart occurring in the skin on the sole of the foot, usually at the base of the toes. *See* wart.

plantigrade *adj.* walking on the entire sole of the foot: a habit of humans and some animals.

plaque *n.* **1.** a layer that forms on the surface of a tooth, principally at its neck, composed of bacteria in an organic matrix. Under certain conditions the plaque may cause *gingivitis, *periodontal disease, or *dental caries. The purpose of oral hygiene is to remove plaque. **2.** a raised patch on the skin, formed by *papules enlarging or coalescing to form an area 2 cm or more across. **3.** a deposit, consisting of a fatty core covered with a fibrous cap, that develops on the inner wall of an artery in atherosclerosis (*see* atheroma). **4.** any flat and often raised patch, for example on mucous membrane, resulting from local damage.

-plasia *suffix denoting* formation; development. Example: *hyperplasia* (excessive tissue formation).

plasm- (plasmo-) *prefix denoting* **1.** blood plasma. **2.** protoplasm or cytoplasm.

plasma (blood plasma) *n.* the straw-colored fluid in which the blood cells are suspended. It consists of a solution of various inorganic salts of sodium, potassium, calcium, etc., with a high concentration of protein (approximately 70 g/liter) and a variety of trace substances.

plasma cells antibody-producing cells found in blood-forming tissue and also in the epithelium of the lungs and gut. They develop in the bone marrow, lymph nodes, and spleen when antigens stimulate B *lymphocytes to produce the precursor cells that give rise to them. Malignant proliferation of plasma cells results in either a *plasmacytoma or multiple *myeloma.

plasmacytoma *n.* a malignant tumor of plasma cells, very closely allied to *myeloma. It usually occurs as a solitary tumor (*solitary myeloma*) of bone or more rarely of soft tissue (*extramedullary plasmacytoma*), but may be multiple (*multiple myeloma*). All of these tumors may produce the abnormal gamma globulins that are characteristic of myeloma, and they may progress to widespread myeloma. The soft tissue tumors often respond to radiotherapy and to such drugs as melphalan and cyclophosphamide; the bone tumors are less responsive. Tumors originating in soft tissue (usually the airways) may spread to bone, producing an appearance on X-ray identical to myeloma deposits; these secondary growths often resolve completely after treatment.

plasmalogen *n.* a phospholipid, found in brain and muscle, similar in structure to *lecithin and *cephalin.

plasmapheresis *n.* a method of removing a quantity of plasma from the blood. Blood is withdrawn from the patient and allowed to settle in a container. The plasma is drawn off the top of the blood, and the blood cells are then transfused back into the patient.

plasmin (fibrinolysin) *n.* an enzyme that digests the protein fibrin. Its function is the dissolution of blood clots (*see* fibrinolysis). Plasmin is not normally present in the blood but exists as an inactive precursor, *plasminogen*.

plasminogen *n.* a substance normally present in the blood plasma that may be activated to form *plasmin. *See* fibrinolysis, tissue-type plasminogen activator.

plasminogen activator an enzyme that converts the inactive substance *plasminogen to the active enzyme *plasmin, which digests blood clots (*see* fibrinolysis). There are two types of plasminogen activators, *tissue-type plasminogen activator (t-PA) and urokinase-like plasminogen activator (u-PA).

plasmoditrophoblast *n.* see syncytiotrophoblast.

Plasmodium *n.* a genus of protozoans (*see* Sporozoa) that live as parasites within the red blood cells and liver cells of humans. The parasite undergoes its asexual development (*see* schizogony) in humans and completes the sexual phase of its development (*see* sporogony) in the stomach and digestive glands of a blood-sucking *Anopheles mosquito. Four species cause *malaria in humans: *P. vivax, P. ovale, P. falciparum,* and *P. malariae.*

plasmolysis *n.* a process occurring in bacteria and plants in which the protoplasm shrinks away from the rigid cell wall when the cell is placed in a *hypertonic solution. This is due to withdrawal of water from the cell by *osmosis.

plaster *n.* adhesive tape used in shaped pieces or as a bandage to keep a dressing in place.

plaster model (in dentistry) an accurate cast of the teeth and jaws made from modified plaster of Paris. A pair of models are used to study the dentition, particularly before treatment. Models are also used to construct dentures, orthodontic appliances, or such restorations as crowns.

plaster of Paris a preparation of gypsum (calcium sulfate) that sets hard when water is added. It is used in various modified forms in dentistry to make *plaster models. It is also used in orthopedics for preparing plaster *casts.

Plastibell device a plastic device that facilitates *circumcision while protecting the glans penis. It is widely used.

plastic lymph a transparent yellowish liquid produced in a wound or other site of inflammation, in which connective tissue cells and blood vessels develop during healing.

plastic surgery a branch of surgery dealing with the reconstruction of deformed or damaged parts of the body. It also includes the replacement of parts of the body that have been lost. If performed simply to improve appearances plastic surgery is called *cosmetic surgery* (or *aesthetic plastic surgery*), but most plastic surgery involves the treatment and repair of disfigurement and disability caused by burns, major accidents, and cancer and the correction of congenital defects, such as cleft lip and cleft palate.

plastron n. the breastbone (*sternum) together with the costal cartilages attached to it.

-plasty *suffix denoting* plastic surgery. Example: *labioplasty* (of the lips).

platelet (thrombocyte) n. a disk-shaped structure, 1–2 μm in diameter, present in the blood. With *Romanovsky stains platelets appear as fragments of pale-blue cytoplasm with a few red granules. They have several functions, all relating to the arrest of bleeding (*see* blood coagulation). There are normally 150–400 $\times 10^9$ platelets per liter of blood. *See also* thrombopoiesis.

platelet-derived growth factor (PDGF) *see* growth factor.

platy- *prefix denoting* broad or flat.

platyhelminth n. *see* flatworm.

platysma n. a broad thin sheet of muscle that extends from below the collar bone to the angle of the jaw. It depresses the jaw.

pledget n. a small wad of dressing material, such as lint, used either to cover a wound or sore or as a plug. It is also used during operations, mounted on an instrument, to wipe away blood or other fluids.

-plegia *suffix denoting* paralysis. Example: *hemiplegia* (of one side of the body).

pleio- (pleo-) *prefix denoting* 1. multiple. 2. excessive.

pleiotropy n. a situation in which a single gene is responsible for more than one effect in the *phenotype. The mutation of such a gene will therefore have multiple effects. —**pleiotropic** *adj.*

pleocytosis n. the presence of an abnormally large number of lymphocytes in the cerebrospinal fluid, which bathes the brain and spinal cord.

pleomastia n. *see* polymastia.

pleomorphism n. the condition in which an individual assumes a number of different forms during its life cycle. The malarial parasite (*Plasmodium*) displays pleomorphism.

pleoptics n. special techniques practiced by orthoptists (*see* orthoptics) for developing normal function of the macula (the most sensitive part of the retina), in people whose macular function has previously been disturbed because of strabismus (squint).

plerocercoid n. a larval stage of certain tapeworms, such as *Diphyllobothrium latum*. It differs from the *cysticercus (another larval form) in being solid and in lacking a cyst or bladder.

plessimeter (pleximeter) n. a small plate of bone, ivory, or other material pressed against the surface of the body and struck with a *plessor in the technique of *percussion.

plessor (plexor) n. a small hammer used to investigate nervous reflexes and in the technique of *percussion.

plethora n. an excessive amount of any bodily fluid, especially blood (*see* hyperemia). —**plethoric** *adj.*

plethysmography n. the process of recording the changes in the volume of a limb caused by alterations in blood pressure. The limb is inserted into a fluid-filled watertight casing (*oncometer*) and the pressure variations in the fluid are recorded.

pleur- (pleuro-) *prefix denoting* 1. the pleura. 2. the side of the body.

pleura n. the covering of the lungs (*visceral pleura*) and of the inner surface of the chest wall (*parietal pleura*). (See illustration.) The covering consists of a closed sac of *serous membrane, which has a smooth shiny moist surface due to the secretion of small amounts of fluid. This fluid lubricates the opposing visceral and parietal surfaces so that they can slide painlessly over each other during breathing. —**pleural** *adj*.

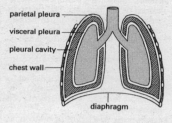

parietal pleura

visceral pleura

pleural cavity

chest wall

diaphragm

The pleura

pleural cavity the space between the visceral and parietal *pleura, which is normally very small because the pleural membranes are in close contact. The introduction of fluid (*pleural effusion*) or gas separates the pleural surfaces and increases the volume of the pleural space.

pleurectomy *n*. surgical removal of part of the *pleura, which is sometimes done to overcome recurrent *pneumothorax or to remove diseased areas of pleura.

pleurisy *n*. inflammation of the *pleura, usually due to pneumonia in the underlying lung. The normally shiny and slippery pleural surfaces lose their sheen and become slightly sticky, so that there is pain on deep breathing and a characteristic "rub" can be heard through a stethoscope. Pleurisy is always associated with some other disease in the lung, chest wall, diaphragm, or abdomen.

pleurocele *n*. herniation of the pleura. *See* hernia.

pleurocentesis (thoracentesis, thoracocentesis) *n*. insertion of a hollow needle into the *pleural cavity through the chest wall in order to withdraw fluid, blood, pus, or air.

pleurodesis *n*. the artificial production of pleurisy by chemical or mechanical means to obliterate the *pleural cavity, in order to prevent recurrent, usually malignant, pleural effusions.

pleurodynia *n*. severe paroxysmal pain arising from the muscles between the ribs. It is often thought to be of rheumatic origin.

pleurolysis (pneumolysis) *n*. surgical stripping of the parietal *pleura from the chest wall to allow the lung to collapse. The procedure was used in the days before effective antituberculous drugs to help tuberculosis to heal.

pleuropneumonia *n*. inflammation involving both the lung and pleura. *See* pleurisy, pneumonia.

pleuropneumonia-like organisms (PPLO) *n*. *see* mycoplasma.

pleurotomy *n*. surgical incision of the pleura. *See* pleurectomy.

pleurotyphoid *n*. *typhoid fever involving the lungs.

pleximeter *n*. *see* plessimeter.

plexor *n*. *see* plessor.

plexus *n*. a network of nerves or blood vessels. *See* brachial plexus.

PLF (serum) *p*lacental *f*ementin: a storage protein levels of which are used for monitoring placental function from conception until delivery.

plica *n*. a fold of tissue; for example, the *plica sublingualis*, the mucous fold in the floor of the mouth. —**plicate** *adj*.

plicamycin *n*. an *antibiotic that prevents the growth of cancer cells. It is used mainly to treat cancer of the testis and is administered by injection. Common side effects are digestive upsets and mouth ulcers and, more seriously, nosebleeds and vomiting of blood. Trade name: **Mithracin**.

plication *n*. a surgical technique in which the size of a hollow organ is reduced by taking tucks or folds in the walls.

ploidy *n*. the status of a cell nucleus in regard to the number of complete chromosome sets it contains, such as diploidy, haploidy, aneuploidy, or polyploidy. An increase in ploidy in the cells of a malignant tumor usually indicates greater aggressiveness and ability to invade.

plombage *n*. **1.** a technique used in surgery for the correction of a *detached retina. A small piece of silicone plastic is sewn on the outside of the eyeball to produce an indentation over the retinal hole to allow the retina to reattach. **2.** the insertion of plastic balls into the pleural cavity to cause collapse of the lung. This was done in the days before effective antituberculous drugs to help tuberculosis to heal.

plumbism n. lead poisoning. See lead[1].

Plummer's disease a hyperfunctioning, usually benign, *adenoma of the thyroid gland, which can be palpated and appears as a "hot nodule" on radioactive thyroid scanning. Treatment is to control the nodule with antithyroid drugs and then remove it surgically or destroy it permanently with radioactive iodine. [H. S. Plummer (1874–1937), US physician]

pluri- prefix denoting more than one; several.

PMS see premenstrual syndrome.

-pnea suffix denoting a condition of breathing. Example: dyspnea (breathlessness).

pneo- prefix denoting breathing; respiration.

pneum- (pneumo-) prefix denoting 1. the presence of air or gas. Example: pneumocolon (within the colon). 2. the lung(s). Example: pneumogastric (relating to the lungs and stomach). 3. respiration.

pneumat- (pneumato-) prefix denoting 1. the presence of air or gas. 2. respiration.

pneumatization n. the presence of air-filled cavities in bone, such as the sinuses of the skull.

pneumatocele n. herniation of lung tissue. See hernia.

pneumatosis n. the occurrence of gas cysts in abnormal sites in the body. Pneumatosis cystoides intestinalis is the occurrence of multiple gas cysts in the wall of the lower intestines. Its cause is unknown; it can be treated by *hyperbaric oxygenation.

pneumaturia n. the presence in the urine of bubbles of air or other gas, due to the formation of gas by bacteria infecting the urinary tract or to an abnormal connection (fistula) between the urinary tract and bowel.

pneumo- prefix. see pneum-.

pneumocephalus (pneumocele) n. the presence of air within the skull, usually resulting from a fracture passing through one of the air sinuses. There may be a leak of cerebrospinal fluid at the site of the fracture, manifested as a watery discharge from the nose. Pneumocephalus can best be detected by plain X-rays of the skull, which show air and a fluid level inside a cavity, or by CT or MRI scanning.

pneumococcus n. (pl. pneumococci) the organism *Streptococcus pneumoniae, which is associated with *pneumonia and pneumococcal meningitis. —**pneumococcal** adj.

pneumoconiosis n. a group of lung diseases caused by inhaling dust. The dust particles must be less than 0.5 μm in diameter to reach the depths of the lung and there is usually a long period after initial exposure before shadows appear on the chest X-ray and breathlessness develops. In practice industrial exposure to coal dust (see anthracosis), silica (see silicosis), and asbestos (see asbestosis) is responsible for most of the cases of pneumoconiosis.

Pneumocystis n. a genus of protozoans. The species P. carinii causes pneumonia in immunosuppressed patients, usually following intensive chemotherapy (see also AIDS). Pneumocystis carinii pneumonia (PCP) can be fatal if untreated, but it can be overcome with high doses of *co-trimoxazole or *pentamidine.

pneumocyte (pneumonocyte) n. a type of cell that lines the walls separating the air sacs (see alveolus) in the lungs. Type I pneumocytes are flat and inconspicuous. Type II pneumocytes are cuboidal and secrete *surfactant.

pneumoencephalography n. a technique used in the X-ray diagnosis of disease within the skull. Air is introduced into the cavities (ventricles) of the brain to displace the cerebrospinal fluid, thus acting as a *contrast medium. X-ray photographs show the size and disposition of the ventricles and the subarachnoid spaces. The technique has largely been superseded by CT and MRI scanning.

pneumograph n. an instrument used to record the movements made during respiration.

pneumohemothorax n. see hemopneumothorax.

pneumohydrothorax n. see hydropneumothorax.

pneumolysis n. see pleurolysis.

pneumon- (pneumono-) prefix denoting the lung(s). Example: pneumonopexy (surgical fixation to the chest wall).

pneumonectomy n. surgical removal of a lung, usually for cancer.

pneumonia n. inflammation of the lung

caused by bacteria, in which the air sacs (*alveoli) become filled with inflammatory cells and the lung becomes solid (*see* consolidation). The symptoms depend on the amount of lung involved and the virulence of the bacteria, but they generally include those of any infection (fever, malaise, headaches, etc.), together with cough and chest pain. Pneumonias may be classified in different ways.

(1) According to the X-ray appearance. *Lobar pneumonia* affects whole lobes and is usually caused by *Streptococcus pneumoniae*, while *lobular pneumonia* refers to multiple patchy shadows in a localized or segmental area. When these multiple shadows are widespread, the term *bronchopneumonia* is used. In bronchopneumonia, the infection starts in a number of small bronchi and spreads in a patchy manner into the alveoli. *Hypostatic pneumonia* develops in dependent parts of the lung in people who are otherwise ill, chilled, or immobilized.

(2) According to the infecting organism. The most common organism is *Streptococcus pneumoniae*, but *Haemophilus influenzae*, *Staphylococcus aureus*, *Legionella pneumophila*, and *Mycoplasma pneumoniae* (among others) may all be responsible for the infection. *See also* atypical pneumonia, viral pneumonia.

(3) According to the clinical and environmental circumstances under which the infection is acquired. These infections are divided into *community-acquired pneumonia*, *hospital-acquired* (*nosocomial*) *pneumonia*, and pneumonias occurring in immunocompromised subjects (including those with AIDS). The organisms responsible for community-acquired pneumonia are totally different from those in the other groups. The bacteria that cause pneumonia are usually sensitive to *antibiotics, and recovery is usually rapid. A vaccine is available for pneumococcal pneumonia. *Compare* pneumonitis.

pneumonitis *n.* inflammation of the lung that is confined to the walls of the air sacs (alveoli) and often caused by viruses or unknown agents. It may be acute and transient or chronic, leading to increasing respiratory disability. It does not respond to antibiotics but corticosteroids may be helpful. *Compare* pneumonia.

pneumonocyte *n. see* pneumocyte.

pneumopericardium *n.* the presence of air within the membranous sac surrounding the heart. *See* hydropneumopericardium.

pneumoperitoneum *n.* air or gas in the peritoneal or abdominal cavity, usually due to a perforation of the stomach or the bowel. Pneumoperitoneum may be induced for diagnostic purposes (e.g. *laparoscopy). A former treatment of tuberculosis was the deliberate injection of air into the peritoneal cavity to allow the tuberculous lung to be rested (*artificial pneumoperitoneum*).

pneumoradiography *n.* X-ray examination of part of the body using a gas, such as air or carbon dioxide, as a *contrast medium. The technique was used to examine the ventricles of the brain (pneumoencephalography). It is now largely obsolete, apart from *double contrast examinations of the bowel.

pneumoretinopexy *n.* a surgical technique in which an inert gas bubble is injected into the eye to press and seal breaks in the retina. When the retina is flat, a laser beam or *cryoretinopexy is applied to cause scarring and permanently seal the tear.

pneumothorax *n.* air in the *pleural cavity. Any breach of the lung surface or chest wall allows air to enter the pleural cavity, causing the lung to collapse. The leak can occur without apparent cause, in otherwise healthy people (*spontaneous pneumothorax*), or result from injuries to the chest (*traumatic pneumothorax*). In *tension pneumothorax* a breach in the lung surface acts as a valve, admitting air into the pleural cavity when the patient breathes in but preventing its escape when he breathes out. This air must be let out by surgical incision.

A former treatment for pulmonary tuberculosis – *artificial pneumothorax* – was the deliberate injection of air into the pleural cavity to collapse the lung and allow the tuberculous areas to heal.

pneumotonometer *n.* an instrument that blows a puff of air at the cornea to cause flattening and hence measure intraocular pressure. It is commonly used by optometrists in tests for glaucoma.

pock *n.* a small pus-filled eruption on the skin characteristic of *chickenpox and *smallpox rashes. *See also* pustule.

pocket n. (in dentistry) see periodontal pocket.

pockmark n. a pitted scar on the skin, especially one left by severe acne.

pod- prefix denoting the foot.

podagra n. gout of the foot, especially the big toe.

podalic version altering the position of a fetus in the uterus so that its feet will emerge first at birth. See also version.

podiatry n. the study and care of the foot, including its normal structure, its diseases, and its treatment. It was formerly called chiropody.

POEMS syndrome a multisystem syndrome, which is mostly reported in Japanese males, consisting of polyneuropathy, organomegaly, endocrine failure, M protein (immunoglobulins) in the plasma, and skin changes, such as thickening, hirsutism, or excess sweating. Each of the components occurs with varying consistency. The cause is not known but it is not thought to be autoimmune in nature.

-poiesis suffix denoting formation; production. Example: hemopoiesis (of blood cells).

poikilo- prefix denoting variation; irregularity.

poikilocyte n. an abnormally shaped red blood cell (*erythrocyte). Poikilocytes may be classified into a variety of types on the basis of their shape; for example elliptocytes (ellipsoid) and schistocytes (semilunar). See also poikilocytosis.

poikilocytosis n. the presence of abnormally shaped red cells (*poikilocytes) in the blood. Poikilocytosis is particularly marked in *myelofibrosis but can occur to some extent in almost any blood disease.

poikiloderma n. a condition in which the skin atrophies and becomes pigmented, giving it a mottled appearance.

poikilothermic adj. cold-blooded: being unable to regulate the body temperature, which fluctuates according to that of the surroundings. Reptiles and amphibians are cold-blooded. Compare homeothermic. —**poikilothermy** n.

pointillage n. a procedure in massage in which the operator's fingers are pressed, fingertip first, deep into the patient's skin. This is done to manipulate underlying structures and break up adhesions that may have formed following injury.

poison n. any substance that irritates, damages, or impairs the activity of the body's tissues. In large enough doses almost any substance acts as a poison, but the term is usually reserved for substances, such as arsenic, cyanide, and strychnine, that are harmful in relatively small amounts.

Poisson distribution see frequency distribution. [S. D. Poisson (1781–1840), French mathematician]

polar body one of the small cells produced during the formation of an ovum from an *oocyte that does not develop into a functional egg cell.

pole n. (in anatomy) the extremity of the axis of the body, an organ, or a cell.

poli- (polio-) prefix denoting the gray matter of the nervous system.

policeman's heel see plantar fasciitis.

polioencephalitis n. a virus infection of the brain causing particular damage to the *gray matter of the cerebral hemispheres and the brainstem. The term is now usually restricted to infections of the brain by the poliomyelitis virus.

polioencephalomyelitis n. any virus infection of the central nervous system affecting the gray matter of the brain and spinal cord. *Rabies is the outstanding example.

poliomyelitis (infantile paralysis, polio) n. an infectious virus disease affecting the central nervous system. The virus is excreted in the feces of an infected person and the disease is therefore most common where sanitation is poor. However, epidemics may occur in more hygienic conditions, where individuals have not acquired immunity to the disease during infancy. Symptoms commence 7–12 days after infection. In most cases paralysis does not occur: in abortive poliomyelitis only the throat and intestines are infected and the symptoms are those of a stomach upset or influenza; in nonparalytic poliomyelitis these symptoms are accompanied by muscle stiffness, particularly in the neck and back. Paralytic poliomyelitis is much less common. The symptoms of the milder forms of the disease are followed by weakness and eventual paralysis of the muscles: in bulbar poliomyelitis the muscles of the respiratory system are involved and breathing is affected.

There is no specific treatment, apart from measures to relieve the symptoms:

cases of bulbar poliomyelitis may require the use of a *respirator. Immunization, using the *Sabin vaccine (taken orally) or the *Salk vaccine (injected), is highly effective. *See also* post-polio syndrome.

poliosis *n.* premature graying of the hair.

poliovirus *n.* one of a small group of RNA-containing viruses causing *poliomyelitis. They are included within the *picornavirus group.

pollen *n.* the fertilizing elements of a flowering plant, a potential allergen source. *See* hay fever.

pollex *n.* (*pl.* **pollices**) the thumb.

pollinosis *n.* a more precise term than *hay fever for an allergy due to the pollen of grasses, trees, or shrubs.

poly- *prefix denoting* **1.** many; multiple. **2.** excessive. **3.** generalized; affecting many parts.

polyarteritis nodosa (periarteritis nodosa) a disease of unknown cause in which there is patchy inflammation of the walls of the arteries. It is one of the *connective tissue diseases. Common manifestations are arthritis, neuritis, asthma, skin rashes, hypertension, kidney failure, and fever. The inflammation is suppressed by corticosteroid drugs (such as prednisolone).

polyarthritis *n.* disease involving several to many joints, either together or in sequence, causing pain, stiffness, swelling, tenderness, and loss of function. *Rheumatoid arthritis is the most common cause.

polychromasia (polychromatophilia) *n.* the presence of certain blue red blood cells (*erythrocytes) seen in blood films stained with *Romanovsky stains, as well as the normal pink cells. The cells that appear blue are juvenile erythrocytes (*see* reticulocyte).

polycoria *n.* a rare congenital abnormality of the eye in which there are one or more holes in the iris in addition to the pupil.

polycystic disease of the kidneys an inherited disorder, transmitted as an autosomal *dominant trait (the gene responsible is located on chromosome no. 16), in which the substance of both kidneys is largely replaced by numerous cysts. Symptoms – including *hematuria, urinary tract infection, and hypertension – appear between the ages of 20 and 40 years and are associated with chronic kidney failure.

polycystic ovary syndrome (PCOS) a hormonal disorder characterized by incomplete development of *graafian follicles in the ovary due to inadequate secretion of *luteinizing hormone; the follicles fail to ovulate and remain as multiple cysts distending the ovary. Further hormone imbalance results in obesity and hirsutism, and the woman is infertile due to the lack of ovulation; this syndrome is known as the *Stein-Leventhal syndrome*. The treatment is administration of appropriate hormones.

polycythemia *n.* an increase in the *packed cell volume (hematocrit) in the blood. This may be due either to a decrease in the total volume of the plasma (*relative polycythemia*) or to an increase in the total volume of the red cells (*absolute polycythemia*). The latter may occur as a primary disease (*see* polycythemia vera) or as a secondary condition in association with various respiratory or circulatory disorders that cause deficiency of oxygen in the tissues and with certain tumors, such as carcinoma of the kidney.

polycythemia vera (erythremia, Vaquez-Osler disease) a disease in which the number of red cells in the blood is greatly increased (*see also* polycythemia). There is often also an increase in the numbers of white blood cells and platelets. Symptoms include headache, thromboses, *cyanosis, *plethora, and itching. Polycythemia vera may be treated by bloodletting, but more severe cases are best treated by radiotherapy or cytotoxic drugs. The cause of the disease is not known.

polydactylism *n. see* hyperdactylism.

polydipsia *n.* abnormally intense thirst, leading to the drinking of large quantities of fluid. This is a symptom typical of diabetes mellitus and diabetes insipidus.

polygene *n.* one of a number of genes that together control a single characteristic in an individual. Each polygene has only a slight effect and the expression of a set of polygenes is the result of their combined interaction. Characteristics controlled by polygenes are usually of a quantitative nature, e.g. height. *See also* multifactorial. —**polygenic** *adj.*

polymastia (pleomastia) *n.* multiple breasts or nipples. These are usually symmetrically arranged along a line between the midpoint of the collar bone and the pelvis (the nipple line).

polymer *n.* a substance formed by the linkage of a large number of smaller molecules known as *monomers*. An example of a monomer is glucose, whose molecules link together to form glycogen, a polymer. Polymers may have molecular weights from a few thousands to many millions. Polymers made up of a single type of monomer are known as *homopolymers*; those of two or more monomers as *heteropolymers*.

polymerase chain reaction (PCR) a technique of molecular genetics in which a particular sequence of DNA can be isolated and amplified sufficiently to enable genetic analysis. The technique may be utilized in the course of *preimplantation diagnosis of genetic disorders and also in the identification of viruses in tissue samples, e.g. *human papillomavirus in cervical smears.

polymorph (polymorphonuclear leukocyte) *n.* any of a group of white blood cells that have lobed nuclei and granular cytoplasm and function as phagocytes. Polymorphs include *eosinophils, *basophils, and *neutrophils.

polymorphism *n.* (in genetics) a condition in which a chromosome or a genetic character occurs in more than one form, resulting in the coexistence of more than one morphological type in the same population.

polymyalgia rheumatica an autoimmune disease causing aching and progressive stiffness of the muscles of the shoulders and hips after inactivity. These symptoms are typically associated with loss of appetite, fatigue, night sweats, and a raised *ESR. The condition is most common in the elderly, rarely occurring before the age of 50 years. The symptoms respond rapidly and effectively to corticosteroid treatment, which must usually be continued for several years. It is often associated with temporal *arteritis.

polymyositis *n.* a generalized disease of the muscles that may be acute or chronic. It particularly affects the muscles of the shoulder and hip girdles, which are weak and tender to the touch. Microscopic examination of the affected muscles shows diffuse inflammatory changes, and relief of the symptoms is obtained with *corticosteroid drugs. The skin may be reddened and atrophic. *See also* dermatomyositis.

polymyxin B an *antibiotic used to treat severe infections caused by gram-negative bacteria, especially *Pseudomonas.* It is usually administered by injection but is also taken by mouth or applied as a solution or ointment for ear and eye infections. The drug may cause mild dizziness. Trade name: **Aerosporin.**

polyneuritis *n.* a disorder involving several of the peripheral nerves, usually in a symmetrical distribution. *See* peripheral neuropathy.

polyneuropathy *n.* *see* peripheral neuropathy.

polynucleotide *n.* a long chain of linked *nucleotides, of which molecules of DNA and RNA are made.

polyopia *n.* the sensation of multiple images of one object. It is sometimes experienced by people with early cataract. *See also* diplopia.

polyorchidism *n.* a congenital abnormality resulting in more than two testes.

polyp (polypus) *n.* a growth, usually benign, protruding from a mucous membrane. Polyps are commonly found in the nose and sinuses, giving rise to obstruction, chronic infection, and discharge. They are often present in patients with allergic rhinitis, in whom they may develop in response to longterm antigenic stimulation. Other sites of occurrence include the ear, the stomach, and the colon, where they may eventually become malignant. *Juvenile polyps* occur in the intestine (usually colon or rectum) of infants or young people; sometimes they are multiple (*juvenile polyposis*). In the latter form there is a risk of malignant change (25% of cases) but most juvenile polyps are benign (*see also* polyposis, Peutz-Jeghers syndrome). Polyps are usually removed surgically (*see* polypectomy).

polypectomy *n.* the surgical removal of a *polyp. The technique used depends upon the site and size of the polyp, but it is often done by cutting across the base using a wire loop (snare) through which is passed a coagulating *diathermy current.

polypeptide *n.* a molecule consisting of three or more amino acids linked together by *peptide bonds. *Protein molecules are polypeptides.

polyphagia *n.* gluttonous excessive eating.

polypharmacy *n.* treatment of a patient with more than one drug.

polyphyletic *adj.* describing a number of individuals, species, etc., that have evolved from more than one ancestral group. *Compare* monophyletic.

polyploid *adj.* describing cells, tissues, or individuals in which there are three or more complete sets of chromosomes. *Compare* diploid, haploid. —**polyploidy** *n.*

polypoid *adj.* having the appearance of a *polyp.

polyposis *n.* a condition in which numerous polyps form in an organ or tissue. *Familial adenomatous polyposis* (*FAP*) is a hereditary disease (caused by a defective dominant gene) in which multiple *adenomas develop in the intestine, usually the large bowel or rectum, at an early age. Because these polyps often become malignant, patients are usually advised to undergo total removal of the colon. *See also* Peutz-Jeghers syndrome. *Compare* pseudopolyposis.

polypus *n. see* polyp.

polyradiculitis (polyradiculopathy) *n.* any disorder of the peripheral nerves (*see* neuropathy) in which the brunt of the disease falls on the nerve roots where they emerge from the spinal cord. An abnormal allergic response in the nerve fibers is thought to be one cause of this condition; the *Guillain-Barré syndrome is an example. Other causes include infections (such as syphilis), herpesviruses, and tumors (such as lymphoma or other forms of cancer).

polyribosome (polysome) *n.* a structure that occurs in the cytoplasm of cells and consists of a group of *ribosomes linked together by *messenger RNA molecules: formed during protein synthesis.

polysaccharide *n.* a *carbohydrate formed from many monosaccharides joined together in long linear or branched chains. Polysaccharides have two important functions: (1) as storage forms of energy, for example *glycogen in animals and humans and *starch in plants; and (2) as structural elements, for example *mucopolysaccharides in animals and humans and *cellulose in plants.

polyserositis *n.* inflammation of the membranes that line the chest, abdomen, and joints, with accumulation of fluid in the cavities. Commonly, the condition is inherited and intermittent and is termed *familial Mediterranean fever.* If complicated by infiltration of major organs by a glycoprotein (*see* amyloidosis) the disease usually proves fatal. Administration of colchicine will prevent attacks in most patients.

polysome *n. see* polyribosome.

polysomnograph *n.* a record of measurements of various bodily parameters during sleep. It is used in the diagnosis of sleep disorders, such as obstructive *sleep apnea.

polyspermia *n.* **1.** excessive formation of semen. **2.** *see* polyspermy.

polyspermy (polyspermia) *n.* fertilization of a single ovum by more than one spermatozoon: the development is abnormal and the embryo dies.

polythelia *n.* a congenital excess of nipples (*see* polymastia).

polyunsaturated *adj.* describing a chemical compound containing two or more double or triple bonds. The term is used specifically to denote a fatty acid or a fat containing many double bonds. *See* unsaturated fatty acid.

polyuria *n.* the production of large volumes of urine, which is dilute and of a pale color. The phenomenon may be due simply to excessive liquid intake or to disease, particularly diabetes mellitus, diabetes insipidus, and kidney disorders.

pompholyx *n.* *eczema of the hands (*see* cheiropompholyx) and feet (*podopompholyx*). Because the horny layer of the skin in these parts is so thick the vesicles typical of eczema cannot rupture, they therefore persist in the skin, looking like rice grains. There is intense itching until the skin eventually peels. There may be secondary infection due to scratching. Pompholyx is most common in early adulthood and attacks occur suddenly, lasting up to six weeks. The disease may be recurrent or persist as a chronic condition.

pons *n.* **1.** *see* pons Varolii. **2.** any portion of tissue that joins two parts of an organ.

pons Varolii (pons) the part of the *brainstem that links the medulla oblongata and the thalamus, bulging forward in front of the cerebellum, from which it is separated by the fourth ventricle. It contains numerous nerve tracts between the cerebral cortex and the spinal cord and several nuclei of gray matter. From its front surface the *trigeminal nerves emerge.

pontic n. (in dentistry) see bridge.

popliteus n. a flat triangular muscle at the back of the knee joint, between the femur and tibia, that helps to flex the knee. —**popliteal** adj.

porcelain n. (in dentistry) a ceramic material used to construct tooth-colored crowns, inlays, or veneers.

pore n. a small opening; for example, sweat pores are the openings of the sweat glands on the surface of the skin.

porencephaly n. an abnormal communication between the lateral *ventricle and the surface of the brain. This is usually a consequence of brain injury or cerebrovascular disease; uncommonly it may be a developmental defect, when it would most likely affect both lateral ventricles.

porocephaliasis n. a rare infestation of the nasal cavities, windpipe, lungs, liver, or spleen by the nymphs of the parasitic arthropod *Porocephalus. Humans become infected on consumption of water or uncooked vegetables contaminated with the parasite's eggs. There may be some abdominal pain while the parasite is in the gut but in many cases there are no symptoms. Porocephaliasis has been occasionally reported in blacks of central Africa.

Porocephalus n. a genus of wormlike arthropods occurring mainly in tropical Africa and India. The legless adults are parasites in the lungs of snakes. The eggs, which are ejected with the snake's bronchial secretions, may be accidentally swallowed by humans. The larva bores through the gut wall and usually migrates to the liver, where it develops into a nymph (see porocephaliasis).

porphin n. a complex nitrogen-containing ring structure and parent compound of the *porphyrins.

porphobilinogen n. a pigment that appears in the urine of individuals with acute *porphyria, causing it to darken if left standing.

porphyria n. one of a group of rare inherited disorders due to *inborn errors of metabolism in which there are deficiencies in the enzymes involved in the biosynthesis of heme. The accumulation of the enzyme's substrate gives rise to symptoms of the disorder. The defect may be derived primarily in the liver (hepatic porphyria) or in the bone marrow (erythropoietic porphyria) or both. Prominent features include the excretion of porphyrins and their derivatives in the urine, which may change color on standing (see porphobilinogen); sensitivity of the skin to sunlight causing chronic inflammation or blistering; inflammation of the nerves (neuritis); mental disturbances; and attacks of abdominal pain. Porphyria cutanea tarda is a hepatic form in which light-exposed areas of the skin are blistered and fragile. Acute intermittent porphyria is a hereditary hepatic porphyria characterized by recurrent attacks of acute abdominal pain, severe constipation, and psychotic behavior. Factors triggering attacks include alcohol and many drugs.

porphyrin n. one of a number of pigments that are derived from *porphin and are widely distributed in living things. All porphyrins form chelates with iron, magnesium, zinc, nickel, copper, and cobalt. These chelates are constituents of *hemoglobin, *myohemoglobin, the *cytochromes, and chlorophyll, and are thus important in many oxidation/reduction reactions in all living organisms. See also protoporphyrin IX.

porphyrinuria n. the presence in the urine of breakdown products of the red blood pigment hemoglobin (porphyrins), sometimes causing discoloration. See porphyria, porphobilinogen.

porta n. the aperture in an organ through which its associated vessels pass. Such an opening occurs in the liver (porta hepatis).

portacaval anastomosis (portacaval shunt) 1. a surgical technique in which the hepatic portal vein is joined to the inferior vena cava. Blood draining from the abdominal viscera is thus diverted past the liver. It is used in the treatment of *portal hypertension, since – by lowering the pressure within the veins of the stomach and esophagus – it prevents serious bleeding into the gastrointestinal tract. 2. any of the natural communications between the branches of the hepatic portal vein in the liver and the inferior vena cava.

portal adj. 1. relating to the portal vein or system. 2. relating to a porta.

portal hypertension a state in which the pressure within the hepatic *portal vein is increased, causing enlargement of the spleen, enlargement of veins in the esophagus (gullet) (which may rupture to cause severe bleeding), and accumulation of fluid in the peritoneal cavity (ascites). The most common cause is *cirrhosis, but other diseases of the liver or thrombosis of the portal vein will also produce it. Treatment is by *diuretic drugs, by surgery to join the portal vein to the inferior vena cava (bypassing the liver; see portacaval anastomosis), or by implanting a *stent in the liver to join portal tract veins to a hepatic vein tributary.

portal pyemia see pylephlebitis.

portal system a vein or group of veins that terminates at both ends in a capillary bed. The best known is the *hepatic portal system*, which consists of the *portal vein and its tributaries (see illustration). Blood is drained from the spleen, stomach, pancreas, and small and large intestines into veins that merge to form the portal vein leading to the liver. Here the portal vein branches, ending in many small capillaries called *sinusoids. These permit the passage into the liver cells of nutrients absorbed by blood from the intestines.

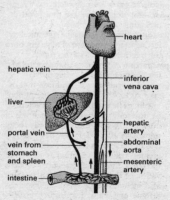

The hepatic portal system

portal vein a short vein, about 8 cm long, forming part of the hepatic *portal system. It receives many tributaries, in-cluding the splenic vein from the spleen and pancreas, the gastric vein from the stomach, the mesenteric vein from the small and large intestines, and the rectal vein from the rectum and anus.

port-wine stain see nevus.

positron n. an electrically charged particle, released in some radioactive decays, that has the same mass as an electron but opposite charge. It has a very short lifetime as it quickly reacts with an electron to produce *gamma rays.

positron emission tomography (PET, positron emission computed tomography, PECT) a technique in *nuclear medicine for *cross-sectional imaging that enables a noninvasive assessment and localization of metabolic activity to be made. Emission of a *positron by a radioisotope results in annihilation of the positron on collision with an electron, and the creation of two gamma rays of known energy traveling in exactly opposite directions. The PET scanner has detectors on each side of the patient to detect the simultaneous arrival of the gamma rays. Images are created using reconstruction *algorithms similar to CT scanning. Fluorodeoxyglucose (FDG), using fluorine-18, is used to examine glucose metabolism, and ammonia, using nitrogen-13, gives information on perfusion. Carbon-11 and oxygen-15 can also be used as radioisotopes for PET scanning. Some diseases result in decreased uptake of the radio-labeled material due to decreased function; others, including many tumors, show increased glucose metabolism and concentrate the isotope avidly. In this way functional activity of the tissues can be compared with anatomical images obtained by CT or MRI scanning. Originally used to study activity in the brain, PET is now also used for investigating the chest and abdomen. See also tomography. Compare computed tomography (CT).

posology n. the science of the dosage of medicines.

Possum n. a device that enables severely paralyzed patients to use typewriters, computers, telephones, and a wide variety of other machines. Modern Possums are operated by micro-switches that require only the slightest movement in any limb. The original device worked by blowing and sucking on a mouthpiece.

The name derives from *patient-operated selector mechanism* (*POSM*).

post- *prefix denoting* **1.** following; after. Example: *postepileptic* (after an epileptic seizure). **2.** (in anatomy) behind. Example: *postoral* (behind the mouth).

postcentral *adj.* **1.** situated behind any center. **2.** situated behind the central fissure of the brain.

postcibal *adj.* occurring after eating.

postcoital contraception prevention of pregnancy after intercourse has taken place. This can be achieved by three methods, which aim to prevent implantation of the fertilized ovum in the uterus: (1) the *Yuzpe method*, which consists of two spaced oral doses of *ethinyl estradiol combined with *levonorgestrel taken within 72 hours of unprotected intercourse; (2) two spaced oral doses of levonorgestrel taken within 72 hours of unprotected intercourse; and (3) insertion of an *IUD within five days of unprotected intercourse.

postcoital test a test used in the investigation of infertility. A specimen of cervical mucus, taken 6–24 hours after coitus, is examined under a microscope. The appearance of 10 or more progressively motile sperms per high-power field in the specimen indicates that there is no abnormal reaction between sperms and mucus. The test should be undertaken in the postovulatory phase of the menstrual cycle.

posterior *adj.* situated at or near the back of the body or an organ. The *posterior chamber* of the eye is the rear section, behind the lens, which is filled with vitreous humor.

postero- *prefix denoting* posterior. Example: *posterolateral* (behind and at the side of).

posteroanterior *adj.* from the back to the front. In radiology it denotes a view in the *coronal plane.

postganglionic *adj.* describing a neuron in a nerve pathway that starts at a ganglion and ends at the muscle or gland that it supplies. In the sympathetic nervous system, postganglionic fibers are *adrenergic, unlike those in the parasympathetic system, which are *cholinergic. *Compare* preganglionic.

postgastrectomy syndrome *see* dumping syndrome.

posthetomy *n.* an obsolete term for *circumcision.

posthitis *n.* inflammation of the foreskin. This usually occurs in association with inflammation of the glans penis (*balanitis; see* balanoposthitis). Pain, redness, and swelling of the foreskin occurs due to bacterial infection. Treatment is by antibiotic administration, and subsequent *circumcision prevents further attacks.

posthumous birth 1. delivery of a child by *cesarean section after the mother's death. **2.** birth of a child after the father's death.

postmature *adj.* describing a baby born after 42 weeks of gestation (calculated from the first day of the last menstrual period). Such a birth can be associated with maternal diabetes or with *anencephaly in the fetus. —**postmaturity** *n.*

postmenopause *n.* the period of a woman's life after the *menopause. The term "menopause" is often used in reference to the postmenopausal period.

postmicturition dribble a *lower urinary tract symptom in which a dribble occurs after voiding has been completed, often after leaving the toilet. It is quite common in men but is not caused by benign prostatic hyperplasia.

postmortem *n. see* autopsy.

postnasal space *see* nasopharynx.

postnatal depression *see* puerperal depression.

postoperative *adj.* following operation: referring to the condition of a patient or to the treatment given at this time.

postpartum *adj.* relating to the period of a few days immediately after birth.

post-polio syndrome a condition that occurs 20 to 40 years after acute *poliomyelitis. The syndrome is characterized by insidious numbness and weakness in muscles that may or may not have been previously affected. It may be caused by loss of nerve cells that have been under greater strain than normal as a result of the polio; there is no evidence of reactivation of the poliovirus. The syndrome also includes other symptoms, such as fatigue and pain, respiratory insufficiency, and difficulty in swallowing, which may be due to secondary mechanical causes. Treatment is with nonfatiguing strengthening exercises and by relief of symptoms. Pacing of physical activities, with work-rest programs, is also helpful.

postprandial adj. occurring after eating.

post-processing n. (in radiology) the electronic manipulation of digitally acquired images (see digitization) following an examination in order to improve diagnostic accuracy.

post-traumatic stress disorder an anxiety disorder caused by the major personal stress of a serious or frightening event, such as an injury, assault, rape, or exposure to warfare or a disaster involving many casualties. The reaction may be immediate or delayed for months. The sufferer experiences the persistent recurrence of images or memories of the event, together with nightmares, insomnia, a sense of isolation, guilt, irritability, and loss of concentration. Emotions may be deadened or depression may develop. The condition usually abates with time, but support and skilled counseling may be needed. More severe cases may be treated by *cognitive therapy and/or *behavior therapy.

postural muscles (antigravity muscles) muscles (principally extensors) that serve to maintain the upright posture of the body against the force of gravity.

postviral fatigue syndrome see chronic fatigue syndrome.

potassium n. a mineral element and an important constituent of the human body. It is the main base ion of intracellular fluid. Together with *sodium, it helps to maintain the electrical potential of the nervous system and is thus essential for the functioning of nerve and muscle. Normal blood levels are between 3.5 and 5 mmols/liter. High concentrations occur particularly in *kidney failure and may lead to *arrhythmia and finally to cardiac arrest. Low values result from fluid loss, e.g. due to vomiting or diarrhea, and this may lead to general muscle paralysis. Symbol: K.

potassium-channel activator any one of a new class of drugs that enhance the movement of potassium ions through the protein channels in cell membranes. In the case of smooth muscle cells, such as those in the walls of arteries, their sensitivity to the normal stimuli to contract is reduced. The result is relaxation of the muscle fibers and widening of the arteries. Potassium-channel activators are used for improving the blood supply to the heart muscle in angina pectoris. Possible side effects include headache, flushing, vomiting, dizziness, and weakness. A currently available member of the class is *nicorandil* (Ikorel).

potassium chloride a salt of potassium used to prevent and treat potassium deficiency, especially during treatment with certain diuretics. It is administered by mouth or injection; some irritation in the digestive system may occur after oral administration. Trade names: **Kaochlor, Kaon-Cl, Kato, Kay Ciel, K-Dur, K-Lease, K-Lor, Klorvess, K-Norm, K-Tab, Micro-K, Slow-K, Ten-K**.

potassium permanganate a salt of potassium used for disinfecting and cleansing wounds and as a general skin *antiseptic. It irritates mucous membranes and is poisonous if taken into the body.

potency n. (in therapeutics) the relationship between the effect of a drug and the dose required to achieve that effect. The higher the potency, the smaller the dose needed to produce a given therapeutic effect.

Potter's syndrome a congenital condition characterized by absence of kidneys, resulting in decreased amniotic fluid (see oligohydramnios) and compression of the fetus. Babies have poorly developed lungs, a characteristic wrinkled and flattened facial appearance, and leg deformities and do not usually survive. The condition is diagnosed by ultrasonography; there is no treatment available. [E. L. Potter (20th century), US pathologist]

Pott's disease *tuberculosis of the backbone. Untreated, it can lead to hunchback deformity. Treatment is with antituberculous drugs and occasionally by surgery. [P. Pott (1714–88), British surgeon]

pouch n. 1. (in anatomy) a small saclike structure, especially occurring as an outgrowth of a larger structure. The *pouch of Douglas* is a pouch of peritoneum occupying the space between the rectum and uterus. 2. (in surgery) a sac created from a loop of intestine and used to replace a section of rectum that has been surgically removed, for example for ulcerative colitis (see ileal pouch), or to replace the bladder after *cystectomy.

poultice (fomentation) n. a preparation of

hot moist material applied to any part of the body to increase local circulation, alleviate pain, or soften the skin to allow matter to be expressed from a boil. Poultices containing kaolin retain heat for a considerable period during use.

Poupart's ligament *see* inguinal ligament. [F. Poupart (1661–1708), French anatomist]

powder *n.* (in pharmacy) a medicinal preparation consisting of a mixture of two or more drugs in the form of fine particles.

pox *n.* **1.** an infectious disease causing a skin rash. **2.** a rash of pimples that become pus-filled, as in *chickenpox and *smallpox.

poxvirus *n.* one of a group of large DNA-containing viruses including those that cause *smallpox (variola) and *cowpox (vaccinia) in humans, and pox and tumors in animals.

PPLO *see* mycoplasma.

PPO *see* Preferred Provider Organization.

Prader orchidometer *see* orchidometer.

Prader-Willi syndrome a congenital condition in which obesity is associated with mental retardation and small genitalia; diabetes mellitus frequently develops in affected individuals. [A. Prader and H. Willi (20th century), Swiss pediatricians]

pravastatin *n.* a drug used to reduce abnormally high levels of cholesterol in the blood (*see* statin). Its action and side effects are similar to those of *atorvastatin and *lovastatin. Trade name: **Pravachol**.

prazepam *n.* an *anxiolytic agent used in the treatment of anxiety disorders and for the short-term relief of the symptoms of anxiety. It is administered orally; side effects are rare but may include dizziness, gastrointestinal upsets, dry mouth, and blurred vision. Trade name: **Centrax**.

praziquantel *n.* an *anthelmintic drug used to eliminate tapeworms, schistosomes, liver flukes, and lung flukes. Praziquantel is administered by mouth. Possible side effects include nausea, abdominal discomfort, fever, sweating, and drowsiness. Trade name: **Biltricide**.

prazosin *n.* a drug used in the treatment of high blood pressure (hypertension) by reducing peripheral vascular resistance. It is administered by mouth; common side effects include dizziness, headache, palpitations, and nausea. Trade name: **Minipress**.

pre- *prefix denoting* **1.** before; preceding. Example: *premenstrual* (before menstruation); *prenatal* (before birth). **2.** (in anatomy) in front of; anterior to. Example: *precardiac* (in front of the heart); *prepatellar* (in front of the patella).

preagonal *adj.* relating to the phenomena that precede the moment of death. *See also* agonal.

precancerous *adj.* describing a nonmalignant condition that is known to become malignant if left untreated. *Leukoplakia of the vulva is known to be a precancerous condition. *See also* metaplasia.

precipitin *n.* any antibody that combines with its antigen to form a complex that comes out of solution and is seen as a precipitate. The antibody-antigen reaction is specific; the precipitin reaction is therefore a useful means of confirming the identity of an unknown antigen or establishing that a serum contains antibodies to a known disease. This test may be performed in watery solution or in a semisolid medium such as agar gel. *See also* agglutination.

precipitinogen *n.* any antigen that is precipitated from solution by a *precipitin.

precision attachment (in dentistry) a special machined joint that holds certain types of partial *dentures in place. The attachment is in two parts, one fixed to the denture and the other fixed to a crown on one of the teeth abutting the denture.

precocious puberty the development at an early age of the physical and physiological changes associated with *puberty. In girls this is usually taken as development of breasts or pubic hair before the age of six or menstruation before the age of eight. In boys development of pubic hair or other adult sexual features below the age of nine is considered to be precocious. In girls 90% of cases have no underlying abnormalities, but in boys approximately half have a serious underlying cause, of which malignant testicular tumors and malignant adrenal tumors are the most common.

precocity *n.* an acceleration of normal development. The intellectually precocious child has a high IQ and may become isolated from his contemporaries or frustrated at school. Mental illness is less common than in those who develop normally. —**precocious** adj.

precordium n. the region of the thorax immediately over the heart. —**precordial** adj.

precuneus n. an area of the inner surface of the cerebral hemisphere on each side, above and in front of the *corpus callosum. See cerebrum.

predisposition n. a tendency to be affected by a particular disease or kind of disease. Such a tendency may be hereditary or may arise because of such factors as lack of vitamins, food, or sleep. See also diathesis.

prednisolone n. a synthetic *corticosteroid used to treat rheumatic diseases, inflammatory and allergic conditions, and some cancers (e.g. leukemia, lymphoma). It is administered by mouth, injected into joints, or applied in creams, lotions, ointments, or drops (to treat skin, eye, or ear conditions). Side effects are those of *cortisone. Trade names: **Delta-Cortef, Orapred, Pediapred, Pred Forte.**

prednisone n. a synthetic *corticosteroid used to treat rheumatic diseases, severe allergic conditions, inflammatory conditions, and leukemia. It is administered by mouth and side effects are those of *cortisone. Trade names: **Cortan, Deltasone, Meticorten, Orasone.**

preeclampsia (pregnancy-induced hypertension) n. high blood pressure developing during pregnancy in a woman whose blood pressure was previously normal. It is often accompanied by excessive fluid retention and less often by the presence of protein in the urine. See also eclampsia.

Preferred Provider Organization (PPO) a group of physicians and hospitals that contracts with an insurer or employer to provide care to patients for a specified fee. Patients are limited to the physicians and hospitals in the group.

prefrontal lobe the region of the brain at the very front of each cerebral hemisphere (see frontal lobe). The functions of the lobe are concerned with emotions, memory, learning, and social behavior. Nerve tracts in the lobe are cut during the operation of prefrontal *leukotomy.

preganglionic adj. describing fibers in a nerve pathway that end in a ganglion, where they form synapses with *postganglionic fibers that continue the pathway to the effector organ, muscle, or gland.

pregnancy n. the period during which a woman carries a developing fetus. Pregnancy lasts for approximately 266 days (or 280 days from the first day of the last menstrual period), from *conception until the baby is born, and the fetus normally develops in the uterus (compare ectopic pregnancy). During pregnancy menstruation is absent, there may be a great increase in appetite, and the breasts increase in size; the woman may also experience *morning sickness. These and other changes are brought about by a hormone (*progesterone) produced at first by the ovary and later by the *placenta. Definite evidence of pregnancy is provided by various *pregnancy tests and by the detection of the heartbeat of the fetus. Medical name: **cyesis**. See also pseudocyesis (phantom pregnancy). —**pregnant** adj.

pregnancy-induced hypertension see preeclampsia.

pregnancy test any of several methods used to demonstrate whether or not a woman is pregnant. A commonly used laboratory test of early pregnancy is based on detection of a hormone, human *chorionic gonadotropin, in the urine. Mixture of a few drops of urine with a test solution containing an antibody that reacts with the hormone gives an almost immediate result. The test becomes positive within a month of conception and false-positive results are very rare. Newer tests using *monoclonal antibodies are more easily interpreted. When carried out on serum rather than urine, these tests give even earlier positive results.

pregnanediol n. a steroid that is formed during the metabolism of the female sex hormone *progesterone. It occurs in the urine during pregnancy and certain phases of the menstrual cycle.

pregnenolone n. a steroid synthesized in the adrenal glands, ovaries, and testes. Pregnenolone is an important intermediate product in steroid hormone synthesis and can – depending on the pathways followed – be converted to corticosteroids (glucocorticoids or mineralocorticoids), androgens, or estrogens.

preimplantation diagnosis prenatal genetic diagnosis of disorders and abnormalities at the earliest stage of embryonic development, i.e. before the embryo is implanted in the uterus. Access to these early embryos requires the removal and *in vitro fertilization of egg cells: three days after fertilization one or two cells are aspirated from the six- to eight-cell embryo; alternatively, tissue is removed from an embryo at five or six days, when it has reached the *blastocyst stage. Isolated cells can then be genetically analyzed, using the *polymerase chain reaction amplification technique to produce enough DNA for genetic diagnosis. Even before pregnancy, this technique can be used to enable a prospective mother to be identified as the carrier of a gene defect, by means of the *mouthwash test. When a defect is detected, *genetic counseling is offered.

premature beat *see* ectopic beat.

premature birth birth of a baby that weighs less than 2500 g (5½ lb). Usually, this is indicative of *preterm birth, but it can be caused by *intrauterine growth retardation. Birth weights of less than 500 g are almost invariably incompatible with life.

premature ejaculation emission of semen (and consequent loss of erection) during the initial stages of preparation for sexual intercourse, before insertion into the vagina or immediately afterward.

premedication *n.* drugs administered to a patient before an operation (usually one in which an anesthetic is used). Premedication usually comprises injection of a *sedative, to calm the patient, together with a drug, such as *atropine, to dry up the secretions of the lungs (which might otherwise be inhaled during anesthesia).

premenstrual syndrome (PMS) a condition of nervousness, irritability, emotional disturbance, headache, bloating, breast tenderness, and/or depression affecting some women for up to about ten days before menstruation. The condition is associated with the accumulation of salt and water in the tissues. It usually disappears soon after menstruation begins. The hormone progesterone is believed to be a causative element and a deficiency of essential fatty acids has also

been observed. Treatments include stress management, salt restriction and low-dose diuretics to relieve fluid retention, simple analgesia for aches and pains, and the contraceptive pill because suppression of ovulation often relieves the symptoms.

premenstruum *n.* the stage of the *menstrual cycle immediately preceding menstruation.

premolar *n.* either of the two teeth on each side of each jaw behind the canines and in front of the molars in the adult *dentition.

premyelocyte *n.* *see* promyelocyte.

prenatal diagnosis (antenatal diagnosis) diagnostic procedures carried out on pregnant women in order to discover genetic or other abnormalities in the developing fetus. Ultrasound scanning (*see* ultrasonography) is the first diagnostic procedure to be performed. Other procedures include estimation of the levels of *alpha-fetoprotein in the mother's serum and the amniotic fluid, chromosome and enzyme analysis of fetal cells obtained by *amniocentesis or, at an earlier stage of pregnancy, by *chorionic villus sampling, and examination of fetal blood obtained by *fetoscopy or *cordocentesis. If the results indicate that the child is likely or certain to be born with severe malformation or abnormality, the possibility of abortion is discussed with the parents. *See also* preimplantation diagnosis.

preoperative *adj.* before operation: referring to the condition of a patient or to treatment, such as sedation, given at this time.

preparedness *n.* (in psychology) a quality of some stimuli that makes them much more likely to give rise to a pathological fear. For example, animals or high places are much more likely to become the subject of a *phobia than are plants or clothes. One theory is that individuals are genetically predisposed to *conditioning of fear to objects that have been a biological threat during the evolution of mankind.

prepatellar bursitis *see* housemaid's knee.

prepubertal *adj.* relating to or occurring in the period before puberty.

prepuce (foreskin) *n.* the fold of skin that grows over the end (glans) of the penis. On its inner surface modified sebaceous glands (*preputial glands*) secrete a lubricating fluid over the glans. The accumulation of this secretion is known as *smegma. The foreskin is often surgically removed in infancy (*see* circumcision). The fold of skin that surrounds the clitoris is also called the prepuce. —**preputial** *adj.*

preputial glands modified sebaceous glands on the inner surface of the *prepuce.

prepyramidal *adj.* **1.** situated in the middle lobe of the cerebellum of the brain, in front of the *pyramid. **2.** describing nerve fibers in tracts that descend from the cerebral cortex to the spinal cord, before the crossing over that occurs at the pyramid of the medulla oblongata.

presby- (presbyo-) *prefix denoting* old age.

presbyacusis *n.* the progressive sensorineural *deafness that occurs with age.

presbyopia *n.* difficulty in reading at the usual distance (about one foot from the eyes) and in performing other close work, due to the decline with age in the ability of the eye to alter its focus to see close objects clearly. This is caused by gradual loss of elasticity of the lens of the eye which thus becomes progressively less able to increase its curvature in order to focus on near objects.

prescription *n.* a written direction from a registered medical practitioner to a pharmacist for preparing and dispensing a drug.

presenility *n.* premature aging of the mind and body, so that a person shows the reduction in mental and physical abilities normally found only in old age. *See also* dementia, progeria. —**presenile** *adj.*

present *vb.* **1.** (of a patient) to come forward for examination and treatment because of experiencing specific symptoms (*presenting symptoms*). **2.** (in obstetrics) *see* presentation.

presentation *n.* the part of the infant's body that is closest to the birth canal and can be felt on inserting the finger into the vagina. Normally, the head presents (*cephalic presentation*). However, the infant's buttocks may present (*see* breech presentation) or, if the baby lies transversely across the womb, the shoulder or arm may present. In *placenta previa, the placenta may lie in front of the presenting part. These abnormal presentations may cause complications during childbirth, and attempts have to be made to correct them.

pressor *n.* an agent that raises blood pressure. *See* vasoconstrictor.

pressure point a point at which an artery lies over a bone on which it may be compressed by finger pressure, to arrest hemorrhage beyond. For example, the femoral artery may be compressed against the pelvic bone in the groin.

pressure sore *see* bedsore.

presymptomatic *adj.* describing or relating to a symptom that occurs before the typical symptoms of a disease. *See also* prodromal.

presystole *n.* the period in the cardiac cycle just preceding systole.

preterm birth birth of a baby before 37 weeks (259 days) of gestation (calculated from the first day of the mother's last menstrual period); dating can also be done by *ultrasonography (*see also* premature birth). Such factors as *preeclampsia, multiple pregnancies (e.g. twins), maternal infection, and cervical incompetence may all result in preterm births, but in the majority of cases the cause is unknown. Conditions affecting preterm babies include *respiratory distress syndrome, feeding difficulties, inability to maintain normal body temperature, *apnea, infection, *necrotizing enterocolitis, and brain hemorrhages. Supportive treatment is provided in an incubator in a neonatal unit; many infants survive with no residual handicap but the shorter the gestation period, the more serious are the problems to be overcome.

prevalence rate a measure of morbidity based on current sickness in a population, estimated either at a particular time (*point prevalence*) or over a stated period (*period prevalence*). It can be expressed either in terms of sick persons or episodes of sickness per 1000 individuals at risk. *Compare* incidence rate.

preventive dentistry the branch of dentistry concerned with the prevention of dental disease. It includes dietary counseling, advice on oral hygiene, and the application of *fluoride and *fissure sealants to the teeth.

preventive medicine the branch of medicine whose main aim is the prevention of disease. This is a wide field, in which workers study problems ranging from the immunization of persons against infectious diseases, such as diphtheria or whooping cough, to finding methods of eliminating *vectors, such as malaria-carrying mosquitoes, to preventing heart attacks.

priapism n. persistent and usually painful erection of the penis that requires decompression. A prolonged erection (i.e. of greater than six hours duration), resulting from administration of *papaverine or a similar drug, can be successfully treated by draining the blood from the corpora cavernosa of the penis and instilling a *vasoconstrictor (e.g. aramine). Priapism may also occur in patients with sickle-cell disease and those on *hemodialysis. An unrelieved priapism results in eventual fibrosis of the spongy tissue of the corpora and no further erections are possible.

prickle cells cells with cytoplasmic processes that form intercellular bridges. The germinative layer of the *epidermis is sometimes called the prickle cell layer.

prickly heat (heat rash) an itchy rash of small raised red spots. It occurs usually on the face, neck, back, chest, and thighs. Infants and obese people are susceptible to prickly heat, which is most common in hot moist weather. It is caused by blockage of the sweat ducts and the only treatment is removal of the patient to a cool (air-conditioned) place. Medical name: **miliaria**.

prilocaine n. a local *anesthetic used particularly in ear, nose, and throat surgery and in dentistry. It is applied in a solution to mucous membranes or injected. High doses may cause methemoglobinemia and cyanosis. Prilocaine is also a constituent of *EMLA cream. Trade name: **Citanest**.

primaquine n. a drug used to treat malaria. It is administered by mouth, usually in combination with other antimalarial drugs, such as *chloroquine. High doses of primaquine may cause blood disorders (such as methemoglobinemia or hemolytic anemia) and digestive upsets.

primary care health care rendered by the physician or other health professional who has first contact with a patient seeking medical treatment. The term is often applied to care provided by internists, pediatricians, general practitioners, or

family practice physicians. *Compare* secondary care, tertiary care.

primary teeth *see* deciduous teeth.

prime vb. (in chemotherapy) to administer small doses of a *cytotoxic drug prior to high-dose chemotherapy and/or radiotherapy. This causes proliferation of the primitive bone marrow cells and aids subsequent regeneration of the bone marrow.

prime mover *see* agonist.

primidone n. an *anticonvulsant drug used to treat major epilepsy. Primidone is administered by mouth; common side effects, which are usually transient, include drowsiness, muscle incoordination, digestive upsets, vertigo, and sight disturbances. Trade names: **Myidone**, **Mysoline**.

primigravida n. a woman experiencing her first pregnancy.

primipara n. a woman who has given birth to one infant capable of survival.

primitive streak the region of the embryo that proliferates rapidly, producing mesoderm cells that spread outward between the layers of ectoderm and endoderm.

primordial adj. (in embryology) describing cells or tissues that are formed in the early stages of embryonic development.

P–R interval the interval on an *electrocardiogram between the onset of atrial activity and ventricular activity. It represents the time required for the impulse from the *sinoatrial node to reach the ventricles.

prion n. an agent that is capable of replication and of causing infection but is of simpler constitution than any virus. Prions are abnormal forms of a normal brain cell protein (PrP). They are produced by mutations in the gene that codes for PrP and are very stable: they are not removed by the normal cellular processes of degradation and are resistant to radiation. They are believed to interact with normal PrP in such a way as to convert it to the abnormal form, which accumulates in the brain. Prions are now widely accepted as being the causal agents of a range of serious diseases including *Creutzfeldt-Jakob disease, *Gerstmann-Sträussler-Scheinker syndrome, and *kuru, all of which are *spongiform encephalopathies. Different mutations in the PrP gene are believed to be responsible for the different forms of these so-called *prion diseases*.

pro- *prefix denoting* **1.** before; preceding. **2.** a precursor. **3.** in front of.

probability *n. see* significance.

proband *n. see* propositus.

probang *n.* a long flexible rod with a small sponge, ball, or tuft at the end, used to remove obstructions from the larynx or esophagus (gullet). A probang is also used to apply medication to these structures.

probe *n.* **1.** a thin rod of pliable metal, such as silver, with a blunt swollen end. The instrument is used for exploring cavities, wounds, *fistulas, or sinus channels. **2. (gene probe)** a radioactively labeled cloned section of DNA that is used to detect identical sections of nucleic acid by means of pairing between complementary bases. *See* Northern blot analysis, Southern blot analysis.

probenecid *n.* a drug that reduces the level of uric acid in the blood (*see* uricosuric drug) and is used chiefly in the treatment of gout. It is administered by mouth; mild side effects, such as digestive upsets, dizziness, and skin rashes, may occur. Trade names: **Benemid**, **Probalan**.

probucol *n.* a drug used to lower *cholesterol levels in the blood in patients with primary hypercholesterolemia who have not responded to diet, weight reduction, and exercise. It acts by increasing the breakdown of low density *lipoproteins and inhibits cholesterol synthesis. It is administered by mouth; side effects include headache, skin rash, diarrhea, and abdominal pain. Trade name: **Lorelco**.

procainamide *n.* a drug that slows down the activity of the heart and is used to control abnormal heart rhythm. It is administered by mouth or injection; side effects may include digestive upsets, dizziness, and allergic reactions. Trade names: **Procan**, **Pronestyl**.

procaine hydrochloride a local *anesthetic administered by injection for *spinal anesthesia. It was formerly used in dentistry. Side effects are uncommon, but allergic reactions may occur. Trade name: **Novocain**.

procarbazine *n.* a drug that inhibits growth of cancer cells by preventing cell division and is used to treat such cancers as Hodgkin's disease. It is administered by mouth; common side effects include loss of appetite, nausea, vomiting, diarrhea, and mouth sores. Trade name: **Matulane**.

process *n.* (in anatomy) a thin prominence or protuberance; for example, any of the processes of a vertebra.

prochlorperazine *n.* an antipsychotic drug used to treat schizophrenia and other mental disorders, migraine, vertigo, nausea, and vomiting. It is administered by mouth, injection, or in suppositories; side effects include drowsiness and dry mouth, and high doses may cause tremors and abnormal muscle movements. Trade name: **Compazine**.

procidentia *n.* the complete downward displacement (*prolapse) of an organ, especially the uterus (*uterine procidentia*), which protrudes from the vaginal opening. Uterine procidentia may result from injury to the floor of the pelvic cavity, the result of childbirth.

proct- (procto-) *prefix denoting* the anus and/or rectum.

proctalgia (proctodynia) *n.* pain in the rectum or anus. In *proctalgia fugax* severe pain suddenly affects the rectum and may last for minutes or hours; attacks may be days or months apart. There is no structural disease and the pain is probably due to muscle spasm (*see* irritable bowel syndrome). Relief is sometimes obtained from a bowel action, inserting a finger into the rectum, or from a hot bath, and it may be prevented by measures used in treating the irritable bowel syndrome.

proctatresia *n. see* imperforate anus.

proctectasia *n.* enlargement or widening of the rectum, usually due to long-standing constipation (*see* dyschezia).

proctectomy *n.* surgical removal of the rectum. It is usually performed for cancer of the rectum and may require the construction of a permanent opening in the colon (*see* colostomy). If the anus is left, an *ileal pouch can be constructed to replace the rectum.

proctitis *n.* inflammation of the rectum. Symptoms are ineffectual straining to empty the bowels (*tenesmus), diarrhea, and often bleeding. Proctitis is invariably present in ulcerative *colitis and sometimes in *Crohn's disease, but may occur independently (*idiopathic proctitis*). Rarer causes include damage by irradiation (for example during radiation therapy for cervical cancer), by *lymphogranuloma venereum, or after a colostomy has rendered the rectum nonfunctional (*disuse proctitis*).

proctocele (rectocele) *n.* bulging or pouching of the rectum, usually a forward protrusion of the rectum into the posterior wall of the vagina in association with prolapse of the uterus. It is repaired by posterior *colporrhaphy.

proctoclysis *n.* an infusion of fluid into the rectum: formerly used to replace fluid but rarely used now.

proctocolectomy *n.* a surgical operation in which the rectum and colon are removed. In *panproctocolectomy* the whole rectum and colon are removed, necessitating either a permanent opening of the ileum (*see* ileostomy) or the construction of an *ileal pouch. This is usually performed for ulcerative *colitis.

proctocolitis *n.* inflammation of the rectum and colon, usually due to ulcerative *colitis. *See also* proctitis.

proctodeum *n.* the site of the embryonic anus, marked by a depression lined with ectoderm. The membrane separating it from the hindgut breaks down in the third month of gestation. *Compare* stomodeum.

proctodynia *n. see* proctalgia.

proctogram *n.* an X-ray photograph of the rectum taken after the introduction into it of a contrast medium. A *defecating proctogram* demonstrates problems of abnormal defecation.

proctology *n.* the study of disorders of the rectum and anus.

proctorrhaphy *n.* a surgical operation to stitch tears of the rectum or anus.

proctoscope *n.* an illuminated instrument through which the lower part of the rectum and the anus may be inspected and minor procedures (such as injection therapy for hemorrhoids) carried out. —**proctoscopy** *n.*

proctosigmoiditis *n.* inflammation of the rectum and the sigmoid (lower) colon. *See also* proctocolitis.

proctotomy *n.* incision into the rectum or anus to relieve *stricture (narrowing) of these canals or to open an imperforate (closed) anus.

procyclidine *n.* an *anticholinergic drug used to reduce muscle tremor and rigidity in parkinsonism. It is administered by mouth; common side effects include dry mouth, blurred vision, and giddiness. Trade name: **Kemadrin**.

prodromal *adj.* relating to the period of time between the appearance of the first symptoms of an infectious disease and the development of a rash or fever. A *prodromal rash* is one preceding the full rash of an infectious disease.

prodrome *n.* a symptom indicating the onset of a disease.

proenzyme (zymogen) *n.* the inactive form in which certain enzymes (e.g. digestive enzymes) are originally produced and secreted. The existence of this inactive form prevents the enzyme from catalyzing biological reactions. It is activated by acid or enzymatic hydrolysis.

proerythroblast *n.* the earliest recognizable precursor of the red blood cell (erythrocyte). It is found in the bone marrow and has a large nucleus and a cytoplasm that stains deep blue with *Romanovsky stains. *See also* erythroblast, erythropoiesis.

Professional Standards Review Organizations (PRSOs) groups of local physicians authorized by a 1972 amendment to the US *Social Security Act to regulate the supply and use of medical care resources in America. Responsibilities of the PRSOs are limited primarily to supervision of federal health care expenditures under the terms of *Medicaid and *Medicare.

profundaplasty *n.* surgical enlargement of the junction of the femoral artery and its deep branch, a common operation to relieve narrowing by atherosclerosis at this point.

profundus *adj.* describing a structure (nerve, vein, artery, muscle) that is deeper from the body surface than another structure and usually lies deep in the tissue.

progeria *n.* a very rare condition in which all the signs of old age appear and progress in a child, so that senility is reached before puberty.

progesterone *n.* a steroid hormone secreted by the *corpus luteum of the ovary, the placenta, and also (in small amounts) by the adrenal cortex and testes. It is responsible for preparing the inner lining (endometrium) of the uterus for pregnancy. If fertilization occurs, it maintains the uterus throughout pregnancy and prevents the further release of eggs from the ovary. *See also* menstrual cycle.

progestogen *n.* one of a group of naturally occurring or synthetic steroid hormones, including *progesterone, that maintain the normal course of pregnancy. Progestogens are used to treat premenstrual tension, *amenorrhea, and abnormal bleeding from the uterus. Because they prevent ovulation, progestogens are a major constituent of contraceptives. Synthetic progestogens may be taken by mouth but the naturally occurring hormone must be given by intramuscular injection or subcutaneous implant, since it is rapidly broken down in the liver.

proglottis *n.* (*pl.* **proglottids** or **proglottides**) one of the segments of a *tapeworm. Mature segments, situated at the posterior end of the worm, each consist mainly of a branched uterus packed with eggs.

prognathism *n.* the state of one jaw being markedly larger than the other and therefore in front of it. —**prognathic** *adj.*

prognosis *n.* an assessment of the future course and outcome of a patient's disease, based on knowledge of the course of the disease in other patients together with the general health, age, and sex of the patient.

progressive supranuclear palsy (Steele-Richardson-Olszewski syndrome) a progressive neurological disorder resulting from degeneration of the motor neurons, basal ganglia, and brainstem. Starting in late middle age, it is characterized by a staring facial expression due to impaired ability to move the eyes up and down, progressing to difficulties in swallowing, speech, balance, and movement and general spasticity. The condition enters the differential diagnosis of *parkinsonism, with which it is often confused in its early stages.

proinsulin *n.* a substance produced in the pancreas from which the hormone *insulin is derived.

projection *n.* (in psychology) the attribution of one's own qualities to other people. In psychoanalytic psychology this is one of the *defense mechanisms; people who cannot tolerate their own feelings (e.g. anger) may cope by imagining that other people have those feelings (e.g. are persecuting).

projective test a way of measuring aspects of personality, in which the subject is asked to talk freely about ambiguous objects. His responses are then analyzed. Examples are the *Rorschach test and the Thematic Apperception Test (in which the subject invents stories about a set of pictures).

prokaryote (procaryote) *n.* any organism that lacks a true nucleus surrounded by a nuclear membrane. The nuclear elements are spread throughout the cytoplasm and division occurs through cell fission. Bacteria are prokaryotes. *Compare* eukaryote.

prokinetic agent an agent that induces movement, especially intestinal activity.

prolactin (lactogenic hormone, luteotropic hormone, luteotropin) *n.* a hormone, synthesized and stored in the anterior pituitary gland, that stimulates milk production after childbirth and also stimulates production of *progesterone by the *corpus luteum in the ovary. In both sexes excessive secretion of prolactin gives rise to abnormal production of milk (galactorrhea).

prolactinoma *n.* a benign tumor (an *adenoma) of the pituitary gland that secretes excessive amounts of prolactin. Symptoms include a loss of sexual drive, amenorrhea or impotence, and sometimes production of milk from the nipples of both men and women. If the tumor is large enough it may compress and damage adjacent structures. Treatment is with *dopamine receptor agonist drugs, such as bromocriptine, as dopamine inhibits prolactin production and may also shrink and harden the tumor, facilitating later surgical removal.

prolapse *n.* downward displacement of an organ or tissue from its normal position, usually the result of weakening of the supporting tissues. Prolapse of the uterus and/or vagina is, in most cases, caused by stretching and tearing of the supporting tissues during childbirth. The cervix may be visible at the vaginal opening or the uterus and vagina may be completely outside the vaginal opening (procidentia). Treatment is by surgical shortening of the supporting ligaments and narrowing of the vagina and vaginal orifice (see also colporrhaphy, colpoperineorrhaphy). In prolapse of the rectum, the rectum descends to lie outside the anus.

prolapsed intervertebral disk (PID) a "slipped disk": protrusion of the pulpy inner material of an *intervertebral disk through the fibrous outer coat, causing pressure on adjoining nerve roots, ligaments, etc. The condition often results from sudden twisting or bending of the backbone or lifting. Pressure on the sciatic nerve root causes *sciatica, and if severe may damage the nerve's function, leading to abnormalities or loss of sensation, muscle weakness, or loss of tendon reflexes. Treatment is by complete bed rest on a firm surface, manipulation, *traction, and analgesics; if these fail, the protruding portion of the disk is surgically removed (see laminectomy, microdiskectomy).

proline n. an *amino acid found in many proteins.

promazine n. a phenothiazine *antipsychotic drug used to relieve agitation, confusion, restlessness, anxiety, nausea, and vomiting and in the treatment of alcoholism and drug withdrawal symptoms. It is administered by mouth or injection; common side effects are drowsiness and dizziness. Trade name: **Sparine**.

promegakaryocyte n. an immature cell, found in the bone marrow, that develops into a *megakaryocyte.

promethazine n. a powerful *antihistamine drug used to treat allergic conditions and – because of its sedative action – insomnia; it is also used as an *antiemetic. Promethazine is administered by mouth or injection; side effects include drowsiness, dizziness, and confusion. Trade name: **Phenergan**.

prominence n. (in anatomy) a projection, such as a projection on a bone.

promontory n. (in anatomy) a projecting part of an organ or other structure.

promoter n. (in oncogenesis) a substance that, in conjunction with an *initiator, leads to the production of a cancer.

prompting n. a technique used in *behavior modification to elicit a response not previously present. The subject is made to engage passively in the required behavior by instructions or by being physically put through the movements. The behavior can then be rewarded (see reinforcement). This is followed by fading, in which the prompting is gradually withdrawn and the reinforcement maintained.

promyelocyte (premyelocyte) n. one of the series of cells that gives rise to the *granulocytes (a type of white blood cell); it develops from the *myeloblast and gives rise to the *myelocyte. It has abundant cytoplasm that, with *Romanovsky stains, appears blue with reddish granules. Promyelocytes are normally found in the blood-forming tissue of the bone marrow but may appear in the blood in a variety of diseases. See also granulopoiesis.

pronation n. **1.** the act of turning the hand so that the palm faces downward. In this position the bones of the forearm (radius and ulna) are rotated. **2.** the act of turning the foot so that the sole faces backward. Compare supination.

pronator n. any muscle that causes pronation of the forearm and hand; for example, the pronator teres, a two-headed muscle arising from the humerus and ulna, close to the elbow, and inserted on the radius.

prone adj. **1.** lying with the face downward. **2.** (of the forearm) in the position in which the palm of the hand faces backward or downward (see pronation). Compare supine.

pronephros n. the first kidney tissue that develops in the embryo. It is not functional and soon disappears. Compare mesonephros, metanephros.

pronucleus n. (pl. **pronuclei**) the nucleus of either the ovum or spermatozoon after fertilization but before the fusion of nuclear material. The pronuclei are larger than the normal nucleus and have a diffuse appearance.

propafenone n. an *antiarrhythmic drug used in the treatment of life-threatening cardiac *arrhythmias. It is administered orally; common side effects include drowsiness, dry mouth, gastrointestinal upsets, and blurred vision. Trade name: **Rythmol**.

propantheline n. an *anticholinergic drug that decreases activity of smooth muscle (see antispasmodic) and is used to treat disorders of the digestive system, including stomach and duodenal ulcers, and enuresis (bed wetting). It is administered by mouth; side effects include dry mouth and blurred vision. Trade name: **Pro-Banthine**.

properdin n. a group of substances in blood plasma that, in combination with *complement and magnesium ions, is capable of destroying certain bacteria and viruses. The properdin complex occurs naturally, rather than as the result of previous exposure to microorganisms, and its activity is not directed against any particular species. *Compare* antibody.

prophase n. the first stage of *mitosis and of each division of *meiosis, in which the chromosomes become visible under the microscope. The first prophase of meiosis takes place in five stages (*see* leptotene, zygotene, pachytene, diplotene, diakinesis).

prophylactic n. an agent that prevents the development of a condition or disease. An example is *nitroglycerin, which is used to prevent attacks of angina.

prophylaxis n. any means taken to prevent disease, such as immunization against diphtheria or whooping cough, or *fluoridation to prevent dental decay in children. —**prophylactic** adj.

propositus (proband) n. the first individual studied in an investigation of several related patients with an inherited or familial disorder.

propoxyphene n. an *analgesic that is used to relieve mild or moderate pain. It is administered by mouth, often in combination with other analgesics, and sometimes causes dizziness, drowsiness, nausea, and vomiting. Trade names: **Darvocet, Darvon**.

propranolol n. a drug (*see* beta blocker) used to treat abnormal heart rhythm, angina, and high blood pressure and also taken to relieve anxiety. It is administered by mouth or injection; common side effects include digestive upsets, insomnia, and lassitude. Trade name: **Inderal**.

proprietary name (in pharmacy) the trade name of a drug: the name assigned to it by the firm that manufactured it. For example, Librium is the proprietary name for chlordiazepoxide.

proprioceptor n. a specialized sensory nerve ending (*see* receptor) that monitors internal changes in the body brought about by movement and mus-

cular activity. Proprioceptors located in muscles and tendons transmit information that is used to coordinate muscular activity (*see* stretch receptor, tendon organ). *See also* mechanoreceptor.

proptometer n. *see* exophthalmometer.

proptosis n. forward displacement of an organ, especially the eye (*see* exophthalmos).

propylthiouracil n. a drug that reduces thyroid activity and is used to treat *thyrotoxicosis and to prepare patients for surgical removal of the thyroid gland. It is administered by mouth; side effects may include rashes and digestive upsets.

prorennin n. *see* rennin.

prosect vb. to dissect a cadaver (or part of one) for anatomical demonstration. —**prosection** n. —**prosector** n.

prosencephalon n. the forebrain.

prosop- (prosopo-) prefix denoting the face. Example: *prosopodynia* (pain in).

prospective study 1. a forward-looking review of a group of individuals in relation to morbidity. 2. *see* cohort study.

prostaglandin n. one of a group of hormonelike substances present in a wide variety of tissues and body fluids (including the uterus, brain, lungs, kidney, and semen). Prostaglandins have many actions; for example, they cause contraction of smooth muscle (including that of the uterus), dilation of blood vessels, and are mediators in the inflammatory process (aspirin and other *NSAIDs act by blocking their production). They are also involved in the production of mucus in the stomach, which provides protection against acid gastric juice; use of NSAIDs reduces this effect and predisposes to peptic ulceration, the principal side effects of these drugs. There are nine classes of prostaglandins (denoted PGA–I), in which individual prostaglandins are denoted by numeral subscripts (e.g. PGE_1). Synthetic prostaglandins are used to induce labor or produce abortion and to treat peptic ulcers, congenital heart disease in newborn babies, and glaucoma.

prostate cancer a malignant tumor (*carcinoma) of the prostate gland, a common form of cancer in elderly men. It may progress slowly over many years and give symptoms similar to those of *benign prostatic hyperplasia. Before it was possible to test for *prostate-specific antigen (PSA), the tumor often had invaded locally, spread to regional lymph nodes, and metastasized to bone before clinical presentation. By checking elevated levels of PSA, prostate cancer can be detected 5–10 years before the tumor would present symptomatically. If the disease is confined to the prostate, the patient may have a radical *prostatectomy, radical radiotherapy, or *brachytherapy; in very old patients, it may be enough to monitor the tumor growth. If the disease is outside the prostate, androgen deprivation therapy may be used; this may be achieved by *LHRH analogues, *antiandrogens, surgical castration, or estrogen therapy.

prostatectomy *n.* surgical removal of the prostate gland. The operation is necessary to relieve retention of urine due to enlargement of the prostate or to reduce *lower urinary tract symptoms thought to be due to *benign prostatic hyperplasia. The operation can be performed through the bladder (*transvesical prostatectomy*) or through the surrounding capsule of the prostate (*retropubic prostatectomy*). In the operation of *transurethral prostatectomy* (*transurethral resection*) the obstructing prostate can be removed through the urethra using a *resectoscope. *Radical* (or *total*) *prostatectomy* is undertaken for the treatment of prostate cancer that is confined to the gland. It entails removal of the prostate together with its capsule and seminal vesicles. Continuity of the urinary tract is achieved by anastomosing the bladder to the divided urethra.

prostate gland a male accessory sex gland that opens into the urethra just below the bladder and vas deferens (see illustration). During ejaculation it secretes an alkaline fluid that forms part of the *semen. The prostate may become enlarged in elderly men (*see* benign prostatic hyperplasia), which may result in obstruction of the neck of the bladder, impairing urination.

prostate-specific antigen (PSA) an enzyme produced by the glandular epithelium of the prostate. Increased quantities are secreted when the gland enlarges, and levels of PSA in the blood are significantly elevated in cancer of the prostate. Although there is no clear "cut-off" level for normality, over 4 ng/ml in the blood is associated with a 20% risk of prostate cancer, even in patients with normal-feeling prostates on rectal examination. Newer PSA assays can measure free PSA and compare it to the total PSA in the blood. Low free:total PSA ratios indicate a greater risk of prostate cancer and improve the discrimination between cancer and benign disease in men with a PSA in the range 4–10 ng/ml. PSA levels tend to be much higher in advanced prostate cancer and the rate of fall on treatment is a good prognostic indicator of response.

prostatic intraepithelial neoplasia (PIN) abnormal cells in the prostate that are not cancer, but are associated with cancer within the prostate. PIN is typically found in prostate biopsies taken because levels of *prostate-specific antigen are elevated, and its presence normally leads to another set of prostate biopsies taken in the future.

prostatism *n.* *see* lower urinary tract symptoms.

prostatitis *n.* inflammation of the prostate gland. This may be due to bacterial infection and can be either acute or chronic. In acute prostatitis the patient has all the symptoms of a urinary infection, including pain in the perineal area, temperature, and shivering. Treatment is by antibiotic administration. In chronic prostatitis, patients commonly complain of pain in the area between the scrotum and the anus, accompanied by *lower urinary tract symptoms. Some of these cases are due to bacterial infection, in which case antibiotics are required. In others, no bacterial infection is demonstrated, although there may be evidence

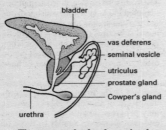

The prostate gland and associated structures (median view)

Labels: bladder, vas deferens, seminal vesicle, utriculus, prostate gland, Cowper's gland, urethra

of inflammation. Treatment in these cases involves the use of alpha blockers, anti-inflammatory agents, and occasionally antibiotics. In some men, vigorous prostate massage performed under a general anesthetic can significantly alleviate symptoms. If urinary obstruction develops, transurethral *prostatectomy is indicated.

prostatorrhea *n.* an abnormal discharge of fluid from the prostate gland. This occurs in some patients with acute *prostatitis, who complain of a profuse discharge from the urethra. The discharge is usually thin and watery and is often sterile on culture. The discharge usually subsides when the underlying prostatitis is controlled.

prosthesis *n.* (*pl.* **prostheses**) any artificial device that is attached to the body as an aid. Prostheses include dentures, artificial limbs, heart valves, implanted pacemakers, cochlear implants, and many other substitutes for parts of the body that are missing or nonfunctional. *Penile prostheses* are malleable, semirigid, or inflatable rods inserted into the corpora cavernosa of the penis to produce rigidity sufficient for vaginal penetration in men with impotence. —**prosthetic** *adj.*

prosthetic dentistry (prosthodontics) the branch of dentistry that is concerned with the provision and fitting of *dentures, *bridges, and implant-retained prostheses.

protamine *n.* one of a group of simple proteins that can be conjugated with nucleic acids to form nucleoproteins. Protamine can also be combined with *insulin and zinc to form *protamine zinc insulin*, which – when injected – is absorbed much more slowly than ordinary insulin and thus reduces the frequency of injections. *See also* isophane insulins.

protanopia *n.* a defect in color vision in which affected persons are sensitive only to blue and yellow and are insensitive to red light and confuse reds, yellows, and greens. *Compare* deuteranopia, tritanopia.

protease *n.* any enzyme that catalyzes the splitting of a protein. *See also* proteolytic enzyme.

protease inhibitor any one of a class of drugs used in the treatment of HIV infection and *AIDS, in combination with other antiviral agents. They act by inhibiting the action of protease, an enzyme produced by HIV that cleaves two precursor proteins into smaller fragments. These fragments are required for viral growth, infectivity, and replication. Protease inhibitors include *indinavir* (Crixivan), *lopinavir* (Kaletra), *nelfinavir* (Viracept), *ritonavir* (Norvir), and *saquinavir* (Fortovase, Invirase). They are administered by mouth; side effects include nausea, vomiting, diarrhea, and rashes.

protein *n.* one of a group of organic compounds of carbon, hydrogen, oxygen, and nitrogen (sulfur and phosphorus may also be present). The protein molecule is a complex structure made up of one or more chains of *amino acids, which are linked by peptide bonds. Proteins are essential constituents of the body; they form the structural material of muscles, tissues, organs, etc., and are equally important as regulators of function, as enzymes and hormones. Proteins are synthesized in the body from their constituent amino acids, which are obtained from the digestion of protein in the diet. Excess protein, not required by the body, can be converted into glucose and used as an energy source.

proteinuria *n.* the presence of protein in the urine. This may indicate the presence of damage to, or disease of, the kidneys. *See also* albuminuria.

proteolysis *n.* the process whereby complex protein molecules, obtained from the diet, are broken down by digestive enzymes in the stomach and small intestine into their constituent amino acids, which are then absorbed into the bloodstream. *See* endopeptidase, exopeptidase. —**proteolytic** *adj.*

proteolytic enzyme a digestive enzyme that causes the breakdown of protein. *See* endopeptidase, exopeptidase.

proteose *n.* a product of the hydrolytic decomposition of protein.

Proteus *n.* a genus of gram-negative rodlike highly motile flagellate bacteria common in the intestines and in decaying organic material. All species can decompose urea. Some species may cause disease in humans: *P. vulgaris* can cause urinary tract infections.

prothrombin *n.* a substance, present in blood plasma, that is the inactive precursor from which the enzyme *thrombin is derived during the process of *blood coagulation. *See also* coagulation factors.

prothrombin time (PT) the time taken for blood clotting to occur in a sample of blood to which calcium and thromboplastin have been added. A prolonged PT (compared with a control sample) indicates a deficiency of *coagulation factors, which – with calcium and thromboplastin – are required for the conversion of prothrombin to thrombin to occur in the final stages of blood coagulation. Measurement of PT is used to control anticoagulant therapy (e.g. with warfarin).

proto- *prefix denoting* **1.** first. **2.** primitive; early. **3.** a precursor.

protodiastole *n.* the short period in the cardiac cycle between the end of systole and the closure of the *aortic valve marking the start of diastole.

proton pump the enzyme in the *oxyntic (parietal) cells of the stomach that causes acid secretion by producing hydrogen ions in exchange for potassium ions.

proton-pump inhibitor a drug that reduces gastric acid secretion by blocking the *proton pump within the *oxyntic (parietal) cells. Proton-pump inhibitors include *esomeprazole, *lansoprazole*, *omeprazole, and *pantoprazole*; they are used for treating gastric and duodenal ulcers, reflux esophagitis, and the hypersecretion caused by *gastrinoma.

protooncogene *n.* a gene in a normal cell that is of identical structure to certain viral genes. Some are important regulators of cell division and damage may change them into *oncogenes.

protopathic *adj.* describing the ability to perceive only strong stimuli of pain, heat, etc. *Compare* epicritic.

protoplasm *n.* the material of which living cells are made, which includes the cytoplasm and nucleus. —**protoplasmic** *adj.*

protoplast *n.* a bacterial or plant cell without its cell wall.

protoporphyrin IX the most common type of *porphyrin found in nature. It is a constituent of hemoglobin, myohemoglobin, most of the cytochromes, and the commoner chlorophylls.

protozoa *n.* a group of microscopic single-celled organisms. Most protozoa are free-living but some are important disease-causing parasites of humans; for example, *Plasmodium*, *Leishmania*, and *Trypanosoma* cause *malaria, *kala-azar, and *sleeping sickness, respectively. *See also* ameba.

protozoan *n.* any organism of the group *protozoa.

protozoology *n.* the study of single-celled animals (*protozoa).

protriptyline *n.* a tricyclic *antidepressant drug used to treat moderate or severe depression, especially in apathetic and withdrawn patients. It is administered by mouth; side effects include dry mouth, blurred vision, fast heartbeat, digestive disturbances, and skin rashes. Trade names: **Triptil**, **Vivactil**.

protrusion *n.* (in dentistry) **1.** forward movement of the lower jaw. **2.** a *malocclusion in which some of the teeth are further forward than usual. *Compare* retrusion.

protuberance *n.* (in anatomy) a rounded projecting part, e.g. the projecting part of the chin (*mental protuberance*).

provitamin *n.* a substance that is not itself a vitamin but can be converted to a vitamin in the body. An example is *beta-carotene, which can be converted into vitamin A.

proximal *adj.* (in anatomy) situated close to the origin or point of attachment or close to the median line of the body. *Compare* distal.

Prozac *n. see* fluoxetine.

PRSOs *see* Professional Standards Review Organizations.

prune belly syndrome (Eagle-Barrett syndrome) a hereditary condition, occurring exclusively in males, characterized by a deficiency of abdominal muscles, complex malformation of the urinary tract, and bilateral undescended testes. The lungs may be underdeveloped. The name derives from the typically wrinkled appearance of the skin over the abdomen.

prurigo *n.* a chronic intensely itchy skin disease of unknown cause in which the characteristic papules are dome-shaped with a tiny vesicle cap, repeated scratching of which leads to crusting and *lichenification. Prurigo may occur in association with hay fever or asthma or start in warm weather. Treatment is unsatisfactory and relapses are frequent. *Prurigo of pregnancy* occurs in 1 in 300 women in the middle trimester of pregnancy, affecting mainly the abdomen and the exterior surfaces of the limbs. It may recur in later pregnancies.

pruritus *n.* itching, caused by local irritation of the skin or sometimes nervous disorders. The condition is mediated by histamine and other vasoactive chemicals and is the predominant symptom of atopic *eczema, *lichen planus, and many other skin diseases. It also occurs in the elderly and may be a manifestation of psychological illness. Perineal itching is common: itching of the vulva in women (*pruritus vulvae*) may be accompanied by itching of the anal region (*pruritus ani*), although the latter is more common in men. Causes of perineal itching include poor hygiene, *candidiasis, *pinworms, and itchy skin diseases (such as eczema). Pruritus also occurs as a symptom of certain systemic disorders, such as chronic renal failure, *cholestasis, and iron deficiency. Treatment of pruritus is determined by the cause.

prussic acid *see* hydrocyanic acid.

PSA *see* prostate-specific antigen.

psammoma *n.* a tumor containing gritty sandlike particles (*psammoma bodies*). It is typical of cancer of the ovary but may also be found in the meninges (the membranes surrounding the brain).

psellism *n.* a deficiency of articulation of speech, such as *stammering.

pseud- (pseudo-) *prefix denoting* superficial resemblance to; false.

pseudarthrosis (nearthrosis) *n.* a "false" joint, formed around a displaced bone end after dislocation. Congenital hip dislocation may result in a pseudarthrosis. A pseudoarthrosis also forms when a fracture fails to unite and the bone ends are separated by fibrous tissue.

pseudoagglutination *n.* the misleading appearance of clumping during an antiserum-antigen test as a result of incorrect temperature or acidity of the solutions used.

pseudocholinesterase *n.* an enzyme found in the blood and other tissues that – like *cholinesterase – breaks down acetylcholine, but much more slowly. Not being localized at nerve endings, it plays little part in the normal breakdown of acetylcholine in synapses and at neuromuscular junctions.

pseudocoxalgia *n.* see Legg-Calvé-Perthes disease.

pseudocrisis *n.* a false crisis: a sudden but temporary fall of temperature in a patient with fever. The pseudocrisis is followed by a return of the fever.

pseudocroup *n.* spasmodic contraction of the larynx that is not caused by inflammation of the glottis or associated with coughing. It occurs particularly in children with rickets.

pseudocryptorchidism *n.* apparent absence of the testes. This is quite common in young boys, who retract their testes into the groin due to involuntary or reflex contraction of the cremasteric muscle of the suspensory cord. The condition is only important in that it needs to be distinguished from true failure of descent of the testes into the scrotum, which requires early surgical treatment (*see* cryptorchidism).

pseudocyesis (phantom pregnancy, false pregnancy) *n.* a condition in which a nonpregnant woman exhibits symptoms of pregnancy, e.g. enlarged abdomen, increased weight, morning sickness, and absence of menstruation. The condition usually has an emotional basis.

pseudocyst *n.* a fluid-filled space without a proper wall or lining, within an organ. A *pancreatic pseudocyst* may develop in cases of chronic pancreatitis or as a complication of acute pancreatitis. As the pseudocyst, which is filled with enzyme-rich pancreatic juice, slowly expands, it may cause episodes of abdominal pain accompanied by a rise in the level of enzymes in the blood. It may be felt by abdominal examination or seen by radiology or ultrasound examination. Treatment is by surgical drainage, usually by the technique of joining the pseudocyst to the stomach (*marsupialization).

pseudodementia *n.* **1.** a condition in which symptoms of *dementia, including memory disorders, are caused by depression rather than organic brain disease. It is most commonly seen in elderly depressed individuals. **2.** *see* Ganser state.

pseudoexfoliation syndrome the appearance of white dandrufflike deposits on structures in the anterior chamber of the eye, which are especially prominent around the pupil margin and on the anterior lens capsule. It is a sign of zonular weakness and indicates an increased risk of secondary glaucoma.

pseudogout *n.* joint pain and swelling, resembling gout, caused by crystals of calcium pyrophosphate in the synovial membrane and fluid. *See also* chondrocalcinosis.

pseudohermaphroditism *n.* a congenital abnormality in which the external genitalia of a male or a female resemble those of the opposite sex; for example, a woman would have enlarged labia and clitoris, resembling a scrotum and penis, respectively.

pseudohypertrophy *n.* increase in the size of an organ or structure caused by excessive growth of cells that have a packing or supporting role but do not contribute directly to its functioning. The result is usually a decline in the efficiency of the organ although it becomes larger. —**pseudohypertrophic** *adj.*

pseudohypoparathyroidism *n.* a syndrome of mental retardation, restricted growth, and bony abnormalities due to a genetic defect that causes lack of response to the hormone secreted by the *parathyroid glands. Treatment with calcium and vitamin D can reverse most of the features. *See also* Albright's syndrome.

pseudologia fantastica the telling of elaborate and fictitious stories as if they were true. Often some facts are woven into the tissue of lies. While not necessarily a symptom of illness, it is sometimes a feature of chronic mental illness and of personality disorders, particularly antisocial personality disorder.

pseudomembrane *n.* a false membrane, consisting of a layer of exudate on the surface of the skin or a mucous membrane. In diphtheria a pseudomembrane forms in the throat.

pseudomembranous colitis *see* Clostridium.

Pseudomonas *n.* a genus of rodlike motile pigmented gram-negative bacteria. Most live in soil and decomposing organic matter; they are involved in recycling nitrogen, converting nitrates to ammonia or free nitrogen. The species *P. aeruginosa* is pathogenic to humans, occurring in pus from wounds; it is associated with urinary tract infections. *P. pseudomallei* is the causative agent of *melioidosis.

pseudomutuality *n.* a disorder of communication within a family in which a superficial pretence of closeness and reciprocal understanding belies a lack of

real feeling. It has been alleged, but not proved, to be a factor in the backgrounds of schizophrenics.

pseudomyxoma *n.* a mucoid tumor of the peritoneum, often seen in association with *myxomas of the ovary. In *pseudomyxoma peritonei* material from a myxoma, usually in the ovary, is spilled into the peritoneal cavity and continues to be produced within the abdomen, often to massive proportions.

pseudoneuritis *n.* a condition that resembles *optic neuritis but is not due to inflammation. The usual cause is blockage of blood vessels in the optic nerve (*ischemic optic neuropathy*).

pseudo-obstruction *n.* obstruction of the alimentary canal without mechanical narrowing of the bowel. It is usually associated with abnormality of the nerve supply to the muscles of the bowel. *See also* ileus, Hirschsprung's disease.

pseudophakia *n.* the state of the eye after the natural lens has been replaced by a plastic lens implanted inside the eye, approximately in the position previously occupied by the natural lens. This is the current form of surgery for cataract. —**pseudophakic** *adj.*

pseudoplegia *n.* paralysis of the limbs not associated with organic abnormalities. *See also* conversion disorder.

pseudopodium *n.* (*pl.* **pseudopodia**) a temporary and constantly changing extension of the body of an ameba or an ameboid cell (*see* phagocyte). Pseudopodia engulf bacteria and other particles as food and are responsible for the movements of the cell.

pseudopolyposis *n.* a condition in which the bowel lining (mucosa) is covered by elevated or protuberant plaques (called *pseudopolyps*) that are not true *polyps but abnormal growths of inflamed mucosa. It is usually found in patients with chronic ulcerative *colitis. The pseudopolyps may be seen with the *sigmoidoscope or colonoscope (*see* colonoscopy), through which they may be sampled for microscopic examination, or by barium enema examination.

pseudopseudohypoparathyroidism *n.* a condition in which all the symptoms of *pseudohypoparathyroidism are present but the patient's response to parathyroid hormone is normal. It is often found in families affected with pseudo-hypoparathyroidism.

pseudotumor cerebri *see* benign intracranial hypertension.

pseudoxanthoma elasticum a hereditary disease in which elastic fibers (*see* elastic tissue) become calcified. The skin becomes lax and yellowish nodules develop in affected areas; this is accompanied by degenerative changes in the blood vessels and *angioid streaks in the retina.

psilosis *n. see* sprue.

psittacosis (parrot disease, ornithosis) *n.* an endemic infection of birds, especially parrots, budgerigars, canaries, finches, pigeons, and poultry, caused by a small intracellular bacterium, *Chlamydia psittaci*. The birds are often asymptomatic carriers. The infection is transmitted to humans by inhalation from handling the birds or by contact with feathers, feces, or cage dust, but person-to-person transmission also occurs. The symptoms include fever, dry cough, severe muscle pain, and headache; occasionally a severe generalized systemic illness results. The condition responds to tetracycline or erythromycin.

psoas (psoas major) *n.* a muscle in the groin that acts jointly with the iliacus muscle to flex the hip joint (see illustration). A smaller muscle, *psoas minor*, has the same action but is often absent.

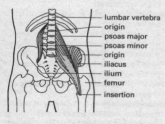

lumbar vertebra
origin
psoas major
psoas minor
origin
iliacus
ilium
femur
insertion

Psoas and iliacus muscles

psoralen *n. see* PUVA.

psoriasis *n.* a chronic skin disease in which itchy scaly red patches form on the elbows, forearms, knees, legs, scalp, and other parts of the body. Psoriasis is one of the most common skin diseases, affecting about 2% of the population, but its cause is not known. The disorder often runs in families and may be brought on by anxiety; it is rare in infants and the elderly, the most common time of onset being in childhood or adolescence. It sometimes occurs in association with arthritis (*see* psoriatic arthritis). Occasionally, the disease may be very severe, affecting much of the skin and causing considerable disability in the patient. While psychological stress may cause an exacerbation of psoriasis, the only significant event that precipitates the disease is a preceding streptococcal infection. Drugs, such as lithium or beta blockers, may occasionally be responsible.

Although there is as yet no cure, treatment of psoriasis has improved greatly in recent years. Tar and *anthralin are still used and topical corticosteroids remain popular. The vitamin D analogue *calcipotriene is a highly effective topical treatment while *PUVA is an effective treatment for moderately severe disease. Systemic therapy, which includes *methotrexate, *retinoids, and *cyclosporine, is reserved for the most severe cases.

psoriatic arthritis arthritis associated with *psoriasis. It occurs in only a small minority of patients with psoriasis but may be painful and disabling. It often affects small joints, such as the terminal joints of the fingers and toes, or the spine (*spondylitis) and sacroiliac joints (*sacroiliitis).

psych- (psycho-) *prefix denoting* **1.** the mind; psyche. **2.** psychology.

psyche *n.* the mind or the soul; the mental (as opposed to the physical) functioning of the individual.

psychedelic *adj.* describing drugs that induce changes in the level of consciousness of the mind. Psychedelic drugs, which include *lysergic acid diethylamide (LSD) and *cannabis, are *hallucinogens and are used legally only for experimental purposes.

psychiatrist *n.* a medically qualified physician who specializes in the study and treatment of mental disorders.

psychiatry *n.* the study of mental disorders and their diagnosis, management, and prevention. —**psychiatric** *adj.*

psychic *adj.* **1.** of or relating to the *psyche. **2.** relating to parapsychological phenomena. **3.** describing a person who is endowed with extrasensory or psychokinetic powers.

psychoanalysis *n.* a school of psychology and a method of treating mental disorders that is based upon the teachings of Sigmund Freud (1856–1939). Psychoanalysis uses the technique of *free association in the course of intensive *psychotherapy in order to bring repressed fears and conflicts to the conscious mind, where they can be dealt with (*see* repression). It stresses the dynamic interplay of unconscious forces and the importance of sexual development in childhood for development of the personality. —**psychoanalyst** *n.* —**psychoanalytic** *adj.*

psychodrama *n.* a form of group psychotherapy in which individuals acquire insight into themselves by acting out situations from their past with other group members. *See* group therapy.

psychogenic *adj.* having an origin in the mind rather than in the body. The term is applied particularly to symptoms and illnesses.

psychogeriatrics *n.* the branch of psychiatry that deals with the mental disorders of old people. —**psychogeriatric** *adj.*

psychokinesis *n.* a supposed ability of some individuals to alter the state of an object by the power of the mind alone, without any physical intervention. *See also* parapsychology.

psycholinguistics *n. see* cognitive psychology.

psychologist *n.* a person who is engaged in the scientific study of the mind. A psychologist may work in a university, in industry, in schools, or in a hospital. A *clinical psychologist* has been trained in aspects of the assessment and treatment of the ill and handicapped. He or she usually works in a hospital, often as one of a multidisciplinary team. An *educational psychologist* has been trained in aspects of the cognitive and emotional development of children. He or she usually works in close association with schools and advises on the management of children.

psychology *n.* the scientific study of behavior and its related mental processes. Psychology is concerned with such matters as memory, rational and irrational thought, intelligence, learning, personality, perceptions, and emotions and their relationship to behavior. Schools of psychology differ in their philosophy and methods. They include the introspectionist Freudian, Jungian, and Adlerian schools and the gestaltist, behaviorist, and cognitive schools; contemporary psychology tends strongly toward the latter (*see* cognitive psychology). The branches of psychology include abnormal, analytic, applied, clinical, comparative, developmental, educational, experimental, geriatric, industrial, infant, physiological, and social psychology and ethology (animal behavior). —**psychological** *adj.*

psychometrics *n.* the measurement of individual differences in psychological functions (such as intelligence and personality) by means of standardized tests. —**psychometric** *adj.*

psychomotor *adj.* relating to muscular and mental activity. The term is applied to disorders in which muscular activities are affected by cerebral disturbance.

psychomotor epilepsy *see* epilepsy.

psychoneuroimmunology *n.* the study of the effects of the mind on the functioning of the immune system, especially in relation to the influence of the mind on susceptibility to disease and the progression of a disease.

psychoneurosis *n.* a *neurosis that is manifested in psychological rather than organic symptoms.

psychopath *n.* a person who behaves in an antisocial way and shows little or no guilt for antisocial acts and little capacity for forming emotional relationships with others. Psychopaths tend to respond poorly to treatment but many improve as they age. *See also* antisocial personality disorder. —**psychopathic** *adj.* —**psychopathy** *n.*

psychopathology *n.* **1.** the study of mental disorders, with the aim of explaining and describing aberrant behavior. *Compare* psychiatry. **2.** the symptoms, collectively, of a mental disorder. —**psychopathological** *adj.*

psychopharmacology *n.* the study of the effects of drugs on mental processes and behavior, particularly *psychotropic drugs.

psychophysiology *n.* the branch of psychology that records physiological measurements, such as the electrical resistance of the skin, the heart rate, the size of the pupil, and the electroencephalogram, and relates them to psychological events. —**psychophysiological** *adj.*

psychosexual development the process by which an individual becomes more mature in his sexual feelings and behavior. Gender identity, sex-role behavior, and choice of sexual partner are the three major areas of development. The phrase is sometimes used specifically for a sequence of stages, supposed by psychoanalytic psychologists to be universal, in which oral, anal, phallic, latency, and genital stages successively occur. These stages reflect the parts of the body on which sexual interest is concentrated during childhood development.

psychosis *n.* a group of mental disorders in which the patient loses contact with reality. The psychoses include *schizophrenia, major disorders of *affect (*see* manic-depressive psychosis), major *paranoid states, and organic mental disorders. Psychotic disorders manifest some of the following: *delusions, *hallucinations, severe thought disturbances, abnormal alteration of mood, poverty of thought, and grossly abnormal behavior. Many cases of psychotic illness respond well to *antipsychotic drugs in that these drugs, while they are being taken, often induce a state of docility, acquiescence, apparent mental normality, and conformity with social norms. —**psychotic** *adj.*

psychosomatic *adj.* relating to or involving both the mind and body: usually applied to illnesses that are caused by the interaction of mental and physical factors. Certain physical illnesses, including asthma, eczema, and peptic ulcer, are thought to be in part a response to psychological and social stresses. Psychological treatments sometimes have a marked effect, but are usually much less effective than physical treatments for such illnesses.

psychosurgery *n.* surgery on the brain to relieve psychological symptoms. The procedure is irreversible and is therefore reserved for the most severe and intractable symptoms, particularly severe chronic anxiety, depression, and untreatable pain. Side effects are common but are less common with modern selective operations. —**psychosurgical** *adj.*

psychotherapy *n.* psychological (as opposed to medical or surgical) methods for the treatment of mental disorders and psychological problems. There are many different approaches to psychotherapy, including *psychoanalysis, *client-centered therapy, *family therapy, and *group therapy. These approaches share the views that the relationship between therapist and client is of prime importance, that the goal is to help personal development and self-understanding generally rather than only to remove symptoms, and that the therapist does not direct the client's decisions. They have all been very widely applied to differing clinical conditions but are of little or no value as treatments of mental illness. *See also* behavior therapy, cognitive therapy, counseling. —**psychotherapeutic** *adj.* —**psychotherapist** *n.*

psychoticism *n.* a dimension of personality derived from psychometric tests, which appears to indicate a degree of emotional coldness and some cognitive impairment.

psychotropic *adj.* describing drugs that affect mood. *Antidepressants, *sedatives, *stimulants, and *antipsychotics are psychotropic.

psychro- *prefix denoting* cold.

psychrophilic *adj.* describing organisms, especially bacteria, that grow best at temperatures of 0–25°C. *Compare* mesophilic, thermophilic.

pterion *n.* the point on the side of the skull at which the sutures between the *parietal, *temporal, and *sphenoid bones meet.

pteroylglutamic acid *see* folic acid.

pterygium *n.* a triangular overgrowth of the cornea, usually the inner side, by thickened and degenerative conjunctiva. It is most commonly seen in people from dry hot dusty climates, and only rarely interferes with vision.

pterygo- *prefix denoting* the pterygoid process of the sphenoid bone. Example: *pterygomaxillary* (of the pterygoid process and the maxilla).

pterygoid process either of two large processes of the *sphenoid bone.

ptomaine *n.* any of various substances produced in decaying foodstuffs and responsible for the unpleasant taste and smell of such foods. These compounds –

which include putrescine, cadaverine, and neurine – were formerly thought to be responsible for food poisoning, but although they are often associated with toxic bacteria they themselves are harmless.

ptosis (blepharoptosis) *n.* drooping of the upper eyelid, for which there are several causes. It may be due to a disorder of the third cranial nerve (*oculomotor nerve), in which case it is likely to be accompanied by paralysis of eye movements causing double vision and an enlarged pupil. When part of *Horner's syndrome, ptosis is accompanied by a small pupil and an absence of sweating on that side of the face. It may be due to *myasthenia gravis, in which the ptosis increases with fatigue and is part of a more widespread fatiguable weakness. Ptosis is associated with the severe pain and other symptoms of a *cluster headache. It may also occur as an isolated congenital feature or as part of a disease of the eye muscles, when it is associated with weak or absent eye movements.

-ptosis *suffix denoting* a lowered position of an organ or part; prolapse. Example: *colpoptosis* (of the vagina).

PTT partial thromboplastin time, also known as activated partial thromboplastin time (*APTT*): a method for estimating the degree of anticoagulation induced by heparin therapy for venous thrombosis.

ptyal- (ptyalo-) *prefix denoting* saliva. Example: *ptyalorrhea* (excessive flow of).

ptyalin *n.* an enzyme (an *amylase) found in saliva.

ptyalism (sialorrhea) *n.* the excessive production of saliva: a symptom of certain nervous disorders, poisoning (by mercury, mushrooms, or organophosphates), or infection (rabies). *Compare* dry mouth.

ptyalography *n. see* sialography.

ptyalolith *n. see* sialolith.

puberty *n.* the time at which the onset of sexual maturity occurs and the reproductive organs become functional (*see* gonadarche). This is manifested in both sexes by the appearance of *secondary sexual characteristics (e.g. deepening of the voice in boys; growth of breasts in girls) and in girls by the start of *menstruation. These changes are brought about by an increase in sex hormone ac-

tivity due to stimulation of the ovaries and testes by pituitary hormones. *See also* adrenarche, androgen, estrogen, precocious puberty. —**pubertal** *adj.*

pubes *n.* **1.** the body surface that overlies the pubis, at the front of the pelvis. It is covered with *pubic hair*. **2.** *see* pubis. —**pubic** *adj.*

pubiotomy *n.* an operation to divide the pubic bone near the symphysis, the front midline where the left and right pubic bones meet. Pubiotomy is now only rarely performed during childbirth if it is necessary to increase the size of an abnormally small pelvis to allow passage of the child and a cesarean section is contraindicated. It is occasionally done in order to facilitate access to the base of the bladder and the urethra during complex urological procedures (e.g. *urethroplasty).

pubis *n.* (*pl.* **pubes**) a bone forming the lower and anterior part of each side of the *hip bone (*see also* pelvis). The two pubes meet at the front of the pelvis at the *pubic symphysis*. *See also* pubes.

Public Health Service (USPHS) the oldest and one of the largest of US federal health agencies. Founded in 1798 to provide medical care for "sick and disabled seamen," the USPHS is now the major health service operating division of the *Department of Health and Human Services and administers eight agencies, including the *Centers for Disease Control and Prevention, the *Food and Drug Administration, the *National Institutes of Health, and the Substance Abuse and Mental Health Services Administration. The agency employs more than 50,000 persons with a total annual budget of nearly 50 billion dollars.

pudendal nerve the nerve that supplies the lowest muscles of the pelvic floor and the anal sphincter. It is often damaged in childbirth, causing incontinence.

pudendum *n.* (*pl.* **pudenda**) the external genital organs, especially those of the female (*see* vulva). —**pudendal** *adj.*

puerperal *adj.* relating to childbirth or the period that immediately follows it.

puerperal depression a state of pathological sadness that sometimes affects a woman soon after the birth of her baby. The condition usually starts suddenly and without warning on the second or third day after delivery and usually resolves in about two months. In most cases the depression is not severe, but in about one case in 1000 it becomes serious enough to require admission to hospital. In these cases careful supervision and treatment are essential as there is a risk that the woman may kill herself or her baby.

puerperal fever blood poisoning (*septicemia) in a mother shortly after childbirth resulting from infection of the lining of the uterus or the vagina, which have been torn or bruised during labor. Increased standards of hygiene in midwifery and the use of such antibiotics as penicillin have reduced the numbers of deaths caused by puerperal fever from the formerly high level almost to nil.

puerperium n. the period of up to about six weeks after childbirth, during which the size of the uterus decreases to normal.

Pulex n. a genus of widely distributed *fleas. *P. irritans*, the human flea, is a common parasite of humans and its bite may give rise to intense irritation and bacterial infection. It is an intermediate host for larvae of the tapeworms *Hymenolepis* and *Dipylidium*, which it can transmit to humans, and it may also be involved in the transmission of plague.

pulicicide (pulicide) n. any chemical agent, for example malathion, used for killing fleas.

pulmo- (pulmon(o)-) *prefix denoting* one or both lungs.

pulmonary adj. relating to, associated with, or affecting the lungs.

pulmonary artery the artery that conveys blood from the heart to the lungs for oxygenation: the only artery in the body containing deoxygenated blood. It leaves the right ventricle and passes upward for 5 cm before dividing into two, one branch going to each lung. Within the lungs each pulmonary artery divides into many fine branches, which end in capillaries in the alveolar walls. *See also* pulmonary circulation.

pulmonary capillary wedge pressure (PCWP) pressure of blood in the left atrium of the heart, which indicates the adequacy of the pulmonary circulation. It is measured using a catheter wedged in the most distal segment of the pulmonary artery. *See also* Swan-Ganz catheter.

pulmonary circulation a system of blood vessels effecting transport of blood between the heart and lungs. Deoxygenated blood leaves the right ventricle by the pulmonary artery and is carried to the alveolar capillaries of the lungs. Gaseous exchange occurs, with carbon dioxide leaving the circulation and oxygen entering. The oxygenated blood then passes into small veins leading to the pulmonary veins, which leave the lungs and return blood to the left atrium of the heart. The oxygenated blood can then be pumped around the body via the *systemic circulation.

pulmonary embolism obstruction of the *pulmonary artery or one of its branches by an *embolus, usually a blood clot derived from *phlebothrombosis of the leg veins (deep vein thrombosis). Large pulmonary emboli result in acute heart failure or sudden death. Smaller emboli cause death of sections of lung tissue, pleurisy, and hemoptysis (coughing of blood). Minor pulmonary emboli respond to the *anticoagulant drugs heparin and warfarin. Major pulmonary embolism is treated by *embolectomy or by dissolution of the blood clot with an infusion of *streptokinase. Recurrent pulmonary embolism may result in *pulmonary hypertension.

pulmonary hypertension a condition in which there is raised blood pressure within the blood vessels supplying the lungs (the pulmonary artery blood pressure is normally much lower than the pressure within the aorta and its branches). Pulmonary hypertension may complicate pulmonary embolism, *septal defects, heart failure, diseases of the mitral valve, and chronic lung diseases. It may also develop without any known cause (*primary pulmonary hypertension*). The right ventricle enlarges and heart failure, fainting, and chest pain occur. The treatment is that of the cause; drugs used to control *hypertension are ineffective.

pulmonary stenosis congenital narrowing of the outlet of the right ventricle of the heart to the pulmonary artery. The defect may be in the pulmonary valve (*valvular stenosis*) or in the outflow tract of the right ventricle below the valve (*infundibular stenosis*). It may be isolated or combined with other heart defects (e.g. *tetralogy of Fallot). Severe pulmonary stenosis may produce angina pectoris, faintness, and heart failure. The defect is corrected by surgery.

pulmonary tuberculosis *see* tuberculosis.

pulmonary vein a vein carrying oxygenated blood from the lung to the left atrium. *See* pulmonary circulation.

pulp *n.* 1. a soft mass of tissue (for example, of the *spleen). 2. the mass of connective tissue in the *pulp cavity*, at the center of a *tooth. It is surrounded by dentine except where it communicates with the rest of the body at the apex. 3. the fleshy cushion on the flexor surface of the fingertip.

pulp capping the procedure of covering an exposed tooth pulp following trauma with a medicament (usually based on calcium hydroxide), which is then covered with a temporary or permanent *restoration.

pulpitis *n.* inflammation of the pulp of a tooth: a frequent cause of toothache.

pulpotomy *n.* a procedure in which part of the pulp of a tooth damaged by trauma or caries is cut back and then covered with a medicament and *restoration.

pulsatile *adj.* characterized by regular rhythmical beating.

pulse *n.* a series of pressure waves within an artery caused by contractions of the left ventricle and corresponding with the heart rate (the number of times the heart beats per minute). It is easily detected on such superficial arteries as the radial artery near the wrist and the carotid artery in the neck. The average adult pulse rate at rest is 60–80 per minute, but exercise, injury, illness, and emotion may produce much faster rates.

pulseless disease *see* Takayasu's disease.

pulseless electrical activity (electromechanical dissociation) the appearance of normal-looking complexes on the electrocardiogram that are, however, associated with a state of *cardiac arrest. It is usually caused by large pulmonary emboli (*see* pulmonary embolism), *cardiac tamponade, tension *pneumothorax, severe disturbance of body salt levels, severe hemorrhage, or hypothermia causing severe lack of oxygen to the heart muscle.

pulsus paradoxus a large fall in systolic blood pressure and pulse volume when the patient breathes in. It is seen in constrictive *pericarditis, pericardial effusion, and asthma.

pulvinar *n.* the expanded posterior end of the *thalamus.

punch-drunk syndrome a group of symptoms consisting of progressive *dementia, tremor of the hands, and epilepsy. It is a consequence of repeated blows to the head that have been severe enough to cause *concussion.

punctum *n.* (*pl.* **puncta**) (in anatomy) a point or small area, especially the *puncta lacrimalia* – the two openings of the tear ducts in the inner corners of the upper and lower eyelids (*see* lacrimal apparatus).

puncture 1. *n.* a wound made accidentally or deliberately by a sharp object or instrument. Puncture wounds need careful treatment because a small entry hole in the skin can disguise serious injury in an underlying organ or tissue. Punctures are also performed for diagnostic purposes, using a hollow needle, in order to withdraw a sample of tissue or fluid for examination; needle punctures are used especially for obtaining tissue samples for the liver, bone marrow, or breast. *See also* lumbar puncture. 2. *vb.* to pierce a tissue with a sharp instrument or needle.

pupil *n.* the circular opening in the center of the *iris, through which light passes into the lens of the eye. —**pupillary** *adj.*

pupillary reflex (light reflex) the reflex change in the size of the pupil according to the amount of light entering the eye. Bright light reaching the retina stimulates nerves of the *parasympathetic nervous system, which cause the pupil to contract. In dim light the pupil opens, due to stimulation of the *sympathetic nervous system. *See also* iris.

purgation *n.* the use of drugs to stimulate intestinal activity and clear the bowels. *See* laxative.

purgative *n. see* laxative.

purine *n.* a nitrogen-containing compound with a two-ring molecular structure. Examples of purines are adenine and guanine, which form the *nucleotides of nucleic acids, and uric acid, which is the end product of purine metabolism.

Purkinje cells nerve cells found in great numbers in the cortex of the cerebellum. The cell body is flask-shaped, with numerous dendrites branching from the neck and extending fanwise among other cells toward the surface and a long axon that runs from the base deep into the cerebellum (see illustration). [J. E. Purkinje (1787–1869), Bohemian physiologist]

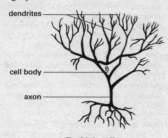

dendrites

cell body

axon

A Purkinje cell

Purkinje fibers *see* atrioventricular bundle. [J. E. Purkinje]

purpura *n.* a skin rash resulting from bleeding into the skin from small blood vessels (capillaries); the individual purple spots of the rash are called *petechiae*. Purpura may be due either to defects in the capillaries (*nonthrombocytopenic purpura*) or to a deficiency of blood platelets (*thrombocytopenic purpura*). Acute *idiopathic thrombocytopenic purpura is a disease of children in which antibodies are produced that destroy the patient's platelets. The child usually recovers without treatment. *See also* Schönlein-Henoch purpura, thrombocytopenia.

purulent *adj.* forming, consisting of, or containing pus.

pus *n.* a thick yellowish or greenish liquid formed at the site of an established infection. Pus contains dead white blood cells, both living and dead bacteria, and fragments of dead tissue. *See also* mucopus, seropus.

pustule *n.* a small pus-containing blister on the skin.

putamen *n.* a part of the lenticular nucleus (*see* basal ganglia).

putrefaction *n.* the process whereby proteins are decomposed by bacteria. This is accompanied by the formation of amines (such as *putrescine* and *cadaverine*) having a strong and very unpleasant smell.

putrescine *n.* an amine formed during *putrefaction.

PUVA (photochemotherapy) *p*soralen + *ul*traviolet *A*: the combination of *psoralen*, a light-sensitive drug, and exposure to long-wave (315–400 nm) ultraviolet light (UVA). It was used in the East in ancient times, using natural sunlight as the light source, for the treatment of *vitiligo. PUVA was introduced into Western medicine in 1973, principally for treating *psoriasis; a number of other conditions also respond. The psoralen is usually taken as tablets but may be administered in a bath. The UVA is administered by means of specially designed light cabinets containing large numbers of fluorescent tubes.

py- (pyo-) *prefix denoting* pus; a purulent condition. Example: *pyoureter* (pus in a ureter).

pyarthrosis *n.* an infected joint filled with pus. Drainage, combined with antibiotic treatment, is necessary, although the joint may already be severely damaged if diagnosis is delayed.

pyel- (pyelo-) *prefix denoting* the pelvis of the kidney. Example: *pyelectasis* (dilation of).

pyelitis *n.* inflammation of the pelvis of the kidney (the part of the kidney from which urine drains into the ureter). This is usually caused by a bacterial infection, which may develop in any condition causing obstruction to the flow of urine. The patient experiences pain in the loins, shivering, and a high temperature. Treatment is by the administration of a suitable antibiotic, together with analgesics and a high fluid intake. Any underlying abnormality of the urinary system must be relieved to prevent further attacks.

pyelocystitis *n.* inflammation of the renal pelvis and urinary bladder (*see* pyelitis, cystitis).

pyelogram *n.* *see* pyelography.

pyelography (urography) *n.* X-ray examination of the pelvis of the kidney using *radiopaque contrast material. In *intravenous urography (excretion urography)* the contrast medium is injected into a vein and is concentrated and excreted by the kidneys (*see* intravenous urogram). In *retrograde pyelography*, fine catheters are passed up the ureter to the kidney at *cystoscopy and contrast material is injected directly into the renal pelvis to allow X-ray examination. The

X-ray pictures obtained from these procedures are called *pyelograms* or *urograms*.

pyelolithotomy *n.* surgical removal of a stone from the kidney through an incision made in the pelvis of the kidney. The incision is usually made into the posterior surface of the pelvis (*posterior pyelotomy*) to gain access to the stone, which can then be lifted clear.

pyelonephritis *n.* bacterial infection of the kidney substance. In *acute pyelonephritis*, the patient has pain in the loins, a high temperature, and shivering. Treatment is by the administration of an appropriate antibiotic, and a full urological investigation is conducted to determine any underlying abnormality and prevent recurrence. In *chronic pyelonephritis*, the kidneys become small and scarred and kidney failure ensues. *Vesicoureteric reflux in childhood is one of the causes.

pyeloplasty *n.* an operation to relieve obstruction at the junction of the pelvis of the kidney and the ureter. *See* hydronephrosis, Dietl's crisis.

pyelotomy *n.* surgical incision into the pelvis of the kidney. This operation is usually undertaken to remove a stone (*see* pyelolithotomy) but is also necessary when surgical drainage of the kidney is required by a catheter or tube.

pyemia *n.* blood poisoning by pus-forming bacteria released from an abscess. Widespread formation of abscesses may develop, with fatal results. *Compare* sapremia, septicemia, toxemia.

Pyemotes *n.* a genus (formerly called *Pediculoides*) of widely distributed tiny predaceous mites. *P. ventricosus* occasionally attacks humans and causes an allergic dermatitis called *grain itch*. This complaint most usually affects those people coming into contact with stored cereal products, such as hay and grain.

pyg- (pygo-) *prefix denoting* the buttocks.

pykno- *prefix denoting* thickness or density.

pyknosis *n.* the process in which the cell nucleus is thickened into a dense mass, which occurs when cells die. —**pyknotic** *adj.*

pyl- (pyle-) *prefix denoting* the portal vein.

pylephlebitis (portal pyemia) *n.* septic inflammation and thrombosis of the hepatic portal vein. This is a rare result of the spread of infection within the abdomen (as from appendicitis). The condition causes severe illness, with fever, liver abscesses, and *ascites. Treatment is by antibiotic drugs and surgical drainage of abscesses.

pylethrombosis *n.* obstruction of the portal vein by a blood clot (*see* thrombosis). It can result from infection of the umbilicus in infants, pylephlebitis, cirrhosis of the liver, and liver tumors. *Portal hypertension is a frequent result.

pylor- (pyloro-) *prefix denoting* the pylorus. Example: *pyloroduodenal* (of the pylorus and duodenum).

pylorectomy *n.* a surgical operation in which the muscular outlet of the stomach (*pylorus) is removed. *See* antrectomy, pyloroplasty.

pyloric stenosis narrowing of the muscular outlet of the stomach (*pylorus). This causes delay in passage of the stomach contents to the duodenum, which leads to repeated vomiting (sometimes of food eaten more than 24 hours earlier), and sometimes visible distension and movement of the stomach. If the condition persists the patient loses weight, becomes dehydrated, and develops *alkalosis. *Congenital hypertrophic pyloric stenosis* occurs in babies about 3–5 weeks old (particularly boys) in which the thickened pyloric muscle can be felt as a nodule. Treatment is by the surgical operation of *pyloromyotomy (Ramstedt's operation). Recovery is usually complete and the condition does not recur. Pyloric stenosis in adults is caused either by a *peptic ulcer close to the pylorus or by a cancerous growth invading the pylorus. Stenosis from peptic ulceration may be treated by healing the ulcer with an *antisecretory drug and dilating the pylorus with a *balloon, or by surgical removal or bypass (*see* gastroenterostomy). Surgery is required for cancerous obstruction.

pyloromyotomy (Ramstedt's operation) *n.* a surgical operation in which the muscle around the outlet of the stomach (pylorus) is divided down to the lining (mucosa) in order to relieve congenital *pyloric stenosis.

pyloroplasty *n.* a surgical operation in which the outlet of the stomach (pylorus) is widened by a form of reconstruction. It is done to allow the contents of the stomach to pass more easily into the duodenum, particularly after *vagotomy to treat peptic ulcers (which would otherwise cause delay in gastric emptying).

pylorospasm n. closure of the outlet of the stomach (pylorus) due to muscle spasm, leading to delay in the passage of stomach contents to the duodenum and vomiting. It is usually associated with duodenal or pyloric ulcers.

pylorus n. the lower end of the *stomach, which leads to the duodenum. It terminates at a ring of muscle – the *pyloric sphincter* – which contracts to close the opening by which the stomach communicates with the duodenum. —**pyloric** adj.

pyo- prefix. see py-.

pyocele n. a swelling caused by an accumulation of pus in a part of the body.

pyocolpos n. the presence of pus in the vagina.

pyocyanin n. an antibiotic substance produced by the bacterium *Pseudomonas aeruginosa* and active principally against gram-positive bacteria.

pyoderma n. any infected skin disease in which pus is produced.

pyoderma gangrenosum an acute destructive ulcerating process of the skin, especially the legs. It may be associated with ulcerative *colitis or *Crohn's disease or with *rheumatoid arthritis or other forms of arthritis affecting many joints. Treatment is with cyclosporine or with high doses of corticosteroids or other immunosuppressants.

pyogenic adj. causing the formation of pus. Pyogenic bacteria include *Staphylococcus aureus*, *Streptococcus hemolyticus*, and *Neisseria gonorrhoeae*.

pyogenic granuloma a common rapidly growing nodule on the surface of the skin; it resembles a red currant or, if large, a raspberry. It is composed of small blood vessels and therefore bleeds readily after the slightest injury. The nodule never becomes malignant and is treated by *curettage and cautery; it may recur and require excision.

pyometra n. the presence of pus in the uterus.

pyometritis n. inflammation of the uterus, with the formation of pus.

pyomyositis n. bacterial or fungal infection of a muscle resulting in painful inflammation.

pyonephrosis n. obstruction and infection of the kidney resulting in pus formation. A kidney stone is the usual cause of the obstruction, and the kidney becomes distended by pus and destroyed by the inflammation, which extends into the kidney substance itself and sometimes into the surrounding tissues (see perinephritis). Treatment is urgent *nephrectomy under antibiotic cover.

pyopneumothorax n. pus and gas or air in the *pleural cavity. The condition can arise if gas is produced by gas-forming bacteria as part of an *empyema or if air is introduced during attempts to drain the pus from an empyema. Alternatively, a *hydropneumothorax may become infected.

pyosalpingitis n. inflammation of a fallopian tube, with the formation of pus.

pyosalpingo-oophoritis n. inflammation of an ovary and fallopian tube, with the formation of pus.

pyosalpinx n. the accumulation of pus in a fallopian tube.

pyosis n. the formation and discharge of pus.

pyothorax n. see empyema.

pyr- (pyro-) prefix denoting 1. fire. 2. a burning sensation. 3. fever.

pyramid n. 1. one of the conical masses that make up the medulla of the *kidney, extending inward from a base inside the cortex toward the pelvis of the kidney. 2. one of the elongated bulging areas on the anterior surface of the *medulla oblongata in the brain, extending downward to the spinal cord. 3. one of the divisions of the vermis of the *cerebellum in the middle lobe. 4. a protrusion of the medial wall of the vestibule of the middle ear.

pyramidal cell a type of neuron found in the *cerebral cortex, with a pyramid-shaped cell body, a branched dendrite extending from the apex toward the brain surface, several dendrites extending horizontally from the base, and an axon running in the white matter of the hemisphere.

pyramidal system a collection of nerve fibers in the central nervous system that extend from the *motor cortex in the brain to the spinal cord and are responsible for initiating movement. In the medulla oblongata the fibers form a *pyramid (hence the name), within which they cross from one side of the brain to the opposite side of the spinal cord; this is called the *decussation of the pyramids*. Damage to the pyramidal system manifests in a specific pattern of weakness in the face, arms, and legs, abnormally brisk reflexes, and an extensor *plantar reflex (Babinski reflex).

pyrantel *n.* an *anthelmintic drug used to treat infestations with intestinal worms, especially roundworms and pinworms. It is administered by mouth. Side effects occur only with large doses and include headache, dizziness, skin rash, and fever. Trade names: **Antiminth, Pin-Rid, Pin-X**.

pyrazinamide *n.* a drug administered by mouth, usually in combination with other drugs, to treat tuberculosis. Side effects may include digestive upsets, joint pains, gout, fever, and rashes, and high doses may cause liver damage. Trade name: **Tebrazid**.

pyret- (pyreto-) *prefix denoting* fever.

pyrexia *n. see* fever.

pyridostigmine *n.* an *anticholinesterase drug used in the treatment of *myasthenia gravis. It is administered by mouth or injection; side effects may include nausea, vomiting, abdominal pain, diarrhea, sweating, and increased salivation. Trade name: **Mestinon**.

pyridoxal phosphate a derivative of vitamin B_6 that is an important *coenzyme in certain reactions of amino acid metabolism. *See* transamination.

pyridoxine *n. see* vitamin B_6.

pyrilamine *n.* an *antihistamine drug administered by mouth or injection to treat allergies and sensitivity reactions and applied as a cream to treat skin allergies and itching. Drowsiness is a common side effect and digestive upsets may occur.

pyrimethamine *n.* a drug administered by mouth for the prevention and treatment of *malaria, either alone or in combination with dapsone. It is also used in the treatment of *toxoplasmosis. Possible side effects include loss of appetite and vomiting, and prolonged use may interfere with red blood cell production. Trade name: **Daraprim**.

pyrimidine *n.* a nitrogen-containing compound with a ring molecular structure. The most common pyrimidines are cytosine, thymine, and uracil, which form the *nucleotides of nucleic acids.

pyrogen *n.* any substance or agent producing fever. —**pyrogenic** *adj*.

pyromania *n.* an excessively strong impulse to set things on fire. —**pyromaniac** *adj.*, *n.*

pyrosis *n. see* heartburn.

pyruvic acid (pyruvate) a compound, derived from carbohydrates, that may be oxidized via a complex series of reactions in the *Krebs cycle to yield carbon dioxide and energy in the form of ATP.

pyrvinium *n.* a drug administered by mouth for the treatment of pinworm infestation. It has low toxicity but may cause nausea and vomiting. It stains the stools a red color. Trade name: **Vanquin**.

pyuria *n.* the presence of pus in the urine, making it cloudy. This is a sign of bacterial infection in the urinary tract.

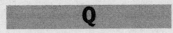

Q

qat *n. see* khat.

Q fever an acute infectious disease of many animals, including cattle, sheep, goats, deer, and dogs, that is caused by a *rickettsia, *Coxiella burnetii*; it can be transmitted to humans primarily through inhalation of infected particles or consumption of contaminated unpasteurized milk but also via ticks, which can act as vectors. After an incubation period of up to three weeks a severe influenza-like illness develops, sometimes with pneumonia. The disease lasts about two weeks; treatment with tetracyclines or chloramphenicol is effective. *See also* typhus.

qinghaosu *n.* a Chinese herbal drug used for 2000 years to treat *malaria. The active ingredient is a sesquiterpene lactone that greatly reduces the number of malarial parasites in the blood.

QRS complex the element of an *electrocardiogram that precedes the *S–T segment and indicates ventricular contraction.

Q–T interval the interval on an *electrocardiogram that contains the deflections that are produced by ventricular contraction.

quadrantanopia *n.* absence or loss of one quarter of the *visual field, i.e. upper nasal (inner), upper temporal (outer), lower nasal (inner), or lower temporal (outer).

quadrate lobe one of the lobes of the *liver.

quadratus *n.* any of various four-sided muscles. The *quadratus femoris* is a flat muscle at the head of the femur, responsible for lateral rotation of the thigh.

quadri- *prefix denoting* four. Example: *quadrilateral* (having four sides).

quadriceps *n.* one of the great extensor muscles of the legs. It is situated in the thigh and is subdivided into four distinct portions: the *rectus femoris* (which also flexes the thigh), *vastus lateralis, vastus*

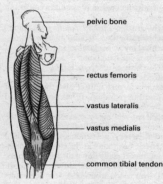

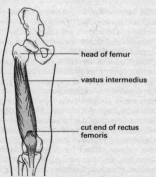

Components of the quadriceps femoris

medialis, and *vastus intermedius* (see illustration).

quadriplegia (tetraplegia) *n.* paralysis affecting all four limbs. —**quadriplegic** *adj.*, *n.*

quantitative digital radiography a method of detecting *osteoporosis. A narrow X-ray beam is directed at the area of interest (usually the spine and hip), which enables a measurement to be made of its calcium content (density). In this way the likelihood of fracture can be assessed and preventive measures considered, e.g. *hormone replacement therapy.

quarantine *n.* the period for which a person (or animal) is kept in isolation to prevent the spread of a contagious disease. The original quarantine was a period of 40 days, but different diseases now have different quarantine periods.

quartan fever *see* malaria.

Queckenstedt test a part of the routine *lumbar puncture procedure. It is used to determine whether or not the flow of cerebrospinal fluid is blocked in the spinal canal. [H. H. G. Queckenstedt (1876–1918), German physician]

quellung reaction a reaction in which antibodies against the bacterium *Streptococcus pneumoniae* combine with the bacterial capsule, which thus becomes swollen and visible to light microscopy.

quickening *n.* the first movement of a fetus in the uterus that is felt by the mother. Quickening is usually experienced after about 16 weeks of pregnancy, although it may occur earlier.

quiescent *adj.* describing a disease that is in an inactive or undetectable phase.

quinacrine *n.* a drug used to treat various infections and infestations, particularly malaria, giardiasis, and teniasis. It is administered by mouth. Digestive upsets and headache may occur and the skin often turns yellow. Trade names: **Atabrine, Mepacrine**.

quinapril *n.* an *ACE inhibitor used to treat high blood pressure, either alone or in combination with thiazide diuretics, and as *adjunct therapy in the treatment of heart failure. It is administered orally; common side effects include dizziness, headache, stomach upset, and nausea. Trade names: **Accupril, Accuretic**.

quinidine *n.* a drug that slows down the activity of the heart and is administered by mouth in order to control abnormal and increased heart rhythm. Digestive upsets and symptoms of *cinchonism may occur as side effects. Trade names: **Cardioquin, Quinaglute, Quinidex, Quinora.**

quinine n. a drug formerly used to prevent and treat *malaria, now largely replaced by more effective, less toxic drugs except in cases of malaria due to *Plasmodium falciparum.* It is administered by mouth or injection; large doses can cause severe poisoning, symptoms of which include headache, fever, vomiting, confusion, and damage to the eyes and ears (*see* cinchonism). Small doses of quinine are used to treat muscular cramps.

quinism n. the symptoms of overdosage or too prolonged treatment with quinine. See cinchonism.

quinolone n. one of a group of chemically related synthetic antibiotics that includes *ciprofloxacin, *nalidixic acid, *ofloxacin, and *enoxacin.* These drugs act by inactivating an enzyme, DNA gyrase, that is necessary for replication of the microorganisms and are often useful for treating infections with organisms that have become resistant to other antibiotics. They are administered by mouth. Possible side effects include nausea, vomiting, diarrhea, abdominal pain, headache, dizziness, and itching. Confusion, joint pains, skin troubles, and tendinitis occasionally occur.

quinsy n. pus in the space between the tonsil and the wall of the pharynx. The patient has severe pain with difficulty opening the mouth (*trismus) and swallowing. Treatment is with antibiotics. Surgical incision of the abscess may be necessary to release the collection of pus. Medical name: **peritonsillar abscess.**

quotidian fever see malaria.

Q wave the downward deflection on an *electrocardiogram that indicates the beginning of ventricular contraction.

R

rabbit fever see tularemia.

rabies (hydrophobia) n. an acute virus disease of the central nervous system that affects all warm-blooded animals and is usually transmitted to humans by a bite from an infected dog. Symptoms appear after an incubation period ranging from 10 days to over a year and include malaise, fever, difficulty in breathing, salivation, periods of intense excitement, and painful muscle spasms of the throat induced by swallowing. In the later stages of the disease the mere sight of water induces convulsions and paralysis; death occurs within 4–5 days. Protection is possible by a rabies vaccine. Daily injections of rabies vaccine, together with an injection of rabies antiserum, may prevent the disease from developing in a person bitten by an infected animal. —**rabid** adj.

racemose adj. resembling a bunch of grapes. The term is applied particularly to a compound gland the secretory part of which consists of a number of small sacs.

rachi- (rachio-) prefix denoting the spine.

rachianesthesia n. *spinal anesthesia.

rachiotomy n. see laminectomy.

rachis n. see backbone.

rachischisis n. see spina bifida.

rachitic adj. afflicted with rickets.

rad n. a former unit of absorbed dose of ionizing radiation. It has been replaced by the *gray.

radial adj. relating to or associated with the radius (a bone in the forearm).

radial artery a branch of the brachial artery, beginning at the elbow and passing superficially down the forearm to the styloid process of the radius at the wrist. It then winds around the wrist and enters the palm of the hand, sending out branches to the fingers.

radial keratotomy an operation for nearsightedness (myopia). Deep cuts into the tissue of the cornea are placed radially around the outer two-thirds of the cornea; this flattens the curvature of the central part of the cornea and reduces the myopia. This procedure, used only for slight degrees of myopia, is being superseded by *excimer laser treatment.

radial nerve an important mixed sensory and motor nerve of the arm, forming the largest branch of the *brachial plexus. It extends downward behind the humerus, supplying muscles of the upper arm, to the elbow, which it supplies with branches, and then runs parallel with the radius. It supplies sensory branches to the base of the thumb and a small area of the back of the hand.

radial reflex flection of the forearm (and sometimes also of the fingers) that occurs when the lower end of the radius is tapped. It is due to contraction of the brachioradialis muscle, which is stimulated by tapping its point of insertion in the radius.

radiation *n.* energy in the form of waves or particles, especially *electromagnetic radiation*, which includes (in order of increasing wavelength), *gamma rays, *X-rays, *ultraviolet rays, visible light, and infrared rays (radiant heat), and the particles.

radiation sickness an acute illness caused by extreme exposure to rays emitted by radioactive substances, e.g. X-rays or gamma rays. Very high doses cause death within hours from destructive lesions of the central nervous system. Lower doses, which may still prove fatal, cause immediate symptoms of nausea, vomiting, and diarrhea followed after a week or more by bleeding and other symptoms of damage to the bone marrow, loss of hair, and bloody diarrhea. Some of these milder symptoms can occur after *radiotherapy during treatment of cancer.

radical treatment vigorous treatment that aims at the complete cure of a disease rather than the mere relief of symptoms. *Compare* conservative treatment.

radicle *n.* (in anatomy) **1.** a small *root. **2.** the initial fiber of a nerve or the origin of a vein. —**radicular** *adj.*

radiculitis *n.* inflammation of the root of a nerve. *See* polyradiculitis.

radio- *prefix denoting* **1.** radiation. **2.** a radioactive substance.

radioactive iodine therapy the administration of an estimated amount of the radioactive isotope iodine-131 as a drink in order to treat an overactive thyroid gland (*see* thyrotoxicosis). The iodine concentrates in the thyroid and thus delivers its beta radiation locally, with little effect on other tissues. The gland will shrink and become euthyroid over the succeeding 8–12 weeks but there is a high incidence of subsequent hypothyroidism (up to 80%), which requires lifetime treatment with thyroxine. The treatment cannot be used if there is any possibility of pregnancy, and the patient must stay away from young children and pregnant women for around ten days after ad-

ministration. Despite these drawbacks, radioactive iodine remains a popular form of treatment for any cause of hyperthyroidism.

radioactivity *n.* disintegration of the nuclei of certain elements, with the emission of energy in the form of alpha, beta, or gamma rays. As particles are emitted, the elements decay into other elements. Naturally occurring radioactive elements include radium and uranium. There are many artificially produced isotopes, including iodine-131 and cobalt-60, which are used in *radiotherapy, and technetium-99m used in *nuclear medicine. *See also* radioisotope. —**radioactive** *adj.*

radioallergosorbent test (RAST) an in-vitro *radioimmunoassay test to determine sensitivity to specific *allergens that cause allergic reactions in hypersensitive persons. The person's serum is mixed with various allergens bound to a radio-labeled substance. If an allergy exists, an antigen–antibody clumping reaction occurs.

radioautography *n. see* autoradiography.

radiobiology *n.* the study of the effects of radiation on living cells and organisms. Studies of the behavior of cancer cells exposed to radiation have important applications in *radiotherapy, revealing why some tumors fail to respond to the treatment; this has led to the development of new radiotherapy techniques that make tumors more susceptible to attack by radiation.

radiodermatitis *n.* inflammation of the skin after exposure to ionizing radiation. This may occur after a short dose of heavy radiation (radiotherapy or atomic explosions) or prolonged exposure to small doses, as may happen accidentally to X-ray workers. The skin becomes dry, hairless, and atrophied, losing its coloring. Infection is common.

radiographer *n.* **1.** (**diagnostic radiographer**) a person trained in the technique of taking X-ray pictures of parts of the body. In modern practice a radiographer may need to be experienced in all other imaging techniques, including *magnetic resonance imaging, *ultrasound, and *nuclear medicine. *See* radiography. **2.** (**therapeutic radiographer**) a person who is trained in the technique of treatment by *radiotherapy.

radiography *n.* diagnostic radiology: traditionally, the technique of examining the body by directing *X-rays through it to produce images (*radiographs*) on photographic film or a *fluoroscope. Increasingly radiography includes the production of images by *computed tomography and *nuclear medicine. It is used to produce images of disease in all parts of the body, to be interpreted by radiologists for physicians and surgeons. It is also widely used in dentistry for detecting dental caries, periodontal disease, periapical disease, the presence and position of unerupted teeth, and disease of the jaws. *See also* radiographer, radiology.

radioimmunoassay *n.* the technique of using radioactive *tracers to estimate the concentration of an antigen, antibody, or other substance in the blood through its ability to bind to the radioactively labeled material. It is widely used in the estimation of hormone levels. For example, radioactive iodine may be used to label the hormone insulin. In some diabetic patients insulin provokes the formation of anti-insulin antibodies, which combine with the insulin. After the injection of the tracer insulin, samples of the patient's blood are analyzed by *electrophoresis or *chromatography, and the antibody components of the blood are tested for the presence of radioactivity.

radioimmunolocalization *n.* a method of identifying the site of a tumor (e.g. colorectal cancer) that relies on its uptake of radioactive isotopes attached to an appropriate anticancer immune cell. As yet this technique is little used in clinical practice.

radioisotope *n.* an *isotope of an element that emits alpha, beta, or gamma radiation during its decay into another element. Artificial radioisotopes, produced by bombarding elements with beams of neutrons, are widely used in medicine as *tracers and as sources of radiation for the different techniques of *radiotherapy.

radiologist *n.* a doctor specialized in the use and interpretation of X-rays and other imaging techniques for the diagnosis of disease. An *interventional radiologist* specializes in the use of imaging to guide *interventional radiology techniques.

radiology *n.* the branch of medicine involving the study of radiographs or other imaging technologies (such as *ultrasound and *magnetic resonance imaging) to diagnose or treat disease. A physician who specializes in this field is known as a *radiologist. *See also* interventional radiology, radiography (diagnostic radiology), radiotherapy (therapeutic radiology).

radiolucent *adj.* having the property of being transparent to X-rays. Radiopacity decreases with atomic number of the element. Radiolucent materials, such as beryllium, are used to construct windows in X-ray tubes to allow the X-rays to escape from the tube. Gases are relatively radiolucent to X-rays and can be used as a negative *contrast medium in X-ray examinations, e.g. in *doublecontrast barium examinations of the bowel or carbon dioxide *angiography.

radionecrosis *n.* death (*necrosis) of tissue, most commonly bone or skin, caused by exposure to ionizing radiation, as in *radiotherapy. It can be induced by subsequent injury or surgery. *See* ionization.

radionuclide *n.* a substance containing a radioactive atomic nucleus. Radionuclides can be used as *tracers for diagnosis in *nuclear medicine.

radiopaque *adj.* having the property of absorbing, and therefore being opaque to, X-rays. Radiopacity increases with atomic weight. Radiopaque materials, such as those containing iodine or barium, are used as *contrast media in radiography. Metallic foreign bodies in tissues are also radiopaque and can be detected by radiography. Such heavy elements as lead and barium can be used in shielding to protect people from unnecessary exposure to ionizing radiation. —**radiopacity** *n.*

radio pill a capsule containing a miniature radio transmitter that can be swallowed by a patient. During its passage through the digestive tract it transmits information about internal conditions (acidity, etc.) that can be monitored by means of a radio receiver near the patient. Such capsules can now contain video cameras and light sources to examine the bowel.

radioscopy *n.* examination of an X-ray

image on a fluorescent screen (see fluoroscope).

radiosensitive adj. describing certain forms of cancer cells that are particularly susceptible to radiation and are likely to be dealt with successfully by radiotherapy.

radiosensitizer n. a substance that increases the sensitivity of cells to radiation. The presence of oxygen and other compounds with a high affinity for electrons will increase radiosensitivity. Chemotherapy drugs such as fluorouracil can be used concurrently with radiotherapy as radiosensitizers.

radiotherapy n. therapeutic radiology: the treatment of disease with penetrating radiation, such as X-rays, beta rays, or gamma rays, which may be produced by machines or given off by radioactive isotopes. Beams of radiation may be directed at a diseased part from a distance (see teletherapy), or radioactive material, in the form of needles, wires, or pellets, may be implanted in the body (see brachytherapy). Many forms of cancer are destroyed by radiation, the chief problem being the risk of damage to normal tissues.

radium n. a radioactive metallic element that emits alpha and gamma rays during its decay into other elements. Gamma radiation was formerly used in *radiotherapy for the treatment of cancer. Because *radon, a radioactive gas, is released from radium, the metal was enclosed in gas-tight containers during use. Radium is stored in lead-lined containers, which give protection from the radiation. Symbol: Ra.

radius n. the outer and shorter bone of the forearm (compare ulna). It partially revolves about the ulna, permitting *pronation and *supination of the hand. The head of the radius articulates with the *humerus. The lower end articulates both with the scaphoid and lunate bones of the *carpus (wrist) and with the ulna (via the ulnar notch on the side of the bone). —**radial** adj.

radix n. see root.

radon n. a radioactive gaseous element that is produced during the decay of *radium. Sealed in small capsules called radon seeds, it is used in *radiotherapy for the treatment of cancer, but has largely been replaced by newer agents

and techniques. It emits alpha and gamma radiation. Symbol: Rn.

rale n. see crepitation.

raloxifene n. a drug used to prevent osteoporosis that develops after the menopause. It mimics the protective action of estrogen in the bones by acting selectively on estrogen receptors; unlike *hormone replacement therapy, it does not relieve menopausal symptoms. It is administered by mouth; side effects include hot flashes, and there is a risk of *thromboembolism and *thrombophlebitis. Trade name: **Evista**.

ramipril n. see ACE inhibitor.

Ramsay Hunt syndrome a form of *herpes zoster affecting the facial nerve, associated with facial paralysis and loss of taste. It also produces pain in the ear and other parts supplied by the nerve. [J. R. Hunt (1872–1937), US neurologist]

Ramstedt's operation see pyloromyotomy. [W. C. Ramstedt (1867–1963), German surgeon]

ramus n. (pl. **rami**) **1.** a branch, especially of a nerve fiber or blood vessel. **2.** a thin process projecting from a bone, e.g. the rami of the *mandible.

Randall's plaque the initial deposit of calcium-loaded material on a renal *pyramid that develops into a kidney stone. [A. Randall (1883–1951), US urologist]

randomized controlled trial see intervention study.

random sample a subgroup of a total population (the so-called universe) selected by a random process ensuring that each member of the universe has an equal chance of being included in the sample. It is sometimes stratified so that separate samples are drawn from each of several layers of the universe, usually on the basis of age, sex, and socioeconomic group. Selection is sometimes facilitated by identifying, in advance, groups of individuals (e.g. townships or neighborhoods) whom it is deemed will together represent the whole (a so-called sampling frame).

ranitidine n. an H_2-receptor antagonist (see antihistamine) that inhibits gastric secretion and is used to treat gastric and duodenal ulcers, gastroesophageal reflux disease, and the *Zollinger-Ellison syndrome. It is administered by mouth, intravenously, and intramuscularly; side effects include headache, rash, and drowsiness. Trade name: **Zantac**.

ranula *n.* a cyst found under the tongue, formed when the duct leading from a salivary or mucous gland is obstructed and distended.

rape *n.* sexual intercourse that is performed by force and without consent. Rape is a criminal act of violence (legal definitions vary from state to state) and victims should be evaluated for trauma and the need for medical and psychological treatment.

raphe *n.* a line, ridge, seam, or crease in a tissue or organ, especially the line marking the junction of two embryologically distinct parts that have fused to form a single structure in the adult. For example, the *raphe of the tongue* is the furrow that passes down the center of the dorsal surface of the tongue.

rarefaction *n.* thinning of bony tissue sufficient to cause decreased density of bone to X-rays, as in osteoporosis.

rash *n.* a temporary eruption on the skin, usually typified by reddening – either discrete red spots or generalized reddening – which may be accompanied by itching. A rash may be a local skin reaction or the outward sign of a disorder affecting the body. Rashes commonly occur with infectious diseases, such as chickenpox and measles, or as a reaction to drugs.

Rasmussen's encephalitis a rare, progressive central nervous system disorder, found most commonly in children, that results in continual focal seizures (*see* epilepsy). The underlying cause is unknown but it may be due to a viral infection. Patients who are unresponsive to medical (antiepileptic) therapy may undergo surgery of the abnormal brain to try and control the seizures. [G. L. Rasmussen (1904–   ), US anatomist]

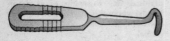

A rib raspatory

raspatory *n.* a filelike surgical instrument used for scraping the surface of bone (see illustration).

RAST *see* radioallergosorbent test.

rat-bite fever (sodoku) a disease, contracted from the bite of a rat, due to infection by either the bacterium *Spirillum minus*, which causes ulceration of the skin and recurrent fever, or by the fungus *Streptobacillus moniliformis*, which causes inflammation of the skin, muscular pains, and vomiting. Both infections respond well to penicillin.

rationalization *n.* (in psychiatry) the explanation of events or behavior in terms that avoid giving the true reasons. For example, a patient may explain not going to a party in terms of being too tired whereas he did not go because he was afraid of meeting new people.

rauwolfia *n.* the dried root of the shrub *Rauwolfia serpentina*, which contains several alkaloids, including *reserpine*. Rauwolfia and its alkaloids lower blood pressure and depress activity of the central nervous system. They were formerly used as tranquilizers and to treat hypertension, but have been replaced by more effective and reliable drugs.

Raynaud's disease a condition of unknown cause in which the arteries of the fingers are unduly reactive and become spastic (*angiospasm* or *vasospasm*) when the hands are cold. This produces attacks of pallor, numbness, and discomfort in the fingers. A similar condition (*Raynaud's phenomenon*) may result from atherosclerosis, connective tissue diseases, ingestion of ergot derivatives, or the frequent use of vibrating tools. Gangrene or ulceration of the fingertips may result from lack of blood to the affected part. Warm gloves and peripheral *vasodilators may relieve the condition. In unresponsive cases *sympathectomy is of value. [M. Raynaud (1834–81), French physician]

reaction formation (in psychoanalysis) a *defense mechanism by which unacceptable unconscious ideas are replaced by the opposite conscious attitude. For instance, a man might make an ostentatious show of affection to a person for whom he has an unconscious hatred.

reactive *adj.* describing mental illnesses that are precipitated by events in the psychological environment.

reactive hypoglycemia a condition of postprandial *hypoglycemia, of varying severity, induced by excessive levels of insulin release from the pancreas. It can be divided into "early" or "late" forms, depending on whether the insulin release occurs less than or more than three hours after the meal. The "early" form is due to the rapid discharge of ingested carbohydrate from the stomach into the small bowel, immediately triggering hyperinsulinemia. It can occur without obvious cause but is most commonly associated with upper-bowel surgery. The "late" form is due to a loss of the early-phase insulin response causing excessive postprandial *hyperglycemia, which then itself triggers an exaggerated insulin response with subsequent hypoglycemia.

reagin *n.* a type of *antibody, formed against an allergen, that has special affinity for cell membranes and remains fixed in various tissues. Subsequent contact with the allergen causes damage to the tissue when the antigen-antibody reaction occurs. The damaged cells, particularly *mast cells, release histamine and serotonin, which are responsible for the local inflammation of an allergy or the very severe effects of anaphylactic shock (*see* anaphylaxis). Reagins belong to the E class of *immunoglobulins.

real-time imaging the rapid acquisition and manipulation of ultrasound information from a scanning probe by electronic circuits to enable images to be produced on TV screens almost instantaneously. The operator can place the scanning probe accurately on the region of interest in order to observe its structure and appreciate moving structures within it (*see* Doppler ultrasonography). Using similar techniques, the instantaneous display of other imaging modalities, such as *computed tomography scanning and *magnetic resonance imaging, can now be achieved. Real-time imaging is useful in guiding *interventional radiology procedures, for example, allowing a needle to be guided accurately as it is passed into the body.

reamer *n.* an instrument used in *endodontics to prepare the walls of a root canal for *root treatment.

receptaculum *n.* the dilated portion of a tubular anatomical part. The *receptaculum* (or *cisterna*) *chyli* is the dilated end of the *thoracic duct, into which lymph vessels from the lower limbs and intestines drain.

receptor *n.* **1.** a cell or group of cells specialized to detect changes in the environment and trigger impulses in the sensory nervous system. All sensory nerve endings act as receptors, whether they simply detect touch, as in the skin, or chemical substances, as in the nose and tongue, or sound or light, as in the ear and eye. *See* exteroceptor, interoceptor, mechanoreceptor, proprioceptor. **2.** a specialized area of a cell membrane, consisting of a specially adapted protein, that can bind with a specific hormone (e.g. *estrogen receptors), neurotransmitter (e.g. *adrenergic receptors), drug, or other chemical, thereby initiating a change within the cell.

recertification *n.* a process by which physicians must prove that they have kept up with the developments in medicine and that they have received continuing education and are competent to practice medicine. Each specialty board controls the specific requirements, such as how often recertification is required, the types of educational credits allowed, and who is permitted to issue such credits.

recess *n.* (in anatomy) a hollow chamber or a depression in an organ or other part.

recessive *adj.* describing a gene (or its corresponding characteristic) whose effect is shown in the individual only when its *allele is the same, i.e. when two such alleles are present (the *double recessive* condition). Many hereditary diseases (including cystic fibrosis) are due to the presence of a defective gene as a double recessive. They are said to show *autosomal recessive* inheritance, since the gene is carried on an autosome (any chromosome other than a sex chromosome). *Compare* dominant. —**recessive** *n.*

recidivism *n.* a tendency to relapse into a previous disease, condition, or behavioral pattern, especially the tendency of an ill person to return to a hospital.

recipient *n.* a person who receives something from a *donor, such as a blood transfusion or a kidney transplant.

recombinant DNA DNA that contains genes from different sources that have been combined by the techniques of *genetic engineering rather than by breeding experiments. Genetic engineering is therefore also known as *recombinant DNA technology.*

record linkage the means by which information about health events from several different sources (e.g. hospital attendance, vaccination, and consultation with general practitioners) are all related to a specific individual in a common file or more usually a computerized record. This contrasts with data in which events only are recorded and two separate individuals treated for the same disease cannot be distinguished from one individual treated on two separate occasions.

recovery position a first-aid position into which an unconscious but breathing patient can be laid to afford maximum protection to the airway. It involves laying the patient on his or her side, with the uppermost leg bent at the knee and hip and the lower arm behind the back to prevent rolling onto the front or back into a position in which the patient could smother or choke.

recreational drug any substance that is taken voluntarily for its effects on the central nervous system rather than for medicinal purposes to alleviate symptoms or treat a disease process. Included in the category are alcohol, barbiturates, amphetamines, narcotics, and, to a degree, caffeine in coffee and cola beverages. *See also* dependence.

recrudescence *n.* a fresh outbreak of a disorder in a patient after a period during which its signs and symptoms had died down and recovery seemed to be taking place.

recruitment *n.* **1.** (in physiology) the phenomenon whereby an increase in the strength of a stimulus or repetition of the stimulus will stimulate increasing numbers of nerve cells to respond. **2.** (in audiology) the phenomenon in which a person with sensorineural *deafness cannot hear quiet sounds but can perceive loud sounds just as loudly as, or even more loudly than, a person with normal hearing. **3.** (in muscle physiology) the orderly increase of activated motor units in voluntary muscle as the need to overcome resistance increases.

rect- (recto-) *prefix denoting* the rectum. Examples: *rectouterine* (relating to the rectum and uterus); *rectovesical* (relating to the rectum and bladder).

rectocele *n. see* proctocele.

rectosigmoid *n.* the region of the large intestine around the junction of the sigmoid colon and the rectum.

rectum *n.* the terminal part of the large *intestine, about 12 cm long, which runs from the sigmoid colon to the anal canal. Feces are stored in the rectum before defecation. —**rectal** *adj.*

rectus *n.* any of several straight muscles. The *rectus muscles of the orbit* are some of the extrinsic *eye muscles. *Rectus abdominis* is a long flat muscle that extends bilaterally along the entire length of the front of the abdomen. The rectus muscles acting together serve to bend the trunk forward; acting separately they bend the body sideways. The *rectus femoris* forms part of the *quadriceps.

recurrent *adj.* (in anatomy) describing a structure, such as a nerve or blood vessel, that turns back on its course, forming a loop.

red blood cell *see* erythrocyte.

redia *n.* (*pl.* **rediae**) the third-stage larva of a parasitic *fluke. Rediae develop within the body of a freshwater snail and undergo a process of asexual reproduction, giving rise to many fourth-stage larvae called *cercariae. *See also* miracidium, sporocyst.

red reflex the red area seen through the pupil as a result of the reflection of light from the retina. It is usually seen on *fundoscopy and sometimes in photographs taken using a flashlight.

reduction *n.* (in surgery) the restoration of a displaced part of the body to its normal position by manipulation or operation. The fragments of a broken bone are reduced before a splint is applied; a dislocated joint is reduced to its normal seating; or a hernia is reduced when the displaced organ or tissue is returned to its usual anatomical site.

reduction division the first division of *meiosis, in which the chromosome number is halved. The term is sometimes used as a synonym for the whole of meiosis.

reduplication *n.* doubling of the heart sounds, which may be heard in healthy individuals and shows variation with respiration due to the slightly asynchronous closure of the heart valves.

reduviid *n.* any one of a group of winged insects (Reduviidae) whose mouthparts

– adapted for piercing and sucking – take the form of a long proboscis that is tucked beneath the head when not in use. Some South American genera, notably *Panstrongylus*, *Rhodnius*, and *Triatoma* (the kissing bugs) are nocturnal bloodsucking insects that transmit the parasite causing *Chagas' disease.

Reduvius *n.* a genus of predatory bloodsucking reduviid bugs. *R. personatus*, widely distributed in Europe, normally preys upon insects but occasionally attacks humans. Its bite causes various allergic symptoms, including rash (*see also* urticaria), nausea, and palpitations.

Reed-Sternberg cell (Sternberg-Reed cell) a large binucleate cell that is characteristic of *Hodgkin's disease. [D. Reed Mendenhall (1874–1964), US pathologist; C. Sternberg (1872–1935), Austrian pathologist]

referred pain (synalgia) pain felt in a part of the body other than where it might be expected. An abscess beneath the diaphragm, for example, may cause a referred pain in the shoulder area, while heart disorders may cause pain in the left arm and fingers. The confusion arises because sensory nerves from different parts of the body share common pathways when they reach the spinal cord.

reflex *n.* an automatic or involuntary activity brought about by relatively simple nervous circuits, without consciousness being necessarily involved. Thus, a painful stimulus such as a pinprick will bring about the reflex of withdrawing the finger before the brain has had time to send a message to the muscles involved. *See* conditioned reflex, patellar reflex, plantar reflex.

reflex arc the nervous circuit involved in a *reflex, being at its simplest a sensory nerve with a receptor, linked at a synapse in the brain or spinal cord with a motor nerve, which supplies a muscle or gland (see illustration). In a simple reflex (such as the *patellar reflex) only two neurons may be involved, but in other reflexes there may be several *interneurons in the arc.

reflexology *n.* a therapy in *complementary medicine based on the theory that reflex points on the feet correspond with all body parts. Firm pressure is applied to the relevant reflex points using the thumb or fingers. Reflexology is said to be able to help with specific illnesses and may also restore the body's natural balance and harmony. It can be used for people of any age and there are very few contraindications.

reflux *n.* a backflow of liquid, against its normal direction of movement. *See also* (reflux) esophagitis, vesicoureteric reflux.

refraction *n.* **1.** the change in direction of light rays when they pass obliquely from one transparent medium to another, of a different density. Refraction occurs as light enters the eye, when it passes from air to the media of the eye, i.e. cornea, aqueous humor, lens, and vitreous humor, to come to a focus on the retina. Errors of refraction, in which light rays do not come to a focus on the retina due to defects in the refracting media or shape of the eyeball, include astigmatism and far- and nearsightedness. **2.** determination of the power of refraction of the eye. This gives the degree to which the eye differs from normal, which determines whether or not the patient needs glasses and, if so, how strong they should be.

refractive error an abnormality of the eye resulting in a blurred image on the retina as a result of abnormal focusing, which can be corrected by glasses, contact lenses, or *refractive surgery. Refractive errors include *myopia, *hyperopia, and *astigmatism.

refractive surgery any surgical procedure

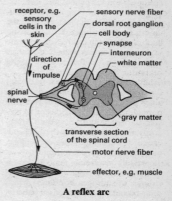

A reflex arc

that has as its primary objective the correction of any refractive error. It includes such procedures as clear lens extraction, *LASIK, *LASEK, photorefractive *keratectomy, and *thermokeratoplasty.

refractometer n. see optometer.

refractory adj. unresponsive: applied to a condition that fails to respond satisfactorily to a given treatment.

refractory period (in neurology) the time of recovery needed for a nerve cell that has just transmitted a nerve impulse or for a muscle fiber that has just contracted. During the refractory period, a normal stimulus will not bring about excitation of the cell, which is undergoing *repolarization.

refrigeration n. lowering the temperature of a part of the body to reduce the metabolic activity of its tissues or to provide a local anesthetic effect.

regimen n. (in therapeutics) a prescribed systematic form of treatment, such as a diet, course of drugs, or special exercises, for curing disease or improving health.

regional ileitis see Crohn's disease.

regression n. 1. (in psychiatry) reversion to a more immature level of functioning. The term may be applied to the state of a patient in the hospital who becomes incontinent and demanding. It may also be applied to a single psychological function; for example, psychoanalysts speak of the *libido regressing to an early stage of development. 2. the stage of a disease during which the signs and symptoms disappear and the patient recovers.

regurgitation n. 1. the bringing up of undigested material from the stomach to the mouth (see vomiting). 2. the flowing back of a liquid in a direction opposite to the normal one, as when blood surges back through a defective valve in the heart after the heart has contracted.

rehabilitation 1. (in *physical medicine) the treatment of an ill, injured, or disabled patient with the aim of restoring normal health and functions or to prevent the disability from getting worse. 2. any means for restoring the independence of a patient after diseases or injury, including employment retraining.

Reifenstein's syndrome male *hypogonadism resulting from a congenital resistance to androgen hormones, which often becomes more obvious at puberty.

Some features of feminization may occur. All features vary widely in severity. [E. C. Reifenstein (1908–75), US endocrinologist]

reiki n. a technique in *complementary medicine based on an ancient healing system rediscovered in the 20th century by a Buddhist monk. It involves a therapist putting his or her hands on or very close to a patient to boost the patient's natural invisible energy fields (reiki mean "universal life force"). It is often used as an adjunct to other therapies and is said to be helpful for many conditions.

reimplantation n. see replantation.

reinforcement n. (in psychology) the strengthening of a conditioned reflex (see conditioning). In classic conditioning this takes place when a conditioned stimulus is presented simultaneously with – or just before – the unconditioned stimulus. In operant conditioning it takes place when a pleasurable event (or reinforcer), such as a reward, follows immediately after some behavior. The reinforcement schedule governs how often and when such behavior is rewarded. Different schedules produce different effects on behavior.

Reissner's membrane the membrane that separates the scala vestibuli and the scala media of the *cochlea of the ear. [E. Reissner (1824–78), German anatomist]

Reiter's syndrome a disease characterized by inflammation of the urethra (see urethritis), conjunctivitis, and polyarthritis, usually affecting young men. Horny areas may develop on the skin. The symptoms resemble those of *gonorrhea. No causative agent has been positively identified, although a virus or Chlamydia may be implicated. [H. Reiter (1881–1969), German physician]

rejection n. 1. (in transplantation) the reaction that occurs in a recipient after transplantation of an *allogeneic or *xenogeneic organ. Antibodies, complement, clotting factors, and platelets are involved in the failure of the graft to survive. Allograft rejection can be prevented by immunosuppressant drugs (such as cyclosporine and corticosteroids) and antibodies against T cells; xenograft rejection is at present beyond therapeutic control. 2. (in psychiatry) the withholding of attention or accep-

rennin

tance of another person, such as a parent withholding affection for a child.

relapse *n.* a return of disease symptoms after recovery had apparently been achieved or the worsening of an apparently recovering patient's condition during the course of an illness.

relapsing fever an infectious disease caused by bacteria of the genus *Borrelia, which is transmitted by ticks or lice and results in recurrent fever. The first episode of fever occurs about a week after infection: it is accompanied by severe headache and aching muscles and joints and lasts 2–8 days. Subsequent attacks are milder and occur at intervals of 3–10 days; untreated, the attacks may continue for up to 12 weeks. Treatment with antibiotics, such as tetracycline or erythromycin, is effective.

relative analgesia a sedation technique, used particularly in dentistry, in which a mixture of *nitrous oxide and oxygen is given. The patient remains conscious throughout; the technique is used to supplement local anesthesia for nervous patients.

relative density *see* specific gravity.

relaxant *n.* an agent that reduces tension and strain, particularly in muscles (*see* muscle relaxant).

relaxation *n.* (in physiology) the diminution of tension in a muscle, which occurs when it ceases to contract: the state of a resting muscle.

relaxation therapy treatment by teaching a patient to decrease his anxiety by reducing the tone in his muscles. This can be used by itself to help people cope with stressful situations or as a part of *desensitization to specific fears.

relaxin *n.* a hormone, secreted by the placenta in the terminal stages of pregnancy, that causes the cervix of the uterus to dilate and prepares the uterus for the action of *oxytocin during labor.

Relenza *n. see* zanamivir.

reline *n.* the procedure by which the fitting surface of a denture is rebased to make it fit a jaw that has undergone resorption since the denture was originally made. The procedure is often necessary for dentures that were fitted immediately after extraction of the teeth.

rem *n.* abbreviation for roentgen equivalent man: a former unit dose of ionizing radiation equal to the dose that gives the same biological effect as that due to one roentgen of X-rays. The rem has been replaced by the *sievert.

REM rapid eye movement: describing a stage of *sleep during which the muscles of the eyeballs are in constant motion behind the eyelids. People woken up during this stage of sleep generally report that they were dreaming at the time.

remedial profession any profession (including occupational therapy, physiotherapy, and speech therapy) in which the therapists use their skills to assist those with a *disability to achieve living and working standards as near normal as possible.

Remicade *n. see* infliximab.

remission *n.* **1.** a lessening in the severity of symptoms or their temporary disappearance during the course of an illness. **2.** a reduction in the size of a cancer and the symptoms it is causing.

remittent fever *see* fever.

renal *adj.* relating to or affecting the kidneys.

renal artery either of two large arteries arising from the abdominal aorta and supplying the kidneys. Each renal artery divides into an anterior and a posterior branch before entering the kidney.

renal cell carcinoma *see* hypernephroma.

renal function tests tests for assessing the function of the kidneys. These include measurements of the specific gravity of urine, creatinine *clearance time, and blood urea levels; intravenous urography (*see* intravenous urogram); and renal angiography.

renal tubule (uriniferous tubule) the fine tubular part of a *nephron, through which water and certain dissolved substances are reabsorbed back into the blood.

reni- (reno-) *prefix denoting* the kidney.

renin *n.* an enzyme released into the blood by the kidney in response to stress. It reacts with a substrate from the liver to produce *angiotensin, which causes constriction of blood vessels and thus an increase in blood pressure. Excessive production of renin results in the syndrome of renal *hypertension.

rennin *n.* an enzyme produced in the stomach that coagulates milk. It is secreted by the gastric glands in an inactive form, *prorennin*, which is activated by hydrochloric acid. Rennin converts caseinogen (milk protein) into insoluble casein in the presence of calcium ions. This ensures that the milk remains in the stomach, exposed to protein-digesting enzymes, for as long as possible. Rennin is present in the largest amounts in the stomachs of young mammals.

renography (isotope renography) *n.* the radiological study of the kidneys by a *gamma camera following the intravenous injection of a radioactive *tracer, which is concentrated and excreted by the kidneys. The radioactive isotope (usually *technetium-99m) emits gamma rays, which are recorded by the camera positioned over the kidneys. A graph of the radioactivity in each kidney over time provides information on its function and rate of drainage. *See* DMSA, MAG3, pentetic acid.

reovirus *n.* one of a group of small RNA-containing viruses that infect both respiratory and intestinal tracts without producing specific or serious diseases (and were therefore termed *r*espiratory *e*nteric *o*rphan viruses). *Compare* echovirus.

repaglinide *n. see* meglitinides.

reperfusion *n.* the restoration of blood flow to an area of the body previously blocked and ischemic. Procedures to open blocked arteries include use of *thrombolytic agents and *angioplasty.

repetitive strain injury pain with associated loss of function in a limb resulting from its repeated movement or sustained static loading. *Tenosynovitis and *tendovaginitis of the wrist associated with typing or operating a computer is the injury most frequently encountered. *See also* carpal tunnel syndrome.

replacement bone a bone that is formed by replacing cartilage with bony material.

replantation *n.* **1.** a developing specialty for the reattachment of severed limbs (or parts of limbs) and other body parts (e.g. the nose). It uses techniques of *microsurgery to rejoin nerves and vessels. **2.** (also **reimplantation**) (in dentistry) the reinsertion of a tooth into its socket after its accidental or deliberate removal. —**replant** *vb.*

replication *n.* the process by which *DNA makes copies of itself when the cell divides. The two strands of the DNA molecule unwind and each strand directs the

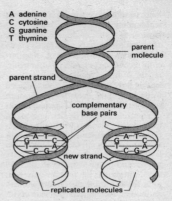

A adenine
C cytosine
G guanine
T thymine

parent molecule

parent strand

complementary base pairs

new strand

replicated molecules

Replication of a DNA molecule

synthesis of a new strand complementary to itself (see illustration).

repolarization *n.* the process in which the membrane of a nerve cell returns to its normal electrically charged state after a nerve impulse has passed. During the passage of a nerve impulse, a temporary change in the molecular structure of the membrane allows a surge of ions across the membrane (*see* action potential). During repolarization ions diffuse back to restore the charge and the nerve becomes ready to transmit further impulses. *See* refractory period.

repositor *n.* an instrument used to return a displaced part of the body – for instance, a prolapsed uterus – to its normal position.

repression *n.* (in *psychoanalysis) the process of excluding an unacceptable wish or an idea from conscious mental life. The repressed material may give rise to symptoms. One goal of psychoanalysis is to return repressed material to conscious awareness so that it may be dealt with rationally.

reproduction rate *see* fertility rate.

reproductive system the combination of organs and tissues associated with the process of reproduction. In males it includes the testes, vasa deferentia, prostate gland, seminal vesicles, urethra, and penis; in females it includes the ovaries, fallopian tubes, uterus, vagina, and vulva. (See illustration.)

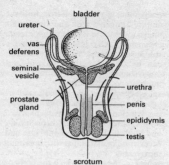

Male reproductive system

Female reproductive system

RES *see* reticuloendothelial system.

resection *n.* surgical removal of a portion of any part of the body. For example, a section of diseased intestine may be removed and the healthy ends sewn together. A *submucous resection* is removal of part of the cartilage septum (central division) of the nose that has become deviated, usually by injury. *Transurethral resection of the prostate* (*TUR* or *TURP*) – an operation that is performed when the prostate gland becomes enlarged – involves the removal of portions of the gland through the urethra using an instrument called a *resectoscope.*

resectoscope *n.* a type of surgical instrument (an *endoscope) used in resection of the prostate or in the removal of bladder tumors.

reserpine *n. see* rauwolfia.

reserve volume the extra volume of air that an individual could inhale or exhale if he is not breathing to the limit of his capacity.

resident *n.* (in a hospital) a licensed physician or surgeon in postgraduate training in a particular specialty, who is responsible for the care of a number of patients with the assistance of interns, whom he instructs. A resident may work with one or more senior surgeons or physicians.

residual volume the volume of air that remains in the lungs after the individual has breathed out as much as he can. This volume is increased in *emphysema.

resistance *n.* **1.** the degree of *immunity that the body possesses: a measure of its ability to withstand disease. **2.** the degree to which a disease or disease-causing organism remains unaffected by antibiotics or other drugs.

resolution *n.* **1.** the stage during which inflammation gradually disappears. **2.** the degree to which individual details can be distinguished by the eye, as through a *microscope.

resonance *n.* the sound produced by wave vibrations transmitted to an organ cavity after *percussion of a body part.

resorcinol *n.* a drug that causes the skin to peel. It has been used in ointments to treat such conditions as acne, but with prolonged use the drug is absorbed into the body, causing underactivity of the thyroid gland (myxedema) and convulsions. Trade names: **Acnomel, Sulforcin**.

resorption *n.* loss of substance through physiological or pathological means.

respiration *n.* the process of gaseous exchange between an organism and its environment. This includes both *external respiration*, which involves *breathing, in which oxygen is taken up by the capillaries of the lung *alveoli and carbon dioxide is released from the blood, and *internal respiration*, during which oxygen is released to the tissues and carbon dioxide absorbed by the blood. Blood provides the transport medium for the gases between the lungs and tissue cells. In addition, it contains the pigment *hemoglobin, which has special affinity for oxygen. Once inside the cell, oxygen is utilized in metabolic processes resulting in the production of energy (*see* ATP), water, and waste materials (including carbon dioxide). *See also* lung. —**respiratory** *adj.*

respirator *n.* **1.** a device used to maintain the breathing movements of paralyzed patients. In the *positive-pressure respirator* air is blown into the patient's lungs via a tube passed either through the mouth into the trachea or through a *tracheostomy. Air is released from the lungs when the pressure from the respirator is relaxed. The *iron lung* is a type of respirator in which the patient is enclosed, except for the head, in an airtight container in which the air pressure is decreased and increased mechanically. This draws air into and out of the lungs, through the normal air passages. The *cuirass respirator* works on a similar principle, but leaves the limbs free. **2.** a face mask for administering oxygen or other gas or for filtering harmful fumes, dust, etc. *See also* artificial respiration.

respiratory distress syndrome (hyaline membrane disease) the condition of a newborn infant in which the lungs are imperfectly expanded. Initial inflation and normal expansion of the lungs requires the presence of a substance (*surfactant) that reduces the surface tension of the air sacs (alveoli) and prevents collapse of the small airways. Without surfactant the airways collapse, leading to inefficient and "stiff" lungs. The condition is most common and serious among preterm infants, in whom surfactant is liable to be deficient. Breathing is rapid, labored, and shallow, and microscopic examinations of lung tissue in fatal cases has revealed the presence of *hyalin material in the collapsed air sacs. The condition is treated by careful nursing, intravenous fluids, oxygen (with or without positive pressure by a *respirator), and administration of surfactant.

respiratory quotient (RQ) the ratio of the volume of carbon dioxide transferred from the blood into the alveoli to the volume of oxygen absorbed into the alveoli. The RQ is usually about 0.8 because more oxygen is taken up than carbon dioxide excreted.

respiratory syncytial virus (RSV) a paramyxovirus (*see* myxovirus) that causes infections of the nose and throat. It is a major cause of bronchiolitis and pneumonia in young children. In tissue cultures infected with the virus, cells merge together to form a conglomerate (*syncytium*). RSV is thought to have a role in *crib deaths. Vulnerable children can be treated with *ribavirin and *palivizumab, but most children just require supportive measures.

respiratory system the combination of organs and tissues associated with *breathing. It includes the nasal cavity, pharynx, larynx, trachea, bronchi, bronchioles, and lungs and also the diaphragm and other muscles associated with breathing movements.

response *n.* the way in which the body or part of the body reacts to a *stimulus. For example, a nerve impulse may produce the response of a contraction in a muscle that the nerve supplies.

response prevention a form of *behavior therapy given for severe *obsessions. Patients are encouraged to abstain from rituals and repetitive acts while they are in situations that arouse anxiety. For example, a hand-washing ritual might be treated by stopping washing while being progressively exposed to dirt. The anxiety then declines, and with it the obsessions.

restenosis *n.* recurrent *stenosis, especially in a heart valve or an artery after corrective surgery or insertion of a stent.

restiform body a thick bundle of nerve fibers that conveys impulses from tracts in the spinal cord to the cortex of the anterior and posterior lobes of the cerebellum.

resting cell a cell that is not undergoing division. *See* interphase.

restless legs syndrome (Ekbom syndrome) a condition in which an irritating sense of uneasiness, restlessness, tiredness, and itching, often accompanied by twitching and pain, is felt in the calves of the legs when sitting or lying down, especially at night. The only relief is walking or moving the legs, which often leads to insomnia. The cause is unknown: it may be inadequate circulation, nerve damage (*see* peripheral neuropathy), deficiency of iron, vitamin B_{12}, or folic acid, or a reaction to antipsychotic or antidepressant drugs. In severe cases treatment with *dopamine receptor agonists or levodopa may be helpful.

restoration *n.* **1.** the act of renewing or reconstruction, or of returning to a former state of health. **2.** (in dentistry) any type of dental *filling or *crown, which is aimed at restoring a tooth to its normal form, function, and appearance.

rest pain pain, usually experienced in the feet, that indicates an extreme degree of *ischemia.

restriction enzyme (restriction endonuclease) an enzyme, obtained from bacteria, that cuts DNA into specific short segments. Restriction enzymes are widely used in *genetic engineering.

resuscitation *n.* the restoration of a person who appears to be dead. It depends upon the revival of cardiac and respiratory function. *See also* artificial respiration, mouth-to-mouth respiration.

retainer *n.* (in dentistry) **1.** a component of a partial *denture that keeps it in place. **2.** an *orthodontic appliance that holds the teeth in position. **3.** a component of a *bridge that is fixed to a natural tooth.

retardation *n.* the slowing up of a process. The term *mental retardation implies a delay in development rather than a qualitative defect. *Psychomotor retardation* is a marked slowing down of activity and speech, which can reach a degree where a patient can no longer care for himself. It is a symptom of severe *depression.

retching *n.* repeated unsuccessful attempts to vomit.

rete *n.* a network of blood vessels, nerve fibers, or other strands of interlacing tissue in the structure of an organ. The *rete testis* is a network of tubules conducting sperm from the seminiferous tubules of the *testis to the vasa efferentia.

retention *n.* inability to pass urine, which is retained in the bladder. The condition may be acute and painful or chronic and painless. *Acute urinary retention (AUR)* can be precipitated by surgery, urinary infection, constipation, and drugs; spontaneous AUR is usually caused by enlargement of the prostate gland in men, although many other conditions may result in obstruction of bladder outflow. Retention is relieved by catheter drainage of the bladder before dealing with the underlying problem. *See also* intermittent self-catheterization.

retention defect (in psychology) a memory defect in which items that have been registered in the memory are lost from storage. It is a feature of *dementia.

reticular activating system the system of nerve pathways in the brain concerned with the level of consciousness – from the states of sleep, drowsiness, and relaxation to full alertness and attention. The system integrates information from all of the senses and from the cerebrum and cerebellum and determines the overall activity of the brain and the autonomic nervous system and patterns of behavior during waking and sleeping.

reticular fibers microscopic, almost nonelastic, branching fibers of *connective tissue that join together to form a delicate supportive meshwork around blood vessels, muscle fibers, glands, nerves, etc. They are composed of a collagen-like protein (*reticulin*) and are particularly common in lymph nodes, the spleen, liver, kidneys, and muscles.

reticular formation a network of nerve pathways and nuclei throughout the *brainstem, connecting motor and sensory nerves to and from the spinal cord, the cerebellum and the cerebrum, and the cranial nerves. It is estimated that a single neuron in this network may have synapses with as many as 25,000 other neurons.

reticulin *n.* a protein that is the major constituent of *reticular fibers.

reticulocyte *n.* an immature red blood cell (erythrocyte). Reticulocytes may be detected and counted by staining living red cells with certain basic dyes that result in the formation of a blue precipitate (*reticulum*) within the reticulocytes. They normally comprise about 1% of the total red cells and are increased (*reticulocytosis*) whenever the rate of red cell production increases.

reticulocytosis *n.* an increase in the proportion of immature red blood cells (reticulocytes) in the bloodstream. It is a sign of increased output of new red cells from the bone marrow.

reticuloendothelial system (RES) a community of cells – *phagocytes – spread throughout the body. It includes *macrophages and *monocytes. The RES is concerned with defense against microbial infection and with the removal of worn-out blood cells from the bloodstream. *See also* spleen.

reticulosis *n.* abnormal overgrowth, usually malignant, of any of the cells of the lymphatic glands or the immune system.

See lymphoma, Hodgkin's disease, Burkitt's lymphoma, mycosis fungoides.

reticulum *n.* a network of tubules or blood vessels. . See endoplasmic reticulum, sarcoplasmic reticulum.

retin- (retino-) *prefix denoting* the retina. Example: *retinopexy* (fixation of a detached retina).

retina *n.* the light-sensitive layer that lines the interior of the eye. The outer part of the retina, next to the *choroid, is pigmented to prevent the passage of light. The inner part, next to the cavity of the eyeball, contains *rods and *cones (light-sensitive cells) and their associated nerve fibers (see illustration). A large number of cones are concentrated in a depression in the retina at the back of the eyeball called the *fovea. —**retinal** *adj.*

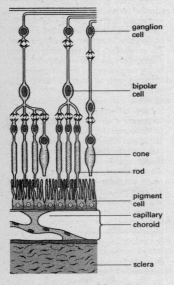

ganglion cell

bipolar cell

cone

rod

pigment cell

capillary

choroid

sclera

The structure of the retina

retinaculum *n.* (*pl.* **retinacula**) a thickened band of tissue that serves to hold various tissues in place. For example, *flexor retinacula* are found over the flexor tendons in the wrist and ankle.

retinal (retinene) *n.* the aldehyde of retinol (*vitamin A). See also rhodopsin.

retinal artery occlusion blockage of an artery supplying blood to the retina, usually as a result of *thrombosis or *embolism. The central retinal artery enters the eye at the optic disk and then divides into branches to supply different parts of the retina. Blockage of the central retinal artery (*central retinal artery occlusion*) usually results in sudden painless loss of vision. Blockage of one of the branches of the central retinal artery (*branch retinal artery occlusion*), usually by emboli, results in *ischemia of the retina supplied by the occluded vessel and related visual field loss.

retinal detachment *see* detached retina.

retinal dialysis separation of the retina from its insertion at the ora serrata (the anterior margin of the retina, lying just posterior to the ciliary body). This acts as a retinal tear and causes a *detached retina.

retinal vein occlusion blockage of a vein carrying blood from the retina. Small branch veins carry blood from different parts of the retina and drain into the central retinal vein, which leaves the eye at the optic disk. Blockage of the central retinal vein (*central retinal vein occlusion*) usually results in sudden painless reduction of vision. Distended veins, hemorrhages, and *cotton-wool spots are seen in the retina and the optic disk may become swollen. The blockage of one branch of the central retinal vein (*branch retinal vein occlusion*) results in painless reduction of vision in the affected area, where engorged veins, hemorrhages, and cotton-wool spots may be seen.

retinene *n. see* retinal.

retinitis *n.* inflammation of the *retina. In practice, the term is often used for conditions now known not to be inflammatory, for example, *retinitis pigmentosa*, a noninflammatory hereditary condition involving progressive degeneration of the retina due to malfunctioning of the retinal pigment epithelium. It starts in childhood with *night blindness and limited peripheral vision and may progress to complete loss of vision. For such conditions the term *retinopathy is becoming more widely used.

retinoblastoma *n.* a rare malignant tumor of the retina, occurring in infants.

retinoid *n.* any one of a group of drugs

derived from vitamin A. They bind to one or more of six specific receptors that are found on many cells. On the skin they act to cause drying and peeling and a reduction in oil (sebum) production. These effects can be useful in the treatment of severe *acne, *psoriasis, *ichthyosis, and other skin disorders. Retinoids include *isotretinoin and *tretinoin; they are administered by mouth or applied as a cream. Possible side effects, which may be serious, include severe fetal abnormalities (if taken by pregnant women), toxic effects on babies (if taken by breast-feeding mothers), liver and kidney damage, excessive drying, redness and itching of the skin, and muscle pain and stiffness.

retinol *n.* see vitamin A.

retinopathy *n.* any disorder of the retina resulting in impairment or loss of vision. It is usually due to damage to the blood vessels of the retina, occurring (for example) as a complication of diabetes (*diabetic retinopathy*), high blood pressure, or AIDS (*AIDS retinopathy*). In diabetic retinopathy, hemorrhaging or exudation may occur, either from damaged vessels into the retina or from new abnormal vessels (*see* neovascularization) into the vitreous humor. Unless treated, this may lead to permanent loss of vision. Treatment may require laser surgery (*photocoagulation).

retinopexy *n.* any surgical procedure used to repair a *detached retina. *See* pneumoretinopexy, cryoretinopexy.

retinoschisis *n.* splitting of the layers of the retina with accumulation of fluid between the layers. This usually progresses very slowly compared with other types of *detached retina.

retinoscope *n.* an instrument used to determine the power of spectacle lens required to correct errors of *refraction of the eye. It is held in the hand and casts a beam of light into the subject's eye. The examiner looks along the beam and sees the reflection it produces in the subject's pupil. By interpreting the way the reflection moves when he moves the instrument, and by altering this by lenses held in his other hand near the subject's eye, he is able to detect far- or nearsightedness or astigmatism and to determine its degree. —**retinoscopy** *n.*

retinotomy *n.* a surgical incision into the retina.

retraction *n.* **1.** (in obstetrics) the failure of the muscle fibers of the uterus to relax after each uterine contraction during labor. The fibers remain at their shorter (contracted) length, which results in a gradual progression of the fetus downward through the pelvis. **2.** (in dentistry) the drawing back of one or more teeth into a better position by an *orthodontic appliance.

retraction ring a depression on the uterine wall marking the junction between the actively contracting muscle fibers of the upper segment of the uterus and the muscle fibers of the lower segment. This depression is not always visible and is normal. In obstructed labor (e.g. contracted pelvis or malposition of the fetus resulting in shoulder presentation), the muscle fibers of the upper segment become shorter and thicker; the muscle fibers of the lower segment, on the other hand, become elongated and thinner. The junction between the two becomes more distinct as it rises into the abdomen from the pelvis. This abnormal ring is known as *Bandl's ring* and is a sign of impending rupture of the lower segment of the uterus, which becomes progressively thinner as Bandl's ring rises upward. Immediate action to relieve the obstruction is then necessary, usually in the form of cesarean section.

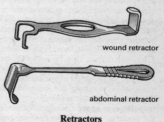

wound retractor

abdominal retractor

Retractors

retractor *n.* a surgical instrument used to expose the operation site by drawing aside the cut edges of skin, muscle, or other tissues. There are several types of retractors for different operations (see illustration).

retro- *prefix denoting* at the back or behind. Examples: *retrobulbar* (at the back of the eyeball); *retroperitoneal* (behind the peritoneum).

retrobulbar neuritis (optic neuritis) inflammation of the optic nerve behind the eye, causing increasingly blurred vision. When the inflammation involves the first part of the nerve and can be seen at the optic disk, it is called *optic papillitis*. Retrobulbar neuritis is one of the symptoms of multiple sclerosis but it can also occur as an isolated lesion, in the absence of any other involvement of the nervous system, with the patient recovering vision completely.

retroflexion *n.* the bending backward of an organ or part of an organ, especially of the abnormal backward bending of the upper part of the uterus in relation to the cervix.

retrograde *adj.* going backward, or moving in the opposite direction to the normal. (*See* [retrograde] pyelography.) *Retrograde amnesia* is a failure to remember events immediately preceding an illness or injury.

retrography *n.* writing in which the words and letters are reversed so that they appear as mirror images. Adoption of this as a consistent style is usually a matter of voluntary choice or is *hysterical; very occasionally it follows brain damage. Mirror-image reversals of single letters are common in children learning to write and in older children whose language abilities are impaired.

retroperitoneal fibrosis (RPF) a condition in which a dense plaque of fibrous tissue develops behind the peritoneum adjacent to the abdominal aorta. The ureters become encased and hence obstructed, causing acute *anuria and renal failure. The obstruction can be relieved by *nephrostomy or the insertion of double J *stents. In the acute phase steroid administration may help, but in established RPF *ureterolysis is required.

retroperitoneal space the region between the posterior parietal *peritoneum and the front of the *lumbar vertebrae. It contains important structures, including the kidneys, adrenal glands, pancreas, lumbar spinal nerve roots, sympathetic ganglia and nerves, and the abdominal *aorta and its major branches.

retropulsion *n.* a compulsive tendency to walk backward. It is a symptom of *parkinsonism.

retrospective study 1. a backward-looking review of the characteristics of a group of individuals in relation to morbidity, embracing certain aspects of *cross-sectional and/or *case control studies. The term is sometimes loosely used as a synonym for such studies. **2.** *see* cohort study.

retroversion *n.* the backward inclination of an organ, especially of the uterus, which is tipped back so that the cervix points toward the pubic symphysis (the bone under the pubic hair) with the base lying in the *pouch of Douglas, against the rectum, instead of on the bladder. It occurs in about 20% of women.

retrovirus *n.* an RNA-containing virus that can convert its genetic material into DNA by means of the enzyme *reverse transcriptase, which enables it to become integrated into the DNA of its host's cells. Retroviruses have been implicated in the development of some cancers and are associated with conditions characterized by an impaired immune system (*HIV is a retrovirus). They are also used as *vectors in gene therapy.

retrusion *n.* (in dentistry) **1.** backward movement of the lower jaw. **2.** a malocclusion in which some of the teeth are further back than usual. *Compare* protrusion.

Rett's syndrome a disorder affecting young girls, in which stereotyped movements (*see* stereotypy) and social withdrawal appear during early childhood. Intellectual development is often impaired and special educational help is needed. [A. Rett (20th century), Austrian pediatrician]

revascularization *n.* **1.** the regrowth of blood vessels following disease or injury so that normal blood supply to an organ, tissue, or part is restored. **2.** the surgical restoration of blood flow to a part by replacing a diseased blood vessel with a graft. *See* coronary revascularization.

reverse transcriptase an enzyme, found mainly in *retroviruses, that catalyzes the synthesis of DNA from RNA. It enables the viral RNA to be integrated into the host DNA. *Reverse transcriptase inhibitors* are antiviral drugs that inhibit this process; they include *zidovudine, *didanosine, *delavirdine, *efavirenz, and *nevirapine, used in the treatment of

HIV infection, and *lamivudine* (Epivir, Zeffix), for treating HIV infection and hepatitis B.

Reye's syndrome a rare disorder occurring in childhood. It is characterized by the symptoms of *encephalitis combined with evidence of liver failure. Often, the symptoms develop in the apparent recovery phase of a viral infection. Treatment is aimed at controlling cerebral *edema and correcting metabolic abnormalities in order to allow spontaneous recovery, but there is still a significant mortality and there may be residual brain damage. The cause is not known, but *aspirin has been implicated and this drug should not be used in children below the age of 12 years unless specifically indicated. [R. D. K. Reye (1912–77), Australian histopathologist]

rhabdomyoma *n.* a rare benign tumor of skeletal muscle or heart muscle.

rhabdomyosarcoma *n.* a rare malignant tumor, usually of childhood, originating in, or showing the characteristics of, striated muscle. *Pleomorphic rhabdomyosarcoma* occurs in late middle age, in the muscles of the limbs. *Embryonal rhabdomyosarcomas*, affecting infants, children, and young adults, are classified as *botryoid* (in the vagina, bladder, ear, etc.), *embryonal* (most common in the head and neck, particularly the orbit); and *alveolar* (at the base of the thumb). The pleomorphic and alveolar types respond poorly to treatment; botryoid tumors are treated with a combination of radiotherapy, surgery, and drugs. The embryonal type, if treated at an early stage, can often be cured with a combination of radiotherapy and drugs (including vincristine, dactinomycin, and cyclophosphamide).

rhagades *pl. n.* cracks or long thin scars in the skin, particularly around the mouth or other areas of the body subjected to constant movement. The fissures around the mouth and nose of babies with congenital syphilis eventually heal to form rhagades.

rhegma *n.* **1.** a tear. **2.** a fracture.

rhegmatogenous *adj.* resulting from a break or tear. For example, *rhegmatogenous detached retina* results as a consequence of a tear in the retina.

rheo- *prefix denoting* **1.** a flow of liquid. **2.** an electric current.

rhesus factor (Rh factor) a group of *antigens that may or may not be present on the surface of the red blood cells; it forms the basis of the rhesus blood group system. Most people have the rhesus factor, i.e. they are *Rh positive*. People who lack the rhesus factor are termed *Rh negative*. Incompatibility between Rh-positive and Rh-negative blood is an important cause of blood transfusion reactions and *hemolytic disease of the newborn. *See also* blood group.

rheumatic fever (acute rheumatism) a disease affecting mainly children and young adults that arises as a delayed complication of infection of the upper respiratory tract with hemolytic streptococci (*see* Streptococcus). The main features are fever, arthritis progressing from joint to joint, reddish circular patches on the skin, small painless nodules formed on bony prominences such as the elbow, abnormal involuntary movements of the limbs and head (*chorea), and inflammation of the heart muscle, its valves, and the membrane surrounding the heart. The condition may progress to *chronic rheumatic heart disease*, with scarring and chronic inflammation of the heart and its valves leading to heart failure, murmurs, and damage to the valves. The initial infection is treated with antibiotics (e.g. penicillin) and bed rest, with aspirin for the joint pain. Following an acute attack, long-term prophylaxis with penicillin is often used to prevent a relapse. Rheumatic fever is becoming much less common in developed countries, probably as a result of antibiotic use.

rheumatism *n.* any disorder in which aches and pains affect the muscles and joints. *See* rheumatoid arthritis, rheumatic fever, osteoarthritis, gout.

rheumatoid arthritis the second most common form of *arthritis (after *osteoarthritis). It typically involves the joints of the fingers, wrists, feet, and ankles, with later involvement of the hips, knees, shoulders, and neck. It is a disease of the synovial lining of joints; the joints are initially painful, swollen, and stiff and are usually affected symmetrically. As the disease progresses the ligaments supporting the joints are damaged and there is erosion of the bone, leading to deformity of the joints. Tendon sheaths can be affected, leading to tendon rupture. Onset can be at any age, and there is a considerable range of severity. Women are at greater risk. Rheumatoid arthritis is an *autoimmune disease, and most patients show the presence of *rheumatoid factor* in their serum. There are characteristic changes on X-ray. In the early stages there is soft tissue swelling and periarticular osteoporosis; late stages are characterized by marginal bony erosions, narrowing of the articular space, articular destruction, and joint deformity.

Treatment is with a variety of drugs, including anti-inflammatory analgesics (*see* NSAID), steroids, *immunosuppressants, *methotrexate, and *gold compounds. Surgical treatment is by excision of the synovium in early cases or by *fusion or joint replacement once bony changes have occurred. (*See also* hip replacement.) The condition may resolve spontaneously, but is usually relapsing and remitting with steady progression. It may finally burn itself out, leaving severely deformed joints.

rheumatology *n.* the medical specialty concerned with the diagnosis and management of disease involving joints, tendons, muscles, ligaments, and associated structures. *See also* physical medicine. —**rheumatologist** *n.*

rhexis *n.* the breaking apart of a blood vessel, organ, or tissue.

Rh factor *see* rhesus factor.

rhin- (rhino-) *prefix denoting* the nose.

rhinencephalon *n.* the parts of the brain, collectively, that in early stages of evolution were concerned mainly with the sense of smell. The rhinencephalon includes the olfactory nerve, olfactory tract, and the regions now usually classified as belonging to the *limbic system.

rhinitis *n.* inflammation of the mucous membrane of the nose. It may be caused by virus infection (*acute rhinitis*; *see* cold) or an allergic reaction (*allergic rhinitis*; *see* hay fever). In *atrophic rhinitis* the mucous membrane becomes thinned and fragile; in *perennial allergic rhinitis* there is overgrowth of, and increased secretion by, the membrane.

rhinolith *n.* a stone (calculus) in the nose, usually formed around a foreign body.

rhinology *n.* the branch of medicine concerned with disorders of the nose and nasal passages.

rhinomycosis *n.* fungal infection of the lining of the nose.

rhinophyma *n.* a bulbous craggy swelling of the nose, usually in men. It is a complication of *rosacea and in no way related to alcohol intake. Surgery may be necessary for cosmetic purposes.

rhinoplasty *n.* reparative or cosmetic surgery of the nose, sometimes using tissue (skin, cartilage, or bone) taken from elsewhere in the body or artificial implants.

rhinorrhea *n.* a persistent watery mucous discharge from the nose, as in the common cold.

rhinoscleroma *n.* the formation of nodules in the interior of the nose and *nasopharynx, which become thickened. It is caused by bacterial infection (with *Klebsiella rhinoscleromatis*).

rhinoscopy *n.* examination of the interior of the nose using a speculum or endoscope.

rhinosinusitis *n.* inflammation of the lining of the nose and paranasal sinuses. Rhinosinusitis is a common condition caused by allergies, infection, immune deficiencies, *mucociliary transport abnormalities, trauma, drugs, or tumors. *See* rhinitis, sinusitis.

rhinosporidiosis *n.* an infection of the mucous membranes of the nose, larynx, eyes, and genitals that is caused by the fungus *Rhinosporidium seeberi* and is characterized by the formation of tiny growths called *polyps. It occurs most commonly in Asia.

rhinovirus *n.* any one of a group of RNA-containing viruses that cause respiratory infections in humans resembling the common cold. They are included in the *picornavirus group.

Rhipicephalus *n.* a genus of hard *ticks widely distributed in the tropics. The dog tick (*R. sanguineus*) can suck the blood of humans and is commonly involved in the transmission of diseases caused by rickettsiae (*see* typhus).

rhiz- (rhizo-) *prefix denoting* a root. Example: *rhizonychia* (the root of a nail).

rhizotomy *n.* a surgical procedure in which selected nerve roots are cut at the point where they emerge from the spinal cord. In *posterior rhizotomy* the posterior (sensory) nerve roots are cut for the relief of intractable pain in the organs served by these nerves. An *anterior rhizotomy* – the cutting of the anterior (motor) nerve roots – is sometimes done for the relief of severe muscle spasm or *dystonia.

Rhodnius *n.* a genus of large bloodsucking bugs (*see* reduviid). *R. prolixus* is important in the transmission of *Chagas' disease in Central America and the northern part of South America.

rhodopsin (visual purple) *n.* a pigment in the retina of the eye, within the *rods, consisting of *retinal* – an aldehyde of retinol (*vitamin A) – and a protein. The presence of rhodopsin is essential for vision in dim light. It is bleached in the presence of light and this stimulates nervous activity in the rods.

rhombencephalon *n. see* hindbrain.

rhomboid *n.* either of two muscles (*rhomboid major* and *rhomboid minor*) situated in the upper part of the back, between the backbone and shoulder blade. They help to move the shoulder blade backward and upward.

rhonchus *n.* (*pl.* **rhonchi**) an abnormal musical noise produced by air passing through narrowed bronchi. It is heard through a stethoscope, usually when the patient breathes out.

rhythm method a contraceptive method in which sexual intercourse is restricted to the *safe period* at the beginning and end of the *menstrual cycle. The safe period is calculated either on the basis of the length of the menstrual cycle or by reliance on the change of body temperature that occurs at ovulation. A third possible indicator is the change that occurs with ovulation in the stickiness of the mucus at the cervix of the uterus. The method depends for its reliability on the woman having uniform regular periods and its failure rate is higher than with mechanical methods, approaching 25 pregnancies per 100 woman-years.

rhytidectomy (rhytidoplasty) *n. see* facelift.

rib *n.* a curved, slightly twisted, strip of bone forming part of the skeleton of the thorax, which protects the heart and lungs. There are 12 pairs of ribs. The head of each rib articulates with one of the 12 thoracic vertebrae of the backbone; the other end is attached to a section of cartilage (*see* costal cartilage). The first seven pairs – the *true ribs* – are connected directly to the sternum by their costal cartilages. The next three pairs – the *false ribs* – are attached indirectly: each is connected by its cartilage to the rib above it. The last two pairs of ribs – the *floating ribs* – end freely in the muscles of the body wall. Anatomical name: **costa**.

ribavirin *n.* an antiviral drug effective against a range of DNA and RNA viruses, including the herpes group, *respiratory syncytial virus, and those causing *hepatitis C, several strains of influenza, and *Lassa fever. It is administered by a small particle aerosol inhaler or by mouth. Possible side effects include breathing difficulty, bacterial pneumonia, and *pneumothorax; it also antagonizes the action of *zidovudine against HIV. Trade names: **Rebetron, Virazole**.

riboflavin *n. see* vitamin B$_2$.

ribonuclease *n.* an enzyme, located in the *lysosomes of cells, that splits RNA at specific places in the molecule.

ribonucleic acid *see* RNA.

ribose *n.* a pentose sugar (i.e. one with free carbon atoms) that is a component of *RNA and several coenzymes. Ribose is also involved in intracellular metabolism.

ribosome *n.* a particle, consisting of RNA and protein, that occurs in cells and is the site of protein synthesis in the cell (*see* translation). Ribosomes are either attached to the *endoplasmic reticulum or free in the cytoplasm as *polysomes. —**ribosomal** *adj.*

ribozyme *n.* an RNA molecule that can act as an enzyme, catalyzing changes to its own molecular structure. Since replication of DNA and RNA cannot occur without enzymes, and since protein enzymes can only be produced by DNA coding, the question arose as to how nucleic acid molecules were able to replicate in the early stages of evolution. The discovery of ribozymes appears to resolve the enigma (before their discovery, it was assumed that all enzymes were proteins). Research is currently being undertaken to exploit the ability of genetically engineered ribozymes to destroy the RNA of HIV (the AIDS virus).

ricin *n.* a highly toxic albumin obtained from castor oil seeds (*Ricinus communis*) that inhibits protein synthesis and becomes attached to the surface of cells, resulting in gastroenteritis, hepatic congestion and jaundice, and cardiovascular collapse. It is lethal to most species, even in minute amounts (1 µg/kg body weight); it is most toxic if injected intravenously or inhaled as fine particles. Ricin is being investigated as a treatment for certain lymphomas, which depends on its delivery to the exact site of the tumor in order to avoid destruction of healthy cells (*see* immunotoxin).

rickets *n.* a disease of children in which the bones do not harden and are malformed due to a deficiency of *vitamin D. Without vitamin D, not enough calcium salts are deposited in the bones to make them rigid. They are therefore softer than normal and bend out of shape. This is particularly noticeable in the long bones, which become bowed, and in the front of the ribcage, where a characteristic rickety "rosary" may become apparent. The deficiency of vitamin D may be dietary or due to lack of exposure to sunlight, which is important in the conversion of vitamin D to its active form. *See also* osteomalacia.

Renal rickets is due to impaired kidney function: the bones are malformed because bone-forming minerals are excreted in the urine.

rickettsiae *pl. n.* (*sing.* **rickettsia**) a group of very small nonmotile spherical or rodlike parasitic bacteria that cannot reproduce outside the bodies of their hosts. Rickettsiae infect arthropods (ticks, mites, etc.), through which they can be transmitted to mammals (including humans), in which they can cause severe illness. The species *Rickettsia akari* causes *rickettsialpox, R. conorii, R. prowazekii, R. tsutsugamushi,* and *R. typhi* cause different forms of *typhus, R. rickettsii* causes *Rocky Mountain spotted fever, and *Coxiella burnetii* causes *Q fever. —**rickettsial** *adj.*

rickettsialpox a disease of mice caused by the microorganism *Rickettsia akari* and transmitted to humans by mites; it produces chills, fever, muscular pain, and a rash similar to that of *chickenpox. The disease is mild and runs its course in 2–3 weeks. *See also* typhus.

ridge *n.* **1.** (in anatomy) a crest or a long narrow protuberance, e.g. on a bone. **2.** (in dental anatomy) *see* alveolus.

Riedel's thyroiditis (Riedel's struma) a rare fibrosing destructive disorder of the thyroid gland that may spread to adjacent tissues and obstruct the airway. It is sometimes associated with fibrosis in other parts of the body, such as the bile duct or *retroperitoneal fibrosis. The treatment is surgical removal. [B. M. C. L. Riedel (1846–1916), German surgeon]

rifabutin an antibacterial agent used in the prevention of *Mycobacterium avium* complex (*see* Mycobacterium) in patients with advanced HIV infection. It is administered orally; side effects include rash, *neutropenia, and gastrointestinal intolerance. Trade name: **Mycobutin**.

rifampin *n.* an *antibiotic used to treat various infections, particularly tuberculosis. It is administered by mouth or injection; digestive upsets and sensitivity reactions sometimes occur. Trade names: **Rifadin, Rimactane**.

Rift Valley fever a virus disease of East Africa transmitted from animals to humans by mosquitoes and causing symptoms resembling those of *influenza.

rigidity *n.* (in neurology) resistance to the passive movement of a limb persisting throughout its range. It is a symptom of *parkinsonism. The smooth resistance through the whole range of movement is called *plastic* or *lead-pipe rigidity*; intermittent resistance with superimposed tremor, as in parkinsonism, is called *cogwheel rigidity. Compare* spasticity.

rigor *n.* **1.** an abrupt attack of shivering and a sensation of coldness, accompanied by a rapid rise in body temperature. This often marks the onset of a fever and may be followed by a feeling of heat, with copious sweating. **2.** *see* rigor mortis.

rigor mortis the stiffening of a body that occurs within some eight hours of death, due to chemical changes in muscle tissue. It starts to disappear after about 24 hours.

riluzole *n.* a drug used to prolong the lives of patients with amyotrophic lateral *sclerosis (*see* motor neuron disease). It is administered by mouth; side effects include nausea, vomiting, and dizziness. Trade name: **Rilutek**.

rima *n.* (in anatomy) a cleft. The *rima glottidis* (or glottis) is the space between the vocal cords.

rimexolone *n.* a *corticosteroid used to

treat inflammation of the eye. It is administered topically as eye drops; side effects include blurred vision, eye irritation, tearing, and sore throat. Trade name: **Vexol**.

ring n. (in anatomy) see annulus.

ring block a circumferential ring of local anesthetic solution used to block the nerves of a digit for purposes of minor surgery (see nerve block). Precautions are necessary to avoid vascular damage leading to gangrene.

Ringer's solution a clear colorless *physiological solution of sodium chloride (common salt), potassium chloride, and calcium chloride prepared with recently boiled pure water. The osmotic pressure of the solution is the same as that of blood serum. Ringer's solution is used for maintaining organs or tissues alive outside the animal or human body for limited periods. Sterile Ringer's solution is injected intravenously to treat dehydration. [S. Ringer (1835–1910), British physiologist]

ringworm (tinea) n. a fungus infection of the skin, particularly the scalp and feet, and occasionally of the nails. Ringworm is caused by various species of the dermatophyte fungi (*Microsporum, Trichophyton,* and *Epidermophyton*) and it also affects animals, a source of infection for humans. Ringworm is highly contagious and can be spread by direct contact or via infected materials. As its name suggests, the infection is ringlike and it causes intense itching. The most common form of ringworm is *athlete's foot* (*tinea pedis*), which affects the skin between the toes. Another common type is ringworm of the scalp (*tinea capitis*), of which there is a severe form – *favus*. Ringworm also affects the groin and thighs (*tinea cruris: see* jock itch) and the skin under a beard (*tinea barbae*). The disease is treated with antifungal agents taken by mouth (such as griseofulvin) or applied locally.

Rinne's test a test to determine whether *deafness is conductive or sensorineural. A vibrating tuning fork is held first in the air, close to the ear, and then with its base placed on the bone (mastoid process) behind the ear. If the sound conducted by air is louder than the sound conducted by bone, the test is positive and the deafness is sensorineural; a negative result, when the sound conducted by the bone lasts longer, indicates conductive deafness. [H. A. Rinne (1819–68), German otologist]

risk factor an attribute, such as a habit (e.g. cigarette smoking) or exposure to some environmental hazard, that causes the individual concerned to have a greater likelihood of developing an illness. The relationship is one of probability and as such can be distinguished from a *causal agent.

risk register a list of infants who have experienced some event in their obstetric and/or perinatal history known to be correlated with a higher than average likelihood of serious abnormality. Such children are subjected to extra surveillance. Problems associated with risk registers include limiting the designation of predisposing conditions in order to contain the number on the register within reasonable proportions and ensuring that children not on the register receive adequate surveillance.

risperidone n. an atypical *antipsychotic drug used in the treatment of schizophrenia and other psychoses in patients unresponsive to conventional antipsychotics. Side effects, which are fewer and less severe than those of the older antipsychotics, include nausea, anxiety, headache, and fatigue. Trade name: **Risperdal**.

risus sardonicus an abnormal grinning expression resulting from involuntary prolonged contraction of facial muscles, as seen in *tetanus.

ritodrine n. see sympathomimetic.

ritonavir n. see protease inhibitor.

Ritter's disease see staphylococcal scalded skin syndrome. [G. Ritter von Rittershain (1820–83), German physician]

rituximab n. a *monoclonal antibody used to treat some types of non-Hodgkin's *lymphoma that have not responded to standard chemotherapy. It is administered by intravenous infusion; side effects include nausea, vomiting, and allergic reactions. Trade name: **Rituxan**.

rivastigmine n. see acetylcholinesterase inhibitor.

river blindness see onchocerciasis.

RNA (ribonucleic acid) a *nucleic acid, occurring in the nucleus and cytoplasm of cells, that is concerned with synthesis of proteins (see messenger RNA, ribosome, transfer RNA, translation). In some viruses RNA is the genetic material. The RNA molecule is a single strand made up of units called *nucleotides.

Rocky Mountain spotted fever (spotted fever, tick fever) a disease of rodents and other small mammals in the US caused by the microorganism *Rickettsia rickettsii* and transmitted to humans by ticks. Symptoms include fever, muscle pains, and a profuse reddish rash like that of measles. If untreated, the disease may be fatal, but treatment with tetracycline or chloramphenicol is effective. *See also* typhus.

rod *n.* one of the two types of light-sensitive cells in the *retina of the eye (*compare* cone). The human eye contains about 125 million rods, which are necessary for seeing in dim light. They contain a pigment, *visual purple* (*rhodopsin*), which is broken down (bleached) in the light and regenerated in the dark. Breakdown of visual purple gives rise to nerve impulses; when all the pigment is bleached (i.e. in bright light), the rods no longer function. *See also* dark adaptation, light adaptation.

rodent ulcer *see* basal cell carcinoma.

roentgen *n.* a unit of exposure dose of X- or gamma-radiation equal to the dose that will produce 2.58×10^{-4} coulomb on all the ions of one sign, when all the electrons released in a volume of air of mass 1 kilogram are completely stopped.

roentgenology *n.* the study of the applications of X-rays (roentgen rays). *Radiology is now the preferred term used in the context of medical application.

rofecoxib *n.* an anti-inflammatory drug (*see* NSAID) that selectively inhibits the enzyme cyclo-oxygenase 2 (*see* COX-2 inhibitor). It is taken by mouth in the treatment of osteoarthritis. Trade name: **Vioxx.**

role playing acting out another person's expected behavior, usually in a contrived situation, in order to understand that person better. It is used in family psychotherapy, in teaching social skills to patients, and also in the training of psychiatric (and other) staff.

Romaña's sign an early clinical sign of *Chagas' disease, appearing some three weeks after infection. There is considerable swelling of the eyelids of one or both eyes. This may be due to the presence of the parasites causing the disease but it may also be an allergic reaction to the repeated bites of their insect carriers. [C. Romaña (20th century), Brazilian physician]

Romanovsky stains a group of stains used for microscopical examination of blood cells, consisting of variable mixtures of thiazine dyes, such as azure B, with eosin. Romanovsky stains give characteristic patterns, on the basis of which blood cells are classified. The group includes the stains of Leishman, Wright, May-Grünwald, and Giemsa. [D. L. Romanovsky (1861–1921), Russian physician]

Romberg's sign a finding on examination suggesting a sensory disorder affecting those nerves that transmit information to the brain about the position of the limbs and joints and the tension in the muscles. The patient is asked to stand upright. Romberg's sign is positive if posture is maintained when the eyes are open but the patient sways and falls when the eyes are closed. [M. Romberg (1795–1873), German neurologist]

rongeur *n.* powerful biting forceps for cutting tissue, particularly bone.

root *n.* 1. (in neurology) a bundle of nerve fibers at its emergence from the spinal cord. The 31 pairs of *spinal nerves have two roots on each side, an anterior root containing motor nerve fibers and a posterior root containing sensory fibers. The roots merge outside the cord to form mixed nerves. 2. (in dentistry) the part of a *tooth that is not covered by enamel and is normally attached to the alveolar bone by periodontal fibers. 3. the origin of any structure, i.e. the point at which it diverges from another structure. Anatomical name: **radix.**

root canal treatment (in *endodontics) the procedure of removing the remnants of the pulp of a tooth, cleaning and shaping the canal inside the tooth, and filling the root canal (*see* root filling). The entire treatment usually extends over several visits. It is used to treat toothache and apical abscesses.

root filling 1. the final stage of *root canal treatment, in which the prepared canal inside a tooth root is filled with a suitable material. **2.** the material used to fill the canal in the root, usually a core of *gutta-percha with a thin coating of sealing cement.

root induction (in *endodontics) a procedure to allow continued root formation in an immature tooth with a damaged pulp.

rooting reflex a primitive reflex present in newborn babies: if the cheek is stroked near the mouth, the infant will turn its head to the same side as the stimulus to suckle.

root resection see apicectomy.

ropinirole n. a *dopamine receptor agonist used to treat Parkinson's disease, either alone or in conjunction with levodopa. It is administered by mouth; side effects include nausea, drowsiness, and swelling (edema) of the legs. Trade name: **Requip.**

Rorschach test a test to measure aspects of personality, consisting of ten inkblots, half of which are in various colors and the other half are in black and white. The responses to the different inkblots are used to derive hypotheses about the subject. The use of the test for the diagnosis of brain damage and schizophrenia is no longer generally supported. *See also* projective test. [H. Rorschach (1884–1922), Swiss psychiatrist]

rosacea n. a chronic inflammatory disease of the face in which the skin becomes abnormally flushed. At times it becomes pustular and there may be an associated *keratitis; hypertrophy of the nose may also occur (see rhinophyma). The disease occurs in both sexes and at all ages but is most common in women in their thirties; the cause is unknown. Treatment with oral tetracycline or. topical metronidazole is very effective.

roseola n. any rose-colored rash, such as occurs in measles, the secondary stage of syphilis, or typhoid fever.

roseola infantum (exanthem subitum) a condition of young children in which a fever lasting for three or four days is followed by a rose-colored maculopapular rash that fades after two days. The most common exanthematous fever in young children, it is caused by human herpesvirus 6.

rosiglitazone n. see thiazolidinediones.

rostellum n. (*pl.* **rostella**) a mobile and retractable knob bearing hooks, present on the head (scolex) of certain *tapeworms, e.g. *Taenia* and *Echinococcus*.

rostrum n. (*pl.* **rostra**) (in anatomy) a beaklike projection, such as that on the sphenoid bone. —**rostral** adj.

rotator n. a muscle that brings about rotation of a part. The *rotatores* are small muscles situated deep in the back between adjacent vertebrae. They help to extend and rotate the vertebrae.

rotavirus n. any member of a genus of viruses that occur in birds and mammals and cause diarrhea (often severe) in children. The viruses are excreted in the feces of infected individuals and are usually transmitted in food prepared with unwashed hands. Rotavirus infection is endemic worldwide.

Rothera's test a method of testing urine for the presence of acetone or acetoacetic acid: a sign of *diabetes mellitus. Strong ammonia is added to a sample of urine saturated with ammonium sulfate crystals and containing a small quantity of sodium nitroprusside. A purple color confirms the presence of acetone or acetoacetic acid. [A. C. H. Rothera (1880–1915), Australian biochemist]

Roth spot a pale area surrounded by hemorrhage sometimes seen in the retina, with the aid of an *ophthalmoscope, in those who have bacterial endocarditis, septicemia, or leukemia. [M. Roth (1839–1915), Swiss physician]

roughage n. see dietary fiber.

rouleau n. (*pl.* **rouleaux**) a cylindrical structure in the blood formed from several red blood cells piled one upon the other and adhering by their rims.

round window see fenestra (rotunda).

roundworm n. see nematode.

RPF see retroperitoneal fibrosis.

RQ see respiratory quotient.

-rrhagia (-rrhage) *suffix denoting* excessive or abnormal flow or discharge from an organ or part. Examples: *hemorrhage* (excessive bleeding); *menorrhagia* (excessive menstrual flow).

-rrhaphy *suffix denoting* surgical sewing; suturing. Example: *herniorrhaphy* (of a hernia).

-rrhea *suffix denoting* a flow or discharge from an organ or part. Example: *rhinorrhea* (from the nose).

-rrhexis *suffix denoting* splitting or rupture of a part. Example: *cardiorrhexis* (of the heart).

RSV see respiratory syncytial virus.

RU-486 *see* mifepristone.

rubefacient *n.* an agent that causes reddening and warming of the skin. Rubefacients, such as methyl salicylate, are often used as *counterirritants for the relief of muscular pain.

rubella *n. see* German measles.

rubeola *n. see* measles.

rubeosis *n.* redness or a red discoloration. *Rubeosis iridis* is a growth of blood vessels onto the iris, usually as a result of ischemia of the eye. This occurs, for example, in diabetic *retinopathy and central *retinal vein occlusion.

rubidium-81 *n.* an artificial radioactive isotope that has a half-life of about four hours and decays into the radioactive gas *krypton-81m, emitting radiations as it does so. It provides a useful source of krypton-81m for use in *ventilation-perfusion scanning. Symbol: ^{81}Rb.

rubor *n.* redness: one of the classic signs of inflammation in a tissue, the other three being *calor (heat), *dolor (pain), and *tumor (swelling). The redness of inflamed tissue is due to the increase in size of the small blood vessels in the area, which therefore contain more blood.

rubrospinal tract a tract of *motor neurons that extends from the midbrain down to different levels in the spinal cord, carrying impulses that have traveled from the cerebral and cerebellar cortex via the nucleus ruber (red nucleus). The tract plays an important part in the control of skilled and dextrous movements.

ruga *n.* (*pl.* **rugae**) a fold or crease, especially one of the folds of mucous membrane that line the stomach.

rule of nines a method for quickly assessing the area of the body covered by burns in order to assist calculation of the amount of intravenous fluid to be given. The body is divided into areas of skin comprising approximately 9% each of the total body surface. These are as follows: each arm = 9%, the head = 9%, each leg = 18%, the back of the torso (including the buttocks) = 18%, the front of the torso = 18%, with the external genitalia making up the final 1%.

rumination *n.* (in psychiatry) an obsessional type of thinking in which the same thoughts or themes are experienced repetitively, to the exclusion of other forms of mental activity. The patient commonly feels depressed and guilty after rumination. Rumination may be distinguished from morbid preoccupation in that the thoughts are irrational and resisted by the patient; they often involve abhorrent or aggressive feelings about events in the remote past and are accompanied by a lack of confidence in memory.

rupture 1. *n. see* hernia. **2.** *n.* the bursting apart or open of an organ or tissue; for example, the splitting of the membranes enclosing an infant during childbirth. **3.** *vb.* (of tissues, etc.) to burst apart or open.

Russell-Silver syndrome a congenital condition characterized by short stature, a triangular face with a small mandible (lower jaw), and asymmetry of the body. [A. Russell (20th century), British pediatrician; H. K. Silver (1918–), US pediatrician]

Russian spring-summer encephalitis an influenza-like viral disease that affects the brain and nervous system and occurs in Russia and central Europe. It is transmitted to humans either through the bite of forest-dwelling ticks of the species *Ixodes persulcatus* or by drinking the milk of infected goats. Infection of the meninges results in paralysis of the limbs and of the muscles of the neck and back. The disease, which is often fatal, can be prevented by vaccination.

Ryle's tube a thin flexible tube of rubber or plastic, inserted through the mouth or nose of a patient and used for withdrawing fluid from the stomach or giving a test meal. [J. A. Ryle (1889–1950), British physician]

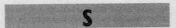

Sabin vaccine an oral vaccine against poliomyelitis, prepared by culture of the virus under special conditions so that it loses its virulence (i.e. it becomes attenuated) but retains its ability to stimulate antibody production. *Compare* Salk vaccine. [A. B. Sabin (1906–93), US bacteriologist]

sac *n.* a pouch or baglike structure. Sacs can enclose natural cavities in the body, e.g. in the lungs (*see* alveolus) or in the *lacrimal apparatus of the eye, or they can be pathological, as in a hernia.

saccades *pl. n.* voluntary rapid movements of the eyes, usually when changing the point of fixation on an object (e.g. when reading).

sacchar- (saccharo-) *prefix denoting* sugar.

saccharide *n.* a carbohydrate. *See also* disaccharide, monosaccharide, polysaccharide.

saccharin *n.* a sweetening agent. Saccharin is 400 times as sweet as sugar and has no energy content. It is very useful as a sweetener in diabetic and low-calorie foods. Saccharin is destroyed by heat and is not therefore used in cooking.

Saccharomyces *n. see* yeast.

saccule (sacculus) *n.* the smaller of the two membranous sacs within the vestibule of the ear: it forms part of the membranous *labyrinth. It is filled with fluid (endolymph) and contains a *macula. This responds to gravity and relays information to the brain about the position of the head.

saccus *n.* a sac or pouch. The *saccus endolymphaticus* is the small sac connected to the saccule and utricle of the inner ear by the *endolymphatic duct.

sacralization *n.* abnormal fusion of the fifth lumbar vertebra with the sacrum.

sacral nerves the five pairs of *spinal nerves that emerge from the spinal column in the sacrum. The nerves carry sensory and motor fibers from the upper and lower leg and from the anal and genital regions.

sacral vertebrae the five vertebrae that are fused together to form the *sacrum.

sacro- *prefix denoting* the sacrum. Examples: *sacrococcygeal* (relating to the sacrum and coccyx); *sacrodynia* (pain in); *sacroiliac* (relating to the sacrum and ilium).

sacroiliitis *n.* inflammation of the sacroiliac joint. Involvement of both of these joints is a common feature of ankylosing *spondylitis and associated rheumatic diseases, including *Reiter's syndrome and *psoriatic arthritis. The resultant low back pain and stiffness may be alleviated by rest and anti-inflammatory analgesics.

sacrum *n.* (*pl.* **sacra**) a curved triangular element of the *backbone consisting of five fused vertebrae (*sacral vertebrae*). It articulates with the last lumbar vertebra above, the coccyx below, and the hip bones laterally. *See also* vertebra.
—**sacral** *adj.*

SAD (seasonal affective disorder) a disorder in which the mood of the affected person is said to change according to the season of the year. Typically, with the onset of winter, there is depression, general slowing of mind and body, excessive sleeping, and overeating. These symptoms resolve with the coming of spring. The phenomenon may partly account for the known seasonal variation in suicide rates. There is evidence that mood is related to light, which suppresses the release of the hormone *melatonin from the pineal gland. Exposure to additional light during the day is said sometimes to relieve symptoms.

saddle joint a form of *diarthrosis (freely movable joint) in which the articulating surfaces of the bones are reciprocally saddle-shaped. It occurs at the carpometacarpal joint of the thumb.

sadism *n.* sexual excitement in response to inflicting or thinking about inflicting pain upon other people. *See also* masochism, sexual deviation. —**sadist** *n.* —**sadistic** *adj.*

safe period the days in each *menstrual cycle when conception is least likely. Ovulation generally occurs at the midpoint of each cycle, and in women with regular periods it is possible to calculate the days at the beginning and end of the cycle when coitus is unlikely to result in pregnancy. *See* rhythm method.

safranin (safranine) *n.* a group of water- and alcohol-soluble basic dyes used to stain cell nuclei and as counterstains for gram-negative bacteria.

sagittal *adj.* describing the dorsoventral plane that extends down the long axis of the body, dividing it into right and left halves (see illustration).

sagittal suture *see* suture (def. 1).

St. Anthony's fire a popular name for inflammation of the skin associated with ergot poisoning. *See* ergotism.

Saint's triad the association between *gallstones, colonic diverticula (*see* diverticulum), and hiatus *hernia. In a patient with dyspepsia it is important to identify which of these conditions, if any, is causing the symptoms. [C. F. M. Saint (1886–1973), South African surgeon]

St. Vitus' dance an archaic name for *Sydenham's chorea.

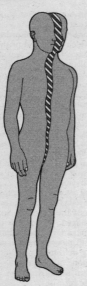

Sagittal plane of section through the body

stituents are water, mucus, buffers, and enzymes (e.g. amylase). The functions of saliva are to keep the mouth moist, to aid swallowing of food, to minimize changes of acidity in the mouth, and to digest starch. *See also* dry mouth. —**salivary** *adj.*

salivary gland a gland that produces *saliva. There are three pairs of salivary glands: the *parotid glands, *sublingual glands, and *submandibular glands (see illustration). They are stimulated by reflex action, which can be initiated by the taste, smell, sight, or thought of food.

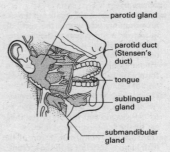

parotid gland

parotid duct (Stensen's duct)

tongue

sublingual gland

submandibular gland

Salivary glands

salaam attacks *see* infantile spasms.

salicylamide *n.* an analgesic drug with effects and uses similar to those of *aspirin. It is administered by mouth and may cause dizziness, sweating, and digestive upsets at high doses.

salicylic acid a drug that causes the skin to peel and destroys bacteria and fungi. It is applied to the skin to treat ulcers, dandruff, eczema, psoriasis, warts, and corns. Skin sensitivity reactions may occur after continued use.

salicylism *n.* poisoning due to an overdose of aspirin or other salicylate-containing compounds. The main symptoms are headache, dizziness, ringing in the ears (tinnitus), disturbances of vision, vomiting, and – in severe cases – delirium and collapse. There is often severe *acidosis.

saline (normal saline) *n.* a solution containing 0.9% sodium chloride. Saline may be used clinically as a diluent for drugs administered by injection and as a plasma substitute.

saliva *n.* the alkaline liquid secreted by the *salivary glands and the mucous membrane of the mouth. Its principal con-

salivary stone *see* sialolith.

salivation *n.* the secretion of saliva by the salivary glands of the mouth, increased in response to the chewing action of the jaws or to the thought, taste, smell, or sight of food. A small but regular flow of saliva is maintained to promote cleanliness in the mouth even when food is not being eaten. *See also* ptyalism.

Salk vaccine a vaccine against poliomyelitis, formed by treating the virus with formalin, which prevents it from causing disease but does not impair its ability to stimulate antibody production. It is administered by injection. *Compare* Sabin vaccine. [J. E. Salk (1914–95), US bacteriologist]

Salmonella *n.* a genus of gram-negative motile rodlike bacteria that inhabit the intestines of animals and humans and cause disease. They ferment glucose, usually with the formation of gas. The species *S. paratyphi* causes *paratyphoid fever, and *S. typhi* causes *typhoid fever. Other species of *Salmonella* cause *food poisoning, gastroenteritis, and septicemia.

salmonellosis *n.* an infestation of the digestive system by bacteria of the genus *Salmonella. See also* food poisoning.

salping- (salpingo-) *prefix denoting* **1.** the fallopian tube. **2.** the auditory tube (meatus).

salpingectomy *n.* the surgical removal of a fallopian tube. The operation involving both tubes is a permanent and completely effective method of contraception (*see* sterilization) since it prevents the egg cells passing from the ovaries to the uterus.

salpingitis *n.* inflammation of a tube, most commonly applied to inflammation of one or both of the fallopian tubes caused by bacterial infection spreading from the vagina or uterus or carried in the blood. In *acute salpingitis* there is a sharp pain in the lower abdomen, which may be mistaken for that of appendicitis, and the infection may spread to the membrane lining the abdominal cavity (*see* peritonitis). In severe cases the tubes may become blocked with scar tissue and the patient will be unable to conceive. The condition is treatable with antibiotics and later, if necessary, by surgical removal of the diseased tube(s).

salpingography *n.* *radiography of one or both fallopian tubes after a *radiopaque substance has been introduced into them via an injection into the uterus. *Standardized selective salpingography* enables occluded tubes, visualized by salpingography, to be restored to patency by means of tubal *catheterization.

salpingolysis *n.* a surgical operation carried out to restore patency to blocked fallopian tubes; it involves the *division and removal of adhesions around the ovarian ends of the tubes.

salpingo-oophoritis *n.* inflammation of a fallopian tube and an ovary.

salpingostomy *n.* the operation performed to restore free passage through a blocked fallopian tube. The blocked portion of the tube is removed surgically and the continuity is then restored. It is performed in women who have been sterilized previously by tubal occlusion (*see* sterilization) and in others whose fallopian tubes have become blocked as a result of pelvic infection.

salt depletion excessive loss of sodium

chloride (common salt) from the body. This may result from sweating, persistent vomiting or diarrhea, or loss of fluid in wounds. The main symptoms are muscular weakness and cramps. Miners and workers in hot climates are particularly at risk, and salt tablets are often taken as a preventive measure.

Salter and Harris classification a method of classifying fractures around the *epiphysis and their prognosis. [R. Salter and R. I. Harris (20th century), Canadian orthopedic surgeons]

Salzmann's degeneration a noninflammatory condition of the cornea resulting in yellow-white nodules under the epithelium in the central area. These may cause symptoms if the epithelium over them breaks down or if they occur in the visual axis. [M. Salzmann (1862–1954), German ophthalmologist]

sanatorium *n.* **1.** a hospital or institution for the rehabilitation and convalescence of patients of any kind. **2.** an institution for patients who have pulmonary tuberculosis. These were prevalent before the antibiotic era.

sandfly *n.* a small hairy fly of the widely distributed genus *Phlebotomus.* Adult sandflies rarely exceed 3 mm in length and have long slender legs. The bloodsucking females of some species transmit various diseases, including *leishmaniasis, *sandfly fever, and *bartonellosis.

sandfly fever (pappataci fever) a viral disease transmitted to humans by the bite of the sandfly *Phlebotomus papatasii.* Sandfly fever occurs principally in countries surrounding the Persian Gulf and the tropical Mediterranean; it occurs during the warmer months, does not last long, and is never fatal. Symptoms resemble those of influenza. There is no specific treatment apart from aspirin and codeine to relieve the symptoms.

sandwich therapy a combination of treatments in which one type of therapy is "sandwiched" between exposures to another therapy. For example, surgical removal of a tumor may be sandwiched between pre- and postoperative courses of radiotherapy. *See also* combined therapy.

sangui- (sanguino-) *prefix denoting* blood.

sanguineous *adj.* **1.** containing, stained, or covered with blood. **2.** (of tissues) containing more than the normal quantity of blood.

sanies *n.* a foul-smelling watery discharge from a wound or ulcer, containing serum, blood, and pus.

SA node *see* sinoatrial node.

saphena *n. see* saphenous vein.

saphenous nerve a large branch of the *femoral nerve that arises in the upper thigh, travels down on the inside of the leg, and supplies the skin from the knee to below the ankle with sensory nerves.

saphenous vein (saphena) either of two superficial veins of the leg, draining blood from the foot. The *long saphenous vein* – the longest vein in the body – runs from the foot, up the medial side of the leg, to the groin, where it joins the femoral vein. The *short saphenous vein* runs up the back of the calf to join the popliteal vein at the back of the knee.

sapr- (sapro-) *prefix denoting* 1. putrefaction. 2. decaying matter.

sapremia *n.* blood poisoning by toxins of saprophytic bacteria (bacteria living on dead or decaying matter). *Compare* pyemia, septicemia, toxemia.

saprophyte *n.* any free-living organism that lives and feeds on the dead and putrefying tissues of animals or plants. *Compare* parasite. —**saprophytic** *adj.*

saquinavir *n. see* protease inhibitor.

sarc- (sarco-) *prefix denoting* 1. flesh or fleshy tissue. 2. muscle.

sarcocele *n.* an obsolete term for a fleshy tumor (sarcoma) of the testis.

Sarcocystis *n.* a genus of parasitic protozoans (*see* Sporozoa) that infect birds, reptiles, and herbivorous mammals. *S. lindemanni*, which occasionally infects humans, forms cylindrical cysts (*sarcocysts*) in the muscle fibers. In heavy infections these cysts can cause tissue degeneration and so provoke muscular pain and weakness. Sarcocysts have, in the few positively diagnosed cases, been located in the heart muscles, arm muscles, and larynx.

sarcoid 1. *adj.* fleshy. 2. *n.* a fleshy tumor.

sarcoidosis (Boeck's disease) *n.* a chronic disorder of unknown cause in which the lymph nodes in many parts of the body are enlarged and small fleshy nodules (*see* granuloma) develop in the lungs, liver, and spleen. The skin, nervous system, eyes, and salivary glands are also commonly affected (*see* uveoparotitis),

and the condition has features similar to *tuberculosis. Recovery is complete with minimal after effects in two-thirds of all cases.

sarcolemma *n.* the cell membrane that encloses a muscle cell (muscle fiber).

sarcoma *n.* any *cancer of connective tissue. These tumors may occur in any part of the body, since they arise in the tissues that make up an organ rather than being restricted to a particular organ. They can arise in fibrous tissue, muscle, fat, bone, cartilage, synovium, blood and lymphatic vessels, and various other tissues. *See also* chondrosarcoma, fibrosarcoma, leiomyosarcoma, liposarcoma, lymphangiosarcoma, osteosarcoma, rhabdomyosarcoma. —**sarcomatous** *adj.*

sarcomatosis *n.* *sarcoma that has spread widely throughout the body, most commonly through the bloodstream. It is treated with drugs, typically one or a combination of the following: cyclophosphamide, vincristine, dactinomycin, methotrexate, or doxorubicin.

sarcomere *n.* one of the basic contractile units of which *striated muscle fibers are composed.

Sarcophaga *n.* a genus of widely distributed nonbloodsucking flies, the flesh flies. Maggots are normally found in carrion or excrement but occasionally females will deposit their eggs in wounds or ulcers giving off a foul-smelling discharge; the presence of the maggots causes a serious *myiasis. Rarely, maggots may be ingested with food and give rise to an intestinal myiasis.

sarcoplasm (myoplasm) *n.* the cytoplasm of muscle cells.

sarcoplasmic reticulum an arrangement of membranous vesicles and tubules found in the cytoplasm of striated muscle fibers. The sarcoplasmic reticulum plays an important role in the transmission of nervous excitation to the contractile parts of the fibers.

Sarcoptes *n.* a genus of small oval mites. The female of *S. scabiei*, the human itch mite, tunnels into the skin, where it lays its eggs. The presence of the mites causes severe irritation, which eventually leads to *scabies.

sarcostyle *n.* a bundle of muscle fibrils.

SARS (severe acute respiratory syndrome) a viral respiratory illness caused by a

virus called SARS-associated corona-
virus (SARS-CoV). Symptoms include
headache, an overall feeling of discomfort and body aches, diarrhea, and dry
cough. Most patients develop pneumonia. SARS was first reported in Asia in
February 2003. Over the following few
months, the illness spread to more than
two dozen countries in North America,
South America, Europe, and Asia. The
SARS global outbreak of 2003 was contained; however, it is possible that the
disease could re-emerge.

sartorius n. a narrow ribbonlike muscle at
the front of the thigh, arising from the
anterior superior spine of the ilium and
extending to the tibia, just below the
knee. The longest muscle in the body,
the sartorius flexes the leg on the thigh
and the thigh on the abdomen.

saturated fatty acid a *fatty acid in which
all the carbon atoms are linked by single
bonds and the molecule is unable to
accept additional atoms (i.e. it cannot
undergo addition reactions with other
molecules). These fats occur mainly in
animal and dairy products, and a diet
high in these foods may contribute to a
high serum cholesterol level, which may
increase the risk of *coronary artery disease. *Compare* unsaturated fatty acid.

satyriasis n. an extreme degree of promis-
cuous heterosexual activity in men.
Compare nymphomania.

saucerization n. **1.** an operation in which
tissue is cut away from a wound to form
a saucerlike depression. It is carried out
to facilitate healing and is commonly
used to treat injuries or disorders in
which bone is infected. **2.** the concave
appearance of the upper surface of a
vertebra that has been fractured by compression.

Sayre's jacket a plaster of Paris cast
shaped to fit around and support the
backbone. It is used in cases where the
vertebrae have been severely damaged
by disease, such as tuberculosis. [L. A.
Sayre (1820–1900), US surgeon]

scab n. a hard crust of dried blood, serum,
or pus that develops during the body's
wound-healing process over a sore, cut,
or scratch.

scabicide n. a drug that kills the mites causing *scabies.

scabies n. a skin infection caused by the
itch mite *Sarcoptes scabiei*. Scabies is

typified by severe itching (particularly
at night), red papules, and often secondary infection. The female mite tunnels in the skin to lay her eggs and the
newly hatched mites pass easily from
person to person by contact. The intense
itching represents a true allergic reaction to the mite, its eggs, and its feces.
Commonly infected areas are the groin,
penis, nipples, and the skin between the
fingers. Local treatment is with *permethrin, *lindane, *malathion, or benzyl
benzoate creams, which kill the mites.
All members of a family may need treatment, and clothing and bedding should
be disinfested.

scala n. one of the spiral canals of the
*cochlea. The *scala media* (*cochlear duct*)
is the central membranous canal, containing the sensory apparatus of the
cochlea; the *scala vestibuli* and *scala tympani* are the two bony canals of the
cochlea.

scald n. a *burn produced by a hot liquid
or vapor, such as boiling water or steam.

scale **1.** n. any of the flakes of dead epidermal cells shed from the skin. **2.** vb. to
scrape deposits of calculus (tartar) from
the teeth (*see* scaler).

scalenus n. one of four paired muscles of
the neck (*scalenus anterior, medius, minimus,* and *posterior*), extending from the
cervical (neck) vertebrae to the first and
second ribs. They are responsible for
raising the first and second ribs in inspiration and for bending the neck forward
and to either side.

**scalenus syndrome (thoracic outlet syn-
drome)** the group of symptoms caused
by the compression of the subclavian
artery and the lower roots of the brachial
plexus against the fibrous and bony
structures of the outlet of the upper thoracic vertebrae. Loss of sensation, wasting, and vascular symptoms may be
found in the affected arm, which also
may be painful.

scaler n. an instrument for removing calculus from the teeth. It may be a hand
instrument or one energized by rapid
ultrasonic vibrations.

scalp n. the part of the skin that covers the
head, exclusive of the face and ears. It is
normally covered with hair.

scalpel n. a small pointed surgical knife
used by surgeons for cutting tissues. It
has a straight handle and usually de-

tachable disposable blades of different shapes.

scan 1. *n.* examination of the body or a part of the body using *ultrasonography, *computed tomography (CT), *magnetic resonance imaging (MRI), or scintigraphy (*see* scintigram). **2.** *n.* the image obtained from such an examination. **3.** *vb.* to examine the body using any of these techniques.

scanning speech a disorder of articulation in which the syllables are inappropriately separated and equally stressed. It is caused by disease of the cerebellum or its connecting fibers in the brainstem.

scaphocephaly *n.* an abnormally long and narrow skull due to premature closure of the suture between the two parietal bones along the top of the skull. —**scaphocephalic** *adj.*

scaphoid bone a boat-shaped bone of the wrist (*see* carpus). It articulates with the trapezium and trapezoid bones in front, with the radius behind, and with the capitate and lunate medially. It is commonly injured in falls.

scaphoid fracture a fracture of the scaphoid bone in the wrist, usually caused by a fall onto the outstretched hand. There is pain and swelling, and movements of the wrist and thumb are painful. Diagnosis is by X-ray, but the fracture may not initially be visible. Treatment is with a cast. Due to the anatomy of its blood supply, healing can take a long time, and bone grafting (*see* graft) and internal fixation may be required for non-*union.

scapul- (scapulo-) *prefix denoting* the scapula.

scapula *n.* (*pl.* **scapulas** *or* **scapulae**) the shoulder blade: a triangular bone, a pair of which form the back part of the shoulder girdle (see illustration). The *spine* on its dorsal (back) surface ends at the *acromion process* at the top of the shoulder. This process turns forward and articulates with the collar bone (*clavicle) at the *acromioclavicular joint*; it overhangs the *glenoid fossa*, into which the humerus fits to form the socket of the shoulder joint. The *coracoid process* curves upward and forward from the neck of the scapula and provides attachment for associated ligaments and muscles. —**scapular** *adj.*

scar *n.* a permanent mark left after wound healing. A *hypertrophic scar* is an abnormal raised scar that tends to settle after a year or so, as distinct from a *keloid, which is not only permanent but tends to extend beyond the original wound.

scarification *n.* the process of making a series of shallow cuts or scratches in the skin to allow a substance to penetrate the body. This was commonly performed during vaccination against smallpox; the vaccine was administered as a droplet left in contact with the scarified area.

scarlatina *n. see* scarlet fever.

scarlet fever a highly infectious disease, mainly of childhood, caused by a strain of *Streptococcus* bacteria that produces toxins. Symptoms begin 2–4 days after exposure and include fever, tonsillitis, and a characteristic widespread scarlet rash. The tongue is also affected; initially covered by a thick white material, it then becomes bright red (the "strawberry tongue"). Treatment with antibiotics shortens the course of the disease and reduces the risk of secondary complications, which include kidney and ear inflammation. Medical name: **scarlatina**. *Compare* German measles.

Scarpa's triangle *see* femoral triangle. [A. Scarpa (1747–1832), Italian anatomist and surgeon]

scat- (scato-) *prefix denoting* feces.

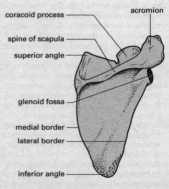

Right scapula (dorsal surface)

scatter diagram (in statistics) *see* correlation.

SCC *see* squamous cell carcinoma.

Scheuermann's disease *osteochondritis involving one or more of the vertebrae. The condition often arises in adolescence and causes spinal pain and *kyphosis. It usually resolves spontaneously without deformity, causing sclerotic change in the affected bone. [H. W. Scheuermann (1877–1960), Danish surgeon]

Schick test a test to determine whether a person is susceptible to diphtheria. A small quantity of diphtheria toxin is injected under the skin; a patch of reddening and swelling shows that the person has no immunity and – if at particular risk – should be immunized. [B. Schick (1877–1967), US pediatrician]

Schiff's reagent aqueous *fuchsin solution decolorized with sulfur dioxide. A blue coloration develops in the presence of aldehydes. [H. Schiff (1834–1915), German chemist]

Schilling test a test used to assess a patient's capacity to absorb vitamin B_{12} from the bowel. Radioactive vitamin B_{12} is given by mouth and urine collected for 24 hours. A normal individual will excrete at least 10% of the original dose over this period; a patient with *pernicious anemia will excrete less than 5%. [R. F. Schilling (1919–   ), US physician]

schindylesis *n.* a form of *synarthrosis (immovable joint) in which a crest of one bone fits into a groove of another.

-schisis *suffix denoting* a cleft or split.

schism *n.* a disorder of relationships within a family, in which parents quarrel and children are made to take sides. It was proposed as a cause of later schizophrenia in the children, but is more likely to be a nonspecific cause of psychological vulnerability.

schisto- *prefix denoting* a fissure; split.

schistoglossia *n.* fissuring of the tongue. Congenital fissures are transverse, whereas those due to disease (such as syphilis) are usually longitudinal.

Schistosoma (Bilharzia) *n.* a genus of blood *flukes, three species of which are important parasites of humans causing one of the most serious of tropical diseases (*see* schistosomiasis). *S. japonicum* is common in the Far East; *S. mansoni* is widespread in Africa, the West Indies, and South and Central America; and *S.*

haematobium occurs in Africa and the Middle East.

schistosomiasis (bilharziasis) *n.* a tropical disease that is caused by blood flukes of the genus *Schistosoma. Eggs present in the stools or urine of infected people undergo part of their larval development within freshwater snails living in water contaminated with human sewage. The disease is contracted when *cercaria larvae, released from the snails, penetrate the skin of anyone bathing in infected water. Adult flukes eventually settle in the blood vessels of the intestine (*S. mansoni* and *S. japonicum*) or bladder (*S. haematobium*); the release of their spiked eggs causes anemia, inflammation, and the formation of scar tissue. Additional intestinal symptoms are diarrhea, dysentery, enlargement of the spleen and liver, and cirrhosis of the liver. If the bladder is affected, blood is passed in the urine and cystitis and cancer of the bladder may develop. The disease is treated with *praziquantel.

schiz- (schizo-) *prefix denoting* a split or division.

schizogony *n.* a phase of asexual reproduction in the life cycle of a sporozoan (protozoan parasite) that occurs in the liver or red blood cells. The parasite grows and divides many times to form a *schizont*, which contains many *merozoites. The eventual release of merozoites of *Plasmodium, the malaria parasite, from the blood cells produces fever in the patient.

schizoid personality a personality characterized by solitariness, emotional coldness to others, inability to experience pleasure, lack of response to praise and criticism, withdrawal into a fantasy world, excessive introspection, and eccentricity of behavior. Some schizophrenics have this personality before their illness, but most schizoid personalities do not become schizophrenic. *See* personality disorder.

schizont *n.* one of the stages that occurs during the asexual phase of the life cycle of a sporozoan. *See* schizogony.

schizonticide *n.* any agent used for killing *schizonts.

schizophrenia *n.* a severe mental disorder (or group of disorders) characterized by a disintegration of the process of thinking, of contact with reality, and of emotional responsiveness. *Delusions and *hallucinations (especially of voices) are usual features, and the patient usually feels that his thoughts, sensations, and actions are controlled by, or shared with, others. He becomes socially withdrawn and loses energy and initiative. The main types of schizophrenia are *simple*, in which increasing social withdrawal and personal ineffectiveness are the major changes; *hebephrenic*, which starts in adolescence or young adulthood (*see* hebephrenia); *paranoid*, characterized by prominent delusions; and *catatonic*, with marked motor disturbances (*see* catatonia). The latter form is now rare.

Schizophrenia commonly – but not inevitably – runs a progressive course. The prognosis has been improved with *antipsychotic drugs and vigorous psychological and social management and rehabilitation. There are strong genetic factors in the causation, and environmental stress can precipitate the illness. —**schizophrenic** *adj.*

schizotypal *adj.* describing a condition characterized by cold aloof feelings, eccentricities of behavior, odd ways of thinking and talking, and occasional short periods of intense illusions, hallucinations, or delusion-like ideas. The condition, known as *borderline schizophrenia*, is similar to some aspects of *schizophrenia and is more common in people who are genetically related to schizophrenics.

Schlemm's canal a channel in the eye, at the junction of the cornea and the sclera, through which the aqueous humor drains. [F. Schlemm (1795–1858), German anatomist]

Schmidt's syndrome the autoimmune destruction of a combination of the thyroid, the adrenals, and the beta cells of the islets of Langerhans, causing type 1 *diabetes mellitus. It is often associated with failure of the ovaries (causing an early menopause), the parathyroids, and the parietal cells of the *gastric glands (causing pernicious anemia). [M. B. Schmidt (1863–1949), German physician]

Schmorl's node (or nodule) a lucent area seen on X-ray of the backbone that denotes extrusion of some nucleus pulposus from an *intervertebral disk into the body of a vertebra. [C. G. Schmorl (1861–1932), German pathologist]

Schönlein-Henoch purpura (Henoch-Schönlein purpura) a blood disease that affects young children; its cause is not known. It is characterized by a purple skin rash due to bleeding into the skin from defective capillaries; abdominal pain; arthritis in major joints; and kidney disturbance. Spontaneous recovery is the usual outcome. Glucocorticoids are often used for treatment. *See also* purpura. [J. L. Schönlein (1793–1864), German physician; E. H. Henoch (1820–1910), German pediatrician]

Schwann cells the cells that lay down the *myelin sheath around the axon of a medullated nerve fiber. Each cell is responsible for one length of axon, around which it twists as it grows, so that concentric layers of membrane envelop the axon. The gap between adjacent Schwann cells forms a *node of Ranvier. [T. Schwann (1810–82), German anatomist and physiologist]

Schwannoma *n. see* neurofibroma.

sciatica *n.* pain felt down the back and outer side of the thigh, leg, and foot. It is usually caused by degeneration of an intervertebral disk, which protrudes laterally to compress a lower lumbar or an upper sacral spinal nerve root. The onset may be sudden, brought on by an awkward lifting or twisting movement. The back is stiff and painful. There may be numbness and weakness in the leg. Bed rest and *NSAIDs will often relieve the pain but surgical treatment, in the form of a *microdiskectomy, is occasionally necessary.

sciatic nerve the major nerve of the leg and the nerve with the largest diameter. It runs down behind the thigh from the lower end of the spine; above the knee joint it divides into two main branches, the *tibial* and *common peroneal nerves*, which are distributed to the muscles and skin of the lower leg.

SCID *see* severe combined immune deficiency.

scintigram *n.* a diagram showing the distribution of radioactive *tracer in a part of the body, produced by recording the flashes of light given off by a *scintillator as it is struck by radiation of different intensities. This technique is called *scintigraphy*. By scanning the body, section by section, a "map" of the radioactivity in various regions is built up, aiding the diagnosis of cancer or other disorders. Such a record is known as a *scintiscan*. These images are now usually obtained using a *gamma camera.

scintillation counter a device to measure and record the fluorescent flashes in a *scintillator exposed to high-energy radiation.

scintillator *n.* a substance that produces a fluorescent flash when struck by high-energy radiation, such as beta or gamma rays. In medicine the most commonly used scintillator is a crystal of thallium-activated sodium iodide, which forms the basis of a *gamma camera. *See also* scintigram.

scintiscan *n. see* scintigram.

scirrhous *adj.* describing carcinomas that are stony hard to the touch. Such a carcinoma (for example of the breast) is known as a *scirrhus*.

scissor leg a disability in which one leg becomes permanently crossed over the other as a result of spasticity of its *adductor muscles or deformity of the hips. The condition occurs in children with brain damage and in adults after strokes. A *tenotomy or injections with *botulinum toxin may reduce the degree of disability.

scissura (scissure) *n.* a cleft or splitting, such as the splitting of the tip of a hair or the splitting open of tissues when a hernia forms.

scler- (sclero-) *prefix denoting* **1.** hardening or thickening. **2.** the sclera. **3.** sclerosis.

sclera (sclerotic coat) *n.* the white fibrous outer layer of the eyeball. At the front of the eye it becomes the cornea. *See* eye. —**scleral** *adj.*

sclerectomy *n.* an operation in which a portion of the sclera (the thick white layer of the eyeball) is removed.

scleredema *n.* a condition characterized by abnormal hardening of the skin, which usually begins with the face and neck and spreads downward over the body. It occurs in association with diabetes mellitus and is usually preceded by an infection, especially a staphylococcal infection. The condition usually disappears spontaneously after a few months.

scleritis *n.* inflammation of the sclera (the white of the eye).

scleroderma *n.* chronic hardening and thickening of the skin, either localized (*see* morphea) or generalized, that results in waxy ivory-colored areas often with pigmented patches. Treatment is unsatisfactory, but spontaneous resolution may occur. The cause is unknown, but scleroderma may well be an *autoimmune disease. Although there is no cure, drugs are available to treat most of its manifestations. *Systemic sclerosis is a related multisystem disorder, which may occur as part of the *CREST syndrome.

scleroma *n.* a hardened patch of skin or mucous membrane, consisting of *granulation tissue.

scleromalacia *n.* thinning of the sclera (white of the eye) as a result of inflammation. The involved area becomes bluish in color. Sometimes the sclera fades away completely in an area, and the underlying tissue (usually the ciliary body) bulges beneath the conjunctiva. This state is known as *scleromalacia perforans*.

scleronychia *n.* hardening and thickening of the nails.

sclerosis *n.* hardening of tissue, usually due to scarring (fibrosis) after inflammation or to aging. It can affect the lateral columns of the spinal cord and the medulla of the brain (*amyotrophic lateral sclerosis* or *Lou Gehrig's disease*), causing progressive muscular paralysis (*see* motor neuron disease). It can also occur in scattered patches throughout the brain and spinal cord (*see* multiple sclerosis) or in the walls of the arteries (*see* arteriosclerosis, atherosclerosis). *See also* tuberous sclerosis.

sclerotherapy *n.* treatment of varicose veins by the injection of an irritant solution. This causes thrombophlebitis, which encourages obliteration of the varicose vein by thrombosis and subsequent scarring. It is also used to treat hemorrhoids and esophageal varices.

sclerotic 1. (sclerotic coat) *n. see* sclera. **2.** *adj.* affected with *sclerosis.

sclerotome *n.* **1.** a surgical knife used in the operation of *sclerotomy. **2.** (in embryology) the part of the segmented mesoderm (*see* somite) in the early embryo that gives rise to all the skeletal tissue of the body. The vertebrae and ribs retain the segmented structure, which is lost in the skull and limbs.

sclerotomy *n.* an operation in which an incision is made in the sclera (white of the eye).

scolex *n.* (*pl.* **scolices**) the head of a *tapeworm. The presence of suckers and/or hooks on the scolex enables the worm to attach itself to the wall of its host's gut.

scoliosis *n.* lateral (sideways) deviation of the backbone, caused by congenital or acquired abnormalities of the vertebrae, muscles, and nerves. Treatment is with spinal braces and, in cases of severe deformity, surgical correction by fusion or *osteotomy. *See also* kyphosis, kyphoscoliosis.

-scope *suffix denoting* an instrument for observing or examining. Example: *gastroscope* (instrument for examining the stomach).

scopolamine (hyoscine) *n.* an *anticholinergic drug that prevents muscle spasm. Scopolamine is used in the treatment of gastric or duodenal ulcers, spasm in the digestive system, and difficult or painful menstruation and also to relax the uterus in labor. It can also be used to calm excitement in some psychiatric conditions, for preoperative medication, for motion sickness, and to dilate the pupil and paralyze the muscles of the eye for examination. It is administered by mouth, injection, or skin patch. Side effects are rare but can include dry mouth, blurred vision, difficulty in urination, and increased heart rate. Trade names: **Isopto Hyoscine**, **Transderm-Scop**.

scorbutic *adj.* affected with scurvy.

scoring system any of various methods in which the application of an agreed numerical scale is used as a means of estimating the degree of a clinical situation, e.g. the severity of an injury, the degree of patient recovery, or the extent of malignancy. Examples include the *Glasgow coma scale, *Apgar score, and the *injury scoring system.

scoto- *prefix denoting* darkness.

scotoma *n.* (*pl.* **scotomata**) a small area of abnormally decreased or absent vision in the visual field, surrounded by normal sight. All people have a *blind spot in the visual field of each eye due to the small area occupied by the optic disk, which is not sensitive to light. Similar islands of total visual loss in other parts of the field are referred to as *absolute scotomata*. A *relative scotoma* is a spot where the vision is decreased but still present.

scotometer *n.* an instrument used for mapping defects in the visual field. *See also* campimetry, perimeter.

scotopic *adj.* relating to or describing conditions of poor illumination. For example, *scotopic vision* is vision in dim light in which the *rods of the retina are involved (*see* dark adaptation).

screening test a test carried out on a large number of apparently healthy people to separate those who probably have a specified disease from those who do not. Examples are the *Guthrie test and cervical smears. Limitations depend on the severity and *frequency distribution of the disease and the efficiency and availability of treatment. Other factors to be taken into account are the safety, convenience, cost, and *sensitivity of the test. *See also* genetic screening.

scrofula *n.* *tuberculosis of lymph nodes, usually those in the neck, causing the formation of abscesses. Untreated, these burst through the skin and form running sores, which leave scars when they heal. Treatment with antituberculous drugs is effective. The disease, which is now rare, most commonly affects young children. —**scrofulous** *adj.*

scrofuloderma *n.* tuberculosis of the skin in which the skin breaks down over suppurating tuberculous glands, with the formation of irregular-shaped ulcers with blue-tinged edges. Treatment is with antituberculous drugs, to which scrofuloderma responds better than *lupus vulgaris, another type of skin tuberculosis.

scrototomy *n.* an operation in which the scrotum is surgically explored, usually undertaken to investigate patients with probable obstructive *azoospermia.

scrotum *n.* the paired sac that holds the testes and epididymides outside the abdominal cavity. Its function is to allow the production and storage of spermatozoa to occur at a lower temperature than that of the abdomen. Further temperature control is achieved by contraction or relaxation of muscles in the scrotum. —**scrotal** *adj.*

scrub typhus (tsutsugamushi disease) a disease, widely distributed in SE Asia, caused by the parasitic microorganism *Rickettsia tsutsugamushi* and transmitted to humans through the bite of mites. Only larval mites of the genus *Trombicula* are involved as vectors. Symptoms include headache, chills, high temperature (104°F), a red rash over most of the body, a cough, and delirium. A small ulcer forms at the site of the bite. Scrub typhus is treated with tetracycline and other broad-spectrum antibiotics. *See also* rickettsiae, typhus.

scruple *n.* a unit of weight used in pharmacy. 1 scruple = 1.295 g (20 grains). 3 scruples = 1 dram.

sculpting *n.* a technique of family psychotherapy, in which all the family members are seen together and one member is asked to arrange the others' physical positions to express their relationships and feelings. *See also* group therapy.

scurf *n. see* dandruff.

scurvy *n.* a disease that is caused by a deficiency of *vitamin C (ascorbic acid). It results from the consumption of a diet devoid of fresh fruit and vegetables (unlike most animals, humans cannot synthesize ascorbic acid and must obtain it from food). The first sign of scurvy is swollen bleeding gums. This may be followed by subcutaneous bleeding and the opening of previously healed wounds; prolonged deficiency of the vitamin may eventually lead to death. Scurvy may result from food faddism or alcoholism; elderly men who live alone are at special risk. Treatment with vitamin C soon reverses the effects.

scybalum *n.* a lump or mass of hard feces.

seasickness *n. see* motion sickness.

seasonal affective disorder *see* SAD.

seat-belt syndrome thoracic injuries that arise from violent contact with a restraining seat belt in motor vehicle accidents occurring at high speeds.

sebaceous cyst 1. (wen) or a pale or flesh-colored dome-shaped cyst that commonly occurs in adults, especially on the face, neck, or trunk. It is firm, with a central dot, and contains keratin not sebum; such cysts are therefore more correctly referred to as *epidermoid cysts*. It is usually removed surgically. **2.** a cyst of the sebaceous glands occurring in multiple form in a rare inherited condition, *steatocystoma multiplex*.

sebaceous gland any of the simple or branched glands in the *skin that secrete an oily substance, *sebum. They open into hair follicles and their secretion is produced by the disintegration of their cells. Some parts of the skin have many sebaceous glands, others few. Activity varies with age: the glands are most active at puberty.

seborrhea *n.* excessive secretion of sebum by the *sebaceous glands. The glands are enlarged, especially on the nose and central face. The condition predisposes to acne and is common at puberty, usually lasting for a few years. Seborrhea is sometimes associated with a kind of *eczema (seborrheic eczema). —**seborrheic** *adj.*

sebum *n.* the oily substance secreted by the *sebaceous glands and reaching the skin surface through small ducts that lead into the hair follicles. Sebum provides a thin film of fat over the skin, which slows the evaporation of water; it also has an antibacterial effect.

second *n.* the *SI unit of time, equal to the duration of 9,192,631,770 periods of the radiation corresponding to the transition between two hyperfine levels of the ground state of the cesium-133 atom. This unit is now the basis of all time measurements. Symbol: s.

secondary care health care provided by medical specialists or hospital staff members for a patient whose primary care was provided by the doctor who first diagnosed or treated the patient. For example, a general practitioner who accepts a patient with an unusual skin condition provides primary care but if he refers the patient to a dermatologist, the skin specialist becomes the source of secondary care. *Compare* tertiary care.

secondary prevention the avoidance or alleviation of the serious consequences of disease by early detection. Best known methods include routine examinations and *screening tests applied to populations regarded as having a high risk of contracting specific diseases.

secondary sexual characteristics the physical characteristics that develop after puberty as a result of sexual maturation. In boys they include the growth of facial and pubic hair and the breaking of the voice. In girls they include the growth of pubic hair and the development of the breasts.

second messenger an organic molecule

that acts within a cell to initiate the response to a signal carried by a chemical messenger (e.g. a hormone) that does not itself enter the cell. Examples of second messengers are *inositol triphosphate and cyclic *AMP.

secretagogue *n.* a substance that stimulates secretion. An example is *pentagastrin, which stimulates the secretion of gastric juice.

secretin *n.* a hormone secreted from the small intestine (duodenum) when acidified food leaves the stomach. Secretin stimulates the secretion of relatively enzyme-free alkaline juice by the pancreas (*see* pancreatic juice) and of bile by the liver.

secretion *n.* **1.** the process by which a gland isolates constituents of the blood or tissue fluid and chemically alters them to produce a substance that it discharges for use by the body or excretes. The principal methods of secretion – *apocrine, *holocrine, and *merocrine – are illustrated in the diagram. **2.** the substance that is produced by a gland.

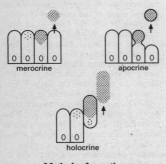

merocrine   apocrine

holocrine

Methods of secretion

secretor *n.* a person in whose saliva and other body fluids are found traces of the water-soluble A, B, or O agglutinogens that determine *blood group.

section *n.* **1.** (in surgery) the act of cutting (the cut or division made is also called a section). For example, an *abdominal section* is performed for surgical exploration of the abdomen (*see* laparotomy). A *transverse section* is a cut made at right angles to a structure's long axis. *See also* cesarean section. **2.** (in imaging) a three-

dimensional reconstruction of body scans obtained by computed tomography or magnetic resonance imaging. These are reconstituted as transverse and sagittal plane sections, less commonly as coronal plane sections. **3.** (in microscopy) a thin slice of the specimen to be examined under a microscope.

sedation *n.* the production of a restful state of mind, particularly by the use of drugs (*see* sedative).

sedative *n.* a drug that has a calming effect, relieving anxiety and tension. Sedatives are *hypnotic drugs administered at lower doses than those needed for sleep (drowsiness is a common side effect). *See also* anxiolytic.

sedimentation rate the rate at which solid particles sink in a liquid under the influence of gravity. *See also* ESR (erythrocyte sedimentation rate).

segment *n.* (in anatomy) a portion of a tissue or organ, usually distinguishable from other portions by lines of demarcation. For example, the uterus consists of *upper* and *lower segments*. The *anterior segment* of the eye is the front portion, including the cornea, anterior chamber, iris, and lens. *See also* somite.

Seidel sign a bright green flow of liquid seen when fluorescein dye is applied to the cornea and viewed with cobalt blue light. It indicates leakage of aqueous humor. [E. Seidel (1882–1948), German ophthalmologist]

seizure *n.* **1.** the sudden attack or onset of a disease. **2.** an epileptic episode or attack; these are usually named for the different kinds of *epilepsy. *See also* convulsion.

Seldinger technique the retrograde passage of a catheter into the aorta via a puncture in the femoral artery. It is used to outline the aorta and its major branches, including the blood vessels of the lower extremities. [S. I. Seldinger (1921–), Swedish radiologist]

selective serotonin reuptake inhibitor *see* SSRI.

selegiline *n.* a selective *MAO inhibitor used in combination with other drugs, in the treatment of parkinsonism. Administered by mouth, selegiline is thought to retard the breakdown of *dopamine. Possible side effects include faintness on standing up, nausea, involuntary movements, and confusion. Trade names: **Carbex, Eldepryl**.

selenium *n.* a *trace element that is an essential component of the enzyme glutathione peroxidase, which catalyzes the oxidation of *glutathione by hydrogen peroxide. It thus has important *antioxidant properties. Dietary deficiency of selenium results in *cardiomyopathy. Symbol: Se.

selenium sulfide a selenium compound with antifungal properties, used to treat *dandruff and scalp infections. It is administered in a shampoo. Trade names: **Exsel, Selsun, Selsun Blue**.

sella turcica a depression in the body of the sphenoid bone that encloses the pituitary gland.

semeiology *n.* see symptomatology.

semen (seminal fluid) *n.* the fluid ejaculated from the penis at sexual climax. Each ejaculate may contain 300–500 million sperm suspended in a fluid secreted by the *prostate gland and *seminal vesicles with a small contribution from *Cowper's glands. It contains fructose, which provides the sperm with energy, and *prostaglandins, which affect the muscles of the uterus and may therefore assist transport of the sperm. —**seminal** *adj.*

semen analysis (seminal analysis) analysis of a specimen of semen, which should be obtained after five days of abstinence from coitus, in order to assess male fertility. Normal values are as follows: volume of ejaculate: 2–6.5 ml; liquefaction complete in 30 minutes; sperm concentration: 20–200 million spermatozoa per ml (*sperm count* refers to the total number of spermatozoa in the ejaculate); motility: 60% moving progressively at 30 minutes to 3 hours; abnormal forms: less than 20%. Analysis of three separate specimens is necessary before confirming the presence of an abnormal result.

semi- *prefix denoting* half.

semicircular canals three tubes that form part of the membranous *labyrinth of the ear. They are concerned with balance and each canal registers movement in a different plane. At the base of each canal is a small swelling (an *ampulla*), which contains a *crista. When the head moves, the fluid (endolymph) in the canals presses on the cristae, which register the movement and send nerve impulses to the brain.

semilunar cartilage one of a pair of crescent-shaped cartilages in the knee joint situated between the femur and tibia.

semilunar valve either of the two valves in the heart situated at the origin of the aorta (*aortic valve*) and the pulmonary artery (*pulmonary valve*). Each consists of three flaps (cusps), which maintain the flow of blood in one direction.

seminal analysis see semen analysis.

seminal fluid see semen.

seminal vesicle either of a pair of male accessory sex glands that open into the vas deferens before it joins the urethra. The seminal vesicles secrete most of the liquid component of *semen.

seminiferous tubule any of the long convoluted tubules that make up the bulk of the *testis.

seminoma *n.* a malignant tumor of the testis, appearing as a swelling, often painless, in the scrotum. It tends to occur in an older age group than the *teratomas. The treatment for localized disease is surgery involving removal of the testis (*see* orchiectomy). Secondary tumors in the lungs can be treated with chemotherapy and radiotherapy to the draining lymph nodes. A similar tumor occurs in the ovary (*see* dysgerminoma).

semipermeable membrane a membrane that allows the passage of some molecules but not others. Cell membranes (*see* cell) are semipermeable. Semipermeable membranes are used clinically in *hemodialysis for patients with kidney failure.

semiprone *adj.* describing the position of a patient lying face downward, but with one or both knees flexed to one side so that the body is not lying completely flat. *Compare* prone, supine.

senescence *n.* the condition of aging, which is often marked by a decrease in physical and mental abilities. —**senescent** *adj.*

senile dementia loss of the intellectual faculties, often associated with behavioral deterioration, beginning for the first time in old age. *See also* dementia.

senna *n.* the dried fruits of certain shrubs of the genus *Cassia*, used as a stimulant *laxative to relieve constipation. It is administered by mouth; side effects do not usually occur, but severe diarrhea may follow large doses. Trade name: **Senokot**.

sensation *n.* a feeling: the result of messages from the body's sensory receptors registering in the brain as information about the environment. Messages from *exteroceptors are interpreted as specific sensations – smell, taste, temperature, pain, etc. – in the conscious mind. Messages from *interoceptors, however, rarely reach the consciousness to produce sensation.

sense *n.* one of the faculties by which the qualities of the external environment are appreciated – sight, hearing, smell, taste, or touch.

sense organ a collection of specialized cells (*receptors), connected to the nervous system, that is capable of responding to a particular stimulus from either outside or inside the body. Sense organs can detect light (the eyes), heat, pain, and touch (the skin), smell (the nose), and taste (the taste buds).

sensibility *n.* the ability to be affected by, and respond to, changes in the surroundings (*see* stimulus). Sensibility is a characteristic of cells of the nervous system.

sensitive *adj.* possessing the ability to respond to a *stimulus. The cells of the retina, for example, are sensitive to the stimulus of light and respond by sending nerve impulses to the brain. Other *receptors are sensitive to different specific stimuli, such as pressure or the presence of chemical substances.

sensitivity *n.* **1.** (in microbiology) the degree to which a disease-causing organism responds to treatment by *antibiotics or other drugs. **2.** (in preventive medicine) a measure of the reliability of a *screening test based on the proportion of people with a specific disease who react positively to the test (the higher the sensitivity the fewer false negatives). This contrasts with *specificity*, which is the proportion of people free from disease who react negatively to the test (i.e. the higher the specificity the fewer the false positives). Although these are theoretically independent variables, most screening tests are so designed that if the sensitivity is increased the specificity is reduced and the number of false positives may rise to wasteful proportions.

sensitization *n.* **1.** alteration of the responsiveness of the body to the presence of foreign substances. In the development of an *allergy, an individual becomes sensitized to a particular allergen and reaches a state of hypersensitivity (*see* hypersensitive). The phenomena of sensitization are due to the production of antibodies. **2.** (in behavior therapy) a form of *aversion therapy in which anxiety-producing stimuli are associated with the unwanted behavior. In *covert sensitization* the behavior and an unpleasant feeling (such as disgust) are evoked simultaneously by verbal cues.

sensory *adj.* relating to the input division of the nervous system, which carries information from *receptors throughout the body toward the brain and spinal cord.

sensory cortex the region of the *cerebral cortex responsible for receiving incoming information relayed by sensory nerve pathways from all parts of the body. Different areas of cortex correspond to different parts of the body and to the various senses. *Compare* motor cortex.

sensory deprivation the state in which there is a major reduction in incoming sensory information. Prolonged sensory deprivation is damaging because the body depends for health and normal function on constant stimulation. The main input sensory channels are the eyes, ears, skin, and nose. If input from all of these is blocked, there is loss of the sense of reality, distortion of time and imagined space, hallucinations, bizarre thought patterns, and other indications of neurological dysfunction. An eye covered for a few months in infancy remains effectively blind for life. Early deprivation of normal hearing can produce severe intellectual and educational damage. Deprivation of the normal contact and stimulation provided for the baby by the mother can cause personality disturbance in later life.

sensory nerve a nerve that carries information inward, from an outlying part of the body toward the central nervous system. Different sensory nerves convey information about temperature, pain, touch, taste, etc., to the brain. *Compare* motor nerve.

sentinel lymph node the first lymph node to show evidence of metastasis of a malignant tumor (e.g. breast cancer) via the lymphatic system. Absence of cancer cells in the sentinel node indicates that more distal lymph nodes will also be free of metastasis.

separation anxiety a state of distress and fear at the prospect of leaving secure surroundings, such as is experienced by some children when they must leave parents to go to school. It is often caused by insecure *attachment.

sepsis n. the putrefactive destruction of tissues by disease-causing bacteria or their toxins.

sept- (septi-) prefix denoting 1. seven. 2. (or **septo-**) a septum, especially the nasal septum. 3. sepsis.

septal defect a hole in the partition (septum) between the left and right halves of the heart. This abnormal communication is congenital due to an abnormality of heart development in the fetus. It may be found between the two atria (see atrial septal defect) or between the ventricles (see ventricular septal defect). A septal defect permits abnormal circulation of blood from the left side of the heart, where pressures are higher, to the right. This abnormal circulation is called a *shunt* and results in excessive blood flow through the lungs. *Pulmonary hypertension develops and *heart failure may occur with large shunts. A heart *murmur is normally present. Large defects are closed surgically but small defects do not require treatment.

septic adj. relating to or affected with *sepsis.

septic arthritis (bacterial arthritis, suppurative arthritis) an acute form of arthritis caused by bacterial infection in a joint. The joint is swollen, hot, and tender, and movement is very restricted and painful. The infecting organism can enter the joint via the bloodstream or from a penetrating injury. Treatment is by *arthrotomy or arthroscopy, irrigation of the joint, and antibiotics. If untreated, the articular cartilage is destroyed, leaving a stiff and deformed joint.

septicemia n. widespread destruction of tissues due to absorption of disease-causing bacteria or their toxins from the bloodstream. The term is also used loosely for any form of *blood poisoning. *Compare* pyemia, sapremia, toxemia.

septum n. (pl. **septa**) a partition or dividing wall within an anatomical structure. For example, the *atrioventricular septum* divides the atria of the heart from the ventricles. —**septal** adj. —**septate** adj.

sequela n. (pl. **sequelae**) any disorder or pathological condition that results from a preceding disease or accident.

sequestration n. 1. the formation of a fragment of dead bone (see sequestrum) and its separation from the surrounding tissue. 2. (in development) a separated part of an organ; a developmental anomaly.

sequestrectomy n. surgical removal of a *sequestrum.

sequestrum n. (pl. **sequestra**) a portion of dead bone formed in an infected bone in chronic *osteomyelitis. It is surrounded by an envelope (*involucrum*) of sclerotic bone and fibrous tissue and can be seen as a dense area within the bone on X-ray. It can cause irritation and the formation of pus, which may discharge through a *sinus, and is usually surgically removed (*sequestrectomy*).

ser- (sero-) prefix denoting 1. serum. 2. serous membrane.

serine n. see amino acid.

seroconvert vb. to produce specific antibodies in response to the presence of an antigen (e.g. a vaccine or a virus). In *AIDS patients *seroconversion* occurs within 4–6 weeks of the initial HIV infection. It is marked by a sore throat, swollen lymph nodes, fever, aches and pains, and fatigue.

serofibrinous adj. describing an exudate of serum that contains a high proportion of the protein fibrin.

serology n. the study of blood serum and its constituents, particularly their contribution to the protection of the body against disease. *See* agglutination, complement fixation, precipitin. —**serological** adj.

sero-negative arthritis an arthritis in which rheumatoid factor is not present in the serum.

seropus n. a mixture of serum and pus, which forms, for example, in infected blisters.

serosa n. see serous membrane.

serositis n. inflammation of a *serous membrane, such as the lining of the thoracic cavity (pleura). *See* polyserositis.

serotherapy n. the use of serum containing known antibodies (see antiserum) to treat a patient with an infection or to confer temporary passive *immunity upon a person at special risk. The use of antisera prepared in animals carries its own risks (for example, a patient may become hypersensitive to horse protein); the risk is reduced if the serum is taken from an immune human being.

serotonin (5-hydroxytryptamine) *n.* a compound widely distributed in the tissues, particularly in the blood platelets, intestinal wall, and central nervous system. It is thought to play a role in inflammation similar to that of *histamine and it is involved in the genesis of a migrainous headache. Drugs that act like serotonin are used in the treatment of migraine (*see* 5HT$_1$ agonist). It also acts as a *neurotransmitter, and its levels in the brain are believed to have an important influence on mood. Drugs that prolong its effects are used as antidepressants (*see* SSRI). As a precursor of *melatonin, serotonin is also involved in regulating the sleep cycle.

serotype *n.* a category into which material is placed based on its serological activity, particularly in terms of the antigens it contains or the antibodies that may be produced against it. Thus bacteria of the same species may be subdivided into serotypes that produce slightly different antigens. The serotype of an infective organism is important when treatment or prophylaxis with a vaccine is being considered.

serous *adj.* **1.** relating to or containing serum. **2.** resembling serum or producing a fluid resembling serum.

serous membrane (serosa) a smooth transparent membrane, which consists of *mesothelium and underlying elastic fibrous connective tissue, lining certain large cavities of the body. The *peritoneum of the abdomen, *pleura of the chest, and *pericardium of the heart are all serous membranes. Each consists of two portions: the *parietal* portion lines the walls of the cavity, and the *visceral* portion covers the organs concerned. The two are continuous, forming a closed sac with the organs essentially outside the sac. The inner surface of the sac is moistened by a thin fluid derived from blood serum, which allows frictionless movement of organs within their cavities. *Compare* mucous membrane.

serpiginous *adj.* having an indented or wavy margin: applied to certain skin lesions.

serratus *n.* any of several muscles arising from or inserted by a series of processes that resemble the teeth of a saw. An example is the *serratus anterior*, a muscle situated between the ribs and shoulder blade in the upper and lateral parts of the thorax. It is the chief muscle responsible for pushing and punching movements.

Sertoli cells cells found in the walls of the seminiferous tubules of the *testis. Compared with the germ cells they appear large and pale. They anchor and probably nourish the developing germ cells, especially the *spermatids, which become partly embedded within them. A *Sertoli cell tumor* is a rare testicular tumor causing *feminization. [E. Sertoli (1842–1910), Italian histologist]

sertraline *n.* an antidepressant drug that acts by prolonging the action of the neurotransmitter serotonin (5-hydroxytryptamine) in the brain (*see* SSRI). It is taken by mouth; side effects may include dizziness, agitation, tremor, nausea, diarrhea, and drowsiness. Trade name: **Zoloft.**

serum (blood serum) *n.* the fluid that separates from clotted blood or blood plasma that is allowed to stand. Serum is essentially similar in composition to *plasma but lacks fibrinogen and other substances that are used in the coagulation process.

serum hepatitis *see* hepatitis.

serum sickness a reaction that sometimes occurs 7–12 days after injection of a quantity of foreign antigen, such as that contained in *antiserum. It is characterized by the deposition of large immune complexes in the arteries, kidneys, and joints, with resultant symptoms of vasculitis, nephritis, and arthritis.

sesamoid bone an oval nodule of bone that lies within a tendon and slides over another bony surface. The patella (kneecap) and certain bones in the hand and foot are sesamoid bones.

sessile *adj.* (of a tumor) attached directly by its base without a peduncle (stalk).

seton *n.* a form of treatment in which a thread is passed through a *fistula and tied in a loop. The seton acts as a wick to drain off pus and can be tightened to open the track. This method can be used to treat high anal fistulas because it has a reduced risk of causing incontinence.

severe acute respiratory syndrome *see* SARS.

severe combined immune deficiency (SCID) a rare disorder that usually manifests itself within the first three months of life by severe bacterial, fungal, and viral infection and *failure to thrive. It is due to reduced numbers of T and B *lymphocytes – white blood cells necessary for fighting infection. Some cases are caused by *adenosine deaminase (ADA) deficiency. The only treatment currently available is a bone-marrow transplant, but *gene therapy offers hope for the future.

Sever's disease *apophysitis caused by pulling at the point of insertion of the Achilles tendon into the calcaneus (heel bone), causing heel pain. [J. W. Sever (20th century), US orthopedic surgeon]

sexarche *n.* the age when a person first engages in sexual intercourse.

sex chromatin *chromatin found only in female cells and believed to represent a single X chromosome in a nondividing cell. It can be used to discover the sex of a baby before birth by examination of cells obtained by *amniocentesis or *chorionic villus sampling. There are two main kinds: (1) the *Barr body*, a small object that stains with basic dyes, found on the edge of the nucleus just inside the nuclear membrane; (2) a drumsticklike appendage to the nucleus in neutrophils (a type of white blood cell).

sex chromosome a chromosome that is involved in the determination of the sex of the individual. Women have two *X chromosomes; men have one X chromosome and one *Y chromosome. *Compare* autosome.

sex hormone any steroid hormone, produced mainly by the ovaries or testes, that is responsible for controlling sexual development and reproductive function. *Estrogens and *progesterone are the female sex hormones; *androgens are the male sex hormones.

sex-limited *adj.* describing characteristics that are expressed differently in the two sexes but are controlled by genes not on the sex chromosomes, e.g. baldness in men.

sex-linked *adj.* describing genes (or the characteristics controlled by them) that are carried on the sex chromosomes, usually the *X chromosome. The genes for certain disorders, e.g. *hemophilia, are carried on the X chromosome; these genes and disorders are described as *X-linked*. Since these sex-linked genes are *recessive, men are more likely to have the diseases since they have only one X chromosome; women can carry the genes but their harmful effects are usually masked by the dominant (normal) alleles on their second X chromosome.

sexology *n.* the study of sexual matters, including anatomy, physiology, behavior, and techniques.

sex ratio the proportion of males to females in a population, usually expressed as the number of males per 100 females. The *primary sex ratio*, at the time of fertilization, is in theory 50% male. The *secondary sex ratio*, found at birth, usually indicates slightly fewer girls than boys.

sexual abuse *see* child abuse, pedophilia.

sexual deviation any sexual behavior regarded as abnormal by society (it is also known as *perversion*, but this has derogatory implications). The deviation may relate to the sexual object (as in *fetishism) or the activity engaged in (for example, *sadism and *exhibitionism). The activity is sexually pleasurable. The definition of what is normal varies with different cultures, and treatment is appropriate only when the deviation causes suffering. Some people may find that *counseling helps them to adjust to their deviation. Others may wish for treatment to change the deviation: *aversion therapy is used, also *conditioning normal sexual fantasies to pleasurable behavior. The only helpful effect of drugs is to reduce sexual drive generally.

sexually transmitted disease (STD) any disease transmitted by sexual intercourse, formerly known as *venereal disease*. STDs include *AIDS, *syphilis, *gonorrhea, *Chlamydia* infection, genital *herpes, and *soft sore. The medical specialty concered with STDs is *genitourinary medicine*.

SGOT (serum glutamic oxaloacetic transaminase) *see* aspartate transaminase.

SGPT (serum glutamic pyruvic transaminase) *see* alanine transaminase.

shaking palsy an archaic name for Parkinson's disease (*see* parkinsonism).

shaping *n.* a technique of *behavior modification used in the teaching of complex skills or in encouraging rare forms of behavior. At first, the therapist rewards actions that are similar to the desired behavior; thereafter the therapist rewards successively closer approximations, until eventually only the desired behavior is rewarded and thereby learned.

sheath *n.* **1.** (in anatomy) the layer of connective tissue that envelops structures such as nerves, arteries, tendons, and muscles. **2.** a *condom.

Sheehan's syndrome a condition in which *amenorrhea and infertility follow a major hemorrhage in pregnancy. It is caused by necrosis (death) of the anterior lobe of the pituitary gland as a direct result of the hemorrhage reducing the blood supply to the gland. *Compare* Asherman syndrome. [H. L. Sheehan (20th century), British pathologist]

Sheridan-Gardiner test a test for detecting visual handicap in children who are too young to be able to read the *Snellen chart. A series of cards, each marked with a single letter of a specific size, is held up at a distance of 6 meters from the child being tested. The child is provided with an identification card containing a selection of letters and is asked to point to the letter that is the same as the one on the card in the distance. The test is suitable for children between the ages of two and seven.

Shigella *n.* a genus of nonmotile rodlike gram-negative bacteria normally present in the intestinal tract of warm-blooded animals and humans. They ferment carbohydrates without the formation of gas. Some species are pathogenic. *S. dysenteriae* is associated with bacillary *dysentery.

shigellosis *n.* an infestation of the digestive system by bacteria of the genus *Shigella*, causing bacillary *dysentery.

shingles *n.* herpes zoster (*see* herpes).

shock *n.* the condition associated with circulatory collapse, when the arterial blood pressure is too low to maintain an adequate supply of blood to the tissues. The patient has a cold sweaty pallid skin, a weak rapid pulse, irregular breathing, dry mouth, dilated pupils, and a reduced flow of urine.

Shock may be due to a decrease in the volume of blood, as occurs after internal or external *hemorrhage, dehydration, burns, or severe vomiting or diarrhea. It may be caused by reduced activity of the heart, as in coronary thrombosis, myocardial infarction, or pulmonary embolism. It may also be due to widespread dilation of the veins so that there is insufficient blood to fill them. This may be caused by the presence of bacteria in the bloodstream (*bacteremic* or *toxic shock*), a severe allergic reaction (*anaphylactic shock*: *see* anaphylaxis), overdosage with such drugs as narcotics or barbiturates, or the emotional shock due to a personal tragedy or disaster (*neurogenic shock*). Sometimes shock may result from a combination of any of these causes, as in *peritonitis. The treatment of shock is determined by the cause.

shoulder *n.* the ball-and-socket joint (*see* enarthrosis) between the glenoid cavity of the *scapula and the upper end (head) of the humerus. It is a common site of dislocation. The joint is surrounded by a capsule closely associated with many tendons: it is the site of many strains and inflammations ("cuff injuries").

shoulder girdle (pectoral girdle) the bony structure to which the bones of the upper limbs are attached. It consists of the right and left *scapulas (*shoulder blades*) and clavicles (collar bones).

shunt *n.* (in medicine) a passage connecting two anatomical channels and diverting blood or other fluid from one to the other. It may occur as a congenital abnormality (as in *septal defects of the heart) or be surgically created. *See also* anastomosis.

SIADH *see* syndrome of inappropriate secretion of antidiuretic hormone.

sial- (sialo-) *prefix denoting* **1.** saliva. **2.** a salivary gland.

sialadenitis *n.* inflammation of a salivary gland.

sialagogue *n.* a drug that promotes the secretion of saliva. *Parasympathomimetic drugs have this action.

sialic acid an amino sugar. Sialic acid is a component of some *glycoproteins, *gangliosides, and bacterial cell walls.

sialography (ptyalography) *n.* a technique

for *X-ray examination of the salivary glands. A series of X-ray images is taken after introducing a quantity of radiopaque *contrast medium through a cannula into the ducts of the *parotid or *submandibular glands in the mouth. It enables the presence of degenerative disease or stones blocking the ducts to be detected.

sialolith (ptyalolith) n. a stone (calculus) in a salivary gland or duct, most often the duct of the submandibular gland. The flow of saliva is obstructed, causing swelling and intense pain. Treatment is primarily by *lithotripsy.

sialorrhea n. see ptyalism.

Siamese twins (conjoined twins) identical twins who are physically joined together at birth. The condition ranges from twins joined only by the umbilical blood vessels (i.e. allantoido-angiopagous twins) to those in whom conjoined heads or trunk are inseparable.

sib n. see sibling.

sibilant adj. whistling or hissing. The term is applied to certain high-pitched abnormal sounds heard through a stethoscope.

sibling (sib) n. one of a number of children of the same parents, i.e. a brother or sister.

sibutramine n. a drug that acts on the central nervous system to suppress the appetite: it inhibits the reuptake of norepinephrine and serotonin. Sibutramine is used in the treatment of obesity; it is prescribed mainly for those with a *body mass index of 30 or over who have failed to respond to standard weight-reduction measures. It is administered by mouth; side effects include dry mouth, constipation, and insomnia. Trade name: **Meridia**.

sickle-cell disease (drepanocytosis) n. a hereditary blood disease that mostly affects people of African ancestry. It occurs when the sickle cell gene has been inherited from both parents and is characterized by the production of an abnormal type of *hemoglobin – sickle-cell hemoglobin (HbS) – in the red blood cells. HbS becomes insoluble when the blood is deprived of oxygen and precipitates, forming elongated crystals that distort the blood cell into the characteristic sickle shape: this process is known as sickling. Sickle cells (drepanocytes) are

rapidly removed from the circulation, leading to anemia and jaundice. There is no satisfactory treatment. Sickle-cell trait occurs when the defective gene is inherited from only one parent. It generally causes no symptoms and confers some resistance to malaria, which accounts for the high frequency of the gene in malarious areas.

sickling n. see sickle-cell disease.

side effect n. an unwanted effect produced by a drug in addition to its desired therapeutic effects. Side effects are often undesirable and may be harmful.

sidero- prefix denoting iron.

sideroblast n. a red blood cell precursor (*erythroblast) in which iron-containing granules can be demonstrated by suitable staining techniques. Sideroblasts may be seen in normal individuals and are absent in iron deficiency. A certain type of anemia (sideroblastic anemia) is characterized by the presence of abnormal ringed sideroblasts. —**sideroblastic** adj.

siderocyte n. a red blood cell in which granules of iron-containing protein (Pappenheimer bodies) can be demonstrated by suitable staining techniques. These granules are normally removed by the spleen and siderocytes are characteristically seen when the spleen is absent.

sideropenia n. iron deficiency. This may result from dietary inadequacy; increased requirement of iron by the body, as in pregnancy or childhood; or increased loss of iron from the body, usually due to chronic bleeding. The most important manifestation of iron deficiency is *anemia, which is readily corrected by iron therapy.

siderophilin n. see transferrin.

siderosis n. the deposition of iron oxide dust in the lungs, occurring in silver finishers, arc welders, and hematite miners. Iron oxide itself is inert, but pulmonary *fibrosis may develop if fibrogenic dusts such as silica are also inhaled.

SIDS (sudden infant death syndrome) see crib death.

siemens n. the *SI unit of electrical conductance, equal to the conductance between two points on a conductor when a potential difference of 1 volt between these points causes a current of 1 ampere to flow between them. Symbol: S.

sievert *n.* the *SI unit of dose equivalent, being the dose equivalent when the absorbed dose of ionizing radiation multiplied by the stipulated dimensionless factors is 1 J kg^{-1}. Since different types of radiation cause different effects in biological tissue, a weighted absorbed dose, called the dose equivalent, is used in which the absorbed dose is modified by multiplying it by dimensionless factors stipulated by the International Commission on Radiological Protection. The sievert has replaced the *rem. Symbol: Sv.

sigmoid- *prefix denoting* the sigmoid colon. Example: *sigmoidotomy* (incision into).

sigmoid colon (sigmoid flexure) the S-shaped terminal part of the descending *colon, which leads to the rectum.

sigmoidectomy *n.* removal of the sigmoid colon by surgery. It is performed for tumors, severe *diverticular disease, or for an abnormally long sigmoid colon that has become twisted (*see* volvulus).

sigmoidoscope *n.* an instrument inserted through the anus in order to inspect the interior of the rectum and sigmoid colon. In its most common form it consists of a steel or chrome tube, 25 cm long and 3 cm in diameter, with some form of illumination and a bellows to inflate the bowel, but flexible fiberoptic instruments ("flexiscopes"), 60 cm long, are now generally used.

sigmoidoscopy *n.* examination of the rectum and sigmoid colon with a *sigmoidoscope. It is used in the investigation of diarrhea or rectal bleeding, particularly to detect colitis or cancer of the rectum. A general anesthetic is sometimes given, especially if the procedure is expected to be painful or uncomfortable, but flexible fiberoptic instruments make this unnecessary.

sign *n.* an indication of a particular disorder that is observed by a physician but is not apparent to the patient. *Compare* symptom.

significance *n.* (in statistics) a relationship between two groups of observations indicating that the difference between them (e.g. between the percentages of smokers and nonsmokers, respectively, who die from lung cancer) is unlikely to have occurred by chance alone. An as-

sumption is made that there is no difference between the two populations from which the two groups come (*null hypothesis*). This is tested, and a calculation indicating that there is a *probability* of less than 5% (P<0.05) that the observed difference or a larger one could have arisen by chance is regarded as being *statistically significant* and the null hypothesis is rejected. Some tests are *parametric*, based on the assumption that the range of observations are distributed by chance in a *normal* or *Gaussian distribution*, where 95% lie within two *standard deviations of the *mean (*Student's t test* to compare means). Nonparametric tests (*Mann-Whitney U tests*) make no assumptions about distribution patterns. *See also* frequency distribution, standard error.

sign of Dance (signe de Dance) a depression elicited by palpation of the right lower quadrant of the abdomen, which is characteristic of *intussusception. [J. B. H. Dance (1797–1832), French physician]

sildenafil *n.* a drug administered orally for the treatment of erectile *impotence. During sexual stimulation, it acts as a selective enzyme inhibitor, causing smooth muscle relaxation and increased blood flow to the corpus cavernosum of the penis, which results in erection. Side effects include headache, facial flushing, dyspepsia, nasal congestion, urinary tract infection, abnormal vision, diarrhea, dizziness, and rash. Because of severe adverse reactions, the drug is contraindicated in patients who are taking any nitrate-based medication, such as *nitroglycerin or *isosorbide. It is administered as needed and at recommended doses has no effect in the absence of sexual stimulation. Trade name: **Viagra**.

silicosis *n.* a lung disease – a form of *pneumoconiosis – produced by inhaling silica dust particles. It affects workers in mineral mining, quarrying, stone dressing, sand blasting, and boiler scaling. Silica stimulates *fibrosis of lung tissue, which produces progressive breathlessness and considerably increased susceptibility to tuberculosis (but not to lung cancer).

silver nitrate a salt of silver with *caustic, *astringent, and *disinfectant properties. It is applied in solutions or creams to destroy warts and to treat skin injuries, including burns. Continued application discolors the skin bluish-black, and ingestion of silver nitrate may cause severe poisoning.

silver sulfadiazine a topical antibacterial preparation used for the treatment and prevention of wound infections following second- and third-degree burns. It is administered as a cream to the burn area; side effects are burning, itching, and rash at the site of application. Trade name: **Silvadene**.

simethicone *n.* a silicone-based material with antifoaming properties, used in the treatment of flatulence and often incorporated into antacid remedies. It is administered orally and has no adverse effects. Trade names: **Gas-X**, **Gas Relief**, **Mylanta Gas**, **Mylicon Drops**.

Simmonds' disease loss of sexual function, loss of weight, and other features of failure of the pituitary gland (*hypopituitarism) caused by trauma or tumors or occurring in women after childbirth complicated by bleeding (postpartum hemorrhage). [M. Simmonds (1885–1925), German physician]

Sims' position the left-sided knees-up position commonly assumed by patients undergoing examinations of the anus and rectum or vagina. [J. M. Sims (1813–83), US gynecologist]

simulator *n.* an X-ray device used in radiotherapy to localize accurately the exact position of the final exposure of radiation before treatment begins.

Simulium *n.* see black fly.

simvastatin *n.* a drug used to reduce abnormally high levels of cholesterol in the blood in patients with hypercholesterolemia (*see* statin). It is administered by mouth; side effects include headache, abdominal pain, and constipation. Trade name: **Zocor**.

sinew *n.* a tendon.

singer's nodule *see* vocal cord nodule.

single payer system a type of health care in which there is only one purchaser of health care services, usually the government. Canada uses the single payer system.

single photon emission computed tomography *see* SPECT scanning.

singultus *n. see* hiccup.

sinistr- (sinistro-) *prefix denoting* left or the left side.

sino- (sinu-) *prefix denoting* **1.** a sinus. **2.** the sinus venosus.

sinoatrial node (SA node) the pacemaker of the heart: a microscopic area of specialized cardiac muscle located in the upper wall of the right atrium near the entry of the vena cava. Fibers of the SA node are self-excitatory, contracting rhythmically at around 70 times per minute. Following each contraction, the impulse spreads throughout the atrial muscle and into fibers connecting the SA node with the *atrioventricular node. The SA node is supplied by fibers of the autonomic nervous system; impulses arriving at the node accelerate or decrease the heart rate.

sinus *n.* **1.** an air cavity within a bone, especially any of the cavities within the bones of the face or skull (*see* paranasal sinuses). **2.** any wide channel containing blood, usually venous blood. *Venous sinuses* occur, for example, in the dura mater and drain blood from the brain. **3.** a pocket or bulge in a tubular organ, especially a blood vessel; for example, the *carotid sinus. **4. (sinus tract)** an infected tract leading from a focus of infection to the surface of the skin or a hollow organ. *See* pilonidal sinus.

sinus arrhythmia a normal variation in the heart rate, which accelerates slightly on inspiration and slows on expiration. It is common in healthy individuals.

sinusitis *n.* inflammation of one or more of the mucous membrane-lined air spaces in the facial bones that communicate with the nose (the paranasal sinuses). It is often associated with inflammation of the nasal lining (*rhinitis) and may be acute or chronic (*see* rhinosinusitis). Symptoms may include pain, purulent discharge from the nose, nasal obstruction, and disturbances of the sense of smell. Many cases are self-limiting. Others require treatment with antibiotics, decongestants, or steroid nose drops. A few cases need surgery, such as sinus washouts, *antrostomy, or *functional endoscopic sinus surgery.

sinusoid *n.* a small blood vessel found in certain organs, such as the adrenal gland and liver. Large numbers of sinusoids occur in the liver. They receive oxygen-rich blood from the hepatic artery and nutrients from the intestines via the portal vein. Oxygen and nutrients diffuse through the capillary walls into the liver cells. The sinusoids are drained by the hepatic veins. *See also* portal system.

sinus venosus a chamber of the embryonic heart that receives blood from several veins. In the adult heart it becomes part of the right atrium.

siphonage *n.* the transfer of liquid from one container to another by means of a bent tube. The procedure is used in gastric *lavage, when the stomach is filled with water through a funnel and rubber tube, and the tube is then bent downward to act as a siphon and empty the stomach of its contents.

Siphunculina *n.* a genus of flies. *S. funicola*, the eye fly of India, feeds on the secretions of the tear glands and in landing on or near the eyes contributes to the spread of *conjunctivitis.

Sipple's syndrome *see* MENS. [J. H. Sipple (1930–), US physician]

sirenomelia *n. see* sympodia.

sito- *prefix denoting* food.

sitz bath a fairly shallow hip bath in which the person is seated. Sitz baths of cold and hot water, rapidly alternated, were formerly used for the treatment of a variety of sexual disorders.

SI units (Système International d'Unités) the internationally agreed system of units now in use for all scientific purposes. Based on the meter-kilogram-second system, SI units have seven base units and two supplementary units. Measurements of all other physical quantities are expressed in derived units, consisting of two or more base units. Tables 1 and 2 (Appendix) list the base units and the derived units having special names; all these units are defined in the dictionary.

Decimal multiples of SI units are expressed using specified prefixes; where possible a prefix representing 10 raised to a power that is a multiple of three should be used. Prefixes are listed in Table 3 (Appendix).

Sjögren's syndrome an autoimmune condition affecting the salivary and lacrimal glands, resulting in a *dry mouth and dryness of the eyes. In the systemic form of the disease other glands may be affected, causing dryness of the airways, vagina, or skin, as well as the joints (pro-ducing a relatively mild form of arthritis) and muscles (which ache), and there may be tiredness and lethargy. Sjögren's syndrome may also occur secondarily to other conditions (e.g. rheumatoid arthritis). Symptomatic treatment, including saliva and tear substitutes, is available. [H. S. C. Sjögren (20th century), Swedish ophthalmologist]

skatole (methyl indole) *n.* a derivative of the amino acid tryptophan, excreted in the urine and feces.

skeletal muscle *see* striated muscle.

skeleton *n.* the rigid framework of connected *bones that gives form to the body, protects and supports its soft organs and tissues, and provides attachments for muscles and a system of levers essential for locomotion. The 206 named bones of the body are organized into the *axial skeleton* (of the head and trunk) and the *appendicular skeleton* (of the limbs). (See illustration.) —**skeletal** *adj.*

skew *n.* a disorder of relationships within a family, in which one parent is overpowering and the other is submissive and there is a general avoidance of anxiety-provoking situations. It was proposed as a specific cause of schizophrenia in the children, but this has not been confirmed.

skew deviation a rare condition of the eyes in which one eye turns down and inward while the other turns up and outward. It is sometimes seen in disorders of the *cerebellum or *brainstem.

skia- *prefix denoting* shadow.

skier's thumb (gamekeeper's thumb) rupture and consequent instability of the ligament on the inside of the thumb between the metacarpal and proximal (first) phalanx, caused by forced abduction of the thumb. Treatment is by surgical repair of the ligament.

skin *n.* the outer covering of the body, consisting of an outer layer, the *epidermis, and an inner layer, the *dermis. Beneath the dermis is a layer of fatty tissue. The skin has several functions. The epidermis protects the body from injury and from invasion by parasites. It also helps to prevent the body from becoming dehydrated. The combination of erectile hairs, *sweat glands, and blood capillaries in the skin form part of the temperature-regulating mechanism of the body. When the body is too hot, loss of heat is increased by sweating and by the dilation of the capillaries. When the body is too cold the sweat glands are inactive, the capillaries contract, and a layer of air is trapped over the epidermis by the erected hairs. The skin also acts as an organ of excretion (by the secretion of *sweat) and as a sense organ (it contains receptors that are sensitive to heat, cold, touch, and pain). The layer of fat underneath the dermis can act as a reservoir of food and water. (See illustration.) Anatomical name: **cutis**.

skin graft a portion of healthy skin cut from one area of the body and used to cover a part that has lost its skin, usually

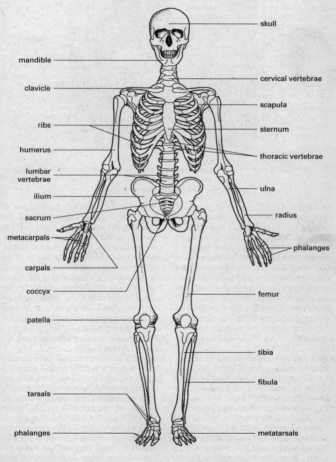

The skeleton

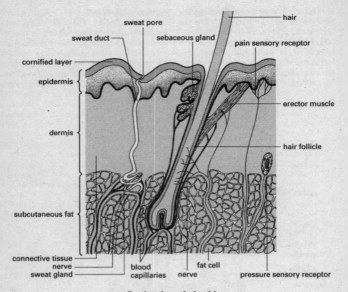

Section through the skin

as a result of injury, burns, or operation. A skin graft is normally taken from another part of the body of the same patient (an *autograft), but occasionally skin may be grafted from one person to another as a temporary healing measure (an *allograft). The full thickness of skin may be taken for a graft (*see* flap) or the surgeon may use three-quarter thickness, thin sheets of skin (*see* split-skin graft), or a pinch skin graft. The type used depends on the condition and size of the damaged area to be treated. The skin graft may be free or attached by a *pedicle.

skull *n.* the skeleton of the head and face, which is made up of 22 bones. It can be divided into the cranium, which encloses the brain, and the face (including the lower jaw (mandible)). (See illustration.) The *cranium* consists of eight bones. The frontal, parietals (two), occipital, and temporals (two) form the vault of the skull (*calvaria*) and are made up of two thin layers of compact bone separated by a layer of spongy bone (*diploë*). The remaining bones of the cranium – the

sphenoid and ethmoid – form part of its base. The 14 bones that make up the face are the nasals, lacrimals, inferior nasal conchae, maxillae, zygomatics, and palatines (two of each), the vomer, and the mandible. All the bones of the skull except the mandible are connected to each other by immovable joints (*see* suture). The skull contains cavities for the eyes (*see* orbit) and nose (*see* nasal cavity) and a large opening at its base (*foramen magnum*) through which the spinal cord passes.

SLE (systemic lupus erythematosus) *see* lupus erythematosus.

sleep *n.* a state of natural unconsciousness, during which the brain's activity is not apparent (apart from the continued maintenance of basic bodily functions, such as breathing) but can be detected by means of an electroencephalogram (EEG). Different stages of sleep are recognized by different EEG wave patterns. Drowsiness is marked by short irregular waves; as sleep deepens the waves become slower, larger, and more irregular. This slow-wave sleep is periodically interrupted by episodes of paradoxical, or *REM (rapid-eye-movement), sleep, when the EEG pattern is similar to that of an awake and alert person. Dreaming occurs during REM sleep. The two states of sleep alternate in cycles of from 30 to 90 minutes, REM sleep constituting about a quarter of the total sleeping time.

sleep apnea *n.* cessation of breathing during sleep, which may be obstructive, due to frustrated efforts to breathe against blocked upper airways, or central, in which there is no evidence of any voluntary effort. *Obstructive sleep apnea* (*OSA*, or *sleep apnea syndrome*) is a serious condition in which airflow from the nose and mouth to the lungs is restricted during sleep. It is defined by the presence of more than five episodes of *apnea per hour of sleep associated with significant daytime sleepiness. Snoring is a feature of the condition but it is not universal. There are significant medical complications of prolonged OSA, including heart failure and high blood pressure. Patients perform poorly on driving simulators, and driving restrictions may be imposed. There are associated conditions in adults: the *hypopnea syndrome and the upper airways resistance syndrome, with less apnea but with daytime somnolence and prominent snoring. In children the cause is usually enlargement of the tonsils and adenoids and treatment is by removing these structures. In adults the tonsils may be implicated but there are often other abnormalities of the *pharynx, and patients are often obese. Treatment may include weight reduction or nasal *continuous positive airways pressure devices, *mandibular advancement splints, or noninvasive ventilation. Alternatively *tonsillectomy, *uvulopalatopharyngoplasty, *laser-assisted uvulopalatoplasty, or *tracheostomy may be required.

sleeping sickness (African trypanosomiasis) a disease of tropical Africa caused by the presence in the blood of the parasitic protozoans *Trypanosoma gambiense* or *T. rhodesiense*. The parasites are transmitted to humans through the bite of *tsetse flies. Initial symptoms include fever, headache, and chills, followed later by enlargement of the lymph nodes, anemia, and pains in the limbs and joints. After a period of several months or even years, the parasites invade the minute blood vessels supplying the central nervous system. This causes drowsiness and lethargy, and ultimately – if untreated – the patient dies. Rhodesian sleeping sickness is the more virulent form of the disease. The drugs *suramin, *eflornithine, and *pentamidine are used to treat the early curable stages of sleeping sickness; drugs containing arsenic (*see* tryparsamide) are administered after the brain is affected. Eradication of tsetse flies helps prevent spread of the infection.

sleep paralysis a terrifying inability to move or speak while remaining fully

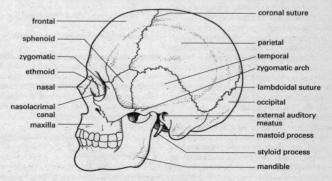

frontal
sphenoid
zygomatic
ethmoid
nasal
nasolacrimal canal
maxilla

coronal suture
parietal
temporal
zygomatic arch
lambdoidal suture
occipital
external auditory meatus
mastoid process
styloid process
mandible

Side view of the skull

alert. It occurs in up to 60% of patients with *narcolepsy and may occur in other conditions, such as severe anxiety.

sleepwalking *n. see* somnambulism.

sling *n.* a bandage arranged to support and rest an injured limb so that healing is not hindered by activity. The most common sling is a *triangular bandage tied behind the neck to support the weight of a broken arm. The arm is bent at the elbow and held across the body.

slipped disk a colloquial term for a *prolapsed intervertebral disk.

slit lamp a device for providing a narrow beam of light, used in conjunction with a special microscope. It can be used to examine minutely the structures within the eye, one layer at a time.

slough *n.* dead tissue, such as skin, that separates from healthy tissue after inflammation or infection.

slow virus one of a group of infective disease agents that resemble viruses in some of their biological properties but whose physical properties (e.g. sensitivity to radiation) suggest that they may not contain nucleic acid. They are now more commonly known as *prions.

SMA *see* spinal muscular atrophy.

small bowel enema (enteroclysis) a technique for examining the jejunum and ileum by passing a tube through the mouth, esophagus, and stomach into the small bowel and directly injecting barium. It gives excellent detail of the lining of the small bowel but is more uncomfortable than a *small bowel meal. It is particularly useful for showing jejunal diseases, such as *celiac disease, as well as tumors and obstructions.

small bowel meal a technique for examining the small bowel. The patient swallows dilute *barium sulfate suspension and then a series of radiographs is taken. It is important that barium reaches the cecum for a complete examination. The technique is particularly useful for showing inflammatory bowel disease, particularly *Crohn's disease.

small-cell lung cancer *see* oat cell.

smallpox *n.* an acute infectious virus disease causing high fever and a rash that scars the skin. Immunization against smallpox has now totally eradicated the disease. Medical name: **variola.** *See also* alastrim, cowpox.

smear *n.* a specimen of tissue or other material taken from part of the body and smeared on a microscope slide for examination. *See* cervical smear.

smegma *n.* the secretion of the glands of the foreskin (*prepuce), which accumulates under the foreskin and has a white cheesy appearance. It becomes readily infested by a harmless bacterium that resembles the tubercle bacillus.

Smith's fracture a fracture just above the wrist, across the lower end of the radius, resulting in forward displacement of the hand and wrist below the fracture. It is the reverse of *Colles' fracture. [R. W. Smith (1807–73), Irish surgeon]

smooth muscle (involuntary muscle) muscle that produces slow long-term contractions of which the individual is unaware. Smooth muscle occurs in hollow organs, such as the stomach, intestine, blood vessels, and bladder. It consists of spindle-shaped cells within a network of connective tissue (see illustration) and is under the control of the autonomic nervous system. *Compare* striated muscle.

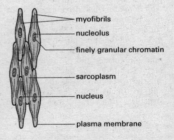

myofibrils
nucleolus
finely granular chromatin
sarcoplasm
nucleus
plasma membrane

Arrangement of smooth muscle cells

snare *n.* an instrument consisting of a wire loop designed to remove polyps, tumors, and other projections of tissue, particularly those occurring in body cavities (see illustration). The loop is used to encircle the base of the tumor and is then pulled tight. *See also* diathermy.

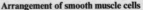

A nasal snare

sneeze 1. *n.* an involuntary violent reflex expulsion of air through the nose and mouth provoked by irritation of the mucous membrane lining the nasal cavity. **2.** *vb.* to produce a sneeze.

Snellen chart the most common chart used for testing sharpness of distant vision (*see* visual acuity). It consists of rows of capital letters, called *test types*, the letters of each row becoming smaller down the chart. The large letter at the top is of such a size that it can be read by a person with normal sight from a distance of 60 meters (200 feet). A normally sighted person can read successive lines of letters from 36, 24, 18, 12, 9, 6, and 5 meters (or approximately 100, 70, 50, 40, 30, 20, and 15 feet), respectively. There is sometimes a line for 4 meters (10 feet). The subject sits 6 meters (20 feet) from the chart and one eye is tested at a time. If he can only read down as far as the 12-meter line, the visual acuity is expressed as 6/12 (20/40). Normally sighted people can read the 6-meter line, i.e. normal acuity is 6/6, or 20/20, and many people read the 5-meter line with ease. A smaller chart on the same principle is available for testing near vision. [H. Snellen (1834–1908), Dutch ophthalmologist]

snoring *n.* noisy breathing while asleep due to vibration of the soft palate, uvula, pharyngeal walls, or epiglottis. In children it is often associated with enlargement of the tonsils and adenoids. Treatments of snoring include weight loss, tobacco and alcohol avoidance, adenoidectomy, tonsillectomy, nasal airway surgery, *uvulopalatopharyngoplasty, and laser *palatoplasty.

snow blindness a painful disorder of the cornea of the eye due to excessive exposure to ultraviolet light reflected from the snow. Recovery usually follows within 24 hours of covering the eyes.

snuffles *n.* **1.** partial obstruction of breathing in infants, caused by the common cold. **2.** (formerly) discharge through the nostrils associated with necrosis of the nasal bones: seen in infants with congenital syphilis.

social medicine *see* community medicine.

Social Security Act a US law established originally in 1935 to provide financial assistance to the needy aged during the era of the Great Depression but amended in later years to cover maternal and child-health services, services to crippled children, financial assistance to the needy blind, and subsidies for state and local public health programs. Major changes since World War II include the 1965 amendments creating *Medicaid and *Medicare. The US Social Security Administration provides for more than 60% of the total annual federal expenditures for public health care.

socket *n.* (in anatomy) a hollow or depression into which another part fits, such as the cavity in the alveolar bone of the jaws into which the root of a tooth fits. *See also* dry socket.

sodium *n.* a mineral element and an important constituent of the human body (average sodium content of the adult body is 4000 mmol). Sodium controls the volume of extracellular fluid in the body and maintains the acid-base balance. It also helps maintain electrical potentials in the nervous system and is thus necessary for the functioning of nerves and muscles. Sodium is contained in most foods and is well absorbed, the average daily intake in the US being 4 g. The amount of sodium in the body is controlled by the kidneys. An excess of sodium leads to the condition of *hypernatremia*, which often results in *edema. This may develop in infants fed on bottled milk, which has a much higher sodium content than human milk. Since babies are less able to remove sodium from the body than adults, the feeding of a high-sodium diet to babies is dangerous and may lead to dehydration. Sodium is also implicated in hypertension: a high-sodium diet is thought to increase the risk of hypertension in later life. Symbol: Na.

sodium bicarbonate a salt of sodium that neutralizes acid and is used to treat stomach and digestive disorders, *acidosis, and sodium deficiency. It is administered by mouth or injection; high doses may cause digestive upsets. *See also* antacid.

sodium chloride common salt: a salt of sodium that is present in all tissues and is important in maintaining the *electrolyte balance of the body. Sodium chloride infusions are the basis of fluid replacement therapy after operations and for conditions associated with salt depletion, including shock and dehydration. Sodium chloride is also a basic constituent of *oral rehydration therapy.

sodium fluoride a salt of sodium used to prevent tooth decay and as a dietary supplement. It is administered by mouth or applied to the teeth as paste or solution. Taken in excess by mouth, it may cause digestive upsets and large doses may cause fluorine poisoning. See also fluoridation. Trade names: **Fluoritab, Pediaflor, Pharmaflur**.

sodium fusidate an *antibiotic used mainly to treat infections caused by *Staphylococcus. It is administered by mouth or injection or applied in an ointment for skin infections; common side effects are mild digestive upsets.

sodium hydroxide (caustic soda) a powerful alkali in widespread use as a cleaning agent. It attacks the skin, causing severe chemical burns that are best treated by washing the area with large quantities of water. When swallowed it causes burning of the mouth and throat, which should be treated by giving water, milk, or other fluid to dilute the stomach contents and by gastric lavage.

sodium hypochlorite a salt of sodium used in solution as an antiseptic and disinfectant. In dentistry a 0.5–5.0% solution is used for washing out infected root canals.

sodium nitrite a sodium salt used, with sodium thiosulfate, to treat cyanide poisoning. It is administered by injection and may cause digestive upsets, dizziness, headache, fainting, and cyanosis. It also has effects similar to *nitroglycerin and has been used to treat angina.

sodium nitroprusside a cyanide-containing drug used in the emergency treatment of high blood pressure. Given by controlled infusion into a vein, it is the most effective known means of reducing dangerously high pressure, but its effects and level in the blood must be closely monitored. It is also used to produce controlled hypotension during surgery. Possible side effects include nausea, vomiting, headache, palpitations, sweating, and chest pain. Trade name: **Nitropress**.

sodium thiosulfate a salt of sodium used, with *sodium nitrite, to treat cyanide poisoning. It is administered by intravenous injection.

sodium valproate see valproic acid.

sodoku n. see rat-bite fever.

sodomy n. sexual intercourse using the anus. This may be homosexual, heterosexual, or between humans and animals. See also sexual deviation.

soft sore (chancroid) a sexually transmitted disease caused by the bacterium Haemophilus ducreyi, resulting in enlargement and ulceration of lymph nodes in the groin. Treatment with sulfonamides is effective.

solarium n. a room in which patients are exposed to either sunlight or artificial sunlight (a blend of visible light and infrared and ultraviolet radiation directed from special lamps).

solar plexus (celiac plexus) a network of sympathetic nerves and ganglia high in the back of the abdomen.

soleus n. a broad flat muscle in the calf of the leg, beneath the *gastrocnemius muscle. The soleus flexes the foot, so that the toes point downward.

soma n. **1.** the entire body excluding the germ cells. **2.** the body as distinct from the mind.

somat- prefix denoting **1.** the body. **2.** somatic.

somatic adj. **1.** relating to the nonreproductive parts of the body. A somatic mutation cannot be inherited. **2.** relating to the body wall (i.e. excluding the viscera), e.g. somatic *mesoderm. Compare splanchnic. **3.** relating to the body rather than the mind.

somatization disorder (Briquet's syndrome) a psychiatric disorder characterized by multiple recurrent changing physical symptoms in the absence of physical disorders that could explain them. The disorder is chronic and is often accompanied by depression and anxiety. It can disrupt personal and family relationships and lead to unnecessary medical and surgical treatment. It is sometimes treated with *cognitive therapy, *psychotherapy, and/or *antidepressants.

somatoform disorders a group of disorders in which there is a history of repeated physical complaints with no physical basis. They include *somatization disorder and hypochondriasis (see hypochondria). Also included (in DSM-IV but not in ICD-10) is *conversion disorder.

somatomedin n. a protein hormone, produced by the liver in response to stimulation by growth hormone, that stimulates protein synthesis and promotes growth. It is biochemically similar to *insulin and has some actions similar to insulin; it is therefore sometimes said to have *insulin-like activity* (*ILA*) or is referred to as *insulin-like growth factor* (*IGF*).

somatopleure n. the body wall of the early embryo, which consists of a simple layer of ectoderm lined with mesoderm. The amnion is a continuation of this structure outside the embryo. *Compare* splanchnopleure.

somatostatin (growth-hormone-release inhibiting factor) n. a hormone, produced by the hypothalamus and some extraneural tissues, including the gastrointestinal tract and pancreas (*see* islets of Langerhans), that inhibits *growth hormone (somatotropin) release by the pituitary gland. Both growth-hormone releasing factor and somatostatin are controlled by complex neural mechanisms related to sleep rhythms, stress, neurotransmitters, blood glucose, and exercise. Its inhibitory effect on gastrointestinal secretions is used to reduce flow from *fistulas from the pancreas or bowel to the body surface. Its effect on reducing abdominal blood flow is used to reduce bleeding from *esophageal varices.

Somatostatin analogues are used to treat acromegaly, caused by overproduction of growth hormone, and to relieve the symptoms caused by hormone-secreting neuroendocrine tumors. They include *lanreotide* and *octreotide* (Sandostatin), which are administered by injection.

somatostatinoma n. a rare tumor of the *islets of Langerhans that produces somatostatin, causing severe effects on gastrointestinal motility. It is an example of an *apudoma.

somatotropin n. *see* growth hormone.

somatotype n. *see* body type.

somite n. any of the paired segmented divisions of *mesoderm that develop along the length of the early embryo. The somites differentiate into voluntary muscle, bones, connective tissue, and the deeper layers of the skin (*see* dermatome, myotome, sclerotome).

somnambulism (noctambulation) n. sleepwalking: walking about and performing other actions in a semiautomatic way during sleep without later memory of doing so. It is common during childhood and may persist into adult life. It can also arise spontaneously or as the result of stress or hypnosis. —**somnambulistic** *adj.*

somniloquence n. talking in one's sleep. *See also* somnambulism.

somnolism n. a hypnotic trance. *See* hypnosis.

Somogyi phenomenon *see* dawn phenomenon. [M. Somogyi (1883–1971), US biochemist]

sonography n. *see* ultrasonography.

sonoplacentography n. the technique of using *ultrasound waves to determine the position of the placenta during pregnancy. This has the advantage over using X-rays in that the fetus is not subjected to possibly harmful radiation. *See also* bedsore.

soporific n. *see* hypnotic.

sorbitol n. a carbohydrate with a sweet taste, used by diabetics as a substitute for cane sugar. It is also used in disorders of carbohydrate metabolism and in drip feeding.

sordes pl. n. the brownish encrustations that form around the mouth and teeth of patients with fevers.

sore n. a lay term for any ulcer or other open wound of the skin or mucous membranes, which may be caused by injury or infection. *See also* bedsore.

sore throat pain at the back of the mouth, most commonly due to bacterial or viral infection of the tonsils (*tonsillitis), larynx (*laryngitis), or pharynx (*pharyngitis). If infection persists, the lymph nodes in the neck may become tender and enlarged (cervical adenitis).

sotalol n. a drug (*see* beta blocker) used to treat abnormal heart rhythm. It is administered by mouth; side effects may include digestive upsets, tiredness, and dizziness. Trade name: **Betapace**.

souffle n. a soft blowing sound heard through the stethoscope, usually produced by blood flowing in vessels.

sound (in surgery) **1.** n. a long rodlike instrument, often with a curved end, used to explore body cavities (such as the bladder) or to dilate *strictures in the urethra or other canals. **2.** vb. to explore a cavity using a sound.

Soundbridge *n. see* implantable hearing aid.

Southern blot analysis a technique for identifying a specific form of DNA in cells. The DNA is extracted from the cells and restriction enzymes used to cut it into small fragments. The fragments are separated and a gene *probe known to match the DNA fragment being sought is used. *Compare* Northern blot analysis, Western blot analysis. [E. M. Southern (1938–), US biologist]

Southey's tubes fine-caliber tubes for insertion into subcutaneous tissue to drain excess fluid. They are rarely used in practice today. [R. Southey (1835–99), British physician]

Spanish fly the blister beetle, *Lytta vesicatoria*: source of the irritant and toxic chemical compound *cantharidin.

sparganosis *n.* a disease caused by the migration of certain tapeworm larvae (*see* sparganum) in the tissues beneath the skin, between the muscles, and occasionally in the viscera and brain. The larvae, which normally develop in frogs and reptiles, are accidentally transferred to humans by eating the uncooked flesh of these animals or by drinking water contaminated with minute crustaceans infected with the tapeworm larvae. The larvae cause inflammation, swelling, and fibrosis of the tissues. Treatment of the condition, common in the Far East, involves intravenous injections of neoarsphenamine and surgical removal of the larvae.

sparganum *n.* the larvae of certain tapeworms, including species of *Diphyllobothrium* and *Spirometra*, which may accidentally infect human beings (*see* sparganosis). They are actually *plerocercoids, but the generic name *Sparganum* is sometimes given to them since they fail to develop into adults and definite classification of the species is not possible from the larvae alone.

spasm *n.* a sustained involuntary muscular contraction, which may occur either as part of a generalized disorder, such as a *spastic paralysis, or as a local response to an otherwise unconnected painful condition. *Carpopedal spasm* affects the muscles of the hands and feet and is caused by reduction in the blood calcium level (often transitory, as in hyperventilation).

spasmo- *prefix denoting* spasm.

spasmodic *adj.* occurring in spasms or resembling a spasm.

spasmolytic *n.* a drug that relieves spasm of smooth muscle, e.g. *aminophylline or *papaverine. Spasmolytics may be used as *bronchodilators to relieve spasm in bronchial muscle, to stimulate the heart in the treatment of angina, or to relieve colic due to spasm of the digestive system.

spasmus nutans a combination of symptoms that includes a slow nodding movement of the head, *nystagmus (involuntary movements of the eyes), and spasm of the neck muscles. It affects infants and it normally disappears within a year or two.

spastic colon *see* irritable bowel syndrome.

spasticity *n.* resistance to the passive movement of a limb that is maximal at the beginning of the movement and gives way as more pressure is applied. It is a symptom of damage to the *pyramidal system in the brain or spinal cord. It is usually accompanied by weakness in the affected limb (*see* spastic paralysis). *Compare* rigidity.

spastic paralysis weakness of a limb or limbs associated with increased reflex activity. This results in resistance to passive movement of the limb (*see* spasticity). It is caused by disease affecting the nerve fibers of the corticospinal tract, which in health not only initiate movement but also inhibit the stretch reflexes to allow the movements to take place. *See also* cerebral palsy.

spatula *n.* an instrument with a blunt blade used to spread ointments or plasters and to mix materials. A flat spatula is used to depress the tongue during examination of the oropharynx.

special hospitals hospitals for the treatment of specific diseases or for the care of mentally ill patients who are also dangerous and must therefore be kept securely.

species *n.* the smallest unit used in the classification of living organisms. Members of the same species are able to interbreed and produce fertile offspring. Similar species are grouped together within one *genus.

specific 1. *n.* a medicine that has properties especially useful for the treatment of a particular disease. **2.** *adj.* (of a disease) caused by a particular microorganism that causes no other disease. **3.** *adj.* of or relating to a species.

specific gravity the ratio, more correctly known as *relative density*, of the density of a substance at 20°C to the density of water at its temperature of maximum density 4°C. Measurement of the specific gravity of urine is one of the tests of renal function.

specificity *n.* (in screening tests) *see* sensitivity.

spectinomycin *n.* an *antibiotic used to treat various infections, particularly gonorrhea. It is administered by injection; side effects may include nausea, dizziness, fever, and rash. Trade name: **Trobicin**.

spectrograph *n.* an instrument (a *spectrometer or *spectroscope) that produces a photographic record (*spectrogram*) of the intensity and wavelength of electromagnetic radiations.

spectrometer *n.* any instrument for measuring the intensity and wavelengths of visible or invisible electromagnetic radiations. *See also* spectroscope.

spectrophotometer *n.* an instrument (a spectrometer) for measuring the intensity of the wavelengths of the components of light (visible or ultraviolet).

spectroscope *n.* an instrument used to split up light or other radiation into components of different wavelengths. The simplest spectroscope uses a prism, which splits white light into the rainbow colors of the visible spectrum.

SPECT scanning (single photon emission computed tomography scanning) (in nuclear medicine) a *cross-sectional imaging technique for observing an organ or part of the body using a *gamma camera; images are produced after injecting a radioactive *tracer. The camera is rotated around the patient being scanned. Using a computer reconstruction *algorithm similar to that of a *computed tomography scanner, multiple "slices" are made through the area of interest. SPECT scanning is used particularly in cardiac nuclear medicine imaging (*see* MUGA scan). It differs from PET scanning in that radioactive decay gives off only a single gamma ray.

specular reflection (in *ultrasonics) the reflection of sound waves from the surface of an internal structure, which can be used to produce a picture of the surface as a sonogram (*see* ultrasonography). A specular reflection contrasts with vaguer diffuse echoes produced by minor differences in tissue density.

speculum *n.* (*pl.* **specula**) a metal instrument for inserting into and holding open a cavity of the body, such as the vagina, rectum, or nasal orifice, in order that the interior may be examined (*see* illustration).

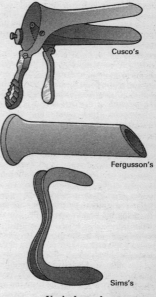

Cusco's

Fergusson's

Sims's

Vaginal specula

speech therapy the rehabilitation of patients who are unable to speak coherently because of congenital causes, accidents, or illness (e.g. stroke). Speech therapists have special training in this field and are licensed by the state.

sperm *n.* a mature male germ cell. *See* spermatozoon.

sperm- (spermi(o)-, spermo-) *prefix denoting* sperm or semen.

spermat- (spermato-) *prefix denoting* **1.** sperm. **2.** organs or ducts associated with sperm.

spermatic artery either of two arteries that originate from the abdominal aorta and travel downward to supply the testes.

spermatic cord the cord, consisting of the *vas deferens, nerves, and blood vessels, that runs from the abdominal cavity to the testicle in the scrotum. The *inguinal canal, through which the spermatic cord passes, becomes closed after the testes have descended.

spermatid *n.* a small cell produced as an intermediate stage in the formation of spermatozoa. Spermatids become embedded in *Sertoli cells in the testis. They are transformed into spermatozoa by the process of spermiogenesis (*see* spermatogenesis).

spermatocele *n.* a cystic swelling in the scrotum containing sperm. The cyst arises from the epididymis (the duct conveying sperm from the testis) and can be felt as a lump above the testis. Needle *aspiration of the cyst reveals a milky opalescent fluid containing sperm. Treatment is by surgical removal.

spermatocyte *n.* a cell produced as an intermediate stage in the formation of spermatozoa (*see* spermatogenesis). Spermatocytes develop from spermatogonia in the walls of the seminiferous tubules of the testis; they are known as either *primary* or *secondary spermatocytes* according to whether they are undergoing the first or second division of meiosis.

spermatogenesis *n.* the process by which mature spermatozoa are produced in the testis (see illustration). *Spermatogonia, in the outermost layer of the seminiferous tubules, multiply throughout reproductive life. Some of them divide by meiosis into *spermatocytes, which produce haploid *spermatids. These are transformed into mature spermatozoa by the process of *spermiogenesis*. The whole process takes 70–80 days.

spermatogonium *n.* (*pl.* **spermatogonia**) a cell produced at an early stage in the formation of spermatozoa (*see* spermatogenesis). Spermatogonia first appear in the testis of the fetus but do not multiply significantly until after puberty. They act as stem cells in the walls of the seminiferous tubules, dividing continuously by mitosis and giving rise to *spermatocytes.

spermatorrhea *n.* the involuntary discharge of semen without orgasm. Semen is usually produced by ejaculation at orgasm and does not normally discharge at other times. If, however, the mechanism of ejaculation is lost, spermatorrhea may occur.

spermatozoon (sperm) *n.* (*pl.* **spermatozoa**) a mature male sex cell (*see* gamete). The tail of a sperm enables it to swim, which is important as a means for reaching and fertilizing the ovum (although muscular movements of the uterus may assist its journey from the vagina). *See also* acrosome, fertilization.

spermaturia *n.* the presence of spermatozoa in the urine. Spermatozoa are occasionally seen on microscopic examination of the urine and their presence is not abnormal. If present in large numbers, the urine becomes cloudy, usually toward the end of micturition. Abnormal ejaculation into the bladder on orgasm (retrograde ejaculation) may occur after *prostatectomy or other surgical procedures or in neurological conditions that destroy the ability of the bladder neck to close on ejaculation.

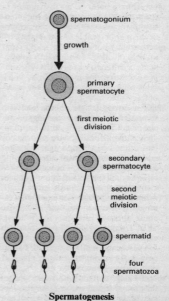

Spermatogenesis

A spermatozoon

(Labels on diagram: acrosome, head, vacuole, nucleus, neck, middle piece, mitochondrial sheath, tail)

sperm count *see* semen analysis.

spermicide *n.* an agent that kills spermatozoa. Creams and jellies containing chemical spermicides are used – in conjunction with a *diaphragm – as contraceptives. —**spermicidal** *adj.*

spermiogenesis *n.* the process by which spermatids become mature spermatozoa within the seminiferous tubules of the testis. *See* spermatogenesis.

spheno- *prefix denoting* the sphenoid bone. Examples: *sphenomaxillary* (relating to the sphenoid and maxillary bones); *sphenopalatine* (relating to the sphenoid bone and palate).

sphenoid bone a bone forming the base of the cranium behind the eyes. It consists of a *body*, containing air spaces continuous with the nasal cavity (*see* paranasal sinuses); two *wings* that form part of the

orbits; and two *pterygoid processes* projecting down from the point where the two wings join the body. *See* skull.

spherocyte *n.* an abnormal form of red blood cell (*erythrocyte) that is spherical rather than disk-shaped. In blood films spherocytes appear smaller and stain more densely than normal red cells. They are characteristic of some forms of hemolytic anemia. Spherocytes tend to be removed from the blood as they pass through the spleen. *See also* spherocytosis.

spherocytosis *n.* the presence in the blood of abnormally shaped red cells (*spherocytes). Spherocytosis may occur as a hereditary disorder (*hereditary spherocytosis*) or be present in certain hemolytic *anemias.

sphincter *n.* a specialized ring of muscle that surrounds an orifice. Contractions of the sphincter partly or completely close the orifice. Sphincters are found, for example, around the anus (*anal sphincter*) and at the opening between the stomach and duodenum (*pyloric sphincter*).

sphincter- *prefix denoting* a sphincter.

sphincterectomy *n.* **1.** the surgical removal of any sphincter muscle. **2.** surgical removal of part of the iris in the eye at the border of the pupil.

sphincterotomy *n.* surgical division of any sphincter muscle. *See also* anal fissure.

sphingomyelin *n.* a *phospholipid that contains sphingosine, a fatty acid, phosphoric acid, and choline. Sphingomyelins are found in large amounts in brain and nerve tissue.

sphingosine *n.* a lipid alcohol that is a constituent of sphingomyelin and cerebrosides.

sphygmo- *prefix denoting* the pulse.

sphygmocardiograph *n.* an apparatus for producing a continuous record of both the heartbeat and the subsequent pulse in one of the blood vessels. The recording can be shown on a moving tape or on an electronic screen.

sphygmograph *n.* an apparatus for producing a continuous record of the pulse in one of the blood vessels, showing the strength and rate of the beats.

sphygmomanometer *n.* an instrument for measuring *blood pressure in the arteries. It consists of an inflatable cuff connected via a rubber tube to a column of

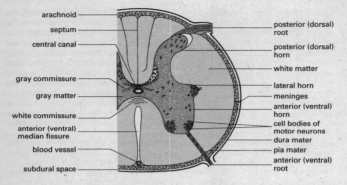

arachnoid
septum
central canal
gray commissure
gray matter
white commissure
anterior (ventral) median fissure
blood vessel
subdural space

posterior (dorsal) root
posterior (dorsal) horn
white matter
lateral horn
meninges
anterior (ventral) horn
cell bodies of motor neurons
dura mater
pia mater
anterior (ventral) root

Transverse section through the spinal cord

mercury with a graduated scale. The cuff is applied to a limb (usually the arm) and inflated to exert pressure on a large artery until the blood flow stops. The pressure is then slowly released and, with the aid of a stethoscope to listen to the pulse, it is possible to determine both the systolic and diastolic pressures (which can be read on the scale).

sphygmophone *n.* a device to record the heartbeat or pulse in the form of amplified sound waves played through a loudspeaker or earphones.

sphygmoscope *n.* a device for showing the heartbeat or pulse as a visible signal, especially a continuous wave signal on a cathode-ray tube.

spica *n.* a bandage wound spirally around an injured limb. At each turn it is given a twist so that the slack material is taken up at the overlap.

spicule *n.* a small splinter of bone.

spina bifida (rachischisis) a developmental defect in which the newborn baby has part of the spinal cord and its coverings exposed through a gap in the backbone. The symptoms may include paralysis of the legs, incontinence, and mental retardation from the commonly associated brain defect *hydrocephalus. Spina bifida is associated with abnormally high levels of *alpha-fetoprotein in the amniotic fluid surrounding the embryo. The condition can be diagnosed at about the 16th week of pregnancy by a maternal blood test and confirmed by *amniocentesis and ultrasound, thus making

termination of the pregnancy possible. The risk of spina bifida is reduced if supplements of *folic acid are taken by women trying to conceive and during the first three months of pregnancy. *See also* neural tube defects.

spina bifida occulta a defect in the bony arch of the spine that (unlike spina bifida) has a normal skin covering; there may be an overlying hairy patch but no protrusion of the cord or its membranes. The condition is usually an incidental finding on X-ray and it is not associated with neurological involvement.

spinal accessory nerve *see* accessory nerve.

spinal anesthesia 1. suppression of sensation in part of the body by the injection of a local anesthetic into the *subarachnoid space. A very fine needle is used to reduce the amount of cerebrospinal fluid that escapes as the needle penetrates the dura. The technique has complications (headache, sepsis, paraplegia). The injection site for spinal anesthetics is most often in the lumbar region of the vertebral column, the needle being inserted between the vertebrae (anywhere between the second and fifth). The extent of the area anesthetized depends upon the amount and strength of local anesthetic injected. Dilute local anesthetic solutions are used when the sensory nerves are targeted rather than the motor nerves. Spinal anesthesia is useful in patients whose condition makes them unsuitable for a general anesthetic, perhaps because of chest infection; to reduce the requirements for general anesthetic drugs; or in circumstances where a skilled anesthesiologist is not readily available to administer a general anesthetic. **2.** loss of sensation in part of the body as a result of injury or disease to the spinal cord. The area of the body affected depends upon the site of the lesion: the lower it is in the cord the less the sensory disability.

spinal column *see* backbone.

spinal cord the portion of the central nervous system enclosed in the vertebral column, consisting of nerve cells and bundles of nerves connecting all parts of the body with the brain. It contains a core of gray matter surrounded by white matter (see illustration). It is enveloped in three layers of membrane, the

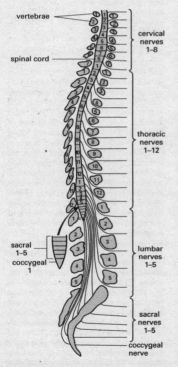

Origins of the spinal nerves (one side only)

*meninges, and extends from the medulla oblongata in the skull to the level of the second lumbar vertebra. From it arise 31 pairs of *spinal nerves.

spinal muscular atrophy (SMA) a hereditary condition in which cells of the spinal cord die and the muscles in the arms and legs become progressively weaker. The gene responsible has been located: in affected children it is inherited as a double *recessive. SMA usually develops between the ages of 2 and 12 years. Eventually, the respiratory muscles are affected and death usually results from respiratory infection. Most affected individuals are wheelchair-bound by the age of 20 and few survive beyond the age of 30. *Infantile spinal muscular atrophy* is an acute aggressive form of the condition (*see* Werdnig-Hoffmann disease).

spinal nerves the 31 pairs of nerves that leave the spinal cord and are distributed to the body, passing out from the vertebral canal through the spaces between the arches of the vertebrae (see illustration). Each nerve has two *roots, an anterior, carrying motor nerve fibers, and a posterior, carrying sensory fibers. Immediately after the roots leave the spinal cord they merge to form a mixed spinal nerve on each side.

spinal shock a state of *shock accompanied by temporary paralysis of the lower extremities that results from injury to the spine and is often associated with *ileus. If the spinal cord is transected, permanent motor paralysis persists below the level of spinal-cord division.

spindle *n.* a collection of fibers seen in a cell when it is dividing. The fibers radiate from the two ends (*poles*) and meet at the center (the *equator*) giving a structure shaped like two cones placed base to base. It plays an important part in chromosome movement in *mitosis and *meiosis and is also involved in division of the cytoplasm.

spine *n.* **1.** a sharp process of a bone. **2.** the vertebral column (*see* backbone). —**spinal** *adj.*

spino- *prefix denoting* **1.** the spine. **2.** the spinal cord.

spinocerebellar degeneration any of a group of inherited disorders of the cerebellum and corticospinal tracts in the brain. They are characterized by *spasticity of the limbs and cerebellar *ataxia.

spiral bandage a bandage wound round a part of the body, overlapping the previous section at each turn.

spiral CT scanning (helical CT scanning) a development of conventional CT scanning (*see* computed tomography) in which the X-ray tube rotates continuously around the patient as he or she passes through the scanner. This enables a much quicker acquisition of images throughout a specified volume of tissue. Since these images are digitally acquired (*see* digitization), *post-processing can produce images in numerous planes, without further exposure of the patient to ionizing radiation.

spiral organ *see* organ of Corti.

Spirillum *n.* a genus of highly motile rigid spiral-shaped bacteria usually found in fresh and salt water containing organic matter. They bear tufts of flagella at one or both ends of the cell. Most species are saprophytes, but *S. minus* causes *rat-bite fever.

spiro- *prefix denoting* **1.** spiral. **2.** respiration.

spirochete *n.* any one of a group of spiral-shaped bacteria that lack a rigid cell wall and move by means of muscular flections of the cell. The group includes the genera *Borrelia, *Leptospira, and *Treponema.

spirograph *n.* an instrument for recording breathing movements. The record (a tracing) obtained is called a *spirogram*. —**spirography** *n.*

spirometer *n.* an instrument for measuring the volume of air inhaled and exhaled. It is used in tests of *ventilation. —**spirometry** *n.*

spironolactone *n.* a synthetic *corticosteroid that inhibits the activity of the hormone *aldosterone and is used as a potassium-sparing *diuretic to treat heart failure, high blood pressure, and fluid retention (edema). It is administered by mouth; side effects may include headache, stomach upsets, drowsiness, breast enlargement (in men), and menstrual disturbances. Trade name: **Aldactone**.

Spitz-Holter valve a one-way valve used to drain cerebrospinal fluid in order to control *hydrocephalus. The device is inserted into the ventricles of the brain and passes via a subcutaneous tunnel to drain into either the right atrium or the peritoneum.

splanch- (splanchno-) *prefix denoting* the viscera.

splanchnic *adj.* relating to the viscera, e.g. splanchnic *mesoderm. *Compare* somatic (def. 2).

splanchnic nerves the series of nerves in the sympathetic system that are distributed to the blood vessels and viscera, passing forward and downward from the chain of sympathetic ganglia near the spinal cord to enter the abdomen and branch profusely.

splanchnocranium *n.* the part of the skull that is derived from the *pharyngeal arches, i.e. the mandible (lower jaw).

splanchnopleure *n.* the wall of the embryonic gut, which consists of a layer of endoderm with a layer of mesoderm outside it. The yolk sac is a continuation of this structure. *Compare* somatopleure.

spleen *n.* a large dark-red ovoid organ situated on the left side of the body below and behind the stomach. It is enclosed within a fibrous capsule that extends into the spongy interior – the *splenic pulp* – to form a supportive framework. The pulp consists of aggregates of *lymphoid tissue (*white pulp*) within a meshwork of *reticular fibers packed with red blood cells (*red pulp*). The spleen is a major component of the *reticuloendothelial system, producing lymphocytes in the newborn and containing *phagocytes, which remove worn-out red blood cells and other foreign bodies from the bloodstream. It also acts as a reservoir for blood and, in the fetus, as a source of red blood cells. Anatomical name: **lien**. —**splenic** *adj.*

splen- (spleno-) *prefix denoting* the spleen. Example: *splenorenal* (relating to the spleen and kidney).

splenectomy *n.* surgical removal of the spleen. This is sometimes necessary in the emergency treatment of bleeding from a ruptured spleen and also in the treatment of some blood diseases. Splenectomy may diminish the immune response to infections.

splenitis *n.* inflammation of the spleen. *See also* perisplenitis.

splenium *n.* the thickest part of the *corpus callosum, rounded and protruding backward over the thalami, the pineal body, and the midbrain.

splenomegaly n. enlargement of the spleen. It commonly occurs in *malaria, *schistosomiasis, and other disorders caused by parasites; in infections; in blood disorders, including some forms of anemia and lack of platelets (*thrombocytopenia); in *leukemia; and in *Hodgkin's disease. *See also* hypersplenism.

splenorenal anastomosis a method of treating *portal hypertension by joining the splenic vein to the left renal vein. *Compare* portacaval anastomosis.

splenunculus n. a small sphere of splenic tissue occurring at a site other than the spleen. Splenunculi are present in many people.

splint n. a rigid support to hold broken bones in position until healing has occurred.

splinter hemorrhage a linear hemorrhage below the nails, usually the result of trauma but also occurring in such conditions as subacute bacterial *endocarditis or severe rheumatoid arthritis.

split-skin graft (Thiersch's graft) a type of skin graft in which thin partial thicknesses of skin are cut in narrow strips or sheets and placed onto the wound area to be healed.

splitting n. a *defense mechanism by which people deal with an emotional conflict by viewing some people as all good and others as all bad: they fail to integrate themselves or other people into complex but coherent images.

spondyl- (spondylo-) *prefix denoting* a vertebra or the spine.

spondylitis n. inflammation of the synovial joints of the backbone. *Ankylosing spondylitis* is a *sero-negative arthritis; 90% of cases carry the tissue-type antigen HLA B27 (*see* HLA system). Ankylosing spondylitis predominantly affects young males and the inflammation affects the joint capsules and their attached ligaments and tendons, principally the intervertebral joints and sacroiliac joints (*see* sacroiliitis). The resultant pain and stiffness of the backbone are treated by analgesics and regular daily exercises. In severe cases the spine becomes completely rigid, through fusion of its joints, and *kyphosis results. *See also* ankylosis.

spondylolisthesis n. a forward shift of one vertebra upon another, usually in the lower back or neck regions, due to a defect in the bone or in the joints that normally bind them together. This may be congenital or develop after injury. The majority of cases in which pain is present are treated with rest and a surgical belt or corset; in a small minority, showing severe disability or pressure on nerve roots, surgical fusion may be required.

spondylosis n. degeneration of the intervertebral disks in the cervical, thoracic, or lumbar regions of the backbone. Symptoms include pain and restriction of movement. Spondylosis produces a characteristic appearance on X-ray, including narrowing of the space occupied by the disk and the presence of *osteophytes; these features of the disease (*radiological spondylosis*) may not be accompanied by any signs and symptoms. Pain is relieved by wearing a collar (when the neck region is affected) or a surgical belt (for the lower spine), which prevents movement. Very severe cases sometimes require surgical fusion.

spondylosyndesis n. surgical fusion of the intervertebral joints of the backbone.

spongiform encephalopathy any one of a group of rapidly progressive degenerative neurological diseases that include scrapie in sheep, bovine spongiform encephalopathy (BSE) in cattle, and *kuru, *Creutzfeldt-Jakob disease, and *Gerstmann-Sträussler-Scheinker syndrome in humans. In humans the spongiform encephalopathies are characterized by rapidly progressive dementia that is associated with myoclonic jerks (*see* myoclonus); on pathological examination the brains of affected individuals show a characteristic cystic degeneration. The diseases are thought to be caused by unconventional transmissible agents (*see* prion).

spongioblast n. a type of cell that forms in the early stages of development of the nervous system, giving rise to *astrocytes and *oligodendrocytes.

spongioblastoma n. *see* glioblastoma.

spontaneous *adj.* arising without apparent cause or outside aid. The term is applied in medicine to certain conditions, such as pathological fractures, that arise in the absence of outside injury; also to recovery from a disease without the aid of specific treatment.

sporadic *adj.* describing a disease that occurs only occasionally or in a few isolated places. *Compare* endemic, epidemic.

spore *n.* a small reproductive body produced by plants and microorganisms. Some kinds of spores function as dormant stages of the life cycle, enabling the organism to survive adverse conditions. Other spores are the means by which the organism can spread vegetatively. *See also* endospore.

sporicide *n.* an agent that kills spores (e.g. bacterial spores). Some disinfectants that liberate chlorine are sporicides, but most germicides are ineffective as spores are very resistant to chemical action. —**sporicidal** *adj.*

sporocyst *n.* the second-stage larva of a parasitic *fluke, found within the tissues of a freshwater snail. A sporocyst develops from a first stage larva (*see* miracidium) and gives rise either to the next larval stage (*see* redia) or daughter sporocysts. The latter develop directly into the final larval stage (*see* cercaria) without the intermediate redia stage.

sporogony *n.* the formation of *sporozoites during the life cycle of a sporozoan. The contents of the zygote, formed by the fusion of sex cells, divide repeatedly and eventually release a number of sporozoites. *Compare* schizogony.

sporotrichosis *n.* a chronic infection of the skin and superficial lymph nodes that is caused by the fungus *Sporothrix schenckii* and results in the formation of abscesses and ulcers. It occurs mainly in the tropics.

Sporozoa *n.* a group of parasitic protozoans that includes *Plasmodium*, the malaria parasite. Most sporozoans do not have cilia or flagella. Sporozoan life cycles are complex and usually involve both sexual and asexual stages. Some sporozoans are parasites of invertebrates, and the parasites are passed to new hosts by means of spores. Sporozoans that parasitize vertebrates are transmitted from host to host by invertebrates, which act as intermediate hosts. For example, the mosquito *Anopheles* is the intermediate host of *Plasmodium*.

sporozoite *n.* one of the many cells formed as a result of *sporogony during the life cyle of a sporozoan. In *Plasmodium* sporozoites are formed by repeated divisions of the contents of the *oocyst inside the body of the mosquito. The released sporozoites ultimately pass into the insect's salivary glands and await transmission to a human host at the next blood meal.

sports injury any injury related to the practice of sport, often resulting from the overuse and stretching of muscles, tendons, and ligaments.

sports medicine a specialty concerned with the treatment of *sports injuries and measures designed to prevent or minimize them (e.g. in the design of sports equipment).

spotted fever *see* meningitis, Rocky Mountain spotted fever, typhus.

sprain *n.* injury to a ligament, caused by sudden overstretching. Since the ligament is not severed, it gradually heals, but this may take several months. Sprains should be treated by cold compresses (ice packs) at the time of injury, and later by restriction of activity.

Sprengel's deformity a congenital abnormality of the scapula (shoulder blade), which is small and positioned high in the shoulder. It is caused by failure of the normal development of this bone. [O. G. K. Sprengel (1852–1915), German surgeon]

sprue (psilosis) *n.* deficient absorption of food due to disease of the small intestine. *Tropical sprue* is seen in people from temperate regions who stay in tropical climates for weeks or months. It is characterized by diarrhea (usually *steatorrhea), inflamed tongue (glossitis), anemia, and weight loss; the lining of the small intestine is inflamed and atrophied, probably because of infection. Treatment with antibiotics and *folic acid is usually effective, but the condition often improves spontaneously on return to a temperate climate. *See also* celiac disease (nontropical sprue), malabsorption.

spud *n.* a blunt needle used for removing foreign bodies embedded in the cornea of the eye.

spur *n.* a sharp projection, especially one of bone.

sputum *n.* material coughed up from the respiratory tract. A sputum-productive cough occurs in many conditions in which examination of the sputum for microorganisms, cells, and other substances are important. The sputum's characteristics, including color, consistency, volume, smell, and the appearance of any solid material within it, often provide information affecting the diagnosis and management of respiratory disease.

squalene *n.* an unsaturated hydrocarbon (a terpene), synthesized in the body, from which *cholesterol is derived.

squama *n.* (*pl.* **squamae**) **1.** a thin plate of bone. **2.** a scale, such as any of the scales from the cornified layer of the *epidermis.

squamo- *prefix denoting* **1.** the squamous portion of the temporal bone. **2.** squamous epithelium.

squamous bone *see* temporal bone.

squamous cell carcinoma (SCC) the second most common form of skin cancer (after *basal cell carcinoma), which usually occurs in late-middle and old age. Sunlight is a common cause but other environmental carcinogens may be responsible. SCC is mainly found on areas exposed to light and is three times more common in men than in women. SCC grows faster than basal cell carcinoma; it spreads locally at first but later may spread to sites distant from its origin (*see* metastasis). Treatment is usually by surgical excision or radiotherapy.

squamous epithelium *see* epithelium.

squint *n. see* strabismus.

SSRI (selective serotonin reuptake inhibitor) any one of a group of *antidepressant drugs that exert their action by blocking the reabsorption of the neurotransmitter *serotonin by the nerve endings in the brain. Their effect is to prolong the action of serotonin in the brain. The group includes *fluoxetine, *paroxetine, and *sertraline. Side effects include agitation and nausea.

stadium *n.* (*pl.* **stadia**) a stage in the course of a disease; for example, the *stadium invasionis* is the period between exposure to infection and the onset of symptoms.

stage *vb.* (in oncology) to classify a primary tumor, by its size and the presence or absence of metastases. In addition to clinical examination, a variety of imaging and surgical techniques may be used to provide a more accurate assessment. Staging tumors is important in defining prognosis and appropriate treatment. *See also* TNM classification.

staghorn calculus a branched stone forming a cast of the collecting system of the kidney and therefore filling the calyces and pelvis. The stone is usually associated with infected urine, the most common organism being *Proteus vulgaris*. The combination of obstruction and infection can cause *pyonephrosis and, if neglected, a *perinephric abscess.

stagnant loop syndrome *see* blind loop syndrome.

stain 1. *n.* a dye used to color tissues and other specimens for microscopical examination. In an *acid stain* the color is carried by an acid radical and the stain is taken up by parts of the specimen having a basic (alkaline) reaction. In a *basic stain* the color, carried by a basic radical, is attracted to parts of the specimen having an acidic reaction. *Neutral stains* have neither acidic nor basic affinities. A *contrast stain* is used to give color to parts of a tissue not affected by a previously applied stain. A *differential stain* allows different elements in a specimen to be distinguished by staining them in different colors. **2.** *vb.* to treat a specimen for microscopical study with a stain.

Stamey procedure an operation devised to cure stress incontinence of urine in women in which specially designed needles are employed to sling or hitch up the neck of the bladder to the anterior abdominal wall with unabsorbable suture material. *See also* colposuspension. [T. A. Stamey, US surgeon]

stammering (stuttering) *n.* halting articulation with interruptions to the normal flow of speech and repetition of the initial consonants of words or syllables (*compare* cluttering). It usually first appears in childhood and the symptoms are most severe when the stammerer is under any psychological stress. It is not a symptom of organic disease and it will usually respond to the reeducation of speech by a trained therapist. Medical name: **dysphemia.** —**stammerer** *n.*

standard deviation (in statistics) a measure of the scatter of observations about their arithmetic *mean, which is calculated from the square root of the *variance* of the readings in the series. The arithmetic sum of the amounts by which each observation varies from the mean must be zero, but if these variations are squared before being summated, a positive value is obtained: the mean of this value is the variance. In practice a more reliable estimate of variance is obtained by dividing the sum of the squared deviations by one *less* than the total number of observations. *See also* significance.

standard error (of a **mean) the extent to which the means of several different samples would vary if they were taken repeatedly from the same population. Differences between means are said to have statistical **significance when they are greater than twice the standard error of those means, since the probability of this difference or a larger one occurring by chance is less than 5%.

stanolone *n.* a synthetic male sex hormone with **anabolic activity, used for its anabolic and antineoplastic actions in inoperable breast cancer.

stanozolol *n.* a synthetic **anabolic steroid used in the treatment of aplastic anemia and osteoporosis and for the prophylaxis of hereditary angioneurotic edema. It is administered by mouth; side effects include edema, decreased production of sperm, and enlarged breasts in males. Trade name: **Winstrol**.

stapedectomy *n.* surgical removal of the third ear ossicle (stapes): part of the treatment for deafness due to **otosclerosis.

stapes *n.* a stirrup-shaped bone in the middle **ear that articulates with the incus and is attached to the membrane of the fenestra ovalis. *See* ossicle.

staphylectomy *n. see* uvulectomy.

staphylococcal scalded skin syndrome (Lyell's disease, Ritter's disease) a potentially serious condition of young infants in which the skin becomes reddened and tender and then peels off, giving the appearance of a scald. The area of skin loss may be quite extensive. The underlying cause is an infection by certain bacteria of the genus **Staphylococcus*. It is contagious and may occur in clusters. Treatment is by antibiotics, but careful nursing is essential to prevent skin damage. Medical name: **toxic epidermal necrolysis**.

Staphylococcus *n.* a genus of gram-positive nonmotile spherical bacteria occurring in grapelike clusters. Some species are saprophytes; others parasites. Many species produce **exotoxins. The species *S. aureus* is commonly present on skin

and mucous membranes; it causes boils and internal abscesses. More serious infections include pneumonia, bacteremia, osteomyelitis, and enterocolitis. Other species produce toxins causing **food poisoning. *See also* MRSA. —**staphylococcal** *adj.*

staphyloma *n.* abnormal bulging of the cornea or sclera (white) of the eye. *Anterior staphyloma* is a bulging scar in the cornea to which a part of the iris is attached. It is usually the site of a healed corneal ulcer that has penetrated right through the cornea; the iris blocks the hole and prevents the further leakage of fluid from the front chamber of the eye. In *ciliary staphyloma* the sclera bulges over the ciliary body as a result of high pressure inside the eyeball. A bulging of the sclera at the back of the eye (*posterior staphyloma*) occurs in some severe cases of nearsightedness.

staphylorrhaphy (palatorrhaphy, uraniscorrhaphy) *n.* surgical suture of a cleft palate.

staple *n.* (in surgery) a piece of metal used to join up pieces of tissue. Staples can be used as an alternative to **sutures for an **anastomosis; stapling machines have been produced for this purpose. *See also* endostapler.

starch *n.* the form in which **carbohydrates are stored in many plants and a major constituent of the diet. Starch consists of linked glucose units and occurs in two forms, α-amylose and *amylopectin*. In α-amylose the units are in the form of a long unbranched chain; in amylopectin they form a branched chain. The presence of starch can be detected using iodine: α-amylose gives a blue color with iodine; amylopectin, a red color. Starch is digested by means of the enzyme **amylase. *See also* dextrin.

Starling's law a law stating that a muscle, including the heart muscle, responds to increased stretching at rest by an increased force of contraction when stimulated. [E. H. Starling (1866–1927), British physiologist]

startle reflex *see* Moro reflex.

starvation *n. see* malnutrition.

stasis *n.* stagnation or cessation of flow; for example, of blood or lymph whose flow is obstructed or of the intestinal contents when onward movement (peristalsis) is hindered.

-stasis *suffix denoting* stoppage of a flow of liquid; stagnation. Example: *hemostasis* (of blood).

static reflex the reflex maintenance of muscular tone for posture.

statin *n.* any one of a class of drugs that inhibit the action of the enzyme *hydroxy-methylglutaryl coenzyme A reductase (HMG-CoA reductase), which is involved in the liver's production of *cholesterol. Statins can lower the levels of low-density *lipoproteins (LDLs) by 25–45% and are used mainly to treat hypercholesterolemia but also to reduce the risk of coronary heart disease in susceptible patients. Muscle inflammation and breakdown is a rare but serious side effect of statins. The class includes *atorvastatin, *fluvastatin, *pravastatin, and *simvastatin.

status asthmaticus a severe and prolonged attack of *asthma, which often does not respond to oral medication. Patients are distressed and very breathless and may die from respiratory failure if not vigorously treated with inhaled oxygen, nebulized or intravenous bronchodilators, and corticosteroid therapy; sedatives are absolutely contraindicated. These patients need hospital care in an intensive care unit.

status epilepticus the occurrence of repeated epileptic seizures without any recovery of consciousness between them. Its control is a medical emergency, since prolonged status epilepticus may lead to the patient's death or long-term disability.

status lymphaticus enlargement of the thymus and other parts of the lymphatic system, formerly believed to be a predisposing cause to sudden death in infancy and childhood associated with hypersensitivity to drugs or vaccines.

STD *see* sexually transmitted disease.

steapsin *n. see* lipase.

stearic acid *see* fatty acid.

steat- (steato-) *prefix denoting* fat; fatty tissue.

steatoma *n.* any cyst or tumor of a sebaceous gland.

steatopygia *n.* the accumulation of large quantities of fat in the buttocks. In the Hottentots of Africa this is a normal condition, thought to be an adaptation that allows fat storage without impeding heat loss from the rest of the body.

steatorrhea *n.* the passage of abnormally increased amounts of fat in the feces (more than 5 g/day) due to reduced absorption of fat by the intestine (*see* malabsorption). The feces are pale, smell offensive, may look greasy, and are difficult to flush away.

steatosis *n.* infiltration of *hepatocytes with fat. This may occur in pregnancy, alcoholism, malnutrition, obesity, hepatitis C infection, or with some drugs.

Steele-Richardson-Olszewski syndrome *see* progressive supranuclear palsy. [J. C. Steele and J. C. Richardson, 20th century Canadian neurologists; J. Olszewski (1913–64), Polish-born Canadian neuropathologist]

stellate fracture a star-shaped fracture of the kneecap caused by a direct blow. The bone may be either split or severely shattered; if the fragments are displaced, the bone may need to be surgically repaired or (rarely) removed (*patellectomy*).

stellate ganglion a star-shaped collection of sympathetic nerve cell bodies in the root of the neck, from which sympathetic nerve fibers are distributed to the face and neck and to the blood vessels and organs of the thorax.

Stellwag's sign apparent widening of the distance between the upper and lower eyelids (the palpebral fissure) caused by retraction of the upper lid and protrusion of the eyeball. It is a sign of exophthalmic *goiter. [C. Stellwag von Carion (1823–1904), Austrian ophthalmologist]

stem cell an undifferentiated cell that is able to renew itself and produce all the specialized cells within an organ. Stem cells occur in many tissues and organs, including the bone marrow (*see* hemopoietic stem cell), muscle, liver, pancreas, etc. *Embryonic stem cells*, in the *blastocyst of the embryo, are capable of producing all the different cell types required by the developing embryo (i.e. they are pluripotent). *See also* umbilical cord blood banked stem cells.

steno- *prefix denoting* **1.** narrow. Example: *stenocephaly* (narrowness of the head). **2.** constricted.

stenopeic *adj.* (in ophthalmology) describing an optical device consisting of an opaque disk punctured with a fine slit or hole (or holes), which is placed in front of the eye in the same position as glasses and enables sharper vision in cases of gross far- or nearsightedness or astigmatism. It sharpens the image formed on the retina because it confines the light reaching the eye to one or more fine beams. The same principle is used in the pinhole camera.

stenosis *n.* the abnormal narrowing of a passage or opening, such as a blood vessel or heart valve. *See* aortic stenosis, carotid artery stenosis, mitral stenosis, pulmonary stenosis, pyloric stenosis.

stenostomia (stenostomy) *n.* the abnormal narrowing of an opening, such as the opening of the bile duct.

Stensen's duct the long secretory duct of the *parotid gland opening in the mouth. [N. Stensen (1838–86), Danish physician]

stent *n.* a tube placed inside the lumen of a duct or canal, such as the ureter, urethra, esophagus, or bile duct, or an artery, to reopen it or keep it open. It may be a simple tube, usually plastic, or an expandable, usually sprung mesh metal, tube. The former is more easily removable, while the latter gives a larger lumen for a given outer diameter. Stents may be used at operation to aid healing of an anastomosis by draining the contents away or placed across an obstruction to maintain an open lumen, e.g. in a bile duct obstructed by a tumor or stricture, or in an artery after *angioplasty to prevent restenosis. *Double J* (or *pigtail*) *stents* are slender catheters with side holes that are passed over a guide wire either through an endoscope or at open operation to drain urine from the kidney pelvis to the bladder via the ureter. On removal of the guide wire, both the upper and lower extremities of the stent assume a J-shape, preventing both upward and downward migration. They are commonly used to splint a damaged ureter and to relieve obstruction.

stepping reflex a primitive reflex in newborn babies that should disappear by the age of two months. If the baby is held in a "walking" position with the feet touching the ground, the feet move in a "stepping" manner. Persistence of this reflex beyond two months is suggestive of *cerebral palsy.

sterco- *prefix denoting* feces.

stercobilin *n.* a brownish-red pigment formed during the metabolism of the *bile pigments biliverdin and bilirubin, which are derived from hemoglobin. Stercobilin is subsequently excreted in the urine or feces.

stercolith *n.* a stone formed of dried compressed feces.

stercoraceous *adj.* composed of or containing feces.

stereognosis *n.* the ability to recognize the three-dimensional shape of an object by touch alone. This is a function of the *association areas of the parietal lobe of the brain. *See also* agnosia.

stereoisomers *pl. n.* compounds that have the same molecular formula but different three-dimensional arrangements of their atoms. The atomic structures of stereoisomers are mirror images of each other.

stereoscopic vision (stereopsis) perception of the shape, depth, and distance of an object as a result of having *binocular vision. The brain receives two distinct images from the eyes, which it interprets as a single three-dimensional image.

stereotactic localization the accurate localization of structures within the body by using three-dimensional measurements. It enables the accurate positioning within the body of radiotherapy beams or sources for the treatment of tumors and of localizing wires for the biopsy of small tumors. *See also* stereotaxy (stereotactic surgery).

stereotaxy (stereotactic surgery) *n.* a surgical procedure in which a deep-seated area in the brain is operated upon after its position has been established very accurately by three-dimensional measurements. The operation may be performed using an electrical current or by heat, cold, or mechanical techniques. *See also* leukotomy.

stereotypy *n.* the constant repetition of a complex action, which is carried out in the same way each time. It is seen in *catatonia and infantile *autism; sometimes it is an isolated symptom in mental retardation. It is more common in patients who live in institutions where they are bored and unstimulated. It can prevent a patient from carrying on normal life, and sometimes causes physical injury to the patient. Drugs, such as *phenothiazines, and behavior therapy are sometimes used in treating the condition.

sterile *adj.* **1.** (of a living organism) barren; unable to reproduce its kind (*see* sterility). **2.** (of inanimate objects) completely free from bacteria, fungi, viruses, or other microorganisms that could cause infection.

sterility *n.* inability to have children, due either to *infertility or (in someone who has been fertile) to a surgical operation as a means of contraception (*see* sterilization). Sterility may be an incidental result of an operation or drug treatment undertaken for other reasons, such as removal of the uterus (*hysterectomy) for cancer.

sterilization *n.* **1.** a surgical operation or any other process that induces *sterility in men or women. In women, hysterectomy and bilateral oophorectomy (surgical removal of both ovaries) are 100% effective and permanent. Alternatively, the fallopian tubes may be removed (*see* salpingectomy) or divided and/or ligated. These operations can be performed through the abdomen or the vagina. The modern technique is to occlude (close) permanently the inner (lower) half of the fallopian tube through a *laparoscope, usually using a clip or a small plastic ring; *diathermy coagulation carries greater dangers (e.g. bowel burns) and is now little used. A more recent method is the use of a rapid-setting plastic introduced into the tubes through a *hysteroscope. Men are usually sterilized by *vasectomy. *See also* castration. **2.** any means of rendering objects, wounds, etc., free of bacteria that would otherwise cause disease. Surgical instruments and dressings can be sterilized by being subjected to steam in an *autoclave. *Disinfectants and *antiseptics are chemicals used to destroy bacteria.

stern- (sterno-) *prefix denoting* the sternum. Example: *sternocostal* (relating to the sternum and ribs).

Sternberg-Reed cell *see* Reed-Sternberg cell.

sternebra *n.* (*pl.* **sternebrae**) one of the four parts that fuse during development to form the body of the sternum.

sternocleidomastoid muscle *see* sternomastoid muscle.

sternohyoid *n.* a muscle in the neck, arising from the sternum and inserted into the hyoid bone. It depresses the hyoid bone.

sternomastoid muscle (sternocleidomastoid muscle) a long muscle in the neck, extending from the mastoid process to the sternum and clavicle. It serves to rotate the neck and flex the head.

sternomastoid tumor a small painless nonmalignant swelling in the lower half of the *sternomastoid muscle, appearing a few days after birth. It occurs when the neck of the fetus is in an abnormal position in the uterus, which interferes with the blood supply to the affected muscle, and it is most common after breech births. The tumor may cause a slight tilt of the head toward the tumor and turning of the face to the other side. This can be corrected by physiotherapy aimed at increasing all movements of the body, but without stretching the neck.

sternotomy *n.* surgical division of the breastbone (sternum), performed to allow access to the heart and its major vessels.

sternum *n.* (*pl.* **sterna**) the breastbone: a flat bone, 15–20 cm long, extending from the base of the neck to just below the diaphragm and forming the front part of the skeleton of the thorax. The sternum articulates with the collar bones (*see* clavicle) and the costal cartilages of the first seven pairs of ribs. It consists of three sections: the middle and longest section – the *body* or *gladiolus* – is attached to the *manubrium at the top and the *xiphoid (or ensiform) process at the bottom. The manubrium slopes back from the body in such a way that the junction between the two parts forms an angle (*angle of Louis* or *sternal angle*). —**sternal** *adj.*

sternutator *n.* an agent that produces sneezing.

steroid *n.* one of a group of compounds having a common structure based on the *steroid nucleus*, which consists of three six-membered carbon rings and one five-membered carbon ring. The naturally occurring steroids include the male and female sex hormones (*androgens and *estrogens), the hormones of the adrenal cortex (*see* corticosteroid), *progesterone, *bile salts, and *sterols. Synthetic steroids have been produced for therapeutic purposes.

sterol *n.* one of a group of *steroid alcohols. The most important sterols are *cholesterol and *ergosterol.

stertor n. a snoring type of noisy breathing heard in deeply unconscious patients.

steth- (stetho-) *prefix denoting* the chest.

stethograph n. an instrument for recording chest movements during breathing. —**stethography** n.

stethometer n. an instrument for measuring the expansion of the chest during breathing.

stethoscope n. an instrument used for listening to sounds within the body, such as those in the heart and lungs (*see* auscultation). A simple stethoscope usually consists of a diaphragm or an open bell-shaped structure (which is applied to the body) connected by rubber or plastic tubes to shaped earpieces for the examiner. More complicated devices may contain electronic amplification systems to aid diagnosis.

sthenia n. a state of normal or greater than normal strength. *Compare* asthenia. —**sthenic** *adj.*

stibophen n. a sodium-containing salt of antimony used as an *anthelmintic primarily to treat *schistosomiasis. It is administered by injection, but because of its toxicity, it is now rarely used.

stigma n. (*pl.* **stigmata**) 1. a mark that characterizes a particular disease, such as the café-au-lait spots characteristic of neurofibromatosis. 2. any spot or lesion on the skin.

stilbestrol n. *see* diethylstilbestrol.

stilet n. *see* stylet.

stillbirth n. birth of a fetus that shows no evidence of life (heartbeat, respiration, or independent movement) at any time later than 24 weeks after conception. The number of such births expressed per 1000 births (live and still) is known as the *stillbirth rate*. Viability is deemed to start at the 24th week of pregnancy and a fetus born dead before this time is known as an *abortion or miscarriage. However, some fetuses born alive before the 24th week may now survive as a result of improved perinatal care. *See* infant mortality rate.

Still's disease chronic arthritis developing in children before the age of 16 years. There are several different forms of arthritis affecting children, and some authorities confine the diagnosis of Still's disease to the following: a disease of childhood marked by arthritis (often involving several joints) with a swinging fever and a transitory red rash. There is sometimes severe illness affecting the entire body and the condition may be complicated by enlargement of the spleen and lymph nodes and inflammation of the pericardium and iris. *See also* juvenile rheumatoid arthritis. [Sir G. F. Still (1868–1941), British physician]

stimulant n. an agent that promotes the activity of a body system or function. *Amphetamines and *caffeine are stimulants of the central nervous system; *doxapram is a respiratory stimulant (*see* analeptic).

stimulator n. any apparatus designed to stimulate nerves and muscles for a variety of purposes. It can be used to stimulate particular areas of the brain or to block pain (as in *transcutaneous electrical nerve stimulation).

stimulus n. (*pl.* **stimuli**) any agent that provokes a response, or particular form of activity, in a cell, tissue, or other structure, which is said to be *sensitive* to that stimulus.

stippling n. a spotted or speckled appearance, such as is seen in the retina in certain eye diseases or in abnormal red blood cells stained with basic dyes.

stirrup n. (in anatomy) *see* stapes.

stitch n. 1. a sharp localized pain, commonly in the abdomen, associated with strenuous physical activity (such as running), especially shortly after eating. It is a form of cramp. 2. *see* suture.

stock culture *see* culture.

Stokes-Adams syndrome (Adams-Stokes syndrome) attacks of temporary loss of consciousness that occur when blood flow ceases due to ventricular *fibrillation or *asystole. This syndrome may complicate *heart block. It is treated by means of a battery-operated *pacemaker. [W. Stokes (1804–78) and R. Adams (1791–1875), Irish physicians]

stoma n. (*pl.* **stomata**) 1. (in anatomy) the mouth or any mouthlike part. 2. (in surgery) the artificial opening of a tube (e.g. the colon or ileum) that has been brought to the abdominal surface (*see* colostomy, ileostomy). *Stoma therapists* are nurses specially trained in the care of these artificial openings and the appliances used with them. —**stomal** *adj.*

stomach *n.* a distensible saclike organ that forms part of the alimentary canal between the esophagus (gullet) and the duodenum (see illustration). It communicates with the former by means of the *cardiac sphincter* and with the latter by the *pyloric sphincter*. The stomach lies just below the diaphragm, to the right of the spleen and partly under the liver. Its function is to continue the process of digestion that begins in the mouth. *Gastric juice, secreted by gastric glands in the mucosa, contains hydrochloric acid and the enzyme *pepsin, which contribute to chemical digestion. This – together with the churning action of the muscular layers of the stomach – reduces the food to a semiliquid partly digested mass that passes on to the duodenum.

stomachic *n.* an agent that stimulates the secretory activity of the stomach, used as a tonic to improve the appetite.

stomat- (stomato-) *prefix denoting* the mouth.

stomatitis *n.* inflammation of the mucous lining of the mouth.

stomatology *n.* the branch of medicine concerned with diseases of the mouth.

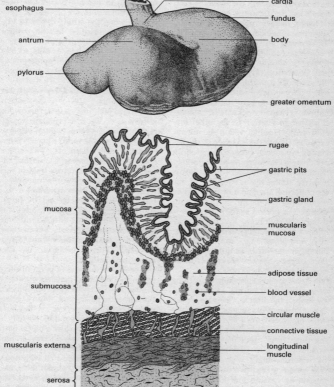

Regions of the stomach seen from the front (above); layers of the stomach wall (below)

stomodeum *n.* the site of the embryonic mouth, marked by a depression lined with ectoderm from which the teeth develop. The membrane separating it from the foregut breaks down by the end of the first month of pregnancy. *Compare* proctodeum.

-stomy (-ostomy) *suffix denoting* a surgical opening into an organ or part. Example: *colostomy* (into the colon).

stone *n. see* calculus.

stool *n.* *feces discharged from the anus.

stop needle a surgical needle with a shank that has a protruding collar to stop it when the needle has been pushed a prescribed distance into the tissue. A stop needle has the eye at the tip.

strabismus (heterotropia) *n.* squint: any abnormal alignment of the two eyes. The strabismus is most commonly horizontal – *convergent strabismus* (*esotropia*) or *divergent strabismus* (*exotropia*) – but it may be vertical (*hypertropia*, in which the eye looks upward, or *hypotropia*, in which it looks downward). In rare cases both eyes look toward the same point but one is twisted clockwise or counterclockwise in relation to the other (*cyclotropia*). Double vision is always experienced, but the image from the deviating eye usually becomes ignored. In cyclotropia the image is not separated from the normal one but rotated across it. Most strabismus is *concomitant*, i.e. the abnormal alignment of the two eyes remains fairly constant, in whatever direction the person is looking. This is usual with childhood squints. Strabismus acquired by injury or disease is usually *incomitant*, i.e. the degree of misalignment varies in different directions of gaze. *See also* cover test, deviation, divergence, heterophoria.

strain 1. *n.* excessive stretching or working of a muscle, resulting in pain and swelling of the muscle. *Compare* sprain. **2.** *n.* a group of organisms, such as bacteria, obtained from a particular source or having special properties distinguishing them from other members of the same species. **3.** *vb.* to damage a muscle by overstretching.

strain gauge a sensitive instrument for measuring tension and alterations in pressure. It is extensively used in medical instruments.

strangulated *adj.* describing a part of the body whose blood supply has been interrupted by compression of a blood vessel, as may occur in a loop of intestine trapped in a *hernia.

strangulation *n.* the closure of a passage, such as the main airway to the lungs (resulting in the cessation of breathing), a blood vessel, or the gastrointestinal tract.

strangury *n.* severe pain in the urethra referred from the base of the bladder and associated with an intense desire to pass urine. It occurs when the base of the bladder is irritated by a stone or an indwelling catheter. It is also noted in patients with an invasive cancer of the base of the bladder or severe *cystitis or *prostatitis, when the strong desire to urinate is accompanied by the painful passage of a few drops of urine.

stratum *n.* a layer of tissue or cells, such as any of the layers of the *epidermis of the skin (the *stratum corneum* is the outermost layer).

strawberry mark (strawberry nevus) *see* nevus.

streak *n.* (in anatomy) a line, furrow, or narrow band. *See also* primitive streak.

Streptobacillus *n.* a genus of gram-negative aerobic nonmotile rodlike bacteria that tend to form filaments. The single species, *S. moniliformis*, is a normal inhabitant of the respiratory tract of rats but causes *rat-bite fever in humans.

streptococcal toxic shock syndrome a bacterial disease characterized by fever, shock, and multiple organ failure. It is similar to the *toxic shock syndrome caused by staphylococci, but in these cases the infecting organisms are *Streptococcus* Type A bacteria. *See also* necrotizing fasciitis.

Streptococcus *n.* a genus of gram-positive nonmotile spherical bacteria occurring in chains. Most species are saprophytes, but some are pathogenic. Many pathogenic species are *hemolytic*, i.e. they have the ability to destroy red blood cells in blood agar. This provides a useful basis for classifying the many different strains. Strains of *S. pyogenes* (the β-hemolytic streptococci) are associated with many infections, including *scarlet fever, and produce many *exotoxins. Strains of the α-hemolytic streptococci are associated with bacterial *endocarditis. The species *S. pneumoniae* (formerly *Diplococcus* *pneumoniae*) – the **pneumococcus* – is associated with pneumonia and pneumococcal **meningitis*. It occurs in pairs, surrounded by a capsule (*see* quellung reaction). *S. mutans* has been shown to cause dental caries. *See also* Lancefield classification, streptokinase. —**streptococcal** *adj.*

streptodornase *n.* an enzyme produced by some hemolytic bacteria of the genus *Streptococcus* that is capable of liquefying pus. *See also* streptokinase.

streptokinase *n.* an enzyme produced by some hemolytic bacteria of the genus **Streptococcus* that is capable of liquefying blood clots. It is injected to treat blockage of blood vessels, including deep vein thrombosis, infarction, and pulmonary embolism. It is also used in combination with streptodornase, applied topically or taken by mouth or injection, to liquefy pus and relieve inflammation. Side effects may include digestive upsets, fever, and hemorrhage. Trade names: **Kabikinase**, **Streptase**.

streptolysin *n.* an **exotoxin* that is produced by strains of streptococci and destroys red blood cells.

Streptomyces *n.* a genus of aerobic mold-like bacteria. Most species live in the soil, but some are parasites of animals, humans, and plants; in humans they cause **Madura* foot. They are important medically as a source of such antibiotics as **streptomycin*, **neomycin*, **dactinomycin*, and **chloramphenicol*.

streptomycin *n.* an **aminoglycoside* antibiotic, derived from the bacterium *Streptomyces griseus*, that is effective against a wide range of bacterial infections; it is administered by intramuscular injection. Because of the emergence of resistant strains, streptomycin is now primarily used in combination with other drugs for treating tuberculosis, brucellosis, and endocarditis. Side effects causing ear and kidney damage may develop in some patients.

stress *n.* any factor that threatens the health of the body or has an adverse effect on its functioning, such as injury, disease, or worry. The existence of one form of stress tends to diminish resistance to other forms. Constant stress brings about changes in the balance of hormones in the body.

stretch receptor a cell or group of cells found between muscle fibers that responds to stretching of the muscle by transmitting impulses to the central nervous system through sensory nerves. Stretch receptors are part of the **proprioceptor* system necessary for the performance of coordinated muscular activity.

stretch reflex (myotatic reflex) the reflex contraction of a muscle in response to its being stretched.

stria *n.* (*pl.* **striae**) (in anatomy) a streak, line, or thin band. The *striae gravidarum* (stretch marks) are the lines that appear on the skin of the abdomen of pregnant women, due to excessive stretching of the elastic fibers. Red or purple during pregnancy, they become white after delivery. The *stria terminalis* is a white band that separates the thalamus from the ventricular surface of the caudate nucleus in the brain.

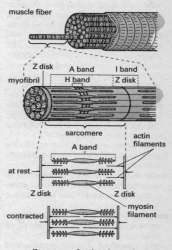

Structure of striated muscle

striated muscle a tissue comprising the bulk of the body's musculature. It is also known as *skeletal muscle*, because it is attached to the skeleton and is responsible for the movement of bones, and *voluntary muscle*, because it is under voluntary control. Striated muscle is composed of parallel bundles of multinucleate fibers (each containing many *myofibrils*), which reveal cross-banding when viewed under the microscope. This effect is due to the alternation of *actin* and *myosin* protein filaments within each myofibril (see illustration). When muscle contraction takes place, the two sets of filaments slide past each other, so reducing the length of each unit (*sarcomere*) of the myofibril. The sliding is caused by a series of cyclic reactions resulting in a change in orientation of projections on the myosin filaments; each projection is first attached to an actin filament but contracts and releases it to become reattached at a different site.

stricture *n.* a narrowing of any tubular structure in the body, such as the esophagus (gullet), bowel, ureter, or urethra. A stricture may result from inflammation, muscular spasm, growth of a tumor within the affected part, or from pressure on it by neighboring organs. For example, a *urethral stricture* is a fibrous narrowing of the urethra, usually resulting from injury or inflammation. The patient has increasing difficulty in passing urine and may develop *retention. The site and length of the stricture is assessed by *urethrography and urethroscopy, and treatment is by periodic dilation of the urethra using *sounds, *urethrotomy, or *urethroplasty. Strictures in the alimentary canal are dilated by *balloon or *stricturoplasty.

stricturoplasty *n.* an operation in which a stricture (usually in the small intestine) is widened by cutting it.

stridor *n.* the noise heard on breathing in when the trachea or larynx is obstructed. It tends to be louder and harsher than *wheeze.

strobila *n.* (*pl.* **strobilae**) the entire chain of segments that make up the body of an adult *tapeworm.

stroke (apoplexy) *n.* a sudden attack of weakness affecting one side of the body. It is the consequence of an interruption to the flow of blood to the brain. An *ischemic stroke* occurs when the flow of blood is prevented by clotting (*see* thrombosis) or by a detached clot, either from the heart or a large vessel, that lodges in an artery (*see* embolism). A *hemorrhagic stroke* results from rupture of an artery wall (*cerebral hemor-

rhage). Prolonged reduction of blood pressure may result in more diffuse brain damage, as after a cardiorespiratory arrest. A stroke can vary in severity from a passing weakness or tingling in a limb (*see* transient ischemic attack) to a profound paralysis, coma, and death.

stroma *n.* **1.** the supportive (connective) tissue of an organ, as opposed to the functional tissue (*parenchyma*); for example, the stroma of the cornea is the transparent fibrous tissue making up the main body of the cornea. **2.** the spongy framework of protein strands within a red blood cell in which the blood pigment hemoglobin is packed.

Strongyloides *n.* a genus of small slender nematode worms that live as parasites in the small intestines of mammals. *S. stercoralis* infects the human small intestine (*see* strongyloidiasis); its larvae, which are passed out in the stools, develop quickly into infective forms.

strongyloidiasis (strongyloidosis) *n.* an infestation of the small intestine with the parasitic nematode worm *Strongyloides stercoralis*, common in humid tropical regions. Larvae, present in soil contaminated with human feces, penetrate the skin of a human host and may produce an itching rash. They migrate to the lungs, where they cause tissue destruction and bleeding, and then via the windpipe and gullet to the intestine. Adult worms burrow into the intestinal wall and may cause ulceration, diarrhea, abdominal pain, nausea, anemia, and weakness. Treatment involves use of the drug *thiabendazole.

strontium *n.* a yellow metallic element, absorption of which causes bone damage when its atoms displace calcium in bone. The radioactive isotope *strontium-90*, which emits beta rays, is used in radiotherapy for the *contact therapy of skin and eye tumors and by injection in the treatment of metastatic prostate cancer. Symbol: Sr.

struma *n.* (*pl.* **strumae**) a swelling of the thyroid gland (*see* goiter). *See also* Riedel's thyroiditis.

struma ovarii a *teratoma of the ovary containing thyroid tissue that becomes overactive and causes *thyrotoxicosis. It is diagnosed by radioiodine scanning showing a high uptake in the pelvis; the treatment is surgical removal of the affected ovary.

strychnine n. a poisonous alkaloid produced in the seeds of the East Indian tree *Strychnos nux-vomica*. In small doses it was formerly widely used in tonics. Poisoning causes painful muscular spasms similar to those of tetanus; the back becomes arched (the posture known as *opisthotonos*) and death is likely to occur from spasm in the respiratory muscles.

S–T segment the segment on an *electrocardiogram that represents the interval preceding the last phase of the *cardiac cycle, when the heart recovers from contraction. The S–T segment is usually raised by acute *ischemia of the heart muscle; it usually returns to normal with recovery.

Student's t test *see* significance. [Pseudonym of W. S. Gosset (1876–1937), British statistician]

stupe n. any piece of material, such as a wad of cotton wool, soaked in hot water (with or without medication) and used to apply a poultice.

stupor n. a condition of near unconsciousness, with apparent mental inactivity and reduced ability to respond to stimulation.

Sturge-Weber syndrome *see* angioma. [W. A. Sturge (1850–1919) and F. P. Weber (1863–1962), British physicians]

stuttering n. *see* stammering.

STYCAR tests Standard (or Screening) Tests for Young Children and Retardates: tests to detect visual problems in children between the ages of six months and five years. They consist of a series of standardized balls, toys, or letters. The tests were developed by the pediatrician Mary Sheridan.

stye n. acute inflammation of a gland at the base of an eyelash, caused by bacterial infection. The gland becomes hard and tender and a pus-filled cyst develops at its center. Styes are treated by bathing in warm water or removal of the eyelash involved. Medical name: **hordeolum**.

stylet (stilet, stylus) n. **1.** a slender probe. **2.** a wire placed in the lumen of a catheter to give it rigidity while the instrument is passed along a body canal (such as the urethra).

stylo- *prefix denoting* the styloid process of the temporal bone. Example: *stylomas-*

toid (relating to the styloid and mastoid processes).

styloglossus n. a muscle that extends from the tongue to the styloid process of the temporal bone. It serves to draw the tongue upward and backward.

stylohyoid n. a muscle that extends from the styloid process of the temporal bone to the hyoid bone. It serves to draw the hyoid bone backward and upward.

styloid process 1. a long slender downward-pointing spine projecting from the lower surface of the *temporal bone of the skull. It provides attachment for muscles and ligaments of the tongue and hyoid bone. **2.** any of various other spiny projections; occurring, for example, at the lower ends of the ulna and radius.

stylus n. **1.** a pencil-shaped instrument, commonly used for applying external medication; for example, to apply silver nitrate to warts. **2.** *see* stylet.

styptic n. *see* hemostatic.

sub- *prefix denoting* **1.** below; underlying. Examples: *subcostal* (below the ribs); *sublingual* (below the tongue); *submandibular* (below the mandible). **2.** partial or slight.

subacute adj. describing a disease that progresses more rapidly than a *chronic condition but does not become *acute.

subacute combined degeneration of the cord the neurological disorder complicating a deficiency of *vitamin B₁₂ and pernicious anemia. There is selective damage to the motor and sensory nerve fibers in the spinal cord, resulting in *spasticity of the limbs and a sensory *ataxia. It may also be accompanied by damage to the peripheral nerves and the optic nerve and by dementia. It is treated by giving vitamin B₁₂ injections.

subacute sclerosing panencephalitis (SSPE) a rare and late complication of *measles characterized by a slow progressive neurological deterioration that is usually fatal. It can occur four to ten years after the initial infection.

subarachnoid hemorrhage sudden bleeding into the subarachnoid space surrounding the brain, which causes severe headache with stiffness of the neck. The usual source of such a hemorrhage is a cerebral *aneurysm that has burst. The diagnosis is confirmed by CT scan or by finding blood-stained cerebrospinal fluid at *lumbar puncture. Identification of the site of the aneurysm, upon which decisions about treatment will be based, is achieved by cerebral *angiography.

subarachnoid space the space between the arachnoid and pia *meninges of the brain and spinal cord, containing circulating cerebrospinal fluid and large blood vessels. Several large spaces within it are known as *cisternae*.

subclavian artery either of two arteries supplying blood to the neck and arms. The right subclavian artery branches from the innominate artery; the left subclavian arises directly from the aortic arch.

subclavian steal syndrome diversion of blood from the vertebral artery to the subclavian artery when the latter is blocked proximally. It causes attacks of diminished consciousness (*syncope).

subclinical *adj.* describing a disease that is suspected but is not sufficiently developed to produce definite signs and symptoms in the patient.

subconscious *adj.* **1.** describing mental processes of which a person is not aware. **2.** (in psychoanalysis) denoting the part of the mind that includes memories, motives, and intentions that are momentarily not present in consciousness but can more or less readily be recalled to awareness. *Compare* unconscious.

subcutaneous *adj.* beneath the skin. A *subcutaneous injection* is given beneath the skin. *Subcutaneous tissue* is loose connective tissue, often fatty, situated under the dermis.

subdural *adj.* below the dura mater (the outermost of the meninges); relating to the space between the dura mater and arachnoid. *See also* hematoma.

subglottis *n.* that part of the *larynx that lies below the vocal cords.

subinvolution *n.* failure of the uterus to return to its normal size during the six weeks following childbirth.

sublimation *n.* the replacement of socially undesirable means of gratifying motives or desires by means that are socially acceptable. *See also* defense mechanism, repression.

subliminal *adj.* subconscious: beneath the threshold of conscious perception.

sublingual gland one of a pair of *salivary glands situated in the lower part of the mouth, one on either side of the tongue. The sublingual glands are the smallest

salivary glands; each gland has about 20 ducts, most of which open into the mouth directly above the gland.

subluxation *n.* partial *dislocation of a joint, so that the bone ends are misaligned but still in contact.

submandibular gland (submaxillary gland) one of a pair of *salivary glands situated below the parotid glands. Their ducts (*Wharton's ducts*) open in two papillae under the tongue, on either side of the frenulum.

submaxillary gland *see* submandibular gland.

submentovertical (SMV) *adj.* denoting an X-ray view of the base of the skull.

submucosa *n.* the layer of loose connective (*areolar) tissue that underlies a mucous membrane; for example, in the wall of the intestine. —**submucosal** *adj.*

subnormality *n.* a former term for *mental retardation.

subphrenic abscess a collection of pus in the space below the diaphragm, usually on the right side, between the liver and diaphragm. Causes include postoperative infection (particularly after the stomach or bowel has been opened) and perforation of an organ (e.g. a perforated peptic ulcer). Prompt treatment by antibiotics may be effective, but more frequently the abscess requires surgical drainage.

substance abuse the nonclinical, or recreational, use of pharmacologically active substances that results in adverse physiological or psychological effects (*see* dependence). Substances commonly abused include alcohol (*see* alcoholism), *amphetamines, *cannabis, *cocaine, *Ecstasy, *heroin, *lysergic acid diethylamide (LSD), and organic solvents (by inhalation).

Substance Abuse and Mental Health Services Administration (SAMHSA) an agency of the US *Public Health Service divison of the *Department of Health and Human Services that, through its numerous programs and funds, works to improve the quality and availability of substance abuse prevention, addiction treatment, and mental health services. SAMHSA comprises three major centers: the Center for Mental Health Services, the Center for Substance Abuse Prevention, and the Center for Substance Abuse Treatment. Established in 1992, this agency replaced the Alcohol, Drug Abuse and Mental Health Administration, which was initiated in 1974.

substitution *n.* **1.** (in psychoanalysis) the replacement of one idea by another: a form of *defense mechanism. **2.** (**symptom substitution**) the supposed process whereby removing one psychological symptom leads to another symptom appearing if the basic psychological cause has not been removed. It is controversial whether this happens.

substitution therapy treatment by providing a less harmful alternative to a drug or remedy that a patient has been receiving. It is used when the patient has become addicted to a drug or is placing too much reliance upon a particular remedy. The patient is weaned off the "hard" drug to which he or she has become addicted by the gradual substitution of a nonaddictive drug with a similar or a sedative effect.

substrate *n.* the specific substance or substances on which a given *enzyme acts. For example, starch is the substrate for salivary amylase; RNA is the substrate for ribonuclease.

subsultus *n.* abnormal twitching or tremor of muscles, such as may occur in feverish conditions.

subtertian fever a form of *malaria resulting from repeated infection by *Plasmodium falciparum* and characterized by continuous fever.

subthalamic nucleus a collection of gray matter, shaped like a biconvex lens, lying beneath the *thalamus and close to the *corpus striatum, to which it is connected by nerve tracts. It has connections with the cerebral cortex and several other nuclei nearby. Stimulation of this nucleus is now being used in the treatment of Parkinson's disease.

subzonal insemination a method of assisting conception in cases of infertility that is caused by the inability of the spermatozoa to penetrate the barriers surrounding the ovum. Using *in vitro fertilization techniques, a small number of spermatozoa (no more than six) are injected through the *zona pellucida into the perivitelline space (which surrounds the egg membrane). If fertilization subsequently occurs, the blastocyst is implanted in the mother's uterus.

succinylcholine *n.* a drug that relaxes voluntary muscle (*see* muscle relaxant). It is administered by intravenous injection and is used mainly to produce muscle relaxation during surgery or mechanical ventilation. Trade name: **Anectine**.

succus *n.* any juice or secretion of animal or plant origin.

succus entericus (intestinal juice) the clear alkaline fluid secreted by the glands of the small intestine. It contains mucus and digestive enzymes, including *enteropeptidase, *erepsin, *lactase, and *sucrase.

succussion *n.* a splashing noise heard when a patient who has a large quantity of fluid in a body cavity, such as the pleural cavity, moves suddenly or is deliberately shaken.

sucralfate *n.* a drug used for the treatment of duodenal ulcer in patients taking nonsteroidal anti-inflammatory drugs. It is only minimally absorbed in the stomach and it acts locally, not systemically, in the duodenum. It is administered by mouth; side effects include constipation, nausea, and skin rash. Trade name: **Carafate**.

sucrase *n.* an enzyme, secreted by glands in the small intestine, that catalyzes the hydrolysis of sucrose into its components (glucose and fructose).

sucrose *n.* a carbohydrate consisting of glucose and fructose. Sucrose is the principal constituent of cane sugar and sugar beet; it is the sweetest of the natural dietary carbohydrates. The increasing consumption of sucrose in the last 50 years has coincided with an increase in the incidence of dental caries, diabetes, coronary heart disease, and obesity.

suction *n.* the use of reduced pressure to remove unwanted fluids or other material through a tube for disposal. Suction is often used to clear secretions from the airways of newly born infants to aid breathing. During surgery, suction tubes are used to remove blood from the area of operation and to decompress the stomach (*nasogastric suction*) and the pleural space of air and blood (*chest suction*).

sudamen *n.* (*pl.* **sudamina**) a white blister caused by sweat collecting in the sweat ducts or in the layers of the skin.

Sudan stains a group of azo compounds used for staining fats. The group includes *Sudan I, Sudan II, Sudan III, Sudan IV,* and *Sudan black.*

sudden infant death syndrome (SIDS) *see* crib death.

Sudek's atrophy (reflex sympathetic dystrophy) pain, swelling, stiffness, and skin changes in a part of the body, most often the hand or foot, caused by overactivity of the sympathetic nervous system following trauma or surgery or occasionally arising spontaneously; a *Colles' fracture is frequently the precipitating cause. In more severe cases the condition progresses over a few months with increasing stiffness, cool shiny skin, and osteoporosis; severe pain may persist. X-rays show patchy rarefaction (thinning) of the bone. Treatment is physiotherapy and sympathetic nerve blocks, often using *guanethidine. The condition can last many months, and in the most severe cases the patient is left with a useless painful limb. [P. H. M. Sudek (1866–1938), German surgeon]

sudor *n.* sweat.

sudorific *n. see* diaphoretic.

suffocation *n.* cessation of breathing as a result of drowning, smothering, etc., leading to unconsciousness or death (*see* asphyxia).

suffusion *n.* the spreading of a flush across the skin surface, caused by changes in the local blood supply.

sugar any *carbohydrate that dissolves in water, is usually crystalline, and has a sweet taste. Sugars are classified chemically as *monosaccharides or *disaccharides. Table sugar is virtually 100% pure *sucrose and contains no other nutrient; brown sugar is less highly refined sucrose. Sugar is used as both a sweetening and preserving agent. *See also* fructose, glucose, lactose.

suggestion *n.* (in psychology) the process of changing people's beliefs, attitudes, or emotions by telling them that they will change. It is sometimes used as a synonym for *hypnosis. *See also* autosuggestion.

suicide *n.* self-destruction as a deliberate act. Distinction is usually made between *attempted suicide,* when death is averted although the person concerned intended to kill himself (or herself), and *parasuicide,* when the attempt is made for reasons other than actually killing oneself. It is estimated that some 85% of at-

tempted suicides are happy to have survived. In the US, deliberate drug overdosing is a common cause of admission to hospital medical wards. *Assisted suicide,* in which a physician aids a terminally ill patient commit suicide, is a recent ethical and controversial issue. In 1997 Oregon became the first state to legally permit physician-assisted suicide for terminally ill patients.

sulcus *n.* (*pl.* **sulci**) **1.** one of the many clefts or infoldings of the surface of the brain. The raised outfolding on each side of a sulcus is termed a *gyrus.* **2.** any of the infoldings of soft tissue in the mouth, for example between the cheek and the alveolus.

sulfacetamide *n.* a drug of the *sulfonamide group that is used in eye drops to treat such infections as conjunctivitis. Transient irritation may occur with higher doses. Trade names: **Bleph-10, Cetamide, Sulamyd, Sulf-10.**

sulfadiazine *n.* a drug of the *sulfonamide group that is used to prevent the recurrence of rheumatic fever and to treat a variety of infections, including toxoplasmosis. It is administered by mouth or injection.

sulfa drug *see* sulfonamide.

sulfamethizole *n. see* sulfonamide.

sulfamethoxazole *n.* a drug of the *sulfonamide group. It is taken by mouth and is effective in the treatment of infections of the respiratory tract (including bronchitis), the urinary and gastrointestinal tracts, and the skin. Sulfamethoxazole is mostly administered in a combined preparation with trimethoprim (*see* cotrimoxazole). Trade name: **Gantanol.**

sulfasalazine *n.* a drug of the *sulfonamide group, used in the treatment of ulcerative colitis and Crohn's disease and (for its anti-inflammatory action) rheumatoid arthritis. It is given by mouth or in the form of suppositories. The most common side effects are nausea, loss of appetite, and raised temperature. Trade name: **Azulfidine.**

sulfinpyrazone *n.* a *uricosuric drug given by mouth for the treatment of chronic gout. The main side effects are nausea and abdominal pain; the drug may also activate a latent duodenal ulcer and it should not be taken by patients with impaired kidney function. Trade name: **Anturane.**

sulfisoxazole n. see sulfonamide.

sulfobromophthalein n. a blue dye used in tests of liver function. A small quantity is injected into the bloodstream, and its concentration in the blood is measured after 5 and then 45 minutes. The presence of more than 10% of the dose in the circulation after 45 minutes indicates that the liver is not functioning normally. Trade name: **Bromsulphalein**.

sulfonamide (sulfa drug) n. one of a group of drugs, derived from sulfanilamide (a red dye), that prevent the growth of bacteria (i.e. they are bacteriostatic). Sulfonamides are usually given by mouth, are rapidly absorbed, and are effective against a variety of infections. Because many sulfonamides are rapidly excreted and very soluble in the urine, they are used to treat infections of the urinary tract.

A variety of side effects may occur with sulfonamide treatment, including nausea, vomiting, headache, and loss of appetite. More severe side effects include *cyanosis, blood disorders, skin rashes, photosensitivity, and fever. Sulfonamides should be avoided in jaundice and kidney disease and in patients allergic to these drugs. Because of increasing bacterial resistance to sulfonamides, and with the development of more effective less toxic antibiotics, the clinical use of these drugs has declined. Those still used include *sulfacetamide, *sulfadiazine, *sulfamethoxazole (combined with trimethoprim in *co-trimoxazole), and *sulfasalazine.

sulfone n. one of a group of drugs closely related to the *sulfonamides in structure and therapeutic actions. Sulfones possess powerful activity against the bacteria that cause leprosy and tuberculosis. The best known sulfone is *dapsone.

sulfonylurea n. one of a group of *oral hypoglycemic drugs, derived from a *sulfonamide, that reduce the level of glucose in the blood. These drugs are given by mouth and are used in the treatment of noninsulin-dependent diabetes mellitus. They include *chlorpropamide, *glipizide, *tolazamide, and *tolbutamide.

sulfur n. a nonmetallic element that is active against fungi and parasites. It is a constituent of ointments and other preparations used in the treatment of skin disorders (such as acne). Symbol: S.

sulfuric acid a powerful corrosive acid, H_2SO_4, widely used in industry. Swallowing the acid causes severe burning of the mouth and throat and difficulty in breathing, speaking, and swallowing. The patient should drink large quantities of milk or water or white of egg; gastric lavage should not be delayed. Skin or eye contact should be treated by flooding the area with water.

sulindac n. a nonsteroidal anti-inflammatory and antipyretic drug used in the treatment of osteoarthritis, rheumatoid arthritis, ankylosing spondylitis, gout, and nonrheumatic inflammatory conditions. It is given by mouth; side effects include skin rash, dizziness, nausea, and headache. Trade name: **Clinoril**.

sumatriptan n. a *$5HT_1$ agonist that is effective in the treatment of acute *migraine by selectively constricting blood vessels to the brain. It is administered by mouth, subcutaneous injection, or nasal spray. Possible side effects include dizziness, drowsiness, fatigue, chest pain, and a rise in blood pressure. Trade name: **Imitrex**.

sunburn n. damage to the skin by prolonged or unaccustomed exposure to the sun's rays, principally UVB (ultraviolet B). Sunburn may vary from reddening of the skin to the development of large painful fluid-filled blisters, which may cause shock if they cover a large area (see burn). Fair-skinned people are more susceptible to sunburn than others. Severe sunburn in childhood is a risk factor for the development of malignant *melanoma in later life.

sunstroke n. see heatstroke.

super- prefix denoting **1.** above; overlying. **2.** extreme or excessive.

superciliary adj. of or relating to the eyebrows (supercilia).

superego n. (in psychoanalysis) the part of the mind that functions as a moral conscience or judge. It is also responsible for the formation of ideals for the *ego. The superego is the result of the incorporation of parental injunctions into the child's mind.

superfecundation n. the fertilization of two or more ova of the same age by spermatozoa from different males. See superfetation.

superfetation *n.* the fertilization of a second ovum some time after the start of pregnancy, resulting in two fetuses of different maturity in the same uterus.

superficial *adj.* (in anatomy) situated at or close to a surface. Superficial blood vessels are those close to the surface of the skin.

superinfection *n.* an infection arising during the course of another infection and caused by a different microorganism, which is usually resistant to the drugs used to treat the primary infection. The infective agent may be a normally harmless inhabitant of the body that becomes pathogenic when other harmless types are removed by the drugs or it may be a resistant variety of the primary infective agent, such as *MRSA (*see also* methicillin).

superior *adj.* (in anatomy) situated uppermost in the body in relation to another structure or surface.

supernumerary *n.* (in dentistry) an additional tooth.

superovulation 1. controlled hyperstimulation of the ovary to produce more follicles with oocytes. Usually induced by *gonadotropin preparations, it is performed in *in vitro fertilization and other procedures of assisted conception in order to improve the pregnancy rates. 2. uncontrolled hyperstimulation of the ovary (*ovarian hyperstimulation syndrome*), an abnormal response of the ovaries leading to multiple follicle production. It may be associated with abdominal pain, ascites, oliguria, or even renal failure. Thromboembolism is the most dangerous complication.

supination *n.* 1. the act of turning the hand so that the palm is uppermost. 2. the act of turning the foot inward so that the medial margin is elevated. *Compare* pronation.

supinator *n.* a muscle of the forearm that extends from the elbow to the shaft of the radius. It supinates the forearm and hand.

supine *adj.* 1. lying on the back or with the face upward. 2. in the position in which the foot or the palm of the hand faces upward. *Compare* prone.

supportive *adj.* (of treatment) aimed at reinforcing the patient's own defense mechanisms in overcoming a disease or disorder.

suppository *n.* a medicinal preparation in solid form suitable for insertion into the rectum or vagina. *Rectal suppositories* may contain simple lubricants (e.g. glycerin); drugs that act locally in the rectum or anus (e.g. corticosteroids, local anesthetics); or drugs that are absorbed and act at other sites (e.g. *bronchodilators). *Vaginal suppositories* are used to treat some gynecological disorders (*see* pessary).

suppression *n.* 1. the cessation or complete inhibition of any physiological activity. 2. treatment that removes the outward signs of an illness or prevents its progress. 3. (in psychology) a *defense mechanism by which a person consciously and deliberately ignores an idea that is unpleasant to him.

suppressor gene a gene that prevents the expression of another (non-allelic) gene.

suppressor T cell a type of T *lymphocyte that prevents an immune response by B cells or other T cells to an antigen.

suppuration *n.* the formation of pus.

suppurative arthritis *see* septic arthritis.

supra- *prefix denoting* above; over. Examples: *supraclavicular* (above the clavicle); *suprahyoid* (above the hyoid bone); *suprarenal* (above the kidney).

supraglottis *n.* that part of the *larynx that lies above the vocal cords and includes the *epiglottis.

supraorbital *adj.* of or relating to the area above the eye orbit.

supraorbital reflex the closing of the eyelids when the supraorbital nerve is struck, due to contraction of the muscle surrounding the orbit (orbicularis oculi muscle).

suprapubic catheter a catheter passed through the abdominal wall above the pubis, usually into a very enlarged bladder with urinary retention. Usually, suprapubic *catheterization is performed only if it is not possible to perform urethral catheterization.

suprarenal glands *see* adrenal glands.

supraventricular tachycardia (SVT) a fast heart beat stemming from an abnormal area in the atria of the heart. It is often benign and relatively easily treated. However, it may be so fast that it reduces the pumping efficiency of the heart, causing a fall in blood pressure or heart failure. *See also* arrhythmia.

supravital staining the application of a

*stain to living tissue, particularly blood cells, removed from the body.

suramin *n.* a nonmetallic drug used in the treatment of *trypanosomiasis. It is usually given by slow intravenous injection. Side effects, which vary in intensity and frequency and are related to the nutritional state of the patient, include nausea, vomiting, shock, and loss of consciousness.

surfactant *n.* a wetting agent: a substance, such as a detergent, that reduces surface tension. A *pulmonary surfactant* is secreted by type II *pneumocytes lining the alveoli of the lungs to prevent the alveolar walls from sticking together. In its absence, as in the immature lungs of premature babies and in some diseases, the lungs tend to collapse. *See* atelectasis, respiratory distress syndrome.

surgeon *n.* a qualified medical practitioner who specializes in surgery.

surgery *n.* the branch of medicine that treats injuries, deformities, or disease by operation or manipulation. *See also* cryosurgery, microsurgery. —**surgical** *adj.*

surgical neck the constriction of the shaft of the *humerus, below the head. It is frequently the point at which fracture of the humerus occurs.

surrogate *n.* (in psychology) a person or object in someone's life that functions as a substitute for another person. In the treatment of sexual problems, when the patient does not have a partner to cooperate in treatment, a surrogate provided by the therapist acts as a sexual partner who gives service to the patient up to and including intercourse. According to psychoanalysts, people and objects in dreams can be surrogates for important individuals in a person's life.

surrogate mother a woman who becomes pregnant (usually by artificial insemination or embryo insertion) following an arrangement made with another party (usually a couple unable themselves to have children) in which she agrees to hand over the child she carries to that party when it is born.

susceptibility *n.* lack of resistance to disease. It is partly a reflection of general health but is also influenced by vaccination or other methods of increasing resistance to specific diseases.

suspensory bandage a bandage arranged to support a hanging part of the body. Examples include a sling used to hold an injured lower jaw in position and a bandage used to support the scrotum in various conditions of the male genital organs.

suspensory ligament a ligament that serves to support or suspend an organ in position. For example, the suspensory ligament of the lens is a fibrous structure attached to the ciliary processes (*see* ciliary body) by means of which the lens of the eye is held in position.

sustentaculum *n.* any anatomical structure that supports another structure. —**sustentacular** *adj.*

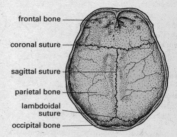

frontal bone

coronal suture

sagittal suture

parietal bone

lambdoidal suture

occipital bone

Sutures of the skull (internal surface of the vault)

suture 1. *n.* (in anatomy) a type of immovable joint, found particularly in the skull, characterized by a minimal amount of connective tissue between the two bones. The cranial sutures include the *coronal suture*, between the frontal and parietal bones; the *lambdoidal suture*, between the parietal and occipital bones; and the *sagittal suture*, between the two parietal bones (see illustration). **2.** *n.* (in surgery) the closure of a wound or incision with material such as silk or catgut, to facilitate the healing process. There is a wide variety of suturing techniques developed to meet the differing circumstances of injuries to and incisions in the body tissues (see illustration). **3.** *n.* the material, including silk, catgut, nylon, any of various polymers, or wire, used to sew up a wound. Some sutures are absorbable. **4.** *vb.* to close a wound by suture.

SVT *see* supraventricular tachycardia.

swab *n.* a pad of absorbent material (such

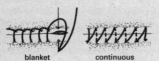

blanket continuous

(skin)

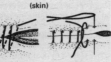

vertical mattress interrupted

purse string (intestine)

Types of surgical suture

as cotton), sometimes attached to a stick or wire, used for cleaning out or applying medication to wounds, operation sites, or body cavities. In operations, gauze swabs are used to clean blood from the site; such swabs are always carefully counted and contain a *radiopaque tag to facilitate identification should it by mischance remain in the body after operation.

swallowing (deglutition) *n.* the process by which food is transferred from the mouth to the esophagus (gullet). Voluntary raising of the tongue forces food backward toward the pharynx. This stimulates reflex actions in which the larynx is closed by the epiglottis and the nasal passages are closed by the soft palate, so that food does not enter the trachea (windpipe). Lastly, food moves down the esophagus by *peristalsis and gravity.

Swan-Ganz catheter a catheter with an inflatable balloon at its tip, which can be inserted into the pulmonary artery via the right chambers of the heart. Inflation of the balloon enables measurement of pressure in the left atrium and hence pul-

monary artery pressure. [H. J. C. Swan (1922–), US cardiologist; W. Ganz (20th century), US engineer]

sweat *n.* the watery fluid secreted by the *sweat glands. Its principal constituents in solution are sodium chloride and urea. The secretion of sweat is a means of excreting nitrogenous waste; at the same time, it has a role in controlling the temperature of the body – the evaporation of sweat from the surface of the skin has a cooling effect. Therefore an increase in body temperature causes an increase in sweating. Other factors that increase the secretion of sweat include pain, nausea, nervousness, and drugs (*diaphoretics). Sweating may be reduced by colds, diarrhea, and certain drugs. Anatomical name: **sudor**.

sweat gland a simple coiled tubular *exocrine gland that lies in the dermis of the *skin. A long duct carries its secretion (*sweat) to the surface of the skin. Sweat glands occur over most of the surface of the body; they are particularly abundant in the armpits, on the soles of the feet and palms of the hands, and on the forehead.

swelling *n.* an abnormal enlargment of a body part or organ that is not due to the proliferation of cells. *See* edema, inflammation.

sycosis *n.* inflammation of the hair follicles caused by bacterial infection. It commonly affects the beard area (*sycosis barbae*) and may cause intense itching. The infection usually spreads unless treated by allowing the beard to grow and applying antibiotic ointments.

Sydenham's chorea a form of *chorea that mainly affects children and adolescents, especially females. It can occur some months after an infection caused by β-hemolytic streptococci (such as rheumatic fever or scarlet fever), causing uncontrolled movements of the muscles of the shoulders, hips, and face (hence the archaic name, *St. Vitus' dance*). Formerly a frightening disease, it is now readily cured by antibiotics. [G. Sydenham (1624–89), English physician]

symbiosis *n.* an intimate and obligatory association between two different species of organism (*symbionts*) in which there is mutual aid and benefit. *Compare* commensal, mutualism, parasite.

symblepharon *n.* a condition in which the

eyelid adheres to the eyeball. It is usually the result of acid or alkali burns to the conjunctiva lining the eyelid and eyeball.

symbolism *n.* (in psychology) the process of representing an object or an idea by something else. Typically, an abstract idea is represented by a simpler and more tangible image. Psychoanalytic theorists hold that conscious ideas frequently act as symbols for unconscious thoughts and that this is particularly evident in dreaming, in *free association, and in the formation of psychological symptoms. According to this theory, a symptom (such as difficulty in swallowing) might be a symbolic representation of an unconscious idea (such as a fantasy of oral intercourse). —**symbolic** *adj.*

symmelia *n.* a developmental abnormality in which the legs appear to be fused.

symmetry *n.* (in anatomy) the state of opposite parts of an organ or parts at opposite sides of the body corresponding to each other.

sympathectomy *n.* the surgical *division of sympathetic nerve fibers. It is done to minimize the effects of normal or excessive sympathetic activity. Most often it is used to improve the circulation to part of the body; less commonly to inhibit excess sweating or to relieve the *photophobia induced by an abnormally dilated pupil of the eye.

sympathetic nervous system one of the two divisions of the *autonomic nervous system, having fibers that leave the central nervous system, via a chain of ganglia close to the spinal cord, in the thoracic and lumbar regions. Its nerves are distributed to the blood vessels, sweat glands, salivary glands, heart, lungs, intestines and other abdominal organs, and the genitals, whose functions it governs by reflex action, in balance with the *parasympathetic nervous system.

sympathin *n.* the name given by early physiologists to the substances released from sympathetic nerve endings, now known to be a mixture of *epinephrine and *norepinephrine.

sympathoblast *n.* a small cell formed in the early development of nerve tissue that eventually becomes a neuron of the sympathetic nervous system.

sympatholytic *adj.* opposing the effects of the sympathetic nervous system. Drugs

such as *guanethidine and *methyldopa block the transmission of impulses along adrenergic nerves; they are used to treat high blood pressure. *Alpha blockers and *beta blockers are other kinds of sympatholytic drugs.

sympathomimetic *adj.* having the effect of stimulating the *sympathetic nervous system. The actions of sympathomimetic drugs are *adrenergic* (resembling those of *norepinephrine). *Alpha-adrenergic stimulants (alpha agonists)* stimulate alpha receptors. They are *vasoconstrictors and include *ephedrine and *phenylephrine, which constrict blood vessels in the mucous membranes and are used in nasal decongestants; *metaraminol; and *apraclonidine and *brimonidine, which are used in the treatment of glaucoma. *Beta-adrenergic stimulants (beta agonists)* such as *albuterol and *terbutaline relax bronchial smooth muscle and are used as *bronchodilators. Some beta agonists (e.g. *dobutamine) stimulate beta receptors in the heart and are therefore used for their *inotropic effects. Others, including *ritodrine* (Yutopar), relax uterine muscle and are used in the treatment of premature labor.

sympathy *n.* (in physiology) a reciprocal influence exercised by different parts of the body on one another.

symphysiotomy *n.* incision into the bone at the front of the pelvis (pubic symphysis) in order to enlarge the diameter of the birth passage and aid delivery of a fetus whose head is too large to pass through the pelvic opening.

symphysis *n.* **1.** a joint in which the bones are separated by fibrocartilage, which

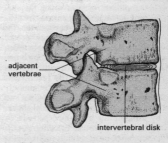

adjacent vertebrae

intervertebral disk

Symphysis between two vertebrae

minimizes movement and makes the bony structure rigid. Examples are the *pubic symphysis* (the joint between the pubic bones of the pelvis) and the joints of the backbone, which are separated by intervertebral disks (see illustration). **2.** the line that marks the fusion of two bones that were separate at an early stage of development, such as the symphysis of the *mandible.

sympodia (sirenomelia) *n.* a developmental abnormality in which there is fusion of the legs with absence of the feet.

symptom *n.* an indication of a disease or disorder noticed by the patient himself. A *presenting symptom* is one that leads a patient to consult a doctor. *Compare* sign.

symptomatology (semeiology) *n.* **1.** the branch of medicine concerned with the study of symptoms of disease. **2.** the symptoms of a disease, collectively.

syn- (sym-) *prefix denoting* union or fusion.

synalgia *n. see* referred pain.

synapse *n.* the minute gap across which *nerve impulses pass from one neuron to the next, at the end of a nerve fiber. Reaching a synapse, an impulse causes the release of a *neurotransmitter, which diffuses across the gap and triggers an electrical impulse in the next neuron. Some brain cells have more than 15,000 synapses. *See also* neuromuscular junction.

synarthrosis *n.* an immovable joint in which the bones are united by fibrous tissue. Examples are the cranial *sutures. *See also* gomphosis, schindylesis.

synchilia (syncheilia) *n.* congenital fusion of the lips.

synchondrosis *n.* a slightly movable joint (*see* amphiarthrosis) in which the surfaces of the bones are separated by hyaline cartilage, as occurs between the ribs and sternum. This cartilage may become ossified in later development, as between the *epiphyses and shaft of a long bone.

syncope (fainting) *n.* loss of consciousness induced by a temporarily insufficient flow of blood to the brain. It commonly occurs in otherwise healthy people and may be caused by an emotional shock, by standing for prolonged periods, or by injury and profuse bleeding. An attack comes on gradually, with lightheadedness, sweating, and blurred vision. Recovery is normally prompt and without any persisting ill effects.

syncytiotrophoblast (plasmoditrophoblast) *n.* that part of the *trophoblast that loses its cellular structure and becomes a *syncytium. This is the invasive part of the trophoblast, which erodes the maternal tissues and forms the villi of the placenta.

syncytium *n.* (*pl.* **syncytia**) a mass of *protoplasm containing several nuclei. Muscle fibers are syncytia. —**syncytial** *adj.*

syndactyly *n.* congenital fusion of the fingers or toes. It varies in severity from no more than marked webbing of two or more fingers to virtually complete union of all the digits. They may be attached along part or all of their length, involving the skin only or including the bone structure. Treatment is surgical separation, and skin grafts may be required.

syndesm- (syndesmo-) *prefix denoting* connective tissue, particularly ligaments.

syndesmology *n.* the branch of anatomy dealing with joints and their components.

syndesmophyte *n.* a vertical outgrowth of bone from a vertebra, seen in ankylosing *spondylitis, *Reiter's syndrome, and *psoriatic arthritis. Fusion of syndesmophytes across the joints between vertebrae contributes to rigidity of the spine, seen in advanced cases of these diseases.

syndesmosis *n.* an immovable joint in which the bones are separated by connective tissue. An example is the articulation between the bases of the tibia and fibula (see illustration).

syndrome *n.* a combination of signs and/or symptoms that forms a distinct clinical picture indicative of a particular disorder.

syndrome of inappropriate secretion of antidiuretic hormone (SIADH) a condition of inappropriately high plasma levels of ADH (*see* vasopressin) with associated water retention, dilutional *hyponatremia, and the production of highly concentrated urine. Renal, adrenal, thyroid, and hepatic function are normal, as is the volume of circulating blood (euvolemia). It is caused by a variety of pathological conditions, usually intrathoracic and intracerebral, and also by a number of drugs, including antidepressants, chemotherapy drugs, and some of the older antidiabetic agents. The treatment involves fluid restriction, treatment (or removal) of the underlying cause (or drug), and, in severe cases, administration of *demeclocycline to reduce the effects of ADH on the kidney. Very rarely, hypertonic saline is given.

syndrome X *see* metabolic syndrome.

synechia *n.* an adhesion between the iris and another part of the eye. An *anterior synechia* is between the iris and the endothelium of the cornea or the part of the sclera that normally hides the extreme outer edge of the iris from view. A *posterior synechia* is between the iris and the lens.

syneresis *n.* **1.** contraction of a blood clot. When first formed, a blood clot is a loose meshwork of fibers containing various blood cells. Over a period of time, this contracts, producing a firm mass that seals the damaged blood vessels. **2.** (in ophthalmology) degenerative shrinkage of the vitreous humor due to aging, usually resulting in *vitreous detachment.

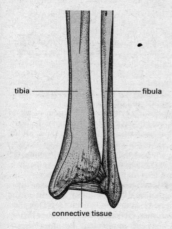

tibia — fibula

connective tissue

A syndesmosis

synergist *n.* **1.** a drug that interacts with another to produce increased activity, which is greater than the sum of the effects of the two drugs given separately. For example sodium aminosalicylate and streptomycin are used together to treat tuberculosis. Some synergists may

have dangerous effects, as when MAO inhibitors enhance the effects of antihistamines. **2.** a muscle that acts with an *agonist in making a particular movement. —**synergism** *n.*

synergistic gangrene gangrene of tissues produced by different bacteria acting together, usually a mixture of aerobic and anaerobic organisms. Particular forms are *Meleney's gangrene* (of the abdominal wall) and *Fournier's gangrene* (of the scrotal area). Synergistic gangrene has a pronounced tendency to spread along fascial planes, causing *necrotizing fasciitis.

synesthesia *n.* a condition in which a secondary subjective sensation (often color) is experienced at the same time as the sensory response normally evoked by the stimulus. For example, the sound of the word "cat" might evoke the color purple.

syngeneic *adj.* describing grafted tissue that is genetically identical to the recipient's tissue, as when the donor and recipient are identical twins.

synoptophore *n. see* amblyoscope.

synostosis *n.* the joining by ossification of two adjacent bones. It occurs, for example, at the *sutures between the bones of the skull.

synovectomy *n.* surgical removal of the synovium of a joint. This is performed in cases of chronic synovitis, such as rheumatoid arthritis, when other measures have been ineffective, in order to reduce pain in the joint and prevent further destruction.

synovia (synovial fluid) *n.* the thick colorless lubricating fluid that surrounds a joint or a bursa and fills a tendon sheath. It is secreted by the synovial membrane.

synovial joint *see* diarthrosis.

synovial membrane (synovium) the membrane, composed of mesothelium and connective tissue, that forms the sac enclosing a freely movable joint (*see* diarthrosis). It secretes the lubricating synovial fluid.

synovioma *n.* a benign or malignant tumor of the synovial membrane. Benign synoviomas occur on tendon sheaths; malignant synoviomas (*synovial sarcomas*) may occur where synovial tissue is not normally found, e.g. in the esophagus.

synovitis *n.* inflammation of the membrane (synovium) that lines a joint capsule, resulting in pain and swelling (arthritis). It is caused by injury, infection, or rheumatic disease. Treatment depends on the underlying cause; to determine this, samples of the synovial fluid or membrane are taken for examination.

synovium *n. see* synovial membrane.

syphilid (syphilide) *n.* the skin rash that appears in the second stage of *syphilis, usually two months to two years after primary infection. Syphilids occur in crops that may last from a few days to several months. They denote a highly infectious stage of the disease.

syphilis *n.* a chronic sexually transmitted disease caused by the bacterium *Treponema pallidum*, resulting in the formation of lesions throughout the body. Bacteria usually enter the body during sexual intercourse, through the mucous membranes of the vagina or urethra, but they may rarely be transmitted through skin wounds or scratches. Bacteria may also pass from an infected pregnant woman across the placenta to the developing fetus, resulting in the disease being present at birth (*congenital syphilis*). The primary symptom – a hard ulcer (*chancre) at the site of infection – forms 2–4 weeks after exposure. Neighboring lymph nodes enlarge about two weeks later. Secondary stage symptoms appear about two months after infection and include fever, malaise, general enlargement of lymph nodes, and a faint red rash on the chest that persists for 1–2 weeks. After months, or even years, the disease enters its tertiary stage with widespread formation of tumorlike masses (*gummas). Tertiary syphilis may cause serious damage to the heart and blood vessels (*cardiovascular syphilis*) or to the brain and spinal cord (*neurosyphilis*), resulting in *tabes dorsalis, blindness, and *general paralysis of the insane. Treatment is with doxycycline, tetracycline, or erythromycin. Syphilis can be diagnosed by several tests. *Compare* bejel. —**syphilitic** *adj.*

syring- (syringo-) *prefix denoting* a tube or long cavity, especially the central canal of the spinal cord.

syringe *n.* an instrument consisting of a piston in a tight-fitting tube that is attached to a hollow needle or thin tube. A syringe is used to give injections, remove material from a part of the body, or to wash out a cavity, such as the outer ear.

syringobulbia *n. see* syringomyelia.

syringocystadenoma *n.* a cystic benign tumor of the sweat glands.

syringoma *n.* multiple benign tumors of the sweat glands, which show as small hard swellings usually on the face, neck, or chest. They can be readily treated by *diathermy.

syringomyelia *n.* a disease of the spinal cord in which longitudinal cavities form within the cord in the cervical (neck) region. The centrally situated cavity (*syrinx*) is especially likely to damage the motor nerve cells and the nerve fibers that transmit the sensations of pain and temperature. Characteristically, there is weakness and wasting of the muscles in the hands with a loss of awareness of pain and temperature. An extension of the cavitation into the lower brainstem is called *syringobulbia*. Cerebellar *ataxia, a partial loss of pain sensation in the face, and weakness of the tongue and palate may occur. Syringomyelia is sometimes associated with an *Arnold-Chiari malformation.

system *n.* (in anatomy) a group of organs and tissues associated with a particular physiological function, such as the *nervous system or *respiratory system.

systemic *adj.* relating to or affecting the body as a whole, rather than individual parts and organs.

systemic circulation the system of blood vessels that supplies all parts of the body. It consists of the aorta and all its branches, carrying oxygenated blood to the tissues, and all the veins draining deoxygenated blood into the vena cava. *Compare* pulmonary circulation.

systemic sclerosis a rare connective-tissue disease affecting many systems in the body, mainly in women (3–6:1) in their forties. Genetic and autoimmune factors may be implicated. Besides *scleroderma, there may be involvement of the lungs, with pulmonary *fibrosis; renal failure and gastrointestinal and myocardial disease also occur. *See also* CREST syndrome.

systole *n.* the period of the cardiac cycle during which the heart contracts. The term usually refers to *ventricular systole*, which lasts about 0.3 seconds. *Atrial sys-*

tole lasts about 0.1 second. —**systolic** *adj.*

systolic pressure *see* blood pressure.

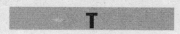

tabes dorsalis (locomotor ataxia) a form of neurosyphilis occurring 5–20 years after the original sexually transmitted infection. The infecting organisms progressively destroy the sensory nerves. Severe stabbing pains in the legs and trunk, an unsteady gait, and loss of bladder control are common. Some patients have blurred vision caused by damage to the optic nerves. Penicillin is used to arrest the progression of this illness. *See also* syphilis, general paralysis of the insane.

tablet *n.* (in pharmacy) a small disk containing one or more drugs, made by compressing a powdered form of the drug(s). It is usually taken by mouth but may be inserted into a body cavity (*see* suppository).

taboparesis *n.* a late effect of syphilitic infection of the nervous system in which the patient shows features of *tabes dorsalis and *general paralysis of the insane.

TAB vaccine a combined vaccine used to produce immunity against the diseases typhoid, paratyphoid A, and paratyphoid B.

tache *n.* a spot, mark, or blemish. An ulcerous blemish covered by a black crust (*tache noire*) is characteristic of the site of infection in certain rickettsial diseases, such as *scrub typhus and tick *typhus.

tachy- *prefix denoting* fast; rapid.

tachycardia *n.* an increase in the heart rate above normal. *Sinus tachycardia* may occur normally with exercise or excitement or it may be due to illness, such as fever. *Arrhythmias may also produce tachycardia (*ectopic tachycardia*). *See* ventricular tachycardia, supraventricular tachycardia.

tachyphylaxis *n.* a decrease in the effects produced by a drug during continuous use or constantly repeated administration, common in drugs that act on the nervous system.

tachypnea *n.* rapid breathing.

tacrine *n.* an acetylcholinesterase inhibitor used to treat mild to moderate Alzheimer's disease. It is administered by mouth; side effects include jaundice and liver function abnormalities. Trade name: **Cognex**.

tacrolimus (FK 506) *n.* a powerful *immunosuppressant drug administered orally or by intravenous infusion to prevent rejection of transplanted organs. It is now also, in the form of an ointment, the first effective noncorticosteroid treatment for atopic *eczema. Side effects include gastrointestinal disturbances, tremor, headache, and kidney impairment. Trade names: **Prograf, Protopic Ointment**.

tactile *adj.* relating to or affecting the sense of touch.

Taenia *n.* a genus of large tapeworms, some of which are parasites of the human intestine. The 4–10 m long beef tapeworm *T. saginata* is the most common tapeworm parasite of humans. Its larval stage (*see* cysticercus) develops within the muscles of cattle and other ruminants, and people become infected on eating raw or undercooked beef. *T. solium*, the pork tapeworm, is 2–7 m long. Its larval stage may develop not only in pigs but also in humans, in whom it may cause serious disease (*see* cysticercosis). *See also* taeniasis.

taeniacide (taenicide) *n.* an agent that kills tapeworms.

taeniafuge *n.* an agent, such as *niclosamide, that eliminates tapeworms from the body of their host.

taeniasis *n.* an infestation with tapeworms of the genus *Taenia*. Humans become infected with the adult worms following ingestion of raw or undercooked meat containing the larval stage of the parasite. The presence of a worm in the intestine may occasionally give rise to increased appetite, hunger pains, weakness, and weight loss. Worms are expelled from the intestine using various *anthelmintics, including niclosamide, dichlorophen, and quinacrine hydrochloride. *See also* cysticercosis.

Takayasu's disease (pulseless disease) progressive occlusion of the arteries arising from the arch of the aorta (including those to the arms and neck), resulting in the absence of pulses in the arms and neck. Symptoms include attacks of unconsciousness (syncope), paralysis of facial muscles, and transient blindness, due to an inadequate supply of blood to the head. [M. Takayasu (1860–1938), Japanese ophthalmologist]

tal- (talo-) *prefix denoting* the ankle bone (talus).

talc *n.* a soft white powder, consisting of magnesium silicate, used in dusting powders and skin applications. Talc used to dust surgical rubber gloves causes irritation of serous membranes, resulting in adhesions, if not washed off prior to an operation.

talipes *n. see* clubfoot.

talus (astragalus) *n.* the ankle bone. It forms part of the *tarsus, articulating with the tibia above, with the fibula to the lateral (outer) side, and with the calcaneus below.

tambour *n.* a recording drum consisting of an elastic membrane stretched over one end of a cylinder. It is used in various instruments for recording changes in air pressure.

tamoxifen *n.* a drug used in the treatment of advanced *breast cancer. It combines with hormone receptors in the tumor to inhibit the effect of estrogens. Side effects are uncommon but include nausea, vaginal bleeding, facial flushing, tumor pain, and hypercalcemia. Tamoxifen is being investigated for its effects in preventing breast cancer in those women considered to be at risk of developing the disease. Trade name: **Nolvadex**.

tampon *n.* a pack of gauze, cotton wool, or other absorbent material used to plug a cavity or canal in order to absorb blood or secretions. A vaginal tampon is commonly used by women to absorb the menstrual flow.

tamponade *n.* **1.** the insertion of a tampon. **2.** abnormal pressure on a part of the body; for example, as caused by the presence of excessive fluid between the pericardium (sac surrounding the heart) and the heart. *See* cardiac tamponade.

tamsulosin *n.* a highly selective *alpha blocker taken by mouth to treat *lower urinary tract symptoms thought to be due to *benign prostatic hyperplasia. Side effects include retrograde ejaculation that is reversible on stopping the drug. Trade name: **Flomax**.

tantalum *n.* a rare heavy metal used in surgery because it is easily molded and does not corrode. For example, tantalum sutures and plates are used for repair of defects in the bones of the skull. Symbol: Ta.

tapetum *n.* **1.** a layer of specialized reflecting cells in the *choroid behind the retina of the eye. **2.** a band of nerve fibers that forms the roof and wall of the lower posterior part of the *corpus callosum.

tapeworm (cestode) *n.* any of a group of flatworms that have a long thin ribbonlike body and live as parasites in the intestines of humans and other vertebrates. The body of a tapeworm consists of a head (*scolex*), a short neck, and a *strobila* made up of a chain of separate segments (*proglottides*). Mature proglottides, full of eggs, are released from the free end of the worm and pass out in the host's stools. Eggs are then ingested by an intermediate host, in whose tissues the larval stages develop (*see* plerocercoid, cysticercus, hydatid). Humans are the primary hosts for some tapeworms (*see* Taenia, Hymenolepis). However, other genera are also medically important (*see* Diphyllobothrium, Dipylidium, Echinococcus).

tapotement (percussion) *n.* a technique used in *massage in which a part of the body is struck rapidly and repeatedly with the hands. Tapotement of the chest wall in bronchitic patients often helps to loosen mucus within the air passages so that it can be coughed up.

tapping *n. see* paracentesis.

tardive dyskinesia a condition characterized by involuntary repetitive movements of the facial muscles and the tongue, usually resembling continued chewing motions, and the muscles of the limbs. It is associated with long-term medication with certain antipsychotic drugs, especially the *phenothiazines, and occurs predominantly in older patients, particularly women.

target cell 1. a cell that is the focus of attack by antibodies, cytotoxic T cells, or natural killer cells or is the object of the action of a specific hormone. **2.** (in hematology) an abnormal form of red blood cell (*erythrócyte) in which the cell assumes the ringed appearance of a "target" in stained blood films. Target cells are a feature of several types of anemia, including those due to iron deficiency, liver disease, and abnormalities in hemoglobin structure.

target organ the specific organ or tissue upon which a hormone, drug, or other substance acts.

tars- (tarso-) *prefix denoting* 1. the ankle; tarsal bones. 2. the edge of the eyelid.

tarsal 1. *adj.* relating to the bones of the ankle and foot (*tarsus). 2. *adj.* relating to the eyelid, especially to its supporting tissue (tarsus). 3. *n.* any of the bones forming the tarsus.

tarsalgia *n.* aching pain arising from the tarsus in the foot.

tarsal glands *see* meibomian glands.

tarsectomy *n.* 1. surgical excision of the tarsal bones of the foot. 2. surgical removal of a section of the tarsus of the eyelid.

tarsitis *n.* inflammation of the eyelid.

tarsoplasty *n. see* blepharoplasty.

tarsorrhaphy *n.* an operation in which the upper and lower eyelids are joined together, either completely or along part of their length. It is performed to protect the cornea or to allow a corneal injury to heal.

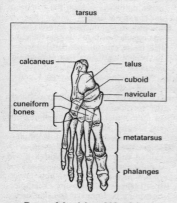

Bones of the right ankle and foot

tarsus *n.* (*pl.* **tarsi**) 1. the seven bones of the ankle and proximal part of the foot (see illustration). The tarsus articulates with the metatarsals distally and with the tibia and fibula proximally. 2. the firm fibrous connective tissue that forms the basis of each eyelid.

tartar *n.* a common term for *calculus, the hard deposit that forms on the teeth.

taste *n.* the sense for the appreciation of the flavor of substances in the mouth. The sense organs responsible are the *taste buds on the surface of the *tongue, which are stimulated when food dissolves in the saliva in the mouth. It is generally held that there are four basic taste sensations – sweet, bitter, sour, and salt – but two others – alkaline and metallic – are sometimes added to this list.

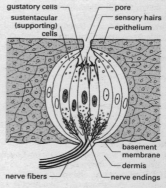

Structure of a taste bud

taste buds the sensory receptors concerned with the sense of taste (see illustration). They are located in the epithelium that covers the surface of the *tongue, lying in the grooves around the papillae, particularly the circumvallate papillae. Taste buds are also present in the soft palate, the epiglottis, and parts of the pharynx. When a taste cell is stimulated by the presence of a dissolved substance, impulses are sent via nerve fibers to the brain. From the anterior two-thirds of the tongue impulses pass via the facial nerve. The taste buds in the posterior third of the tongue send impulses via the glossopharyngeal nerve.

taurine *n.* an amino acid that is a constituent of the *bile salt taurocholate and also functions as a *neurotransmitter in the central nervous system.

taurocholic acid *see* bile acids.

taxane *n.* any of a group of *cytotoxic

drugs formerly extracted from a species of yew tree (*Taxus*) but now synthesized or produced by biotechnological methods. These drugs interact with tubulin, a protein involved in cell division, and have been found to exercise control on the growth of certain cancers. Taxanes include *docetaxel* (Taxotere), used for treating advanced breast cancer and non-small-cell lung cancer, and *paclitaxel*.

taxis *n.* (in surgery) the returning to a normal position of displaced bones, organs, or other parts by manipulation only, unaided by mechanical devices.

Taxol *n. see* paclitaxel.

Tay-Sachs disease (amaurotic familial idiocy) an inherited disorder of lipid metabolism (*see* lipidosis) in which abnormal accumulation of lipid in the brain leads to blindness, mental retardation, and death in infancy. The gene responsible for the disorder is *recessive, and the disease can now be largely prevented by genetic counseling in communities known to be affected. [W. Tay (1843–1927), British physician; B. Sachs (1858–1944), US neurologist]

TB *see* tuberculosis.

T cell *n. see* lymphocyte, cytotoxic T cell, helper T cell, suppressor T cell.

TCR T-cell receptor: an important component of the surface of T *lymphocytes, by which antigen is recognized.

tear gas any of the several kinds of gas used in warfare and by the police to produce temporary incapacitation. Most tear gases produce stinging pain in the eyes and streaming from the eyes and nose. *See also* CS gas.

tears *pl. n.* the fluid secreted by the lacrimal glands (*see* lacrimal apparatus) to keep the front of the eyeballs moist and clean. Tears contain *lysozyme, an enzyme that destroys bacteria. Irritation of the eye, and sometimes emotion, cause excessive production of tears. *See also* blinking.

technetium-99m *n.* an isotope of the artificial radioactive element technetium. It emits gamma radiation only, with no beta particles, at a convenient energy for detection by a *gamma camera and has a short half-life. For these reasons it is widely used in *nuclear medicine as a *tracer for the examination of many organs (*see* scintigram). Symbol: Tc-99m.

tectospinal tract a tract that conveys nerve impulses from the midbrain, across the midline as it descends, to the spinal cord in the cervical (neck) region. It contains important *motor neurons.

tectum *n.* the roof of the *midbrain, behind and above the *cerebral aqueduct. From the nerve tissue protrude two pairs of rounded swellings called the *superior* and *inferior colliculi*, which contain cells concerned with reflexes involving vision and hearing, respectively.

teeth *pl. n. see* tooth.

teething *n.* the entire physiological process involved in the eruption of the *deciduous teeth. It normally begins between the ages of six and eight months and takes about two years for the complete set of 20 teeth to appear.

tegmen *n.* (*pl.* **tegmina**) a structure that covers an organ or part of an organ. For example the *tegmen tympani* is the bony roof of the middle ear.

tegmentum *n.* the region of the *midbrain below and in front of the *cerebral aqueduct. It contains the nuclei of several cranial nerves, the *reticular formation, and other ascending and descending nerve pathways linking the forebrain and the spinal cord.

teichopsia *n.* shimmering colored lights, accompanied by blank spots in the visual field (*transient scotomata*), often seen at the beginning of an attack of migraine. *See* aura.

tel- (tele-, telo-) *prefix denoting* **1.** end or ending. **2.** distance.

tela *n.* any thin weblike tissue, particularly the *tela choroidea*, a folded double layer of *pia mater, containing numerous small blood vessels, that extends into several of the *ventricles of the brain.

telangiectasis *n.* (*pl.* **telangiectases**) a localized collection of distended blood capillary vessels. It is recognized as a red spot, sometimes spidery in appearance, that blanches on pressure. Telangiectases may be found in the skin or the lining of the mouth, gastrointestinal, respiratory, and urinary passages. The condition in which multiple telangiectases occur is termed *telangiectasia*. It may be seen as an inherited condition associated with a bleeding tendency (*hemorrhagic telangiectasia*). Accessible bleeding telangiectases (e.g. in the nose) may be obliterated by cauterization.

telangiitis *n.* inflammation of the smallest blood vessels (*see* angiitis).

teleceptor *n.* a sensory *receptor that is capable of responding to distant stimuli. An example is the eye, which is capable of detecting changes and happenings at a great distance.

telegony *n.* the unsubstantiated theory that mating with one male has an effect on the offspring of later matings with other males.

telemedicine *n.* the use of the telephone or the Internet in the diagnosis and treatment of patients by seeking advice, or a second opinion, from experts at a distant hospital. For example in *telepathology* digital pictures of microscope slides can be sent by the Internet to a pathologist in another laboratory. Using telemedicine, a paramedic can access a consultant in an emergency department for the appropriate treatment in difficult cases.

telencephalon *n. see* cerebrum.

teleradiology *n.* the process of transmitting and receiving medical images, to and from distant sites, via modem, cable, or satellite over telephone lines.

teletherapy *n.* a form of *radiotherapy in which penetrating radiation is directed at a patient from a distance. Originally radium was used as the radiation source; today artificial radioactive isotopes, such as cobalt-60, are used. *See* linear accelerator.

telmisartan *n. see* angiotensin II antagonist.

telocentric *n.* a chromosome in which the centromere is situated at either of its ends. —**telocentric** *adj.*

telodendron *n.* one of the branches into which the *axon of a neuron divides at its destination. Each telodendron finishes as a terminal *bouton*, which takes part in a *synapse or a *neuromuscular junction.

telogen *n. see* anagen.

telomere *n.* the end of a chromosome, which consists of repeated sequences of DNA that perform the function of ensuring that each cycle of DNA replication has been completed. Each time a cell divides some sequences of the telomere are lost; eventually (after 60–100 divisions in an average cell) the cell dies. Replication of telomeres is directed by *telomerase*, an enzyme consisting of RNA and protein that is inactive in nor-

mal cells. Its presence in tumors is linked to the uncontrolled multiplication of cancer cells.

telophase *n.* the final stage of *mitosis and of each of the divisions of *meiosis, in which the chromosomes at each end of the cell become long and thin and the nuclear membrane reforms around them. The cytoplasm begins to divide.

temazepam *n.* a *benzodiazepine used for the treatment of insomnia associated with difficulty falling asleep, frequent nocturnal awakenings, or early morning awakening. It is given by mouth; common side effects include drowsiness, dizziness, and loss of appetite. Trade name: **Restoril**.

temperature *n.* **1.** the degree of heat or cold as perceived by the body senses. **2.** *see* body temperature. **3.** *Informal.* a fever.

temple *n.* the region of the head in front of and above each ear.

temporal *adj.* of or relating to the temple.

temporal arteritis *see* arteritis.

temporal artery a branch of the external carotid artery that supplies blood mainly to the temple and scalp.

temporal bone either of a pair of bones of the cranium. The *squamous* portion forms part of the side of the cranium. The *petrous* part contributes to the base of the skull and contains the middle and inner ears. Below it are the *mastoid process, *styloid process, and zygomatic process (*see* zygomatic arch). *See also* skull.

temporalis *n.* a fan-shaped muscle situated at the side of the head, extending from the temporal fossa to the mandible. This muscle lifts the lower jaw, thus closing the mouth.

temporal lobe one of the main divisions of the *cerebral cortex in each hemisphere of the brain, lying at the side within the temple of the skull and separated from the frontal lobe by a cleft, the *lateral sulcus*. Areas of the cortex in this lobe are concerned with the appreciation of sound and spoken language.

temporal lobe epilepsy *see* epilepsy.

temporo- *prefix denoting* **1.** the temple. **2.** the temporal lobe of the brain.

temporomandibular joint the articulation between the *mandible and the *temporal bone: a hinge joint (*see* ginglymus).

temporomandibular joint syndrome a condition in which the patient has painful temporomandibular joints, tenderness in the muscles that move the jaw, clicking of the joints, and limitation of jaw movement. Stress, resulting in clenching the jaws and grinding the teeth, is thought to be a causal factor.

tenaculum *n.* **1.** a sharp wire hook with a handle. The instrument is used in surgical operations to pick up pieces of tissue or the cut end of an artery. **2.** a band of fibrous tissue that holds a part of the body in place.

tendinitis *n.* inflammation of a tendon. It occurs most commonly after excessive overuse but is sometimes due to bacterial infection (e.g. *gonorrhea) or associated with a generalized rheumatic disease (e.g. *rheumatoid arthritis, ankylosing spondylitis). Treatment is by rest, achieved sometimes by splinting the adjacent joint, and corticosteroid injection into the tender area around the tendon. Tendinitis at the insertion of the supraspinatus muscle is a frequent cause of pain and restricted movement in the shoulder. *See also* jumper's knee, tennis elbow. *Compare* tenosynovitis.

tendon *n.* a tough whitish cord, consisting of numerous parallel bundles of collagen fibers, that serves to attach a muscle to a bone. Tendons are inelastic but flexible; they assist in concentrating the pull of the muscle on a small area of bone. Some tendons are surrounded by *tendon sheaths* – tubular double-layered sacs lined with synovial membrane and containing synovial fluid. Tendon sheaths enclose the flexor tendons at the wrist and ankle, where they minimize friction and facilitate movement. *See also* aponeurosis. —**tendinous** *adj.*

tendon organ (Golgi tendon organ) a sensory *receptor found within a tendon that responds to the tension or stretching of the tendon and relays impulses to the central nervous system. Like stretch receptors in muscle, tendon organs are part of the *proprioceptor system.

tendonosis *n.* a degenerative condition of a tendon, most commonly the patellar tendon. Overuse is a causal factor.

tendon transfer plastic surgery in which the tendon from an unimportant muscle is used to replace the damaged tendon of an important muscle. A common tendon used is the palmaris longus tendon of the forearm.

tendovaginitis (tenovaginitis) *n.* inflammatory thickening of the fibrous sheath containing one or more tendons, usually caused by repeated minor injury. It usually occurs at the back of the thumb (*de Quervain's tendovaginitis*) and results in pain on using the wrists. Treatment is by rest, injection of cortisone into the tendon sheath, and, if these fail, surgical incision of the sheath.

tenesmus *n.* a sensation of the desire to defecate, which is continuous or recurs frequently, without the production of significant amounts of feces (often small amounts of mucus or blood alone are passed). This uncomfortable symptom may be due to *proctitis, prolapse of the rectum, rectal tumor, or *irritable bowel syndrome.

tenia *n.* (*pl.* **teniae**) a flat ribbonlike anatomical structure. The *teniae coli* are the longitudinal ribbonlike muscles of the colon.

teniposide (VM-26) *n.* an *antineoplastic drug used in the treatment of certain cancers, particularly in childhood, including acute lymphoblastic leukemia, non-Hodgkin's lymphoma, and neuroblastoma. It is similar to *etoposide. Trade name: **Vumon**.

tennis elbow a painful inflammation of the tendon at the lower end of the *humerus at the elbow joint, caused by overuse of the forearm muscles. Treatment is by rest, massage, and local corticosteroid injection. If symptoms do not subside, surgery may be required. *See also* tendinitis. *Compare* golfer's elbow.

teno- *prefix denoting* a tendon.

Tenon's capsule the fibrous tissue that lines the orbit and surrounds the eyeball. [J. R. Tenon (1724–1816), French surgeon]

tenoplasty *n.* surgical repair of a ruptured or severed tendon.

tenorrhaphy *n.* the surgical operation of uniting the ends of divided tendons by suture.

tenosynovitis (peritendinitis) *n.* inflammation of a tendon sheath, producing pain, swelling, and an audible creaking on movement. It may result from a bacterial infection or occur as part of a rheumatic disease causing *synovitis.

tenotomy *n.* surgical *division of a tendon. This may be necessary to correct a joint deformity caused by tendon shortening or to reduce the imbalance of forces caused by an overactive muscle in a spastic limb. *See also* scissor leg.

tenovaginitis *n. see* tendovaginitis.

TENS *see* transcutaneous electrical nerve stimulation.

tensor *n.* any muscle that causes stretching or tensing of a part of the body.

tent *n.* **1.** an enclosure of material (usually transparent plastic) around a patient in bed, into which a gas or vapor can be passed as part of treatment. An *oxygen tent* is relatively inefficient as a means of administering oxygen; a face mask or intranasal oxygen is used when possible. **2.** a piece of dried vegetable material, usually a seaweed stem, shaped to fit into an orifice, such as the cervical canal. As it absorbs moisture it expands, providing a slow but forceful means of dilating the orifice.

tented diaphragm the radiological sign of a raised diaphragm, which is indicative of *peritonitis.

tentorium *n.* a curved infolded sheet of *dura mater that dips inward from the skull and separates the cerebellum below from the occipital lobes of the cerebral hemispheres above.

terat- (terato-) *prefix denoting* a monster or congenital abnormality.

teratogen *n.* any substance, agent, or process that induces the formation of developmental abnormalities in a fetus. Known teratogens include such drugs as *thalidomide and alcohol, such infections as German measles and cytomegalovirus, and irradiation (e.g. with X-rays and other ionizing radiation). *Compare* mutagen. —**teratogenic** *adj.*

teratogenesis *n.* the process leading to developmental abnormalities in the fetus.

teratology *n.* the study of developmental abnormalities and their causes.

teratoma *n.* a tumor composed of a number of tissues not usually found at that site. Teratomas most frequently occur in the testis and ovary, possibly derived from remnants of embryological cells that have the ability to differentiate into many types of tissue. *Malignant teratoma of the testis* is found in young men: it is more common in patients with a history of undescended testis. Like *seminoma, it frequently occurs as a painless swelling of one testis (pain is not a good

indication that the swelling is benign). Treatment is by *orchiectomy avoiding an incision into the scrotum. The tumor can spread to lymph nodes, lungs, and bone, treatment of which may involve the use of chemotherapy drugs, such as vinblastine, bleomycin, cisplatin, and etoposide, with a high rate of cure even in metastatic disease. Teratomas often produce *alpha-fetoprotein, beta human chorionic gonadotropin, or both; the presence of these substances (*tumor markers) in the blood is a useful indication of the amount of tumor and the effect of treatment.

teratospermia *n. see* oligospermia.

terbinafine *n.* an antifungal drug used to treat severe ringworm and other fungal infections of the scalp, groin, feet, fingernails, and toenails. It is administered by mouth or topically; possible side effects of oral treatment include nausea, abdominal pain, and allergic skin rashes. Trade name: **Lamisil**.

terbutaline *n.* a *bronchodilator drug (*see* sympathomimetic) used in the treatment of asthma, bronchitis, and other respiratory disorders. It may be given by mouth, injection, or inhalation; common side effects include nervousness and dizziness. Trade names: **Brethaire**, **Brethine**, **Bricanyl**.

terconazole *n.* a synthetic antifungal drug used in the treatment of candidiasis. It is administered as a vaginal cream or as suppositories; side effects include headache, fever, and localized burning and itching. Trade name: **Terazol**.

teres *n.* either of two muscles of the shoulder, extending from the scapula to the humerus. The *teres major* draws the arm toward the body and rotates it inward; the *teres minor* rotates the arm outward.

terfenadine *n.* a nonsedating antihistamine formerly used for the treatment of the symptoms of hay fever, such as sneezing, itching, and tearing, and other allergic conditions. The drug was withdrawn from the US market in 1998 because of serious cardiac side effects.

terminal dribble a *lower urinary tract symptom in which the flow of urine does not end quickly, but dribbles slowly toward an end. This must be distinguished from *postmicturition dribble, which occurs after voiding has been completed.

terpene *n.* any of a group of unsaturated

hydrocarbons, many of which are found in plant oils and resins and are responsible for the scent of these plants (e.g. mint). Larger terpenes include vitamin A, squalene, and the carotenoids.

tertian fever *see* malaria.

tertiary care the specialized, highly technical level of health care provided usually by large, sophisticated research and teaching facilities where doctors and support staff are uniquely qualified to treat rare or unusual disorders that do not respond to therapy that is available at general hospitals or from *secondary care physicians.

tesla *n.* the *SI unit of magnetic flux density, equal to a density of 1 weber per square meter. Symbol: T.

testicle *n.* either of the pair of male sex organs within the scrotum. It consists of the *testis and its system of ducts (the vasa efferentia and epididymis).

testis *n.* (*pl.* **testes**) either of the pair of male sex organs that produce spermatozoa and secrete the male sex hormone *androgen under the control of *gonadotropins from the pituitary gland. The testes of the fetus form within the abdomen but descend into the *scrotum in order to maintain a lower temperature that favors the production and storage of spermatozoa. The bulk of the testis is made up of long convoluted *seminiferous tubules* (see illustration), in which the spermatozoa develop (*see* spermatogenesis). The tubules also contain *Sertoli cells, which may nourish developing sperm cells. Spermatozoa pass from the testis to the *epididymis to complete their development. The *interstitial* (*Leydig*) *cells*, between the tubules, are the major producers of androgen.

test meal a standard meal given to stimulate secretion of digestive juices, which can then be withdrawn by tube and measured as a test of digestive function. A *fractional test meal* was a gruel preparation to stimulate gastric secretion, whose acid content was measured. This has been replaced by tests using secretory stimulants. The *Lundh test meal* is a meal of oil and protein to stimulate pancreatic secretion, which is withdrawn from the duodenum and its trypsin content measured as a test of pancreatic function.

testosterone *n.* the principal male sex hormone (*see* androgen).

test-tube baby a baby born to a woman as a result of fertilization of one of her ova by sperm outside her body. *See* in vitro fertilization.

tetan- (tetano-) *prefix denoting* **1.** tetanus. **2.** tetany.

tetanolysin *n.* a toxin produced by tetanus bacilli in an infected wound, causing the local destruction of tissues.

tetanospasmin *n.* a toxin produced by tetanus bacilli in an infected wound. The toxin diffuses along nerves, causing paralysis, and may reach the spinal cord and brain, causing violent muscular spasms and the condition of lockjaw.

tetanus (lockjaw) *n.* an acute infectious disease, affecting the nervous system, caused by the bacterium *Clostridium tetani*. Infection occurs by contamination of wounds by bacterial spores. Bacteria multiply at the site of infection and produce a toxin that irritates nerves so that they cause spasmodic contraction of muscles. Symptoms appear 4–25 days after infection and consist of muscle stiffness, spasm, and subsequent rigidity, first in the jaw and neck, then in the back, chest, abdomen, and limbs; in severe cases the spasm may affect the whole body, which is arched backward (*see* opisthotonos). High fever, convulsions, and extreme pain are common. If respiratory muscles are affected, a *tra-

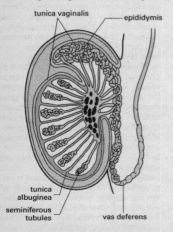

tunica vaginalis — epididymis

tunica albuginea

seminiferous tubules — vas deferens

Longitudinal section through a testis

cheostomy or intubation and ventilation are essential to avoid death from asphyxia. Mortality is high in untreated cases but prompt treatment is effective. An attack does not confer immunity. Immunization against tetanus is effective but temporary. —**tetanic** *adj.*

tetany *n.* spasm and twitching of the muscles, particularly those of the face, hands, and feet. Tetany is caused by a reduction in the blood calcium level, which may be due to underactive parathyroid glands, rickets, or *alkalosis.

tetra- *prefix denoting* four.

tetracycline *n.* **1.** one of a group of *antibiotic compounds that are derived from cultures of *Streptomyces* bacteria. These drugs, which include *chlortetracycline, *doxycycline, *oxytetracycline, and tetracycline, are effective against a wide range of bacterial infections. They are usually given by mouth to treat various conditions, including respiratory tract infections, syphilis, and acne. Side effects such as nausea, vomiting, and diarrhea are fairly common. In addition, suppression of normal intestinal bacteria may make the patient susceptible to infection with tetracycline-resistant organisms. Tetracyclines should not be administered after the fourth month of pregnancy and their use should be avoided in young children to prevent unsightly staining of the permanent teeth. **2.** a particular antibiotic of the tetracycline group. Trade names: **Achromycin, Robitet, Sumycin, Tetracap, Topicycline.**

tetrad *n.* (in genetics) **1.** the four cells resulting from meiosis after the second telophase. **2.** the four chromatids of a pair of homologous chromosomes (*see* bivalent) in the first stage of meiosis.

tetradactyly *n.* a congenital abnormality in which there are only four digits on a hand or foot.

tetrahydrocannabinol *n.* a derivative of marijuana that has antiemetic activity and also produces euphoria. These two properties are utilized in the prevention of chemotherapy-induced sickness.

tetrahydrozoline *n.* a drug that constricts blood vessels and is used to relieve minor eye irritation. *See* vasoconstrictor. Trade names: **Murine Plus, Tetrasine, Visine.**

tetralogy of Fallot a form of congenital heart disease in which there is *pulmonary stenosis, enlargement of the right ventricle, a ventricular *septal defect, and in which the origin of the aorta lies over the septal defect. The affected child is blue (cyanosed) and frequently squats. The defect is corrected surgically (*see* Blalock-Taussig operation). [E. L. A. Fallot (1850–1911), French physician]

tetraplegia *n. see* quadriplegia.

tetrodotoxin *n.* puffer-fish toxin, one of the most powerful known nerve toxins with a mortality of about 50%. There is no known antidote.

T-group *n.* a group of people who meet in order to increase their sensitivity and their skills in human relationships by discussing themselves and their relationships. Such groups are sometimes formed in the training of psychiatric staff (the "T" stands for training).

thalam- (thalamo-) *prefix denoting* the thalamus. Example: *thalamolenticular* (relating to the thalamus and lenticular nucleus of the brain).

thalamencephalon *n.* the structures, collectively, at the anterior end of the brainstem, comprising the *epithalamus, *thalamus, *hypothalamus, and subthalamus, all of which are concerned with the reception and processing of information entering from sensory nerve pathways.

thalamic syndrome a condition resulting from damage to the thalamus, often by a stroke, that is characterized by severe intractable pain and hypersensitivity in the area of the body served by the damaged brain region. It is extremely resistant to treatment.

thalamotomy *n.* an operation on the brain in which a lesion is made in a precise part of the *thalamus. It has been used to control psychiatric symptoms of severe anxiety and distress, in which cases the lesion is made in the dorsomedial nucleus of the thalamus, which connects with the frontal lobe. *See also* psychosurgery.

thalamus *n.* (*pl.* **thalami**) one of two egg-shaped masses of gray matter that lie deep in the cerebral hemispheres on each side of the forebrain. The thalami are relay stations for all the sensory messages that enter the brain, before they are transmitted to the cortex. All sensory pathways, except that for the sense of smell, are linked to nuclei within the thalamus, and it is here that the conscious awareness of messages as sensations – temperature, pain, touch, etc. – probably begins.

thalassemia (Cooley's anemia) *n.* an hereditary blood disease, widespread in the Mediterranean countries, Asia, and Africa, in which there is an abnormality in the protein part of the *hemoglobin molecule. The affected red cells cannot function normally, leading to anemia. Other symptoms include enlargement of the spleen and abnormalities of the bone marrow. Individuals inheriting the disease from both parents are severely affected (*thalassemia major*), but those inheriting it from only one parent are usually symptom-free. Patients with the major disease are treated with repeated blood transfusions or bone marrow transplantation. The disease can be detected by prenatal diagnosis.

thalassotherapy *n.* treatment by remedial bathing in seawater.

thalidomide *n.* a drug that was formerly widely used as a sedative. If taken during the first three months of pregnancy, it was found to cause fetal abnormalities involving limb malformation and was withdrawn as a sedative in 1962. Recently, however, thalidomide has been found to be effective in treating certain cancers and other disorders (including *Behçet's syndrome).

thallium *n.* a leadlike element that has several dangerously poisonous compounds. The poison is cumulative and causes liver and nerve damage and bone destruction. The person's hair is likely to fall out and does not grow again. Treatment is by administration of *chelating agents. Symbol: Tl.

thallium scan a method of studying blood flow through the heart muscle (myocardium) and diagnosing myocardial *ischemia using an injection of the radioisotope thallium-201. Defects of perfusion, such as a recent infarct, emit little or no radioactivity and are seen as "cold spots" when an image is formed using a gamma camera and computer. Exercise may be used to provoke "cold spots" in patients for the diagnosis of ischemic heart disease.

thallium-technetium isotope subtraction imaging a technique used to image the *parathyroid glands. Technetium is taken up only by the thyroid gland, but thallium is taken up by both the thyroid and parathyroid glands. *Digital subtraction of the two isotopes leaves an image of the parathyroid glands alone. It is an accurate technique (90%) for the identification of *adenomas of the parathyroid glands secreting excess hormone.

theca *n.* a sheathlike surrounding tissue. For example, the *theca folliculi* is the outer wall of a *graafian follicle.

theine *n.* the active volatile principle found in tea (*see* caffeine).

thelarche *n.* the process of breast development, which occurs as a normal part of *puberty. Isolated premature breast development in girls is not uncommon and is almost always benign.

thenar *n.* **1.** the palm of the hand. **2.** the fleshy prominent part of the hand at the base of the thumb. *Compare* hypothenar. —**thenar** *adj.*

theobromine *n.* an alkaloid, occurring in cocoa, coffee, and tea, that has a weak diuretic action and dilates coronary and other arteries. It was formerly used to treat angina.

theophylline *n.* an alkaloid, occurring in the leaves of the tea plant, that has a diuretic effect and relaxes smooth muscles, especially that of the bronchi. Theophylline preparations, particularly *aminophylline, are used mainly to control bronchial asthma. Trade names: **Slo-bid, Slo-Phyllin, Theo-24, Theo-Dur, Theolair, Uniphyl.**

therapeutic index the ratio of a dose of a therapeutic agent that produces damage to normal cells to the dose necessary to have a defined level of anticancer activity. It indicates the relative efficacy of a treatment against tumors.

therapeutics *n.* the branch of medicine that deals with different methods of treatment and healing (*therapy*), particularly the use of drugs in the cure of disease.

therm *n.* a unit of heat equal to 100,000 British thermal units. 1 therm = 1.055×10^8 joules.

therm- (thermo-) *prefix denoting* **1.** heat. **2.** temperature.

thermalgesia (thermoalgesia) *n.* an abnormal sense of pain that is felt when part of the body is warmed. It is a type of *dysesthesia and is a symptom of partial damage to a peripheral nerve or to the fiber tracts conducting temperature sensation to the brain.

thermoanesthesia n. absence of the ability to recognize the sensations of heat and coldness. When occurring as an isolated sensory symptom it indicates damage to the spinothalamic tract in the spinal cord, which conveys the impulses of temperature to the thalamus.

thermocautery n. the destruction of unwanted tissues by heat (see cauterize).

thermocoagulation n. the coagulation and destruction of tissues by cautery.

thermography n. a technique for measuring and recording the heat produced by different parts of the body using photographic film sensitive to infrared radiation. The picture produced is called a *thermogram*. The heat radiated from the body varies in different parts according to the flow of blood through the vessels; thus areas of poor circulation produce less heat. On the other hand a tumor with an abnormally increased blood supply may be revealed on the thermogram as a "hot spot." The technique was formerly used in the diagnosis of tumors of the breast (*mammothermography*) before the development of more sensitive techniques (see mammography).

thermokeratoplasty n. the application of heat to the periphery of the cornea in order to shrink the cornea and thus change its refractive power. This refractive procedure is used to correct farsightedness (hyperopia) and presbyopia.

thermoluminescent dosimeter (TLD) a radiation *dosimeter that utilizes the ability of activated sodium fluoride to luminesce in proportion to the radiation dose to which it is exposed when it is heated. It is now a common form of radiation dosimeter for personnel monitoring.

thermolysis n. (in physiology) the dissipation of body heat by such processes as the evaporation of sweat from the skin surface.

thermometer n. a device for registering temperature. A *clinical thermometer* consists of a sealed narrow-bore glass tube with a bulb at one end. It contains mercury, which expands when heated and rises up the tube. The tube is calibrated in degrees, and is designed to register temperatures between 35°C (95°F) and 43.5°C (110°F). An *oral thermometer* is

placed in the mouth; a *rectal thermometer* is inserted into the rectum.

thermophilic adj. describing organisms, especially bacteria, that grow best at temperatures of 48–85°C. Compare mesophilic, psychrophilic.

thermophore n. any substance that retains heat for a long time, such as kaolin, which is often used in hot poultices.

thermoreceptor n. a sensory nerve ending that responds to heat or to cold. Such *receptors are scattered widely in the skin and in the mucous membrane of the mouth and throat.

thermotaxis n. the physiological process of regulating or adjusting body temperature.

thermotherapy n. the use of heat to alleviate pain and stiffness in joints and muscles and to promote an increase in circulation. *Diathermy provides a means of generating heat within the tissues themselves.

thiabendazole n. an *anthelmintic used to treat infestations of pinworms and other intestinal worms. It is administered orally and may cause vomiting, vertigo, and gastric discomfort. Trade name: **Mintezol.**

thiamine n. see vitamin B_1.

thiazide diuretic see diuretic.

thiazolidinediones pl. n. a group of *oral hypoglycemic drugs, including *pioglitazone* (Actos) and *rosiglitazone* (Avandia), used in the treatment of type 2 *diabetes mellitus. These drugs act by reducing resistance of the body to its own insulin and should be taken in combination with *metformin.

Thiersch's graft see split-skin graft. [K. Thiersch (1822–95), German surgeon]

thigh n. the part of the lower limb situated between the hip and the knee.

thioguanine n. a drug that prevents the growth of cancer cells and is used in the treatment of leukemia. It is given by mouth and commonly reduces the numbers of white blood cells and platelets. Other side effects include nausea, vomiting, loss of appetite, and jaundice. Trade name: **Tabloid.**

thiopental n. a short-acting *barbiturate. It is given by intravenous injection to produce general *anesthesia or as a premedication prior to surgery. Possible complications of thiopental anesthesia include respiratory depression, laryngeal spasm, and thrombophlebitis. The drug is not used when respiratory obstruction is present. Trade name: **Pentothal**.

thiophilic *adj.* growing best in the presence of sulfur or sulfur compounds. The term is usually applied to bacteria.

thioridazine *n.* a phenothiazine *antipsychotic used in the treatment of a wide range of mental, behavioral, and emotional disturbances, including schizophrenia. The drug is given by mouth; side effects include faintness, dizziness, dry mouth, and impairment of sexual function. Trade name: **Mellaril**.

thiotepa *n.* a *cytotoxic drug. It is given by injection to treat cancer of the breast, ovary, or bladder, lymphoma, and sarcoma. The most serious side effects are on the blood-forming tissues, resulting in a reduction in white blood cells and platelets. Headache, nausea, and vomiting may also occur. Trade name: **Thioplex**.

thioxanthene *n.* see antipsychotic.

thiothixene *n.* an *antipsychotic drug used in the treatment of manifestations of psychotic disorders. It is administered by mouth and intramuscularly; side effects include drowsiness, hypotension, and skin rash. Trade name: **Navane**.

third-party payer the source of payment (or reimbursement for payment) of charges for hospital or medical services when the patient does not make direct payment. A third-party payer may be an insurance company, a government agency, an employer, or a philanthropic organization. Most major medical care costs in the US are paid by third parties; minor expenses, such as prescription drug costs, usually are covered by direct payment as out-of-pocket expenditures by the patient, although many third parties are now paying a part or all of these expenses as well. The patient and the doctor, or other provider of health care, represent the other two parties in third-party payment arrangements.

thirst *n.* a sensation associated with the body's need for water. The sensory nerve endings for thirst are located in the *pharynx.

thorac- (thoraco-) *prefix denoting* the thorax or chest.

thoracectomy *n.* an operation in which the chest cavity is opened (thoracotomy) and a rib or part of a rib is removed.

thoracentesis *n.* see pleurocentesis.

thoracic cavity the chest cavity. *See* thorax.

thoracic duct one of the two main trunks of the *lymphatic system. It receives lymph from both legs, the lower abdomen, left thorax, left side of the head, and left arm and drains into the left brachiocephalic vein.

thoracic vertebrae the 12 bones of the *backbone to which the ribs are attached. They lie between the cervical (neck) and lumbar (lower back) vertebrae and are characterized by the presence of facets for articulation with the ribs. *See also* vertebra.

thoracocentesis *n.* see pleurocentesis.

thoracoplasty *n.* a former treatment for pulmonary tuberculosis involving surgical removal of parts of the ribs, thus allowing the chest wall to fall in and collapse the affected lung.

thoracoscope *n.* an instrument used to inspect the *pleural cavity. —**thoracoscopy** *n.*

thoracotomy *n.* surgical opening of the chest cavity to inspect or operate on the heart, lungs, or other structures within.

thorax *n.* the chest: the part of the body cavity between the neck and the diaphragm. The skeleton of the thorax is formed by the sternum, costal cartilages, ribs, and thoracic vertebrae. It encloses the lungs, heart, esophagus, and associated structures. *Compare* abdomen. —**thoracic** *adj.*

thought-stopping *n.* a technique of *behavior therapy used in the treatment of obsessional thoughts. Attention is voluntarily withdrawn from these thoughts and focused on some other vivid image or engrossing activity.

threadworm *n.* see pinworm.

threonine *n.* an *essential amino acid. *See also* amino acid.

threshold *n.* (in neurology) the point at which a stimulus begins to evoke a response, and therefore a measure of the sensitivity of a system under particular conditions. A *thermoreceptor that responds to an increase in temperature of only two degrees is said to have a much lower threshold than one that will only respond to a change in temperature of ten degrees or more. In this example the threshold can be measured directly in terms of degrees.

thrill n. a vibration felt on placing the hand on the body. A heart murmur that is felt by placing the hand on the chest wall is said to be accompanied by a thrill.

-thrix suffix denoting a hair or hairlike structure.

throat n. the front part of the neck; the *pharynx.

thromb- (thrombo-) prefix denoting 1. a blood clot (thrombus). 2. thrombosis. 3. blood platelets.

thrombasthenia n. a hereditary blood disease in which the function of the *platelets is defective although they are present in normal numbers. The manifestations are identical to those of thrombocytopenic *purpura.

thrombectomy n. a surgical procedure in which a blood clot (thrombus) is removed from an artery or vein (see endarterectomy, phlebothrombosis).

thrombin n. a substance (*coagulation factor) that acts as an enzyme, converting the soluble protein fibrinogen to the insoluble protein fibrin in the final stage of *blood coagulation. Thrombin is not normally present in blood plasma, being derived from an inactive precursor, *prothrombin*. Trade name: **Thrombostat**.

thromboangiitis obliterans see Buerger's disease.

thrombocyte n. see platelet.

thrombocythemia n. a disease in which there is an abnormal proliferation of the cells that produce blood *platelets (*megakaryocytes), leading to an increased number of platelets in the blood. This may result in an increased tendency to form clots within blood vessels (thrombosis); alternatively the function of the platelets may be abnormal, leading to an increased tendency to bleed. Treatment is by radiotherapy, *cytotoxic drugs, *interferon, or drugs that inhibit *megakaryocyte maturation.

thrombocytopenia n. a reduction in the number of *platelets in the blood. This results in bleeding into the skin (thrombocytopenic *purpura), spontaneous bruising, and prolonged bleeding after injury. Thrombocytopenia may result from failure of platelet production or excessive destruction of platelets. —**thrombocytopenic** adj.

thrombocytosis n. an increase in the number of *platelets in the blood. It may occur in a variety of diseases, including chronic infections, cancers, and certain blood diseases and is likely to cause an increased tendency to form blood clots within vessels (thrombosis).

thromboembolism n. the condition in which a blood clot (thrombus), formed at one point in the circulation, becomes detached and lodges at another point. It is most commonly applied to the association of phlebothrombosis and *pulmonary embolism (*pulmonary thromboembolic disease*).

thromboendarterectomy n. see endarterectomy.

thromboendarteritis n. thrombosis complicating *endarteritis, seen in temporal *arteritis, *polyarteritis nodosa, and syphilis. It may cause death of part of the organ supplied by the affected artery.

thrombokinase n. see thromboplastin.

thrombolysis n. the dissolution of a blood clot (thrombus) by the infusion of a *fibrinolytic agent into the blood. It may be used in the treatment of *phlebothrombosis, *pulmonary embolism, and *coronary thrombosis. See also tissue-type plasminogen activator.

thrombolytic adj. describing an agent that breaks up blood clots (thrombi). See fibrinolytic, tissue-type plasminogen activator.

thrombophilia n. an inherited or acquired condition that predisposes individuals to *thrombosis.

thrombophlebitis n. inflammation of the wall of a vein (see phlebitis) with secondary *thrombosis occurring within the affected segment of vein. Pregnant women are more prone to thrombophlebitis because of physiological changes in the blood and the effects of pressure within the abdomen. It may involve superficial or deep veins of the legs (the latter being less common in pregnancy than the former). Thrombophlebitis of the femoral vein may produce *phlegmasia alba dolens* (painful white leg), which was a common accompaniment to puerperal fever (now fortunately rare). Deep vein thrombosis (see phlebothrombosis) may precede *pulmonary embolism.

thromboplastin (thrombokinase) n. a substance formed during the earlier stages of *blood coagulation. It acts as an enzyme, converting the inactive substance prothrombin to the enzyme *thrombin.

thrombopoiesis *n.* the process of blood *platelet production. Platelets are formed as fragments of cytoplasm that are shed from giant cells (*megakaryocytes) in the bone marrow by a budding process.

thrombosis *n.* a condition in which the blood changes from a liquid to a solid state and produces a blood clot (*thrombus*). Thrombosis may occur within a blood vessel in diseased states. Thrombosis in an artery obstructs the blood flow to the tissue it supplies: obstruction of an artery to the brain is one of the causes of a *stroke and thrombosis in an artery supplying the heart – a *coronary thrombosis – will result in a heart attack (*see* myocardial infarction). Thrombosis can also occur in a vein (*deep vein thrombosis*; *see* phlebothrombosis), and it may be associated with inflammation (*see* thrombophlebitis). The thrombus may become detached from its site of formation and carried in the blood to lodge in another part (*see* embolism).

thromboxane *n.* any of a group of compounds that are synthesized by platelets and are extremely potent vasoconstrictors.

thrombus *n.* a blood clot (*see* thrombosis).

thrush *n. see* candidiasis.

thumb *n.* the first digit on the radial side of the hand. It can oppose the other four fingers of the hand.

thym- (thymo-) *prefix denoting* the thymus.

thymectomy *n.* surgical removal of the thymus.

-thymia *suffix denoting* a condition of the mind. Example: *cyclothymia* (marked alternation of mood).

thymic aplasia failure of development of the *thymus. This was formerly thought to predispose to hypersensitivity reactions (*see* hypersensitive) and to infection and so to death in childhood (*see* status lymphaticus), a concept no longer held.

thymidine *n.* a compound containing thymine and the sugar ribose. *See also* nucleoside.

thymine *n.* one of the nitrogen-containing bases (*see* pyrimidine) occurring in the nucleic acids DNA and RNA.

thymitis *n.* inflammation of the thymus

(the mass of lymphatic tissue behind the breastbone).

thymocyte *n.* a lymphocyte within the *thymus.

thymoma *n.* a benign or malignant tumor of the *thymus. It is sometimes associated with *myasthenia gravis, a chronic disease in which muscles tire easily. Surgical removal of the tumor may result in improvement of the muscle condition, but the response is often slow.

thymus *n.* a bilobed organ in the root of the neck, above and in front of the heart. The thymus is enclosed in a capsule and divided internally by cross walls into many lobules, each full of T lymphocytes (white blood cells associated with antibody production). In relation to body size the thymus is largest at birth. It doubles in size by puberty, after which it gradually shrinks, its functional tissue being replaced by fatty tissue. In infancy the thymus controls the development of *lymphoid tissue and immune response to microbes and foreign proteins (accounting for allergic response, autoimmunity, and rejection of organ transplants). T lymphocytes migrate from the bone marrow to the thymus, where they mature and differentiate until activated by antigen. —**thymic** *adj.*

thyro- *prefix denoting* the thyroid gland. Example: *thyroglossal* (relating to the thyroid gland and tongue).

thyrocalcitonin *n. see* calcitonin.

thyrocele *n.* a swelling of the thyroid gland. *See* goiter.

thyroglobulin *n.* a protein in the thyroid gland from which the *thyroid hormones (thyroxine and triiodotyrosine) are synthesized.

thyrohyoid *adj.* relating to the thyroid cartilage and hyoid bone. The *thyrohyoid ligaments* form part of the *larynx; contraction of the *thyrohyoid muscle* raises the larynx.

thyroid acropachy a rarely seen but well-documented alteration in the shape of the nails resembling *clubbing but unique to Graves' disease (*see* thyrotoxicosis). It is often associated with formation of new bone seen on X-rays of the hands and wrists, which is said to resemble bubbles along the surface of the bones.

thyroid antibodies autoantibodies against the thyroid gland, which cause *Hashimoto's disease. They are of two types: *microsomal*, against thyroid cytoplasm; and *anti-thyroglobulin*, against thyroid colloid (*see* thyroid gland).

thyroid cartilage the main cartilage of the *larynx, consisting of two broad plates that join at the front to form a V-shaped structure. The thyroid cartilage forms the *Adam's apple* in front of the larynx.

thyroidectomy *n.* surgical removal of the thyroid gland. In *partial thyroidectomy*, only the diseased part of the gland is removed; in *subtotal thyroidectomy*, a method of treating *thyrotoxicosis, the surgeon removes 90% of the gland.

thyroid gland a large *endocrine gland situated in the base of the neck (see illustration). It consists of two lobes, one on either side of the trachea, that are joined by an *isthmus* (sometimes a third lobe extends upward from the isthmus). The thyroid gland consists of a large number of closed follicles inside which is a jelly-like colloid, which contains the principal active substances that are secreted by the gland. The thyroid gland is concerned with regulation of the metabolic rate by the secretion of *thyroid hormone, which is stimulated by *thyroid-stimulating hormone from the pituitary gland and requires trace amounts of iodine. The *C cells of the thyroid gland secrete *calcitonin.

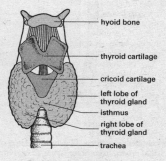

hyoid bone

thyroid cartilage

cricoid cartilage

left lobe of thyroid gland

isthmus

right lobe of thyroid gland

trachea

Position of the thyroid gland

thyroid hormone an iodine-containing substance, synthesized and secreted by the thyroid gland, that is essential for normal metabolic processes and mental and physical development. There are two thyroid hormones, *triiodothyro-

nine and *thyroxine, which are formed from *thyroglobulin. Lack of these hormones gives rise to *cretinism in infants and *myxedema in adults. Excessive production of thyroid hormones gives rise to *thyrotoxicosis.

thyroiditis *n.* inflammation of the thyroid gland. *Acute thyroiditis* is due to bacterial infection; *chronic thyroiditis* is commonly caused by an abnormal immune response (*see* autoimmunity) in which lymphocytes invade the tissues of the gland. *See* Hashimoto's disease.

thyroid-stimulating hormone (TSH, thyrotropin) a hormone, synthesized and secreted by the anterior pituitary gland under the control of *thyrotropin-releasing hormone, that stimulates activity of the thyroid gland. Defects in TSH production lead to over- or undersecretion of *thyroid hormones.

thyroid storm a life-threatening condition due to a severe worsening of previously undiagnosed or inadequately treated *thyrotoxicosis. It often follows infections, childbirth, nonthyroid surgery, or trauma but can occur without an obvious cause. The presenting features are fever, severe agitation, nausea and vomiting, diarrhea, and abdominal pains. An accelerated heart rate and irregularity of the heart rhythm can cause heart failure, and psychotic episodes or coma can result. Blood tests will reveal hyperthyroidism and may also show altered liver function, high blood sugar, high calcium levels, a high white blood cell count, and often anemia. Treatment is with intravenous fluids, oxygen, antithyroid drugs (such as *carbimazole or *propylthiouracil), high-dose iodide solution (*see* Lugol's iodine), high-dose steroids, and beta blockers. The patient must be cooled and given antipyretics, such as aspirin or acetaminophen. Any underlying cause must also be treated.

thyroplasty *n.* a surgical procedure performed on the thyroid cartilage of the larynx to alter the characteristics of the voice.

thyrotomy *n.* surgical incision of either the thyroid cartilage in the neck or of the thyroid gland itself.

thyrotoxicosis *n.* the syndrome due to excessive amounts of thyroid hormones in the bloodstream, causing a rapid heartbeat, sweating, tremor, anxiety, increased appetite, loss of weight, and intolerance of heat. Causes include simple overactivity of the gland, a hormone-secreting benign tumor or carcinoma of the thyroid, and *Graves' disease* (*exophthalmic goiter*), in which there are additional symptoms, including swelling of the neck (*goiter*) due to enlargement of the gland and protrusion of the eyes (*exophthalmos*). Treatment may be by surgical removal of the thyroid gland, *radioactive iodine therapy to destroy part of the gland, or by the use of drugs (e.g. *carbimazole or *propylthiouracil) that interfere with the production of thyroid hormones. —**thyrotoxic** *adj.*

thyrotoxic periodic paralysis a condition in which attacks of sudden weakness and flaccidity occur in patients with *thyrotoxicosis, seen most often in Asian males. The attacks last from hours to days; they can be prevented by potassium supplements and subsequent treatment of the thyrotoxicosis.

thyrotropin *n. see* thyroid-stimulating hormone.

thyrotropin-releasing hormone (TRH) a hormone from the hypothalamus (in the brain) that acts on the anterior pituitary gland to stimulate the release of *thyroid-stimulating hormone. TRH may be given by intravenous injection to test thyroid gland function and to estimate reserves of thyroid-stimulating hormone in the pituitary.

thyroxine *n.* one of the hormones synthesized and secreted by the thyroid gland (*see* thyroid hormone). A preparation of thyroxine (levothyroxine) can be administered by mouth to treat underactivity of the thyroid gland (*see* cretinism, myxedema).

TIA *see* transient ischemic attack.

tibia *n.* the shin bone: the inner and larger bone of the lower leg (see illustration). It articulates with the *femur above, with the *talus below, and with the *fibula to the side (at both ends); at the lower end is a projection, the medial *malleolus, forming part of the articulation with the talus.

tibialis *n.* either of two muscles in the leg, extending from the tibia to the metatarsal bones of the foot. The *tibialis anterior* turns the foot inward and flexes the toes backward. Situated be-

hind it, the *tibialis posterior* extends the toes and inverts the foot.

tibial torsion a normal variation in posture in which there is an in-toe gait due to mild internal rotation of the tibia. The condition is often apparent in infancy when the child starts walking and resolves spontaneously with time. Usually symmetrical, it is associated with normal mobility and is pain-free.

tibia vara *see* Blount disease.

tibio- *prefix denoting* the tibia. Example: *tibiofibular* (relating to the tibia and fibula).

tic *n.* a repeated and largely involuntary movement varying in complexity from the twitch of a muscle to elaborate well-coordinated actions. Simple tics occur in about a quarter of all children and usually disappear within a year. Tics most often become prominent when the individual is exposed to emotional stress. *See also* Gilles de la Tourette syndrome.

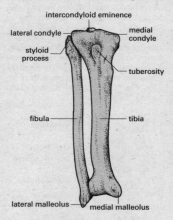

Right tibia and fibula

ticarcillin *n.* a *penicillin-type antibiotic that is used in combination with *clavulanate potassium against the bacteria *Pseudomonas aeruginosa*, *Proteus* species, and *Escherichia coli* in the treatment of severe systemic infections, septicemia, and infections of the genitourinary tract and respiratory tract. The drug is administered intravenously or intramuscularly and side effects are similar to those of other broad-spectrum antibiotics. Trade name: **Timentin**.

tic douloureux *see* neuralgia.

tick *n.* a bloodsucking parasite belonging to the order of arthropods (Acarina) that also includes the *mites. Tick bites can cause serious skin lesions and occasionally paralysis (*see* Ixodes, Amblyomma), and certain tick species transmit *typhus, *Lyme disease, and *relapsing fever. Dimethyl phthalate is used as a tick repellent. There are two families: Argasidae (soft ticks), including *Ornithodoros*, with mouthparts invisible from above and no hard shield (*scutum*) on the dorsal surface; and Ixodidae (hard ticks), including *Dermacentor*, *Haemaphysalis*, and *Rhipicephalus*, with clearly visible mouthparts and a definite scutum.

tick fever any infectious disease transmitted by ticks, especially *Rocky Mountain spotted fever.

Tietze's syndrome (costochondritis) a painful swelling of a rib in the region of the chest, over the junction of bone and cartilage. The cause is unknown and the condition usually resolves without treatment, but in some cases local injections of corticosteroids are needed. [A. Tietze (1864–1927), German surgeon]

time sampling (in psychology) a way of recording behavior in which the presence or absence of particular kinds of behavior is noted during each of several fixed prearranged periods of time. *See also* event sampling.

timolol *n.* a *beta blocker used in the treatment of high blood pressure (hypertension), long-term prophylaxis after an acute myocardial infarction, and *glaucoma. It is administered by mouth or in solution as eye drops; side effects include decreased heart rate, hypotension, and dizziness. Trade names: **Betimol, Blocadren, Timolide, Timoptic**.

tincture *n.* an alcoholic extract of a drug derived from a plant.

tinea *n. see* ringworm.

Tinel's sign a method for checking the regeneration of a nerve: usually used in patients with *carpal tunnel syndrome. Direct tapping over the sheath of the nerve elicits a distal tingling sensation (*see* paresthesia), which indicates the beginning of regeneration. [J. Tinel (1879–1952), French neurosurgeon]

tinnitus *n.* the sensation of sounds (buzzing, ringing, roaring, etc.) in the ears or head in the absence of an external sound source. It can occur with any form of hearing loss or with normal hearing. It is thought to be due to a misinterpretation of signals in the central auditory pathways of the brain. The signals that are misinterpreted can arise in any part of the auditory system and may result from ordinary age-related hair cell loss in the *cochlea; wax (*cerumen) blocking the ear canal; damage to the eardrum; diseases of the inner ear, such as *Ménière's disease; drugs, such as aspirin and quinine; and abnormalities of the auditory nerve and its connections within the brain. Treatment includes the correction of any underlying condition, counseling, *cognitive therapy, relaxation techniques, sound therapy (*see* white noise instrument), and use of *hearing aids. A unified method of treatment that makes use of all of these components is referred to as *tinnitus retraining therapy*.

tinnitus masker the former name for a *white noise instrument.

tintometer *n.* an instrument for measuring the depth of color in a liquid. The color can then be compared with those on standard charts so that the concentration of a particular compound in solution can be estimated.

tissue *n.* a collection of cells specialized to perform a particular function. The cells may be of the same type (e.g. in nervous tissue) or of different types (e.g. in connective tissue). Aggregations of tissues constitute organs.

tissue culture the culture of living tissues, removed from the body, in a suitable medium supplied with nutrients and oxygen. *Tissue engineering*, in which skin, cartilage, and other connective-tissue cells are cultured on a *fibronectin "mat" to create new tissues, is being explored for use in tissue grafting for patients with burns, sports injuries, etc.

tissue-type plasminogen activator (t-PA, TPA) a natural protein found in the body, now manufactured by genetic engineering (*see* alteplase). It is used to break up a thrombus (*see* thrombolysis). t-PA requires the presence of *fibrin as a cofactor and is able to activate *plasminogen on the fibrin surface, which distinguishes it from the other plasminogen activators *streptokinase and *urokinase. It is used in the treatment of deep vein thrombosis, pulmonary embolism, acute myocardial infarction, and other thrombotic conditions.

tissue typing determination of the HLA profiles of tissues (see HLA system) to assess their compatibility. It is the most important predictor of success or failure of a transplant operation.

titer n. (in immunology) the extent to which a sample of blood serum containing antibody can be diluted before losing its ability to cause agglutination of the relevant antigen. It is used as a measure of the amount of antibody in the serum.

titubation n. a rhythmical nodding movement of the head, sometimes involving the trunk. Occasionally, the use of this term is extended to include a stumbling gait.

TLD see thermoluminescent dosimeter.

T lymphocyte n. see lymphocyte.

TNF see tumor necrosis factor.

TNM classification a classification formulated by the American Joint Committee on Cancer in collaboration with the *UICC for the extent of spread of a cancer. T refers to the size of the tumor, N the presence and extent of lymph node involvement, and M the presence of distant spread (metastasis).

tobacco n. the dried leaves of the plant *Nicotiana tabacum* or related species, used in smoking and as snuff. Tobacco contains the stimulant but poisonous alkaloid *nicotine, which enters the bloodstream during smoking. The volatile tarry material also released during smoking contains chemicals known to produce cancer in animals (see carcinogen).

tobramycin n. an antibiotic used to treat septicemia, external eye infections, and lower respiratory, urinary, skin, abdominal, and central nervous system infections. Tobramycin is administered by intravenous or intramuscular injections or by inhalation, or is applied by ointment or solution to the eye. Kidney damage or hearing impairment may occur with high doses or prolonged use. Trade names: **TOBI**, **Tobrex**.

tocainide n. an *antiarrhythmic drug used to treat life-threatening cardiac arrest due to ventricular *fibrillation. It is ad-

ministered by mouth. Possible side effects include nausea, vomiting, dizziness, tremor, and reduced white blood cell production. Trade name: **Tonocard**.

toco- *prefix denoting* childbirth or labor.

tocolytic agent a drug used to delay preterm labor, such as *magnesium sulfate, *progesterone, or ritodrine (see sympathomimetic).

tocopherol n. see vitamin E.

tocophobia n. a profound fear of childbirth. There are two types: *primary tocophobia*, which develops in adolescence and causes many women to avoid childbirth altogether; and *secondary tocophobia*, which occurs after a traumatic delivery and can stop a woman having another child. Women are more at risk from tocophobia if they have had any of the following: a history of rape or sexual abuse; harrowing memories of educational videos during adolescence; a history of depression; or experience of panic attacks.

Todd's paralysis (Todd's palsy) transient paralysis of a part of the body that has previously been involved in a focal epileptic seizure (see epilepsy). [R. B. Todd (1809–60), British physician]

tolazamide n. a drug administered by mouth in the treatment of noninsulin-dependent diabetes. Side effects include nausea, loss of appetite, diarrhea, weakness, and lethargy. Trade name: **Tolinase**.

tolbutamide n. a drug given by mouth in the treatment of noninsulin-dependent diabetes mellitus. It acts directly on the pancreas to stimulate insulin production and is particularly effective in elderly patients with mild diabetes. Side effects are similar to those of the *sulfonamides and include skin reactions and transient jaundice. Trade name: **Orinase**.

tolerance n. the reduction or loss of the normal response to a drug or other substance that usually provokes a reaction in the body. *Drug tolerance* may develop after taking a particular drug over a long period of time. In such cases increased doses are necessary to produce the desired effect. Some drugs that cause tolerance also cause *dependence. See also glucose tolerance test, immunological tolerance, tachyphylaxis.

tolnaftate n. an antifungal drug applied topically as a cream, powder, or solution in the treatment of various fungal infections of the skin, including ringworm. It is not effective in candidiasis. Trade names: **Aftate, Desenex, Tinactin**.

tolterodine *n.* an anticholinergic drug used to treat *detrusor overactivity giving rise to the *lower urinary tract symptoms of frequency, urgency, or urge incontinence. Trade name: **Detrol**.

toluidine blue a dye used in microscopy for staining *basophilic substances in tissue specimens.

-tome *suffix denoting* a cutting instrument. Example: *microtome* (instrument for cutting microscopical sections).

tomo- *prefix denoting* **1.** section or sections. **2.** surgical operation.

tomography *n.* the technique of rotating a radiation detector around the patient so that the image obtained gives additional three-dimensional information. In plain film tomography the source of X-rays and the photographic film move around the patient to produce an image of structures at a particular depth within the body, bringing them into sharp focus, while deliberately blurring structures above and below them. In *computed tomography (CT) this technique produces an image of a slice through the body at a particular level. The visual record of this technique is called a *tomogram. See also* pantomography, positron emission tomography, SPECT scanning.

-tomy (-otomy) *suffix denoting* a surgical incision into an organ or part. Example: *gastrotomy* (into the stomach).

tone *n. see* tonus.

tongue *n.* a muscular organ attached to the floor of the mouth. It consists of a *body* and a *root*, which is attached by muscles to the hyoid bone below, the styloid process behind, and the palate above. It is covered by mucous membrane, which is continuous with that of the mouth and pharynx. On the undersurface of the tongue a fold of mucous membrane, the *frenulum linguae*, connects the midline of the tongue to the floor of the mouth. The surface of the tongue is covered with minute projections (*papillae*), which give it a furred appearance (see illustration). *Taste buds are arranged in grooves around the papillae, particularly the fungiform and circumvallate papillae. The tongue has

three main functions. It helps in manipulating food during mastication and swallowing; it is the main organ of taste; and it plays an important role in the production of articulate speech. Anatomical name: **glossa**.

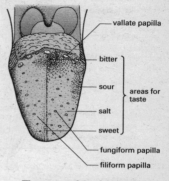

The upper surface of the tongue

tongue-tie *n.* a disorder of young children in which the tongue is anchored in the floor of the mouth more firmly than usual. No treatment is required unless the condition is extreme and associated with forking of the tongue, in which case surgery may be necessary.

tonic 1. *adj.* **a.** relating to normal muscle tone. **b.** marked by continuous tension (contraction), as in a tonic muscle *spasm. **2.** *n.* a medicinal substance taken to increase vigor and liveliness and produce a feeling of well-being. Beneficial effects of tonics are probably due to their placebo action.

tonicity *n.* **1.** the normal state of slight contraction, or readiness to contract, of healthy muscle fibers. **2.** the effective osmotic pressure of a solution. *See* hypertonic, hypotonic, osmosis.

tonic neck reflex (asymmetric tonic neck reflex) a normal reflex that is present from birth but should disappear by six months of age. If the infant is lying on its back and the head is turned to one side, the arm and leg on the side to which the head is turned should straighten, and the arm and leg on the opposite side should flex. The position prevents the infant from rolling over until adequate motor

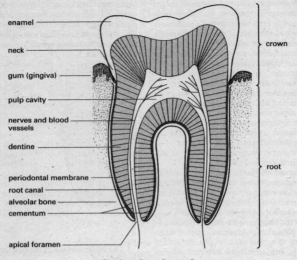

enamel

neck

gum (gingiva)

pulp cavity

nerves and blood
vessels

dentine

periodontal membrane

root canal

alveolar bone

cementum

apical foramen

crown

root

Section of a molar tooth

and neurologic development occurs. Persistence of the reflex beyond six months is suggestive of *cerebral palsy.

tonic pupil (Adie's pupil) a pupil that is dilated as a result of damage to the nerves supplying the ciliary muscle and iris. It reacts poorly to light but contracts normally for near vision, with slow redilation of the pupil on refixation at a distance. The most common characteristic of the tonic pupil is its extreme sensitivity to dilute 0.1% pilocarpine drops, which cause marked constriction of a tonic pupil but have little effect on a normal pupil. *See also* Adie's syndrome.

tono- *prefix denoting* **1.** tone or tension. **2.** pressure.

tonofibril *n.* a tiny fiber occurring in bundles in the cytoplasm of cells that lie in contact, as in epithelial tissue. Tonofibrils are concerned with maintaining contact between adjacent cells. *See* desmosome.

tonography *n.* measurement of the pressure within the eyeball in such a way as to allow a record to be made on a chart of variations in pressure occurring over a period of several minutes.

tonometer *n.* an instrument for measuring

pressure or tension, especially intraocular pressure (an *ophthalmotonometer*). There are several types. The *applanation tonometer* measures the pressure required to flatten a known area of the cornea. A high pressure is required when the pressure inside the eye is increased, and vice versa. The *Goldmann applanation tonometer* flattens a corneal area of 3 mm^2. *See also* glaucoma.

tonsil *n.* a mass of *lymphoid tissue on either side of the back of the mouth. It is concerned with protection against infection. The term usually refers to either of the *palatine tonsils*, but below the tongue is another pair, the *lingual tonsils*. *See also* adenoids (pharyngeal tonsils).

tonsillectomy *n.* surgical removal of the tonsils.

tonsillitis *n.* inflammation of the tonsils due to bacterial or viral infection, causing a sore throat, fever, and difficulty in swallowing. If tonsillitis due to streptococcal infection is not treated (by antibiotics) it may lead to *rheumatic fever or *nephritis.

tonsillotomy *n.* surgical incision of a tonsil or removal of part of a tonsil.

tonus (tone) *n.* the normal state of partial

contraction of a resting muscle, maintained by reflex activity.

tooth n. (pl. **teeth**) one of the hard structures in the mouth used for cutting and chewing food. Each tooth is embedded in a socket in part of the jawbone (mandible or maxilla) known as the *alveolar bone* (or *alveolus*), to which it is attached by the *periodontal membrane. The exposed part of the tooth (*crown*) is covered with *enamel and the part within the bone (*root*) is coated with *cementum; the bulk of the tooth consists of *dentine enclosing the *pulp (see illustration). The group of embryological cells that gives rise to a tooth is known as the *tooth germ*.

There are four different types of tooth (*see* canine, incisor, premolar, molar). *See also* dentition.

tooth extraction *see* extraction.

toothpaste n. a paste used for cleaning the teeth. It contains a fine abrasive and a suitable flavoring to promote use. Most toothpastes contain *fluoride salts, which help to prevent *dental caries. Some contain antimicrobials to counteract dental *plaque.

topagnosis n. inability to identify a part of the body that has been touched. It is a symptom of disease in the parietal lobes of the brain. The normal ability to localize touch is called *topognosis*.

tophus n. (pl. **tophi**) a hard deposit of crystalline uric acid and its salts in the skin, cartilage (especially of the ears), or joints; a feature of *gout.

topical adj. local: used for the route of administration of a drug that is applied directly to the part being treated (e.g. to the skin or eye).

topo- *prefix denoting* place; position; location.

topography n. the study of the different regions of the body, including the description of its parts in relation to the surrounding structures. —**topographical** *adj.*

topoisomerase inhibitor any one of a class of *cytotoxic drugs that work by blocking the action of topoisomerase I, an enzyme that promotes the uncoiling of the DNA double helix, which is a necessary preliminary to replication. These drugs include *irinotecan* (Camptosar), used for treating advanced colorectal cancer; and *topotecan* (Hycamtin), for treating ad-

vanced ovarian cancer. They are administered by intravenous infusion; side effects include delayed but severe diarrhea and reduction in blood-cell production by the bone marrow.

topotecan n. *see* topoisomerase inhibitor.

TORCH syndrome *t*oxoplasmosis, *o*ther agents, *r*ubella, *c*ytomegalovirus, *h*erpes simplex: a group of infections that may be seen in newborns due to the causative agent having crossed the placental barrier during pregnancy.

Torkildsen shunt an operation in which a *shunt is created between the lateral *ventricle of the brain and the *cisterna magna to bypass a block of the cerebral *aqueduct and thus relieve *hydrocephalus. Originally this was achieved by means of an external indwelling catheter, but later techniques use an internal catheter, which reduces the risk of septic complications. [A. Torkildsen (20th century), Norwegian neurosurgeon]

tormina n. *see* colic.

torpor n. a state of sluggishness and diminished responsiveness: a characteristic of certain mental disorders and a symptom of certain forms of poisoning or metabolic disorder.

torsion n. twisting. Abnormal twisting of a testis within the scrotum or of a loop of bowel in the abdomen may impair blood and nerve supplies to these parts and cause severe damage.

torticollis (**wryneck**) n. an irresistible turning movement of the head that becomes more persistent, so that eventually the head is held continually to one side. This is a form of *dystonia. The spasm of the muscles is often painful and the patient is sensitive about his appearance. It may be caused by a birth injury to the sternomastoid muscle (*see* sternomastoid tumor). Relief may be obtained by cutting the motor nerve roots of the spinal nerves in the neck region or by injection of the affected muscles with *botulinum toxin.

toruloma n. a tumorlike lesion in the lungs resulting from *cryptococcosis.

torulosis n. *see* cryptococcosis.

Tourette's syndrome (TS) *see* Gilles de la Tourette syndrome.

tourniquet n. a device to press on an artery and prevent flow of blood through it, usually a cord, rubber tube, or tight bandage bound around a limb. Tourniquets are no longer recommended as a first-aid measure to stop bleeding from a wound because of the danger of reducing the supply of oxygen to other tissues (direct pressure on the wound itself is considered less harmful). However, a temporary tourniquet to increase the distension of veins when a sample of blood is being taken does no harm.

tow *n.* the teased-out short fibers of flax, hemp, or jute, used in swabs for cleaning, in *packs or *stupes for the application of poultices, and for a variety of other purposes.

Towne's projection a *posteroanterior X-ray film to show the entire skull and mandible. [E. B. Towne (1883–1957), US otolaryngologist]

tox- (toxi-, toxo-, toxic(o)-) *prefix denoting* **1.** poisonous; toxic. **2.** toxins or poisoning.

toxemia *n.* blood poisoning that is caused by toxins formed by bacteria growing in a local site of infection. It produces generalized symptoms, including fever, diarrhea, and vomiting. *Compare* pyemia, sapremia, septicemia.

toxic *adj.* having a poisonous effect; potentially lethal.

toxicity *n.* the degree to which a substance is poisonous. *See also* LD_{50}.

toxicology *n.* the study of poisonous materials and their effects on living organisms. —**toxicologist** *n.*

toxicosis *n.* the deleterious effects of a toxin; poisoning: includes any disease caused by the toxic effects of any substances.

toxic shock syndrome a condition characterized by sudden onset, high fever, vomiting, diarrhea, skin rash, and ultimately by acute *shock and hypotension due to *septicemia. It is caused by toxin from strains of staphylococci usually combined with the presence of a retained foreign body (such as a tampon or IUD). More than two organ systems are always involved. Treatment is with supportive care, such as fluid and electrolyte replacement, and antibiotics, such as penicillin or a cephalosporin. The condition can be life-threatening if not treated aggressively. *See also* streptococcal toxic shock syndrome.

toxin *n.* a poison produced by a living organism, especially by a bacterium (*see* endotoxin, exotoxin). In the body toxins act as *antigens, and special *antibodies (*antitoxins*) are formed to neutralize their effects.

Toxocara *n.* a genus of large nematode worms that are intestinal parasites of vertebrates. *T. canis* and *T. cati*, the common roundworms of dogs and cats, respectively, have life cycles similar to that of the human roundworm, *Ascaris lumbricoides*. *See* toxocariasis.

toxocariasis (visceral larva migrans) *n.* an infestation with the larvae of the dog and cat roundworms, *Toxocara canis* and *T. cati*. Humans, who are not the normal hosts, become infected on swallowing eggs of *Toxocara* present on hands or in food and drink contaminated with the feces of infected domestic pets. The larvae, which migrate around the body, cause destruction of various tissues; the liver becomes enlarged and the lungs inflamed (*see* pneumonitis). Symptoms may include fever, joint and muscle pains, vomiting, an irritating rash, and convulsions. Larvae can also lodge in the retina of the eye where they cause inflammation and *granuloma. The disease, widely distributed throughout the world, primarily affects children. Severe cases are treated with thiabendazole.

toxoid *n.* a preparation of the poisonous material (toxin) that is produced by dangerous infective organisms, such as those of tetanus and diphtheria, and has been rendered harmless by chemical treatment while retaining its antigenic activity. Toxoids are used in *vaccines.

Toxoplasma *n.* a genus of crescent-shaped sporozoans that live as parasites within the cells of various tissues and organs of vertebrate animals, especially birds and mammals, and complete their life cycle in a single host, the cat. *T. gondii* infects sheep, cattle, dogs, and humans, sometimes provoking acute illness (*see* toxoplasmosis).

toxoplasmosis *n.* a disease of mammals and birds caused by *Toxoplasma gondii*, which is transmitted to humans via undercooked meat, contaminated soil, or by direct contact (especially in food or drink contaminated with the feces of infected cats). Generally, symptoms are mild (swollen lymph nodes and an influenza-like illness), but severe infection can occur in patients whose immune systems are compromised. *Congenital toxoplasmosis* occurs when a woman infected during pregnancy transmits the organism to her fetus. Although most babies are unaffected or have very mild disease, some can have severe malformations of the skull and eyes or active infection in the liver. It can also cause stillbirth. Infection can be detected by blood tests in the mother. Treatment is with sulfonamides and pyrimethamine.

t-PA (TPA) *see* tissue-type plasminogen activator.

trabecula *n.* (*pl.* **trabeculae**) **1.** any of the bands of tissue that pass from the outer part of an organ to its interior, dividing it into separate chambers. For example, trabeculae occur in the penis. **2.** any of the thin bars of bony tissue in spongy *bone. **3.** the hypertrophied bands of bladder-wall muscle that are found in bladder outflow obstruction. —**trabecular** *adj.*

trabeculectomy *n.* an operation for glaucoma, one part of which is the removal of a small segment of tissue from part of the wall of *Schlemm's canal. This area is known as the *trabecular meshwork*. Trabeculectomy allows aqueous fluid to filter out of the eye under the conjunctiva, thus reducing the pressure inside the eye.

trabeculoplasty *n.* a method used to selectively destroy parts of the *trabecular meshwork* (*see* trabeculectomy) and thus reduce intraocular pressure in the treatment of glaucoma. This may be achieved by means of a laser, as in *argon laser trabeculoplasty*.

trace element an element that is required in minute concentrations for normal growth and development (*see* micronutrient). Trace elements include fluorine (*see* fluoride), manganese, zinc, copper, *iodine, cobalt, *selenium, molybdenum, chromium, and silicon. They may serve as *cofactors or as constituents of complex molecules (e.g. cobalt in vitamin B_{12}).

tracer *n.* a substance that is introduced into the body and whose progress can subsequently be followed so that information is gained about metabolic processes. Radioactive tracers, which are substances labeled with *radionuclides,

give off radiation that can be detected on a *scintigram or with a *gamma camera. They are used for a variety of purposes in *nuclear medicine. *See* MUGA scan, positron emission tomography, SPECT scanning.

trache- (tracheo-) *prefix denoting* the trachea.

trachea *n.* the windpipe: the part of the air passage between the *larynx and the main *bronchi, i.e. from just below the Adam's apple, passing behind the notch of the *sternum (breastbone) to behind the angle of the sternum. The upper part of the trachea lies just below the skin, except where the thyroid gland is wrapped around it. —**tracheal** *adj.*

tracheal tugging a sign that is indicative of an *aneurysm of the aortic arch: a downward tug is felt on the windpipe when the finger is placed in the midline at the root of the neck.

tracheitis *n.* inflammation of the *trachea, usually secondary to bacterial or viral infection in the nose or throat. Tracheitis causes soreness in the chest and a painful cough and is often associated with bronchitis. In babies it can cause asphyxia, particularly in *diphtheria. Treatment includes appropriate antibacterial drugs, humidification of the inhaled air or oxygen, and mild sedation to relieve exhaustion due to persistent coughing.

tracheostomy (tracheotomy) *n.* a surgical operation in which a hole is made into the *trachea through the neck to relieve obstruction to breathing, as in diphtheria. A curved metal, plastic, or rubber tube is usually inserted through the hole and held in position by tapes tied round the neck. It may be possible for the patient to speak by occluding the opening with his fingers. The tube must be kept clean and unblocked. Tracheostomy is also used in conjunction with artificial respiration, when it serves not only to secure the airway but also provides a route for sucking out secretions and protects the airway against the inhalation of pharyngeal contents. *See also* minitracheostomy.

tracheotomy *n. see* tracheostomy.

trachoma *n.* a chronic contagious eye disease – a severe form of *conjunctivitis – caused by the viruslike bacterium *Chlamydia trachomatis*; it is common in tropical regions. The conjunctiva of the eyelids becomes inflamed, leading to discharge of pus. If untreated, the conjunctiva becomes scarred and shrinks, causing the eyelids to turn inward so that the eyelashes scratch the cornea (*see* trichiasis); blindness usually follows. Treatment with tetracyclines is effective in the early stages of the disease.

tract *n.* **1.** a group of nerve fibers passing from one part of the brain or spinal cord to another, forming a distinct pathway, e.g. the spinothalamic tract, pyramidal tract, and corticospinal tract. **2.** an organ or collection of organs providing for the passage of something, e.g. the digestive tract.

traction *n.* the application of a pulling force, especially as a means of counteracting the natural tension in the tissues surrounding a broken bone (*see* countertraction), to produce correct alignment of the fragments. Considerable force, exerted with weights, ropes, and pulleys, may be necessary to ensure that a broken femur is kept correctly positioned during the early stages of healing. Traction is also used for the treatment of back pain by physiotherapists.

tractotomy *n.* a neurosurgical operation for the relief of intractable pain. The nerve fibers that carry painful sensation to consciousness travel from the spinal cord through the brainstem in the spinothalamic tracts. This procedure is designed to sever the tracts within the medulla oblongata. *See also* cordotomy.

tragus *n.* the projection of cartilage in the *pinna of the outer ear that extends back over the opening of the external auditory meatus.

trait *n.* any condition or characteristic that is genetically inherited. *See also* dominant, recessive, genotype.

TRAM flap *transverse rectus abdominis myocutaneous *flap: a piece of tissue (skin, muscle, and fat) dissected from the abdomen and used to reconstruct the breast after mastectomy.

trance *n.* a state in which reaction to the environment is diminished although awareness is not impaired. It can be caused by hypnosis, meditation, catatonia, conversion disorder, drugs (such as hallucinogens), and religious ecstasy.

tranexamic acid a drug that prevents the breakdown of blood clots in the circulation (*fibrinolysis) by blocking the activation of plasminogen to form *plasmin, i.e. it is an *antifibrinolytic* drug. It is administered by mouth as an antidote to overdosage by *fibrinolytic drugs and to control severe bleeding, for example in hemophiliacs, or after surgery, or to treat menorrhagia. Possible side effects include nausea and vomiting. Trade name: **Cyklokapron**.

tranquilizer *n.* a drug that produces a calming effect, relieving anxiety and tension. *Antipsychotic drugs (formerly known as *major tranquilizers*), such as the phenothiazines (e.g. *chlorpromazine and *trifluoperazine) and *haloperidol, are used to treat severe mental disorders (psychoses), including schizophrenia and mania. *Anxiolytic drugs (formerly known as *minor tranquilizers*), such as the benzodiazepines (e.g. *chlordiazepoxide and *diazepam) and *meprobamate, are used to treat neuroses and to relieve anxiety and tension due to various causes. Some drowsiness and dizziness are side effects of most tranquilizers, and prolonged use may result in *dependence.

trans- *prefix denoting* through or across. Example: *transurethral* (through the urethra).

transaminase (aminotransferase) *n.* an enzyme that catalyzes the transfer of an amino group from an amino acid to an α-keto acid in the process of *transamination. Examples are *aspartate transaminase (AST), which catalyzes the transamination of glutamate and oxaloacetate to α-ketoglutarate and aspartate, and *alanine transaminase (ALT), converting glutamate and pyruvate to α-ketoglutarate and alanine.

transamination *n.* a process involved in the metabolism of amino acids in which amino groups ($-NH_2$) are transferred from amino acids to certain α-keto acids, with the production of a second keto acid and amino acid. The reaction is catalyzed by enzymes (*see* transaminase), which require pyridoxal phosphate as a coenzyme.

transcervical resection of the endometrium an operation, which is performed under local anesthetic, in which the membrane lining the uterus (*see* endometrium) is cut away by a form of *electrosurgery using a *resectoscope, which is introduced through the cervix. Like *endometrial ablation, the procedure is used as an alternative to hysterectomy to treat abnormally heavy menstrual bleeding since it results in fewer complications and shorter stays in the hospital.

transcription n. the process in which the information contained in the *genetic code is transferred from DNA to RNA: the first step in the manufacture of proteins in cells. See messenger RNA, translation.

transcutaneous electrical nerve stimulation (TENS) the introduction of pulses of low-voltage electricity into tissue for the relief of pain. It is effected by means of a small portable battery-operated unit with leads connected to electrodes attached to the skin; the strength and frequency of the pulses, which prevent the passage of pain impulses to the brain, can be adjusted by the patient. TENS is used mainly for the relief of rheumatic pain; as a method of producing pain relief in labor, it is less frequently used than epidural anesthesia, which has a much wider application for pain relief in obstetrics.

transducer n. a device used to convert one form of signal into another, allowing its measurement or display to be made appropriately. For example, an *ultrasound probe converts reflected ultrasound waves into electronic impulses, which can be displayed on a TV monitor.

transduction n. the transfer of DNA from one bacterium to another by means of a *bacteriophage (phage). Some bacterial DNA is incorporated into the phage. When the host bacterium is destroyed, the phage infects another bacterium and introduces the DNA from its previous host, which may become incorporated into the new host's DNA.

transection n. 1. a cross-section of a piece of tissue. 2. cutting across the tissue of an organ (see also section).

transesophageal echocardiography see echocardiography.

transfection n. the direct transfer of DNA molecules into a cell.

transferase n. an enzyme that catalyses the transfer of a group (other than hydrogen) between a pair of substrates.

transference n. (in psychoanalysis) the process by which a patient comes to feel and act toward the therapist as though he or she were somebody from the patient's past life, especially a powerful parent. The patient's transference feelings may be of love or of hatred, but they are inappropriate to the actual person of the therapist. *Countertransference* is the reaction of the therapist to the patient, which is similarly based on past relationships.

transferrin (siderophilin) n. a *glycoprotein, found in the blood plasma, that is capable of binding iron and thus acts as a carrier for iron in the bloodstream.

transfer RNA a type of RNA whose function is to attach the correct amino acid to the protein chain being synthesized at a *ribosome. See also translation.

transformation zone the area of the *cervix of the uterus where the squamous epithelium, which covers the vaginal portion of the cervix, joins with the columnar epithelium, which forms the lining (endocervix) of the cervical canal.

transfusion n. 1. the injection of a volume of blood obtained from a healthy person (the *donor*) into the circulation of a patient (the *recipient*) whose blood is deficient in quantity or quality, through accident or disease. Direct transfusion from one person to another is rarely performed; usually packs of carefully stored blood of different *blood groups are kept in *blood banks for use as necessary. During transfusion the blood is allowed to drip, under gravity, through a needle inserted into one of the recipient's veins. Blood transfusion is routine during major surgical operations in which much blood is likely to be lost. 2. the administration of any fluid, such as plasma or saline solution, into a patient's vein by means of a *drip. See also autotransfusion.

transient ischémic attack (TIA) the result of temporary disruption of the circulation to part of the brain due to *embolism, *thrombosis to brain arteries, or spasm of the vessel walls. The symptoms may be similar to those of a *stroke but patients recover within 24 hours.

transillumination n. the technique of shining a bright light through part of the body to examine its structure. Transillumination of the sinuses of the skull is a means of detecting abnormalities.

transitional cell carcinoma a form of cancer that affects the *urothelium*, which lines the urinary collecting system of the kidney, ureters, bladder, and most of the urethra. It is the most common type of bladder cancer.

translation *n.* (in cell biology) the manufacture of proteins in a cell, which takes place at the ribosomes. The information for determining the correct sequence of amino acids in the protein is carried to the ribosomes by *messenger RNA, and the amino acids are brought to their correct position in the protein by *transfer RNA.

translocation *n.* (in genetics) a type of chromosome mutation in which part of a chromosome is transferred to another part of the same chromosome or to a different chromosome. This changes the order of the genes on the chromosomes and can lead to serious genetic disorders, e.g. chronic myeloid leukemia.

transmethylation *n.* the process whereby an amino acid donates its terminal methyl ($-CH_3$) group for methylation of other compounds. Methionine is the principal methyl donor in the body and the donated methyl group may subsequently be involved in the synthesis of such compounds as choline or creatinine or in detoxification processes.

transmigration *n.* the act of passing through or across, e.g. the passage of blood cells through the intact walls of capillaries and venules (*see* diapedesis).

transmission *n.* the passage or transfer of a thing or condition from one organism or part of the body to another, such as the transfer of a neural impulse from one nerve cell to another, a disease from person to person, or an inherited trait from parent to offspring.

transmyocardial revascularization a form of laser surgery that is being evaluated in the treatment of coronary artery disease. At *diastole, a laser positioned over the left ventricle fires beams that create minute channels, about 1 mm in diameter, through the thickness of the ventricle. When the ventricle contracts, oxygenated blood is forced into the channels and supplies the damaged muscle; the blood clots at the surface of the heart, thus preventing leakage.

transplantation *n.* the implantation of an organ or tissue (*see* graft) from one part of the body to another or from one person (called the donor) to another (the recipient). Success for transplantation depends on the degree of compatibility between donor and graft: it is greatest for *autografts (self-grafts), less for *allografts (between individuals of the same species), and least for *xenografts (between different species; *see* xenotransplantation). Skin and bone grafting are examples of transplantation techniques in the same individual. A kidney transplant involves the grafting of a healthy kidney from a donor to replace the diseased kidney of the recipient: renal transplantation is the second most common example of human transplant surgery using allografts (after corneal grafts – *see* keratoplasty). Bone marrow, heart, heart–lung, and liver transplants are also very successful, and pancreatic·transplantation is now being performed. A few patients have undergone laryngeal transplantation following *laryngectomy. Transplanting organs or tissues between individuals is a difficult procedure because of the natural rejection processes in the recipient of the graft. Special treatment (e.g. with *immunosuppressant drugs) is needed to prevent graft rejection.

transposition *n.* the abnormal positioning of a part of the body so that it is on the opposite side to its normal site in the body. For example, it may involve the heart (*see* dextrocardia).

transposition of the great vessels a congenital abnormality of the heart in which the aorta arises from the right ventricle and the pulmonary artery from the left ventricle. Life is impossible unless there is an additional abnormality, such as a septal defect, that permits the mixing of blood between the pulmonary and systemic (aortic) circulations. Few of those untreated survive infancy and childhood, but the defect may be improved or corrected surgically.

transrectal ultrasonography (TRUS) a technique of *ultrasonography for examining the prostate gland and seminal vesicles by placing an ultrasound probe through the anus to lie directly behind these structures in the rectum. Because of the close proximity of the probe, excellent detail is seen. The technique enables biopsies of the prostate to be taken in a systematic manner in the diagnosis of cancer. *See also* vesiculography.

transsexualism *n.* the condition of one who firmly believes that he (or she) belongs to the sex opposite to his (or her) biological gender. The roots of such a belief usually go back to childhood. Children with such beliefs are treated with encouragement to engage in the activities appropriate to their biological sex and to work through their difficulties in psychotherapy. Adults with such beliefs can seldom be persuaded to change them; surgical sex reassignment is sometimes justifiable, to make the externals of the body conform to the individual's view of himself (or herself). —**transsexual** *adj.*, *n.*

transudation *n.* the passage of a liquid through a membrane, especially of blood through the wall of a capillary vessel. The liquid is called the *transudate*.

transuretero-ureterostomy *n.* the operation of connecting one ureter to the other in the abdomen. The damaged or obstructed ureter is cut above the diseased or damaged segment and joined end-to-side to the other ureter.

transurethral resection of the prostate (TUR, TURP) *see* resection.

transurethral vaporization of the prostate (TUVP) a new technique that vaporizes (rather than resects) prostate tissue; it is associated with less bleeding during the procedure. TUVP is used to treat *lower urinary tract symptoms thought to be due to benign prostatic hyperplasia or urinary retention.

transvaginal ultrasonography *ultrasonography using a vaginal probe instead of an abdominal transducer. It allows the use of a higher frequency, thus providing superior resolution and therefore a more detailed anatomy of the female pelvis and an earlier and more accurate identification of fetal structures.

transverse *adj.* (in anatomy) situated at right angles to the long axis of the body or of an organ.

transverse process the long projection from the base of the neural arch of a *vertebra.

transvestism (cross-dressing) *n.* dressing in a manner normally associated with the opposite sex, which may occur in both heterosexual and homosexual people. Cross-dressing may be practiced by transsexuals (*see* transsexualism), in whom it is not sexually arousing. Other transvestites are fetishistic, and in these cross-dressing is sexually arousing and may lead to masturbatory or other sexual behavior. Treatment may be by behavioral techniques, such as *aversion therapy, but is not always needed. *See also* sexual deviation. —**transvestite** *n.*

Trantas' dots clumps of degenerating eosinophils and epithelial cells seen clinically as slightly elevated grayish-white dots on the superior *limbus of the conjunctiva in cases of allergic conjunctivitis. [A. Trantas (1867–1960), Greek ophthalmologist]

tranylcypromine *n.* an antidepressant drug – one of the *MAO inhibitors – given by mouth for the treatment of severe mental depressive states. Common side effects include restlessness, insomnia, giddiness, and a fall in blood pressure. Trade name: **Parnate**.

trapezium *n.* a bone of the wrist (*see* carpus). It articulates with the scaphoid bone behind, the first metacarpal in front, and the trapezoid and second metatarsal on either side.

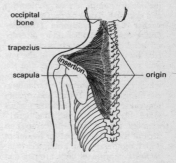

Left trapezius muscle

trapezius *n.* a flat triangular muscle covering the back of the neck and shoulder. It is important for movements of the scapula and it also draws the head backward to either side.

trapezoid bone a bone of the wrist (*see* carpus). It articulates with the second metatarsal bone in front, with the scaphoid bone behind, and with the trapezium and capitate bones on either side.

trastuzumab *n.* a *monoclonal antibody used to treat types of breast cancer that are positive for *HER2: the drug binds to these receptors on the tumor. It is administered by intravenous infusion; side effects include chills, fever, and allergic reactions. Trade name: **Herceptin**.

trauma *n.* **1.** a physical wound or injury, such as a fracture or blow. *Trauma scores* are numerical systems for assessing the severity and prognosis of serious injuries. **2.** (in psychology) an emotionally painful and harmful event. Theorists have speculated that some events (such as birth) are always traumatic. Symptoms of neurosis may follow an overwhelmingly stressful event, such as battle or serious injury. —**traumatic** *adj.*

traumatic fever a fever resulting from a serious injury.

traumatology *n.* accident surgery: the branch of surgery that deals with wounds and disabilities arising from injuries.

travel sickness *see* motion sickness.

trazodone *n.* a drug used in the treatment of depression with and without anxiety. It is administered by mouth; side effects include dry mouth, nausea, excitement, and skin rash. Trade name: **Desyrel**.

Treacher Collins syndrome (Treacher Collins deformity) a hereditary disorder of facial development. It is characterized by underdevelopment of the jaw and zygomatic (cheek) bones and the precursors of the ear fail to develop, which results in a variety of ear and facial malformations. The ear abnormality may cause deafness. [E. Treacher Collins (1862–1919), British ophthalmologist]

treatment field *n.* (in radiotherapy) an area of the body selected for treatment with radiotherapy. For example, a *mantle field* comprises the neck, armpits, and central chest, for the radiotherapy of Hodgkin's disease. Radiation is administered to the defined area by focusing the beam of particles that is emitted by the radiotherapy machine and shielding the surrounding area of the body.

trematode *n. see* fluke.

tremor *n.* a rhythmical alternating movement that may affect any part of the body. The *physiological tremor* is a feature of the normal mechanism for maintaining posture. It may be more apparent in states of fatigue or anxiety or when the thyroid gland is overactive. *Essential tremor* is slower and particularly affects the hands. It can be embarrassing and inconvenient but it is not accompanied by any other symptoms. A similar tremor may also occur in several members of one family or in elderly people. Propranolol reduces the intensity of essential tremor. *Primary orthostatic tremor* affects the legs when standing still, causing unsteadiness if the position is maintained. *Resting tremor* is a prominent symptom of *parkinsonism. An *intention tremor* occurs when a patient with disease of the cerebellum tries to touch an object. The closer the object is approached the wilder become the movements.

trench foot (immersion foot) blackening of the toes and the skin of the foot due to death of the superficial tissues and caused by prolonged immersion in cold water or exposure to damp and cold.

Trendelenburg position a special operating-table posture for patients undergoing surgery of the pelvis or for patients with shock or to reduce blood loss in operations on the legs. The patient is laid on his back with the pelvis higher than the head, inclined at an angle of about 45°, with knees bent. [F. Trendelenburg (1844–1924), German surgeon]

trephine *n.* a surgical instrument used to remove a circular area of tissue, usually from the cornea of the eye (in the operation of penetrating *keratoplasty) or from bone (for microscopical examination). It consists of a hollow tube with a serrated cutting edge. It is used during the preliminary stages of craniotomy.

Treponema *n.* a genus of anaerobic spirochete bacteria. All species are parasitic and some cause disease in animals and humans: *T. carateum* causes *pinta, *T. pallidum* *syphilis, and *T. pertenue* *yaws.

treponematosis *n.* any infection caused by spirochete bacteria of the genus *Treponema. See* pinta, syphilis, yaws.

tretinoin *n.* a drug used in the treatment of acne vulgaris. Tretinoin is administered topically by cream, gel, or liquid; side effects include blistering, altered pigmentation, and increased sensitivity to sunlight. It is also administered orally (as *Vesanoid*) to treat acute promyelocytic leukemia. Trade name: **Retin-A**.

TRH *see* thyrotropin-releasing hormone.

triad *n.* (in medicine) a group of three united or closely associated structures or three symptoms or effects that occur together. A *portal triad* in a portal canal of the liver consists of a branch of the portal vein, a branch of the hepatic artery, and an interlobular bile tubule.

triage *n.* a system whereby a group of casualties or other patients is sorted according to the seriousness of their injuries or illnesses so that treatment priorities can be allocated between them. In emergency situations it is designed to maximize the number of survivors.

triamcinolone *n.* a synthetic corticosteroid hormone that reduces inflammation but does not cause salt and water retention. It is used for treating a wide range of inflammatory and allergic conditions, including arthritis, eczema, psoriasis, asthma, and hay fever. It is administered by mouth, injection, nasal spray, and topically; common side effects include dizziness, headache, somnolence, muscle weakness, and a fall in blood pressure, particularly on the sudden withdrawal of treatment. Trade names: **Azmacort**, **Mycogen**, **Nasacort**.

triamterene *n.* a potassium-sparing *diuretic that is given by mouth and produces an effect within two hours. It causes the loss of sodium and chloride from the kidneys and is used in the treatment of various forms of fluid retention (edema). Common side effects include nausea, vomiting, weakness, reduced blood pressure, and digestive disorders. Trade name: **Dyrenium**.

triangle *n.* (in anatomy) a three-sided structure or area; for example, the *femoral triangle.

triangular bandage a piece of material cut or folded into a triangular shape and used for making an arm sling or holding dressings in position.

Triatoma *n.* a genus of bloodsucking bugs (*see* reduviid). *T. infestans* is important in transmitting *Chagas' disease in Argentina, Uruguay, and Chile.

triazolam *n.* a drug used for the short-term treatment of insomnia associated with difficulty falling asleep, frequent nocturnal awakenings, or early morning awakening. It is administered by mouth; side effects include drowsiness, nausea

and vomiting, and headache. Trade name: **Halcion**.

triceps *n.* a muscle with three heads of origin, particularly the *triceps brachii*, which is situated on the back of the upper arm and contracts to extend the forearm. It is the *antagonist of the *brachialis.

trich- (tricho-) *prefix denoting* hair or hair-like structures.

trichiasis *n.* a condition in which the eyelashes rub against the eyeball, producing discomfort and sometimes ulceration of the cornea. It may result from inflammation of the eyelids, which makes the lashes grow out in abnormal directions, or when scarring of the conjunctiva (lining membrane) turns the eyelid inward. It accompanies all forms of *entropion.

Trichinella *n.* a genus of minute parasitic nematode worms. The adults of *T. spiralis* live in the small intestine of humans, where the females release large numbers of larvae. These bore through the intestinal wall and can cause disease (*see* trichinosis). The parasite can also develop in pigs and rats.

trichiniasis *n. see* trichinosis.

trichinosis (trichiniasis) *n.* a disease of cold and temperate regions caused by larvae of the nematode worm *Trichinella spiralis*. Humans contract trichinosis after eating imperfectly cooked meat infected with the parasite's larval cysts. Larvae, released by females in the intestine, penetrate the intestinal wall and cause diarrhea and nausea. They migrate around the body and may cause fever, vertigo, delirium, and pains in the limbs. The larvae eventually settle within cysts in the muscles, and this may result in pain and stiffness. Trichinosis, rarely a serious disease, is treated with thiabendazole.

trichlormethiazide *n.* a thiazide *diuretic used in the treatment of hypertension. It is administered orally; common side effects include dizziness, dry mouth, irregular heartbeat, and nausea. Trade name: **Metahydrin, Naqua, Trichlorex**.

trichloroacetic acid an *astringent used in solution for a variety of skin conditions. It is also applied topically to produce sloughing, especially for the removal of warts.

trichobezoar *n.* hairball; a mass of swallowed hair in the stomach. It may be the patient's own hair or animal hairs. *See* bezoar.

Trichocephalus *n. see* whipworm.

trichoglossia *n.* hairiness of the tongue, due to the growth of fungal organisms infecting its surface.

trichology *n.* the study of hair.

Trichomonas *n.* a genus of parasitic flagellate protozoans that move by means of a wavy membrane, bearing a single flagellum, projecting from the body surface. *T. vaginalis* often infects the vagina, where it may cause severe irritation and a foul-smelling discharge (*see* vaginitis), and sometimes also the male *urethra; it can be transmitted during sexual intercourse. *T. hominis* and *T. tenax* live in the large intestine and mouth, respectively. *See also* trichomoniasis.

trichomoniasis *n.* **1.** an infection of the digestive system by the protozoan *Trichomonas hominis*, causing dysentery. **2.** an infection of the vagina due to the protozoan *Trichomonas vaginalis*, causing inflammation of genital tissues with vaginal discharge (*see* vaginitis). It can be transmitted to males in whom it causes urethral discharge. Treatment is with *metronidazole.

trichomycosis *n.* any hair disease caused by infection with a fungus.

Trichophyton *n.* a genus of fungi, parasitic in humans, that frequently infect the skin, nails, and hair and cause *favus and *ringworm. *See also* dermatophyte.

trichorrhexis *n.* a condition in which the hairs break or split easily. It may be due to a hereditary condition or it may occur as a consequence of repeated physical or chemical injury. The latter condition may follow the use of heat or bleach on the hair or be caused by persistent rubbing. *Trichorrhexis nodosa* is characterized by the appearance of minute white nodes, which are sites on the cortex of the hair shaft that have fractured and split into strands, weakening the hair and causing it to break at these points.

trichosis *n.* any abnormal growth or disease of the hair.

Trichosporon *n.* a genus of fungi, parasitic in humans, that infect the scalp and beard (*see* piedra).

trichotillomania *n.* loss of hair caused by a person persistently rubbing or pulling it.

trichromatic *adj.* describing or relating to the normal state of color vision, in which

a person is sensitive to all three of the primary colors (red, green, and blue) and can match any given color by a mixture of these three. *Compare* dichromatic, monochromat.

trichuriasis *n.* an infestation of the large intestine by the *whipworm *Trichuris trichiura*; it occurs principally in humid tropical regions. Humans acquire the infection by eating food contaminated with the worms' eggs. Symptoms, including bloody diarrhea, anemia, weakness, and abdominal pain, are evident only in heavy infestations. Trichuriasis can be treated with various anthelmintics, including thiabendazole and piperazine salts.

Trichuris *n. see* whipworm.

tricuspid atresia a rare form of congenital heart disease in which there is no communication between the right atrium and the right ventricle. Affected babies present with *cyanosis, breathlessness, particularly on feeding, and *failure to thrive. Diagnosis is by *echocardiography. Treatment involves surgical intervention, but the prognosis is often poor.

tricuspid valve the valve in the heart between the right atrium and right ventricle. It consists of three cusps that channel the flow of blood from the atrium to the ventricle and prevent any backflow.

tricyclic antidepressant *see* antidepressant.

tridactyly *n.* a congenital abnormality in which there are only three digits on a hand or foot.

trientine *n.* a *chelating agent that removes excess copper from the body, used in the treatment of patients with *Wilson's disease who are intolerant to *penicillamine. It is administered orally; side effects include anemia, joint pain, skin rash, and swollen glands. Trade name: **Syprine**.

trifluoperazine *n.* an *antipsychotic drug with uses and effects similar to those of *chlorpromazine. Common side effects include drowsiness, dizziness, dryness of mouth, muscular spasm and tremor, and amenorrhea. Trade name: **Stelazine**.

triflupromazine *n.* a *phenothiazine derivative used as an *antipsychotic and *antiemetic agent. It is prescribed in the treatment of schizophrenia and other psychotic disorders and for the control of severe agitation, hiccups, and nausea and vomiting. It is administered orally or by injection; common side effects include restlessness, blurred vision, difficulty seeing at night, and dry mouth. Trade name: **Vesprin**.

trifocal lenses lenses in which there are three segments. The upper provides a clear image of distant objects; the lower is used for reading and close work; and the middle one for the intermediate distance. Musicians sometimes find the middle segment useful for reading the score during a performance.

trigeminal nerve the fifth and largest *cranial nerve (V), which is split into three divisions: the ophthalmic, maxillary, and mandibular nerves (see illustration). The motor fibers are responsible for controlling the muscles involved in chewing, while the sensory fibers relay information about temperature, pain, and touch from the whole front half of the head (including the mouth) and also from the meninges.

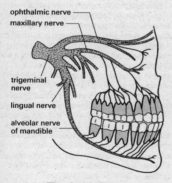

ophthalmic nerve
maxillary nerve
trigeminal nerve
lingual nerve
alveolar nerve of mandible

The trigeminal nerve

trigeminal neuralgia (tic douloureux) *see* neuralgia.

trigeminy *n.* a condition in which the heartbeats can be subdivided into groups of three. The first beat is normal, but the second and third are premature beats (*see* ectopic beat).

trigger finger an impairment in the ability to extend a finger, resulting either from a nodular thickening in the flexor tendon or a narrowing of the flexor tendon sheath. On unclenching the fist, the affected finger (usually the third or fourth)

at first remains bent and then, on overcoming the resistance, suddenly straightens (triggers). Treatment is by incision of the tendon sheath or injection of steroid around the tendon.

triglyceride *n.* a lipid or neutral *fat consisting of glycerol combined with three fatty-acid molecules. Triglycerides are synthesized from the products of digestion of dietary fat: they are the form in which fat is stored in the body. A high concentration of triglycerides in the blood, in the form of lipoproteins, predisposes to coronary heart disease.

trigone *n.* a triangular region or tissue, such as the triangular region of the wall of the bladder that lies between the openings of the two ureters and the urethra.

trigonitis *n.* inflammation of the trigone (base) of the urinary bladder. This can occur as part of a generalized *cystitis or it can be associated with inflammation in the urethra, prostate, or cervix (neck) of the uterus. The patient experiences an intense desire to pass urine frequently; treatment includes the clearing of any underlying infection by antibiotic administration.

trigonocephaly *n.* a deformity of the skull in which the vault of the skull is sharply angled just in front of the ears, giving the skull a triangular shape. —**trigonocephalic** *adj.*

trihexyphenidyl hydrochloride (benzhexol) *n.* an *anticholinergic drug that has actions and side effects similar to those of *atropine. Taken by mouth, it is used mainly to reduce muscle spasm in parkinsonism. Trade names: **Artane**, **Trihexane**.

triiodothyronine *n.* one of the hormones synthesized and secreted by the thyroid gland (*see* thyroid hormone). A preparation of triiodothyronine (*liothyronine) is administered by mouth or injection for treating underactivity of the thyroid.

trimeprazine *n.* an *antihistamine drug (a *phenothiazine derivative) that also possesses sedative properties. Given by mouth, it is mainly used in the treatment of pruritus (itching), *urticaria, and as a preoperative medication, especially in children. Common side effects include drowsiness, dizziness, dryness of mouth, muscular tremor and incoordination, and confusion. Trade name: **Temaril**.

trimester *n.* (in obstetrics) any one of the three successive three-month periods (the *first*, *second*, and *third trimesters*) into which a pregnancy may be divided.

trimethadione *n.* an *anticonvulsant drug given by mouth, alone or in conjunction with other drugs, in the treatment of epilepsy. Trimethadione is highly toxic and, in addition to producing nausea, vertigo, visual disturbances, and skin reactions, it can affect the bone marrow and cause anemia. Trade name: **Tridione**.

trimethobenzamide *n.* a drug used for the treatment of nausea and vomiting. It is administered by mouth and rectally; side effects include headache, diarrhea, and drowsiness. Trade names: **Tebamide**, **Tigan**.

trimethoprim *n.* an antibacterial drug that is active against a range of microorganisms. Taken by mouth, it is used mainly in the treatment of chronic urinary-tract infections and respiratory-tract infections. Long-term treatment may cause anemia due to deficiency of folic acid, with which the drug interacts. Trimethoprim is sometimes administered in a combined preparation with sulfamethoxazole (*see* co-trimoxazole) but is now more usually prescribed alone, because of the severity of the side effects of cotrimoxazole. Trade names: **Proloprim**, **Septra**, **Trimpex**.

trimipramine *n.* a tricyclic *antidepressant drug that also possesses sedative properties. It is given by mouth for the treatment of acute or chronic mental depression. Common side effects include drowsiness, dizziness, dry mouth, and a fall in blood pressure. Trade name: **Surmontil**.

trinitrophenol *n.* *see* picric acid.

triose *n.* a carbohydrate with three carbon units: for example, glyceraldehyde.

trioxsalen *n.* an agent used in combination with ultraviolet A irradiation (*see* PUVA) for the treatment of *vitiligo. It is administered orally; common side effects include nausea and itchy, red, or sore skin. Trade name: **Trisoralen**.

triploid *adj.* describing cells, tissues, or individuals in which there are three complete chromosome sets. *Compare* haploid, diploid. —**triploid** *n.*

triprolidine *n.* an *antihistamine drug used

to treat hay fever or other allergies and, in combination with other drugs, to relieve the symptoms of the common cold. Trade names: **Actifed**, **Sudafed**.

triquetrum (triquetral bone) *n.* a bone of the wrist (*see* carpus). It articulates with the ulna behind via cartilage, and with the pisiform, hamate, and lunate bones in the carpus.

trismus *n.* spasm of the jaw muscles, keeping the jaws tightly closed. This is the characteristic symptom of *tetanus but it also occurs less dramatically as a sensitivity reaction to certain drugs and in disorders of the *basal ganglia.

trisomy *n.* a condition in which there is one extra chromosome present in each cell in addition to the normal (diploid) chromosome set. A number of chromosome disorders are caused by trisomy, including *Down's syndrome and *Klinefelter's syndrome. —**trisomic** *adj.*

tritanopia *n.* a rare defect of color vision in which affected persons are insensitive to blue light and confuse blues and greens. *Compare* deuteranopia, protanopia.

tritium *n.* an isotope of hydrogen that emits beta particles (electrons) during its decay. It has been used as a *tracer in the investigation of metabolic diseases. Symbol: T or ^{3}H.

trocar *n.* an instrument used combined with a *cannula to draw off fluids from a body cavity (such as the peritoneal cavity). It comprises a metal tube containing a removable shaft with a sharp three-cornered point; the shaft is withdrawn after the trocar has been inserted into the cavity.

trochanter *n.* either of the two protuberances that occur below the neck of the *femur.

troche *n.* a medicinal lozenge, taken by mouth, used to treat conditions of the mouth or throat and also of the alimentary canal.

trochlea *n.* an anatomical part having the structure or function of a pulley; for example the groove at the lower end of the *humerus or the fibrocartilaginous ring in the frontal bone (where it forms part of the orbit), through which the tendon of the superior oblique eye muscle passes. —**trochlear** *adj.*

trochlear nerve the fourth *cranial nerve (IV), which supplies the superior oblique muscle, one of the muscles responsible for movement of the eyeball in its socket. The action of the trochlear nerve is coordinated with that of the *oculomotor and *abducens nerves.

trochoid joint (pivot joint) a form of *diarthrosis (freely movable joint) in which a bone moves around a central axis, allowing rotational movement. An example is the joint between the atlas and axis vertebrae.

Troisier's sign enlargement of the lymph node at the base of the neck on the left side (*Troisier's node*), which indicates metastatic spread from an abdominal malignant growth, usually a carcinoma of the stomach. [C. E. Troisier (1844–1919), French physician]

Trombicula *n.* a genus of widely distributed mites – the harvest mites. The six-legged parasitic larvae (chiggers) are common in fields during the autumn and frequently attack humans, remaining attached to the skin for several days while feeding on the lymph and digested skin tissues. Their bite causes intense irritation and a severe dermatitis. Various repellents, e.g. benzyl benzoate, can be applied to clothing. *Trombicula* larvae are responsible for transmitting scrub typhus in southeast Asia.

tromethamine *n.* a drug that reduces the acidity of body fluids. It is given by intravenous injection in conditions of acidosis to adjust the pH of the blood to normal levels. Side effects include respiratory depression, lowered blood glucose, and reaction at site of injection. Trade name: **THAM**.

troph- (tropho-) *prefix denoting* nourishment or nutrition.

trophoblast *n.* the tissue that forms the wall of the *blastocyst. At implantation it forms two layers, an inner cellular layer (*cytotrophoblast*) and an outer syncytial layer (*plasmoditrophoblast*), which forms the outermost layer of the placenta and attains direct contact with the maternal bloodstream.

trophozoite *n.* a stage in the life cycle of the malarial parasite (*Plasmodium*) that develops from a merozoite in the red blood cells. The trophozoite, which has a ring-shaped body and a single nucleus, grows steadily at the expense of the blood cell; eventually its nucleus and cytoplasm undergo division to form a *schizont containing many merozoites.

-trophy *suffix denoting* nourishment, development, or growth Example: *dystrophy* (defective development).

-tropic *suffix denoting* **1.** turning toward. **2.** having an affinity for; influencing. Example: *inotropic* (muscle).

tropical abscess (amebic abscess) an abscess of the liver caused by infection with *Entamoeba histolytica. See* (amebic) dysentery.

tropical medicine the study of diseases more commonly found in tropical regions than elsewhere, such as *malaria, *leprosy, *trypanosomiasis, *schistosomiasis, and *leishmaniasis.

tropical ulcer (Naga sore) a skin disease prevalent in wet tropical regions. A large open sloughing sore usually develops at the site of a wound or abrasion. The ulcer, commonly located on the feet and legs, is often infected with spirochetes and bacteria and may extend deeply and cause destruction of muscles and bones. Treatment involves the application of mild antiseptic dressings and intramuscular doses of *penicillin. Skin grafts may be necessary in more serious cases. The exact cause of the disease has not yet been determined.

tropicamide *n.* an *anticholinergic drug used in the form of eye drops to dilate the pupil so that the inside of the eye can more easily be examined or operated upon. Trade names: **Mydriacyl, Opticyl, Tropicacyl**.

tropocollagen *n.* the molecular unit of *collagen. It consists of a helix of three collagen molecules: this arrangement confers on the fibers structural stability and resistance to stretching.

Trousseau's sign spasmodic contractions of muscles, especially the muscles of mastication, in response to nerve stimulation (e.g. by tapping). It is a characteristic sign of hypocalcemia (*see* tetany). [A. Trousseau (1801–67), French physician]

truncus *n.* a *trunk: a main vessel or other tubular organ from which subsidiary branches arise.

truncus arteriosus the main arterial trunk arising from the fetal heart. It develops into the aorta and pulmonary artery.

trunk *n.* **1.** the main part of a blood vessel, lymph vessel, or nerve, from which branches arise. **2.** the body excluding the head and limbs.

TRUS *see* transrectal ultrasonography.

truss *n.* a device for applying pressure to a hernia to prevent it from protruding. It usually consists of a pad attached to a belt with straps or spring strips and it is worn under the clothing.

trypanocide *n.* an agent that kills trypanosomes and is therefore used to treat infestations caused by these parasites (*see* trypanosomiasis). The principal trypanocides are arsenic-containing compounds.

Trypanosoma *n.* a genus of parasitic protozoans that move by means of a long trailing flagellum and a thin wavy membrane, which project from the body surface. Trypanosomes undergo part of their development in the blood of a vertebrate host. The remaining stages occur in invertebrate hosts, which then transmit the parasites back to the vertebrates. *T. rhodesiense* and *T. gambiense*, which are transmitted through the bite of *tsetse flies, cause *sleeping sickness in Africa. *T. cruzi*, carried by *reduviid bugs, causes Chagas' disease in South America.

trypanosomiasis *n.* any disease caused by the presence of parasitic protozoans of the genus *Trypanosoma*. The two most important diseases are *Chagas' disease (South American trypanosomiasis) and *sleeping sickness (African trypanosomiasis).

tryparsamide *n.* a drug used in the treatment of trypanosomiasis (sleeping sickness). Usually given by injection, it penetrates the cerebrospinal fluid and is highly active against the infective organism (*Trypanosoma gambiense*).

trypsin *n.* an enzyme that continues the digestion of proteins by breaking down peptones into smaller peptide chains (*see* peptidase). It is secreted by the pancreas in an inactive form, trypsinogen, which is converted in the duodenum to trypsin by the action of the enzyme enteropeptidase.

trypsinogen *n. see* trypsin.

tryptophan *n.* an *essential amino acid. *See also* amino acid.

TSAB thyroid-stimulating antibody. TSABs are implicated in the causes of *thyroiditis.

tsetse *n.* a large bloodsucking fly of tropical Africa belonging to the genus *Glossina*. Tsetse flies, which have slender forwardly projecting biting mouthparts, feed during the day on humans and other mammals. They transmit the blood parasites that cause *sleeping sickness. *G. palpalis* and *G. tachinoides*, which are found along river banks, transmit *Trypanosoma gambiense*; *G. morsitans*, *G. swynnertoni*, and *G. pallidipes*, which are found in savannah country, transmit *T. rhodesiense*.

TSH *see* thyroid-stimulating hormone.

tsutsugamushi disease *see* scrub typhus.

tubal *adj.* relating to or affecting a fallopian tube.

tubal occlusion blocking of the fallopian tubes. This is achieved by surgery as a means of *sterilization; it is also a result of *pelvic inflammatory disease.

tubal pregnancy *see* ectopic pregnancy.

tube *n.* (in anatomy) a long hollow cylindrical structure, e.g. a *fallopian tube.

tuber *n.* (in anatomy) a thickened or swollen part. The *tuber cinereum* is a part of the brain situated at the base of the hypothalamus, connected to the stalk of the pituitary gland.

tubercle *n.* **1.** (in anatomy) a small rounded protuberance on a bone. **2.** the specific nodular lesion of *tuberculosis.

tubercular *adj.* having small rounded swellings or nodules, not necessarily caused by tuberculosis.

tuberculid *n.* a papular lesion in the skin, probably due to an allergic reaction to tuberculosis infection.

tuberculin *n.* a protein extract from cultures of tubercle bacilli, used to test whether a person has had or been in contact with tuberculosis. In the *Mantoux test* a quantity of tuberculin is injected beneath the skin and a patch of inflammation appearing in the next 48–72 hours is regarded as a positive reaction, meaning that a degree of immunity is present.

tuberculoma *n.* a mass of cheeselike material resembling a tumor, seen in some cases of *tuberculosis. Tuberculomas are found in a variety of sites, including the lung or brain, and a single mass may be the only clinical evidence of disease. Treatment is by surgical excision, together with antituberculous drugs.

tuberculosis (TB) *n.* an infectious disease caused by the bacillus *Mycobacterium tuberculosis* (first identified by Koch in 1882) and characterized by the formation of nodular lesions (*tubercles*) in the tissues.

In *pulmonary tuberculosis* – formerly known as *consumption* and *phthisis* (wasting) – the bacillus is inhaled into the lungs where it sets up a primary tubercle and spreads to the nearest lymph nodes (the *primary complex*). Natural immune defenses may heal it at this stage; alternatively, the disease may smolder for months or years and fluctuate with the patient's resistance. Many people become infected but show no symptoms. They can, however, act as carriers, transmitting the bacillus by coughing and sneezing. Symptoms of the active disease include fever, night sweats, weight loss, and the spitting of blood. In some cases the bacilli spread from the lungs to the bloodstream, setting up millions of tiny tubercles throughout the body (*miliary tuberculosis*), or migrate to the meninges to cause tuberculous *meningitis. Bacilli entering by the mouth, usually in infected cows' milk, set up a primary complex in abdominal lymph nodes, leading to *peritonitis, and sometimes spread to other organs, joints, and bones (*see* Pott's disease).

Tuberculosis is curable by various combinations of the antibiotics *streptomycin, *ethambutol, *isoniazid (INH), *rifampin, and *pyrazinamide. Preventive measures include the detection of carriers by X-ray screening of vulnerable populations and inoculation with *BCG vaccine of those with no immunity to the disease (the *tuberculin test identifies which people require vaccination). There has been a resurgence of tuberculosis in recent years in association with HIV infection. The number of patients with multidrug resistant TB has also increased due to patients not completing drug courses. Many centers have introduced *direct observed therapy* (DOT) with nurse practitioners to administer drugs.

tuberose *see* tuberous.

tuberosity *n.* a large rounded protuberance on a bone. For example, there is a tuberosity at the upper end of the tibia.

tuberous (tuberose) *adj.* knobbed; having nodules or rounded swellings.

tuberous sclerosis (Bourneville's disease, epiloia) an hereditary disorder in which the brain, skin, and other organs are studded with small plaques or tumors: eye involvement includes retinal tumors, optic nerve gliomas, and eyelid neuromas. Symptoms include epilepsy and mental retardation.

tubo- *prefix denoting* a tube, especially a fallopian tube or eustachian tube.

tuboabdominal *adj.* relating to or occurring in a fallopian tube and the abdomen.

tubocurarine *n.* a drug given by intravenous injection to produce relaxation of voluntary muscles before surgery and convulsive therapy (*see* muscle relaxant), and in the diagnosis of myasthenia gravis. Toxic side effects are usually only seen with overdosage, when respiratory failure due to paralysis of respiratory muscles may occur.

tubo-ovarian *adj.* relating to or occurring in a fallopian tube and an ovary.

tubotympanal *adj.* relating to the tympanic cavity and the *eustachian tube.

tubule *n.* (in anatomy) a small cylindrical hollow structure. *See also* renal tubule, seminiferous tubule.

tuftsin *n.* a tetrapeptide derived from IgG (*see* immunoglobulin), produced mainly in the spleen, that stimulates *neutrophil activity (phagocytosis). Levels of tuftsin are reduced after *splenectomy, resulting in diminished resistance to infection, especially by encapsulated organisms.

tularemia (rabbit fever) *n.* a disease of rodents and rabbits, caused by the bacterium *Francisella tularensis*, that is transmitted to humans by deer flies (*see* Chrysops), by direct contact with infected animals, by contamination of wounds, or by drinking contaminated water. Symptoms include an ulcer at the site of infection, inflamed and ulcerating lymph nodes, headache, aching pains, loss of weight, and a fever lasting several weeks. Treatment with chloramphenicol, streptomycin, or tetracycline is effective.

tulle gras a soft dressing consisting of open-woven silk (or other material) impregnated with a waterproof soft paraffin wax.

tumbu fly a large nonbloodsucking fly, *Cordylobia anthropophaga*, widely distributed in tropical Africa. The female fly lays eggs on ground contaminated with urine or excreta or on clothing tainted with sweat or urine. The maggots are normally parasites of rats, but if they come into contact with humans they penetrate the skin, producing boil-like swellings (*see also* myiasis). The maggots can be gently eased out by applying oil to the swellings.

tumefaction *n.* the process in which a tissue becomes swollen and tense by accumulation within it of fluid under pressure.

tumescence *n.* a swelling, or the process of becoming swollen, usually because of an accumulation of blood or other fluid within the tissues.

tumid *adj.* swollen.

tumor *n.* **1.** any abnormal swelling in or on a part of the body. The term is usually applied to an abnormal growth of tissue, which may be *benign or *malignant. *Compare* cyst. **2.** swelling: one of the classic signs of *inflammation in a tissue, the other three being *calor (heat), *rubor (redness), and *dolor (pain). The swelling of an inflamed area is due to the leakage from small blood vessels of clear protein-containing fluid, which accumulates between the cells.

tumor-associated antigen a protein produced by cancer cells. Its presence in the blood can be revealed by means of a simple blood test, which could provide a basis for the diagnosis of malignant melanoma and other cancers at their earliest – and most treatable – stages of development.

tumor-infiltrating lymphocyte a lymphoid cell that can infiltrate solid tumors. Such cells can be cultured in vitro, in the presence of *interleukin-2, and have been used as vehicles for *tumor necrosis factor in gene therapy trials for cancer.

tumor marker a substance produced by a tumor that can be used to monitor the size of the tumor and the effects of treatment. An example is *alpha-fetoprotein, which is used to monitor treatment of testicular teratomas.

tumor necrosis factor (TNF) either of two proteins, TNF-α or TNF-β, that function as *cytokines. Among their many actions is destruction of tumor cells. The gene encoding TNF has been used in gene therapy trials for cancer.

Tunga *n.* a genus of sand fleas found in tropical America and Africa. The fertilized female of *T. penetrans*, the chigoe or jigger, burrows beneath the skin of the foot, where it becomes enclosed in a swelling of the surrounding tissues and causes intense itching and inflammation. Surgical removal of the fleas is recommended.

tunica *n.* a covering or layer of an organ or part; for example, a layer of the wall of a blood vessel (*see* adventitia, intima, media). The *tunica albuginea* is a fibrous membrane comprising one of the covering tissues of the ovary, penis, and testis.

tunnel *n.* (in anatomy) a canal or hollow groove. *See also* carpal tunnel.

tunnel vision a visual-field defect in which only the central area of the *visual field remains. It occurs in advanced *glaucoma.

TUR, TURP (transurethral resection of the prostate) *see* resection.

turbinate bone *see* nasal concha.

turbinectomy *n.* the surgical removal of one of the bones forming the nasal cavity (nasal conchae, or turbinate bones).

turgescence *n.* a swelling, or the process by which a swelling arises in tissues, usually by the accumulation of blood or other fluid under pressure.

turgor *n.* a state of being swollen or distended.

Turkel's needle a specially designed needle for purposes of transrectal prostatic biopsy.

Turner's syndrome a genetic defect in women in which there is only one X chromosome instead of the usual two. Affected women are infertile: they have female external genitalia but no ovaries and therefore no menstrual periods (*see* amenorrhea). Characteristically they are short and have variable developmental defects, which may include webbing of the neck. [H. H. Turner (1892–1970), US endocrinologist]

turricephaly *n. see* oxycephaly.

tussis *n.* the medical name for *coughing.

TUVP *see* transurethral vaporization of the prostate.

twilight state a condition of disturbed consciousness in which the individual can still carry out some normal activities but is impaired in his awareness and has no memory of what he has done. It is encountered after epileptic attacks, in alcoholism, and in organic states of confusion. It may be associated with other symptoms, such as physical and mental slowing, episodes of rage, and hallucinations. Twilight states last only for a short time, commonly a few hours.

twins *n.* two individuals who are born at the same time and of the same parents. *Fraternal* (or *dizygotic*) *twins* are the result of the simultaneous fertilization of two egg cells; they may be of different sexes and are no more alike than ordinary siblings. *Identical* (or *monozygotic*) *twins* result from the fertilization of a single egg cell that then divides to give two separate fetuses. They are of the same sex and otherwise genetically identical; any differences in their appearance are due to environmental influences. *See also* Siamese twins.

tylosis *n.* the development of a callus on the skin, especially the palms and soles (*see* callosity). It occurs early in life and is inherited as an autosomal *dominant. It is associated with oral leukoplakia and with esophageal cancer.

tympan- (tympano-) *prefix denoting* 1. the eardrum. Example: *tympanectomy* (surgical excision of). 2. the middle ear.

tympanic cavity *see* middle ear.

tympanic membrane (eardrum) the membrane at the inner end of the external auditory meatus, separating the outer and middle ears. It is formed from the outer wall of the lining of the tympanic cavity and the skin that lines the external auditory meatus. When sound waves reach the ear the tympanum vibrates, transmitting these vibrations to the malleus – one of the auditory *ossicles in the middle ear – to which it is attached.

tympanites (meteorism) *n.* distension of the abdomen with air or gas: the abdomen is resonant (drumlike) on *percussion. Causes include intestinal obstruction, *irritable bowel syndrome, and *aerophagia.

tympanoplasty *n.* surgical repair of defects of the eardrum and middle ear ossicles. *See* myringoplasty.

tympanotomy *n. see* myringotomy.

tympanum *n.* the *middle ear (tympanic cavity) and/or the eardrum (*tympanic membrane).

typhlitis *n. Obsolete.* inflammation of the cecum: formerly a common diagnosis of the condition now recognized as appendicitis.

typhlosis *n.* an obsolete term for *blindness.

typho- *prefix denoting* 1. typhoid fever. 2. typhus.

typhoid fever an infection of the digestive system by the bacterium *Salmonella typhi*, causing general weakness, high temperature, a rash of red spots on the chest and abdomen, chills, sweating, and in serious cases inflammation of the spleen and bones, delirium, and erosion of the intestinal wall leading to hemorrhage. It is transmitted through food or drinking water contaminated by the feces or urine of patients or carriers. In most cases recovery occurs naturally but treatment with such antibiotics as ampicillin, amoxicillin, ciprofloxacin, or chloramphenicol reduces the severity of symptoms. Vaccination with *TAB vaccine provides temporary immunity. *Compare* paratyphoid fever.

typhus (spotted fever) *n.* any one of a group of infections caused by *rickettsiae and characterized by severe headache, a widespread rash, prolonged high temperature, and delirium. They all respond to treatment with chloramphenicol or tetracyclines. *Epidemic typhus* (also known as *classic* or *louse-borne typhus*) is caused by infection with *Rickettsia prowazekii* transmitted by lice. It was formerly very prevalent in overcrowded unsanitary conditions (as during wars and famines), with a mortality rate approaching 100%. *Endemic typhus* (*murine* or *flea-borne typhus*) is a disease of rats due to *Rickettsia mooseri*; it can be transmitted to humans by rat fleas, causing a mild typhus fever. There are also several kinds of *tick typhus* (in which the rickettsiae are transmitted by ticks), including *Rocky Mountain spotted fever, and typhus transmitted by mites (*see* rickettsialpox, scrub typhus).

tyramine *n.* an amine naturally occurring in cheese. It has a similar effect in the body to that of *epinephrine. This effect can be dangerous in patients taking *MAO inhibitors (antidepressants), in whom blood pressure may become very high. Cheese is therefore not advised when such drugs are prescribed.

Tyroglyphus *n. see* Acarus.

tyrosine *n. see* amino acid.

tyrosinemia *n.* an *inborn error of metabolism in which there is build-up of the amino acid tyrosine in the body that in

severe cases may lead to liver failure.
Treatment consists of a diet low in tyrosine and *phenylalanine and high in vitamin C.

tyrosinosis *n.* an inborn defect of metabolism of the amino acid tyrosine causing excess excretion of parahydroxyphenylpyruvic acid in the urine, giving it abnormal reducing power.

U

ubiquinone *n.* a *coenzyme (formerly called *coenzyme Q*) that acts as an electron transfer agent in the mitochondria of cells (*see* electron transport chain).

UGH syndrome *uv*eitis associated with *glaucoma and *hyphema. This is an uncommon inflammatory condition occurring as a complication of intraocular lens *implants.

UICC Union international contre le cancer: an international body promoting cancer prevention and treatment. It produces respected texts on the most important types of cancer.

ulcer *n.* a break in the skin extending to all its layers, or in the mucous membrane lining the alimentary tract, that fails to heal and is often accompanied by inflammation. Of the many types of skin ulcer, the most common is the *venous* (or *hypostatic*) *ulcer* of the leg, known incorrectly as a *varicose ulcer*, which is caused by increased venous pressure and usually occurs in older women; *bedsores (decubitus ulcers), due to pressure; and ulcers due to malignant growth (*see* basal cell carcinoma). For ulcers of the alimentary tract, *see* aphtha, duodenal ulcer, gastric ulcer, peptic ulcer.

ulcerative colitis inflammation and ulceration of the colon and rectum. *See* colitis.

ulcerative gingivitis acute painful gingivitis with ulceration, in which the tissues of the gums are rapidly destroyed. Occurring mainly in debilitated patients, it is associated with anaerobic microorganisms (*see* Fusobacterium, Bacteroides) and is accompanied by an unpleasant odor. Treatment is with *metronidazole and a careful and thorough regimen of oral hygiene supplemented with oxidizing mouthwashes. In the past ulcerative

gingivitis has been called *Vincent's angina*; in its severe form it is known as *noma.

ule- (ulo-) *prefix denoting* **1.** scars; scar tissue. **2.** the gums.

ulna *n.* the inner and longer bone of the forearm (see illustration). It articulates with the humerus and radius above and with the radius and indirectly with the wrist bones below. At its upper end is the *olecranon process and *coronoid process; at the lower end is a coneshaped *styloid process*. —**ulnar** *adj.*

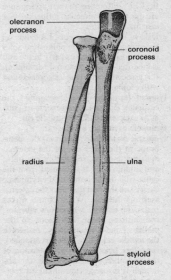

Right ulna and radius (front view)

ulnar artery a branch of the brachial artery arising at the elbow and running deep within the muscles of the medial side of the forearm. It passes into the palm of the hand, where it unites with the arch of the radial artery and gives off branches to the hand and fingers.

ulnar nerve one of the major nerves of the arm and forearm. It originates in the neck, from spinal roots of the last cervical and first thoracic divisions, and runs down the inner side of the arm to behind the elbow. In the forearm it supplies the muscles with motor nerves; lower it divides into several branches that supply the skin of the palm and fourth and fifth fingers.

ultra- *prefix denoting* **1.** beyond. **2.** an extreme degree (e.g. of large or small size).

ultracentrifuge *n.* a *centrifuge that works at extremely high speeds of rotation: used for separating large molecules, such as proteins.

ultradian *adj.* denoting a biological rhythm or cycle that occurs more frequently than once in 24 hours. *Compare* circadian, nyctohemeral.

ultrafiltration *n.* filtration under pressure. In the kidney, blood undergoes ultrafiltration to remove the unwanted water, urea, and other waste material that goes to make up urine.

ultramicroscope *n.* a microscope for examining particles suspended in a gas or liquid under intense illumination from one side. Light is scattered or reflected from the particles, which can be seen through the eyepiece as bright objects against a dark background.

ultramicrotome *n.* an instrument for cutting extremely thin sections of tissue (not more than 0.1 μm thick) for electron microscopy. *See also* microtome.

ultrasonics *n.* the study of the uses and properties of sound waves of very high frequency (*see* ultrasound). —**ultrasonic** *adj.*

ultrasonography (sonography) *n.* the use of *ultrasound to produce images of structures in the human body. The ultrasound probe sends out a short pulse of high-frequency sound and detects the reflected waves (echoes) occurring at interfaces within the organs. The direction of the pulse can then be moved across the area of interest with each pulse to build up a complete image. Scans may produce a single stationary image similar to a photograph (static) or multiple sequential images similar to a video (*real-time imaging). The ultrasound waves are transmitted from – and echoes detected by – piezoelectric crystals contained within the scanning probe (*see* transducer). As far as is known, there are no adverse effects from the use of ultrasound at diagnostic energies. Ultrasound waves are blocked by gas, as in the lungs and bowel, which can obscure underlying structures. The detail seen increases with the frequency of the ultra-

sound but the depth of penetration decreases. Ultrasonography is extensively used in obstetrics (for example, in the diagnosis of pregnancy, assessment of gestational age, diagnosis of *malpresentations and *hydatidiform moles, and detection of fetal abnormalities). It is also used to examine the abdominal organs, urinary tract, blood vessels, muscles, and tendons. More specialized techniques include *echocardiography, *transvaginal ultrasonography, *transrectal ultrasonography (TRUS), *intraoperative ultrasound (IOUS), endoscopic ultrasound, and transesophageal echocardiography examinations.

ultrasound (ultrasonic waves) *n.* sound waves of extremely high frequency (above 20,000 Hz), inaudible to the human ear. Ultrasound, usually in the range of 2–20 MHz, can be used to produce images of the interior of the human body, in the same way that X-rays can be used to build up pictures but with the advantages that the patient is not submitted to potentially harmful ionizing radiation and that structures not opaque to X-rays can be seen (*see* ultrasonography). The vibratory effect of these sound waves can also be used to break up stones in the kidney or elsewhere (*see* lithotripsy) and in the treatment of rheumatic conditions and cataract (*see* phacoemulsification). Ultrasonic instruments are used in dentistry to remove *calculus from the surfaces of teeth and to remove debris from the root canals of teeth in *root canal treatment.

ultrasound marker the appearance, on *ultrasound examination of a pregnant woman, of a particular physical abnormality in the fetus at a specific stage in fetal development. Such markers suggest the presence of specific chromosomal or developmental abnormalities. For example, the *nuchal marker* – a dark area in the neck region of the fetus – is one of the markers for Down's syndrome (*see* nuchal thickness scanning).

ultraviolet rays invisible short-wavelength radiation beyond the violet end of the visible spectrum. Sunlight contains ultraviolet rays, which are responsible for the production of both suntan and – on overexposure – sunburn. The dust and gases of the earth's atmosphere absorb most of the ultraviolet rays in sunlight (*see* ozone). If this did not happen, the intense ultraviolet radiation from the sun would be lethal to living organisms.

umbilical cord the strand of tissue connecting the fetus to the placenta. It contains two arteries that carry blood to the placenta and one vein that returns it to the fetus. It also contains remnants of the *allantois and *yolk sac and becomes ensheathed by the *amnion.

umbilical cord blood banked stem cells *stem cells collected from umbilical-cord blood at birth, which can be stored indefinitely and used if that particular baby or a blood-compatible sibling ever develops an illness (such as leukemia) that could be treated by cord-blood stem-cell transplantation. This facility is now available in the US and the UK.

umbilicus (omphalus) *n.* the navel: a circular depression in the center of the abdomen marking the site of attachment of the *umbilical cord in the fetus. —**umbilical** *adj.*

umbo *n.* a projecting center of a round surface, especially the projection of the inner surface of the eardrum to which the malleus is attached.

unciform bone *see* hamate bone.

uncinate seizure a form of temporal lobe *epilepsy in which hallucinations of taste and smell and inappropriate chewing movements are prominent features.

unconscious *adj.* **1.** in a state of unconsciousness. **2.** describing those mental processes of which a person is not aware. **3.** (in psychoanalysis) denoting the part of the mind that includes memories, motives, and intentions that are not accessible to awareness and cannot be made conscious without overcoming resistances. *Compare* subconscious.

unconsciousness *n.* a condition of being unaware of one's surroundings, as in sleep, or of being unresponsive to stimulation. An unnatural state of unconsciousness may be caused by factors that produce reduced brain activity, such as lack of oxygen, head injuries, poisoning, blood loss, and many diseases, or it may be brought about deliberately during general *anesthesia. *See also* coma.

uncus *n.* any hook-shaped structure, especially a projection of the lower surface of the cerebral hemisphere that is composed of cortex belonging to the temporal lobe.

undecylenic acid an antifungal agent, applied to the skin in the form of powder, ointment, lotion, or aerosol spray for the treatment of such infections as athlete's foot. Trade names: **Cruex**, **Desenex**.

undine *n.* a small rounded container, usually made of glass, for solutions used to wash out the eye. It has a small neck for filling and a long tapering spout with a narrow outlet to deliver a fine stream of fluid to the eye.

undulant fever *see* brucellosis.

ungual *adj.* relating to the fingernails or toenails (ungues).

unguentum (in pharmacy) *n.* an ointment.

unguis *n.* a fingernail or toenail. *See* nail.

uni- *prefix denoting* one.

unicellular *adj.* describing organisms or tissues that consist of a single cell. Unicellular organisms include the protozoans, most bacteria, and some fungi.

unilateral *adj.* (in anatomy) relating to or affecting one side of the body or one side of an organ or other part.

union *n.* (in a fractured bone) the successful result of healing of a fracture, in which the previously separated bone ends have become firmly united by newly formed bone. Failure of union (*nonunion*) may result if the bone ends are not immobilized or from infection or bone diseases. *Compare* malunion.

Union international contre le cancer *see* UICC.

unipolar *adj.* (in neurology) describing a neuron that has one main process extending from the cell body. *Compare* bipolar.

urachus *n.* the remains of the cavity of the *allantois, which usually disappears during embryonic development. In the adult it normally exists in the form of a solid fibrous cord connecting the bladder with the umbilicus, but it sometimes persists abnormally as a patent duct. —**urachal** *adj.*

uracil *n.* one of the nitrogen-containing bases (*see* pyrimidine) occurring in the nucleic acid RNA.

uracil mustard (uramustine) a *cytotoxic drug used in the treatment of various forms of cancer, particularly chronic lymphatic leukemia. It is administered orally and is highly toxic; common side effects are nausea, vomiting and diarrhea, and depression of bone marrow function.

uran- (urano-) *prefix denoting* the palate.

uraniscorrhaphy *n. see* staphylorrhaphy.

uratemia *n.* the presence in the blood of sodium urate and other urates, formed by the reaction of uric acid with bases. In *gout, uratemia leads to deposition of urates in various parts of the body.

uraturia *n.* the presence in the urine of urates (salts of uric acid). Abnormally high concentrations of urates in urine occur in *gout.

urea *n.* the main breakdown product of protein metabolism. It is the chemical form in which unrequired nitrogen is excreted by the body in the urine. Urea is formed in the liver from ammonia and carbon dioxide in a series of enzyme-mediated reactions (the *urea cycle*). Accumulation of urea in the bloodstream together with other nitrogenous compounds is due to kidney failure and gives rise to *uremia.

urease *n.* an enzyme that catalyses the hydrolysis of urea to ammonia and carbon dioxide.

urecchysis *n.* the escape of uric acid from the blood into spaces in the connective tissue.

uremia *n.* the presence of excessive amounts of urea and other nitrogenous waste compounds in the blood. These waste products are normally excreted by the kidneys in urine; their accumulation in the blood occurs in kidney failure and results in lethargy, drowsiness, nausea, vomiting, and eventually (if untreated) death. Treatment may require *hemodialysis on a kidney machine. —**uremic** *adj.*

ureter *n.* either of a pair of tubes, 25–30 cm long, that conduct urine from the pelvis of kidneys to the bladder. The walls of the ureters contain thick layers of smooth muscle, which contract to force urine into the bladder, between an outer fibrous coat and an inner mucous layer. —**ureteral, ureteric** *adj.*

ureter- (uretero-) *prefix denoting* the ureter or ureters. Example: *ureterovaginal* (relating to the ureters and vagina).

ureterectomy *n.* surgical removal of a ureter. This usually includes removal of the associated kidney as well (*see* nephroureterectomy). If previous nephrectomy has been performed to re-

move a kidney destroyed by *vesicoureteric reflux or because of a tumor of the renal pelvis, subsequent ureterectomy may be necessary to cure reflux into the stump of the ureter or tumor in the ureter, respectively.

ureteritis *n.* inflammation of the ureter. This usually occurs in association with inflammation of the bladder (*see* cystitis), particularly if caused by *vesicoureteric reflux. Tuberculosis of the urinary tract can also cause ureteritis, which progresses to *stricture formation.

ureterocele *n.* a cystic swelling of the wall of the ureter at the point where it passes into the bladder. It is associated with stenosis of the opening of the ureter and it may cause impaired drainage of the kidney with dilation of the ureter and *hydronephrosis. If urinary obstruction is present, the ureterocele should be dealt with surgically.

ureteroenterostomy *n.* an artificial communication, surgically created, between the ureter and the bowel. In this form of urinary diversion, which bypasses the bladder, the ureters are attached to the sigmoid colon (*see* ureterosigmoidostomy).

ureterolithotomy *n.* the surgical removal of a stone from the ureter (*see* calculus). The operative approach depends upon the position of the stone within the ureter. If the stone occupies the lower portion of the ureter, it may be extracted by *cystoscopy, thus avoiding open surgery.

ureterolysis *n.* an operation to free one or both ureters from surrounding fibrous tissue causing an obstruction.

ureteroneocystostomy *n.* the surgical reimplantation of a ureter into the bladder. This is most commonly performed to cure *vesicoureteric reflux. The ureter is reimplanted obliquely through the bladder wall to act as a valve and prevent subsequent reflux. The operation is usually referred to as an *antireflux procedure* or simply *reimplantation of ureter*.

ureteronephrectomy *n. see* nephroureterectomy.

ureteroplasty *n.* surgical reconstruction of the ureter using a segment of bowel or a tube of bladder (*see* Boari flap). This is necessary if a segment of ureter is damaged by disease or injury.

ureteropyelonephritis *n.* inflammation involving both the ureter and the renal pelvis (*see* ureteritis, pyelitis).

ureteroscope *n.* a rigid or flexible instrument that can be passed into the ureter and up into the pelvis of the kidney. It is most commonly used to visualize a stone in the ureter and remove it safely under direct vision with a stone basket or forceps. Larger stones need to be fragmented before removal with an ultrasound or *lithotripsy probe, lithoclast, or lasers. Ureteroscopy can also be used to visualize tumors in the ureter, and a flexible ureteroscope can be passed into the kidney to visualize and treat tumors or stones.

ureteroscopy *n.* the inspection of the lumen of the ureter with a *ureteroscope.

ureterosigmoidostomy *n.* the operation of implanting the ureters into the sigmoid colon (*see* ureteroenterostomy). This method of permanent urinary diversion may be used after *cystectomy or to bypass a diseased or damaged bladder. The urine is passed together with the feces, and continence depends upon a normal anal sphincter. The main advantage of this form of diversion is the avoidance of an external opening and appliance to collect the urine; the disadvantages include possible kidney infection and acidosis with long-term development of new tumors in 10% of cases.

ureterostomy *n.* the surgical creation of an external opening into the ureter. This usually involves bringing the ureter to the skin surface so that the urine can drain into a suitable appliance (*cutaneous ureterostomy*). The divided dilated ureter can be brought through the skin to form a spout, but ureters of a normal size need to be implanted into a segment of bowel used for this purpose (*see* ileal conduit) to avoid narrowing and obstruction.

ureterotomy *n.* surgical incision into the ureter. The most common reason for performing this incision is to allow removal of a stone (*see* ureterolithotomy).

urethr- (urethro-) *prefix denoting* the urethra.

urethra *n.* the tube that conducts urine from the bladder to the exterior. The female urethra is quite short (about 3.5 cm) and opens just within the *vulva, between the clitoris and vagina. The male urethra is longer (about 20 cm) and runs through the penis. As well as urine, it receives the secretions of the male accessory sex glands (prostate and Cowper's glands and seminal vesicles) and spermatozoa from the *vas deferens; thus, it also serves as the ejaculatory duct.

urethritis *n.* inflammation of the urethra. This may be due to gonorrhea (*specific urethritis*), another sexually transmitted infection, often infection with *Chlamydia trachomatis (nongonococcal urethritis*; or *nonspecific urethritis*), or to the presence of a catheter in the urethra. The symptoms are those of urethral discharge with painful or difficult urination (*dysuria). Treatment of urethritis is by administration of appropriate antibiotics after the causative organisms have been isolated from the discharge. Untreated or severe disease results in a urethral *stricture.

urethrocele *n.* prolapse of the urethra into the vaginal wall causing a bulbous swelling to appear in the vagina, particularly on straining. The condition is associated with previous childbirth. Treatment usually involves surgical repair of the lax tissues to give better support to the urethra and the vaginal wall.

urethrography *n.* a technique for X-ray examination of the urethra. *Contrast medium is introduced into the urethra so that its outline and any narrowing or other abnormalities may be observed in X-ray images (*urethrograms*). In *ascending urethrography* contrast medium is injected up the urethra using a special syringe and penile clamp. In *descending urethrography* (or *micturating cystourethrography*, *MCU*), X-rays of the urethra can be taken during the passing of water-soluble contrast material previously inserted into the bladder in order to demonstrate disorders of micturition, particularly bladder emptying.

urethroplasty *n.* surgical repair of the urethra, especially a urethral *stricture. The operation entails the insertion of a flap or patch of skin from the scrotum or perineum into the urethra at the site of the stricture, which is laid widely open. The operation can be performed in one stage, although two stages are usual in the reconstruction of a posterior urethral stricture (*see* urethrostomy). *Transpubic urethroplasty* is performed to repair a ruptured posterior urethra following a fractured pelvis. Access to the damaged urethra is achieved by partial removal of the pubic bone.

urethrorrhaphy *n.* surgical restoration of the continuity of the urethra. This may be required following laceration of the urethra.

urethrorrhea *n.* a discharge from the urethra. This is a symptom of *urethritis.

urethroscope *n.* an *endoscope, consisting of a fine tube fitted with a light and lenses, for examination of the interior of the male urethra, including the prostate region. —**urethroscopy** *n.*

urethrostenosis *n.* a *stricture of the urethra.

urethrostomy *n.* the operation of creating an opening of the urethra in the perineum in men. This can be permanent, to bypass a severe *stricture of the urethra in the penis, or it can form the first stage of an operation to cure a stricture of the posterior section of the urethra (*urethroplasty).

urethrotomy *n.* the operation of cutting a *stricture in the urethra. It is usually performed with a *urethrotome*. This instrument, a type of *endoscope, consists of a sheath down which is passed a fine knife, which is operated by the surgeon viewing the stricture down an illuminated telescope.

urgency *n.* a *lower urinary tract symptom in which there is a desire to pass urine urgently; this may or may not be associated with incontinence (urge incontinence).

-uria *suffix denoting* **1.** a condition of urine or urination. Example: *polyuria* (passage of excess urine). **2.** the presence of a specified substance in the urine. Example: *hematuria* (blood in).

uric acid a nitrogen-containing organic acid that is the end product of nucleic acid metabolism and is a component of the urine. Crystals of uric acid are deposited in the joints of people with *gout.

uricosuric drug a drug, such as *probenecid or *sulfinpyrazone, that increases the amount of *uric acid excreted in the urine. Uricosuric drugs are used to treat gout and other conditions in which the levels of uric acid in the blood are increased, as during treatment with some *diuretics. Uricosuric drugs are sometimes administered with certain antibiotics (such as penicillin) to maintain high blood levels of the antibiotic, since uricosuric drugs block their excretion.

uridine *n.* a compound containing uracil and the sugar ribose. *See also* nucleoside.

uridrosis *n.* the presence of excessive amounts of urea in the sweat; when the sweat dries, a white flaky deposit of urea may remain on the skin. The phenomenon occurs in *uremia.

urin- (urino-, uro-) *prefix denoting* urine or the urinary system.

urinalysis *n.* the analysis of *urine, using physical, chemical, and microscopical tests, to determine the proportions of its normal constituents and to detect alcohol, drugs, sugar, or other abnormal constituents.

urinary bladder *see* bladder.

urinary diversion any of various techniques for the collection and diversion of urine away from its usual excretory channels, after the bladder has been removed (*see* cystectomy) or bypassed. These techniques include *ureterosigmoidostomy and the construction of an *ileal conduit. *Continent diversion*, usually after cystectomy, may be achieved by constructing a reservoir or pouch from a section of small or large intestine or a combination of both. This can be emptied by catheterization via a small *stoma and has the advantage over an ileal conduit in that a urinary drainage bag is not required.

urinary tract the entire system of ducts and channels that conduct urine from the kidneys to the exterior. It includes the ureters, the bladder, and the urethra.

urination (micturition) *n.* the periodic discharge of urine from the bladder through the urethra. It is initiated by voluntary relaxation of the sphincter muscle below the bladder and maintained by reflex contraction of the muscles of the bladder wall. *See also* incontinence.

urine *n.* the fluid excreted by the kidneys, which contains many of the body's waste products. It is the major route by which the end products of nitrogen metabolism – *urea, *uric acid, and *creatinine – are excreted. The other major constituent is sodium chloride. Over 100 other substances are usually present, but only in trace amounts. Analysis of urine (*see* urinalysis) is commonly used in the diagnosis of diseases (for example, there are high levels of urinary glucose in diabetes and of ketone bodies in ketonuria); immunological analysis of urine is the basis of most *pregnancy tests.

uriniferous tubule *see* renal tubule.

urinogenital *adj. see* urogenital.

urinometer *n.* a hydrometer for measuring the specific gravity of urine.

urobilinogen *n.* a colorless product of the reduction of the *bile pigment bilirubin. Urobilinogen is formed from bilirubin in the intestine by bacterial action. Part of it is reabsorbed and returned to the liver; part of it is excreted in the feces (a trace may also appear in the urine). When exposed to air, urobilinogen is oxidized to a brown pigment, *urobilin*.

urocele *n.* a cystic swelling in the scrotum, containing urine that has escaped from the urethra. This may arise following urethral injury. Immediate treatment is to divert the urine by suprapubic *cystotomy, local drainage of the swelling, and antibiotic administration.

urochezia *n.* the passage of urine through the rectum. This may follow a penetrating injury involving both the lower urinary tract and the bowel.

urodynamics *n.* the recording of pressures within the bladder by the use of special equipment that can also record urethral sphincter pressures. Simultaneously, abdominal pressure is usually recorded with a catheter in the rectum, vagina, or ileal conduit. It is an essential investigation in the study of urinary incontinence. In some men, urodynamic studies are necessary to determine if their *lower urinary tract symptoms are caused by bladder outflow obstruction or *detrusor instability.

urogenital (urinogenital) *adj.* of or relating to the organs and tissues concerned with excretion and reproduction, which are anatomically closely associated.

urogenital sinus the duct in the embryo that receives the ureter and mesonephric and paramesonephric ducts and opens to the exterior. The innermost portion forms most of the bladder and the remainder forms the urethra with its asso-

ciated glands. Part of it may also contribute to the vagina.

urogram *n.* an X-ray of the urinary tract or any part of it. It is usually obtained after the intravenous injection of a radio-opaque substance, as in an *intravenous urogram, but the contrast medium can also be introduced percutaneously or, in the case of the bladder, transurethrally (for a *cystogram*; *see* cystography).

urography *n.* radiological examination of the urinary tract or any part of it after the introduction of a contrast medium. *See* cystography, pyelography, urethrography.

urokinase *n.* an enzyme produced in the kidney and also present in blood and urine that is capable of breaking up blood clots (*see* thrombolysis). It activates *plasminogen directly to plasmin, which dissolves fibrin thrombi. It is produced by tissue culture techniques for clinical use. When injected, it has a short half-life, which makes it more useful in certain cases. It is used in the treatment of pulmonary embolism, deep vein thrombosis, acute myocardial infarction, and other causes of thrombosis. *See also* plasminogen activator. Trade name: **Abbokinase**.

urolith *n.* a stone in the urinary tract. *See* calculus.

urology *n.* the branch of medicine concerned with the study and treatment of diseases of the urinary tract. —**urological** *adj.* —**urologist** *n.*

uroporphyrin *n.* a porphyrin that plays an intermediate role in the synthesis of *protoporphyrin IX. It is excreted in significant amounts in the urine in porphyria.

ursodiol *n.* a drug (a *bile acid) used to dissolve cholesterol gallstones; it is administered by mouth. Side effects are infrequent but include diarrhea and indigestion. Trade name: **Actigall**.

urticaria (hives, nettle rash) *n.* an acute or chronic allergic reaction, resulting from the release of *histamine by *mast cells, in which red round wheals develop on the skin, ranging in size from small spots to several inches across. These itch intensely and may last for hours or days; the cause is sensitivity to certain foods, such as shellfish or strawberries, or other allergens. Sometimes urticaria may affect areas other than the skin, causing swelling on the tongue and lips: this serious variety, *angioedema*, needs urgent medical attention. Urticaria can be prevented by taking antihistamines regularly. *Cholinergic urticaria* is a condition in which very small wheals are brought on by heat, exercise, or emotion.

USAN United States Adopted Name: the US generic name for any compound to be used as a drug. The names are determined by the USAN Council, which works in conjunction with the pharmaceutical manufacturers of the drugs, and then submitted to the World Health Organization for designation of an *INN.

United States Public Health Service (USPHS) *see* Public Health Service.

unsaturated fatty acid a *fatty acid in which one (*monounsaturated*) or many (*polyunsaturated*) of the carbon atoms are linked by double bonds that are easily split in chemical reactions so that other substances can connect to them. These fats occur in fish and plant-derived foods, and a diet high in unsaturated fats is associated with low serum cholesterol levels. *Compare* saturated fatty acid.

USP *United States Pharmacopeia*: a compendium of pharmaceutical preparations, published by the United States Pharmacopeia Convention, that contains descriptions, uses, dosage information, and other information for nearly four thousand drugs, as well as dietary supplements and other health care products. The *USP* establishes state-of-the-art standards to ensure the quality of pharmaceuticals for human and veterinary use.

USPHS *see* (United States) Public Health Service.

uter- (utero-) *prefix denoting* the uterus. Examples: *uterocervical* (relating to the cervix (neck) of the uterus); *uterovaginal* (relating to the uterus and vagina); *uterovesical* (relating to the uterus and bladder).

uterine *adj.* of or relating to the uterus.

uterography *n.* *radiography of the uterus.

utero-ovarian *adj.* relating to or occurring in the uterus and an ovary.

uterosalpingography (hysterosalpingography) *n.* *radiography of the interior of the uterus and the fallopian tubes following injection of a *radiopaque fluid.

uterus (womb) *n.* the part of the female reproductive tract that is specialized to allow the embryo to become implanted in its inner wall and to nourish the growing fetus from the maternal blood. The nonpregnant uterus is a pear-shaped organ, about 7.5 cm long. It is suspended in the pelvic cavity by means of peritoneal folds (ligaments) and fibrous bands. The upper part is connected to the two *fallopian tubes and the lower part joins the vagina at the cervix. The uterus has an inner mucous lining (*see* endometrium) and a thick muscular wall (*myometrium). During childbirth, the myometrium undergoes strong contractions to expel the fetus through the cervix and vagina. In the absence of pregnancy the endometrium undergoes periodic development and degeneration (*see* menstrual cycle). —**uterine** *adj.*

uterus didelphys (double uterus) a congenital condition that results from incomplete midline fusion of the two *paramesonephric (Müllerian) ducts during early embryonic development. The usual result is a double uterus with one or two cervices and a single vagina. Complete failure of fusion results in a double uterus with double cervices and two separate vaginas.

utricle (utriculus) *n.* **1.** the larger of the two membranous sacs within the vestibule of the ear: it forms part of the membranous *labyrinth. It is filled with fluid (endolymph) and contains a *macula. This responds to gravity and relays information to the brain about the position of the head. **2.** a small sac (the *prostatic utricle*) extending out of the urethra of the male into the substance of the prostate gland.

uvea (uveal tract) *n.* the vascular pigmented layer of the eye, which lies beneath the outer layer (sclera). It consists of the *choroid, *ciliary body, and *iris. —**uveal** *adj.*

uveal tract *see* uvea.

uveitis *n.* inflammation of any part of the uveal tract of the eye, either the iris (*iritis*), ciliary body (*cyclitis*), or choroid (*choroiditis*). Inflammation confined to the iris and ciliary body, which are commonly inflamed together, is called *anterior uveitis* or *iridocyclitis* (*see also* Fuchs' heterochromic cyclitis); that confined to the choroid is termed *posterior* *uveitis.* In general, the causes of anterior and posterior uveitis are different; anterior uveitis (unlike choroiditis) usually is painful, with clusters of inflammatory cells (keratic precipitates) adhering to the inner surface of the cornea. All types may lead to visual impairment, and uveitis is an important cause of blindness. In most cases the disease appears to originate in the uveal tract itself, but it may occur secondarily to disease of other parts of the eye, particularly of the cornea and sclera.

Treatment consists of the use of drugs that suppress the inflammation, combined with measures to relieve the discomfort and more specific drug treatment if a specific cause of the uveitis is found. The drugs may be given as drops, injections, or tablets, often in combination.

uveoparotitis (uveoparotid fever) *n.* inflammation of the iris, ciliary body, and choroid regions of the eye (the uvea) and swelling of the parotid salivary gland: one of the more common varieties of the chronic disease *sarcoidosis.

uvula *n.* a small soft extension of the soft palate that hangs from the roof of the mouth above the root of the tongue. It is composed of muscle, connective tissue, and mucous membrane.

uvulectomy (staphylectomy) *n.* surgical removal of the uvula.

uvulitis *n.* inflammation of the uvula.

uvulopalatopharyngoplasty *n.* a surgical operation to remove the uvula, part of the soft palate, and the tonsils in the treatment of snoring and obstructive *sleep apnea.

V

VAC a *cytotoxic drug regimen that includes *vincristine, *dactinomycin, and *cyclophosphamide.

vaccination *n.* a means of producing immunity to a disease by using a *vaccine, or a special preparation of antigenic material, to stimulate the formation of appropriate antibodies. The name was applied originally only to treatment with vaccinia (cowpox) virus, which gives protection not only against cowpox itself but also against the related smallpox. However, it is now used synonymously with *inoculation* as a method of *immunization against any disease. Vaccination is often carried out in two or three stages, because separate doses are less likely to cause unpleasant side effects. A vaccine is usually given by injection but may be introduced into the skin through light scratches; for some diseases (such as polio), oral vaccines are available.

vaccine *n.* a special preparation of antigenic material that can be used to stimulate the development of antibodies and thus confer active *immunity against a specific disease or number of diseases. Many vaccines are produced by culturing bacteria or viruses under conditions that lead to a loss of their virulence but not of their antigenic nature. Other vaccines consist of specially treated toxins (*toxoids) or of dead bacteria that are still antigenic. Examples of live but attenuated (weakened) organisms in vaccines are those against tuberculosis, rabies, smallpox, and influenza (in the form of a nasally administered vaccine, FluMist). Dead organisms are used against cholera and typhoid; precipitated toxoids are used against diphtheria and tetanus. *See* immunization.

vaccinia *n. see* cowpox.

vaccinoid *adj.* resembling a local infection with vaccinia (cowpox) virus.

vacuole *n.* a space within the cytoplasm of a cell, formed by infolding of the cell membrane, that contains material taken in by the cell. White blood cells form vacuoles when they surround and digest bacteria and other foreign material.

vacuum extractor (ventouse) a suction cup that can be attached to the head of a fetus and then steadily pulled, in order to aid delivery.

vagin- (vagino-) *prefix denoting* the vagina.

vagina *n.* the lower part of the female reproductive tract: a muscular tube, lined with mucous membrane, connecting the cervix of the uterus to the exterior. It receives the erect penis during coitus: semen is ejaculated into the upper part of the vagina and from there the sperm must pass through the cervix and uterus in order to fertilize an ovum in the fallopian tube. The wall of the vagina is sufficiently elastic to allow the passage of the newborn child. —**vaginal** *adj.*

vaginismus *n.* sudden and painful contraction of the muscles surrounding the vagina, usually in response to the *vulva or vagina being touched. Sexual intercourse may be impeded, and the condition may be associated with fear of or aversion to coitus. Other causative factors include vaginal injury or ulceration, dryness or shrinkage of the lining membrane of the vagina, and inflammation of the vagina or bladder. *See also* dyspareunia.

vaginitis *n.* inflammation of the vagina, which may be caused by infection (commonly with *Trichomonas vaginalis*), dietary deficiency, or poor hygiene. There is often itching (*see* pruritus), increased vaginal discharge, and pain on passing urine. Vaginitis may indicate the presence of sexually transmitted disease. *Postmenopausal* (or *atrophic*) *vaginitis* is caused by a deficiency of female sex hormones.

vaginoplasty (colpoplasty) *n.* a tissue-grafting operation on the vagina.

vaginoscope *n. see* colposcope.

vago- *prefix denoting* the vagus nerve.

vagotomy *n.* the surgical cutting of any of the branches of the vagus nerve. This is usually performed to reduce secretion of acid and pepsin by the stomach in order to cure a peptic ulcer. *Truncal vagotomy* is the cutting of the main trunks of the vagus nerve; in *selective vagotomy* the branches of the nerve to the gallbladder and pancreas are left intact. *Highly selective* or *proximal vagotomy* is the cutting of the branches of the vagus nerve to the body of the stomach, leaving the branches to the outlet (pylorus) intact: this makes additional surgery to permit emptying of the stomach contents unnecessary. Following surgery, patients may experience *postvagotomy diarrhea* after a meal (*compare* dumping syndrome).

vagus nerve the tenth *cranial nerve (X), which supplies motor nerve fibers to the muscles of swallowing and parasympathetic fibers to the heart and organs of the chest cavity and abdomen. Sensory branches of the vagus carry impulses from the viscera and the sensation of taste from the mouth.

valacyclovir *n.* an antiviral drug used to treat genital herpes and shingles. Like acyclovir, it is a *DNA polymerase inhibitor. Trade name: **Valtrex**.

valgus *adj.* describing any deformity that displaces the hand or foot away from the midline. *See* clubfoot (talipes valgus), hallux valgus, knock knee (genu valgum). *Compare* varus.

validity *n.* an indication of the extent to which a clinical sign or test is a true indicator of disease. Reduced validity can arise if the tests produce different results when conducted several times on the same person under identical conditions (i.e. *reduced reproducibility, reliability*, or *repeatability*). This may be because the same observer gets different results on successive occasions (*intraobserver error*) or because a series of different observers fail to obtain the same result (*interobserver error*). Such errors may arise because of a true difference in observation and/or interpretation or because of a preconceived notion (often unconscious) by the observer, which influences either his judgment or the tone and manner with which he questions the patient. *Compare* intervention study.

valine *n.* an *essential amino acid. *See also* amino acid.

Valium *n. see* diazepam.

vallecula *n.* a furrow or depression in an organ or other part. On the undersurface of the cerebellum a vallecula separates the two hemispheres.

valproic acid an *anticonvulsant drug used for the treatment of simple and complex absence seizures and in combination therapy for multiple seizure types. It is administered by mouth; side effects include sedation, nausea, and vomiting. Trade name: **Depakene**.

Valsalva maneuver any forced exhalation or straining against a closed airway, such as exhaling with the mouth and nostrils closed to clear the ears and to test the patency of the *eustachian tube. This action increases the pressure in the eustachian tube and middle ear, causing the *tympanic membrane to move outward so that the subject hears a popping sound. [A. M. Valsalva (1666–1723), Italian anatomist]

valsartan *n. see* angiotensin II antagonist.

valve *n.* a structure found in some tubular organs or parts that restricts the flow of fluid within them to one direction only. Valves are important structures in the heart, veins, and lymphatic vessels. Such a valve consists of two or three *cusps fastened like pockets to the walls of the vessel. Blood flowing in the correct direction flattens the cusps to the walls, but when flow is reversed the cusps become filled with blood or lymph and dilate to block the opening (see illustration). *See also* mitral valve, tricuspid valve, semilunar valve.

(A)

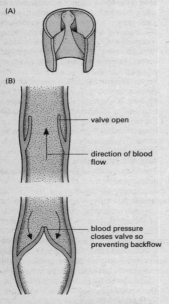

(B)

valve open

direction of blood flow

blood pressure closes valve so preventing backflow

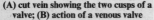

(A) cut vein showing the two cusps of a valve; (B) action of a venous valve

valvotomy (valvulotomy) *n.* surgical cutting through a valve. The term is usually used to describe the operation to relieve obstruction caused by stenosed valves in the heart. In *percutaneous balloon valvotomy* the narrowed valves are opened up by *balloon dilation, the balloon being introduced on a catheter passed up a great vessel.

valvula *n.* (*pl.* **valvulae**) a small valve. The *valvulae conniventes* are circular folds of mucous membrane in the small intestine.

valvulitis *n.* inflammation of one or more valves, particularly the heart valves.

Valvulitis may be acute or chronic and is most often due to rheumatic fever (*see* endocarditis).

valvuloplasty *n.* the surgical reconstruction of a heart valve affected by stenosis or incompetence.

vancomycin *n.* an *antibiotic, derived from the bacterium *Streptomyces orientalis*, that is effective against most gram-positive organisms (e.g. streptococci and staphylococci). It is given by intravenous infusion for infections (including endocarditis) due to strains that are resistant to other antibiotics. It usually has a low toxicity but may cause deafness and blood disorders. Trade names: **Vancocin**, **Vancoled**.

van den Bergh's test a test to determine whether excess bilirubin in the blood is conjugated or unconjugated, and therefore whether jaundice in a patient is due to *hemolysis or to disease of the liver or bile duct. A sample of serum is mixed with sulfanilic acid, hydrochloric acid, and sodium nitrite. The immediate appearance of a violet color is called a *direct reaction* and indicates that the jaundice is due to liver damage or obstruction of the bile duct. If the color appears only when alcohol is added, this is an *indirect reaction* and points to hemolytic jaundice or a congenital unconjugated hyperbilirubinemia (*see* Gilbert's syndrome). [A. A. H. van den Bergh (1869–1943), Dutch physician]

vanillylmandelic acid (VMA) a metabolite of *catecholamines excreted in abnormal amounts in the urine in conditions of excess catecholamine production, such as *pheochromocytoma. The measurement of VMA levels in a 24-hour urine sample is still used as a screening test for this condition, although this is being replaced by the direct measurement of urinary catecholamines. Urinary levels may be misleadingly high if foodstuffs with vanillin or the drug levodopa are taken before the test.

vaporizer *n.* a piece of equipment for producing an extremely fine mist of liquid droplets by forcing a jet of liquid through a narrow nozzle with a jet of air. Vaporizers are used to produce aerosols of various medications for use in inhalation therapy.

Vaquez-Osler disease *see* polycythemia vera. [L. H. Vaquez (1860–1936), French physician; Sir W. Osler (1849–1919), Canadian physician]

variable *n.* (in biostatistics) a characteristic (e.g. morbidity, life style, or habit) relating to a single individual or group. *Qualitative variables* are descriptive characteristics, such as sex, race, or occupation; *quantitative variables* relate to a numerical scale and are subdivided into *discrete variables*, found only at fixed points (e.g. number of children), and *continuous variables*, found at any point on a scale (e.g. weight).

variance *n.* *see* standard deviation.

varicectomy *n.* *see* phlebectomy.

varicella *n.* *see* chickenpox.

varices *pl. n.* *see* varicose veins.

varicocele *n.* a collection of dilated veins in the spermatic cord, more commonly affecting the left side of the scrotum than the right. It usually produces no symptoms apart from occasional aching discomfort. In some cases varicocele is associated with a poor sperm count (*see* oligospermia) sufficient to cause infertility. Surgical correction or radiological embolization of the varicocele in such patients (*varicocelectomy*) usually results in a considerable improvement in the quality and motility of the sperm, but may or may not improve the number of pregnancies and live births thereafter.

varicose veins veins that are distended, lengthened, and tortuous. The superficial veins (saphenous veins) of the legs are most commonly affected; other sites include the esophagus (*esophageal varices) and testes (*varicocele). There is an inherited tendency to varicose veins but obstruction to blood flow is responsible in some cases. Complications including thrombosis, *phlebitis, and hemorrhage may occur. Treatment includes elastic support and *sclerotherapy, but *avulsion (stripping) or excision (*phlebectomy) is required in some cases. Medical name: **varices**.

varicotomy *n.* incision into a varicose vein (*see* phlebectomy).

variola *n.* *see* smallpox.

varioloid 1. *n.* before smallpox was eradicated, a mild form of the disease in people who had previously had smallpox or had been vaccinated against it. **2.** *adj.* resembling smallpox.

varix *n.* (*pl.* **varices**) a single *varicose vein.

varus *adj.* describing any deformity that displaces the hand or foot toward the midline. *See* bowlegs (genu varum), clubfoot (talipes varus), hallux varus. *Compare* valgus.

vas *n.* (*pl.* **vasa**) a vessel or duct.

vas- (vaso-) *prefix denoting* **1.** vessels, especially blood vessels. **2.** the vas deferens.

vasa efferentia (*sing.* **vas efferens**) the many small tubes that conduct spermatozoa from the testis to the epididymis. They are derived from some of the excretory tubules of the *mesonephros.

vasa vasorum *pl. n.* the tiny arteries and veins that supply the walls of blood vessels.

vascular *adj.* relating to or supplied with blood vessels.

vascularization *n.* the development of blood vessels (usually capillaries) within a tissue.

vascular system *see* cardiovascular system.

vasculitis *n.* *see* angiitis.

vas deferens (*pl.* **vasa deferentia**) either of a pair of ducts that conduct spermatozoa from the *epididymis to the *urethra on ejaculation. It has a thick muscular wall, the contraction of which assists in ejaculation.

vasectomy *n.* the surgical operation of severing the duct (vas deferens) connecting the testis to the seminal vesicle and urethra. Vasectomy of both ducts causes sterility and is an increasingly popular means of birth control. Vasectomy does not affect sexual desire or potency.

vaso- *prefix. see* vas-.

vasoactive *adj.* affecting the diameter of blood vessels, especially arteries. Examples of vasoactive agents are emotion, pressure, carbon dioxide, and temperature. Some exert their effect directly, others via the *vasomotor center in the brain.

vasoactive intestinal peptide *see* VIP.

vasoconstriction *n.* a decrease in the diameter of blood vessels, especially the arteries. This results from activation of the *vasomotor center in the brain, which brings about contraction of the muscular walls of the arteries and hence an increase in blood pressure.

vasoconstrictor *n.* an agent that causes narrowing of the blood vessels and thus a decrease in blood flow. Examples are *metaraminol, *methoxamine, and *phenylephrine. Vasoconstrictors are used to raise the blood pressure in disorders of circulation, shock, or severe bleeding and to maintain blood pressure during surgery. Some vasoconstrictors (e.g. *xylometazoline) have a rapid effect when applied to mucous membranes and may be used to relieve nasal congestion. If blood pressure rises too quickly, headache and vomiting may occur. A vasoconstrictor is often added to local anesthetic solutions used in dentistry to prolong their effectiveness.

vasodilation n. an increase in the diameter of blood vessels, especially arteries. This results from activation of the *vasomotor center in the brain, which brings about relaxation of the arterial walls and a consequent lowering of blood pressure.

vasodilator n. a drug that causes widening of the blood vessels and therefore an increase in blood flow. Vasodilators are used to lower blood pressure in cases of hypertension. *Coronary vasodilators*, such as *nitroglycerin and *pentaerythritol, increase the blood flow through the heart and are used to relieve and prevent angina. Large doses of coronary vasodilators cause such side effects as flushing of the face, severe headache, and fainting. *Peripheral vasodilators*, such as *alpha blockers and *cyclandelate, affect the blood vessels of the limbs and are used to treat conditions of poor circulation, such as acrocyanosis, chilblains, and Raynaud's disease.

vasoepididymostomy n. the operation of joining the vas deferens to the epididymis in a side-to-side manner in order to bypass an obstruction to the passage of sperm from the testis. The obstruction, which may be congenital or acquired, is usually present in the midportion or tail of the epididymis. Vasoepididymostomy is therefore usually performed by anastomosing the head of the epididymis to a longitudinal incision in the lumen of the adjacent vas.

vasography n. X-ray imaging of the vas deferens. A *contrast medium is injected either into the exposed vas deferens at surgery, using a fine needle, or by inserting a catheter into the ejaculatory duct (which discharges semen from the vesicle into the vas deferens) via an *endoscope. The technique is used in the investigation of *azoospermia to look for blockages in the vas.

vasoligation n. the surgical tying of the vas deferens (the duct conveying sperm from the testis). This is performed to prevent infection spreading from the urinary tract and causing recurrent *epididymitis. It is sometimes performed at the time of *prostatectomy to prevent the complication of epididymitis in the postoperative period.

vasomotion n. an increase or decrease in the diameter of blood vessels, particularly the arteries. *See* vasoconstriction, vasodilation.

vasomotor adj. controlling the muscular walls of blood vessels, especially arteries, and therefore their diameter.

vasomotor center a collection of nerve cells in the medulla oblongata that receives information from sensory receptors in the circulatory system (*see* baroreceptor) and brings about reflex changes in the rate of the heartbeat and in the diameter of blood vessels, so that blood pressure can be adjusted. The vasomotor center also receives impulses from elsewhere in the brain, so that emotion (such as fear) may also influence the heart rate and blood pressure. The center works through *vasomotor nerves of the sympathetic and parasympathetic systems.

vasomotor nerve any nerve, usually belonging to the autonomic nervous system, that controls the circulation of blood through blood vessels by its action on the muscle fibers within their walls or its action on the heartbeat. The *vagus nerve slows the heart and reduces its output, but sympathetic nerves increase the rate and output of the heart and increase blood pressure by causing the constriction of small blood vessels at the same time.

vasomotor symptoms subjective sensations experienced by women around the time of the *menopause, often described as explosions of heat, mostly followed by profuse sweating and sometimes preceded by an undetermined sensation with waking at night. Objective signs are sudden reddening of the skin on the head, neck, and chest and profuse sweating. Physiological changes include peripheral vasodilation, *tachycardia with normal blood pressure, and raised skin temperature with normal body temperature.

vasopressin (antidiuretic hormone, ADH) *n.* a hormone, released by the pituitary gland, that increases the reabsorption of water by the kidney, thus preventing excessive loss of water from the body. Vasopressin also causes constriction of blood vessels. It is administered by injection to treat *diabetes insipidus and *esophageal varices and for the prevention and treatment of postoperative abdominal distension. Trade name: **Pitressin**.

vasopressor *adj.* stimulating the contraction of blood vessels and therefore bringing about an increase in blood pressure.

vasospasm *n. see* Raynaud's disease.

vasotomy *n.* a surgical incision into the vas deferens (the duct conveying sperm from the testis). This is usually undertaken to allow catheterization of the vas and the injection of radiopaque contrast material for X-ray examination (*see* vasography), to test for patency of the duct in patients with *azoospermia.

vasovagal *adj.* relating to the action of impulses in the *vagus nerve on the circulation. The vagus reduces the rate at which the heart beats, and so lowers its output.

vasovagal attack excessive activity of the vagus nerve, causing slowing of the heart and a fall in blood pressure, which leads to fainting. *See* syncope.

vasovasostomy *n.* the surgical operation of reanastomosing the vas deferens after previous vasectomy: the reversal of vasectomy, undertaken to restore fertility.

vasovesiculitis *n.* inflammation of the *seminal vesicles and *vas deferens. This usually occurs in association with *prostatitis and causes pain in the perineum, groin, and scrotum and a high temperature. On examination, the vasa and seminal vesicles are thickened and tender. Treatment includes administration of antibiotics.

vastus *n.* any of three muscles (*vastus intermedius*, *vastus lateralis*, and *vastus medialis*) that form part of the *quadriceps muscle of the thigh.

vector *n.* **1.** an animal, usually an insect or a tick, that transmits parasitic microorganisms – and therefore the diseases they cause – from person to person or from infected animals to human beings. Mosquitoes, for example, are vectors of malaria, filariasis, and yellow fever. **2.** an agent used to insert a foreign gene or DNA fragment into a bacterial or other cell in *genetic engineering and *gene therapy. Viruses, especially retroviruses, are often used as vectors: once inside the host cell, the virus can replicate and thus produce copies (*clones) of the gene.

vectorcardiography *n. see* electrocardiography.

vegetation *n.* (in pathology) an abnormal outgrowth from a membrane, fancied to resemble a vegetable growth. In ulcerative endocarditis, such outgrowths, consisting of *fibrin with enmeshed blood cells, are found on the membrane lining the heart valves.

vegetative *adj.* **1.** relating to growth and nutrition rather than to reproduction. **2.** functioning unconsciously; autonomic.

vehicle *n.* (in pharmacy) any substance that acts as the medium in which a drug is administered. Examples are sterile water, isotonic sodium chloride, and dextrose solutions.

vein *n.* a blood vessel conveying blood toward the heart (the principal veins are illustrated overleaf). All veins except the *pulmonary vein carry deoxygenated blood from the tissues, via the capillaries, to the vena cava. The walls of veins consist of three tissue layers, but these are much thinner and less elastic than those of arteries (see illustration). Veins contain *valves that assist the flow of blood back to the heart. Anatomical name: **vena**. —**venous** *adj.*

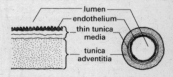

Transverse section through a vein

velamen (velamentum) *n.* a covering membrane.

vellus *n.* the fine hair that occurs on the body before puberty is reached.

velum *n.* (in anatomy) a veillike covering. The *medullary velum* is either of two thin layers of tissue that form part of the roof of the fourth ventricle of the brain.

vena *n.* (*pl.* **venae**) *see* **vein**.
vena cava (*pl.* **venae cavae**) either of the two main veins conveying deoxygenated blood from the other veins to the right atrium of the heart. The *inferior vena cava*, formed by the union of the right and left common iliac veins, receives blood from parts of the body below the diaphragm. The *superior vena cava*, originating at the junction of the two bra-

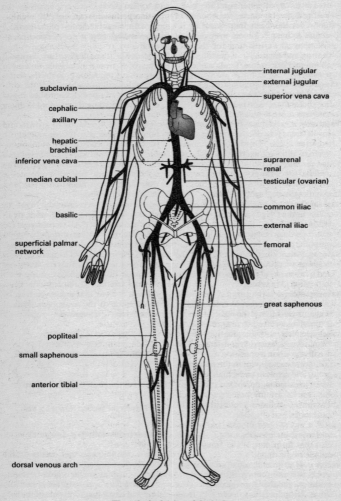

internal jugular
external jugular
superior vena cava

subclavian
cephalic
axillary
hepatic
brachial
inferior vena cava
median cubital

suprarenal
renal
testicular (ovarian)

basilic

common iliac
external iliac
femoral

superficial palmar
network

great saphenous

popliteal
small saphenous

anterior tibial

dorsal venous arch

The principal veins of the body

chiocephalic veins, drains blood from the head, neck, thorax, and arms.

vene- (veno-) *prefix denoting* veins.

veneer *n.* a facing of *composite resin or *porcelain applied to the surface of a tooth to give improved shape and/or color. The tooth requires minimal preparation and the facing is retained by enamel that has been treated by the *acid-etch technique. Veneers are a more conservative way of treating discolored teeth than by *crowns.

venene *n.* a mixture of two or more *venoms: used to produce antiserum against venoms (*antivenene*).

venereal disease (VD) *see* sexually transmitted disease.

venesection *n. see* phlebotomy.

venipuncture (venepuncture) *n.* the puncture of a vein for any therapeutic purpose, for example, to extract blood for laboratory tests. *See also* phlebotomy.

veno- *prefix. see* vene-.

venoclysis *n.* the continuous infusion into a vein of saline or other solution.

venography (phlebography) *n.* imaging of veins in a particular region of the body. Traditionally, a *radiopaque contrast medium is injected slowly into a vein and X-ray photographs (*venograms*) taken as the compound is carried toward the heart. Damage, obstruction, or abnormal communication with other vessels will be seen where the medium does not fill the vein properly or apparently leaks from it. A common usage is in demonstrating deep vein *thrombosis in the legs. Increasingly ultrasound is now used in imaging the veins, both with color Doppler venography (*see* Doppler ultrasound) and *compression venography. *See also* angiography.

venom *n.* the poisonous material produced by snakes, scorpions, spiders, and other animals for injecting into their prey or enemies. Some venoms produce no more than local pain and swelling; others produce more general effects and can prove lethal.

venosclerosis *n. see* phlebosclerosis.

ventilation *n.* the passage of air into and out of the respiratory tract. The air that reaches only as far as the conducting airways cannot take part in gas exchange and is known as *dead space ventilation* – this may be reduced by performing a *tracheostomy. In the air sacs of the lungs (alveoli) gas exchange is most efficient when matched by adequate blood flow (*perfusion). Ventilation/perfusion imbalance (ventilation of underperfused alveoli or perfusion of underventilated alveoli) is an important cause of *anoxia and *cyanosis.

ventilation–perfusion scanning (V/Q scanning) a *nuclear medicine technique in which two different isotopes are used, one inhaled (usually *xenon-133 or *krypton-81m), to examine lung ventilation, and one injected, to examine lung perfusion. In *pulmonary embolism, the area of lung supplied by the blocked artery is not being perfused with blood – a perfusion defect – but has normal ventilation. This technique is highly sensitive for pulmonary embolism.

ventilator *n.* **1.** a device to ensure a supply of fresh air. **2.** equipment that is manually or mechanically operated to maintain a flow of air into and out of the lungs of a patient who is unable to breathe normally. A *self-inflating bag* is a device for delivering emergency artificial ventilation by means of a tight-fitting face mask, a *laryngeal mask, or an endotracheal tube (*see* intubation). It consists of a stiff plastic bag, which is squeezed to deliver its gas contents into the patient's airway; when the pressure is released, it is reinflated from the atmosphere or an attached oxygen supply. Flow into and out of the bag is controlled by a system of simple valves. With an attached oxygen supply, high concentrations of oxygen can be given. *See also* respirator.

ventouse *n. see* vacuum extractor.

ventral *adj.* relating to or situated at or close to the front of the body or to the anterior part of an organ.

ventricle *n.* **1.** either of the two lower chambers of the *heart, which have thick muscular walls. The left ventricle, which is thicker than the right, receives blood from the pulmonary vein via the left atrium and pumps it into the aorta. The right ventricle pumps blood received from the venae cavae (via the right atrium) into the pulmonary artery. **2.** one of the four fluid-filled cavities within the brain. The paired first and second ventricles (*lateral ventricles*), one in each cerebral hemisphere, communicate with the third ventricle in the midline between them. This in turn leads through a narrow channel, the *cerebral aqueduct*, to the fourth ventricle in the hindbrain, which is continuous with the spinal canal in the center of the spinal cord. *Cerebrospinal fluid circulates through all the cavities of the brain. —**ventricular** *adj.*

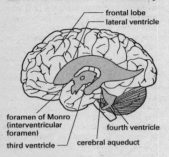

Ventricles of the brain (side view)

ventricul- (ventriculo-) *prefix denoting* a ventricle (of the brain or heart).

ventricular folds *see* vocal cords.

ventricular septal defect (VSD) a congenital defect of the heart in which there is a hole in the partition (septum) separating the two ventricles (*see* septal defect); it is the most common congenital heart disease. In 25% of patients there are other defects present. 50% of VSDs close spontaneously. If the hole is large, blood is diverted to the lungs at a greater pressure than usual and *pulmonary hypertension can occur, which becomes irreversible and progressive. Early surgical intervention can prevent this.

ventricular tachycardia (VT) a dangerously fast beating of the heart stemming from an abnormal focus of electrical activity in the *ventricles. The electricity does not pass through the heart along the usual channels and as a result the contraction of the heart muscle is often not as efficient as normal, which can result in a sudden drop in blood pressure or even *cardiac arrest. Left untreated it will prove ultimately fatal. *See also* arrhythmia.

ventriculitis *n.* inflammation in the ventricles of the brain, usually caused by infection. It may result from the rupture of a cerebral abscess into the cavity of the

ventricle or from the spread of a severe form of *meningitis from the subarachnoid space.

ventriculoatriostomy *n.* an operation for the relief of raised pressure due to the build-up of cerebrospinal fluid that occurs in *hydrocephalus. Using a system of catheters, the fluid is drained into the jugular vein in the neck.

ventriculography *n.* X-ray examination of the ventricles of the brain after the introduction of a contrast medium, such as air or radiopaque material. This procedure has been replaced by *computed tomography and *magnetic resonance imaging.

ventriculoscopy *n.* observation of the ventricles of the brain through a fiberoptic instrument. *See* endoscope, fiberoptics.

ventriculostomy *n.* an operation to introduce a hollow needle (cannula) into one of the lateral ventricles (cavities) of the brain. This may be done to relieve raised intracranial pressure, to obtain cerebrospinal fluid from the ventricle for examination, or to introduce antibiotics or contrast material for X-ray examination.

ventro- *prefix denoting* **1.** ventral. **2.** the abdomen.

ventrosuspension (ventrofixation) *n.* surgical fixation of a displaced uterus to the anterior abdominal wall. This may be achieved by shortening the round ligaments at their attachment to the uterus or to the abdominal wall.

venule *n.* a minute vessel that drains blood from the capillaries. Many venules unite to form a vein.

verapamil *n.* a *calcium antagonist used in the treatment of essential hypertension, angina, and arrhythmia. It is administered by mouth; side effects include constipation, nausea, and hypotension. Trade names: **Calan, Isoptin, Verelan.**

verbigeration *n.* repetitive utterances of the same words over and over again. This is a kind of *stereotypy affecting speech and is most common in institutionalized schizophrenics.

vermicide *n.* a chemical agent used to destroy parasitic worms living in the intestine. *Compare* vermifuge.

vermiform appendix *see* appendix.

vermifuge *n.* any drug or chemical agent used to expel worms from the intestine.

See also anthelmintic. *Compare* vermicide.

vermilion *n.* the normally pink-red part of the lip. The *vermilion border* is the intersection of the skin and the pigmented lip.

vermis *n.* the central portion of the *cerebellum, lying between its two lateral hemispheres and immediately behind the pons and the medulla oblongata of the hindbrain.

vermix *n.* the vermiform *appendix.

vernal conjunctivitis *conjunctivitis of allergic origin that occurs seasonally during warm weather, often associated with hay fever or other forms of *atopy.

Verner-Morrison syndrome *see* VIPoma. [J. V. Verner (1927–), US physician; A. B. Morrison (1922–), Irish pathologist]

vernier *n.* a device for obtaining accurate measurements of length, to 1/10th, 1/100th, or smaller fractions of a unit. It consists of a fixed graduated main scale against which a shorter vernier scale slides. The vernier scale is graduated into divisions equal to nine-tenths of the smallest unit marked on the main scale. The vernier scale is often adjusted by means of a screw thread. A reading is taken by observing which of the markings on the scales coincide.

vernix caseosa the layer of greasy material that covers the skin of a fetus or newborn baby. It is produced by the oil-secreting glands of the skin and contains skin scales and fine hairs.

verruca *n. see* wart.

verrucous carcinoma an *indolent preinvasive wartlike carcinoma of the oral cavity, which is associated with chewing tobacco.

version *n.* a maneuver to alter the position of a fetus in the womb to aid delivery. For example, the fetus may be turned from a transverse to a longitudinal position or from a buttocks-first to a head-first presentation (*see* cephalic version).

vertebra *n.* (*pl.* **vertebrae**) one of the 33 bones of which the *backbone is composed. Each vertebra typically consists of a *body*, or *centrum*, from the back of which arises an arch of bone (the *neural arch*) enclosing a cavity (the *vertebral canal*, or *foramen*) through which the spinal cord passes. The neural arch bears

one *spinous process* and two *transverse processes*, providing anchorage for muscles, and four *articular processes*, with which adjacent vertebrae articulate (see illustration). Individual vertebrae are bound together by ligaments and *intervertebral disks. —**vertebral** *adj.*

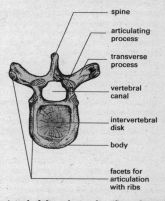

spine

articulating process

transverse process

vertebral canal

intervertebral disk

body

facets for articulation with ribs

A typical thoracic vertebra (from above)

vertebral column *see* backbone.

vertigo *n.* a disabling sensation in which the affected individual feels that either he or his surroundings are in a state of constant movement. It is most often a spinning sensation but there may be a feeling that the ground is tilting. It is a symptom of disease either in the *labyrinth of the inner ear or in the *vestibular nerve or its nuclei in the brainstem, which are involved in the sense of balance. *See also* benign paroxysmal positional vertigo.

vesical *adj.* relating to or affecting a bladder, especially the urinary bladder.

vesicant *n.* an agent that causes blistering of the skin.

vesicle *n.* **1.** a very small blister in the skin, often no bigger than a pinpoint, that contains a clear fluid (serum). Vesicles occur in a variety of skin disorders, including eczema and herpes. **2.** (in anatomy) any small bladder, especially one filled with fluid. —**vesicular** *adj.*

vesico- *prefix denoting* the urinary bladder. Example: *vesicovaginal* (relating to the bladder and vagina).

vesicofixation *n. see* cystopexy.

vesicostomy n. the surgical creation of an artificial channel between the bladder and the skin surface for the passage of urine. It is sometimes combined with closure of the urethra.

vesicoureteric reflux the backflow of urine from the bladder into the ureters. This is due to defective valves (which normally prevent reflux). Infection is conveyed to the kidneys, causing recurrent attacks of acute *pyelonephritis and scarring of the kidneys in childhood. Children with urinary infection must be investigated for reflux by *cystoscopy; if the condition does not settle with antibiotic therapy, corrective surgery must be performed.

vesicovaginal fistula an abnormal communication between the bladder and the vagina causing urinary incontinence. This may result from surgical damage to the bladder during a gynecological operation (e.g. hysterectomy) or radiation damage following radiotherapy for pelvic malignancy. In developing countries it is often caused by necrosis resulting from prolonged obstructed labor.

vesicular breathing see breath sounds.

vesiculectomy n. surgical removal of a *seminal vesicle. This operation, which is rarely undertaken, may be performed for a tumor of the seminal vesicles.

vesiculitis n. inflammation of the seminal vesicles. See vasovesiculitis.

vesiculography n. any technique for imaging the seminal vesicles. This used to be performed by injecting a *contrast medium into the vas deferens during *vasography. More commonly direct injection is now performed during *transrectal ultrasonography (TRUS), which enables sperm to be sampled at the same examination. *Magnetic resonance imaging is a good technique for imaging the seminal vesicles with no radiation exposure. Both these techniques are useful for investigation of patients with *azoospermia.

vesiculopapular adj. describing a skin condition typified by having both vesicles (blisters) and papules (raised spots).

vesiculopustular adj. describing a skin condition that has both vesicles (blisters) and pustules (pus-filled blisters).

vessel n. a tube conveying a body fluid, especially a blood vessel or a lymphatic vessel.

vestibular glands the two pairs of glands that open at the junction of the vagina and vulva. The more posterior of the two are the *greater vestibular glands* (*Bartholin's glands*); the other pair are the *lesser vestibular glands*. Their function is to lubricate the entrance to the vagina during coitus.

vestibular nerve the division of the *vestibulocochlear nerve that carries impulses from the semicircular canals, utricle, and saccule of the inner ear to the brain, conveying information about the body's posture and movements in space and allowing coordination and balance.

vestibule n. (in anatomy) a cavity situated at the entrance to a hollow part. The vestibule of the ear is the cavity of the bony *labyrinth that contains the *saccule and *utricle – the organs of equilibrium.

vestibulocochlear nerve (acoustic nerve, auditory nerve) the eighth cranial nerve (VIII), responsible for carrying sensory impulses from the inner ear to the brain. It has two branches, the *vestibular nerve* and the *cochlear nerve*. The cochlear nerve carries impulses from the spiral *cochlea and is therefore the nerve of hearing, while the vestibular nerve serves equilibrium, carrying impulses from the semicircular canals, utricles, and saccules with information about posture, movement, and balance.

vestigial adj. existing only in a rudimentary form. The term is applied to organs whose structure and function have diminished during the course of evolution until only a rudimentary structure exists.

viable adj. capable of surviving. The term is applied to a fetus from about the 24th week of gestation, at which stage it can survive, although some fetuses now survive birth at an even earlier age.

Viagra n. see sildenafil.

vibrator n. a machine used to generate vibrations of different frequencies, which have a stimulating effect when applied to different parts of the body. A vibrator may also be used to loosen thick mucus in the sinuses or air passages.

Vibrio n. a genus of gram-negative motile comma-shaped bacteria that are widely distributed in soil and water. Most species are saprophytic but some are parasites, including *V. cholerae*, which causes *cholera.

vibrissa *n.* (*pl.* **vibrissae**) a stiff coarse hair, especially one of the stiff hairs that lie just inside the nostrils.

vicarious *adj.* describing an action or function performed by an organ not normally involved in the function. For example, *vicarious menstruation* is a rare disorder in which monthly bleeding occurs from places other than the vagina, such as the sweat glands, breasts, nose, or eyes.

vidarabine (adenine arabinoside) *n.* an antiviral drug used as an ophthalmic ointment to treat viral infections of the eye. Possible side effects include irritation and sensitivity of the eyes to light. Trade name: **Vira-A**.

video- *prefix denoting* the use of a video camera to view and record moving images. *See* videofluoroscopy.

videofluoroscopy *n.* the technique of viewing and recording real-time X-ray investigation using a video camera (*see* real-time imaging). This enables the moving images to be reviewed at a later time, by individual frames or in slow motion.

videokeratography *n. see* corneal topography.

videokymography *n.* a method of studying the vibration of the *vocal cords of the larynx using high-speed digital photography. *See* laryngeal stroboscopy.

video-otoscope *n.* a small *endoscope connected to a digital camera for examining the outer ear and eardrum.

vigabatrin *n. see* anticonvulsant.

villus *n.* (*pl.* **villi**) one of many short fingerlike processes that project from some membranous surfaces. Numerous *intestinal villi* line the small *intestine. Each contains a network of blood capillaries and a *lacteal. Their function is to absorb the products of digestion and they greatly increase the surface area over which this can take place. *Chorionic villi* are folds of the *chorion (the outer membrane surrounding a fetus) from which the fetal part of the *placenta is formed. They provide an extensive area for the exchange of oxygen, carbon dioxide, food, and waste products between maternal and fetal blood. *See also* arachnoid villus, chorionic villus sampling.

vinblastine *n.* a *vinca alkaloid that is given by intravascular injection, mainly in the treatment of cancers of the lymphatic system, such as Hodgkin's disease. It is highly toxic, since it also acts on normal tissues; common side effects include nausea, vomiting, diarrhea, and depression of bone marrow function. Trade name: **Velban**.

vinca alkaloid one of a group of antimitotic drugs (*see* cytotoxic drug) derived from the periwinkle (*Vinca rosea*). Vinca alkaloids are usually administered intravenously and are used especially to treat leukemias and lymphomas; they include *vinblastine, *vincristine, and *vindesine.

Vincent's angina an obsolete term for *ulcerative gingivitis. [H. Vincent (1862–1950), French physician]

vincristine *n.* a *vinca alkaloid with uses and side effects similar to those of vinblastine. It is usually used with other drugs in combination therapy. Trade names: **Oncovin**, **Vincasar**, **Vincrex**.

vinculum *n.* (*pl.* **vincula**) a connecting band of tissue. The *vincula tendinum* are threadlike bands of synovial membrane that connect the flexor tendons of the fingers and toes to their point of insertion on the phalanges.

vindesine *n.* a *vinca alkaloid with similarities to *vinblastine and *vincristine. Additional side effects include alopecia and peripheral neuropathy. Trade name: **Eldisine**.

vinorelbine tartrate an *antineoplastic drug (a semisynthetic *vinca alkaloid) used mainly in the treatment of *non-small-cell lung cancer as well as some other cancers, including breast and ovarian cancer and Hodgkin's disease. It is administered intravenously; side effects include nausea and vomiting, thinned or brittle hair, constipation or diarrhea, and fatigue. Trade name: **Navelbine**.

VIP (vasoactive intestinal peptide) a peptide hormone that is produced by cells of the pancreas. Large amounts of this hormone cause severe diarrhea (*see* VIPoma).

VIPoma *n.* a usually malignant tumor of islet cells of the pancreas that secrete *VIP. The presence of excess amounts of this hormone causes severe diarrhea ("pancreatic cholera" or the *Verner-Morrison syndrome*), with loss of potassium and bicarbonate and a low level of stomach acid. The treatment is surgical removal of the tumor.

viral hepatitis see hepatitis.

viral pneumonia an acute infection of the lung caused by any one of a number of viruses, such as *respiratory syncytial virus, adenovirus, parainfluenza, influenza A and B, and enteroviruses. It is characterized by headache, fever, muscle pain, and a cough that produces a thick sputum. The pneumonia often occurs with or subsequent to a systemic viral infection. Treatment is by supportive care, but antibiotics are administered if a bacterial infection is superimposed.

viremia n. the presence of virus particles in the blood.

virilism n. the development in a female of a combination of increased body hair, muscle bulk, and deepening of the voice (*masculinization) and male psychological characteristics.

virilization n. the most extreme result of excessive androgen production (*hyperandrogenism) in women. It is characterized by temporal balding, a male body form, muscle bulk, deepening of the voice, enlargement of the clitoris, and *hirsutism. Virilization in prepubertal boys may be caused by some tumors (see Leydig tumor).

virology n. the science of viruses. See also microbiology.

virulence n. the disease-producing (pathogenic) ability of a microorganism. See also attenuation.

virus n. a minute particle that is capable of replication but only within living cells. Viruses are too small to be visible with a light microscope and too small to be trapped by filters. They infect animals, plants, and microorganisms (see bacteriophage). Each consists of a core of nucleic acid (DNA or RNA) surrounded by a protein shell. Some bear an outer lipid capsule. Viruses cause many diseases, including the common cold, influenza, measles, mumps, chickenpox, herpes, AIDS, poliomyelitis, and rabies. Antibiotics are ineffective against them, but *antiviral drugs are effective against certain viral diseases and many others are controlled by means of vaccines. —**viral** adj.

viscera pl. n. (sing. **viscus**) the organs within the body cavities, especially the organs of the abdominal cavities (stomach, intestines, etc.). —**visceral** adj.

visceral arch see pharyngeal arch.

visceral cleft see pharyngeal cleft.

visceral pouch see pharyngeal pouch.

viscero- prefix denoting the viscera.

viscid (viscous) adj. sticky, gummy, or gelatinous.

viscodissection n. a surgical technique in which a *viscoelastic material is used to dissect and separate layers of tissue.

viscoelastic adj. both viscous and elastic; especially describing any gel-like material used in ophthalmic surgery to help maintain the shape of ocular tissues as well as lubricate and minimize trauma. Viscoelastic material is commonly used in intraocular surgery, such as cataract surgery.

viscus n. see viscera.

visual acuity sharpness of vision: the degree to which a person is able to distinguish and resolve detail. Visual acuity depends on how well objects are illuminated and upon such factors as practice and motivation, but the essential requirements are a healthy retina and the ability of the eye to focus incoming light to form a sharp image on the retina. Acuity of distant vision is often expressed as a Snellen score (see Snellen chart); acuity of near vision as a Jaeger score (see Jaeger test types).

visual field the area in front of the eye in any part of which an object can be seen without moving the eye. With both eyes open and looking straight forward it is possible to see well-illuminated objects placed anywhere in front of the eyes, although the eyebrows and eyelids reduce the extent of the field somewhat. This is the binocular visual field. With only one eye open, the field is uniocular and is restricted inward by the nose. If the object is small or poorly illuminated, it will not be seen until it is moved closer to the point at which the eye is actually looking, i.e. nearer to the center of the visual field. Similarly, colored objects are not seen so far away from the center as are white objects of the same size and brightness. This is because the retina is not uniformly sensitive to light of different colors or intensities (see rod, cone): retinal sensitivity increases toward its center (the *macula). Thus, although there is an absolute visual field beyond which things cannot be seen, no matter how large or bright they are, a relative field exists for objects of different brightness, size, and color. The most common visual field loss is due to *glaucoma. *See also* campimetry, perimeter.

visual purple *see* rhodopsin.

vital capacity the maximum volume of air that a person can exhale after maximum inhalation. It is usually measured on an instrument called a *spirometer*.

vital center any of the collections of nerve cells in the brain that act as governing centers for different vital body functions – such as breathing, heart rate, blood pressure, temperature control, etc. – making reflex adjustments according to the body's needs. Most lie in the hypothalamus and brainstem.

Vitallium *n*. *Trademark*. an alloy of chromium and cobalt that is used in instruments, prostheses, surgical appliances, and dentures.

vital staining (intravital staining) the process of staining a living tissue by injecting a stain into the organism. *Compare* supravital staining.

vital statistics *see* biostatistics.

vitamin *n*. any of a group of substances that are required, in very small amounts, for healthy growth and development: they cannot be synthesized by the body and are therefore essential constituents of the diet. Vitamins are divided into two groups, according to whether they are soluble in water or fat. The water-soluble group includes the vitamin B complex and vitamin C and are not stored in the body; the fat-soluble vitamins are A, D, E, and K and are stored in the body. Lack of sufficient quantities of any of the vitamins in the diet results in specific vitamin deficiency diseases.

vitamin A (retinol) a fat-soluble vitamin that occurs preformed in foods of animal origin (especially milk products, egg yolk, and liver) and is formed in the body from the pigment *beta-carotene, present in some vegetable foods (for example cabbage, lettuce, and carrots). Retinol is essential for growth, vision in dim light, and the maintenance of soft mucous tissue. A deficiency causes stunted growth, *night blindness, *xerophthalmia, *keratomalacia, and eventual blindness. The recommended daily intake is 750 µg retinol equivalents for

an adult (1 µg retinol equivalent = 1 µg retinol or 6 µg β-carotene).

vitamin B any one of a group of water-soluble vitamins that, although not chemically related, are often found together in the same kinds of food (milk, liver, cereals, etc.) and all function as *coenzymes. *See* vitamins B₁, B₂, B₆, B₁₂, biotin, folic acid, niacin, pantothenic acid.

vitamin B₁ (thiamine, aneurin) a vitamin of the B complex that is active in the form of *thiamine pyrophosphate*, a coenzyme in decarboxylation reactions in carbohydrate metabolism. A deficiency of vitamin B₁ leads to *beriberi. Good sources of the vitamin are cereals, beans, meat, potatoes, and nuts. The recommended daily intake is 1 mg for an adult.

vitamin B₂ (riboflavin) a vitamin of the B complex that is a constituent of the coenzymes *FAD (flavine adenine dinucleotide) and *FMN (flavine mononucleotide). Riboflavin is therefore important in tissue respiration. A deficiency of riboflavin causes a condition known as *ariboflavinosis, which is not usually serious. Good sources of riboflavin are liver, milk, and eggs. The recommended daily intake for an adult is 1.7 mg.

vitamin B₆ (pyridoxine) a vitamin of the B complex from which the coenzyme *pyridoxal phosphate, involved in the transamination of amino acids, is formed. The vitamin is found in most foods and a deficiency is therefore rare.

vitamin B₁₂ (cyanocobalamin) a vitamin of the B complex. The form of vitamin B₁₂ with coenzyme activity is *5-deoxyadenosyl cobalamin*, which is necessary for the synthesis of nucleic acids, the maintenance of *myelin in the nervous system, and the proper functioning of *folic acid, another B vitamin. The vitamin can be absorbed only in the presence of *intrinsic factor*, a protein secreted in the stomach. A deficiency of vitamin B₁₂ affects nearly all the body tissues, particularly those containing rapidly dividing cells. The most serious effects of a deficiency are *pernicious anemia and degeneration of the nervous system. Vitamin B₁₂ is manufactured only by certain microorganisms and is contained only in foods of animal origin. Good sources are liver, fish, and eggs. The daily recommended adult intake is 3–4 µg.

vitamin C (ascorbic acid) a water-soluble vitamin with *antioxidant properties that is essential in maintaining healthy connective tissues and the integrity of cell walls. It is necessary for the synthesis of collagen. A deficiency of vitamin C leads to *scurvy. The recommended daily intake is 30 mg for an adult; rich sources are citrus fruits and vegetables.

vitamin D a fat-soluble vitamin that enhances the absorption of calcium and phosphorus from the intestine and promotes their deposition in the bone. It occurs in two forms: *ergocalciferol* (*vitamin D_2, calciferol*), which is manufactured by plants when the sterol ergosterol is exposed to ultraviolet light, and *cholecalciferol* (*vitamin D_3*), which is produced by the action of sunlight on 7-dehydrocholesterol, a sterol widely distributed in the skin. A deficiency of vitamin D, either from a poor diet or lack of sunlight, leads to decalcified bones and the development of *rickets and *osteomalacia. Good sources of vitamin D are liver and fish oils. The recommended daily intake is 10 µg for a child up to five years and 2.5 µg thereafter. Vitamin D is toxic and large doses must therefore be avoided.

vitamin E any of a group of chemically related fat-soluble compounds (*tocopherols* and *tocotrienols*) that have *antioxidant properties and are thought to stabilize cell membranes by preventing oxidation of their unsaturated fatty acid components. The most potent of these is α-tocopherol. Good sources of the vitamin are vegetable oils, eggs, butter, and wholemeal cereals. It is fairly widely distributed in the diet and a deficiency is therefore unlikely. There is evidence to suggest that vitamin E supplements (400–800 mg/day) reduce the risk of coronary thrombosis in patients with heart disease.

vitamin K a fat-soluble vitamin occurring in two main forms: *phytonadione* (of plant origin) and *menaquinone* (of animal origin). It is necessary for the formation of *prothrombin in the liver, which is essential for blood clotting, and it also regulates the synthesis of other clotting factors. A dietary deficiency does not often occur because the vitamin

is synthesized by bacteria in the large intestine and is widely distributed in green leafy vegetables and meat.

vitelliform degeneration (Best's disease, congenital macular degeneration) degeneration of the *macula of the eye that is inherited as a dominant characteristic and usually starts in childhood. There is widespread abnormality of retinal pigment epithelium (*see* retina) with the accumulation of a yellowish material, especially in the macular area.

vitellus *n.* the yolk of an ovum.

vitiligo *n.* a condition in which areas of skin lose pigmentation and symmetrical white or pale *macules appear. It affects all races, but is more conspicuous in dark-skinned people. Vitiligo is an autoimmune disease and may occur with other such diseases (e.g. thyroid disease or *alopecia areata). It is usually progressive, although spontaneous repigmentation may occur. Treatment with *PUVA may be effective in darker-skinned people; pale-skinned sufferers can best be helped by using potent sunscreens or by cosmetic camouflage.

vitrectomy *n.* the removal of the whole or part of the vitreous humor of the eye, including vitreous hemorrhage. It is often necessary in surgery to repair a *detached retina.

vitreous detachment the separation of the *vitreous humor from the underlying retina. This is a normal aging process, but it is also more common in such conditions as diabetes and severe myopia. It can sometimes cause a tear in the retina and lead to a *detached retina.

vitreous humor (vitreous body) the transparent jellylike material that fills the chamber behind the lens of the eye.

viviparous *adj.* describing animal groups (including most mammals) in which the embryos develop within the body of the mother so that the young are born alive rather than hatch from an egg. —**viviparity** *n.*

vivisection *n.* a surgical operation on a living animal for experimental purposes.

VMA *see* vanillylmandelic acid.

vocal cord nodule (singer's nodule) a pearly white nodule that may develop on the vocal cords of people who use their voice excessively or in those with poor vocal technique.

vocal cords (vocal folds) the two folds of

tissue which protrude from the sides of the *larynx to form a narrow slit (glottis) across the air passage (see illustration). Their controlled interference with the expiratory air flow produces audible vibrations that make up speech, song, and all other vocal noises. Alterations in the vocal cords themselves or in their nerve supply by disease interferes with phonation.

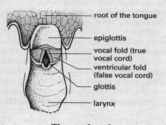

root of the tongue

epiglottis

vocal fold (true vocal cord)

ventricular fold (false vocal cord)

glottis

larynx

The vocal cords

vocal fremitus *see* fremitus.

vocal resonance the sounds heard through the stethoscope when the patient speaks ("ninety nine"). These are normally just audible but become much louder (*bronchophony*) if the lung under the stethoscope is consolidated, whereupon they resemble the sounds heard over the trachea and main bronchi. Vocal resonance is lost over pleural fluid except at its upper surface, when it has a bleating quality and is called *egophony. See also* pectoriloquy.

voice *n.* audible sound produced by phonation, that is, by vocal cord interaction with the exhaled airstream. An abnormal voice can be a symptom of illness, a disorder of communication, or *psychogenic.

volar *adj.* relating to the palm of the hand or the sole of the foot (the *vola*).

Volkmann's contracture fibrosis and shortening of muscles due to inadequate blood supply. It is a complication that arises if the blood supply is interrupted by pressure on the blood vessels from a fracture fragment, or from raised pressure due to *compartmental syndrome, or by pressure from constricting bandages and plaster casts. [R. von Volkmann (1830–89), German surgeon]

volsella *n. see* vulsella.

volt *n.* the *SI unit of electric potential, equal to the potential difference between two points on a conducting wire through which a constant current of 1 ampere flows when the power dissipated between these points is 1 watt. Symbol: V.

voluntary admission entry of a patient into a psychiatric hospital with his (or her) agreement.

voluntary hospital a hospital that is owned or operated by a religious organization or community association to provide health-care facilities on a nonprofit basis. Voluntary hospitals in the US evolved from a sense of obligation by wealthy public-spirited citizens to provide better health care for the indigent sick persons in urban areas. In recent years the role of voluntary hospitals has changed from one of caring primarily for charity patients to one of serving all members of a community. At the same time, the practice of charging higher fees to patients able to afford them in order to compensate for the expense of caring for charity patients has generally been eliminated because of the availability of government funds and refusal of insurance companies to reimburse policyholders charged the higher fees.

voluntary muscle *see* striated muscle.

volvulus *n.* twisting of part of the digestive tract, usually leading to partial or complete obstruction and sometimes reducing the blood supply, causing gangrene. A volvulus may untwist spontaneously or by manipulation, but surgical exploration is usually performed. *Gastric volvulus* is a twist of the stomach, usually in a hiatus *hernia. *Small-intestinal volvulus* is twisting of part of the bowel around an *adhesion. *Sigmoid volvulus* is a twist of the sigmoid colon, usually when this loop is particularly long. *Compound volvulus* (or *ileosigmoid knotting*) involves both the small and the large bowel.

vomer *n.* a thin plate of bone that forms part of the nasal septum (*see* nasal cavity). *See also* skull.

vomica *n.* **1.** an abnormal cavity in an organ, usually a lung, sometimes containing pus. **2.** the abrupt expulsion from the mouth of a large quantity of pus or decaying matter originating in the throat or lungs.

vomit 1. *vb.* to eject the contents of the

stomach through the mouth (see vomiting). **2.** n. the contents of the stomach ejected during vomiting. Medical name: **vomitus**.

vomiting n. the reflex action of ejecting the contents of the stomach through the mouth. Vomiting is controlled by a special center in the brain that may be stimulated by drugs (e.g. *apomorphine) acting directly on it; or by impulses transmitted through nervous pathways either from the stomach (e.g. after ingesting irritating substances or in stomach diseases, such as peptic ulceration or pyloric stenosis), the intestine (e.g. in intestinal obstruction), or from the inner ear (in motion sickness). The stimulated vomiting center sets off a chain of nerve impulses producing coordinated contractions of the diaphragm and abdominal muscles, relaxation of the muscle at the entrance to the stomach, etc., causing the stomach contents to be expelled. See also bulimia. Medical name: **emesis**.

von Hippel-Lindau disease an inherited syndrome in which *hemangioblastomas, particularly in the cerebellum, are associated with renal and pancreatic cysts, *angiomas in the retina, cancer of the kidney cells, and red birthmarks. [E. von Hippel (1867–1939), German ophthalmologist; A. Lindau (1892–1958), Swedish pathologist]

von Recklinghausen's disease 1. a syndrome due to excessive secretion of *parathyroid hormone (hyperparathyroidism), characterized by the loss of mineral from bones, which become weakened and fracture easily, and formation of kidney stones. Medical name: **osteitis fibrosa**. **2.** see neurofibromatosis. [F. D. von Recklinghausen (1833–1910), German pathologist]

von Willebrand's disease an inherited disorder of the blood characterized by episodes of spontaneous bleeding similar to *hemophilia, except that it affects either sex. It is due to a variety of abnormalities of the von Willebrand factor, a glycoprotein necessary for normal platelet function. This results in a bleeding tendency. The most common type of von Willebrand's disease is inherited as an autosomal *dominant trait; some types are inherited as autosomal *recessive traits. [A. von Willebrand (1870–1949), Swedish physician]

voxel n. short for "volume element," the volume of tissue in a body that is represented by a *pixel in a cross-sectional image. It depends on the slice thickness of the original scan.

voyeurism n. the condition of obtaining sexual pleasure by watching other people undressing or having sexual relations. See also sexual deviation. —**voyeur** n.

VSD see ventricular septal defect.

VT see ventricular tachycardia.

vulsella (volsella) n. surgical forceps with clawlike hooks at the ends of both blades.

vulv- (vulvo-) prefix denoting the vulva.

vulva n. the female external genitalia. Two pairs of fleshy folds – the labia majora and labia minora – surround the openings of the vagina and urethra and extend forward to the clitoris (see illustration). See also vestibular glands.

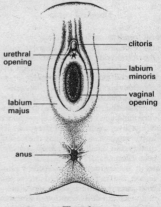

The vulva

vulvectomy n. surgical removal of the external genitals (vulva) of a woman. Simple vulvectomy involves excision of the labia majora, labia minora, and clitoris and is carried out for a nonmalignant growth. Radical vulvectomy is a much more extensive operation carried out for a malignant growth. It involves wide excision of the labia majora and minora and the clitoris in addition to complete removal of all regional lymph nodes on both sides. The skin covering these areas is also removed, leaving an extensive raw area that is allowed to heal by *granulation.

vulvitis *n.* inflammation of the vulva, which is often accompanied by intense itching (*see* pruritus). (*see* pruritus, vaginitis).

W

Waardenburg's syndrome an inherited form of deafness accompanied by a characteristic white forelock of hair and multiple colors within the irises of the eyes. It is inherited as an autosomal *dominant disease, i.e. the children of an affected parent have a 50% chance of inheriting the disorder, although severity is variable. The gene responsible has been identified. [P. J. Waardenburg (1886–1979), Dutch ophthalmologist]

wafer *n.* a thin sheet made from moistened flour, formerly used to enclose a powdered medicine that is taken by mouth.

WAGR syndrome *W*ilms' tumor (*see* nephroblastoma), *a*nirida, *g*enitourinary abnormalities, and mental *r*etardation: a condition due to a deletion of part of the short arm of chromosome 11.

Waldeyer's ring the ring of lymphoid tissue that is formed by the tonsils. [H. W. G. von Waldeyer (1836–1921), German anatomist]

walking distance the measured distance that a patient can walk before he or she is stopped by pain in the muscles, usually the calf muscles. It is a useful estimate of the degree of impairment of the blood supply. *See* claudication.

walk-in patient a patient who enters a hospital or other health facility and requests medical care without a prior appointment.

Wallerian degeneration degeneration of a ruptured nerve fiber that occurs within the nerve sheath distal to the point of severance. [A. V. Waller (1816–70), British physician]

warfarin *n.* an *anticoagulant used mainly in the treatment of coronary or venous thrombosis to reduce the risk of embolism. It is given by mouth or injection. The principal toxic effect is local bleeding, usually from the gums and other mucous membranes. Trade name: **Coumadin**.

wart *n.* a small (often hard) benign growth on the skin, caused by infection with the *human papillomavirus. Warts are common in young people, usually occurring on the face, fingers, hands, elbows, and knees. There are several types. *Common warts* are firm horny papules, 1–10 mm in diameter, found mainly on the hands. Most will clear spontaneously within two years. *Plantar warts* (or *verrucas*) occur on the soles of the feet and are often tender. *Plane warts* are flat and skin-colored – and therefore difficult to see; they are usually found on the face and may be present in very large numbers. *Genital warts* are frequently associated with other genital infections and affected women have an increased risk of developing cervical cancer. Treatment of warts is with OTC (over-the-counter) remedies, such as lactic and salicylic acids, but *cryotherapy with liquid nitrogen is probably more effective. Occasionally curettage and cautery are used; surgical excision is never indicated.

Warthin's tumor (adenolymphoma) a tumor of the parotid salivary glands, containing epithelial and lymphoid tissues with cystic spaces. [A. S. Warthin (1866–1931), US pathologist]

Wassermann reaction formerly, the most commonly used test for the diagnosis of *syphilis. [A. P. von Wassermann (1866–1925), German bacteriologist]

wasting *n.* loss of body mass. This may be generalized, as in the process of deterioration, usually seen in the severely ill or elderly, in which there is extreme weight loss as well as decreased physical and mental vigor and activity; or localized, as seen in muscle loss in those who are bedridden or paralyzed.

water bed a bed with a flexible water-containing mattress. The surface of the bed adapts itself to the patient's posture, which leads to greater comfort and fewer bedsores.

water brash *n.* a sudden filling of the mouth with dilute saliva. This often accompanies dyspepsia, particularly if there is nausea.

water-deprivation test a test for *diabetes insipidus in which fluid and food intake is withheld completely for (usually) 24 hours, with regular measurement of plasma and urinary *osmolality and body weight. In a normal person the output of *vasopressin will be increased in order to concentrate the urine as the plasma osmolality rises; correspondingly, the urine osmolality also rises and its volume diminishes. A patient with diabetes insipidus, however, will not achieve this: the urine osmolality will remain low and of high volume while the patient steadily dehydrates. The test must be abandoned if the patient loses 3% of body weight.

Waterhouse-Friderichsen syndrome acute hemorrhage in the adrenal glands with hemorrhage into the skin associated with the sudden onset of acute bacteremic *shock. It is usually caused by meningococcal septicemia (see meningitis). [R. Waterhouse (1873–1958), British physician; C. Friderichsen (20th century), Danish physician]

Waters' projection a *posteroanterior X-ray film to show the maxillae, maxillary sinuses, and zygomatic bones. [C. A. Waters (1888–1961), US radiologist]

watt n. the *SI unit of power, equal to 1 joule per second. In electrical terms it is the energy expended per second when a current of 1 ampere flows between two points on a conductor between which there is a potential difference of 1 volt. 1 watt = 10^7 ergs per second. Symbol: W.

weal n. see wheal.

weber n. the *SI unit of magnetic flux, equal to the flux linking a circuit of one turn that produces an electromotive force of 1 volt when reduced uniformly to zero in 1 second. Symbol: Wb.

Weber-Christian disease see panniculitis. [F. P. Weber (1863–1962), British physician; H. A. Christian (1876–1951), US physician]

Weber's test a hearing test in which a vibrating tuning fork is placed at the midpoint of the forehead. A normal individual hears it equally in both ears, but if one ear is affected by conductive *deafness the sound appears louder in the affected ear. If one ear has a sensorineural deafness the sound appears louder in the unaffected ear. [F. E. Weber (1832–91), German otologist]

web space the soft tissue between the bases of the fingers and toes.

Wechsler scales standardized scales for the measurement of *intelligence quotient (IQ) in adults and children. They are administered by a psychologist. See intelligence test. [D. Wechsler (1896–1981), US psychologist]

Wegener's granulomatosis an autoimmune disease predominantly affecting the nasal passages, lungs, and kidneys, characterized by *granuloma formation in addition to arteritis. It is usually fatal but can be controlled (sometimes for years) with steroids, cyclophosphamide, or azathioprine. [F. Wegener (1907–90), German pathologist]

Weil-Felix reaction a diagnostic test for typhus. A sample of the patient's serum is tested for the presence of antibodies against the organism Proteus vulgaris. Although this relatively harmless organism is not the cause of typhus, it possesses certain antigens in common with the causative agent of the disease and can therefore be used instead of it in laboratory tests. Typhus is suspected if antibodies are found to be present. [E. Weil (1880–1922), German physician; A. Felix (1887–1956), Czech bacteriologist]

Weil's disease see leptospirosis. [A. Weil (1848–1916), German physician]

Weiss ring a ringlike opacity on the posterior vitreous surface, arising as a result of a posterior *vitreous detachment. It is seen as a ring-shaped *floater.

Welch's bacillus see Clostridium. [W. H. Welch (1850–1934), US pathologist]

wen n. see sebaceous cyst.

Werdnig-Hoffmann disease an hereditary disorder – a severe form of *spinal muscular atrophy – in which the cells of the spinal cord begin to die between birth and the age of six months, causing a symmetrical muscle weakness. Affected infants become floppy and progressively weaker; respiratory and facial muscles become affected. Children usually die by the age of 20 months from respiratory failure and there is no treatment. *Genetic counseling is required for parents of an affected child as each of their subsequent children has a one in four chance of being affected. [G. Werdnig (1844–1919), Austrian neurologist; J. Hoffmann (1857–1919), German neurologist]

Wermer's syndrome see MENS. [P. Wermer, US physician]

Werner's syndrome a rare genetic disorder resulting in premature aging that starts at adolescence. Growth may be retarded and affected individuals may suffer from a thin skin, arterial disease, leg ulcers, and diabetes. Treatment is limited to the management of complications, such as diabetes. The gene responsible codes for an enzyme involved in the mechanisms of DNA replication and repair, which in affected individuals is defective. [C. W. O. Werner (1879–1936), German physician]

Wernicke's encephalopathy mental confusion or delirium occurring in combination with paralysis of the eye muscles, *nystagmus, and an unsteady gait. It is caused by a deficiency of vitamin B$_1$ (thiamine) and is most commonly seen in alcoholics and in patients with persistent vomiting or an unbalanced diet. Treatment with thiamine relieves the symptoms. [K. Wernicke (1848–1905), German neurologist]

Wertheim's hysterectomy an extensive operation performed for cancer of the uterus or ovary, in which the uterus, fallopian tubes, ovaries, upper vagina, broad ligaments, and regional lymph nodes are removed. [E. Wertheim (1864–1920), Austrian gynecologist]

Western blot analysis a technique for the detection of specific proteins. After separation by *electrophoresis, the proteins are bound to radioactively labeled antibodies and identified by X-ray. *Compare* Northern blot analysis, Southern blot analysis.

West Nile fever a viral disease caused by the West Nile virus (a *flavivirus), which is spread by the *Culex pipiens* mosquito. It causes encephalitis, with influenza-like symptoms, enlarged lymph nodes, and a bright red rash on the chest and abdomen. In patients with a weakened immune system (such as the elderly) it can progress to convulsions, coma, and paralysis.

Wharton's duct the secretory duct of the submandibular *salivary gland. [T. Wharton (1614–73), English physician]

Wharton's jelly the mesoderm tissue of the umbilical cord, which becomes converted to a loose jellylike *mesenchyme surrounding the umbilical blood vessels.

wheal (weal) *n.* a temporary red or pale raised area of the skin, often accompanied by severe itching. Wheals are caused by scratching or rubbing the skin and are sometimes the sign of a local or general allergy (*see* urticaria). *See also* dermatographism.

wheeze *n.* an abnormal breathing sound, such as whistling, squeaking, or puffing, mainly during expiration. Wheezes occur as a result of narrowing of the airways, such as that resulting from *bronchospasm or increased secretion and retention of sputum; they are commonly heard in patients with asthma or chronic bronchitis. *Compare* stridor.

whiplash injury damage to the ligaments, vertebrae, spinal cord, or nerve roots in the neck region, caused by sudden jerking back of the head and neck, often in occupants of a car hit from behind. Whiplash is an injury to the soft tissues causing pain and stiffness in the neck. Treatment is with a soft surgical collar for a short period, and physiotherapy can help. Symptoms occasionally last for many months or years.

Whipple's disease a rare disease, occurring only in males, in which absorption of digested food in the intestine is reduced. As well as symptoms and signs of *malabsorption, there is usually skin pigmentation and arthritis. Diagnosis is made by *jejunal biopsy; microorganisms have been found in the mucosa, and the disease usually responds to prolonged antibiotic treatment. [G. H. Whipple (1878–1976), US pathologist]

Whipple's operation *see* pancreatectomy. [A. O. Whipple (1881–1963), US surgeon]

Whipple's triad a combination of three clinical features that indicate the presence of an *insulinoma: (1) attacks of fainting, dizziness, and sweating on fasting; (2) severe hypoglycemia present during the attacks; (3) relief from the attacks achieved by administering glucose. [A. O. Whipple]

whipworm *n.* a small parasitic whiplike nematode worm, *Trichuris trichiura* (*Trichocephalus dispar*), that lives in the large intestine. Eggs are passed out of the body with the feces and human infection (*see* trichuriasis) results from the consumption of water or food contaminated with fecal material. The eggs hatch in the small intestine but mature worms migrate to the large intestine.

Whitaker's test a direct percutaneous renal infusion test to investigate obstruction of the ureter causing *hydronephrosis.

white blood cell see leukocyte.

white finger the appearance of a finger resulting from spasm of the vessels of the finger. It occurs in *Raynaud's disease but can also be attributed to the long-term use of percussion implements.

whitehead n. see milium.

white leg see thrombophlebitis.

white matter nerve tissue of the central nervous system that is paler in color than the associated *gray matter because it contains more nerve fibers and thus larger amounts of the insulating material *myelin. In the brain the white matter lies within the gray layer of cerebral cortex; in the spinal cord it is between the arms of the X-shaped central core of gray matter.

white noise instrument a device, resembling a small hearing aid, that produces sounds of many frequencies at equal intensities and is used in the treatment of tinnitus. It was formerly known as a *tinnitus masker*.

whitlow n. see felon.

WHO see World Health Organization.

whoop n. a noisy convulsive drawing in of the breath following the spasmodic coughing attack characteristic of *whooping cough.

whooping cough an acute infectious disease, primarily affecting infants and young children, due to infection of the mucous membranes lining the air passages by the bacterium *Bordetella pertussis*. After an incubation period of 1–2 weeks there is a "catarrhal" stage in which mild fever, coughing, and loss of appetite gradually develop and persist for 1–2 weeks. The cough becomes paroxysmal: series of short coughs followed by involuntary drawing in of the breath, which produces the whooping sound. Bleeding from the nose and mouth and vomiting often occur after a paroxysm. This stage lasts about two weeks and the child is infectious throughout. Over the following 2–3 weeks symptoms slowly decline but the cough may persist for many weeks. The most common complication is pneumonia, but bronchiectasis and convulsions due to *asphyxia or bleeding into the brain tissue may also occur. Immunization reduces the incidence (the disease often occurs in epidemics) and severity of the disease: the vaccine is usually given in a combined form (see DPT vaccine). An attack usually also confers immunity. Medical name: **pertussis**.

Widal reaction an *agglutination test for the presence of antibodies against the *Salmonella* organisms that cause typhoid fever. It is thus a method of diagnosing the presence of the disease in a patient and also a means of identifying the organisms in infected material. [G. F. I. Widal (1862–1929), French physician]

Williams syndrome a hereditary condition, caused by a defect (a *deletion) in chromosome 7, marked by a characteristic "elfin" facial appearance (including large eyes, a wide mouth, and small chin), *hypercalcemia, short stature, mental retardation, and *aortic stenosis. Most affected children are highly sociable and have unusual conversational ability, using a rich and complex vocabulary. The condition can be diagnosed prenatally. [J. C. P. Williams (20th century), British cardiologist]

Wilms' tumor see nephroblastoma. [M. Wilms (1867–1918), German surgeon]

Wilson's disease an *inborn error of copper metabolism in which there is a deficiency of *ceruloplasmin (which normally forms a nontoxic complex with copper). The free copper may be deposited in the liver, causing jaundice and cirrhosis, or in the brain, causing mental retardation and symptoms resembling *parkinsonism. There is a characteristic brown ring in the cornea (the *Kayser-Fleischer ring*). If the excess copper is removed from the body by regular treatment with *penicillamine and *trientine, both mental and physical development may be normal. Medical name: **hepatolenticular degeneration**. [S. A. K. Wilson (1878–1936), British neurologist]

windigo n. a delusion of having been transformed into a *windigo*, a mythical monster that eats human flesh. It is often quoted as an example of a syndrome confined to one culture (that of some Inuit and North American Indian tribes, such as the Cree).

windowing n. a technique of image manipulation commonly used in *cross-sectional imaging to manipulate a *gray scale image. Typically there is too much data obtained in a scan to see on a single image: the radiologist therefore chooses the window level centered on the density of the tissue of interest and a window width wide enough to include the densities of all the tissues that need to be seen. Tissues denser than this window usually appear white, and tissues darker appear black. Sometimes several different images of the same scan are required at different window settings to see adequately all the necessary detail (for example, window settings to observe the lung are different from those for the bones or the soft tissues in the chest on CT). *See also* Hounsfield unit.

windpipe *n. see* trachea.

wisdom tooth the third *molar tooth on each side of either jaw, which erupts normally around the age of 20.

witch hazel (hamamelis) a preparation made from the leaves and bark of the tree *Hamamelis virginiana*, used as an *astringent, especially for the treatment of sprains and bruises.

withdrawal *n.* **1.** (in psychology) the removal of one's interest from one's surroundings. *Thought withdrawal* is the experience of one's thoughts being removed from one's head, which is characteristic of *schizophrenia. **2.** *see* coitus interruptus.

withdrawal symptoms *see* dependence.

Wohlfahrtia *n.* a genus of nonbloodsucking flies. Females of *W. magnifica* and *W. vigil* deposit their parasitic maggots in wounds and the openings of the body. This causes *myiasis, particularly in children.

Wolff-Chaikoff effect the inhibition of thyroid hormone production by administration of large doses of iodide. This occurs at a critical dosage level below which the addition of iodide to an iodine-deficient individual results in increased production of thyroid hormone. The effect is transient in individuals with normal thyroids but may persist in thyroiditis; it can be utilized medically to induce a hypothyroid state, for example in patients with *thyroid storm (see Lugol's iodine). [L. Wolff (1898–1972), US cardiologist; I. L. Chaikoff (20th century), US physiologist]

wolffian body *see* mesonephros. [K. F. Wolff (1733–94), German anatomist]

wolffian duct the mesonephric duct (*see* mesonephros).

Wolff-Parkinson-White syndrome a congenital abnormality of heart rhythm caused by the presence of an accessory conduction pathway between the atria and ventricles (*see* atrioventricular bundle). It results in premature excitation of one ventricle and is characterized by an abnormal wave (*delta wave*) at the start of the *QRS complex on the electrocardiogram. [L. Wolff; Sir J. Parkinson (1885–1976), British physician; P. D. White (1886–1973), US cardiologist]

Wolfram syndrome (DIDMOAD syndrome) a rare syndrome consisting of a combination of *diabetes insipidus, *diabetes mellitus, *optic atrophy, and *deafness.

womb *n. see* uterus.

Wood's light ultraviolet light filtered through a nickel oxide prism, which causes fluorescence in skin and hair affected by some fungal and bacterial infections and is therefore useful in diagnosis. For example, *erythrasma fluoresces coral pink, while scalp ringworm caused by *Microsporum* species fluoresces green. [R. W. Wood (1868–1955), US physician]

word blindness *see* alexia.

Workmen's Compensation Laws legislation designed to ensure prompt medical care and cash benefits to workers injured in connection with a job or cash benefits to the family of a worker killed in an accident "arising out of and in the course of employment." Each state is allowed to provide its own Workmen's Compensation Laws but no state's laws cover all jobs and in some states employers are not required to participate in the compensation system. However, employers who choose not to participate are forbidden from using the system as a defense against the claims of an injured worker. Most state Workmen's Compensation Laws include coverage for occupational diseases but do not permit claims for injuries due to worker misconduct, such as intoxication on the job or negligence.

Workmen's Compensation payments are financed in three ways: through a private insurance company, by an approved self-insurance program, or through a state fund.

World Health Organization (WHO) an international organization, membership of which is open to every country, with subscription according to means; health issues are discussed and policies evolved mainly through working groups, including acknowledged authorities, and published reports. Staff are seconded by invitation to advise on self-help to solve problems (especially infectious disease control). WHO handles information on the internationally *notifiable diseases, publishes the *International Classification of Diseases, and awards fellowships to enable health staff from poorer countries to obtain further training.

worm *n.* any member of several groups of soft-bodied legless animals, including flatworms, nematode worms, earthworms, and leeches, that were formerly thought to be closely related and classified as a single group – Vermes.

wormian bone one of a number of small bones that occur in the cranial sutures.

wound *n.* a break in the structure of an organ or tissue caused by an external agent. Bruises, grazes, tears, cuts, punctures, and burns are all examples of wounds.

wrist *n.* **1.** the joint between the forearm and hand. It consists of the proximal bones of the *carpus, which articulate with the radius and ulna and the metacarpals. **2.** the whole region of the wrist joint, including the carpus and lower parts of the radius and ulna.

wrist drop paralysis of the muscles that raise the wrist, which is caused by damage to the *radial nerve. This may result from compression of the nerve against the humerus in the upper arm or from selective damage to the nerve, which is a feature of lead poisoning (*see* lead[1]).

wryneck *n. see* torticollis.

Wuchereria *n.* a genus of white threadlike parasitic worms (*see* filaria) that live in the lymphatic vessels. *W. bancrofti* is a tropical and subtropical species that causes *elephantiasis, lymphangitis, and chyluria. The immature forms concentrate in the lungs during the day. At night they become more numerous in the blood vessels of the skin, from which they are taken up by bloodsucking mosquitoes, acting as carriers of the diseases they cause.

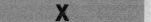

X

xanthelasma *n.* one or more yellow deposits of fatty material in the skin around the eyes. In elderly people it is quite common and of no more than cosmetic importance, but severe cases may be seen in certain disorders of fat metabolism (hyperlipidemia). The deposits may be removed by careful use of saturated trichloroacetic acid.

xanthemia *n. see* carotenemia.

xanthine *n.* a nitrogenous breakdown product of the purines adenosine and guanine. Xanthine is an intermediate product of the breakdown of nucleic acids to uric acid.

xanthinuria *n.* excess of the purine derivative *xanthine in the urine, usually the result of an inborn defect of metabolism. It is both rare and symptomless.

xantho- *prefix denoting* yellow color.

xanthochromia *n.* yellow discoloration, such as may affect the skin (for example, in jaundice) or the cerebrospinal fluid (when it contains the breakdown products of hemoglobin from red blood cells that have entered it).

xanthoma *n.* (*pl.* **xanthomata**) a yellowish swelling, nodule, or plaque in the skin associated with any of various disorders of lipid metabolism. There are several types of xanthoma. *Tuberous xanthomata* are found on the knees and elbows; *tendon xanthomata* involve the extensor tendons of the hands and feet and the Achilles tendon. Crops of small yellow papules at any site are known as *eruptive xanthomata*, while larger flat lesions are called *plane xanthomata*.

xanthomatosis *n.* the presence of multiple small fatty tumors in the skin, the eyes, and the internal organs due to an excess of fats in the blood (hyperlipidemia). *See* xanthoma.

xanthophyll *n.* a yellow pigment found in green leaves. An example of a xanthophyll is *lutein*.

xanthopsia *n.* yellow vision: the condition in which all objects appear to have a yellowish tinge. It is sometimes experienced in digitalis poisoning.

X chromosome the sex chromosome present in both sexes. Women have two X chromosomes and men have one. Genes for some important genetic disorders, including *hemophilia, are carried on the X chromosomes; these genes are described as *sex-linked. *Compare* Y chromosome.

xeno- *prefix denoting* different; foreign; alien.

xenodiagnosis *n.* a procedure for diagnosing infections transmitted by insect carriers. Uninfected insects of the species known to carry the disease in question are allowed to suck the blood of a patient suspected of having the disease. A positive diagnosis is made if the disease parasites appear in the insects. This method has proved invaluable for diagnosing Chagas' disease, using reduviid bugs (the carriers), since the parasites are not always easily detected in blood smears.

xenogeneic *adj.* described grafted tissue derived from a donor of a different species.

xenograft (heterograft) *n.* a living tissue graft that is transplanted from an animal of one species to another of a different species. For example, attempts have been made to graft animal organs into humans. *Bioengineering techniques are now available to produce animals whose *MHC (major histocompatibility complex) is compatible with that of another species. *See also* xenotransplantation. *Compare* allograft.

xenon-133 *n.* a radioactive isotope that has a half-life of about five days and is used in ventilation scanning of the lungs in *nuclear medicine (*see* ventilation-perfusion scanning). It gives off beta particles, which are responsible for the relatively high radiation dose compared to *krypton-81m. Symbol: Xe-133.

xenophobia *n.* excessive fear of strangers and foreigners. *See* phobia.

Xenopsylla *n.* a genus of tropical and subtropical fleas, with some 40 species. The rat flea, *X. cheopis*, occasionally attacks humans and can transmit plague from an infected rat population; it also transmits murine typhus and two tapeworms, *Hymenolepis nana* and *H. diminuta*.

xenotransplantation *n.* the *transplantation of organs from one species to another. Experimental work into the feasibility of transplanting pig organs into human beings is under way. It in-

cludes the genetic manipulation of pig embryos to produce animals whose organs produce a human cell-surface protein and would therefore not be rejected at transplantation.

xero- *prefix denoting* a dry condition.

xeroderma *n.* a mild form of the hereditary disorder *ichthyosis, in which the skin develops slight dryness and forms bran-like scales. It is common in the elderly. *Xeroderma pigmentosum* is a rare genetically determined disorder (*see* genodermatosis) in which there is an inherited defect in the mechanism that repairs damage to DNA brought about by ultraviolet radiation (*see* DNA repair); this leads to multiple skin cancers. Affected individuals must avoid any exposure to sunlight.

xerophthalmia *n.* a progressive disease of the eye due to deficiency of vitamin A. The cornea and conjunctiva become dry, thickened, and wrinkled. This may progress to *keratomalacia and eventual blindness.

xeroradiography *n.* X-ray imaging produced by exposing an electrically charged plate and then dusting it with a fine blue powder. The powder is then transferred to paper. This technique has been superseded by *computerized radiography.

xerosis *n.* abnormal dryness of the conjunctiva, the skin, or the mucous membranes. Xerosis affecting the conjunctiva is due not to decreased production of tears, but to changes in the membrane itself, which becomes thickened and gray in the area exposed when the eyelids are open.

xerostomia *n.* dryness of the mouth resulting from diminished secretion of saliva. *See* dry mouth. *Compare* ptyalism.

xiphi- (xipho-) *prefix denoting* the xiphoid process of the sternum. Example: *xiphocostal* (relating to the xiphoid process and ribs).

xiphisternum *see* xiphoid process.

xiphoid process (xiphoid cartilage) *n.* the lowermost section of the breastbone (*see* sternum): a flat pointed cartilage that gradually ossifies until it is completely replaced by bone, a process not completed until after middle age. It does not articulate with any ribs. Also called: **en-**

siform process, ensiform cartilage, xiphisternum.

X-linked disease *see* sex-linked.

X-linked lymphoproliferative syndrome (XLP syndrome, Duncan's disease) a hereditary disorder of the immune system caused by a defective *sex-linked gene carried on an *X chromosome. There is uncontrolled proliferation of B *lymphocytes in response to infection by the Epstein-Barr virus, which can lead to fulminating hepatitis or lymphoma. This condition is due to a defect in a gene, *SAP*, which encodes a signaling molecule found in the cytoplasm of cells.

XLP syndrome *see* X-linked lymphoproliferative syndrome.

X-rays *n.* electromagnetic radiation of extremely short wavelength (beyond the ultraviolet), which passes through matter to varying degrees depending on its density. X-rays are produced when high-energy beams of electrons strike matter. They are distinguishable from gamma rays, produced during radioactive decay. Both are used in diagnostic *radiology (*see* radiography, nuclear medicine) and *radiotherapy. Great care is needed to avoid unnecessary exposure, because the radiation is harmful to all living things (*see* ionization, radiation sickness). Heavy elements, such as lead and barium, tend to stop X-rays and can be used to shield people from unwanted exposure to ionizing radiation.

X-ray screening the use of an image intensifier to produce *real-time imaging on a TV monitor during an X-ray examination. It is widely used in angiography and *interventional radiology to guide procedures. *See* videofluoroscopy.

XX the designation for the normal sex chromosome complement in females. *See also* X chromosome.

XY the designation for the normal sex chromosome complement in males. *See also* X chromosome, Y chromosome.

xylene (dimethylbenzene) *n.* a liquid used for increasing the transparency of tissues prepared for microscopic examination after they have been dehydrated. *See* clearing.

xylitol *n.* a five-carbon sugar alcohol obtained by the reduction of the sugar *xylose and used as an artificial sweetener and sugar substitute in diabetic diets.

xylometazoline *n.* a *sympathomimetic drug that constricts blood vessels (*see* vasoconstrictor). It is rapidly acting and long lasting and is applied topically as a nasal decongestant in the relief of the common cold and sinusitis. Toxic effects are rare. Trade name: **Otrivin**.

xylose *n.* a pentose sugar (i.e. one with five carbon atoms) that is involved in carbohydrate interconversions within cells. It is used as a diagnostic aid for intestinal function. Trade name: **Xylo-Pfan**.

xysma *n.* material, such as pieces of membrane, found in the feces, especially in patients with diarrhea.

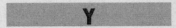

YAG laser yttrium–aluminum–garnet laser: a type of *laser used for cutting tissue, for example in lens *capsulotomy or *iridotomy.

yawning *n.* a reflex action in which the mouth is opened wide and air is drawn into the lungs and then slowly released. It is a result of drowsiness, fatigue, or boredom.

yaws (pian, frambesia) *n.* a tropical infectious disease caused by the spirochete *Treponema pertenue* in the skin and its underlying tissues. Yaws occurs chiefly in conditions of poor hygiene. It is transmitted by direct contact with infected persons and their clothing and possibly also by flies of the genus *Hippelates*. The spirochetes enter through abrasions on the skin. Initial symptoms include fever, pains, and itching, followed by the appearance of small tumors, each covered by a yellow crust of dried serum, on the hands, face, legs, and feet. These tumors may deteriorate into deep ulcers. The final stage of yaws, which may appear after an interval of several years, involves destructive and deforming lesions of the skin, bones, and periosteum (*see also* gangosa, goundou). Yaws, which commonly affects children, is prevalent in hot humid lowlands of equatorial Africa, tropical America, the Far East, and the West Indies. It responds well to treatment with antibiotics, such as penicillin G benzathine.

Y chromosome a sex chromosome that is present in men but not in women; it is believed to carry the genes for maleness. *Compare* X chromosome.

yeast *n.* any one of a group of fungi in which the body (mycelium) consists of individual cells, which may occur singly, in groups of two or three, or in chains. Yeasts reproduce by budding and by the formation of sexual spores (in the case of the perfect yeasts) or asexual spores (in the case of the imperfect yeasts). The group includes baker's yeast (*Saccharomyces*), which ferments carbohydrates to produce alcohol and carbon dioxide and is important in brewing and bread-making. Some yeasts are a commercial source of proteins and of vitamins of the B complex. Yeasts that cause disease in humans include *Candida, *Cryptococcus,* and *Malassezia.*

yellow fever an infectious disease, caused by an *arbovirus, occurring in tropical Africa and the northern regions of South America. It is transmitted by mosquitoes, principally *Aëdes aegypti.* The virus causes degeneration of the tissues of the liver and kidneys. Symptoms, depending on severity of infection, include chill, headache, pains in the back and limbs, fever, vomiting, constipation, a reduced flow of urine (which contains high levels of albumin), and *jaundice. Yellow fever may prove fatal, but recovery from a first attack confers subsequent immunity. The disease is treated with fluid replacement and can be prevented by vaccination.

yellow spot *see* macula (lutea).

Yersinia *n.* a genus of aerobic or facultatively anaerobic gram-negative bacteria that are parasites of animals and humans. The species *Y. pestis* causes bubonic *plague, and *Y. enterocolitica* causes intestinal infections.

yohimbine *n.* an alkaloid with *sympatholytic effects: it lowers blood pressure and controls arousal and anxiety and has been used to treat both physical and psychogenic impotence.

yolk (deutoplasm) *n.* a substance, rich in protein and fat, that is laid down within the egg cell as nourishment for the embryo. It is absent (or nearly so) from the eggs of mammals (including humans) whose embryos absorb nutrients from their mother.

yolk sac (vitelline sac) the membranous sac, composed of mesoderm lined with endoderm, that lies ventral to the embryo. It is one of the *extraembryonic membranes. Its initially wide communication with the future gut is later reduced to a narrow duct passing through the *umbilicus. It probably assists in transporting nutrients to the early embryo and is one of the first sites where blood cells are formed.

Y-plasty *n.* a type of surgical incision made in the shape of a "Y," used to reduce shortening of scar tissue at the site of the wound and maintain elasticity of the adjacent skin.

yttrium-90 *n.* an artificial radioactive isotope of the element yttrium, used in *radiotherapy.

Z

zafirlukast *n. see* leukotriene receptor antagonist.

zalcitabine *n.* a drug, similar to *didanosine, that is used to prolong the lives of patients with AIDS and HIV infection. Zalcitabine is administered by mouth. Possible side effects include reversible nerve damage, ulceration of the gullet, skin rashes, severe pancreatitis, nausea, vomiting, and headache. Trade name: **Hivid**.

zanamivir *n.* an antiviral drug that acts by inhibiting the action of neuraminidase in viruses. This enzyme destroys the receptor sites on the surface of the host cells. Zanamivir is used for the treatment of influenza A and B. To be effective, the drug must be taken within 48 hours of the onset of symptoms. Administered by inhalation, it is liable to cause tightening of the bronchial tubes and this may be dangerous in people with asthma. Trade name: **Relenza**.

zein *n.* a protein found in corn.

zidovudine (AZT) *n.* an antiviral drug used in the treatment of AIDS and HIV infection. The drug slows the growth of HIV infection in the body, but is not curative. It is administered by mouth and intravenously; the most common side effects are nausea, headache, and insomnia, and zidovudine may damage the blood-forming tissues of the bone marrow. Trade name: **Retrovir**.

Ziehl-Neelsen stain an acid-fast *carbolfuchsin stain used specifically for identifying the tubercle bacillus. [F. Ziehl (1857–1926), German bacteriologist; F. K. A. Neelsen (1854–94), German pathologist]

Zieve's syndrome a combination of severe *hyperlipidemia, hemolytic *anemia, and *jaundice seen in susceptible individuals taking alcohol to excess. [L. Zieve (1915–   ), US physician]

zinc n. a *trace element that is a cofactor of many enzymes. Deficiency rarely arises with a balanced diet but may occur in alcoholics and those with kidney disease; symptoms include lesions of the skin, esophagus, and cornea and (in children) retarded growth. Symbol: Zn.

zinc chloride a *caustic substance having strong *astringent properties. It is used as a solution for cleansing wounds and ulcers and also as a mouthwash and deodorant; in paste form it is the main component of zinc dental cement. Toxic effects are essentially due to poisoning by ingestion.

zinc oxide a mild *astringent that is used in various skin conditions, usually in combination with other substances. It is applied as a cream, an ointment, a dusting powder, or a paste, sometimes in the form of an impregnated bandage.

zinc sulfate an *astringent applied in a lotion for the treatment of ulcers of the skin and mouth and to assist in the healing of wounds. It is also used in eye drops and, occasionally, as an emetic or as zinc replacement. Trade names: **Verazinc**, **Zincate**.

zinc undecylenate (zinc undecenoate) an antifungal agent with uses similar to those of *undecylenic acid.

zoacanthosis n. inflammation of the skin caused by retention of foreign substances, such as insect stingers or animal hairs.

Zollinger-Ellison syndrome a rare disorder in which there is excessive secretion of gastric juice due to high levels of circulating *gastrin, which is produced by a pancreatic tumor (see gastrinoma) or an enlarged pancreas. The high levels of stomach acid cause diarrhea and peptic ulcers, which may be multiple, in unusual sites (e.g. jejunum), or which quickly recur after *vagotomy or partial *gastrectomy. Treatment with an H_2-receptor antagonist (see antihistamine) or *proton-pump inhibitor, by removal of the tumor (if benign), or by total gastrectomy is usually effective. [R. M. Zollinger (1903–92) and E. H. Ellison (1918–70), US physicians]

zolmitriptan n. see $5HT_1$ agonist.

zona pellucida the thick membrane that develops around the mammalian oocyte within the ovarian follicle. It is penetrated by at least one spermatozoon at fertilization and persists around the *blastocyst until it reaches the uterus. See ovum.

zonula n. see zonule.

zonule (zonula) n. (in anatomy) a small band or zone; for example the zonule of Zinn (zonula ciliaris) is the suspensory ligament of the eye. —**zonular** adj.

zonulolysis n. dissolution of the suspensory ligament of the lens of the eye (the zonule of Zinn), which facilitates removal of the lens in cases of cataract. A small quantity of a solution of an enzyme that dissolves the zonule without damaging other parts of the eye is injected behind the iris a minute or two before the lens is removed. This technique is not used for modern cataract surgery.

zoo- prefix denoting animals.

zoograft n. tissue from an animal that is transplanted into a human. See also allograft, xenograft.

zoonosis n. an infectious disease of animals that can be transmitted to humans. See anthrax, brucellosis, cat-scratch fever, cowpox, glanders, Q fever, Rift Valley fever, rabies, rat-bite fever, toxoplasmosis, tularemia, typhus.

zoophilism n. sexual attraction to animals, which may be manifested in stroking and fondling animals or in sexual intercourse (bestiality). —**zoophilic** adj.

zoophobia n. excessively strong fear of animals. See phobia.

zoopsia n. visual hallucinations of animals. These can occur in any condition causing hallucinations but are most typical of *delirium tremens.

zootoxin n. any poisonous substance produced by an animal, such as the venom from snakes, spiders, or scorpions.

zoster n. herpes zoster. See herpes.

Z-plasty n. a type of surgical incision made in the shape of a "Z," used to reduce shortening of scar tissue at the site of the wound and maintain elasticity of the adjacent skin.

zwitterion n. an ion that bears a positive and a negative charge. Amino acids can yield zwitterions.

zyg(o)- prefix denoting union, joined, or a junction.

zygoma n. see zygomatic arch, zygomatic bone.

zygomatic arch (zygoma) the horizontal arch of bone on either side of the face, just below the eyes, that is formed by connected processes of the zygomatic and temporal bones. See skull.

zygomatic bone (zygoma, malar bone) either of a pair of bones that form the prominent part of the cheeks and contribute to the orbits. See skull.

zygote n. the fertilized ovum before *cleavage begins. It contains both male and female pronuclei.

zygotene n. the second stage of the first prophase of *meiosis, in which the homologous chromosomes form pairs (bivalents).

zym- (zymo-) prefix denoting **1.** an enzyme. **2.** fermentation.

zymogen n. see proenzyme.

zymology n. the science of the study of yeasts and fermentation.

zymolysis n. the process of *fermentation or digestion by an enzyme.

zymosis n. **1.** the process of *fermentation, brought about by yeast organisms. **2.** the changes in the body that occur in certain infectious diseases, once thought to be the result of a process similar to fermentation. —**zymotic** adj.

zymotic disease an old name for a contagious disease, which was formerly thought to develop within the body following infection in a process similar to the fermentation and growth of yeast.

APPENDIX

TABLE 1. BASE AND SUPPLEMENTARY SI UNITS

Physical quantity	Name of unit	Symbol for unit
length	meter	m
mass	kilogram	kg
time	second	s
electric current	ampere	A
thermodynamic temperature	kelvin	K
luminous intensity	candela	cd
amount of substance	mole	mol
*plane angle	radian	rad
*solid angle	steradian	sr

*supplementary units

TABLE 2. SI UNITS WITH SPECIAL NAMES

Physical quantity	Name of unit	Symbol for unit
frequency	hertz	Hz
energy	joule	J
force	newton	N
power	watt	W
pressure	pascal	Pa
electric charge	coulomb	C
electric potential difference	volt	V
electric resistance	ohm	Ω
electric conductance	siemens	S
electric capacitance	farad	F
magnetic flux	weber	Wb
inductance	henry	H
magnetic flux density (magnetic induction)	tesla	T
luminous flux	lumen	lm
illuminance (illumination)	lux	lx
absorbed dose	gray	Gy
activity	becquerel	Bq
dose equivalent	sievert	Sv

TABLE 3. DECIMAL MULTIPLES AND SUBMULTIPLES TO BE USED WITH SI UNITS

Submultiple	Prefix	Symbol		Multiple	Prefix	Symbol
10^{-1}	deci-	d		10^{1}	deca-	da
10^{-2}	centi-	c		10^{2}	hecto-	h
10^{-3}	milli-	m		10^{3}	kilo-	k
10^{-6}	micro-	μ		10^{6}	mega-	M
10^{-9}	nano-	n		10^{9}	giga-	G
10^{-12}	pico-	p		10^{12}	tera-	T
10^{-15}	femto-	f		10^{15}	peta-	P
10^{-18}	atto-	a		10^{18}	exa-	E
10^{-21}	zepto-	z		10^{21}	zetta-	Z
10^{-24}	yocto-	y		10^{24}	yotta-	Y